Textbook of Gynaecology

in

cont

Fif

OTHER BOOKS BY THE SAME AUTHOR

- Textbook of Obstetrics
- A Guide to Clinical Obstetrics and Gynaecology
- Emergencies in Manipulative and Operative Obstetrics

Textbook of Gynaecology

including

contraception

Fifth Edition

D C Dutta MBBS, DGO, MO(CAL)
Professor and Head, Dept of Obstetrics and Gynaecology
Nilratan Sircar Medical College and Hospital, Kolkata, India

Edited by

Hiralal Konar
(HONS; GOLD MEDALLIST)
MBBS (CAL), MD (PGI), DNB (INDIA)
MNAMS, FACS (USA), FRCOG (LONDON)

Professor, Obstetrics and Gynaecology
Nilratan Sircar Medical College and Hospital, Kolkata, India

One time Rotation Registrar in Obstetrics, Gynaecology, and Oncology
Northern and Yorkshire Region, Newcastle-upon-Tyne, UK
Examiner of MBBS, DGO, and MD of different Indian universities
and National Board of Examination, New Delhi

New Central Book Agency

KOLKATA • DELHI • PUNE • ERNAKULAM

Textbook of Gynaecology

Publisher

NEW CENTRAL BOOK AGENCY (P) LTD

- 8/1 Chintamoni Das Lane, Kolkata 700 009
- 4262/3 1st Floor, Flat Nos. 105 & 106
  Ansari Road, Daryaganj, New Delhi 110 002
- Shop Nos. 3 & 4, Vinayak Towers
  681/B Budhwar Peth, Appa Balwant Chowk
  Pune 411 002
- GSS Shopping Complex (1st Floor)
  Opposite College Post Office
  Convent Road, Ernakulam 682 035

Typesetter: New Central Book Agency (P) Ltd, 8/1 Chintamoni Das Lane, Kolkata 700 009

Printer: New Central Book Agency (P) Ltd, Web-Offset Division, Dhulagarh, Sankrail, Howrah

Cover Designer: Soumen Paul

Cover Printer: Liba Graphics, Kolkata 700 046

Technical Editor: Dr Mita Sen, MBBS

Project Supervisor: Nochiel Radhakrishnan

Project Team: Prasenjit Halder, Mrs S Dutta, Subir Pal, Suman Dutta, and Prabir Ghosh

ISBN 81-7381-041-9

1st Published	: 1989	Revised Reprint : 1990
2nd Edition	: 1994	Reprint : 1996 Revised Reprint : 1997 Reprint : 1999 and 2000
3rd Edition	: 2001	Reprint : 2002
4th Edition	: 2003	Reprint : 2005 and 2006
5th Edition	: 2008	(Thoroughly revised, enlarged, and updated) **Revised Reprint : 2009**

Price: **Rs. 650.00** (in India, Pakistan, Bangladesh, Nepal, and Sri Lanka) **US $40** (other Countries)

dedicated
to the
students of gynaecology
— past and present

Contents

Preface to the Fifth Edition

Within the span of seventeen years, Dutta's widely acclaimed Textbook of Gynaecology has stepped into its fifth edition. Dutta's text is well-known for its continuity and timely incorporation of advancing information. The new cover of this fifth edition is the prime indicator of the new direction in the progress of science and clinical practice. This fifth edition is in fully coloured format to meet the changing needs of the readers. The coloured format is for the readers' convenience. It helps to highlight the core knowledge (must-know area) and also to present the high quality photographs, anatomical drawings, and imaging studies. The text has been enriched with tables, diagrams, boxes, charts, and algorithms which could be reproduced easily. Key points at the end of each chapter are for quick and easy revision. All these modalities and the thoroughly improved layout are targeted to confer easy understanding and bring clarity to the subject. The state-of-the art in Dutta's text lies in the presentation which is simple, lucid, clear, and concise. Above all, it provides a balanced distillation of evidence-based information upon which a student, trainee resident, a practitioner, and a nurse can fully depend.

Recent research necessitated major changes in all the chapters in this treatise. Chapters on reproductive endocrinology (Chapters 7, 8, 16, 28, 31, 33), menopause (Chapter 6), diagnostic and imaging technologies (Chapter 9), oncology (Chapters 22, 23), urogynaecology (Chapters 24, 25), contraception (Chapter 29) have either been thoroughly revised or exhaustively rewritten. New topics, for example adolescent gynaecology (Chapter 32), sexual dysfunction (Chapter 33), gene therapy (Chapter 30) have been incorporated. Chapters in general gynaecology have been extensively updated. For example, the chapter on pelvic organ prolapse (Chapter 15), has been rewritten, based upon the latest concept of pelvic anatomy and the new concepts of correction. Operative gynaecology (Chapter 34) is meant to provide the basic principles of commonly performed gynaecologic surgery so as to guide an apprentice. More emphasis has been given on case selection (indications) and complications of the operation. The chapter on endoscopic (laparoscopic and hysteroscopic) surgery (Chapter 35) has been rewritten as it has gained its place to a large extent. The chapter on practical gynaecology (Chapter 36) consists of several hundreds of questions along with answers, explanations and high quality photographs and plates of imaging studies. This chapter is designed to help the students while preparing the clinical and oral part of the examination. The self-assessment questionnaire having objective structured clinical examination (OSCE) format is to improve the clinical competence of the students. The total information given in the chapter 36 amounts to a "mini-textbook-cum-colour atlas" in gynaecology.

Dutta's text is a thorough review of gynaecology with medical advances up to the time of publication. Considering the mass of new information, to remain concise proved difficult. I did my best, even with the use of different type size, to accommodate the information thought to be relevant. Consistency and uniformity of information for all the chapters have been maintained.

The marathon task of editing such a comprehensive text is stupendous. My aim with this book has always been to help the students, residents, and the clinicians to remain updated with the knowledge that has passed the test of clinical relevancy.

While editing such a magnum opus, I have, naturally, consulted many outstanding teachers in the profession, a multitude of eminent authors and many current evidence-based studies—the legacy is gratefully acknowledged. The editor expresses his sincere thanks to many of his esteemed colleagues throughout the country and abroad for their valued suggestions, criticisms, and contribution of photographs which have been duly acknowledged.

The editor also acknowledges sincerely the support of all the students (undergraduate and postgraduate) of different medical institutions in this country for their opinion and criticisms that have helped to improve the text. As before, the editor always welcomes the views of students and teachers who regularly write to us offering valuable suggestions and new ideas on our e-mails: ncbapvt.ltd@eth.net; ncba@cal2.vsnl.net.in.

The editor is specially grateful to Dr K M Gun, MD, FRCOG, FRCS, Prof. (Retd) for his contribution on the topic "Amenorrhoea", Dr B N Chakravorty, MD, FRCOG, DSc, Prof. (Retd), Director, Institute of Reproductive Medicine, Kolkata, for his contribution on the topics "Reproductive endocrinology","Infertility", "Intersex", and "Hormones in gynaecology". The editor wishes to express his sincere thanks to Dr Subir Kumar Dutta, MD, Professor (Retd), Dept of Pathology and Bacteriology, University College of Medicine, Kolkata, for the microphotographs depicted throughout the text.

Dr (Mrs) Mita Sen, MBBS (Ahmedabad) deserves special appreciation for her sincere help throughout. Special thanks are due to Mrs Shilpi Dutta, for her patience in correcting the proofs. Computing the text and layout with different type faces, tables and flow charts, colours, and the entire supervision of the book were done by Mr Nochiel Radhakrishnan. His untiring efforts gave the book a new and novel ornamentation, for which he deserves special credit. Mr Prasenjit Halder needs much appreciation for the sketches and anatomic drawings that have enriched this text. The editor thanks sincerely all the members of New Central Book Agency (P) Ltd, who have laboured untiringly in this project to make it a success. Mrs Madhusri Konar, MA, BEd, deserves full credit for her sincere and patient secretarial job as ever. The editor wishes to thank Mr Amitabha Sen, BCom, MBA, LLB, Director, New Central Book Agency (P) Ltd, for the generous support given throughout and for his sincere effort to bring out the book within the stipulated time.

Lastly, I am grateful to all who have taught me, most of all the patients and my beloved students.

I do hope this comprehensive textbook will continue to be of immense value to the students as ever. According to the author's desire, the book is, therefore, dedicated once again to the ***students of gynaecology —past and present***.

Makar Sankranti, 15 January 2008
P 13, New C I T Road
Kolkata 700 014

HIRALAL KONAR

Preface to the First Edition

Since my publication of Textbook of Obstetrics about 5 years back, I have been pressed hard by my esteemed colleagues and the students all over the country and abroad to write a textbook on gynaecology of similar style to fill up the deficit. Initially, I was hesitant to proceed with the stupendous task but considering the fact that a compact, comprehensive and practical-oriented fundamental book in gynaecology is not available to the undergraduates, I have decided to comply with their request.

The book has been written in a lucid language in author's own style. Extensive diagrams, photographs, and flow-charts (schemes) have been depicted throughout the text to give clarity of the subject. Due attention has been paid to project the fundamental principles and practice of gynaecology. As such, more emphasis has been given on medical gynaecology. But for that, indications, limitations, and principles of techniques of operations have received adequate consideration. The book is thus made invaluable not only to the medical students but also the practising physicians and students of Nursing.

The author wishes to acknowledge gratitude to his esteemed colleague Dr N. Chowdhury, MBBS, DGO, MO (Cal), for his contribution to the topic "Hormone Therapy in Gynaecological practice". Dr Santosh Kr. Paul, MBBS, DGO, MO (Cal), Prof. Dept of Obst. and Gynae., NRS Medical College, Calcutta, deserves full appreciation for his contribution in a lucid way to the topic "Radiotherapy and Chemotherapy in Gynaecology". The author has much pleasure in expressing grateful thanks to Dr B N Chakrabarty, MBBS, DGO, MO (Cal), FRCOG (Eng) and Dr K M Gun, MBBS, DGO, MO (Cal), FRCOG (Eng), FRCS (Edin), FACS (USA), for their valued suggestions as and when required and their contribution of photographs to enrich the text. I gratefully record my thanks to Dr Subir Kumar Dutta, MBBS, DCP, MD (Path. & Bact.), Prof. Dept of Pathology and Bacteriology, University College of Medicine, Calcutta, for the microphotographs depicted throughout the text. The author records his thanks to Dr SM Dali, Prof. of Obst. and Gynae. and Dr Bhola Rijal, Associate Prof. of Obst. and Gynae. of Teaching Hospital and Dr (Mrs) Dibya S Malla, Director, Maternity Hospital, Kathmandu, Nepal, for their contribution of few outstanding photographs to enrich the text.

The author expressed much pleasure all the time to the House Surgeons, Internees and students of Nilratan Sircar Medical College, Calcutta, for the help they have rendered in preparation of the final drafts of the manuscripts, check up of the proofs and compiling the index. Their help is invaluable and unforgettable and without which the book could never have been published.

The author wishes to thank Mr Biren Das for his exhaustive number of drawings and flow-charts which enrich the lucidity of the book. The author also thanks Mr Ranjit Sen for preparation of photographs (black and white) depicted throughout the text. The author have much pleasure in expressing his appreciation to Mr Bimal Bhattacharya, MSc, LLB (Cal), DSW, DHE, Lecturer, Health Education and Family Welfare, Post-partum Unit, NRS Medical College, Calcutta, for the patience shown in dealing with correction of manuscripts and proofs.

In preparing the textbook, the author has utilised the knowledge of number of stalwarts in his profession and consulted many books and publications. The author wishes to express his appreciation and gratitude to all of them including the related authors and publishers.

The author expresses his sincere thanks to his publishers 'New Central Book Agency' for their sincere efforts in publishing the book within the stipulated period.

The author still confesses that as a teacher he has learnt a lot from the students and more so while writing this book and as such he could not think to dedicate the book to any one else than the *students of gynaecology, past and present*.

Mahalaya, 29 September 1989

P 49 New CIT Road
Calcutta 700 014

D C DUTTA

Anatomy of the Female Pelvic Organs

1

EXTERNAL GENITALIA
(Syn. Vulva, pudendum)

The vulva includes mons veneris, labia majora, labia minora, clitoris, vestibule and conventionally the perineum. These are all visible on external examination. It is therefore bounded anteriorly by the mons veneris, laterally by the labia majora and posteriorly by the perineum (Fig. 1.1).

MONS VENERIS (MONS PUBIS)

It is the pad of subcutaneous adipose connective tissue lying in front of the pubis and in the adult female, is covered by hair.

LABIA MAJORA

The vulva is bounded on each side by the elevation of skin and subcutaneous tissue which form the labia majora. They are continuous where they join medially to form the posterior commissure in front of the anus. The inner surface of the labia majora are hairless. The labia majora are covered with squamous epithelium and contain sebaceous glands, sweat glands and hair follicles. Beneath the skin, there are dense connective tissue and adipose tissue. The adipose tissue is richly supplied with venous plexus which may produce haematoma, if injured during childbirth. **The labia majora are homologous with the scrotum in the male.** The round ligaments terminate at its anterior third.

LABIA MINORA

Labia minora are two thick folds of skin, devoid of fat, on either side just within the labia majora. Except in the parous women, they are only exposed when the labia majora are separated. Anteriorly, they are divided to enclose the clitoris and unite with each other in front and behind the clitoris to form the prepuce and frenulum respectively. The lower portion of the labia minora fuses across the midline to form a fold of skin known as fourchette. It is usually injured during childbirth. **Between the fourchette and the vaginal orifice is the fossa navicularis. The labia minora do not contain hair follicle.** The folds contain connective tissues, numerous sebaceous glands, erectile muscle fibres and numerous vessels and nerve endings. **It is homologous with the ventral aspect of the penis.**

CLITORIS

Clitoris is a small cylindrical erectile body, measuring about 2.5 cm situated in the most anterior part of the vulva. It consists of glans, a body and two crura. The glans is covered by squamous epithelium and is richly supplied with nerves. The vessels of the clitoris are connected with the vestibular bulb and are liable to be injured during childbirth. **Clitoris is an analogue to the penis in the male,** but it differs basically in being entirely separate from the urethra. It is attached to the under surface of the symphysis pubis by the suspensory ligament.

VESTIBULE

Vestibule is a triangular space bounded anteriorly by the clitoris, posteriorly by the fourchette and on either side by labium minus. **There are four openings into the vestibule (Fig. 1.1).**

Urethral opening

The opening is situated in the midline, just in front of the vaginal orifice about 1-1.5 cm below the pubic arch. The paraurethral ducts open either on the

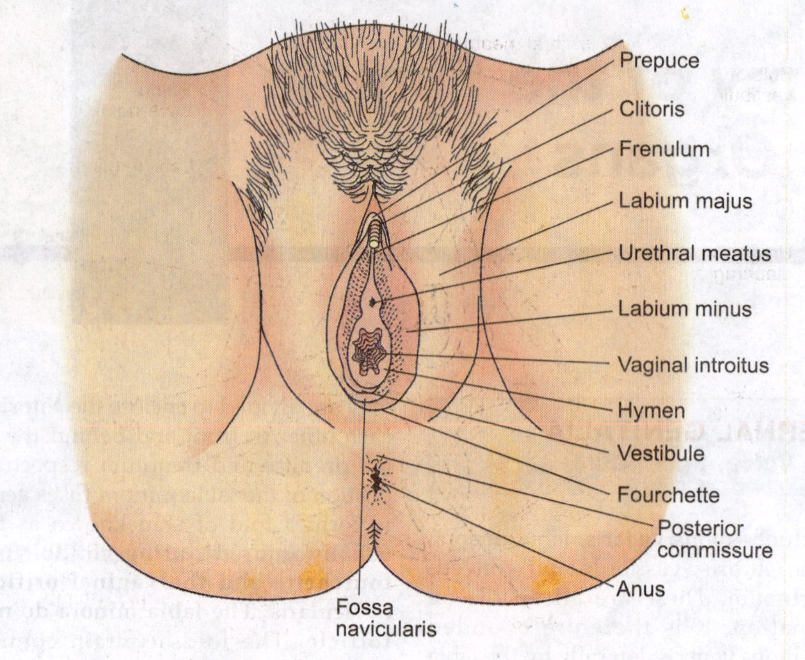

Fig. 1.1. The virginal vulva

posterior wall of the urethral orifice or directly into the vestibule.

Vaginal orifice and hymen

The vaginal orifice lies in the posterior end of the vestibule and is of varying size and shape. In virgins and nulliparae, the opening is closed by the labia minora but in parous, it may be exposed. It is incompletely closed by a septum of mucous membrane, called hymen. The membrane varies in shape but is usually circular or crescentic in virgins. The hymen is usually ruptured at the consummation of marriage. During childbirth, the hymen is extremely lacerated and is later represented by cicatrised nodules of varying sizes, called the **caruncula myrtiformes**. On both sides, it is lined by stratified squamous epithelium.

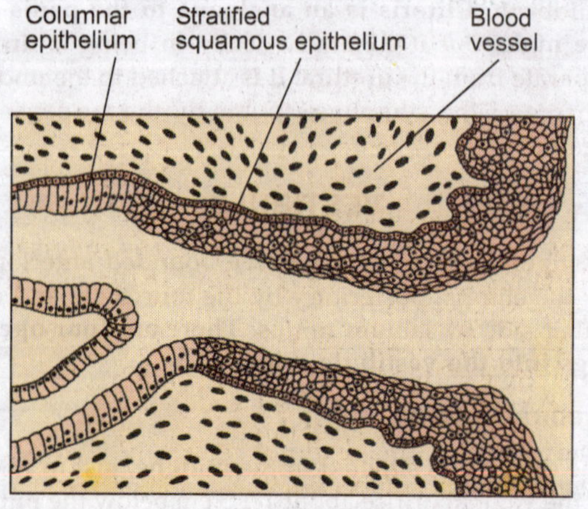

Fig. 1.2. Mucous lining of Bartholin's duct

Opening of Bartholin's ducts

The Bartholin's glands are situated in the superficial perineal pouch, close to the posterior end of the vestibular bulb. They are pea sized, of about 0.5 cm and yellowish white in colour. During sexual excitement, it secretes abundant alkaline mucus which helps in lubrication. Contraction of bulbocavernosus helps to squeeze the secretion. The glands are compound racemose variety and are lined by columnar epithelium. **Each gland has got a duct which measures about 2 cm** and opens into the vestibule outside the hymen at the junction of the anterior two-third and posterior one-third in the groove between the hymen and the labium minus. **The duct is lined by columnar epithelium** but **near its opening by stratified**

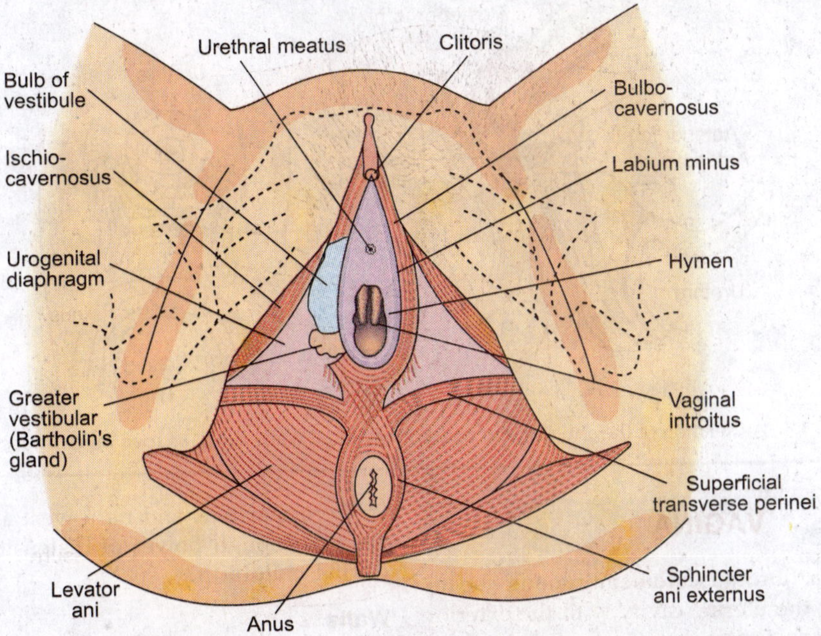

Fig. 1.3. Exposition of superficial perineal pouch with vestibular bulb and Bartholin's gland

squamous epithelium (Fig. 1.2). **The Bartholin's gland corresponds to the bulbourethral gland of male.**

VESTIBULAR BULB

These are bilateral elongated masses of erectile tissues situated beneath the mucous membrane of the vestibule. Each bulb lies on either side of the vaginal orifice in front of the Bartholin's gland and is incorporated within the bulbocavernosus muscles. **They are homologous to the single bulb of the penis and corpus spongiosum in the male.** They are likely to be injured during childbirth with brisk haemorrhage (Fig. 1.3).

PERINEUM

The details of the anatomy of perineum are described later in the chapter (p. 19).

Blood supply of the vulva

Arteries : (a) Branches of internal pudendal artery — the chief being labial, transverse perineal, artery to the vestibular bulb and deep and dorsal arteries to the clitoris. (b) Branches of femoral artery — superficial and deep pudendal.

Veins : The veins form plexuses and drain into — (a) internal pudendal vein, (b) vesical or vaginal venous plexus and (c) long saphenous vein. Varicosities during pregnancy are not uncommon and may rupture spontaneously causing visible bleeding or haematoma formation.

Nerve supply of the vulva

The supply is through bilateral spinal somatic nerves. Anterosuperior part is supplied by the cutaneous branches from the ilioinguinal and genital branch of genitofemoral nerve (L_1 and L_2) and the posteroinferior part by the pudendal branches from the posterior cutaneous nerve of thigh ($S_{2,3,4}$). Between these two groups, the vulva is supplied by the labial and perineal branches of the pudendal nerve ($S_{2,3,4}$).

INTERNAL GENITAL ORGANS

The internal genital organs in female include vagina, uterus, Fallopian tubes and the ovaries. These organs are placed internally and require special instruments for inspection.

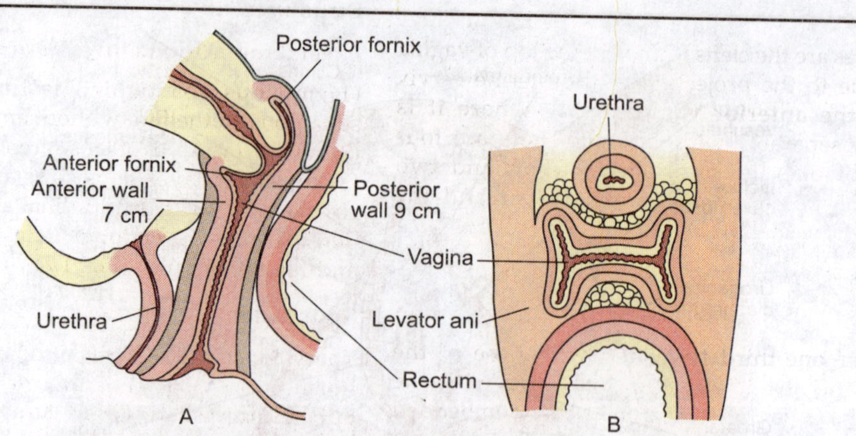

Fig. 1.4. A. Relation of the anterior and posterior vaginal wall. B. 'H' shaped on cross section

VAGINA

The vagina is a fibromusculomembranous sheath communicating the uterine cavity with the exterior at the vulva. It constitutes the excretory channel for the uterine secretion and menstrual blood. It is the organ of copulation and forms the birth canal of parturition. The canal is directed upwards and backwards forming an angle of 45° with the horizontal in erect posture. The long axis of the vagina almost lies parallel to the plane of the pelvic inlet and at right angles to that of the uterus. The diameter of the canal is about 2.5 cm, being widest in the upper part and narrowest at its introitus. It has got enough power of distensibility as evident during childbirth.

Walls

Vagina has got an anterior, a posterior and two lateral walls. The anterior and posterior walls are apposed together but the lateral walls are comparatively stiffer specially at its middle, as such it looks 'H' shaped on transverse section. **The length of the anterior wall is about 7 cm and that of the posterior wall is about 9 cm (Fig. 1.4)**. The upper end of vaginalis above the pelvic floor.

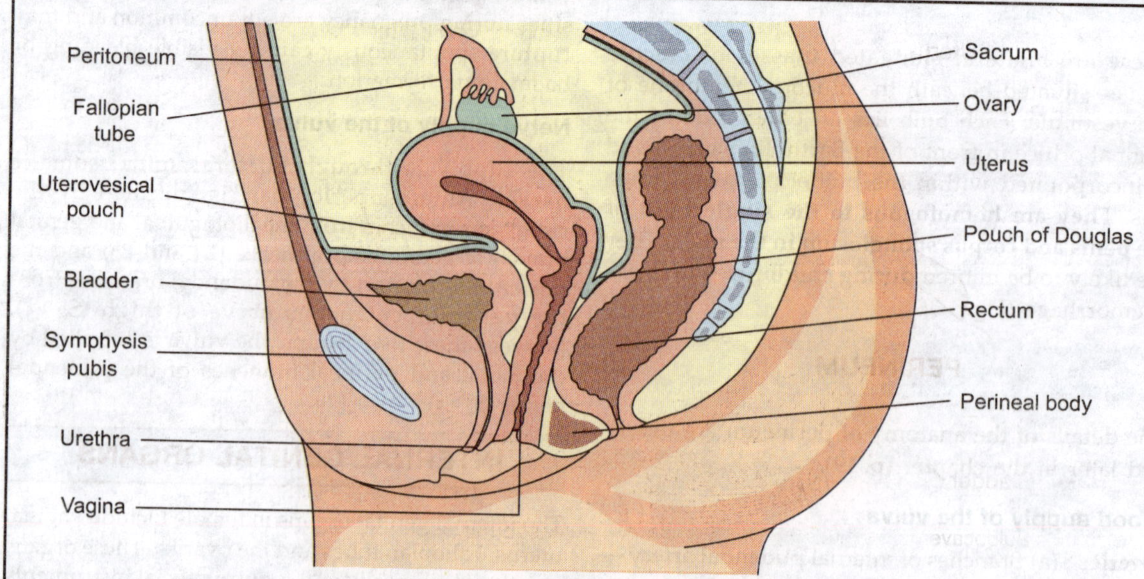

Fig. 1.5. Mid-sagittal section of the female pelvis showing relative position of the pelvic organs

Fornices

The fornices are the clefts formed at the top of vagina (vault) due to the projection of the uterine cervix through the anterior vaginal wall, where it is blended inseparably with its wall. There are four fornices — one anterior, one posterior and two lateral; the posterior one being deeper and the anterior, most shallow one.

Relations

Anterior

The upper one-third is related with base of the bladder and the lower two-thirds are with the urethra, the lower half of which is firmly embedded with its wall (Fig. 1.4).

Posterior

The upper one-third is related with the pouch of Douglas, the middle-third with the anterior rectal wall separated by rectovaginal septum and the lower-third is separated from the anal canal by the perineal body (Fig. 1.5).

Lateral walls

The upper one-third is related with the pelvic cellular tissue at the base of broad ligament in which the ureter and the uterine artery lie approximately 2 cm from the lateral fornices. The middle-third is blended with the levator ani and the lower-third is related with the bulbocavernosus muscles, vestibular bulbs and Bartholin's glands (Fig. 1.6).

Structures

Layers from within outwards are

(1) mucous coat which is lined by stratified squamous epithelium without any secreting glands; (2) submucous layer of loose areolar vascular tissues; (3) muscular layer consisting of indistinct inner circular and outer longitudinal and (4) fibrous coat derived from the endopelvic fascia which is tough and highly vascular (Fig. 1.7).

Epithelium

The vaginal epithelium is under the action of sex hormones. **At birth and upto 10-14 days,** the epithelium is stratified squamous under the influence of maternal oestrogen circulating in the newborn. Thereafter upto prepuberty and in postmenopause, the epithelium becomes thin, consisting of few layers only.

From puberty till menopause, the vaginal epithelium is stratified squamous and devoid of any gland. Three distinct layers are defined — basal cells, intermediate cells and superficial cornified cells. The intermediate and superficial cells contain glycogen under the influence of oestrogen. These cells become continuous with those covering the vaginal portion of the cervix and extend upto the squamocolumnar junction at the external os. The superficial cells exfoliate constantly and more so in inflammatory or neoplastic condition. Replacement of the superficial cells occurs from the basal cells. When the

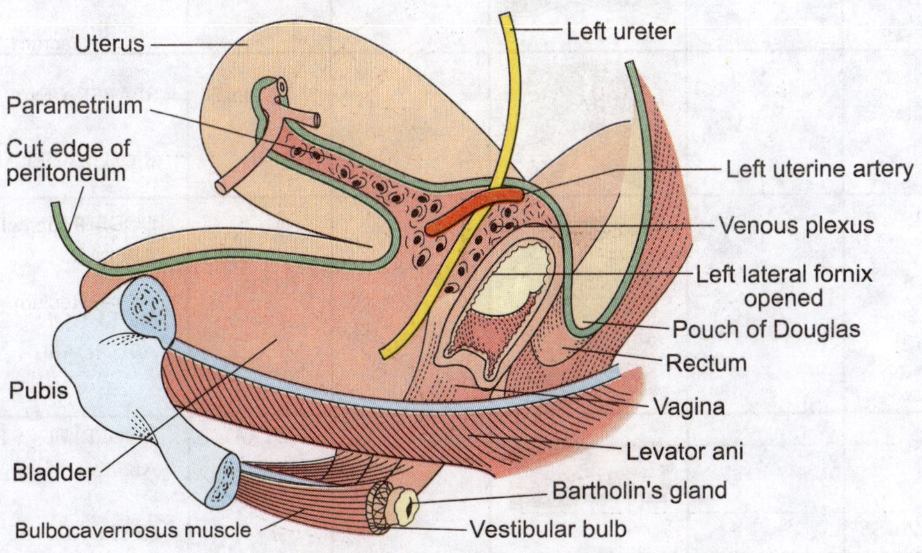

Fig. 1.6. Lateral relation of vagina

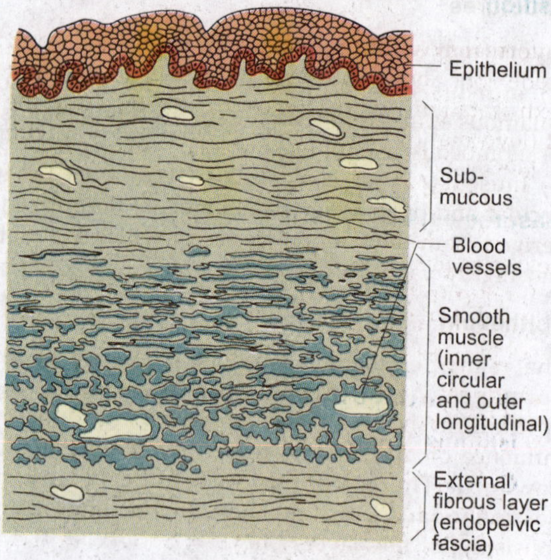

Fig. 1.7. Structure of vaginal wall

epithelium is exposed to the dry external atmosphere, keratinisation occurs. **Unlike skin, it does not contain hair follicle, sweat and sebaceous gland.**

Secretion

The vaginal secretion is very small in amount sufficient to make the surface moist. Normally, it may be little excess in mid menstrual or just prior to menstruation, during pregnancy and during sexual excitement. **The secretion is mainly derived from** the glands of the cervix, uterus, transudation of the vaginal epithelium and Bartholin's glands (during sexual excitement).

	OESTROGEN	EPITHELIUM	GLYCOGEN	pH	FLORA
BIRTH TO 2 WEEKS	+	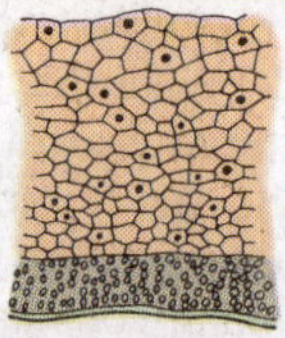	+	ACID 4 - 5	STERILE ↓ DODERLEIN'S BACILLI SECRETION ABUNDANT
2 WEEKS TO PREPUBERTY	–	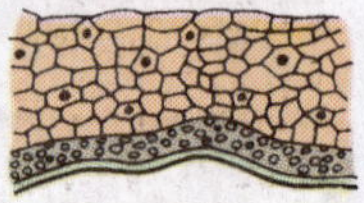	–	ALKALINE >7	DODERLEIN'S BACILLI ABSENT SECRETION SCANT
PUBERTY	APPEARS	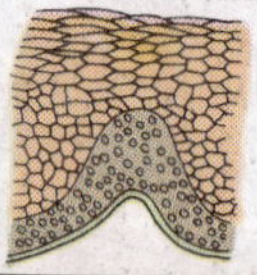	– → +	ALKALINE ↓ ACID	SPARSE, COCCAL ↓ RICH BACILLARY
REPRODU-CTIVE PERIOD	++	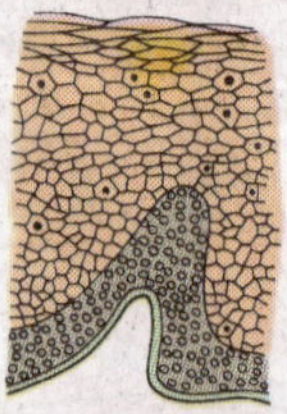	+	ACID 4 - 5	DODERLEIN'S BACILLI APPEAR SECRETION ABUNDANT
POST MENOPAUSE	+ → –	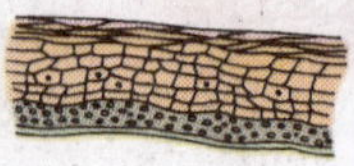	–	NEUTRAL OR ALKALINE 6 – >7	DODERLEIN'S BACILLI ABSENT SECRETION SCANT

Fig. 1.8. Oestrogenic effect on vaginal epithelium and flora at different ages

The pH is acidic and varies during different phases of life and menstrual cycle. Conversion of glycogen in the exfoliated squamous cells to lactic acid by the **Doderlein's bacilli** is dependent on oestrogen. As such, the pH is more towards acidic during childbearing period and ranges **between 4 to 5.5 with average of 4.5.** The pH is highest in upper vagina because of contaminated cervical secretion (alkaline). The **vaginal secretion consists** of tissue fluid, epithelial debris, some leucocytes (never contains more than an occasional pus cell), electrolytes, proteins and lactic acid (in a concentration of 0.75 per cent). Apart from Doderlein's bacilli, it contains many a pathogenic organism including *Cl. welchii*. **The glycogen content is highest** in the vaginal fornix to the extent of 2.5 – 3 mg and is lowest in the lower-third being 0.6 – 0.9 mg per cent.

Doderlein's bacillus : It is a rod-shaped gram-positive bacillus which grows anaerobically on acid media. It appears in the vagina 3-4 days after birth and disappears after 10-14 days. It appears again at puberty and disappears after menopause. It probably comes from the intestine. Its presence is dependent to oestrogen and its function is to convert the glycogen present in the vaginal mucosa into lactic acid so that the vaginal pH is maintained towards acidic side. This acid pH prevents growth of the other pathogenic organisms (Fig. 1.8).

Blood supply

The arteries involved are :

(1) cervicovaginal branch of the uterine artery, (2) vaginal artery — a branch of anterior division of internal iliac or in common origin with the uterine, (3) middle rectal and (4) internal pudendal. These anastomose with one another and form two azygos arteries — anterior and posterior.

Veins drain into internal iliac and internal pudendal veins.

Nerve supply

The vagina is supplied by sympathetic and parasympathetic from the pelvic plexus. The lower part is supplied by the pudendal nerve.

THE UTERUS

The uterus is a hollow pyriform muscular organ situated in the pelvis between the bladder in front and the rectum behind (Fig. 1.5).

Position

Its normal position is one of the anteversion and anteflexion. The uterus usually inclines to the right (dextrorotation) so that the cervix is directed to the left (levorotation) and comes in close relation with the left ureter.

Measurements and parts

The uterus measures about 8 cm long, 5 cm wide at the fundus and its walls are about 1.25 cm thick. Its weight varies from 50-80 gm. It has got the following parts (Fig. 1.9).

- **Body or corpus**
- **Isthmus**
- **Cervix**

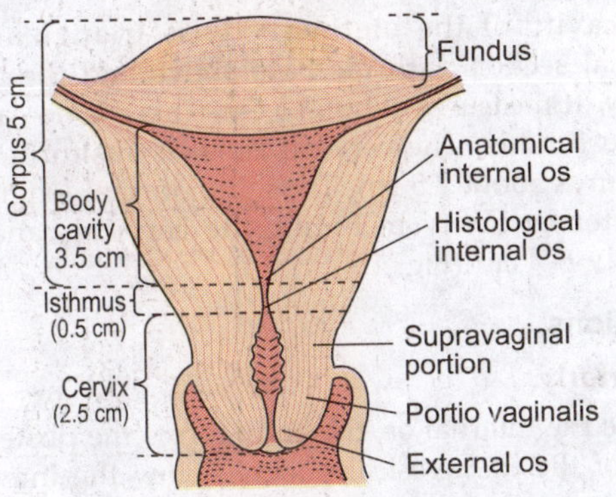

Fig. 1.9. Coronal section showing different parts of uterus

Body or corpus

The body is further divided into fundus — the part which lies above the openings of the uterine tubes. The body proper is triangular and lies between the openings of the tubes and the isthmus. The superolateral angles of the body of the uterus project outwards from the junction of the fundus and body and are called the cornua of the uterus. The uterine tube, round ligament and ligament of the ovary are attached to each cornu.

Isthmus

The isthmus is a constricted part measuring about 0.5 cm situated between the body and the cervix. It is limited above by the anatomical internal os and below by the histological internal os (Aschoff). Some consider isthmus as a part of the lower portion of the body of the uterus.

Cervix

The cervix is the lowermost part of the uterus. It extends from the histological internal os and ends at external os which opens into the vagina after perforating the anterior vaginal wall. It is almost cylindrical in shape and measures about 2.5 cm in length and diameter. It is divided into a supravaginal part — the part lying above the vagina and a vaginal part which lies within the vagina, each measuring 1.25 cm. **In nulliparous**, the vaginal part of the cervix is conical with the external os looking circular, **whereas in parous,** it is cylindrical with the external os having bilateral slits. The slit is due to invariable tear of the circular muscles surrounding the external os and gives rise to anterior and posterior lips of the cervix.

Cavity

The cavity of the uterine body is triangular on coronal section with the base above and the apex below. It measures about 3.5 cm. There is no cavity in the fundus. The cervical canal is fusiform and measures about 2.5 cm. Thus, the normal length of the uterine cavity including the cervical canal is usually 6-7 cm (Fig. 1.9).

Relations

Anteriorly

Above the internal os, the body forms the posterior wall of the uterovesical pouch. Below the internal os, it is separated from the base of the bladder by loose areolar tissue.

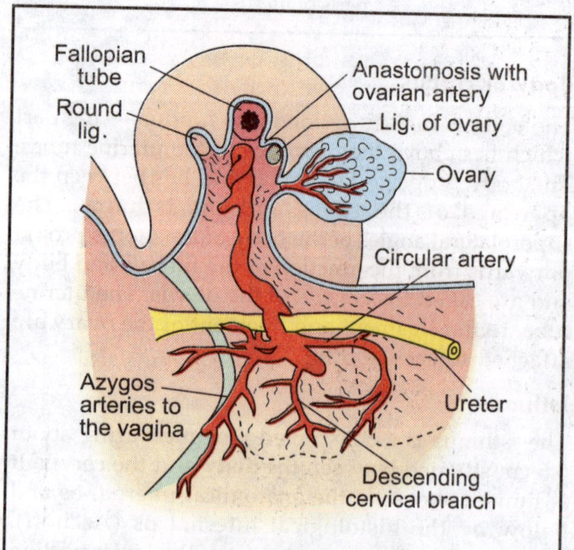

Fig. 1.10. The relation of the ureter to the uterine artery

Posteriorly

It is covered with peritoneum and forms the anterior wall of the pouch of Douglas containing coils of intestine.

Laterally

The double folds of peritoneum of the broad ligament are attached laterally between which the uterine artery ascends up. Attachment of the Mackenrodt's ligament extends from the internal os down to the supravaginal cervix and lateral vaginal wall. About 1.5 cm away at the level of internal os, a little nearer on the left side is the crossing of the uterine artery and the ureter. **The uterine artery crosses from above and in front of the ureter,** soon before the ureter enters the ureteric tunnel (Fig. 1.10).

Structures

Body

The wall consists of 3 layers from outside inwards :

- ***Perimetrium*** — It is the serous coat which invests the entire organ except on the lateral borders. The peritoneum is intimately adherent to the underlying muscles.

- ***Myometrium*** — It consists of thick bundles of smooth muscle fibres held by connective tissues and are arranged in various directions. During pregnancy, however, three distinct layers can be identified — outer longitudinal, middle interlacing and the inner circular.

- ***Endometrium*** — The mucous lining of the cavity is called endometrium. As there is no submucous layer, the endometrium is directly apposed to the muscle coat. It consists of lamina propria and surface epithelium. The surface epithelium is a single layer of ciliated columnar epithelium. The lamina propria contains stromal cells, endometrial glands, vessels and nerves. The glands are simple tubular and lined by mucus secreting non-ciliated columnar epithelium which penetrate the stroma and sometimes even enter the muscle coat. All the components are changed during menstrual cycles (see Ch. 8). The endometrium is changed to decidua during pregnancy.

Cervix

The cervix is composed mainly of fibrous connective tissues. The smooth muscle fibres average 10-15 per cent. Only the posterior surface has got peritoneal coat (Fig. 1.5).

Epithelial lining of the cervix

Endocervical canal and glands

There is a median ridge on both the anterior and posterior surface of the canal from which transverse folds radiate. This arrangement is called arbor vitae uteri. The canal is lined by single layer of tall columnar epithelium with basal nuclei. Those placed over the top of the folds are ciliated. There are patches of cubical basal or reserve cells underneath the columnar epithelium. These cells may undergo squamous metaplasia or may replace the superficial cells (see p. 309).

The glands which dip into the stroma are of complex racemose type and are lined by secretory columnar epithelium. There is no stroma unlike the corpus and the lining epithelium rests on a thin basement membrane. The change in the epithelium and the glands during menstrual cycle and pregnancy are not so much as those in the endometrium.

Portio vaginalis

It is covered by stratified squamous epithelium and extends right upto the external os where there is abrupt change to columnar type.

The transitional zone (transformation zone) may be of 1-10 mm width with variable histological features. The zone consists of endocervical stroma and glands covered by squamous epithelium. **The zone is not static but changes with hormone level of oestrogen.** The site is constantly irritated not only by hormones but also by infection and trauma. Thus, **there is more chance of severe dysplasia, carcinoma *in situ* or even invasive carcinoma at this zone (Fig. 1.11)** **(see p. 312)**.

Secretion

The endometrial secretion is scanty and watery. The physical and chemical properties of the cervical secretion change with menstrual cycles and with pregnancy. The cervical glands secrete an alkaline mucus with **pH 7.8**. The mucus is rich in fructose, glycoprotein and mucopolysaccharides. It also contains sodium chloride. The fructose has got nutritive function to the spermatozoa. Under oestrogenic stimulation, glycoprotein network is arranged parallel to each other thus facilitating sperm ascent. Progesterone produces interlacing bridges thereby preventing sperm penetration. Cervical mucus contributes significantly to the normal vaginal discharge. A part forms the mucus plug which functionally closes the cervical canal and has got bacteriolytic property.

Pelvic peritoneum in relation to the uterus

This is described later in the chapter.

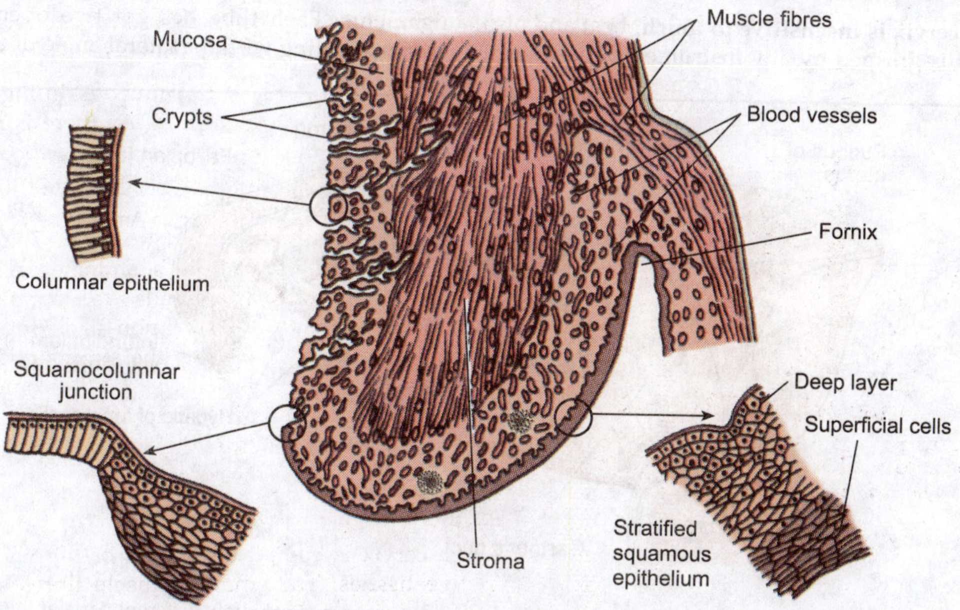

Fig. 1.11. Character of the lining epithelium of the cervix

Blood Supply

Arterial supply

The arterial supply is from the uterine artery — one on each side. The artery arises directly from the anterior division of the internal iliac or in common with superior vesical artery. The other sources are ovarian and vaginal arteries to which the uterine arteries anastomose. **The uterine artery crosses the ureter anteriorly about 1.5 cm away at the level of internal os** before it ascends up along the lateral border of the uterus in between the leaves of broad ligament. The internal supply of the uterus is shown in Fig. 2.1.

Veins

The venous channels correspond to the arterial course and drain into internal iliac veins.

Nerve supply

The nerve supply of the uterus is derived principally from the sympathetic system and partly from the parasympathetic system. Sympathetic components are from T_5 and T_6 (motor) and T_{10} to L_1 spinal segments (sensory). The somatic distribution of uterine pain is that area of the abdomen supplied by T_{10} to L_1. The parasympathetic system is represented on either side by the pelvic nerve which consists of both motor and sensory fibres from S2, S3, S4 and ends in the ganglia of Frankenhauser which lies on either sides of the cervix.

The cervix is insensitive to touch, heat and also when it is grasped by any instrument. The uterus, too is insensitive to handling and even to incision over its wall.

Changes of uterus with age

At birth, the uterus lies in the false pelvis; the cervix is much longer than the body. **In childhood,** the proportion is maintained but reduced to 2 : 1. **At puberty,** the body is growing faster under the action of ovarian steroids (oestrogens) and the proportion is reversed to 1 : 2 and following childbirth, it becomes even 1 : 3. **After menopause** the uterus atrophies; the overall length is reduced; the walls become thinner, less muscular but more fibrous (Fig. 5.1).

Position of the uterus

The normal position of the uterus is anteversion and anteflexion. **The anteversion relates** the long axis of the cervix to the long axis of vagina which is about 90°. **Anteflexion relates** the long axis of the body to the long axis of the cervix and is about 120°. In about 15-20 per cent, normally the uterus remains in retroverted position. In erect posture, the internal os lies on the upper border of the symphysis pubis and the external os lies at the level of ischial spines.

FALLOPIAN TUBE

(Syn : Uterine tube)

The uterine tubes are paired structures, measuring about 10 cm (4") and are situated in the medial three-fourth of the upper free margin of the broad ligaments. Each tube has got two openings, one communicating with the lateral angle of the uterine

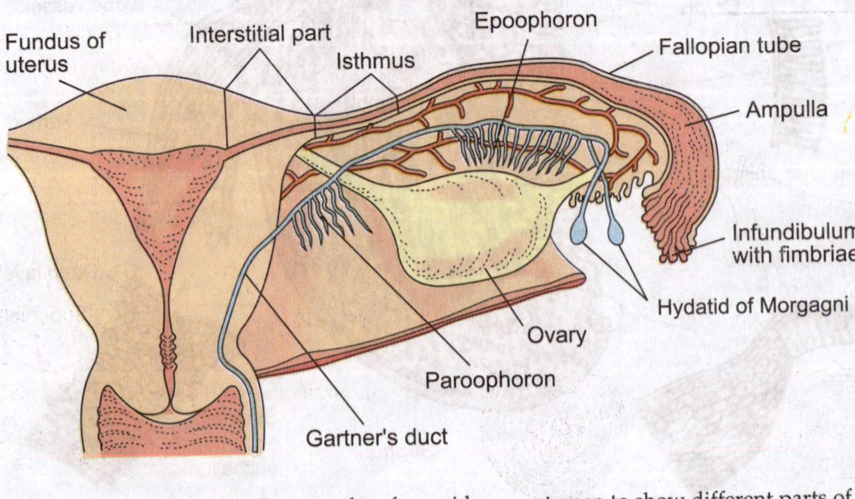

Fig. 1.12. Half of uterine cavity and Fallopian tube of one side are cut open to show different parts of the tube. The vestigial structures in the broad ligament are shown

cavity, called uterine opening and measures 1 mm in diameter, the other is on the lateral end of the tube, called pelvic opening or abdominal ostium and measures about 2 mm in diameter (Fig. 1.12).

Parts

There are four parts, from medial to lateral they are — (1) intramural or interstitial lying in the uterine wall and measures 1.25 cm ($^1/_2$") in length and 1 mm in diameter; (2) isthmus almost straight and measures about 2.5 cm (1") in length and 2.5 mm in diameter; (3) ampulla — tortuous part and measures about 5 cm (2") in length which ends in wide; (4) infundibulum measuring about 1.25 cm ($^1/_2$") long with a maximum diameter of 6 mm. The abdominal ostium is surrounded by a number of radiating fimbriae, one of these is longer than the rest and is attached to the outer pole of the ovary called ovarian fimbria (Fig. 1.13).

Structures

It consists of 3 layers :

(1) Serous — consists of peritoneum on all sides except along the line of attachment of mesosalpinx.

(2) Muscular — arranged in two layers — outer longitudinal and inner circular.

(3) Mucous membrane is thrown into longitudinal folds. It is lined by columnar epithelium, partly ciliated, others secretory non-ciliated and 'Peg cells'. The epithelium rests on delicate vascular reticulum of connective tissue. There is no submucous layer nor any glands. Changes occur in the tubal epithelium during menstrual cycle but are less pronounced and there is no shedding (Fig. 1.13).

Functions

The important functions of the tubes are — (1) Transport of gametes (2) to facilitate fertilization and (3) survival of zygote through its secretion.

Blood supply

Arterial supply is from the uterine and ovarian. Venous drainage is through the pampiniform plexus into the ovarian veins.

Nerve supply

The nerve supply is derived from the uterine and ovarian nerves. The tube is very much sensitive to handling.

THE OVARY

The ovaries are paired sex glands or gonads in female which **are concerned with** :

(i) Germ cell maturation, storage and its release.
(ii) Steroidogenesis.

Each gland is oval in shape and pinkish grey in colour and the surface is scarred during reproductive period. It measures about 3 cm in length, 2 cm in breadth and 1 cm in thickness. Each ovary presents two ends — tubal and uterine, two borders — mesovarium and free posterior and two surfaces — medial and lateral.

The ovaries are intraperitoneal structures. In nulliparae, the ovary lies in the ovarian fossa on the

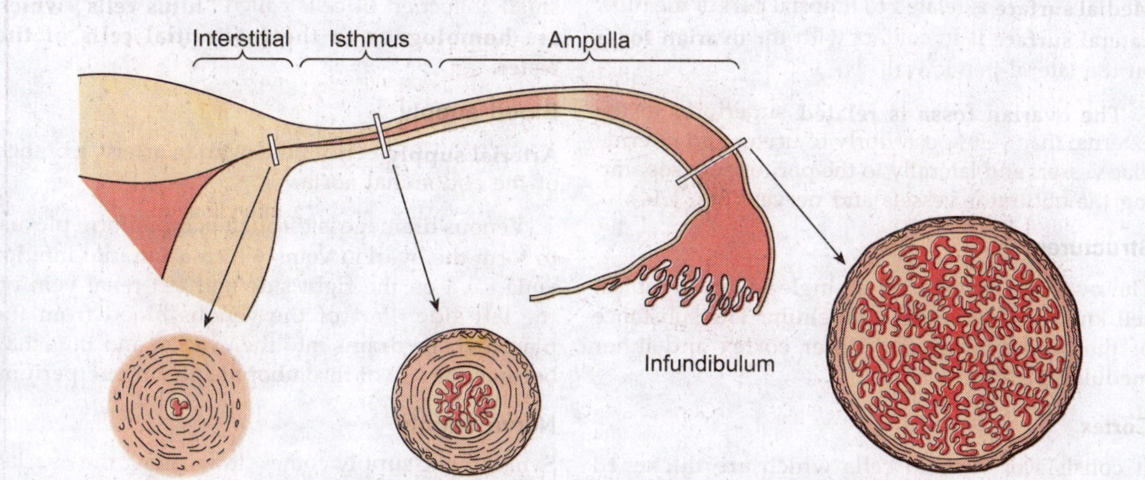

Fig. 1.13. Cut section of the tube showing complex mucosal pattern

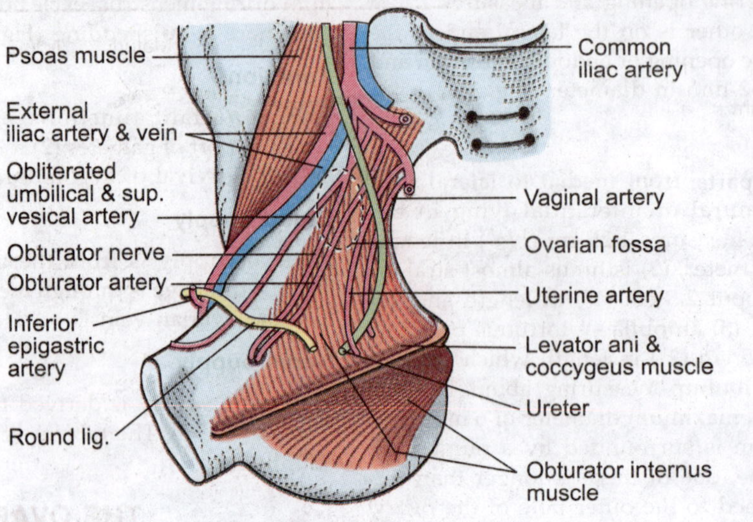

Fig. 1.14. The ovarian fossa with the structures in the lateral pelvic wall

lateral pelvic wall. **The ovary is attached** to the posterior layer of the broad ligament by the mesovarium, to the lateral pelvic wall by infundibulopelvic ligament and to the uterus by the ovarian ligament.

Relations

Mesovarium or anterior border — A fold of peritoneum from the posterior leaf of the broad ligament is attached to the anterior border through which the ovarian vessels and nerves enter the hilum of the gland. **Posterior border** is free and is related with tubal ampulla. It is separated by the peritoneum from the ureter and the internal iliac artery. **Medial surface** is related to fimbrial part of the tube. **Lateral surface** is in contact with the **ovarian fossa** on the lateral pelvic wall.

The ovarian fossa is related superiorly to the external iliac vein, posteriorly to ureter and internal iliac vessels and laterally to the peritoneum separating the obturator vessels and nerves (Fig. 1.14).

Structures

The ovary is covered by a single layer of cubical cell known as germinal epithelium. The substance of the gland consists of outer cortex and inner medulla (Fig. 1.15).

Cortex

It consists of stromal cells which are thickened beneath the germinal epithelium to form tunica albuginea. During reproductive period (i.e. from puberty to menopause), the cortex is studded with numerous follicular structures, called the functional units of the ovary in various phases of their development. These are related to sex hormone production and ovulation. **The structures include** primordial follicles, maturing follicles, Graafian follicles and corpus luteum. Atresia of the structures results in formation of atretic follicles or corpus albicans (Fig. 1.15). The structural changes during ovular cycle are described in the Chapter 8 (p. 81).

Medulla

It consists of loose connective tissues, few unstriped muscles, blood vessels and nerves. There are small collection of cells called **"hilus cells" which are homologous to the interstitial cells of the testes.**

Blood supply

Arterial supply is from the ovarian artery, a branch of the abdominal aorta.

Venous drainage is through pampiniform plexus, to form the ovarian veins which drain into inferior vena cava on the right side and left renal vein on the left side. Part of the venous blood from the placental site drains into the ovarian and thus may become the site of thrombophlebitis in puerperium.

Nerve supply

Sympathetic supply comes down along the ovarian artery from T_{10} segment. Ovaries are sensitive to manual squeezing.

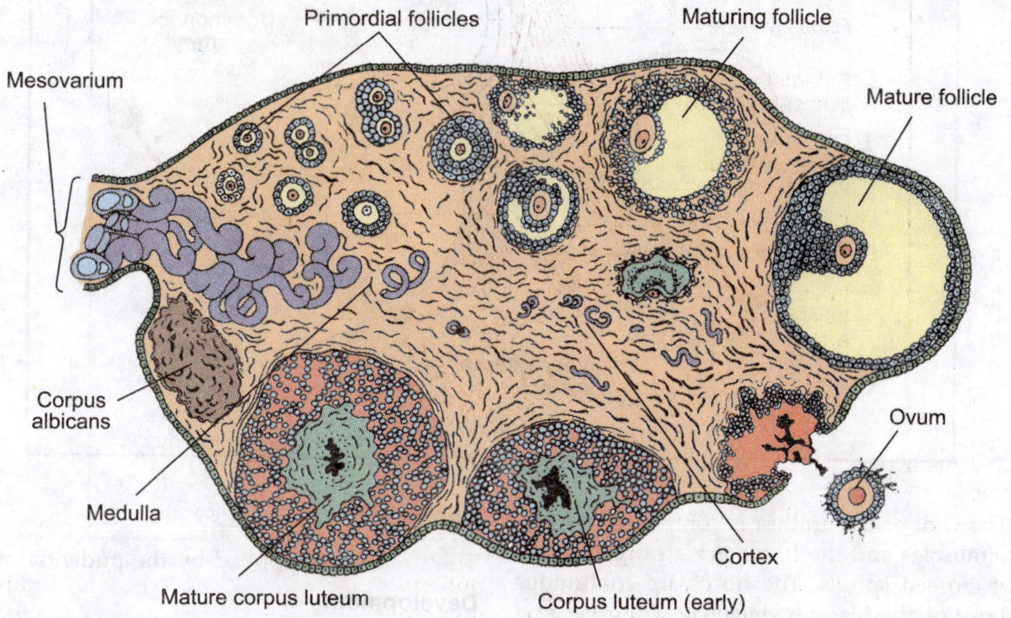

Fig. 1.15. Histological structures of the ovary

FEMALE URETHRA

The female urethra extends from the neck of the bladder to the external urethral meatus. **It measures about 4 cm and has a diameter of about 6 mm.**

The bladder base forms an angle with the posterior wall of the urethra called posterior urethrovesical-angle (PUV) which normally measures 100°. The urethra runs downwards and forwards in close proximity of the anterior vaginal wall. About 1 cm from the lower end, it pierces the triangular ligament. It ultimately opens into the vestibule about 2.5 cm below the clitoris.

Relations

Posteriorly

It is related to the anterior vaginal wall to which it is loosely separated in the upper two-third but firmly adherent in the lower-third.

Anteriorly

It is related to the posterior aspect of symphysis pubis. The upper two-third is separated by loose areolar tissue; the lower one-third is attached on each side of the pubic rami by fibrous tissue called — pubourethral ligament.

Laterally

(i) As it passes through the triangular ligament, it is surrounded by compressor urethra.

(ii) Whether the medial fibres of puborectalis get attached to the urethra while passing by its sides to get attached to lateral vaginal walls is debatable.

(iii) Bulbocavernosus and vestibular bulb.

Glands

Numerous tubular glands called paraurethral glands open into the lumen through ducts. Of these, two are longer and called Skene's ducts which open either on the posterior wall just inside the external meatus or into the vestibule. **Skene's glands are homologous to the prostate in the male.**

Sphincters

The following sphincters are described :

(1) At the urethrovesical junction, there is intricate decussation of the involuntary muscles. This has the effect of forming anterior and posterior slings which function as an involuntary internal sphincter. This is the lissosphincter. When the detrusor muscle actively contracts, the slings relax → funnelling of the bladder neck → urine flows into the urethra (Fig. 1.16).

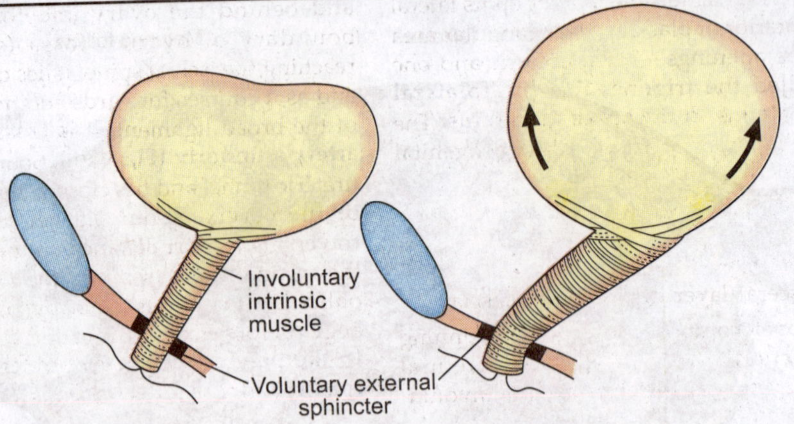

Fig. 1.16. Urethral sphincters

(2) The wall of the urethra is composed of involuntary muscles and the fibres are arranged in the form of crossed spirals. The fibres are continuous with those of the bladder detrusor. The tone and elasticity of these muscles keep it close except during micturition.

(3) Sphincter urethra in the urogenital diaphragm. This sphincter allows the voluntary arrest of urine flow.

(4) Although debatable, puborectalis part of levator ani which surrounds the lower-third of the urethra acts as an external sphincter.

(5) Superficial perineal muscles, bulbocavernosus and ischiocavernosus form an accessory external sphincter.

Structures

Mucous membrane is lined by transitional epithelium except at the external urethral meatus where it becomes stratified squamous. Submucous coat is vascular. Muscle coat is composed of involuntary muscles and the fibres are arranged in the form of crossed spirals.

Blood supply

Arterial supply

Proximal part is supplied by the inferior vesical branch and the distal part by a branch of internal pudendal artery.

The veins drain into vesical plexus and into internal pudendal veins.

Lymphatics (see p. 30).

Nerves

The urethra is supplied by the pudendal nerve.

Development

The urethra is developed from the vesicourethral portion of the cloaca.

Applied Anatomy

(i) Because of shortness and its close proximity to the vagina and anus, the infection is likely which commonly spreads upwards to involve the bladder. (ii) Because of close proximity of the anterior vaginal wall, the urethra may be injured during the process of childbirth. (iii) The paraurethral glands are the sites of infection and occasional development of benign adenoma or malignant changes.

THE URINARY BLADDER

The bladder is a hollow muscular organ with considerable power of distension. Its capacity is about 450 ml (15 oz) but can retain as much as 3-4 litres of urine. When distended, it is ovoid in shape. It has got : (1) an apex, (2) superior surface, (3) base, (4) two inferolateral surfaces and (5) neck which is continuous with the urethra. **The base and the neck remain fixed even when the bladder is distended.**

Relations

The superior surface is related with the peritoneum of the uterovesical pouch (Fig. 1.5). The base is related with the supravaginal cervix and the anterior fornix. The ureters, after crossing the pelvic floor at the sides of the cervix, enter the bladder on its lateral angles. In the interior of bladder, the triangular area marked by three openings — two ureteric and one urethral, is called the trigone. The **inferolateral surfaces are related with the space of Retzius**. The neck rests on the superior layer of the urogenital diaphragm.

Structures

From outside inwards :

(1) Outer visceral layer of the pelvic fascia.

(2) Muscle layer composed of muscles running in various directions. Near the internal urethral opening, the circular muscle fibres provide involuntary sphincter.

(3) Mucous coat is lined by transitional epithelium with no gland. **There is no submucous coat.**

Blood supply

The arterial supply is through superior and inferior vesical arteries. The veins drain into vesical and vaginal plexus and thence to internal iliac veins.

Lymphatics

Lymphatics drain into external and internal iliac lymph nodes.

Nerve supply

The sympathetic supply is from the pelvic plexus and the parasympathetic via the pelvic plexus from the nervi erigentes ($S_{2,3,4}$). **The parasympathetic** produces contraction of the detrusor muscles and relaxation of the internal sphincter (nerve of evacuation). Sympathetic conveys afferent painful stimuli of over-distension.

Development

The urinary bladder is developed from the upper part of the urogenital sinus.

PELVIC URETER

The pelvic ureter extends from its crossing over the pelvic brim upto its opening into the bladder. **It measures about 13 cm in length and has a diameter of 5 mm.**

Course and relations

The ureter enters the pelvis in front of the bifurcation of the common iliac artery over the sacroiliac joint behind the root of the mesentery on the right side and the apex of the mesosigmoid on the left side. As it courses downwards in contact with the peritoneum, it lies anterior to the internal iliac artery and behind the ovary and forms the posterior boundary of ovarian fossa (see Fig. 1.14).. On reaching the ischial spine, it lies over the pelvic floor and as it courses forwards and medially on the base of the broad ligament, **it is crossed by the uterine artery anteriorly (Fig. 1.10)**. Soon, it enters into the ureteric tunnel and lies close to the supravaginal part of the cervix, about 1.5 cm lateral to it. After traversing a short distance on the anterior fornix of the vagina, it courses into the wall of the bladder obliquely for about 2 cm by piercing the lateral angle before it opens into the base of the trigone. **In the pelvic portion, the ureter is comparatively constricted :**

(a) Where it crosses the pelvic brim.

(b) Where crossed by the uterine artery.

(c) In the intravesical part.

Structures

From outside inwards — (1) Fibres derived from the visceral layer of the pelvic fascia. (2) Muscle coat consisting of three layers — outer and inner longitudinal and intermediate circular. (3) Mucous layer lined by transitional epithelium.

Blood supply

The ureter has got segmental supply from nearly all the visceral branches of the anterior division of the internal iliac artery. The venous drainage corresponds to the arteries.

Lymphatics

The lymphatics from the lower part drain into the external and internal iliac lymph nodes and the upper part into the lumbar lymph nodes.

Nerve supply

Sympathetic supply is from the hypogastric and pelvic plexus; parasympathetic from the sacral plexus.

Development

The ureter is developed as an ureteric bud from the caudal end of the mesonephric duct.

Applied Anatomy

- **The ureter is recognised by the following features :**

  (i) Pale glistening appearance.

  (ii) Longitudinal vessels on the surface.

  (iii) Peristalsis.

- **The ureter is likely to be damaged** during pelvic surgery (see p. 408).

Abdominal hysterectomy

The common sites of ureteric injury are — (i) Infundibulopelvic ligament. (ii) By the side of the cervix (clamping the cardinal ligament along with descending cervical artery). (iii) Vaginal angle as the ureter traverses along the anterior fornix. (iv) During pelvic peritonisation (ureter lies in the posterior leaf of the peritoneum).

The chances of injury are more in cases of endometriosis, pelvic inflammation or broad ligament tumour. Injury is more common during reclamping than primary clamping.

Radical hysterectomy

Direct injury is not common. Sloughing necrosis may occur due to stripping the ureter off the peritoneum → devitalisation → sloughing.

RECTUM

The rectum commences at the level of the third piece of the sacrum in continuation of pelvic colon and ends in anal canal. It measures 12-15 cm. The rectum follows the curve of the sacrum. It curves twice to the left and once to the right before it passes down to continue as anal canal.

Peritoneal coverings

Rectum is covered anteriorly and laterally in its upper-third, only anteriorly in the middle-third. Whole of the posterior surface and the entire lower-third remain uncovered.

Relations

Anteriorly :

(i) The part of the rectum covered by peritoneum is related to the posterior wall of the pouch of Douglas.

(ii) The ampulla is related to the posterior vaginal wall separated by rectovaginal septum.

(iii) The lower part is related to the perineal body.

Posteriorly : Rectum is related to the sacrum and coccyx from which intervened by loose areolar tissue, sacral nerve trunks and middle sacral vessels.

Laterally : Rectum is related to uterosacral ligament, pelvic plexus of nerves and ureter. Near the anorectal junction, it is related to puborectalis part of levator ani. Below the muscle, it is related to ischiorectal fossa.

Structures

Rectum is surrounded by rectal fascia. Muscle coat consists of outer longitudinal and inner circular fibres. Submucous layer is loose and contains venous plexuses. Mucous membrane is lined by columnar epithelium.

ANAL CANAL

The anal canal measures about 2.5 cm. It is directed backwards almost at right angles to the ampulla and at the site of insertion of puborectalis part of levator ani. It ends at the anal orifice. At the junction of the upper two-third and lower one-third is the white line (Hilton's line).

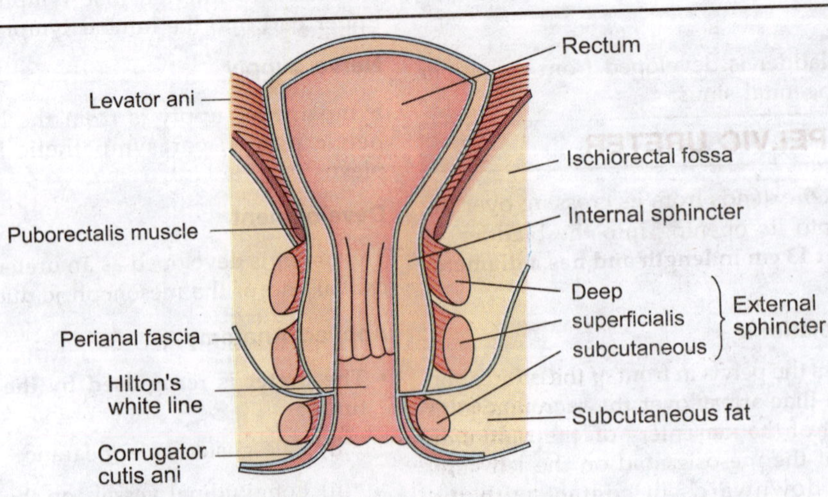

Fig. 1.17. Rectum and anal canal with anal structures

Relations

Anteriorly, it is related to perineal body and posteriorly to the anococcygeal body.

Anal sphincters

The anal canal has got two sphincters.

• Involuntary internal sphincter is formed by thickening of circular layer of the upper two-third of the anal canal.

• Voluntary sphincter ani externus which surrounds the entire length of the canal, **consists of three parts** :

(i) Subcutaneous part—It is attached to the skin.

(ii) Superficial part — It starts from the perineal body and is inserted posteriorly to the tip of the coccyx.

(iii) Deep part — It is separated from the sphincter ani internus by levator ani (Fig. 1.17).

Lining epithelium

The upper two-third is lined by columnar epithelium but the lower-third with stratified squamous epithelium.

Blood supply of rectum and anal canal

Arterial supply is from :

(i) Superior rectal — branch of inferior mesenteric artery.

(ii) Middle rectal — branch of internal iliac artery.

(iii) Inferior rectal — branch of the internal iliac artery.

Venous drainage

The rectum and upper-third of the anal canal drain via superior rectal veins to portal circulation. The lower-third of the anal canal drains on both sides into inferior rectal veins (systemic system).

Lymphatics of rectum and anal canal

The lymphatics from the rectum and upper-third of the anal canal drain into internal iliac and pre-aortic nodes, while the lower-third of the anal canal drains into the superficial inguinal nodes.

Nerve supply of rectum and anal canal

The rectum and the upper two-third of the anal canal are supplied by autonomic through pelvic plexuses. The lower-third of the anal canal is supplied by inferior haemorrhoidal nerve.

Development of rectum and anal canal

The rectum and the upper two-third of the anal canal are developed from the dorsal part of cloaca (endoderm). The lower one-third of the anal canal is developed from the anal pit (ectoderm).

PELVIC MUSCLES

The most important muscle supporting the pelvic organs is the levator ani which forms the pelvic floor. The small muscles of the perineum also have got some contribution in the support.

PELVIC FLOOR

(Syn : Pelvic diaphragm)

Pelvic floor is a muscular partition which separates the pelvic cavity from the anatomical perineum. It consists of three sets of muscles on either side — **pubococcygeus, iliococcygeus and ischiococcygeus. These are collectively called levator ani.** Its upper surface is concave and slopes downwards, backwards and medially and is covered by parietal layer of pelvic fascia. The inferior surface is convex and is covered by anal fascia. The muscle with the covering fascia is called the **pelvic diaphragm**. **Levator ani** is a strong and fatigue resistant striated muscle. It is stug like a hammock around the midline pelvic effluents (urethra, vagina and anal canal : Fig. 1.18).

Origin

Each levator ani arises from the back of the pubic rami, from the condensed fascia covering the obturator internus **(white line)** and from the inner surface of the ischial spine.

Insertion

The **pubococcygeus** — The fibres pass backwards, downwards and medially and are inserted as followers. (a) The posterior fibres are inserted into the anococcygeal raphe and tip of the coccyx. (b) **Puborectalis** — these fibres wind round the anorectal junction and are continuous with the similar fibres of the opposite side forming a 'U'-shaped loop known as *Puborectal sling.* (c) **Puboanalis** — these fibres run between the sphincter and externus and internus and are inserted in the wall of the anal canal along the longitudinal fibres. (d) Pubovaginalis — these anterior fibres pass by the side of vagina and are inserted into the perineal body (Fig. 1.18).

Coccygeus (Ischiococcygeus) is triangular in

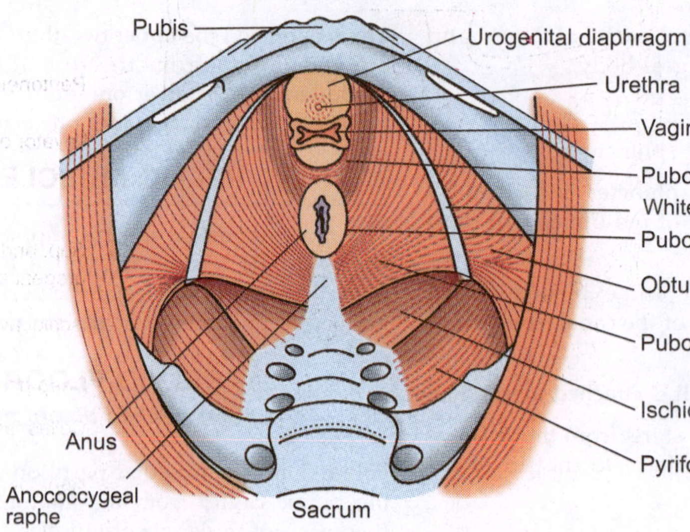

Fig. 1.18. Levator ani muscles viewed from above

shape. It arises from the apex of the ischial spine and the sacrospinous ligament and is inserted by its base into the sides of the upper two pieces of the coccyx and the last piece of sacrum (Fig. 1.18).

Anococcygeal raphe also known as **levator plate**, is a layered musculo-fibrous tissue. It extends from the anorectal junction to the tip of the coccyx. It comprises from above downwards : (i) Presacral fascia, (ii) tendinous plate of pubococcygeus, (iii) muscular raphe of ilio coccygeus and (iv) superficial fibres of sphincter ani externus muscles (Fig. 1.18).

Gaps

There are two gaps in the midline — (1) The anterior one is called **hiatus urogenitalis** which is bridged by the muscles and fascia of urogenital triangle and pierced by the urethra and vagina. (2) The posterior one is called **hiatus rectalis,** transmitting the rectum.

Structure in relation to pelvic floor

The superior surface is related with the following :

(1) Pelvic organs from anterior to posterior are bladder, vagina and rectum.

(2) Pelvic cellular tissues between the pelvic peritoneum and upper surface of the levator ani which fill all the available spaces.

(3) Ureter lies on the floor in relation to the lateral vaginal fornix. **The uterine artery lies above and the vaginal artery lies below it.**

(4) Pelvic nerves.

The inferior surface is related to the anatomical perineum.

Nerve supply

The muscle is supplied by the 3rd and 4th sacral nerve, inferior rectal nerve and a perineal branch of pudendal nerve ($S_{2,3,4}$).

Functions

(1) To support the pelvic organs — The pubovaginalis which forms a 'U'-shaped sling, supports the vagina which in turn supports the other pelvic organs — bladder and uterus. Weakness or tear of this sling during parturition is responsible for prolapse of the organs concerned.

(2) Counteracts the downward thrust of increased intra-abdominal pressure and guards the hiatus urogenitalis.

(3) Facilitates anterior internal rotation of the presenting part when it presses on the (puborectal sling) pelvic floor.

(4) Puborectalis plays an ancillary role to the action of the external anal sphincter.

(5) Ischiococcygeus helps to stabilise the sacroiliac and sacrococcygeal joints.

(6) To steady the perineal body.

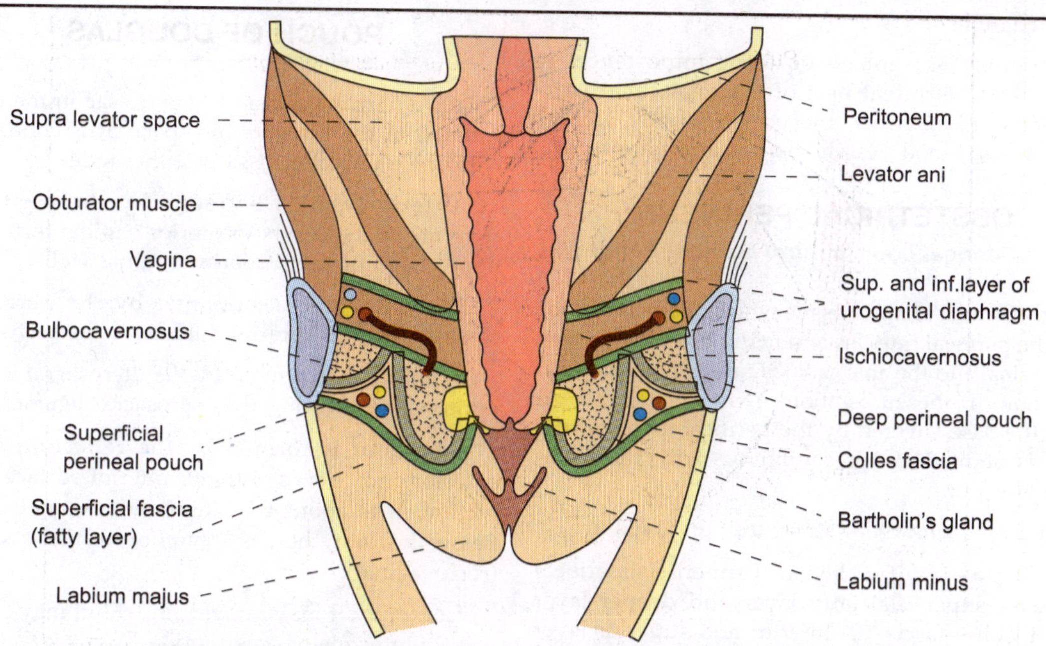

Fig. 1.19. Schematic diagram showing the pelvic muscles, fascia and cellular tissue as seen from the front

Pelvic floor during pregnancy and parturition

During pregnancy, levator muscles hypertrophy, become less rigid and more distensible. Due to water retention, it swells up and sags down. In the second stage, the pubovaginalis and puborectalis relax and the levator ani is drawn up over the advancing presenting part in the second stage. Failure of the levator ani to relax at the crucial moment may lead to extensive damage of the pelvic structures. The effect of such a displacement is to elongate the birth canal which is composed solely of soft parts below the bony outlet. The soft canal has got deep lateral and posterior walls and its axis is in continuation with the axis of the bony pelvis.

PERINEUM

Anatomical perineum

Anatomically, the perineum is bounded above by the inferior surface of the pelvic floor, below by the skin between the buttocks and thighs. Laterally, it is bounded by the ischiopubic rami, ischial tuberosities and sacrotuberous ligaments and posteriorly, by the coccyx. The diamond-shaped space of the bony pelvic outlet is divided into two triangular spaces with the common base formed by the free border of the urogenital diaphragm. The anterior triangle is called the urogenital triangle which fills up the gap of the hiatus urogenitalis and is important from the obstetric point of view. The posterior one is called the anal triangle.

Urogenital triangle

It is pierced by the terminal part of the vagina and the urethra. The small perineal muscles are situated in two compartments formed by the ill-defined fascia. The compartments are superficial and deep perineal pouch. **The superficial pouch** is formed by the deep layer of the superficial perineal fascia (Colles fascia) and inferior layer of the urogenital diaphragm (perineal membrane). **The contents are** (Figs. 1.3 and 1.19) superficial transverse perinei (paired), bulbocavernosus covering the bulb of the vestibule, ischiocavernosus (paired) covering the crura of the clitoris and the Bartholin's gland (paired). The **deep perineal pouch** is formed by the inferior and superior layer of the urogenital diaphragm — together called urogenital diaphragm or triangular ligament. Between the layers there is a potential space of about 1.25 cm. **The contents are** the following muscles — deep transverse perinei (paired) and sphincter urethrae membranaceae. Both the pouches contain vessels and nerves (Fig. 1.19).

Anal triangle

The triangle has got no obstetric importance. It contains the terminal part of the anal canal with sphincter ani externus, anococcygeal body, ischiorectal fossa, blood vessels, nerves and lymphatics.

OBSTETRICAL PERINEUM

(Syn : Perineal body, central point of perineum)

The pyramidal-shaped tissue where the pelvic floor and the perineal muscles and fascia meet in between the vaginal and the anal canal is called the obstetrical perineum. It measures about 4 cm × 4 cm (1 1/2") with the base covered by the perineal skin and the apex is pointed and is continuous with the rectovaginal septum.

The musculofascial structures involved are :

- **Fascia** — (1) Two layers of superficial perineal fascia — superficial fatty layer and deeper layer called Colles fascia. (2) Inferior and superior layer of urogenital diaphragm, together called triangular ligament.
- **Muscles** — (1) Superficial and deep transverse perinei (paired). (2) Bulbospongiosus. (3) Levator ani — pubococcygeus part (paired) situated at the junction of the upper two-third and lower one-third of the vagina. (4) Sphincter ani externus (few fibres)

Importance :

(1) It helps to support the levator ani which is placed above it.

(2) By supporting the posterior vaginal wall, it indirectly supports the anterior vaginal wall, bladder and the uterus.

(3) It is vulnerable to injury during childbirth.

(4) Deliberate cutting of the structures during delivery is called episiotomy.

PELVIC PERITONEUM

Traced anteriorly, the peritoneum covering the superior surface of the bladder reflects over the anterior surface of the uterus at the level of the internal os. The pouch, so formed, is called **uterovesical pouch**. The peritoneum thereafter, is firmly attached to the anterior and posterior walls of the uterus and upper one-third of the posterior vaginal wall where from it is reflected over the rectum. The pouch, so formed, is called **pouch of Douglas** (Fig. 1.6).

POUCH OF DOUGLAS

This is a narrow peritoneal cul-de-sac in the pelvis situated in the rectouterine space. It is continuous with the pararectal fossa of either side.

Anteriorly, it is bounded by the peritoneal covering of the cervix, posterior vaginal fornix and upper-third of the posterior vaginal wall.

Posteriorly, it is bounded by the peritoneal covering on the anterior surface of the rectum.

Laterally, it is limited by the uterosacral folds of peritoneum covering the uterosacral ligaments.

The floor is formed by the reflection of the anterior peritoneum onto the anterior surface of the rectum. It is about 6-7 cm above the anal orifice. Below the floor, there is a thin fibrous tissue septum (rectovaginal).

Contents : It may remain empty but may contain coils of intestine or omentum.

Surgical importance

- As it is the most dependent part of the peritoneal cavity, intraperitoneal blood or pus usually settles down to the pouch to produce either pelvic haematocele or pelvic abscess.
- Herniation of the pouch through the posterior fornix may occur producing the clinical entity of enterocele.
- Vaginal ligation is done through opening the pouch.
- Culdoscopy, culdocentesis or at time pneumoperitoneum may be done through the pouch.
- Nodules deposited in the pouch can help in the clinical diagnosis of pelvic malignancy, endometriosis or genital tuberculosis.

BROAD LIGAMENT

The double fold of peritoneum which extends from the lateral border of the uterus to the lateral pelvic wall of pelvis is called broad ligament. These are two, one on each side. These, truly are not ligaments (Fig. 1.12).

Each broad ligament consists of two layers, anterior and posterior. The layers are continuous at its upper free border embracing the Fallopian tube. The lower part of the broad ligament is wider from before backwards and the layers are reflected above the pelvic diaphragm. The anterior leaf is reflected forwards at the level of the internal os as utero-vesical pouch. The posterior leaf descends a little down to cover the upper-third of the posterior vaginal wall to form the posterior layer of the pouch of Douglas.

Parts

INFUNDIBULOPELVIC LIGAMENT
(Syn : Suspensory ligament of the ovary)

It includes the portion of the broad ligament which extends from the infundibulum of the Fallopian tube to the lateral pelvic wall. It contains ovarian vessels and nerves and lymphatics from the ovary, Fallopian tube and body of the uterus.

Mesovarium : The ovary is attached to the posterior layer of the broad ligament by a fold of peritoneum called mesovarium (ovarian mesentery). Through this fold, ovarian vessels, nerves and lymphatics enter and leave the hilum. The ovary is not enclosed within the broad ligament (Fig. 1.10).

Mesosalpinx : The part of the broad ligament between the Fallopian tube and the level of attachment of the ovary is the mesosalpinx. It contains utero-ovarian anastomotic vessels and vestigial remnants (Fig. 1.12).

Mesometrium : The part of the broad ligament below the mesosalpinx is called mesometrium. It is the longest portion which is related with the lateral border of the uterus.

Contents

Each broad ligament contains :

- Fallopian tube
- Uterine and ovarian arteries with their branches, including the anastomotic branches between them and corresponding veins.
- Nerves and lymphatics from the uterus, Fallopian tube and ovary.
- Proximal part of the round ligament which raises a peritoneal fold on the anterior leaf.
- Ovarian ligament which raises a peritoneal fold on the posterior leaf.
- Parametrium containing loose areolar tissue and fat. The terminal part of the ureter, uterine artery, paracervical nerve and lymphatic plexus are lying at the base of the broad ligament.
- Vestigial structures such as — duct of Gartner, epoophoron and paroophoron.

Development

The broad transverse fold which is established as the two müllerian ducts approach each other is developed into broad ligament.

Function

Along with the loose areolar tissue (packing material), it has got steadying effect to maintain the uterus in position.

PELVIC FASCIA AND CELLULAR TISSUE

PELVIC FASCIA

For descriptive purpose, the pelvic fascia is grouped under the heading that covers the pelvic wall, the pelvic floor and the pelvic viscera.

Fascia on the pelvic wall

The fascia is very tough and membranous. It covers the obturator internus and pyriformis and gets attached to the margins of the bone. The pelvic nerves lie external to the fascia but the vessels lie internal to it.

Fascia on the pelvic floor

The fascia is not tough but loose. The superior and the inferior surfaces are covered by the parietal layer of the pelvic fascia which runs down from the white line to merge with the visceral layer of the pelvic fascia covering the anal canal (Fig. 1.19).

Fascia covering the pelvic viscera

The fascia is not condensed and often contains loose areolar tissue to allow distension of the organs.

PELVIC CELLULAR TISSUE

The cellular tissue lies between the pelvic peritoneum and the pelvic floor and fills up all the available empty spaces. It contains fatty and connective tissues and unstriped muscle fibres. **Collectively it is known as endopelvic fascia.** Its distribution round the vaginal vault, supravaginal part of the cervix and into the layers of the broad ligament is called **parametrium**. Condensation occurs specially near the cervicovaginal junction to form ligaments which extend from the viscera to the pelvic walls on either side. **The deep endopelvic connective tissue condenses to form** (i) Uterosacral ligaments. (ii) Cardinal ligaments. (iii) Pubocervical ligament. (iv) Rectovaginal septum. (v) Pubovesical fascia.

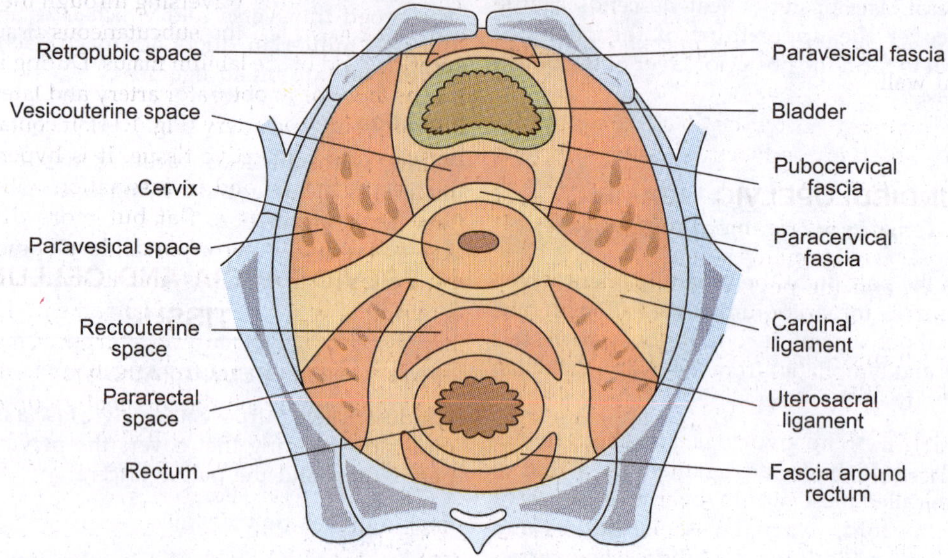

Fig. 1.20. The main supporting ligaments of the uterus viewed from above

MACKENRODT'S LIGAMENTS

(Syn : Cardinal ligament, transverse cervical)

Origin : Condensation of parietal fascia covering the obturator internus.

Insertion : Lateral supravaginal cervix and upper part of lateral vaginal wall in a fan-shaped manner. This insertion is continuous with the endopelvic and paricervical fascial ring.

Content : Uterosacral plexus of autonomic nerves, uterine artery and vein, smooth muscle fibre. **Distal part of ureter passes under the uterine artery within the upper part of the cardinal ligament.** It is situated inferior to the uterosacral ligament with which it is blended (Fig. 1.20).

Function : (i) Lateral stabilisation to the cervix at the level of ischial spine. (ii) Primary vascular conduits of the uterus and vagina.

UTEROSACRAL LIGAMENTS

Origin : Periosteum of sacral vertebra 2, 3 and 4.

Insertion : Posterolateral surface of the cervix at the level of internal os. Here it blends with the endopelvic fascial ring. These are formed by condensation of peritoneum.

Content : Uterosacral plexus of autonomic nerves. Smooth muscle and minimal vessels.

Function : These are the primary proximal suspensory ligaments of the uterovaginal complex. They hold the cervix posteriorly at the level of the ischial spines. Uterus is thus maintained anteflexed and the vagina is suspended over the levator plate.

PUBOCERVICAL FASCIA (BLADDER PILLAR)

Origin : Back of the pubic bone and the arcus tendinous fascia laterally.

Insertion : Anterolateral supravaginal cervix and blends with the pericervical ring of endopelvic fascia and the cardinal ligaments.

Content : Artery and veins of the bladder pillar.

Function : These ligaments are poorly developed. They serve mainly as vascular conduit and provide less cervical stabilisation force.

Vesicovaginal Septum : It is a fibroelastic connective tissue with some smooth muscle fibres.

Extension : Laterally, it extends from pubic tubercles, pubic arch. Arcus tendinous fascia (white line) and centrally to the pubocervical ring, blending with the pubocervical and cardinal ligaments and pelvic visceral fascia.

Function : It supports the bladder and the anterior vaginal wall.

Rectovaginal septum (Fascia of Denonvilliers'). It is also a fibroelastic connective tissue with few smooth muscle fibres.

Extension : Laterally, it extents from arcus tendinous, uterosacral ligaments and fuses with the perineal body, and the pericervical ring centrally. It also act as the visceral fascia of the rectum.

Function : It supports the posterior vaginal wall, stabilises the rectum and the perineum.

Pericervical ring : See Fig. 1.20.

Importances of the pelvic cellular tissue and their condensation :

- To support the pelvic organs.
- To form protective sheath for the blood vessels and the terminal part of the ureter.
- Infection spreads along the track, so formed outside the pelvis to the perinephric region along the ureter, to the buttock along the gluteal vessels, to the thigh along the external iliac vessels and to the groin along the round ligament.
- Marked hypertrophy occurs during pregnancy to widen up the spaces.

ROUND LIGAMENTS

These are paired, one on each side. Each measures about 10-12 cm. It is attached at the cornu of the uterus below and in front of the Fallopian tube. It courses beneath the anterior leaf of the broad ligament to reach the internal abdominal ring (Figs. 1.10 and 1.14). After traversing through the inguinal canal, it fuses with the subcutaneous tissue of the anterior third of the labium majus. During its course it runs anterior to obturator artery and lateral to the inferior epigastric artery (Fig. 1.14). It contains plain muscles and connective tissue. It is hypertrophied during pregnancy and in association with fibroid. Near the uterus, it is flat but more distally, it becomes round. It corresponds developmentally to the gubernaculum testis and is morphologically continuous with the ovarian ligament. The blood supply is from the utero-ovarian anastomotic vessels. The lymphatics from the body of the uterus pass along it to reach the inguinal group of nodes. While it is not related to maintain the uterus in anteverted position but its shortening by operation is utilised to make the uterus anteverted.

Embryologically, it corresponds with gubernaculum testis. In the fetus, there is a tubular process of peritoneum continuing with the round ligament into the inguinal region. This process is called canal of Nuck. It is analogous to the processus vaginalis which precedes to descent of the testis.

OVARIAN LIGAMENTS

These are paired, one on each side. Each one is a fibromuscular cord-like structure which attaches to the inner pole of the ovary and to the cornu of the uterus posteriorly below the level of the attachment of the Fallopian tube (Fig. 1.12). It lies beneath the posterior leaf of the broad ligament and measures about 2.5 cm in length. **Morphologically, it is continuous with the round ligament and together are the homologue to the gubernaculum testis.**

KEY POINTS

- The labia majora contain sebaceous, sweat glands and hair follicles.
- The labia minora are devoid of fat and do not contain hair follicle.
- There are four openings in the vestibule—vaginal orifice, urethral opening, opening of paired Bartholin's ducts. Rarely, paraurethral ducts open into the vestibule.
- Bartholin's gland is situated in the superficial perineal pouch and measures about 0.5 cm. The duct measures 2 cm. The gland is compound racemose and lined by columnar epithelium. The duct is lined by columnar epithelium except near the opening, where it is lined by stratified squamous epithelium.
- The length of the anterior vaginal wall is 7 cm and that of posterior wall is 9 cm. Ureter lies about 2 cm from the lateral fornix. Vagina is lined by stratified squamous epithelium. It has no glands. The pH ranges between 4-5.5. Doderlein bacillus is gram-positive anaerobic organism. The glycogen content is highest in the vaginal fornix being 2.5-3 mg. per cent.
- Uterus measures 8 cm and weighs 50-80 gm. Isthmus is bounded above by the anatomical internal os and below by the histological internal os. Isthmus measures 0.5 cm. Normal length of uterine cavity is 6-7 cm. Uterine artery crosses the ureter anteriorly from above. The epithelium, called endometrium is ciliated columnar type. The glands are simple tubular. There is no submucous layer. Cervical canal is lined by tall columnar epithelium. The cervical glands are compound racemose type.
- Fallopian tube has got 4 parts — interstitial (1 mm diameter), isthmus, ampullary (fertilisation takes place) and infundibulum (6 mm diameter). It is lined by ciliated columnar epithelium, secretory non-ciliated epithelium and 'peg' cells. The tube measures 10 cm.
- Ovary is attached to the posterior leaf of the broad ligament by the mesovarium. The ovarian fossa is related posteriorly to ureter. The cortex is studded with follicular structures and the medulla contains hilus cells which are homologous to the interstitial cells of the testes.
- Female urethra measures 4 cm with a diameter of 6 mm. Posterior urethrovesical angle measures 100°. Mucous coat is lined by transitional epithelium. There is no submucous coat.
- Pelvic part of the female ureter measures 13 cm with a diameter of 5 mm. It lies close to the supravaginal part of the cervix (1.5 cm). It is comparatively constricted (i) where it crosses the brim, (ii) where crossed by the uterine artery and (iii) in the intravesical part. The ureter is likely to be damaged during hysterectomy at the infundibulopelvic ligament, by the side of the cervix, at the vaginal angle and during posterior peritonisation.
- Superficial perineal pouch is formed by the deep layer of the superficial perineal fascia and inferior layer of the urogenital diaphragm. The deep perineal pouch is formed by the inferior and superior layer of the urogenital diaphragm. Obstetrical perineum is the fibromuscular structure, pyramidal-shaped with the base covered by the perineal skin and situated in between the vaginal and anal canal. It measures 4 cm × 4 cm.
- Broad ligament has got four parts — infundibulopelvic ligament, mesovarium, mesosalpinx and mesometrium. Broad ligament contains Fallopian tube, round ligament, ovarian ligament, parametrium, utero-ovarian anastomotic vessels, nerves, lymphatics of the uterus, tubes and ovaries and vestigial structures — duct of Gartner, epoophoron and paroophoron.
- Round ligament measures 10-12 cm. One end is attached to cornu of the uterus and the other end terminates in the anterior third of the labium majus.

Blood Vessels, Lymphatic Drainage and Innervation of Pelvic Organs

2

THE PELVIC BLOOD VESSELS

• **Arterial supply** • **Venous drainage**

ARTERIAL SUPPLY

Sources

- Anterior division of internal iliac artery.
- Ovarian artery.
- Superior rectal artery.

Internal iliac artery

Internal iliac artery is one of the bifurcation of the common iliac artery. The bifurcation occurs over the sacroiliac articulation. It measures about 2 cm. Ureter lies anteriorly and the internal iliac vein posteriorly. It soon divides into anterior and posterior divisions. Only the anterior division supplies the pelvic viscera. The branches are schematically mentioned overleaf.

Uterine artery

Origin : The uterine artery arises either directly from the internal iliac artery or in common with the obliterated umbilical artery.

Course : It runs downwards and forwards along the lateral pelvic wall almost in the same direction as the ureter until it reaches the base of the broad ligament. It then turns medially and crosses the ureter anteriorly from above and at right angle to it; about 1.5-2 cm lateral to, at the level of internal os. On reaching the side of the uterus, it runs upwards and takes a spiral course along the lateral uterine wall between the layers of broad ligament. It ultimately anastomoses end on with the tubal branch of the ovarian artery in the mesosalpinx.

Branches

The following branches are given off :

- Ureteric — as it cross it.
- Descending cervical.
- Circular artery to the cervix — This is formed by anterior and posterior branches of the artery to the cervix of both sides.
- Segmental arcuate arteries — These are the branches from the ascending part. These pierce about one-third of the myometrium and then divide into anterior and posterior branches. These anastomose with the corresponding branches of the opposite side in the midline. Thus, the middle of the uterus is comparatively avascular. From the arcuate arteries, a series of radial arteries arise almost at right angles which stretch through the entire length of the myometrium. Near the myoendometrial junction, the radial arteries are divided into —

(a) short basal artery — supplies the basal endometrium, and

(b) spiral artery which proceeds as far as superficial portion of the endometrium and ends finally in extensive capillary plexuses (Fig. 2.1).

- Fundal branch.
- Twigs to round ligament.
- Tubal branch.
- Ovarian anastomotic branch.

Vaginal artery

Origin : The vaginal artery arises either from the uterine artery or directly from the anterior division of the internal iliac artery. It is in relation to the lateral fornix and then runs down along the lateral wall of the vagina. Numerous transverse branches

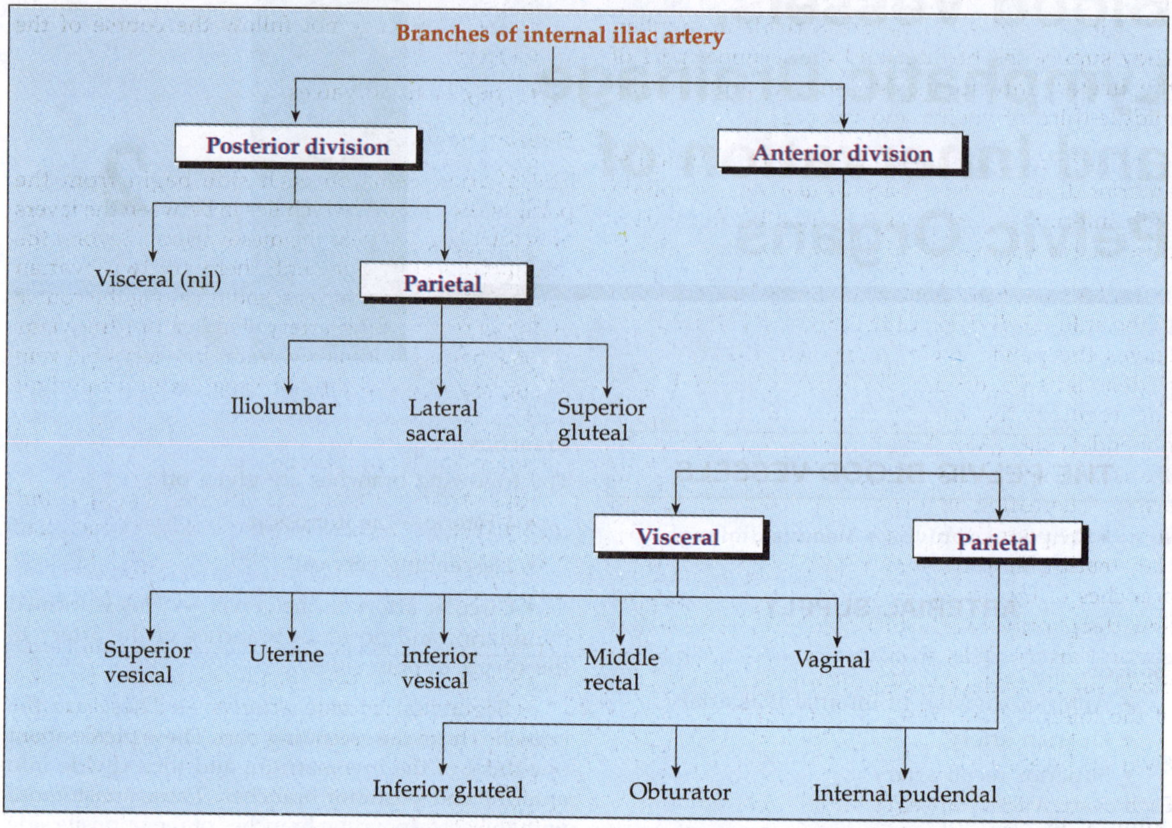

are sent off anteriorly and posteriorly which anastomose with the similar branches of the other side to form azygos arteries of the vagina — one anterior and one posterior.

Other arteries contributing to azygos arteries are : (i) descending cervical, (ii) circular artery to the cervix, (iii) inferior vesical and (iv) internal pudendal.

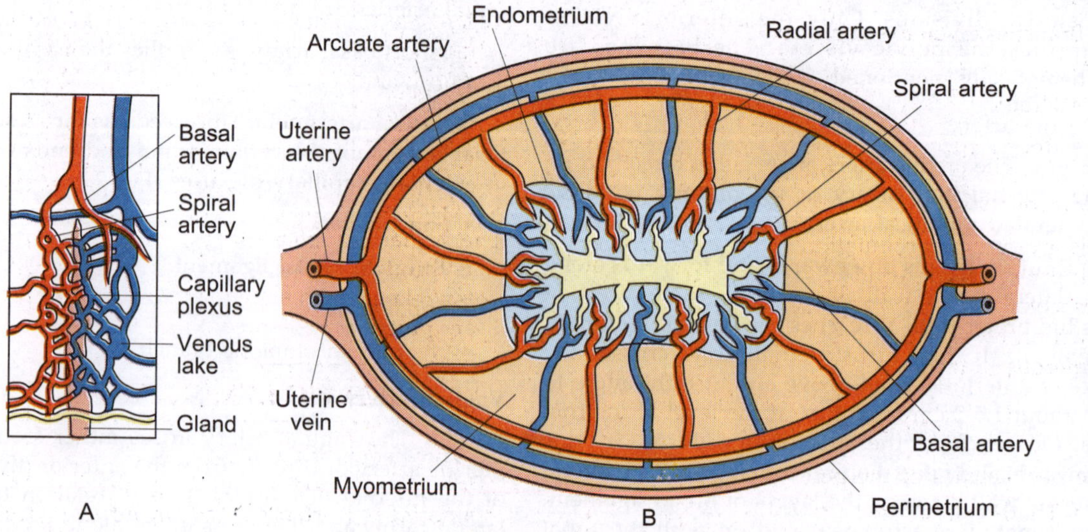

Fig. 2.1. Internal blood supply of the uterus

Vesical arteries : These are variable in number. They supply the bladder and the terminal part of the ureter. Inferior vesical artery supplies the middle-third of vagina and urethra.

Middle rectal : It arises either directly from the anterior division of the internal iliac or in common with inferior vesical artery. It supplies the lower-third of the vagina.

Pudendal artery : It is one of the parietal branches of the anterior division of the internal iliac artery. It leaves the pelvic cavity along with its vein and pudendal nerve through the greater sciatic foramen and reenters the ischiorectal fossa to lie in the pudendal canal (Alcock's canal) after winding round the ischial spine. Here, it gives off inferior rectal artery. Thereafter, it sends numerous branches to supply the perineal and vulval structures including the vestibular bulb and clitoris. The terminal branches of the artery anastomose with superficial and deep pudendal arteries — branches of the femoral artery. This will help in maintaining the blood supply of the bladder when the vesical branch of the internal iliac artery is ligated.

Ovarian artery

Each ovarian artery arises from the front of the aorta, a little below the renal artery. It enters the pelvic cavity after crossing the external iliac vessels. It then runs medially along the infundibulopelvic ligament to enter the mesovarium. As it enters the hilum of the ovary, it breaks up into numerous branches to supply the organ.

Branches given to structures other than the ovary are :

- Ureter
- Uterine tube
- Round ligament
- Uterine anastomotic

Superior rectal artery

This artery is a continuation of the inferior mesenteric artery and descends down to the base of pelvic mesocolon. It then divides into two and each courses down on either side of the rectum to supply it by numerous branches.

PELVIC VEINS

The peculiarities of the pelvic veins are :

- There is a tendency to form plexuses.
- The plexuses anastomose freely with each other.
- The veins may not follow the course of the artery.
- They have no valves.

Ovarian veins

The ovarian veins on each side begin from the pampiniform plexus which lies in between the layers of broad ligament near the mesovarium. Beyond the infundibulopelvic ligament, there are two ovarian veins on each side which ascend up along the course of the corresponding artery. Higher up, the veins become one and ultimately drains into left renal vein on the left side and inferior vena cava on the right side.

Uterus, vagina and bladder

Venous drainage from the uterine, vaginal and vesical plexuses chiefly drain into internal iliac vein.

Rectum

Venous drainage from the rectal plexus drains via superior rectal vein into the inferior mesenteric vein. The middle and inferior rectal veins drain into the internal pudendal vein and thence to the internal iliac vein.

Applied anatomy

- The free anastomosis between the superior rectal veins of the portal, the middle and inferior rectal veins of the systemic system explains the liver metastases from the genital organs.
- The uterine veins communicate with the vaginal plexus; thus accounting for vaginal metastases in endometrial carcinoma or choriocarcinoma.
- A free communication between pelvic plexuses with the sacral and lumbar channels of the vertebral venous plexus explains not only the development of vertebral metastases but also explains the intracranial malignant metastases bypassing the lungs through jugular vein. This collateral pathway is also related with supine hypotension syndrome in late pregnancy.

PELVIC LYMPHATICS

The knowledge of the lymphatic channels and the draining lymph nodes from the genital organs is of paramount importance either in inflammatory or specially in malignant diseases. The following groups of nodes are involved.

Inguinal nodes (Fig. 2.2)

Superficial : There are two groups. One lying horizontally and parallel to the inguinal ligament and the other is placed vertically along the long saphenous vein.

Superficial group receive afferents from gluteal region, anterior abdominal wall below the umbilicus, vulva, perineum, vagina below the hymen, anal canal below the Hilton's line and cornu of the uterus (along the round ligament). The efferents from the superficial inguinal lymph nodes drain into the deep inguinal nodes and external iliac lymph nodes passing through the inguinal canal.

Deep inguinal lymph nodes — These nodes receive afferents from deep femoral vessels, glans clitoris and few from superficial inguinal nodes. They are 5–6 in number and lie on the medial side of the femoral vein. The uppermost gland of this group is called the **gland of Cloquet or the gland of Rosenmüller,** which lies beneath the inguinal ligament in the femoral canal. Efferents from the deep nodes pass through the femoral canal and drain to the **external iliac nodes**.

Parametrial node

It is of small size, inconsistently present in the parametrium near the crossing of the ureter with the uterine artery.

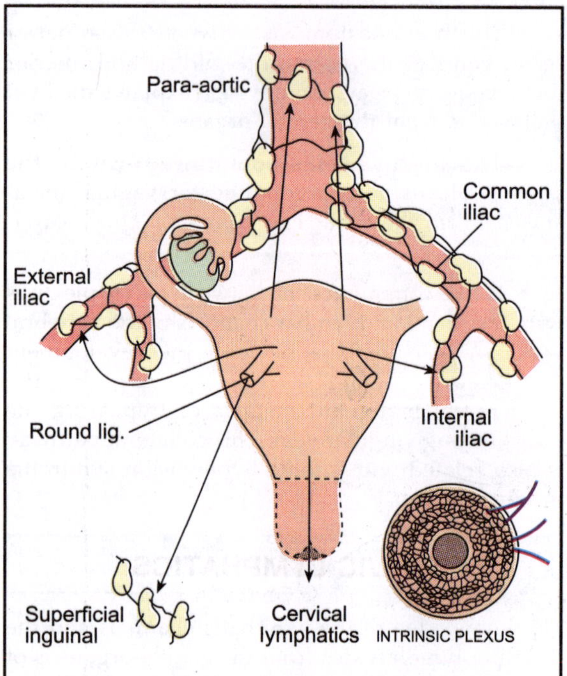

Fig. 2.2. Schematic representation of the lymphatic drainage of the body of uterus

Internal iliac nodes receive afferents from all the pelvic viscera, deeper perineum, muscles of the thigh and buttock. These glands receive the afferents from the obturator (obturator canal) and the sacral nodes (along the median and lateral sacral vessels).

External iliac nodes

There are three groups : (i) Lateral — lateral to external iliac artery (ii) Middle (anterior) — in between the artery and vein (iii) Medial — medial to the vein. These glands receive drainage from the cervix, upper vagina, bladder, lower abdominal wall and from the inguinal nodes. Afferents are from internal iliac, inferior epigastric, circumflex iliac and obturator nodes. The efferents ultimately drain into the **common iliac group. In carcinoma cervix, the medial and middle groups are involved.**

Common iliac lymph nodes are arranged in three groups : (i) Lateral (ii) Intermediate (iii) Medial. They receive **afferents** from external and internal iliac nodes and send **efferents** to the lateral aortic nodes.

Sacral group

It consists of two sets of glands; one lateral group, which lies lateral to the rectum and a medial group lying in front of the sacral promontory. The lymphatics from these groups pass on either to the inferior lumbar group or to the common iliac group.

Lumbar group

It consists of two sets of glands — (1) Inferior group which lies in front of the aorta below the origin of inferior mesenteric artery. (2) Superior group which lies near the origin of the ovarian artery. These two groups receive all the lymph from the pelvic organs. Thereafter, it passes up to cisterna chyli situated over the body of 12th thoracic vertebra. The lymph is finally carried upwards via the **thoracic duct which opens into the left subclavian vein at its junction with left internal jugular vein.**

LYMPHATICS OF THE CORPUS (Fig. 2.2)

Intrinsic plexus

Two plexuses are demonstrated : (i) Basal layer of the endometrium (ii) Subserosal layer. The lymphatics from the basal layer run through the myometrium in close relation to the blood vessels to reach the subserosal plexus.

Extrinsic drainage

(i) From the fundus and the adjoining part of the body → along ovarian lymphatics → superior lumbar (para-aortic) group of glands.

(ii) From the cornu → along the round ligament → superficial inguinal (horizontal group).

(iii) Rest of the body of uterus → external iliac group.

(iv) Adjacent to cervix → into cervical lymphatics.

LYMPHATICS OF THE CERVIX (Fig. 2.3)

The lymphatics from the cervix drain into the following lymph nodes coursing along the uterine veins.

Primary groups are :

1. Parametrial group — inconsistent.
2. Internal iliac group.
3. Obturator group.
4. External iliac — anterior and medial group.
5. Sacral group.

Secondary group :

The lymphatics from all the primary groups drain into common iliac and superior lumbar group.

LYMPHATICS FROM THE FALLOPIAN TUBE AND OVARY

The intrinsic plexuses of the Fallopian tube are situated in the mucosal and subperitoneal layers. The afferents from these plexuses pass up along with ovarian lymphatics to superior lumbar group. There is free anastomosis between the ovarian lymphatics of each side across the uterosacral ligament or via the subperitoneal lymphatic plexus of the fundus of the uterus.

LYMPHATICS OF THE VAGINA

The intrinsic plexuses are situated in the mucosal and muscle layers. (i) Upper two-thirds drain into the glands like those of the cervix. (ii)Lower one-third drains into inguinal and at times into external iliac nodes.

LYMPHATICS OF THE VULVA (Fig. 2.4)

There are dense lymphatic plexuses in the dermis of the vulva which intercommunicate with those of subcutaneous tissue (see p. 323).

- The lymphatics of each side freely communicate with each of them.
- The lymphatics hardly cross beyond the labiocrural fold.

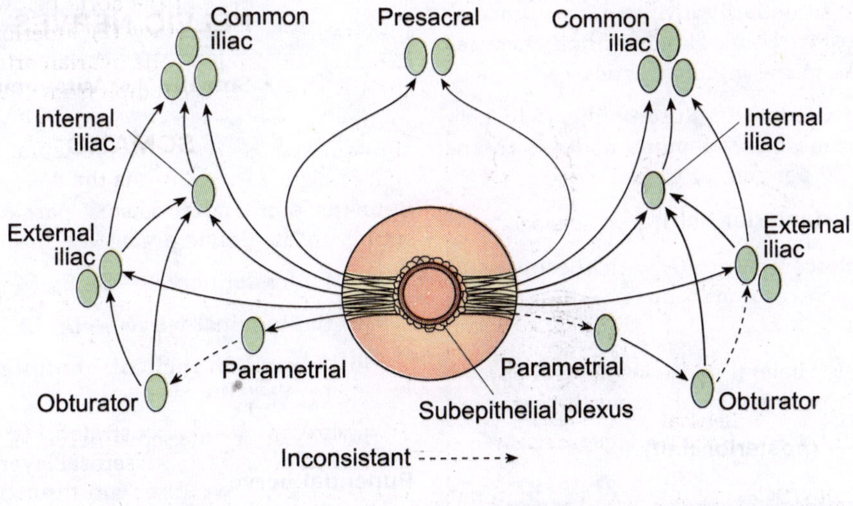

Fig. 2.3. Schematic representation of the lymphatic drainage of the cervix

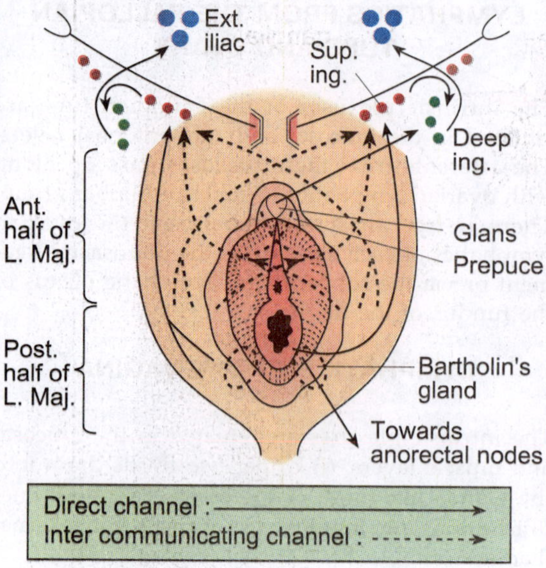

Fig. 2.4. Schematic representation of the vulval lymphatics

- The vulval lymphatics also anastomose with the lymphatics of the lower-third of the vagina and drain into external iliac nodes.
- Lymphatics from the deep tissues of the vulva accompany the internal pudendal vessels to the internal iliac nodes.
- Superficial inguinal lymph nodes are the primary lymph nodes that act as the sentinel nodes of the vulva. Deep inguinal lymph nodes are secondarily involved. It is unusual to find positive pelvic glands without metastatic disease in the inguinal nodes.
- Gland of Cloquet or Rosenmüller which is the upper most deep femoral nodes is absent in about 50 per cent of cases.

Labia majora — (anterior half)

Lymphatics intercommunicate with the opposite side in the region of mons veneris → Superficial inguinal nodes.

Thus, there is bilateral and contralateral spread of metastasis in malignancy affecting the areas.

Labia majora — (posterior half)

Drains into → Superficial inguinal → Deep inguinal → External iliac.

Labia minora and prepuce of clitoris

Intercommunicating with the lymphatics of the opposite side in the vestibule and drains into superficial inguinal.

Glans of clitoris

Drains directly into the deep inguinal glands and external iliac.

Bartholin's glands

The lymphatics drain into superficial inguinal and anorectal nodes.

Node of Cloquet

It was previously thought to be the main relay node through which the efferents from the superficial inguinal nodes pass to the external iliac nodes. Recent study shows its insignificant involvement in vulval malignancy and thus, it is not considered to be the relay node. The efferents from the superficial inguinal may reach the external iliac group bypassing the node of Cloquet.

LYMPHATICS OF BLADDER AND URETHRA

Bladder

The lymphatics drain into hypogastric group of glands → external iliac.

Urethra

Upper half drains like that of bladder; lower half drains into superficial inguinal node.

PELVIC NERVES

• Somatic • Autonomic

SOMATIC

Both the motor and sensory part of the somatic supply to the pelvic organs are through :

(i) Pudendal nerve — S_2, S_3, S_4.

(ii) Ilio-inguinal nerve — L_1, L_2.

(iii) Genital branch of genitofemoral nerve L_1, L_2.

(iv) Posterior cutaneous nerve of thigh.

Pudendal nerve

The sensory component supplies the skin of the

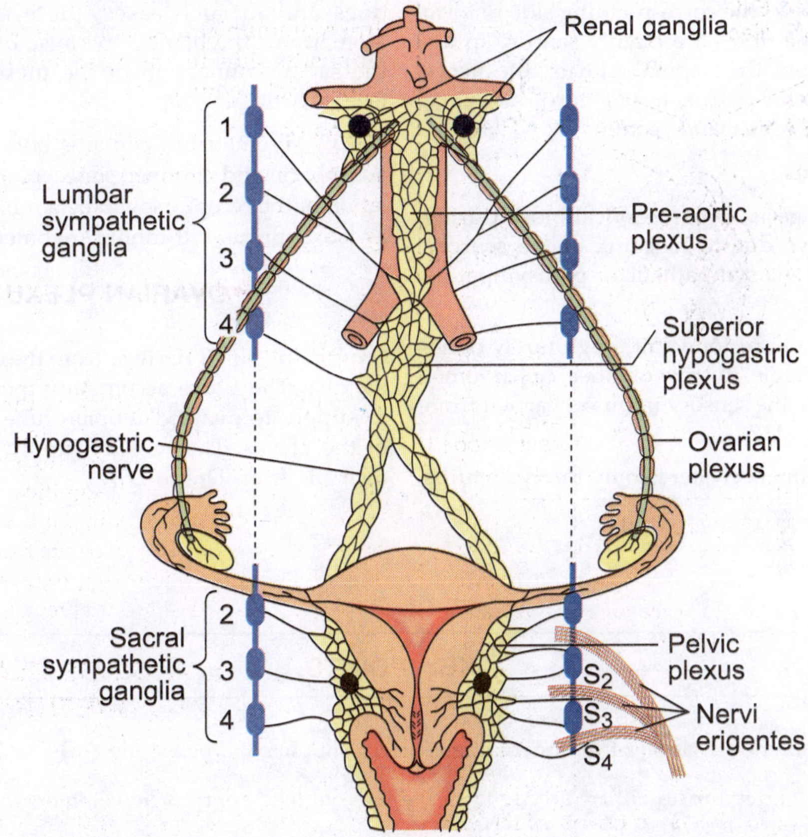

Fig. 2.5. Diagram showing nerve supply of the internal genital organs

vulva, external urethral meatus, clitoris, perineum and lower vagina. The motor fibres supply all the voluntary muscles of the perineal body, levator ani and sphincter ani externus. Levator ani, in addition, receives direct supply from S_3 and S_4 roots.

While the anterior half of vulval skin is supplied by the ilio-inguinal and genital branch of genito-femoral nerves, the posterior part of the vulva including the perineum is supplied by the posterior cutaneous nerve of thigh.

AUTONOMIC

The autonomic supply is principally from the sympathetic and partly from the parasympathetic systems.

Sympathetic

The sympathetic system carries both the sensory and motor fibres. The motor fibres arise from the segments D_5 and D_6 and the sensory fibres from the segments D_{10} to L_1. The fibres from the pre-aortic plexus of the sympathetic system are continuous with those of the superior hypogastric plexus. This plexus lies in front of 5th lumbar vertebra and more often wrongly called presacral nerve. While passing over the bifurcation of aorta, it divides into right and left hypogastric nerves. The hypogastric nerve joins the pelvic parasympathetic nerve of the corresponding side and forms the pelvic plexus (right and left) or inferior hypogastric plexus or Frankenhauser plexus. This plexus lies in the loose cellular tissue, posterolateral to the cervix below the uterosacral folds of peritoneum. The pelvic plexus then continues along the course of the uterine artery as paracervical plexus (Fig. 2.5).

Parasympathetic

The parasympathetic fibres (nervi erigentes) are

derived from the S_2, S_3 and S_4 nerves and join the hypogastric nerve of the corresponding side to form pelvic plexus. The fibres are mainly sensory to the cervix. Thus, from the vaginal plexus, the nerve fibres pass on to the uterus, upper-third of vagina, urinary bladder, ureter and rectum.

Applied Anatomy

(i) Epidural analgesia or paracervical block during labour is effective due to blocking of the sensory impulses carried via sympathetic or parasympathetic fibres.

(ii) Presacral neurectomy, although rarely done, either for intractable dysmenorrhoea or endometriosis is to divide the sensory impulses carried from the uterus (see p. 177).

(iii) While ordinary hysterectomy rarely disturbs the paracervical plexus, but the radical hysterectomy does and in such cases, there may be marked atonicity of the bladder because of the division of the sacral connection of the uterovaginal plexus (see p. 336).

(iv) Myometrium contains both alpha and beta adrenergic and cholinergic receptors. Strong stimulation of the receptors with beta mimetic drugs, such as isoxsuprine will inhibit myometrial activity.

OVARIAN PLEXUS

Ovarian plexus is derived from the coeliac and renal ganglia. The fibres accompany the ovarian vessels to supply to ovary, Fallopian tube and the fundus of the uterus. The sensory supply of the tube and ovary is from D_{10} to D_{12}.

KEY POINTS

- Only the anterior division of the internal iliac artery supplies the pelvic viscera.
- The uterine artery arises either directly from the internal iliac artery or in common with obliterated umbilical artery.
- Vaginal artery arises either from the uterine artery or directly from the anterior division of internal iliac artery. The azygos arteries (two) are formed by vaginal, descending cervical, inferior vesical and internal pudendal arteries.
- The ovarian artery arises from the aorta below the renal artery. The ovarian veins drain into inferior vena cava on the right side and into the left renal vein on the left side.
- The free anastomosis between the superior rectal veins of the portal, the middle and inferior rectal veins of the systemic system explains the liver metastases from the genital organs.
- The gland of Cloquet lies beneath the inguinal ligament in the femoral canal.
- From the cornu of the uterus, the lymphatics course along the round ligament to superficial inguinal group of glands.
- Levator ani is supplied by pudendal nerve and receives direct supply from S_3 and S_4 nerve roots.
- The motor fibres of the sympathetic arise from the segments D_5 and D_6 and the sensory fibres from the segments D_{10} to L_1.
- The parasympathetic fibres are derived from the S_2, S_3 and S_4 nerves.
- The sensory supply of the tube and ovary is from D_{10} to D_{12}.
- Myometrium contains both alpha and beta adrenergic and cholinergic receptors.

Development of Genital Organs and Gonads

3

DEVELOPMENT OF EXTERNAL GENITAL ORGANS

The external genital organs start developing almost simultaneously with the development of the internal genital organs. The site of origin is from the **urogenital sinus (Fig. 3.1)**. The endodermal cloaca is divided by a coronally oriented vertical partition, known as **Urorectal septum.** The urorectal septum contains a pair of **paramesonephric ducts** close to the midline and a pair of **mesonephric ducts** laterally. The dorsal part of the endodermal cloaca, thus formed, differentiates to form the **rectum and anal canal**. The ventral portion, known as **Urogenital sinus,** differentiates into three parts (Fig. 3.4).

(a) **Upper-vesicourethral part** forms the **mucous membrane of the bladder except the trigonal area.** It also contributes to the major part of **female urethra.**

(b) **Middle-pelvic part of urogenital sinus** : It receives the united caudal end of the two paramesonephric ducts in the midline. Derivatives of this part differentiates into the epithelium of the vagina, Bartholin's gland and the hymen.

(c) **The lower-phallic part of the urogenital sinus:** It is lined by the bilaminar urogenital membrane (see below). It contributes to **vestibule of vagina**.

The site of fusion between the urorectal septum and the cloacal membrane is the **primitive perineal body.**

The part of the cloacal membrane in front of the primitive perineal body is called **urogenital membrane** and the part behind is called **anal membrane.** When the urogenital membrane ruptures, the genital folds do not reunite in female (e.f. male). They persist as **labia minora**. The perineal cleft persists as **vestibule**, into which the urethra and the vagina open. The ectodermal swelling, one on either side and lateral to the genital fold is

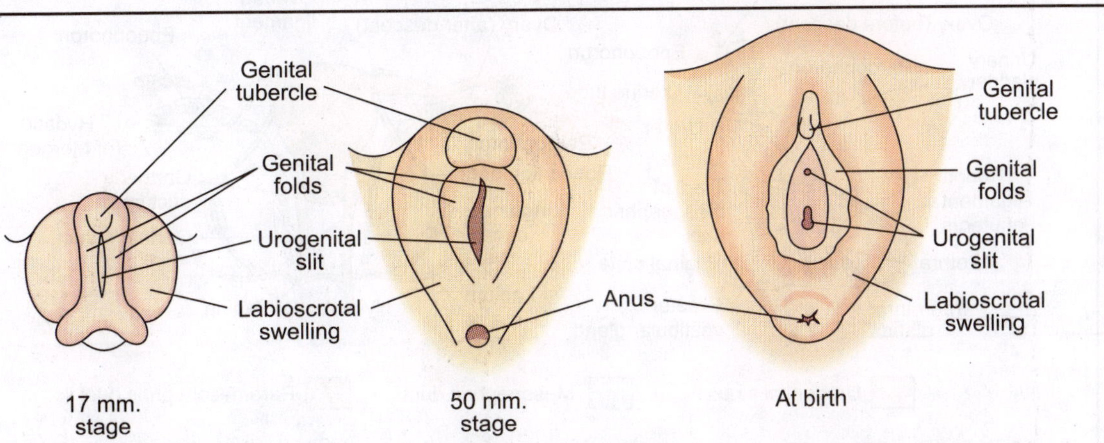

Fig. 3.1. Diagrammatic representation showing differentiation of the female external genitalia

called **labioscrotal swelling**. Eventually they form the **labia majora**.

The genital folds meet at the cephalic end of the cloacal membrane to form an elevation. This elevation is known as **genital tubercle** which ultimately differentiates into the **clitoris**.

Development upto this stage is the same in the male and the female (50 mm C.R. length, 10 weeks).

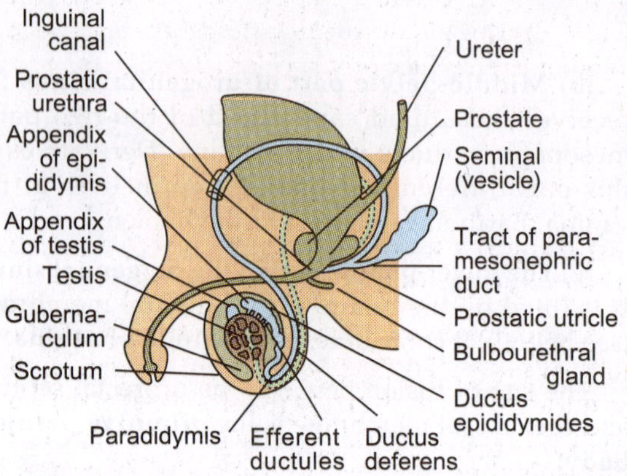

Fig. 3.2. Diagrammatic representation showing development of male reproductive systems from the primitive genital ducts. Vestigial structures are also shown (see p. 38).

If the gonads become ovaries, the external genitalia will attain the female characteristics (Table 3.1).

- **Clitoris** is developed from the genital tubercle.
- **Labia minora** are developed from the genital folds.
- **Labia majora** are developed from the genital swellings.
- **The Bartholin's glands** are developed as outgrowths from the caudal part of the urogenital sinus and correspond to the bulbourethral glands of male.
- **The vestibule :** The inferior portion of the pelvic part (Fig. 3.4D) and whole of the phallic part of the urogenital sinus expand to form the **vestibule** of the vagina (at about 5th month). It receives the openings of urethra, the vagina and Bartholin's ducts (Fig. 3.1).

DEVELOPMENT OF INTERNAL GENITAL ORGANS

- **Fallopian tubes**
- **Uterus**
- **Broad ligaments**
- **Vagina**

The major part of the female genital tract develops from the **Müllerian ducts**. The duct forms one on each side as an ingrowth of coelomic epithelium in the lateral aspect of mesonephros at about 5-6 weeks (10 mm CR length). The ingrowth forms a groove

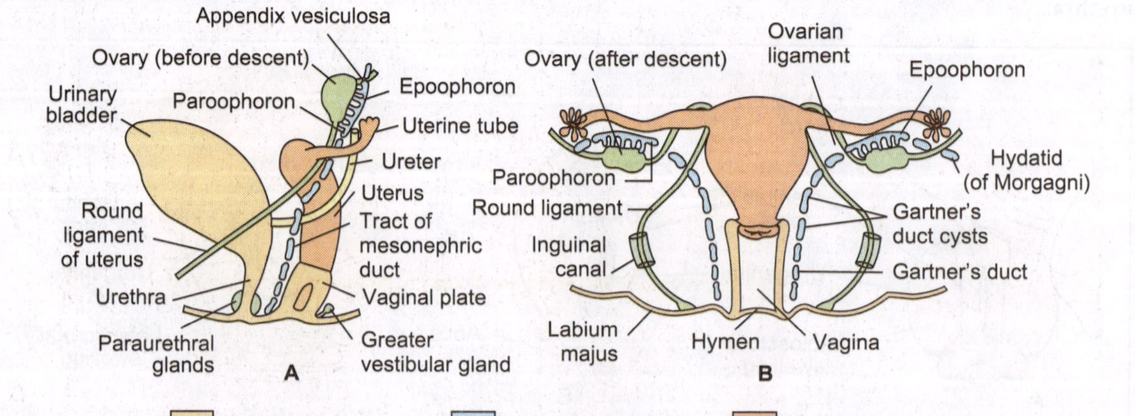

Fig. 3.3. Diagrammatic representation showing development of female reproductive systems from the primitive genital ducts. Vestigial structures are also shown. A. Female fetus at 12 weeks B. Newborn female

and then a tube which goes beneath the surface. While it grows downwards, it has developed three parts — (1) cranial vertical, (2) middle horizontal and (3) caudal vertical after crossing the Wolffian duct anteriorly. In the absence of **androgen** (testosterone) and **Anti-Müllerian Hormone (AMH)**, as in a normal female, there is further growth and development of the Müllerian duct system with regression of the Wolffian ducts (Fig. 3.3 and 3.6).

FALLOPIAN TUBES

Fallopian tube is developed from **upper vertical part and the adjoining the horizontal of the Müllerian duct.** The coelomic opening of the duct becomes the **abdominal ostium.**

UTERUS

Uterus is developed by the fusion of the **intermediate horizontal and the adjoining vertical part of the Müllerian ducts** which begins at 7-8 weeks (22 mm C.R. length) and completes by 12th week. Cervix is developed from the fused lower vertical parts of the two paramesonephric ducts. The cervix is differentiated from the corpus by 10th week. The intervening septum disappears during the 5th month of intrauterine life. The lining epithelium and the glands of the uterus and cervix are developed from the coelomic epithelium. Myometrium and endometrial stroma are developed from the **mesoderm of the paramesonephric ducts.**

BROAD LIGAMENT

When the Müllerian ducts approach each other in the midline, a broad transverse fold is established. It extends from the lateral side of the fused Müllerian ducts upto the lateral pelvic walls which is named as Broad ligament. All the vestigial remnants of mesonephric tubules, i.e. **epoophoron** (situated above the ovary), **paroophoron** (between ovary and uterus) and the duct, remnant as **Gartner's duct** are found in the broad ligament in the mesosalpinx (Fig. 3.3). **Kobelt's tubules** on the outer set are said to be of pronephric origin (Fig. 1.12).

VAGINA

Development of vagina is composite, partly from the Müllerian (paramesonephric) ducts and partly from the urogenital sinus.

The **paramesonephric ducts** develop at about **sixth week,** as an invagination of coelomic epithelium lateral to each mesonephric (Wolffian) duct. Each paramesonephric duct passes ventral to the corresponding mesonephric duct and then meet its counterpart from the opposite side in the midline (Fig. 3.4D). The lower vertical parts of the two paramesonephric (Müllerian) ducts pass caudal wards in the urorectal septum and meet each other. Around 9th week, the solid caudal tip of the fused vertical parts of the Müllerian ducts project blindly

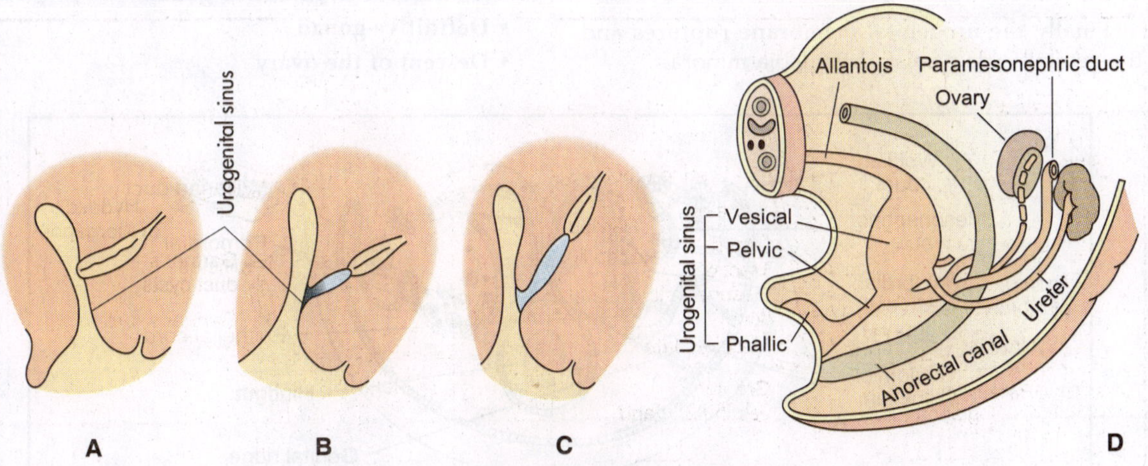

Fig. 3.4. Schematic representation of the development of vagina

A. Formation of Müllerian tubercle. B. Earliest development of vaginal plate. C. Further development of the vaginal plate. D. Further development of the paramesonephric ducts, urogenital sinus, permanent (metanephric) kidney and degenerations of mesonephric ducts.

into the dorsal wall of the urogenital sinus as **Müllerian tubercles (Fig. 3.3).**

The paramesonephric ducts shortly undergo fusion with each other and the partition between them disappears. The united lower vertical parts form the **uterovaginal canal** and the fused Müllerian tubercles form the **Müllerian eminence.** The **unfused cranial part** of each paramesonephric duct forms the uterine tube and the distal open end forms the abdominal ostium.

The endodermal cells from the dorsal wall of the urogenital sinus proliferate and form the **sinovaginal bulb** (Fig. 3.4). These endodermal cells further proliferate and extend cranially into the central axis to form a solid plate, called **vaginal plate.** This vaginal plate as elongates increases the distance between the urogenital sinus (below) at the cervix (above).

At about 20 weeks the vaginal plate undergoes canalisation with the disintegration of the central cells. The upper end of the canal forms the vaginal fornices and communicates with the cervical canal and uterine cavity.

Central cells of the Müllerian eminence disintegrate, so that the vaginal canal now opens into the urogenital sinus. The tissue at the periphery persists as **hymen.** It is lined by sinus epithelium (endodermal origin) on either side with a thin mesoderm in between. Thus whole of the vagina is lined by endoderm of the urogenital sinus and the muscle in the wall is derived from the mesoderm of the Müllerian ducts.

Finally the urogenital membrane ruptures and the genital folds persist as the labia minora.

Eventually the vaginal segment grows and is extended between the paramesonephric derived cervix at the top and the sinus derived vestibule at the bottom.

SUMMARY

Vagina is developed mainly from the Müllerian ducts and partly from the urogenital sinus.

Upper three-fifth above the hymen develop from the fused uterovaginal canal of the Müllerian ducts.

(a) Mucous membrane is developed from the endoderm of the canalised (vaginal plate) sinovaginal bulb.

(b) The musculature is developed from the mesoderm of the fused caudal vertical part of the Müllerian ducts.

(c) The hymen is developed from the junction of the Müllerian tubercle (mesodermal) and the urogenital sinus (endodermal).

Lower one-fifth below the hymen is developed entirely from the urogenital sinus.

Vaginal introitus is developed from the ectoderm of the genital folds after rupture of the bilaminar urogenital membrane.

DEVELOPMENT OF THE OVARY

- **Site**
- **Sources**
- **Indifferent or primitive gonad**
- **Definitive gonad**
- **Descent of the ovary**

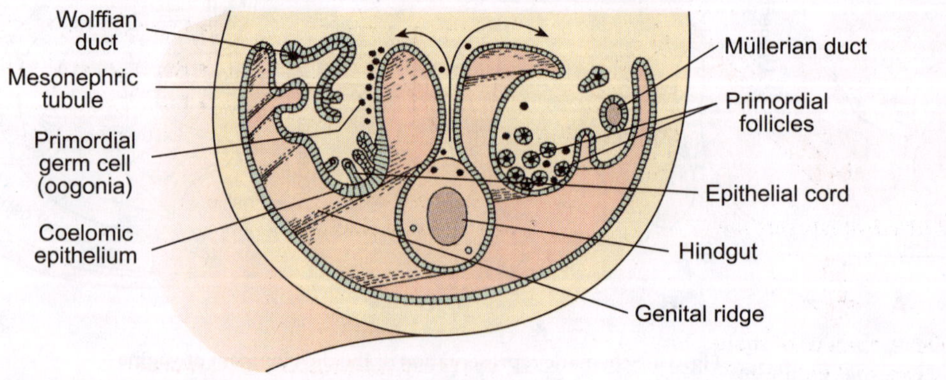

Fig. 3.5. The development of the ovary with migration of the germ cells into the genital ridge

Site

The ovary is developed on either side from the genital or gonadal ridge. This ridge is formed in a four-week embryo between the dorsal mesentery and mesonephros by the multiplication of the coelomic epithelium along with condensation of the underlying mesenchyme.

Sources

The cortex and the covering epithelium are developed from the coelomic epithelium and the medulla from the mesenchyme. **The germ cells are of endodermal origin**. They migrate from the **yolk sac** to the genital ridge along the dorsal mesentery by amoeboid movement between 20 and 30 days. The germ cells undergo a number of rapid mitotic divisions and differentiate into oogonia. **The number of oogonia reaches its maximum at 20th week numbering about 7 million.** The mitotic division gradually ceases and the majority enter into the prophase of the first meiotic division and are called **primary oocytes**. These are surrounded by flat cells (granulosa cells) and are called primordial follicles. At birth, there is no more mitotic division and all the oogonia are replaced by primary oocytes. **The estimated number at birth is about 2 million (Fig. 3.5).**

Indifferent or Primitive Gonad

Initially, the gonads do not acquire male or female morphological characteristics until the **seventh week of development**. Around the time of arrival of germ cells, the coelomic epithelium of the genital ridge proliferates. The irregular cords of cells (primitive sex cords) invaginate the underlying mesenchyme. These cords of cells surround the primordial germ

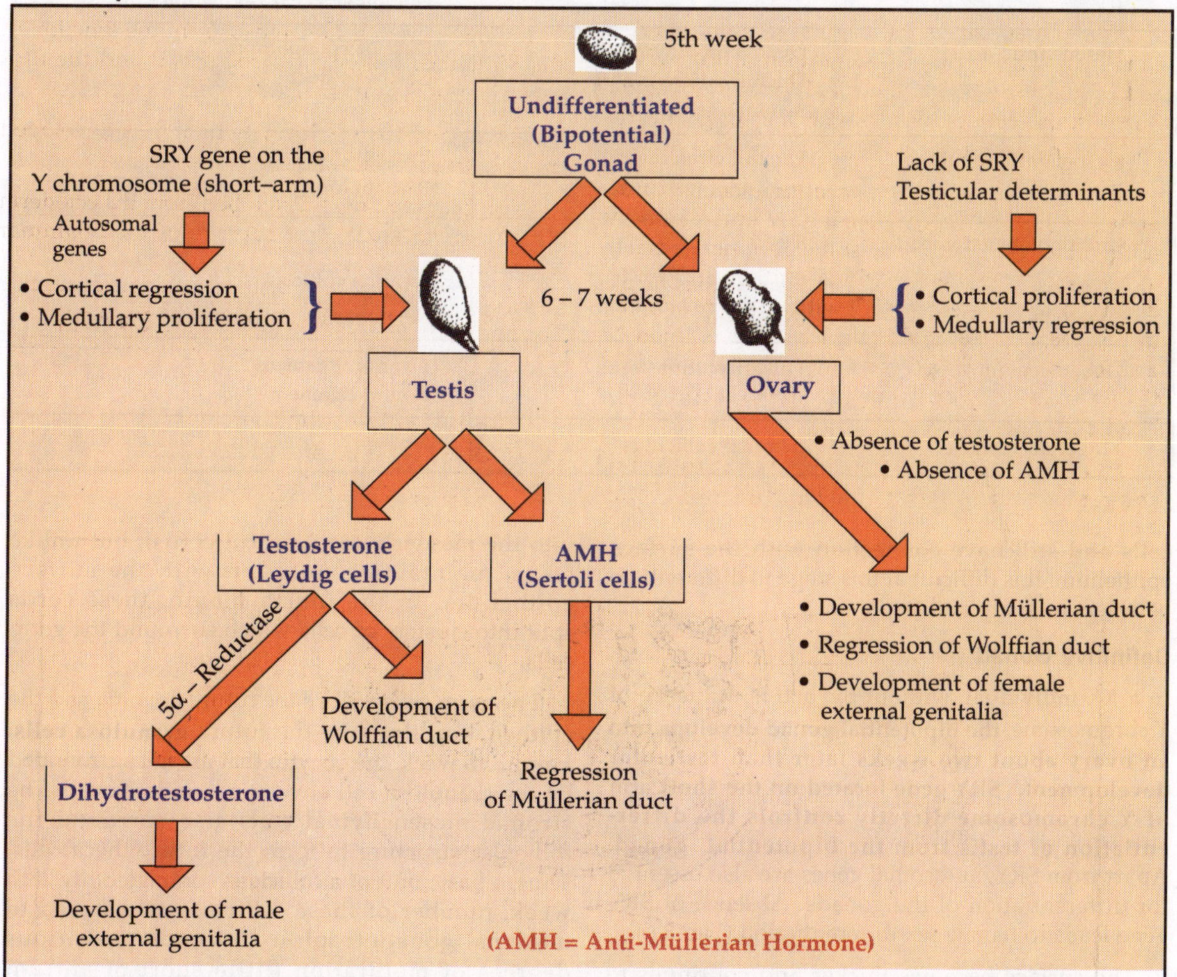

Fig. 3.6. Schematic representation of the development of the reproductive systems in the male and female

Table 3.1
Male and female derivatives of embryonic urogenital structures

Embryonic structure	Derivatives	
	Male (Fig. 3.2)	**Female (Fig. 3.3)**
Labioscrotal swelling	Scrotum	Labia majora
Urogenital folds	Ventral aspect of penis	Labia minora
Genital tubercle	Penis	Clitoris
Urogenital sinus	Urinary bladder Urethra except navicular fossa Prostate gland Prostatic utricle Bulbourethral glands	Urinary bladder, urethra Urethral and paraurethral glands Vagina Bartholin's glands
Paramesonephric duct	Appendix of testes	Hydatid of Morgagni, Uterus, Cervix Fallopian tubes, vagina(muscular wall)
Mesonephric duct	Ductus epididymis Ductus differens and Seminal vesicles	Duct of epoophoron Gartner's duct
Mesonephric tubules	Ductuli efferentes Paradidymis	Epoophoron Paroophoron
Undifferentiated gonad Cortex Medulla	Testis Seminiferous tubules Rete testis	Ovary Ovarian follicles Rete ovarii
Gubernaculum	Gubernaculum testis	Ovarian ligament Round ligament
Müllerian tubercle	Seminal colliculus	Hymen

cells and still have connection with the surface epithelium. It is difficult at this stage to differentiate between an ovary and testis.

Definitive Gonad

In a XX individual, without the active influence of Y chromosome, **the bipotential gonad develops into an ovary about two weeks later than testicular development. SRY gene located on the short arm of Y chromosome directly controls the differentiation of testis from the bipotential gonad.** Apart from SRY, autosomal genes are also essential for differentiation of the gonads. Absence of SRY gene leads to female sex differentiation (Fig. 3.6).

The surface becomes thicker and continues to proliferate extensively. It sends down cords of cells into the mesenchyme (cortical cords), but unlike testis, maintains connection with the surface epithelium. In the fourth month, these cords split into clusters of cells which surround the germ cells.

The germ cells will be the future oogonia and the epithelial cells will be the future **granulosa cells.** From 20th week, the oocytes that are not surrounded by the granulosa cell envelope, are destroyed. The stromal mesenchymal cells also surround the follicular structure to form the future theca cells. Thus, a basic unit of a follicle is completed. By 28th week, number of these follicles are exposed to maternal gonadotrophin and undergo various degrees of maturation (little short of antrum formation) and atresia.

Descent of the Ovary

The cranial part of the genital ridge becomes the infundibulopelvic ligament (Fig. 3.3). From the lower pole of the ovary, genital ligament (gubernaculum) is formed which is attached to the external genitalia. The genital ligament gets attached as it comes close to Müllerian ducts (angle of the developing uterus). The part between **the ovary and the Müllerian attachment is the ovarian ligament and the part between the cornu of the uterus to the end is the round ligament. The ovaries descend during the seventh to ninth month and at birth, they are situated at the pelvic brim.**

KEY POINTS

- The external genital organs start developing almost simultaneously with the development of the internal genital organs.
- Clitoris is developed from the genital tubercle, labia minora from the genital folds and labia majora from the genital swellings.
- Bartholin's glands are developed from the caudal part of the urogenital sinus.
- Major part of the vagina is developed from urogenital sinus.
- SRY (sex-determining region of the Y chromosome) gene directly controls the testicular differentiation from the bipotential gonad. SRY gene encodes the testicular determining factor (TDF) which induces the differentiation. Testicular development is an active event whereas ovarian development is a default pathway due to absent SRY gene.
- An individual with absent SRY gene, though the chromosomal complement is 46, XY, the gonado-ductal development is towards female (XY gonadal dysgenesis).
- The ovary is developed from the gonadal ridge. The cortex and the covering epithelium are developed from the coelomic epithelium and the medulla from the mesenchyme. The germ cells are endodermal in origin and migrate from the yolk sac to the genital ridge. The number of oogonia reaches its maximum at 20th week numbering about 7 million. The estimated number at birth is about 2 million.
- The bipotential gonad develops into an ovary about two weeks later than the testicular development.
- The cranial end of the genital ridge becomes the infundibulopelvic ligament.
- The ovary is developed from the middle part of the genital ridge.
- The part of the gubernaculum (genital ligament) between the lower pole of the ovary and the Müllerian attachment is the ovarian ligament. The part between the cornu of the uterus (Müllerian attachment) to the end (external genitalia) is the round ligament.
- The ovaries descend during seventh to ninth month and at birth, they are situated at the pelvic brim.
- The paramesonephric duct in female differentiates into Fallopian tube, uterus and cervix. The mesonephric duct in male gives rise to epididymis, vas deferens and seminal vesicles. The sinovaginal bulbs, which grow out from the posterior aspect of the urogenital sinus, differentiates into vagina. The genital tubercle differentiates into clitoris (female) or penis (male). The urinary bladder develops from the urogenital sinus.
- Urinary bladder develops from the upper vesico urethral part of the urogenital sinus except the trigone.
- A cyst of the vagina, specially on the anterolateral vaginal wall, is usually Gartner's duct cyst (embryonic cyst).

Congenital Malformation of Female Genital Organs

4

Introduction

From the embryological considerations, the following facts can be deduced.

- Developmental anomalies of the external genitalia along with ambiguity of sex are usually genetic in origin.

- Major anatomic defect of the genital tract is usually associated with urinary tract abnormality and normal gonadal function.

- While minor abnormality escapes attention, it is the moderate or severe form which will produce gynaecologic and obstetric problem.

DEVELOPMENTAL ANOMALIES OF THE EXTERNAL GENITALIA

PERINEAL OR VESTIBULAR ANUS

The entity is detected at birth. The usual anal opening site is evidenced by anal pit. The anal opening is situated either close to the posterior end of the vestibule or in the vestibule. Rarely, it is situated in the vagina (congenital rectovaginal fistula). The opening is usually sufficiently big and continence is present. There is no problem in future reproduction. The delivery should be by caesarean section (see p. 46).

If there are features of obstruction or the opening is situated high in the vagina, pull through operation is to be done bringing the anal end to the anal pit with prior colostomy.

ECTOPIC URETER

The additional ureteric opening is usually in the vestibule close to the urethra or in the vagina. The main symptom is uncontrollable wetness. Partial nephrectomy and ureterectomy may be indicated or implantation of the ectopic ureter into the bladder may be done.

VAGINAL ABNORMALITIES

The significant abnormalities include :

- **Narrow introitus**
- **Hymen abnormality**
- **Septum**
- **Agenesis**
- **Associated abnormalities.**

NARROW INTROITUS

The existence is revealed after marriage. Dyspareunia may be the first complaint or it may be detected during investigation of infertility. Treatment is effective by manual stretching under general anaesthesia or by surgical enlargement (Perineoplasty/ Fenton's operation — see p. 562).

HYMEN ABNORMALITY

Gross hymenal abnormality of significance is **imperforate hymen.** It is due to failure of disintegration of the central cells of the **Müllerian eminence** that projects into the **urogenital sinus** (p. 35). The existence is almost always unnoticed until the girl attains the age of 14-16. As the uterus is functioning normally, the menstrual blood is pent up inside the vagina behind the hymen (cryptomenorrhoea). Depending upon the amount of blood so accumulated, it first distends the vagina (haematocolpos). The uterus is next involved and the cavity dilated (haematometra). In the late and neglected cases, the tubes may also be distended after the fimbrial ends becoming closed by adhesions (haematosalpinx) (Fig. 4.1).

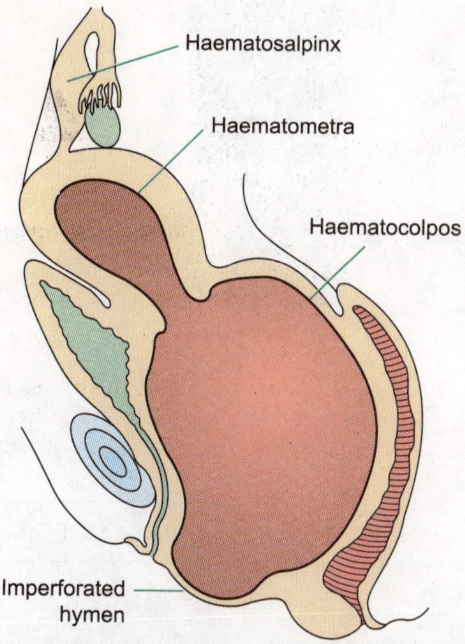

Fig. 4.1. Haematocolpos and haematometra due to imperforate hymen. Note the elongation of the urethra due to distension of the vagina by blood

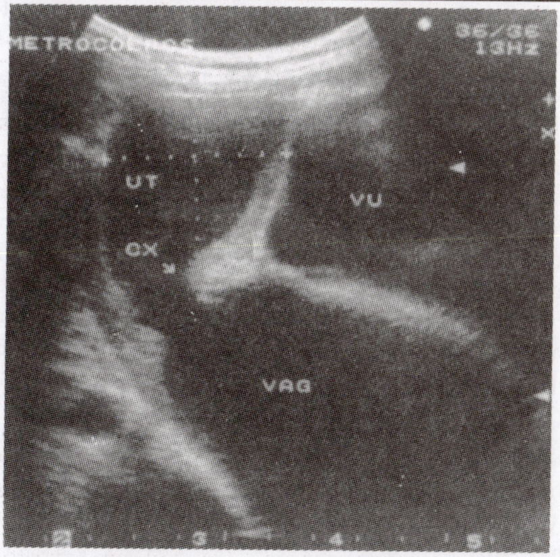

Fig. 4.2. Ultrasonographic view of haematometra and haematocolpos in a girl with imperforate hymen

Clinical features

The girl is aged about 14-16. The chief complaints are periodic lower abdominal pain which may be continuous, primary amenorrhoea and urinary symptoms like frequency, dysuria or even retention of urine. In fact, in significant cases the presenting feature may be the retention of urine. **The cause of retention is due to elongation of the urethra** (Fig. 4.1).

Abdominal examination reveals a suprapubic swelling which may be uterine or full bladder. Prior catheterisation reveals the true state.

Vulval inspection reveals a tense bulging membrane of bluish colouration (Fig. 4.3). In majority however, it is not the true hymen but the obstructing membrane is a transverse vaginal septum close to the inner aspect of the hymen. Rectal examination reveals the bulged vagina. **Ultrasonography** can make the diagnosis of **haematometra** and **haematocolpos** (Fig. 4.2).

In newborn (usually within one week of birth), accumulated mucus behind the imperforate membrane gives the clinical entity of mucocolpos. The secretion is either from the desquamated vaginal epithelial cells or from the cervical glands.

Treatment

Cruciate incision is made in the hymen. The quadrants of the hymen are partially excised not too close to the vaginal mucosa. Spontaneous escape of dark tarry coloured blood is allowed (Fig. 4.4).

Pressure from above should not be given. Internal examination should not be done. The patient is put to bed with the head end raised. Antibiotic should be given. The residual pathology, if any, may be detected by internal examination after the next period is over.

VAGINAL SEPTUM

Transverse vaginal septa are due to faulty fusion or canalisation of the urogenital sinus and the Müllerian ducts. About 45% occur in the upper vagina, 40% in mid vagina and 15% in the lower vagina. Septum located in the lower vagina is often complete and the signs and symptoms are similar to that imperforate hymen (p. 40). The principles of surgical treatment are the same. Septum in the upper vagina is often perforated. Incision of a complete (imperforate) septum becomes easy when the upper vagina is distended. This reduces the risk of injury to adjacent organs. Otherwise abdominovaginal approach (see p. 42) is made.

Longitudinal septum of the vagina may be present when the distal parts of the Müllerian ducts fail to fuse. It may be associated with double uterus

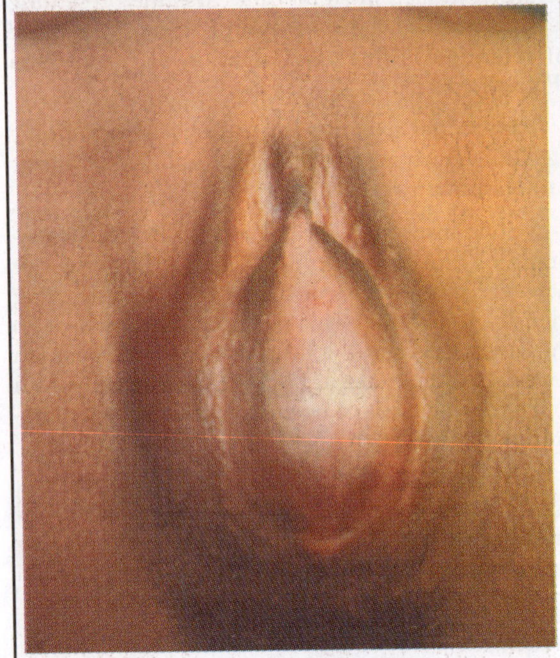

Fig. 4.3. Tense bulging of the hymen in haematocolpos

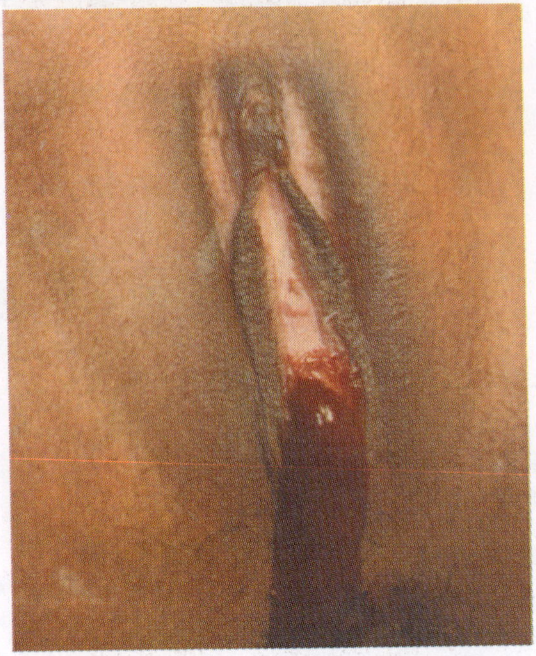

Fig. 4.4. Spontaneous escape of dark tarry blood following incision

and double cervix. It may be asymptomatic and needs no treatment. But it may cause dyspareunia or may obstruct delivery. In such circumstances, the septum is to be excised.

AGENESIS OF VAGINA

PARTIAL AGENESIS OF UPPER VAGINA

A segment of vagina may be atretic in the upper-third. It is often associated with hypoplasia or even absence of cervix. Uterus may be normal and functioning or malformed. Primary amenorrhoea (cryptomenorrhoea), periodic lower abdominal pain and presence of lower abdominal mass (as felt per abdomen or per rectum) point to the diagnosis. Conventional treatment is hysterectomy. Currently abdominovaginal approach is made to establish communication between the uterovaginal canal above and the newly created vagina below. Prosthesis is used to prevent restenosis. The result is however not always satisfactory though successful pregnancy and live birth have been reported. When hysterectomy is considered, ovaries should be conserved. This gives the benefit of endogenous oestrogen. Assisted reproductive technology would be the option, when desired, using a surrogate uterus.

COMPLETE AGENESIS

Complete agenesis of the vagina is almost always associated with absence of uterus. There is, however, presence of healthy gonads and Fallopian tubes. The patient is phenotypically female, with normal female karyotype pattern.The entity is often associated with urinary tract (40%) and skeletal (12%) malformation. This is called **Mayer-Rokitansky-Küster-Hauser syndrome.** The patient usually seeks advice for primary amenorrhoea and dyspareunia.

If the patient wishes to marry or has dyspareunia, reconstructive operation is done (vaginoplasty). The principles of surgery are mentioned in page 437.

ASSOCIATED ABNORMALITIES

Associated abnormalities with —

(a) **Vesicovaginal fistula** is formed when the Müllerian eminence ruptures into the vesicourethral part of the cloaca instead of the pelvic part of the urogenital sinus (Fig. 3.4D).

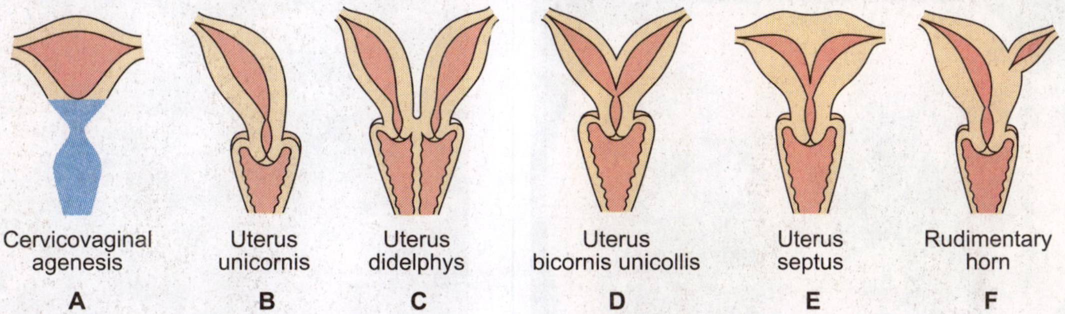

Fig. 4.5. Malformations of the Müllerian ducts

(b) **Rectovaginal fistula** when the müllerian eminence opens in the dorsal segment of the endodermal cloaca.

(c) **Persistent urogenital sinus** with various irregularities of urethral and vaginal orifices in the sinus.

UTERINE ANOMALIES

Uterine anomalies are often associated with vaginal maldevelopment.

American Fertility Society (AFS) Classification of müllerian anomalies (1988) are (Fig. 4.5) :

Class I : Müllerian Agenesis/Hypoplasia — segmental, **Class II** : Unicornuate uterus, **Class III** : Didelphys uterus, **Class IV** : Bicornuate uterus, **Class V** : Septate uterus, **Class VI** : Arcuate uterus and **Class VII** : Diethyl stilboestrol (DES) related abnormality.

- **Failure of development of one or both Müllerian ducts**

The absence of both ducts leads to absence of uterus including oviducts. There is absence of vagina as well. Primary amenorrhoea is the chief complaint.

The absence of one duct leads to a unicornuate uterus with a single oviduct.

- **Failure of recanalisation of the Müllerian ducts**

Agenesis of the upper vagina or of the cervix — This may lead to haematometra as the uterus is functioning (discussed above).

- **Failure of fusion of Müllerian ducts**

In majority, the presence of deformity escapes attention. In some, the detection is made accidentally during investigation of infertility or repeated pregnancy wastage. In others, the diagnosis is made during D + E operation, manual removal of placenta or during caesarean section.

Types of fusion anomalies (Fig. 4.5)

- **Arcuate (18%)** — The cornual parts of the uterus remains separated. The uterine fundus looks concave with heart-shaped cavity outline (Fig. 4.6D).
- **Uterus didelphys (8%)** — There is complete lack of fusion of the Müllerian ducts with a double uterus double cervix and a double vagina (Fig. 4.5C).
- **Uterus bicornis (26%)** — There is varying degrees of fusion of the muscle walls of the two ducts.
  - *Uterus bicornis bicollis* — There are two uterine cavities with double cervix with or without vaginal septum.
  - *Uterus bicornis unicollis* — There are two uterine cavities with one cervix. The horns may be equal or one horn may be rudimentary and have no communication with the developed horn (Figs 4.5D and 4.6F).
- **Septate uterus (35%)** — The two Müllerian ducts fused together but there is persistence of septum in between the two either partially (subseptate) or completely (Figs. 4.5E and 4.6A and B).
- **Uterus unicornis (10%)** — Failure of development of one Müllerian duct (Figs. 4.5B and 4.6E).
- **DES–related abnormality (Fig. 4.6C)** is due to DES exposure during intrauterine life. Varieties of malformations are included, e.g. **Vagina** : Adenosis, Adenocarcinoma. **Cervix** : Cockscomb cervix, Cervical collar. **Uterus** : Hypoplasia, T-shaped cavity, Uterine synechae. **Fallopian tube** : Cornual budding, Abnormal fimbriae.

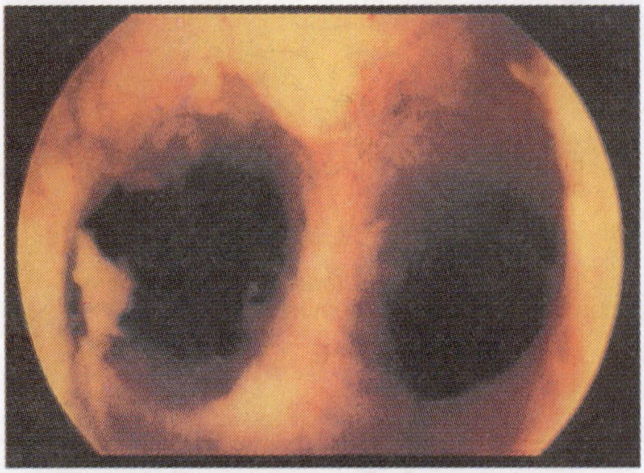

Fig. 4.6A. Hysteroscopic view of a septate uterus

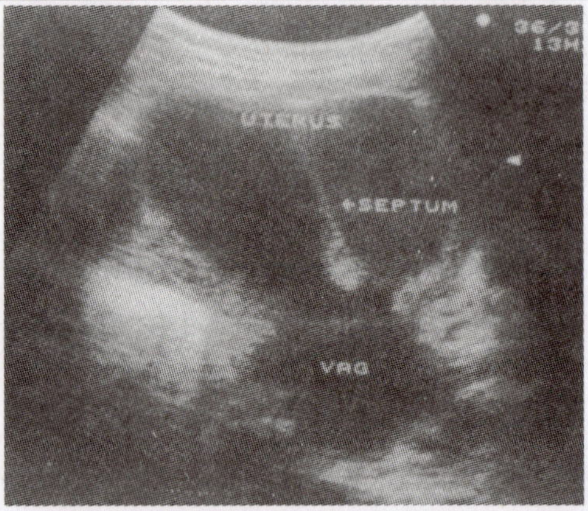

Fig. 4.6B. Ultrasonographic view of a septate uterus

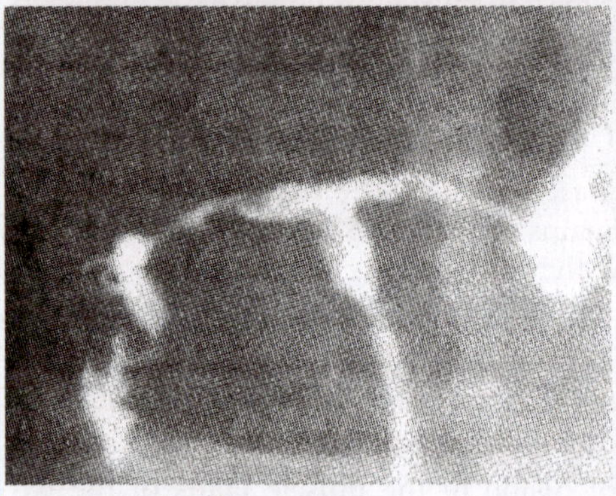

Fig. 4.6C. Hysterographic view of T-shaped hypoplastic uterus — consistent with inutero exposure to DES (p. 43)

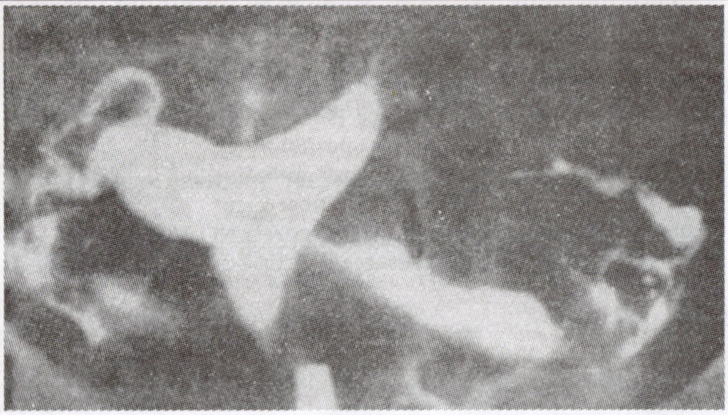

Fig. 4.6D. Hysterographic view of an arcuate uterus confirmed by laparoscopy

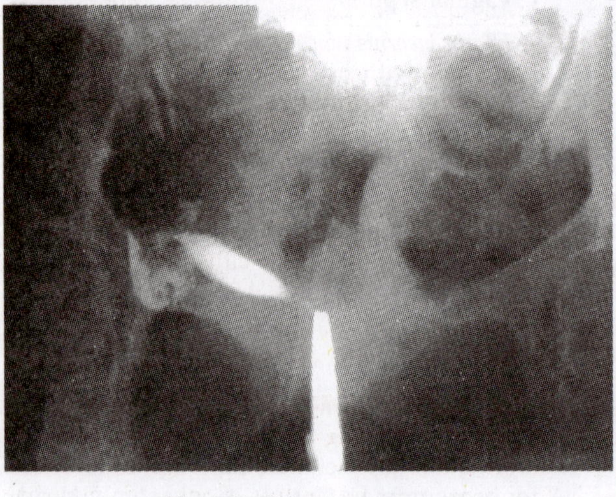

Fig. 4.6E. Unicornuate uterus

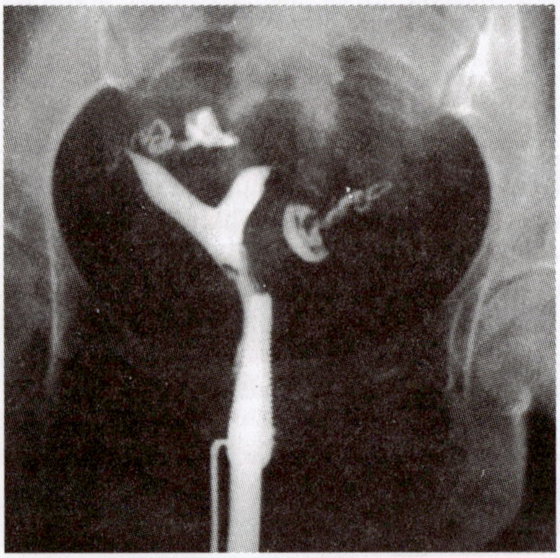

Fig. 4.6F. Bicornuate uterus confirmed by laparoscopy

Fig. 4.6. Hysteroscopic (A), Ultrasonographic (B) & Hysterographic diagnosis of congenital malformations of uterus (C, D, E and F).

Clinical features

As previously mentioned, the condition may not produce any clinical manifestation.

Gynaecological

(i) Infertility and dyspareunia are often related in association with vaginal septum.

(ii) Dysmenorrhoea in bicornuate uterus or due to cryptomenorrhoea (pent up menstrual blood in rudimentary horn).

(iii) Menorrhagia — due to increased surface area in bicornuate uterus.

Obstetrical

(i) Midtrimester abortion which may be recurrent.

(ii) Cornual pregnancy — with inevitable rupture around 16th week — if pregnancy occurs in the rudimentary horn.

(iii) Increased incidence of malpresentation — transverse lie in arcuate or subseptate, breech in bicornuate, unicornuate or complete septate uterus.

(iv) Preterm labour, IUGR, IUD.

(v) Prolonged labour — due to incordinate uterine action.

(vi) Obstructed labour — obstruction by the non-gravid horn of the bicornuate uterus or rudimentary horn.

(vii) Retained placenta and postpartum haemorrhage where the placenta is implanted over the uterine septum.

Diagnosis

Internal examination reveals septate vagina and two cervices. Passage of a sound can diagnose two separate cavities. In fact in significant number of cases, the clinical diagnosis is made during uterine curettage, manual removal of placenta or caesarean section. For exact diagnosis of the malformation, internal as well as external architecture of the uterus must be visualised. For this reason several investigations in **different combinations** are done, such as **hysterography (p. 559), hysteroscopy (p. 587), laparoscopy (p. 117), ultrasonography (vaginal probe) (Fig. 4.6B) and magnetic resonance imaging (MRI)**. Ultrasonography and MRI are noninvasive procedures. Urological tract is also evaluated at the same time. The renal tract abnormality in association with Müllerian abnormality is about 40 per cent. Skeletal system anomaly (12 per cent) is also associated.

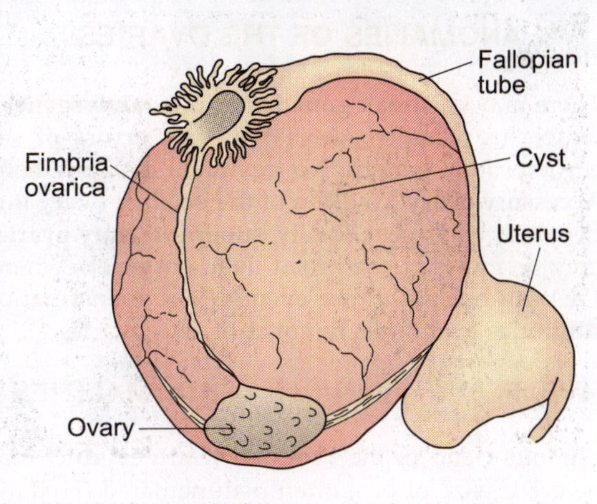

Fig. 4.7. Parovarian cyst

Treatment

Mere presence of any uterine malformation *per se* is not an indication of surgical intervention. Better obstetric outcome in septate uterus (86%), bicornuate uterus (50%) and unicornuate uterus (40%) has been mentioned. Didelphic uterus has high successful pregnancy outcome (64%) without metroplasty. Other causes of infertility or recurrent fetal loss must be excluded. Rudimentary horn should be excised. Unification operation (bicornuate/septate uterus) is therefore indicated in an otherwise unexplained cases. Abdominal metroplasty could be done either by excising the septum (Strassman, Jones and Jones) or by incising the septum (Tompkins). Success rate of abdominal metroplasty in terms of live birth is high (5–75%).

Hysteroscopic metroplasty is becoming popular these days. Resection of the septum can be done either by a resectoscope or by laser (see p 562). Advantages are : (a) High success rate (80-89%); (b) Short hospital stay; (c) Reduced postoperative morbidity (infection or adhesions); (d) Subsequent chance of vaginal delivery is high compared to abdominal metroplasty where caesarean section is mandatory.

ABNORMALITIES OF THE FALLOPIAN TUBES

The tubes may be unduly elongated; may have accessory ostia or diverticula. Rarely, the tube may be absent on one side. These conditions may lower the fertility or favour ectopic pregnancy.

ANOMALIES OF THE OVARIES

There may be **streak gonads** or gonadal dysgenesis which are usually associated with errors of sex chromosomal pattern. No treatment is of any help. **Accessory ovary** (division of the original ovary into two) may be present. Rarely, **supernumerary ovaries** may be found in the broad ligament or elsewhere. This can explain a rare event where menstruation continues even after removal of two ovaries.

WOLFFIAN REMNANT ABNORMALITIES

The outer end of the Wolffian (Gartner) duct may be cystic, size of pea, often pedunculated (Hydatid of Morgagni) and attached near the outer end of the tube. The tubules of the Gartner's duct may be cystic, the outer ones are Kobelt's tubules, the middle set, the epoophoron and the proximal set, the paroophoron. Small cyst may arise from any of the tubules. **A cystic swelling from the Gartner duct** may appear in the anterolateral wall of the vagina confusing with cystocele.

PAROVARIAN CYST

It arises from the vestigial remnants of Wolffian tissue situated in the mesosalpinx between the tube and the ovary. This can attain a big size. The cyst is unilocular; the wall is thin and contains clear translucent fluid. The ovarian fimbria with the ovary is stretched over the cyst (Fig. 4.7). The wall consists of connective tissue lined by single layer of low columnar epithelium.

OTHER ABNORMALITIES

1. LABIA MINORA : ***Labial fusion*** : (a) True — due to developmental defect (b) Inflammatory (see p. 525).

2. LABIA MAJORA : (a) Hyperplastic or hypoplastic labia. (b) Abnormal fusion in adrenogenital syndrome (see p. 424).

3. CLITORIS : ***Clitorial hypertrophy***—often associated with various intersex problems (see p. 424).

4. PERINEUM : Perineum differentiates from the area of contact between the urorectal septum (mesoderm) and the dorsal wall of cloaca (endoderm) at about 7th week. This site of contact between the two is the perineal body. Malformations of the perineum are rare. Imperforate anus, anal stenosis or fistula are the result of abnormal development of the urorectal septum (p. 40). This is due to the posterior deviation the septum as it approach the cloacal membrane. Anal agenesis and fistula is rare. **The anal fistula may open into the posterior aspect of the vestibule of the vagina** (anovestibular fistula p. 40).

KEY POINTS

- Developmental anomalies of the external genitalia along with ambiguity of sex are usually genetic in origin.
- The clinical features with imperforate hymen usually appear at 14-16 years. Retention of urine may be the first symptom. Cruciate incision of the hymen is the treatment.
- Major anatomic defect of the genital tract is usually associated with normal gonadal function and urinary tract abnormalities.
- While minor abnormality escapes attention, it is the moderate or severe form which will produce gynaecologic and obstetric problems.
- For exact diagnosis of malformation both the internal and external architecture of the uterus must be viewed.

  Failure of fusion of Müllerian ducts may lead to arcuate, bicornuate, septate or didelphys uterus.

  While gynaecological symptoms are far and few but at times, they may produce infertility or obstetric problems like recurrent miscarriage, cornual pregnancy, preterm labour or even obstructed labour.

  Presence of uterine malformation *per se* is not an indication of surgical correction. Unification operation is indicated in otherwise unexplained cases of infertility or repeated pregnancy wastage. Hysteroscopic metroplasty has got many advantages (p. 45).
- Vaginal agenesis is most commonly due to Rokitansky — Küster-Hauser Syndrome. In such a case urologic (40%) and skeletal (12%) anomalies are associated.
- Nearly 15-20% of women with recurrent miscarriage are associated with malformation of the uterus.

Puberty Normal and Abnormal

5

PUBERTY

Definition

Puberty in girls is the period which links childhood to adulthood. It is the **period of gradual development of secondary sexual characters.** There are profound biological, morphological and psychological changes which lead to full sexual maturity and eventually fertility.

Morphological changes

As described by Tanner and Marshall, **five** important physical changes are evident during puberty. **These are breast, pubic and axillary hair growth, growth in height and menstruation.** Most of the changes occur gradually but only the menarche can be dated. Moreover, there is lot of variation in the timing of the events. **The most common order is beginning of the growth spurt → breast budding (thelarche) → pubic and axillary hair growth (adrenarche) → peak growth in height → menstruation (menarche).** All these changes are usually completed between the age of 10 and 16 years.

Important controlling factors for onset of puberty are genetic, nutrition, body weight, psychologic state, social and cultural background, exposure to light and others. A girl, living in urban areas with good nutrition, adequate body weight and whose mother and sisters have early menarche, start puberty early. Blind girls start menarche early.

ENDOCRINOLOGY IN PUBERTY

The levels of gonadal steroids and gonadotrophins are low until the age of 6-8 years. This is mainly due to the negative feedback effect of oestrogen to the hypothalamic pituitary system (Gonadostat). The gonadostat remains very sensitive (6-15 times) to the negative feedback effect, even though the level of oestradiol is very low (10 pg/ml) during that time. As puberty approaches this negative feedback effect of oestrogen is gradually lost (see p. 71). This results in some significant changes in the endocrine function of the girl.

- **Hypothalamopituitary gonadal axis**

GnRH pulses from hypothalamus results in pulsatile gonadotrophin secretion (first during the night then by the day time).

$$GnRH \rightarrow FSH, LH \rightarrow Estradiol$$

The tonic and episodic secretion of gonadotrophins in prepubertal period is gradually changed to one of cyclic release in postpubertal period (details in p. 75, Fig. 7.6).

- **Thyroid gland** plays an active role in the hypothalamo-pituitary-gonadal axis.

- **Adrenal glands** (Adrenarche) increase their activity of sex steroid synthesis (androstenedione, DHA, DHAS) from about 7 years of age. Increased sebum formation, pubic and axillary hair and change in voice are primarily due to adrenal androgen production.

- **Gonadarche :** Increased amplitude and frequency of GnRH → ↑ secretion of FSH and LH → ovarian follicular development → ↑ oestrogen. Gonadal oestrogen is responsible for the development of uterus, vagina, vulva and also the breasts (see p. 49).

- **Leptin,** a peptide, secreted in the adipose tissue is also involved in pubertal changes and menarche (see p. 441).

Menarche

The onset of first menstruation in life is called menarche. It may occur anywhere between 10 and 16 years, the **peak time being 13 years**. There is endometrial proliferation due to ovarian oestrogen but when the level drops temporarily, the endometrium sheds and bleeding is visible. It denotes an intact hypothalamo-pituitary-ovarian axis, functioning ovaries, presence of responsive endometrium to the endogenous ovarian steroids and the presence of a patent uterovaginal canal. The **first period is usually anovular**. The ovulation may be irregular for a variable period following menarche and may take about 2 years for regular ovulation to occur. The menses may be irregular to start with.

Growth

Growth in height in an adolescent girl is mainly due to hormones. The important hormones are growth hormone, oestrogen and insulin like growth factor-1 (IGF-1). The bone or skeletal age is determined by X-ray of hand or knee.

Genital organ changes

Ovaries change their shape, the elongated shape becomes bulky and oval. The ovarian bulk is due to

Tanner Stages of Pubertal Development in Girls

Stage	Breast	Pubic hair
Stage I	Prepubertal state, elevation of papilla only.	No pubic hair present.
Stage II	Breast buds and papilla slightly elevated, and areola begins to enlarge. (Median age : 9.8 years).	Sparse, long hair on either side of labia majora. (Median age : 10.5 years).
Stage III	Further enlargement of entire breast tissue.	Darker, coarser and curly hair over the mons pubis.
Stage IV	Secondary mound of areola and papilla projecting above the breast tissue. (Median age : 12.1 years).	Adult type hair covering the mons only. (Median age : 12.0 years).
Stage V	Areola recessed to general contour of breast. (Median age : 14.6 years).	Adult hair with an inverse triangle distribution (female escutcheon) covering the medial thighs. (Median age : 13.7 years).

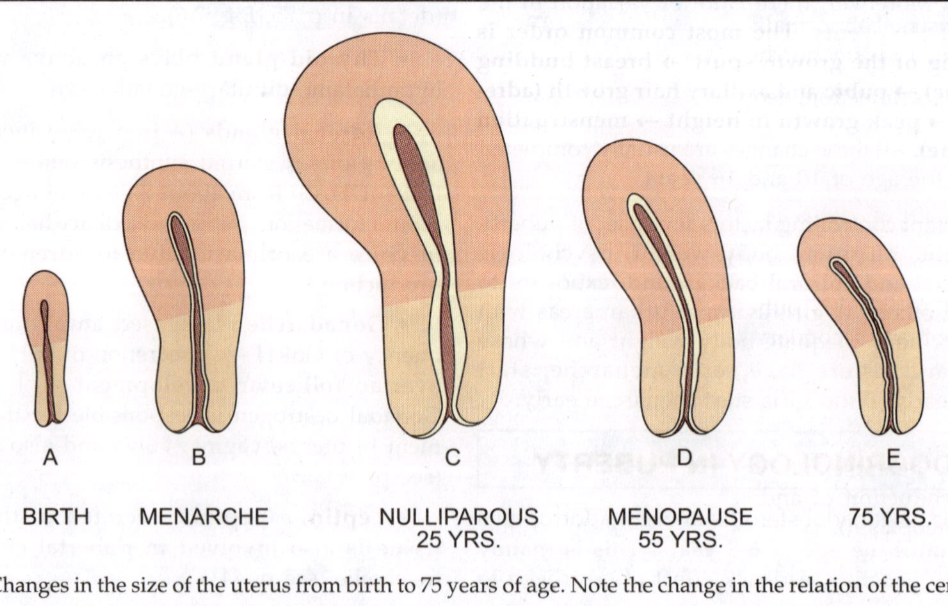

Fig. 5.1. Changes in the size of the uterus from birth to 75 years of age. Note the change in the relation of the cervix to the body

follicular enlargement at various stages of development and proliferation of stromal cells.

The uterine body and the cervix ratio at birth is about 1 : 2, the ratio becomes 1 : 1 when menarche occurs. Thereafter, the enlargement of the body occurs rapidly, so that the ratio soon becomes 2 : 1 (Fig. 5.1).

The vaginal changes are more pronounced. A few layers of thin epithelium in a child become stratified epithelium of many layers. The cells are rich in glycogen due to oestrogen. Doderlein's bacilli appear which convert glycogen into lactic acid; the vaginal pH becomes acidic, ranging between 4-5.

The vulva is more reactive to steroid hormones.

The mons pubis and the labia minora increase in size.

Breast changes are pronounced. Under the influence of oestrogen, there is marked proliferation of duct systems and deposition of fat. The breast becomes prominent and round. Under the influence of progesterone, the development of acini increases considerably.

Tanner staging : According to Tanner, breast and pubic hair development at puberty are divided into five stages (see table on p. 48).

Common disorders of puberty

- Precocious puberty.
- Delayed puberty.
- Menstrual abnormalities (amenorrhoea, menorrhagia, dysmenorrhoea).
- Others (infection, neoplasm, hirsutism etc.) see Ch. 32.

PRECOCIOUS PUBERTY

Definition

The term precocious puberty is reserved for girls who exhibit any secondary sex characteristics before the age of 8 or menstruate before the age of 10.

Precocious puberty may be isosexual where the features are due to excess production of oestrogen. It may be heterosexual where features are due to excess production of androgen (from ovarian and adrenal neoplasm).

Types or causes

The causes are tabulated in the Table 5.1.

Table 5.1 : Causes of precocious puberty

GnRH dependent – 80% (complete, central, isosexual or true)
Constitutional — commonest
Juvenile primary hypothyroidism
Intracranial lesions — trauma, tumour or infection
Incomplete :
Premature thelarche
Premature puberche
Premature menarche
GnRH independent (precocious pseudopuberty or peripheral)
(Excess oestrogen or androgen)
Ovary :
Granulosa cell tumour
Theca cell tumour
Leydig cell tumour
Chorionic epithelioma
Androblastoma
McCune – Albright syndrome
Adrenal :
Hyperplasia
Tumour
Liver :
Hepatoblastoma
Iatrogenic :
Oestrogen or androgen intake

Aetiopathology

Constitutional

It is due to premature activation of hypothalamo-pituitary ovarian axis. There is secretion of gonadotrophins and gonadal steroids due to premature release of GnRH. Bone maturation is accelerated, leading to premature closure of the epiphysis and curtailed stature. If menstruation occurs, they may be ovulatory. The changes in puberty progress in an orderly sequence.

Intracranial lesions

Meningitis, encephalitis, craniopharyngioma, neurofibroma or any tumour — hypothalamic or pineal gland.

McCune – Albright syndrome is characterised by sexual precocity, multiple cystic bone lesions (polyostotic fibrous dysplasia), endocrinopathies and café-au-lait spots on the skin. Sexual precocity is due to early and excessive oestrogen production from the ovaries. FSH, LH levels are low. There may be associated hyperthyroidism, hyperparathyroidism and acromegaly.

Premature thelarche

It is the isolated development of breast tissue before the age of 8 and commonly between 2 and 4 years of age. Either one or both the breasts may be enlarged. There is no other feature of precocious puberty. It generally requires no treatment.

Premature pubarche

Premature pubarche is isolated development of axillary and or pubic hair prior to the age of 8 without other signs of precocious puberty. The premature hair growth may be due to unusual sensitivity of endorgans to the usual low level of hormones in the blood during childhood. Rarely, there may be signs of excess androgen production due to adrenal hyperplasia or tumour or androgenic ovarian tumour (Leydig cell tumour, androblastoma, etc.).

Premature menarche

Premature menarche is an isolated event of cyclic vaginal bleeding without any other signs of secondary sexual development. The cause remains unclear but may be related to unusual endocrine sensitivity of the endometrium to the low level of oestrogens.

Chorionic epithelioma, hepatoblastoma are the ectopic sources of human chorionic gonadotrophin and may cause sexual precocity.

Diagnosis

True precocious

Constitutional type is the commonest one but the rare one is to be kept in mind. The diagnosis is made by :

- History of early menarche of mother and sisters.
- The pubertal changes occur in orderly sequence.
- Tanner stages.
- No cause could be detected.

The basic investigations, to confirm or to exclude some pathologic lesions, include :

- X-ray hand and wrist (non-dominant) for bone age. Acceleration of growth is one of the earliest clinical features of precocious puberty.
- Pelvic sonography to exclude ovarian pathology.
- Skull X-ray, CT scan or MRI brain — to exclude intracranial lesion.
- Serum hCG, FSH, LH.
- Thyroid profile (TSH, T_4).
- Serum estradiol, testosterone, 17 OH progesterone, dehydroepiandrosterone (DHEA).
- Electroencephalogram.

Premature thelarche

- Somatic growth pattern is not accelerated.
- Bone age is not advanced.
- Nipple development is absent.
- Vaginal smear shows negative oestrogen effect.

Premature puberche

It may be due to adrenal or ovarian mischief. As such, the investigations are directed accordingly.

- An ovarian enlargement may not be palpable clinically. Examination under anaesthesia or sonography is helpful.

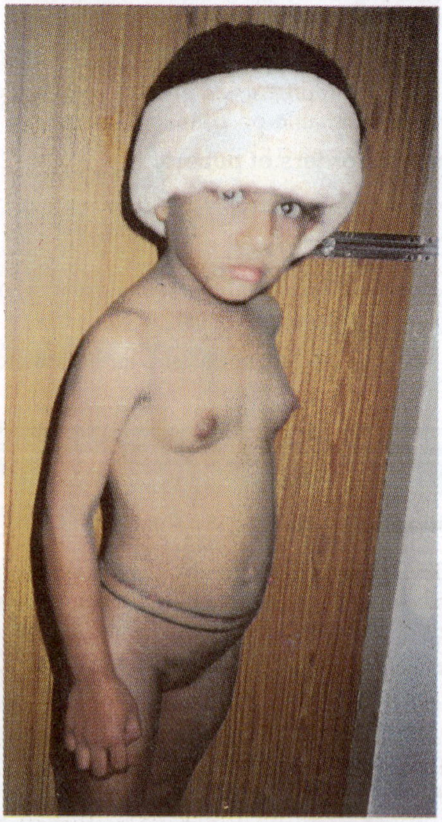

Fig. 5.2. Precocious puberty in a girl aged 4 years [*By courtesy* : Prof. B. N. Chakraborty, IRM, Kolkata]

- IVP or CT scan is required to detect adrenal tumour.
- Estimations of serum 17 α-hydroxy-progesterone, DHEA-S and serum testosterone are to be done in suspected cases of adrenal mischief — hyperplasia or tumour.

If nothing abnormal is detected, then the diagnosis of idiopathic pubarche is made.

Premature menarche

The other causes of vaginal bleeding such as foreign body or injury has to be excluded. If the bleeding is cyclic, the diagnosis is confirmed.

Remarks

Investigations must be carried out to rule out any pathology in the CNS, ovary and adrenal. It should be borne in mind that even in cases when no cause can be detected in any of the types mentioned, the periodic evaluation at 6 monthly intervals is to be made to detect any life-threatening pathology at the earliest.

TREATMENT

The treatment depends upon the cause. The exogenous oestrogen therapy or its inadvertent intake should be stopped forthwith. Cortisone therapy for adrenal hyperplasia and surgery to remove the adrenal or ovarian tumour eliminate the excess source of either androgen or oestrogen. The intracranial tumour requires neurosurgery or radiotherapy. Primary hypothyroidism needs thyroid replacement therapy.

Constitutional or idiopathic type

The goals are :

- To reduce gonadotrophin secretions.
- To suppress gonadal steroidogenesis or counteract the peripheral action of sex steroids.
- To decrease the growth rate to normal and slowing the skeletal maturation.
- To protect the girl from sex abuse.

The drugs used are :

- **GnRH agonist therapy** arrests the pubertal precocity and growth velocity significantly. The agonists suppress the premature activation of hypothalamopituitary axis due to down regulation and thereby diminished oestrogen secretion. **GnRH agonist therapy is the drug of choice in cases with GnRH dependent precocious puberty.** Therapy should be started as soon as the diagnosis is established. GnRH agonist therapy suppresses FSH, LH secretion, reverses the ovarian cycle, establishes amenorrhoea, causes regression of breast, pubic hair changes and other secondary sexual characteristics. This drug should be continued till the median age of puberty (p. 48).

Dose : Buserelin nasal spray 100 μg daily. It can slow down the process of skeletal maturation. Depot forms (goserelin or leuprolide) once a month can be used (see p. 500). Dose is adjusted to maintain the serum oestradiol below 10 pg/ml.

- **Medroxy progesterone acetate** — 30 mg daily orally or 100-200 mg. IM weekly to suppress gonadal steroids. It can suppress menstruation and breast development but cannot change the skeletal growth rate.
- **Cyproterone acetate** — It acts as a potent progestogen, having agonist effects on progesterone receptors.

Dose — 70-100 mg/m^2/day orally for 10 days starting from 5th day of cycle.

- **Danazol** — It produces amenorrhoea and arrest breast development. But there is no effect on growth rate or skeletal maturation.

Duration of therapy :

The drugs should be used upto the age of 11 years. However, individualisation is to be done.

Prognosis

Prognosis vary considerably depending on the aetiology. Overall prognosis is good with primary hypothyroidism, adrenal or ovarian tumours following treatment. For the CNS group, prognosis depends on neurological involvement and treatment outcome. Apart from the short stature due to accelerated bone maturation, **the idiopathic group** have got a normal menstrual pattern in future. The fertility rate is also expected to be normal.

DELAYED PUBERTY

Puberty is said to be delayed when the breast tissue and/or pubic hair have not appeared by 13-14 years or menarche appears as late as 16 years. The normal upper age limit of menarche is 15 years.

Table 5.2
Causes of delayed puberty

- **Hypergonadotrophic hypogonadism** (see p. 434)
  - Gonadal dysgenesis, 45 XO
  - Pure gonadal dysgenesis 46 XX, 46 XY
  - Ovarian failure 46 XX
- **Hypogonadotrophic hypogonadism** (see p. 433)
  - Constitutional delay
  - Chronic illness, malnutrition
  - Primary hypothyroidism
  - Isolated gonadotrophin deficiency (Kallmann's syndrome)
  - Intracranial lesions – tumours : craniopharyngioma, pituitary adenomas
- **Eugonadism**
  - Anatomical causes (see ch. 4)
    Müllerian agenesis
    Imperforate hymen
    Transverse vaginal septum
  - Androgen insensitivity syndrome

TREATMENT

Treatment is directed according to the aetiology. Assurance, improvement of general health and treatment of any illness may be of help in non-endocrinal causes. Cases with hypogonadism may be treated with cyclic oestrogen. Unopposed oestrogen 0.3 mg (conjugated oestrogen) daily is given for first 6 months. Then combined oestrogen and progestin, sequential regimen is started (see p. 56). Cases of hypergonadotrophic hypogonadism should have chromosomal study to exclude intersexuality (see p. 423).

PUBERTY MENORRHAGIA

Menstrual abnormality in adolescents are common. The periods may be heavy, irregular or scanty initially. Eventually the majority of these teenaged girls establish a normal cycle and are fertile.

The important causes of menorrhagia are :

(i) **Dysfunctional uterine bleeding** (95%). Anovulatory cycles → unopposed oestrogen → Endometrial hyperplasia → prolonged and heavy periods (see p. 183).

(ii) **Endocrine dysfunction** :

- Polycystic Ovary Syndrome (PCOS, p. 440).
- Hypo or Hyperthyroidism.

(iii) **Haematological** :

- Idiopathic thrombocytopenic purpura (p. 181).
- Von-Willebrand's disease (p. 181).
- Leukaemia.

(iv) **Pelvic tumours** :

- Fibroid uterus (p. 262).
- Sarcoma botryroides (p. 355).
- Oestrogen producing ovarian tumour (p. 370).

(v) **Pregnancy complications** (abortion).

Diagnosis is made by careful history taking and thorough clinical examination.

Evaluation is specially indicated if the menstrual interval is < 22 days or > 44 days, lasts longer than one week or the bleeding is too heavy that anaemia develops.

Investigations are planned according to the clinical diagnosis. Investigations include : routine haematological examination including bleeding time, clotting time, platelet count. Thyroid profile (TSH, T_3, T_4), clotting profile, and imaging study of the pelvis by ultrasonography may be needed. EUA and uterine curettage are rarely needed to exclude any pelvic pathology (pregnancy complications). The curetted material is sent for histopathological study.

Management : The girl needs adequate explanation, reassurance and psychological support. Rest and correction of anaemia are helpful in majority of the cases.

Therapy with haematinics or even blood transfusion may be needed. In refractory cases, progestogens such as medroxyprogesterone acetate or norethisterone 5 mg thrice daily is given till bleeding stops. Usually the bleeding is controlled within 3-7 days. Medication is continued for 21 days. The condition usually becomes normal following 2-3 courses and then normal cycles resume. In emergency, conjugated equine oestrogen 20-40 mg IV is given every 6-8 hours. Once the bleeding is controlled, combined oral pills are started.

Regular menstrual cycle will be established once the hypothalamo-pituitary-ovarian axis is matured.

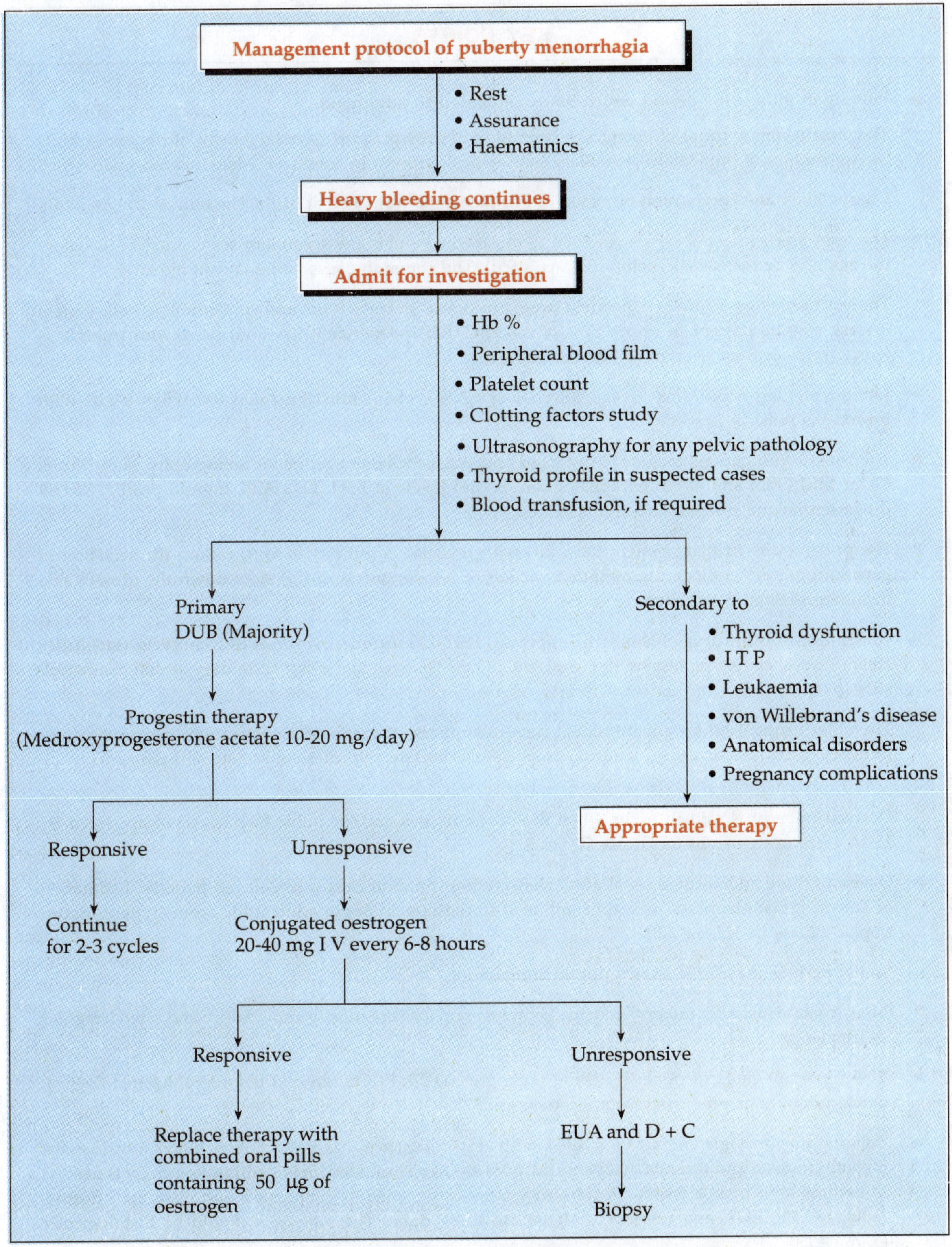

Fig. 5.3. Management protocol of puberty menorrhagia

KEY POINTS

- Puberty in girls is the period which binds childhood to adulthood.

  The most common order of changes is beginning of growth spurt → enlargement of the breast buds → Appearance of pubic hair → Axillary hair → peak growth in height → Menstruation (menarche).

  Uterine body and cervix ratio becomes 1 : 1 at menarche from 1 : 2 at birth. The ratio is 2 : 1 in adult.

- The term precocious puberty is reserved to those who exhibit any secondary sex characteristic before the age of 8 or menstruate before the age of 10. The common cause being constitutional.

  The exact aetiology of GnRH dependent (true) precocious puberty is not known. Central nervous system disease may be present in nearly 30% of cases. GnRH independent (pseudo) precocious puberty is mostly related to an ovarian or adrenal pathology.

- Life-threatening neoplasms (ovary, adrenal or CNS system) must be ruled out when a girl with precocious puberty is seen.

- The basic investigations include X-ray hand and wrist for bone age, pelvic sonography, skull X-ray, CT or MRI brain and electroencephalogram. Serum levels of FSH, LH, hCG, thyroid profile, 17 OH progesterone and testosterone are measured.

- The primary aim of management for a girl with precocious puberty is to (i) reduce the secretion of gonadotrophins. (ii) block the peripheral action of sex steroids and (iii) slow down the growth rate including skeletal maturation.

- GnRH agonist is the drug of choice. It suppresses FSH, LH secretion, reverses ovarian cycle, establishes amenorrhoea, causes regression of breast, pubic hair changes and other secondary sexual characteristics (p. 51).

  The other drugs used for constitutional type to suppress the premature activation of hypothalamo-pituitary–gonadal axis are — medroxyprogesterone acetate, cyproterone acetate and danazol.

- Delayed puberty is said to occur when the breast tissues and/or pubic hair have not appeared by 13-14 years or menarche as late as 17 years.

- Ovarian failure and chromosomal anomalies are the common causes of delayed puberty. Estimation of serum gonadotrophins is important to differentiate hypogonadotrophic from hypergonadotrophic causes (see Table 5.2).

- Initial periods may be excessive due to anovulation.

- Menstruation just after puberty and just before menopause are mostly anovulatory and often irregular in frequency.

- The important cases of puberty menorrhagia are : DUB, PCOS, thyroid disorders, haematological, pelvic tumours or pregnancy complications (p. 52).

- Pubertal menorrhagia should be treated with rest, assurance, haematinics and blood transfusions. Hypothyroidism and thrombocytopenic purpura are to be excluded. Pelvic ultrasonography is needed to exclude any organic lesion. In refractory cases, progestins or conjugated oestrogen are effective failing which, EUA and uterine curettage are to be done. The materials should be histologically examined.

Menopause

6

Definition

Menopause means *permanent cessation of menstruation at the end of reproductive life due to loss of ovarian follicular activity. It is the point of time when last and final menstruation occurs.*

The clinical diagnosis is confirmed following stoppage of menstruation (amenorrhoea) for twelve consecutive months without any other pathology. As such, a woman is declared to have attained menopause only retrospectively. Premenopause refers to the period prior to menopause, postmenopause to the period after menopause and perimenopause to the period around menopause (40-55 years).

Climacteric is the phase of aging process during which a woman passes from the reproductive to the non-reproductive stage. This phase covers 5-10 years on either side of menopause.

Premenopause is the part of the climacteric before menopause, when the menstrual cycle is likely to be irregular.

Postmenopause is the phase of life that comes after the menopause.

Age of menopause

Age at which menopause occurs is genetically predetermined. The age of menopause is not related to age of menarche or age at last pregnancy. It is also not related to number of pregnancy, lactation, use of oral pill, socio-economic condition, race, height or weight. Thinner women have early menopause. However, cigarette smoking and severe malnutrition may cause early menopause. The age of menopause ranges between 45-55 years, average being 50 years.

Clinical importance

Due to increased life expectancy, specially in affluent society, about one-third of life span will be spent during the period of oestrogen deprivation stage with long-term symptomatic and metabolic complications.

ENDOCRINOLOGY OF CLIMACTERIC AND MENOPAUSE

Hypothalamopituitary gonadal axis

Few years prior to menopause, along with depletion of the ovarian follicles, the follicles become resistant to pituitary gonadotrophins. As a result, effective folliculogenesis is impaired with diminished oestradiol production. There is a significant fall in the level of serum estradiol from 50-300 pg/ml before menopause to 10-20 pg/ml after menopause. **This decreases the negative feedback effect on hypothalamopituitary axis resulting increase in FSH. The increase in FSH is also due to diminished inhibin.** Inhibin, a peptide, is secreted by the granulosa cells of the ovarian follicle. The increase of LH occurs subsequently.

Disturbed folliculogenesis during this period may result in anovulation, oligo-ovulation, premature corpus luteum or corpus luteal insufficiency. The sustained level of oestrogens may even cause endometrial hyperplasia and clinical manifestation of menstrual abnormalities prior to menopause.

The mean cycle length is significantly shorter. This is due to shortening of the follicular phase of the cycle. Luteal phase length remaining constant.

Ultimately, no more follicles are available and even some exist, they are resistant to gonadotrophins. Oestradiol production drops down to the optimal level of 20 pg/ml → no endometrial growth → absence of menstruation.

Oestrogens

Following menopause, the predominant oestrogen is oestrone and to a lesser extent oestradiol. Serum level of oestrone (30-70 pg/ml) is higher than that of oestradiol (10-20 pg/ml). The major source of oestrone is peripheral conversion (aromatisation) of androgens from adrenals (mainly) and ovaries. The aromatisation occurs at the level of muscle and adipose tissue. The trace amount of oestradiol is derived from peripheral conversion of oestrone and androgens. Compared to oestradiol, oestrone is biologically less (about one-tenth) potent.

With times, the sources fail to supply the precursors of oestrogen and about 5-10 years after menopause, there is a sharp fall in oestrogen and also the trophic hormones. The woman is said to be in a state of true menopause.

Androgens

After menopause, the stromal cells of the ovary continue to produce androgens because of increase in LH. The main androgens are androstenedione and testosterone. Though the secretion of androgens from postmenopausal ovary are more, their peripheral levels are reduced due to conversion of androgens to oestrone in adipose tissue. However, the cumulative effect is a decrease in oestrogen : androgen ratio. This results in increased facial hair growth and change in voice.

As the obese patient converts more androgens into oestrone, they are less likely to develop symptoms of oestrogen deficiency and osteoporosis. But, they are vulnerable to endometrial hyperplasia and endometrial carcinoma.

Progesterone

A trace amount of progesterone detected is probably adrenal in origin.

Gonadotrophins

The secretions of both FSH and LH are increased due to **absent negative feedback effect of oestradiol and inhibin** or due to enhanced responsiveness of pituitary to GnRH. Rise in FSH is about 10-20 fold where as that of LH is about 3 fold. GnRH pulse section is increased both in frequency and amplitude. During menopause there is fall in the level of prolactin and inhibin. Ultimately, due to physiologic aging GnRH and both FSH, LH decline along with decline of oestrogens.

Organ changes

Ovaries shrink in size, become wrinkled and white. There is thinning of the cortex with increase in medullary components. There is abundance of stromal cells which have got secretory activity.

Fallopian tubes show feature of atrophy. The muscle coat becomes thinner, the cilia disappear and the plicae become less prominent.

The uterus becomes smaller and the ratio between the body and the cervix reverts to the 1 : 1 ratio. The endometrium becomes thin and atrophic. In some women, however, with high endogenous oestrogens, the endometrium may be proliferative or even hyperplastic. The cervical secretion becomes scanty.

The vagina becomes narrower due to gradual loss of elasticity. The vaginal epithelium becomes thin. The rugae progressively flatten. There is no glycogen. Doderlein's bacillus is absent. The vaginal pH becomes alkaline. Maturation Index (parabasal, intermediate and superficial cells) is 10/85/5.

The vulva shows features of atrophy. The labia becomes flattened and the pubic hair becomes scantier. The end result is a narrow introitus.

Breast fat is reabsorbed and the glands atrophy. The nipples decrease in size. Ultimately, the breasts become flat and pendulous.

Bladder and urethra undergo similar changes to those of the vagina. The epithelium becomes thin and is more prone to damage and infection. There may be dysuria, frequency, urge or even stress incontinence.

Loss of muscle tone leads to pelvic relaxation, uterine descent and anatomic changes in the urethra and neck of the bladder. The pelvic cellular tissues become scanty and the ligaments supporting the uterus and vagina lose their tone. As such preexisting weakness gets aggravated.

BONE METABOLISM

Normally bone formation (osteoblastic activity) and bone resorption (osteoclastic activity) are in balance depending on many factors (age, endocrine, nutrition and genetic). Following menopause there is loss of bone mass by about 3-5 per cent per year. This is due to deficiency of oestrogen. Osteoporosis is a condition where there is reduction in bone mass but bone mineral to matrix ratio is normal. Postmenopausal woman runs a high risk for fracture of bones due to osteoporosis. Parathyroid hormone (PTH) and IL-I are involved in osteoporosis. Oestrogen prevents osteoporosis by several mechanisms. It inhibits osteoclastic activity and inhibits release of IL-I by monocytes. Oestrogen increases absorption of calcium from the gut, stimulates calcitonin secretion from the C cells of the thyroid and increases 1, 25 dihydroxy vitamin D. All these lead to increased bone mineralisation.

CARDIOVASCULAR SYSTEM

Risk of cardiovascular disease is high in postmenopausal women **due to deficiency of oestrogen**. **Oestrogen prevents cardiovascular disease by several ways.** It increases HDL (particularly HDL 2) and decreases LDL and total cholesterol. It inhibits platelet and macrophage (foam cell) aggregation at the vascular intima. It stimulates the release of nitric oxide (NO) and prostacycline from vascular endothelium to dilate the blood vessels. It prevents atherosclerosis by its **antioxidant property**.

MENSTRUATION PATTERN PRIOR TO MENOPAUSE

Any of the following patterns are observed :

(i) Abrupt cessation of menstruation (rare).

(ii) Gradual decrease in both amount and duration. It may be spotting or delayed and ultimately lead to cessation.

(iii) Irregular with or without excessive bleeding. One should exclude genital malignancy prior to declare it as the usual premenopausal pattern.

MENOPAUSAL SYMPTOMS

In majority, apart from cessation of menstruation, no more symptoms are evident. In some women symptoms appear. **The important symptoms and the health concerns of menopause are :**

- Vasomotor symptoms.
- Urogenital atrophy.
- Osteoporosis and fracture.
- Cardiovascular disease.
- Cerebrovascular disease.
- Psychological changes.
- Skin and Hair.
- Sexual dysfunction.
- Dementia and cognitive decline.

Vasomotor symptoms : The characteristic symptom of menopause is "hot flush". **Hot flush is characterised by sudden feeling of heat followed by profuse sweating.** There may also be the symptoms of palpitation, fatigue and weakness. The physiologic changes with hot flushes are **perspiration** and **cutaneous vasodilatation**. Both these two functions are under central thermoregulatory control. Low oestrogen level is a prerequisite for hot flush. Hot flush coincides with GnRH pulse secretion. It may last for 1-10 minutes, and may be at times unbearable. Sleep may be disturbed due to night sweats. The **thermoregulatory centre in association with GnRH centre in the hypothalamus is involved in the aetiology of hot flush.** Gonadotrophins are thought be involved.

Genital and urinary system : Steroid receptors have been identified in the mucous membrane of urethra, bladder, vagina and the pelvic floor muscles. Oestrogen plays an important role to maintain the epithelium of vagina, urinary bladder and the urethra. Oestrogen deficiency produces atrophic epithelial changes in these organs. This may cause dyspareunia.

Vagina : Minimal trauma may cause vaginal bleeding. Dyspareunia, vaginal infections, dryness, pruritus and leucorrhoea are also common. **The urinary symptoms are :** urgency, dysuria and recurrent urinary tract infection and stress incontinence.

Sexual dysfunction : Oestrogen deficiency is often associated with decreased sexual desire. This may be due psychological changes (depression anxiety) as well as atrophic changes of the genitourinary system.

Skin and hair : There is thining, loss of elasticity and wrinkling of the skin. Skin collagen content and thickness decrease by 1-2 per cent per year. *"Purse String"* wrinkling around the month and *"Crow feet"* around the eyes are the characteristics. Oestrogen receptors are present in the skin and maximum are present in the facial skin. Oestrogen replacement can prevent this skin loss during menopause. After menopause, there is some loss of pubic and axillary hair and slight balding. This may be due to low level of oestrogen with normal level of testosterone.

Psychological changes : There is increased frequency of anxiety, headache, insomnia, irritability dysphasia and depression. They also suffer from dementia, mood swing and inability to concentrate. Oestrogen increases opioid (neurotransmitter) activity in the brain and is known to be important for memory.

Dementia : Oestrogen is thought to protect the function of central nervous system. Dementia and mainly Alzheimer disease are more common in postmenopausal women.

Osteoporosis and fracture : Following menopause there is decline in collagenous bone matrix resulting in osteoporotic changes. Bone mass loss and microarchitectural deterioration of bone tissue occurs primarily in trabecular bone (vertebra, distal radius) and in cortical bones. Bone loss increases to 5 per cent per year during menopause. **Osteoporosis** may be **primary (Type 1)** due to oestrogen loss, age, deficient nutrition (calcium, vit. D) or hereditary. It may be **secondary (Type 2)** to endocrine abnormalities (parathyroid, diabetes) or medication (see p. 60). Osteoporosis may lead to back pain, loss of height and kyphosis. Fracture of bones is a major health problem. Fracture may involve the vertebral body, femoral neck, or distal forearm (Colles' fracture). Morbidity and mortality in elderly women following fracture is high.

Detection of osteoporosis : Computed tomography (CT) and specially the Dual-ene rgy X-ray absorptiometry (DEXA) are reliable methods to assess the bone mineral density. Total radiation exposure is high with CT than DEXA.

Biochemical parameters to detect bone loss are measurement of urinary calcium/creatinine and hydroxyproline/creatinine ratios.

Cardiovascular and cerebrovascular effects : Oxidation of LDL and foam cell formation cause vascular endothelial injury, cell death and smooth muscle proliferation. All these lead to vascular atherosclerotic changes, vasoconstriction and thrombus formation (see p. 57).

Risks of ischaemic heart disease, coronary artery disease and strokes are increased.

DIAGNOSIS OF MENOPAUSE

1. Cessation of menstruation for consecutive 12 months during climacteric.
2. Appearance of menopausal symptoms 'hot flush' and 'night sweats'.
3. Vaginal cytology – showing maturation index of at least 10/85/5 (Features of low oestrogen).
4. Serum oestradiol : < 20 pg/ml.
5. Serum FSH and LH : > 40 mIU/ml (three values at weeks interval required).

MANAGEMENT

Prevention

Spontaneous menopause is unavoidable. However, **artificial menopause** induced by surgery (bilateral oophorectomy) or by radiation (gonadal) during reproductive period can to some extent be preventable or delayed.

Counselling : Every woman with postmenopausal symptoms should be adequately explained about the physiologic events. This will remove her fears, and minimise or dipel the symptoms of anxiety, depression and insomnia. Reassurance is essential.

TREATMENT

Non-hormonal Treatment

- Nutritious diet — balanced with calcium and protein is helpful.
- Supplementary calcium — daily intake of 1-1.5 gm can reduce osteoporosis and fracture.
- Exercise — weight bearing exercises, walking, jogging.
- Vitamin D — Supplementation of vitamin D_3 (400-800 IU/day) along with calcium can reduce osteoporosis and fractures. Exposure to sunlight enhances synthesis of cholecalciferol (Vitamin D_3) in the skin.
- Cessation of smoking and alcohol.
- **Biphosphonates** prevent osteoclastic bone resorption. Commonly used drugs are etidronate and alendronate. Alendronate is more potent. Ibandronate and risedronate are also effective and have less side effects. Biphosphonates when used alone cannot prevent hot flushes, atrophic changes and cardiovascular disease. It is taken in empty stomach. Nothing should be taken by mouth for at least 30 minutes after oral dosing. Patient should remain upright for 30 minutes. Side effects include gastric and oesophageal ulceration.
- **Fluoride** prevents osteoporosis and increases bone matrix. It is given at a dose of 1 mg/kg for short-term only. Calcium supplementation should be continued. Long-term therapy induces side effects (brittle bones).

• **Calcitonin** inhibits bone resorption. Simultaneous therapy with calcium and vitamin D should be given. It is given either by nasal spray (200 IU daily) or by injection (S.C.) (50-100 IU daily). It is suitable when oestrogen therapy is contraindicated.

• **Selective oestrogen receptor modulators (SERMs)** are tissue specific in action. Of the many SERMs, **raloxifene** has shown to increase bone mineral density, reduce serum LDL and to raise HDL2 level. Raloxifene inhibits the oestrogen receptors at the breast and endometrial tissues. **Risks of breast cancer and endometrial cancer are therefore reduced. Raloxifene does not improve hot flushes or urogenital atrophy.** Risks of venous thromboembolism is increased.

• **Clonidine**, an alpha adrenergic agonist may be used to reduce the severity and duration of hot flushes. It is helpful where oestrogen is contraindicated in hypertension.

• **Thiazides** reduce urinary calcium excretion. It increases bone density specially when combined with oestrogen.

• **Paroxetine,** a selective serotonin reuptake inhibitor, is effective to reduce hot flushes both the frequency and severity.

• **Gabapentine** is an analogue of gamma-aminobutyric acid. It is found also to be effective.

• **Phytoestrogens** containing isoflavones are found to lower the incidence of vasomotor symptoms, osteoporosis and cardiovascular disease.

• **Soy protein** is also found effective to reduce vasomotor symptoms. Soy protein acts as SERMS.

HORMONE REPLACEMENT THERAPY (HRT)

The HRT is indicated in menopausal women to overcome the short-term and long-term consequences of oestrogen deficiency.

Indication of Hormone Replacement Therapy

(i) Relief of menopausal symptoms (see p. 57).

(ii) Prevention of osteoporosis (see p. 58).

(iii) To maintain the quality of life in menopausal years.

Special group of women to whom HRT should be prescribed :

• Premature ovarian failure

• Gonadal dysgenesis

• Surgical or radiation menopause

BENEFITS OF HORMONE REPLACEMENT THERAPY (HRT)

• Improvement of vasomotor symptoms (70-80%).

• Improvement urogenital atrophy.

• Increase in bone mineral density (2-5%).

• Decreased risk in vertebral and hip fractures (25-50%).

• Reduction in colorectal cancer (20%).

• Possibly cardio protection.

Table 6.1
RISK FACTORS FOR OSTEOPOROSIS IN A WOMAN

• Family history.
• Age — elderly.
• Race — Asian, White race.
• Lack of oestrogen.
• Body weight — Low BMI.
• Early menopause — Surgical, radiation.
• Dietary — ↓ Calcium and ↓ Vitamin D, ↑ Caffeine, ↑ Smoking.
• Sedentary habit.
• Drugs—Heparin, corticosteroids, GnRH analogues.
• Diseases—Thyroid disorders, hyperparathyroidism malabsorption, multiple myeloma.

HRT and Osteoporosis : The major cause of postmenopausal osteoporosis appears to be an increase in bone resorption. HRT prevents bone loss and stimulate new bone formation. Oestrogen is found to play a direct role, as receptors have been found in the osteoblasts. Women receiving HRT should supplement their diet with an extra 500 mg of calcium daily. **Total daily requirement of calcium in postmenopausal women is 1.5 gm.**

HRT is thought to be cardiovascular protective. LDL on oxidation produces vascular endothelial injury and foam cell (macrophage) formation. These endothelial changes ultimately lead to intimal smooth muscle proliferation and atherosclerosis. Oestrogen prevents oxidation of LDL, as it has got **antioxidant properties.**

Table 6.2 : Risk factors for cardiovascular disease

• Hypertension	• Smoking habit
• Familial hyperlipidaemia	• Impaired glucose tolerance

In postmenopausal women there is some amount of insulin resistance and hyperinsulinaemia. Hyperinsulinaemia induces atherogenesis. Oestrogen improve glucose metabolism.

RISKS OF HORMONE REPLACEMENT THERAPY

(a) **Endometrial cancer :** When oestrogen is given alone to a woman with intact uterus, it causes endometrial proliferation, hyperplasia and carcinoma. It is therefore advised that a progestogen should be added to ERT to counter balance such risks.

(b) **Breast cancer :** Combined oestrogen and progestin replacement therapy, increases the risk of breast cancer slightly (R.R 1.26). Adverse effects of hormone therapy are related to the dose and duration of therapy.

(c) **Venous Thromboembolic (VTE) disease** has been found to be increased with the use of combined oral oestrogen and progestin. Transdermal oestrogen use does not have the same risk compared to oral oestrogen.

(d) **Coronary Heart Disease (CHD)** : Combined HRT therapy shows a relative hazard (R.R, 1.29) of CHD. Hypertension has not been observed to be a risk of HRT.

(e) **Lipid metabolism** : An increased incidence of gallbladder disease has been observed following ERT due to rise in cholesterol (in bile).

(f) **Dementia, Alzheimer** disease are increased.

Table 6.3 : CONTRAINDICATIONS TO HRT

- Undiagnosed genital tract bleeding
- Oestrogen dependent neoplasm in the body
- History of venous thromboembolism
- Active liver disease
- Gallbladder disease

AVAILABLE PREPARATIONS FOR HORMONE REPLACEMENT THERAPY

The principal hormone used in HRT is oestrogen. This is ideal for a woman who had her uterus removed (hysterectomy) already. But a woman with an intact uterus, only oestrogen therapy leads to endometrial hyperplasia and even endometrial carcinoma. Addition of progestins for last 12-14 days each month can prevent this problem. **Commonly used oestrogens** are conjugated oestrogen (0.625-1.25 mg/day) or micronised oestradiol (1-2 mg/day). **Progestins** used are medroxyprogesterone acetate (2.5-5 mg/day), micronised progesterone (100-300 mg/day) or dydrogesterone (5-10 mg/day).

Considering the risks, hormone therapy should be used with the lowest effective dose and for a short period of time. Low dose oral conjugated oestrogen 0.3 mg daily is effective and has got minimal side effects. Dose interval may be modified as daily for initial 2-3 months then it may be changed to every other day for another 2-3 months and then every third day for the next 2-3 months. It may be stopped thereafter if symptoms are controlled.

Oral oestrogen regime

Oestrogen — conjugated equine oestrogen 0.3 mg or 0.625 mg is given daily for woman who had hysterectomy.

Oestrogen and cyclic progestin

For a woman with intact uterus oestrogen is given continuously for 25 days and progestin is added for last 12-14 days.

Continuous oestrogen and progestin therapy

Continued combined therapy can prevent endometrial hyperplasia. There may be irregular bleeding with this regimen.

- **Subdermal implants** : Implants are inserted subcutaneously over the anterior abdominal wall using local anaesthesia. 17 β oestradiol implants 25 mg, 50 mg or 100 mg are available and can be kept for 6 months. This method is suitable in patients after hysterectomy. Implants maintain physiological E_2 to E_1 ratio.

- **Percutaneous oestrogen gel** : 1 gm applicator of gel, delivering 1 mg of oestradiol daily, is to be applied onto the skin over the anterior abdominal wall or thighs. Effective blood level of oestradiol (90-120 pg/ml) can be maintained.

- **Transdermal patch** : It contains 3.2 mg of 17 β oestradiol, releasing about 50 μg of oestradiol in 24 hours. Physiological level of E_2 to E_1 is maintained. It should be applied below the waist line and **changed twice a week.** Skin reaction, irritation and itching have been noted with their use.

- **Vaginal cream** : Conjugated equine vaginal oestrogen cream 1.25 mg daily is very effective specially when associated with atrophic vaginitis. It also reduces urinary frequency, urgency and recurrent infection. Women with symptoms of uro-genital atrophy and urinary symptoms and who do not like to have systemic HRT, are suitable for such treatment.

• **Progestins**: Patients with history of breast carcinoma, or endometrial carcinoma, progestins may be used. It may be effective in suppressing hot flushes and it prevents osteoporosis. Medroxy progesterone acetate 2.5–5 mg/day can be used.

LNG-IUS (see p. 459) with daily release of 10 microgram (see below) of levonorgestrel per 24 hours, it protects the endometrium from hyperplasia and cancer. At the same time it has got no systemic progestin side effects. Oestrogen can be given by any route. It can serve as contraception and HRT when given in a perimenopausal women.

• **Tibolone**: Tibolone is a steroid (19-nortesto-sterone derivative) having weakly oestrogenic, progestogenic and androgenic properties. It prevents osteoporosis, atrophic changes of vagina and hot flushes. It increases libido. Endometrium is atrophic. A dose of 2.5 mg per day is given.

Table 6.4

MONITORING PRIOR TO AND DURING HRT

A base level parameter of the following and their subsequent check up (at least annually) are mandatory.

- Physical examination including pelvic examination.
- Blood pressure recording.
- Breast examination (see p. 538) and Mammography (see p. 538).
- Cervical cytology (p. 106).
- Pelvic ultrasonography (TVS) to measure endometrial thickness (normal< 5 mm).

Any irregular bleeding should be investigated throughly (endometrial biopsy, hysteroscopy).

Ideal serum level of oestradiol should be 100 pg/ml during HRT therapy. Serum level of oestradiol is useful to monitor the HRT therapy rather than that of serum FSH.

Duration of HRT use

Generally, use of HRT for a short period of 3-5 years have been advised. Reduction of dosage should be done as soon as possible. Menopausal women should maintain optimum nutrition, ideal body weight and perform regular exercise.

Individual woman should be given informed choice as regard the relative merits and possible risks of continuing HRT.

PROGRESS IN HORMONE REPLACEMENT THERAPY

Low Dose HRT — Women with intact uterus with 0.3 mg conjugated equine oestrogen (CEE) and Medroxy Progesterone acetate (MPA) 1.5 mg is found effective to control the vasomotor symptoms. Similarly 1 mg of oestradiol and norethisterone acetate 0.5 mg orally, are also effective and have significant bone sparing effect. Progestogen is added in the HRT to minimise the adverse effects of oestrogen. **Hormone therapy should be used with lowest effective dose and for the short period of time as possible.** Dose interval may be modified (see above) before stopping the therapy. To minimise the systemic adverse effects of progestogen, Levonorgestrel intrauterine delivery system (LNG-IUS) is being used. It is primarily used as a contraceptive (p. 459). Oestrogen component is delivered by oral or by transdermal route or as an implant. A small size LNG-IUS has been developed that releases 10 μg LNG per day. This reduced size LNG-IUS is suitable for the postmenopausal women as the size of the uterus is also small.

ABNORMAL MENOPAUSE

Premature

If the menopause occurs at or below the age of 40, it is said to be premature (details in p. 444). Often, there is familial diathesis. Treatment by substitution therapy is of value (details in p. 451).

Delayed menopause

If the menopause fails to occur even beyond 55 years it is called delayed.

The common causes are constitutional, uterine fibroids, diabetes mellitus and oestrogenic tumour of the ovary. The cases should not be neglected. In the absence of palpable pelvic pathology, diagnostic curettage should be done and an early decision of hysterectomy should be taken in the face of increased incidence of endometrial carcinoma.

ARTIFICIAL MENOPAUSE

Permanent cessation of ovarian function done by artificial means, e.g. surgical removal of ovaries or by radiation is called artificial menopause.

Surgical

Menstruating women who have bilateral oophorectomy, experience menopausal symptoms (see p. 61). It is sometimes more troublesome than natural menopause.

Radiation

The ovarian function may be suppressed by external gamma radiation in women below the age of 40. The castration is not permanent. The menstruation may resume after 2 years and even conception is possible. Intracavity introduction of radium can cause castration effect by destroying the endometrium and also by depressing the ovarian function. The menopausal symptoms are not so intense as found in surgical menopause or menopause following external radiation.

KEY POINTS

- Menopause means permanent cessation of menstruation at the end of reproductive life due to ovarian follicular inactivity. The average age being 50 years.
- Mean age of menopause is about 50 years and it is genetically predetermined. It is not related to the number of pregnancies, race, socioeconomic conditions, education, height, weight, age at menarche or age of last childbirth.
- There is gradual elevated levels of first the FSH and then LH. Simultaneously, oestradiol levels fall to optimal 20 pg/ml when menopause sets in. There is increased androgen secretion from the ovarian stroma and from the adrenal. A trace amount of progesterone is adrenal in origin.
- The initial endocrine change with the onset of menopause is decreased ovarian inhibin production and increase in pituitary FSH release. The amount of oestrogen replacement in menopause is not dependent upon the level of FSH.
- Diagnosis is from the classic symptom of 'hot flush' and confirmed by elevated FSH levels to > 100 mIU/ml and serum oestradiol < 20 pg/ml.

  HRT ensures potential benefits and minimises the risks. It is beneficial in symptomatic women.
- In menopause there is depletion of ovarian follicles with degeneration of granulosa and theca cells. Stromal cells produce androgens, which are converted to oestrogens in peripheral body fat. Obese postmenopausal women, have higher levels of oestrone, less hot flushes and osteoporosis. But risk of developing endometrial cancer is high for them.

  Benefits of HRT are : Improvement in vasomotor symptoms, urogenital atrophy, increase in BMD, reduced risk of vertebral and hip fractures, reduction colorectal cancer and possibly cardioprotection (see p. 59). Oestrogen reduces the risk of late onset Alzheimer's disease.

  Risks of HRT are : Endometrial cancer, breast cancer, VTE and coronary heart disease (see p. 60).

  For a woman with intact uterus, progestin (for last 12-14 days) must be combined with oestrogen. Otherwise unopposed oestrogen therapy will increase the risk of endometrial hyperplasia and adenocarcinoma. Oestrogen without a progestin is recommended for a postmenopausal women who had hysterectomy.

  Contraindications to HRT include undiagnosed genital tract bleeding, oestrogen dependent neoplasm in the body, history of venous thromboembolism, active liver disease and gallbladder disease (see p. 60).

  Oestrogen may be administered orally, subdermal implants, vaginal cream, percutaneous gel or by transdermal patch.

  Provided the women is monitored during the period of therapy (see Table 6.4), HRT can be continued as long as the benefits are desired. However, low dose and short period of therapy (3-5 years) is currently recommended.
- **Indications of oestrogen therapy in menopause are** : presence of vasomotor symptoms, prevention of atrophic vaginitis, urethritis and osteoporosis.
- Soy extracts help to prevent hot flushes but have no effect on vaginal epithelium or bone.
- LDL cholesterol increases the risk of coronary artery disease (CAD) while HDL protects CAD. Estrogen therapy decreases LDL cholesterol and increases HDL.
- **Premature menopause** is one when the mens stops at or below the age of 40.
- **Delayed menopause** is one when menopause fails to occur even beyond 55 years.

Neuroendocrinology in Relation to Reproduction

7

The neuroendocrine mechanisms are the basic factors in the reproductive cycle. A transducer concept has been evolved in which the specialised neural cells of the hypothalamus function as the final common pathway to guide the appropriate anterior pituitary hormonal response.

HYPOTHALAMUS

Hypothalamus plays an important role in the neuroendocrine regulation. Three well-defined areas are demarked — (i) supraoptic area, (ii) tuberal region and (iii) mamillary region. Each region is further subdivided into areas, or nuclei (Fig. 7.1).

Both a tonic and a cyclic centre are located within the hypothalamus resulting in changes in GnRH production.

Connections

- Cortical
- Pituitary

Cortical

During recent years, the neural connection between the higher cortical centres and the hypothalamus has been well-established. Apart from this there are numerous output connections to pituitary gland as well other areas of the CNS, e.g. amygdala, hippocampus (limbic system), the thalamus and the pons

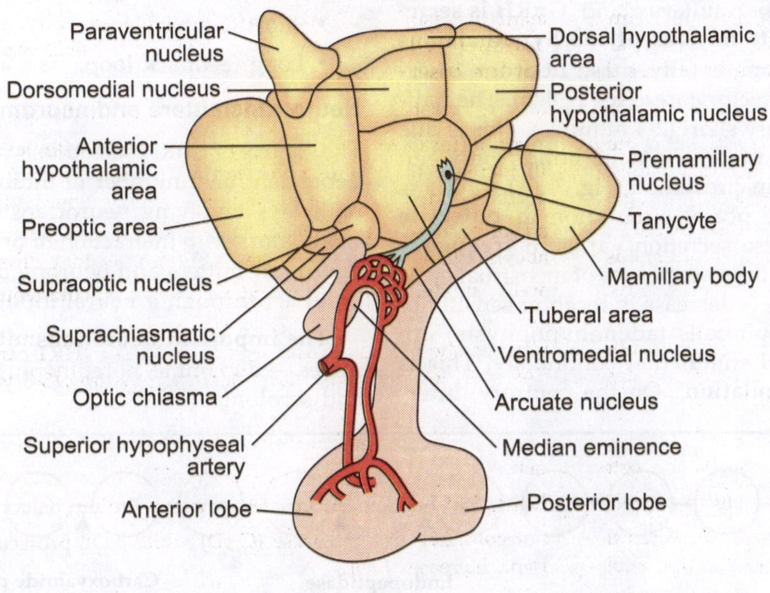

Fig. 7.1. Anatomy of the hypothalamus and pituitary

(Fig. 7.6). Through this system, the ovarian and consequently the menstrual cycle are affected by various emotional and environmental factors.

Pituitary

The hypothalamus is connected with the anterior lobe of the pituitary (adenohypophysis) through a special hypothalamo-pituitary portal system of vessels. However, it is directly connected with the posterior lobe of the pituitary (neurohypophysis) by the supraoptic and paraventricular nuclei (Fig. 7.1).

Secretions

The hypothalamus produces a series of specific releasing and inhibiting hormones which have got effect on the production of the specific pituitary hormones. These hormones are synthesized by the hypothalamic neurons and are released at the nerve endings around the tuber cinereum. Thereafter, these are drained to the pituitary through the hypothalamo-pituitary portal system of vessels.

1. Gonadotrophin releasing hormone (GnRH)

The GnRH is also named as *luteinising hormone releasing hormone* (LHRH). **GnRH is a decapeptide** and is concerned with the release, synthesis and storage of both the gonadotrophins (FSH and LH) from the anterior pituitary. The divergent patterns of FSH and LH in response to a single GnRH are due to modulating influence of the endocrine environment specially the feedback effects of steroids on anterior pituitary gland. **GnRH is secreted by the arcuate nucleus of the hypothalamus (Fig. 7.1).** Developmentally these neurons originated from the olfactory area (see p. 445). The half-life of GnRH is very short (2-4 minutes). This is due to the cleavage of amino acid bonds between 5-6, 6-7 and 9-10 in circulation (Fig. 7.1A). GnRH is secreted into the portal circulation in **pulsatile fashion**. This pulse secretion varies in **frequency and amplitude** at different phases of menstrual cycle (see below). There is decrease in receptor sensitivity when gonadotroph cells (adenohypophysis) are exposed to GnRH stimulation continually. This is called **'down regulation'**. On the contrary, intermittent exposure of GnRH to gonadotrophs, increase the receptor sensitivity. This is called **'up-regulation'**. This variable response of anterior pituitary gonadotrophs to GnRH have been utilised in different clinical situation to get therapeutic benefits (see p. 500).

2. Prolactin inhibitory factor (PIF)

Prolactin secretion from the anterior pituitary seems to be under chronic inhibition by PIF. **Dopamine is the physiological inhibitor.**

3. Thyrotrophin releasing hormone (TRH)

The hormone TRH, a tripeptide stimulates the release of not only the thyrotrophin but also prolactin from the pituitary.

4. Corticotrophin releasing hormone (CRH)

It is a tetradecapeptide.

5. Other secretions are — growth hormone releasing hormone (GHRH) and melanocytic releasing factor.

CONTROL OF GnRH SECRETION

The neurohormonal control of GnRH secretion is modulated by four ways :

- Neurotransmitters and neuromodulators.
- Peptides.
- Ultrashort feedback loop.
- Short feedback loop.
- Long feedback loop.

Neurotransmitters and neuromodulators

The control of GnRH secretion is highly complex and dependent on a number of inhibitory or excitatory pathways involving neurotransmitters and neuromodulators with interaction of ovarian steroids. The neurotransmitters and neuromodulators within the brain act through a neural input.

The important neurotransmitters are catecholamines — dopamine, norepinephrine (noradrenaline) and serotonin.

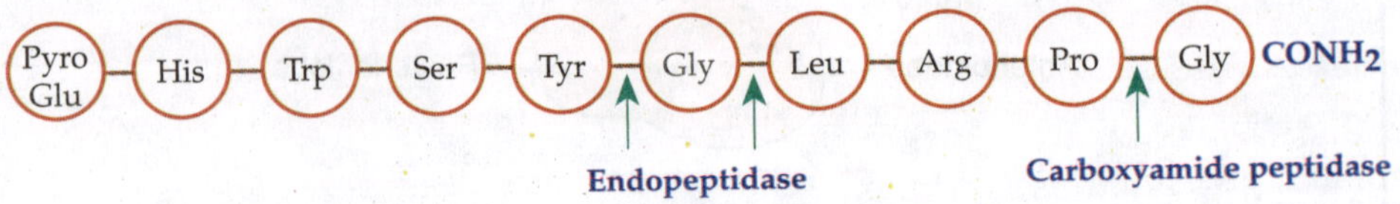

Fig. 7.1A. Gonadotrophin releasing hormone (GnRH)

Neurotransmitters and neuromodulators in the control of GnRH secretion

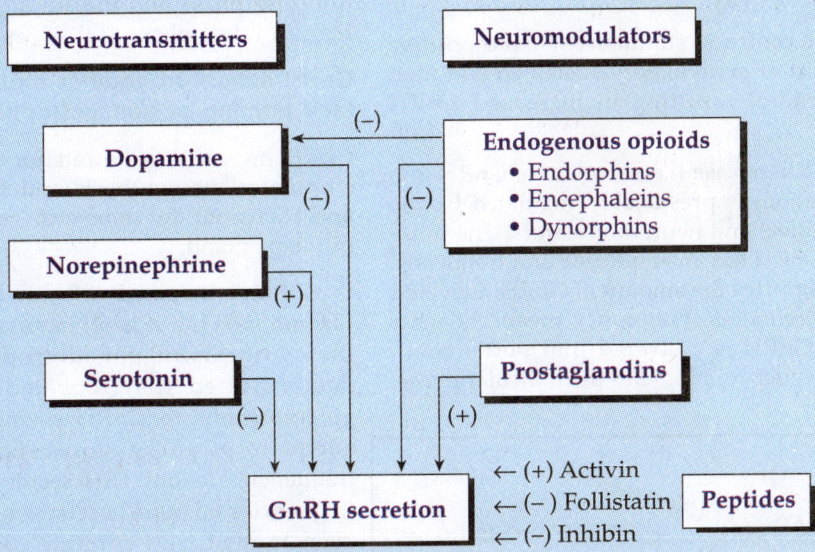

Norepinephrine exerts a stimulatory effect on the release of GnRH, while **dopamine** exerts its inhibitory effect. **Serotonin** plays an inhibitory role in GnRH release.

Catecholamines are capable of changing the frequency of GnRH pulse. Thus, pharmacological agents, psychological factors which affect the brain catecholamines, are likely to affect the pulsatile release of GnRH.

The principal neuromodulators are endogenous opioids, peptides and prostaglandins.

Endogenous opioids

The important endogenous opioids are endorphins, encephaleins and dynorphins. They inhibit GnRH release and thereby inhibit gonadotrophin secretion.

The endorphins may suppress both the dopamine and GnRH pathway leading to increase in prolactin secretions. Increased endogenous opioids has been actively implicated in hypothalamic amenorrhoea and elevated prolactin levels observed in association with stress and exercise. **Prostaglandin E** produced locally, increases the release of GnRH.

Role of peptides — a number of peptides like activin, inhibin and follistatin are produced by GnRH from pituitary cells as well as from the granulosa cells of the ovary. Activin stimulates but follistatin inhibits GnRH secretion. Inhibin blocks GnRH receptors.

Ultrashort feedback loop

It refers to autoregulation of the releasing hormone of the hypothalamus on its own synthesis. If the GnRH production is more, it will suppress and if it is less, it will stimulate its own production.

GnRH can regulate the concentration of its own pituitary receptors.

Short feedback loop (gonadotrophins)

It relates to the secretion of the GnRH by the interplay between the neurotransmitters and the pituitary gonadotrophins. FSH and LH are believed to exert negative feedback effect on hypothalamic production of GnRH.

Long feedback loop (sex steroid hormones)

The secretion of the hypothalamus (GnRH) and pituitary (FSH, LH) are influenced by the sex steroids. Sex steroids exert their inhibitory effect throughout except in preovulatory period, when a high and sustained level of oestradiol exerts a stimulatory effect in the release of GnRH through catechol oestrogen.

Nature of secretion

The secretion and release of GnRH are tonic, cyclic and pulsatile.

The tonic centre is controlled primarily by the negative feedback of sex steroids, probably via dopaminergic activity.

The cyclic centre is stimulated by the positive feedback effect of preovulatory sustained and high rise of oestradiol resulting in increased GnRH secretion.

The pulsatile release (i.e. secretion of GnRH into portal circulation) is presumably regulated by the neurotransmitters and neuromodulators. The pulse secretion of GnRH has an amplitude and frequency. **Amplitude signifies** the amount of GnRH delivered into portal circulation. **Frequency means** at what interval the GnRH is delivered into portal circulation. The frequency is rapid in the follicular phase, about one pulse per hour and lower in the luteal phase about one pulse every 2-3 hours. In the follicular phase and the amplitude is low but it is high in luteal phase.

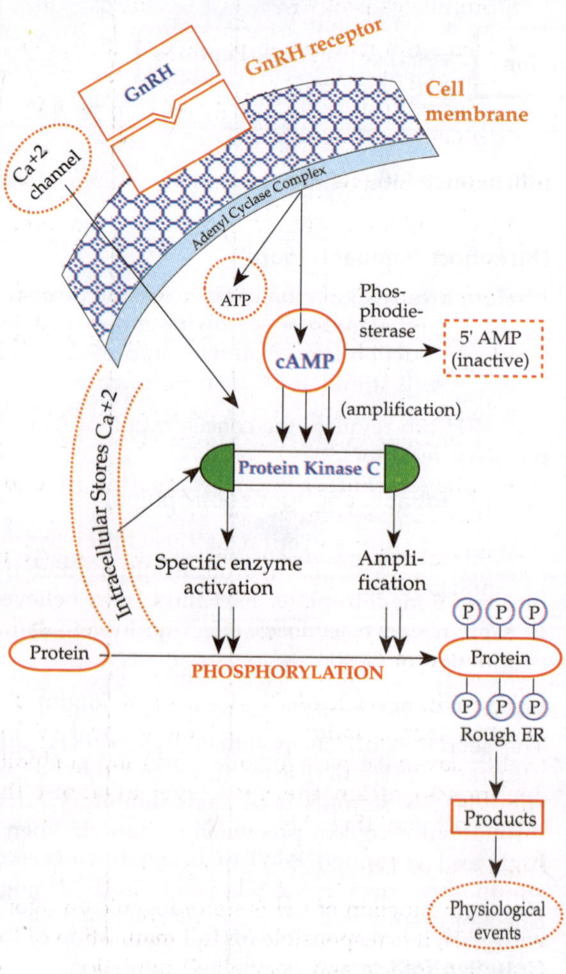

Fig. 7.2. Schematic representation of hormone GnRH receptor signal activation

GnRH action on anterior pituitary (self priming of gonadotrophs)

GnRH, on reaching the anterior lobe of the pituitary, stimulates the synthesis and release of both LH and FSH from the same cell (gonadotrophs) in the pituitary gland.

GnRH is involved not only in release of stored LH and FSH but it is of importance in maintaining the synthesis of gonadotrophins. It has been demonstrated that repeated exposure of the gonadotrophs to GnRH seems essential for the adequate pituitary stores. Lower GnRH pulse frequencies favour FSH secretion and the higher frequencies favour LH secretion. This response has been termed 'self priming'. It has got a cyclic relationship and is greatest with the higher levels of oestrogen. Oestrogen preferentially induces more LH than FSH release.

Physiological control mechanism of gonadotrophin release

There are two pools of gonadotrophins. One is readily releasable by the initial exposure to GnRH (primary pool) and a second one – called reserve pool (secondary pool). GnRH makes this larger reserve pool to be more readily released by a subsequent repeated exposure. Thus, this is suggestive of a transfer of gonadotrophins from one pool to the other.

Mechanism of action of GnRH on pituitary cell (Fig. 7.2)

GnRH binds to the specific receptors on the cell membrane of the gonadotrophs. Within a second, there is activation of the enzyme, adenyl cyclase which catalyses the conversion of ATP to cyclic AMP (cAMP). cAMP-receptor protein complex then activates protein kinase C. Intracellular free Ca^{++} concentration increases. Protein kinase C causes phosphorylation and activation of specific enzymes. Ca^{++}, protein kinase C and cAMP then interact to stimulate the release of stored FSH and LH and their subsequent biosynthesis.

However, if GnRH continues to be infused, gonadotrophin secretion is inhibited, probably because the receptors are saturated and are unable to stimulate the release of second messenger. This is known as **desensitisation or down regulation.**

PITUITARY

The pituitary gland lies in a bony cavity called sella turcica. The gland, principally consists of two parts — the anterior pituitary (adenohypophysis) and the posterior pituitary (neurohypophysis).

ANTERIOR PITUITARY

The anterior pituitary is a large, compact and highly vascular gland. It consists of cells arranged in nests or columns. The cells are of two types :

(a) Chromophobes or parent cells — these are small cells without affinity for any dye.

(b) Chromophils — these are larger cells which stain easily.

(i) Acidophils or eosinophils or alpha cells which stain red with eosin. These cells produce growth hormone and lactogenic hormone (prolactin).

(ii) Basophils or beta cells which stain blue with haematoxylin.

These beta cells are of three types. **The oval ones produce gonadotrophins;** the angular ones produce thyrotrophin and the lightly granulated ones produce corticotrophin.

Secretions from anterior pituitary

I. Gonadotrophins

There are two gonadotrophic hormones secreted from the anterior pituitary — (a) Follicle stimulating hormone (FSH) and (b) Luteinising hormone (LH).

Site of secretion and chemical nature

The mechanisms of hormone synthesis, storage and release of the anterior pituitary hormones are poorly understood. While pulsatile stimulation of hypothalamic GnRH is required by the pituitary for the synthesis and release of gonadotrophins, ovarian hormones determine the cyclic pattern of FSH and LH as they occur in normal cycle. FSH and LH are secreted from the beta cells in a pulsatile fashion in response to pulsatile GnRH. **These are water-soluble glycoproteins** of high molecular weight. They have got two subunits. The amino acid composition of the α subunits of FSH, LH and human chorionic gonadotrophins (hCG) are similar. The hormone specificity being determined by the difference between the β subunits.

Functions of FSH

The function of FSH is predominantly morphogenic, related to the growth and maturation of the Graaffian follicle. In conjunction with LH, it is also involved in maturation of oocyte, ovulation and steroidogenesis.

- **Morphological effects**
- **Biochemical effects**

Morphological effects of FSH

- FSH rescues follicles from apoptosis.
- Stimulates formation of follicular vesicles (antral follicle).
- Stimulates proliferation of granulosa cells.
- Helps full maturation of the Graaffian follicle (dominant follicle) as it converts the follicular microenvironment from androgen dominated to oestrogen dominated (see p. 82).

Biochemical effects of FSH

- Synthesizes its own receptors in the granulosa cells.
- Synthesizes LH receptors in the theca cells.
- Synthesizes LH receptors in the granulosa cells.
- Induces aromatisation to convert androgens to oestrogens in granulosa cells (see p. 68).
- Enhances autocrine and paracrine function (IGF-II, IGF-I) in the follicle.
- Stimulates granulosa cells to produce activin and inhibin.
- Stimulates plasminogen activator necessary for ovulation.

The FSH level tends to rise soon following the onset of menstruation and attains its peak at the twelfth day of the cycle (preovulatory) and gradually declines to attain the base level at about the eighteenth day (Fig. 7.5).

Functions of LH

The main function of LH is steroidogenic but along with FSH, it is responsible for full maturation of the Graaffian follicle and oocyte and ovulation.

- **Biochemical effects**
- **Morphological effects**

Biochemical effects (steroidogenic) of LH

- Activation of LH receptors in the theca cells which stimulates the enzymes necessary for androgen production → diffuse into the granulosa cells → oestrogens.
- Luteinisation of the granulosa cells → to secrete progesterone.
- Synthesizes prostaglandins.

Morphological effects of LH

- Stimulates resumption of meiosis with extrusion of first polar body (p. 80).
- Helps in the physical act of ovulation (p. 83).
- Formation and maintenance of corpus luteum.

LH levels remain almost static throughout the cycle except at least 12 hours prior to ovulation, when it attains its peak, called LH surge (Fig. 7.5).

II. Prolactin

Prolactin is secreted from the alpha cells and **is a polypeptide**.

Its role in the human reproductive physiology is not clearly understood. Its role in the maintenance of corpus luteum in human is not well-documented, but the fact remains that there is high incidence of anovulation in women with elevated plasma prolactin levels (see p. 445 and 548).

III. Thyrotrophic hormone (TSH)

TSH (thyroid stimulating hormone) is produced by the beta cells. It acts on the thyroid gland and regulate the production of thyroxine. It has got α and β subunits like those of FSH and LH, with functions of β subunits being different. Abnormal TSH secretion is associated with menstrual and ovulatory dysfunction.

IV. Adrenocorticotrophic hormone (ACTH)

ACTH is also secreted by the beta cells. It stimulates the production of corticosteroids in the adrenal cortex.

V. Somatotrophin or growth producing hormone

It is secreted from the alpha cells of the pituitary and acts directly on the skeletal system.

VI. Melanocyte stimulating hormone (MSH)

It is clearly linked with ACTH. The hormone is increased during puberty and in pregnancy. It is probably responsible for the pigmentary changes during those periods.

POSTERIOR PITUITARY

The hormones oxytocin and vasopressin are formed in the hypothalamus and transported within the neurons in the hypothalamo-hypophyseal tract. Both the hormones are bound to polypeptides called neurophysins. **Oxytocin** is a nonapeptide. It is produced by the paraventricular nucleus of the hypothalamus. Oxytocin acts on the myometrial contractile system, specially during labour and also causes contraction of the myoepithelial cells in the breast ductules during lactation.

Arginine-vasopressin is also a nonapeptide, with two amino acid composition different from that of oxytocin. It is produced by the supraoptic nucleus. It regulates plasma osmolality and circulating blood volume.

OVARY

The gross anatomy (ch. 1) and the structure of the functional unit of the ovary (ch. 8) are described in the appropriate chapters. **The functions of the ovary** are ovulation and production of hormones (steroidogenesis). The ovulation is dealt in the chapter 8.

OVARIAN STEROIDOGENESIS

The principal hormones secreted from the ovaries are — (i) oestrogens, (ii) progesterone, (iii) androgens and (iv) inhibin.

Oestrogens

Site of production

The oestrogen is predominantly oestradiol (E_2) and to a lesser extent oestrone. The sites of production in the ovary are :

- Predominant sites are granulosa cells of the follicles and from the same cells after luteinisation to form corpus luteum.
- Small quantity is also produced from the theca cells and ovarian stroma.

Mechanism of steroid hormone production (Fig. 7.3 and 7.4A)

Two cell, two gonadotrophin, concept of ovarian steroidogenesis establishes the fact that two cells **(theca cells and granulosa cells)** produce different hormones under the influence of **two gonadotrophins (LH and FSH)**.

During the **follicular phase**, under the influence

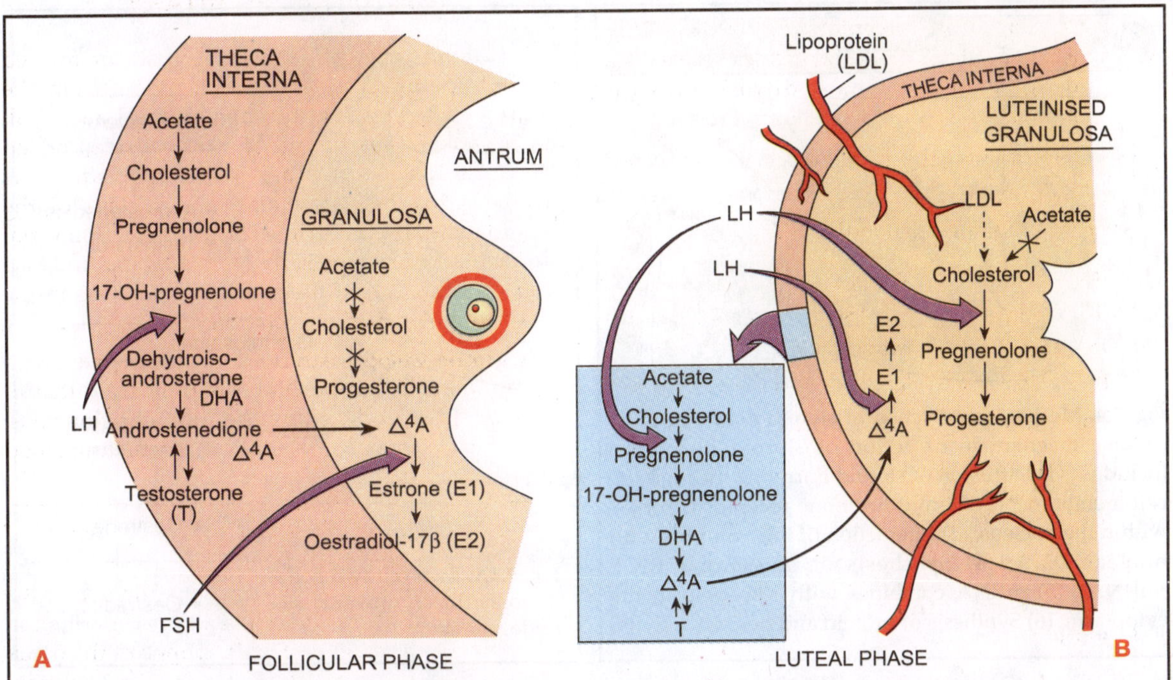

Fig. 7.3. Schematic representation of the ovarian steroidogenesis (Two cell, two gonadotrophin 7.3A and Two cell, one gonadotrophin 7.3B concept)

of LH, androgens (androstenedione and testosterone) are produced in the theca cells. These androgens diffuse into the granulosa cells where they are aromatised under the influence of FSH to oestrogens — oestradiol predominantly and to lesser extent oestrone (Figs 7.3, 7.4 and 7.4A).

After ovulation, progesterone is synthesized in the luteinised granulosa cells under the influence of LH. The precursor-LDL is available to the site after vascularisation of the granulosa cells following ovulation. During luteal phase, androstenedione produced by the theca luteal cells diffuses into the granulosa luteal cells (Fig. 7.3B) to be converted into estradiol by LH. During follicular phase, it is the FSH that enhances aromatase activity in the granulosa cells. Whereas during the luteal phase it is the LH that enhances the aromatase activity in the luteinised granulosa cells for the conversion of androstenedione to estradiol. Therefore, during luteal phase, a two cell (theca luteal and granulosa luteal) — one gonadotrophin (LH) system works for oestradiol biosynthesis.

Metabolism

The oestrogens are bound to albumin (30%) and sex hormone binding globulin (SHBG) in 69 per cent and the remaining free 1 per cent is biologically active. Unlike trophic hormones, steroid hormones enter the cell and mediate action via receptors within the nucleus as shown diagrammatically in Figure 7.4 to produce specific response.

Following this, the oestrogens are quickly inactivated by converting to oestriol. Of the three classic oestrogens, **oestradiol is the most potent,** being ten times as potent as oestrone which is ten times as potent as oestriol.

The oestriol is conjugated in the liver with glucuronic acid. The conjugated oestrogen is excreted partly in the bile and partly in the urine. The bile fractions on reaching the intestine are broken down by microorganisms and then reabsorbed as active hormones (enterohepatic circulation). The disturbances of liver function or of the intestinal flora can thus alter this mechanism with consequent disturbances of menstrual cycles.

Amount of oestrogen production and blood level (see Table 7.2)

Total daily production of oestradiol is estimated to be about 50 µg during the early follicular phase reaching 150-300 µg at ovulation.

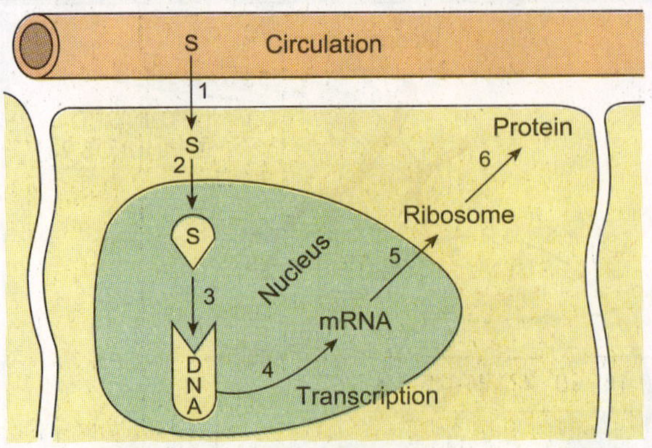

Fig. 7.4. Mechanism of action of steroid hormone : The precise mechanism of action of steroid hormones includes : (1) Diffusion of steroid hormone through the cell membrane; (2) Steroid hormone receptor complex within the nucleus; (3) Interaction of this complex with nuclear DNA; (4) Synthesis of messenger RNA (mRNA); (5) mRNA combines with ribosome in the cytoplasm; (6) Synthesis of protein and desired activity.

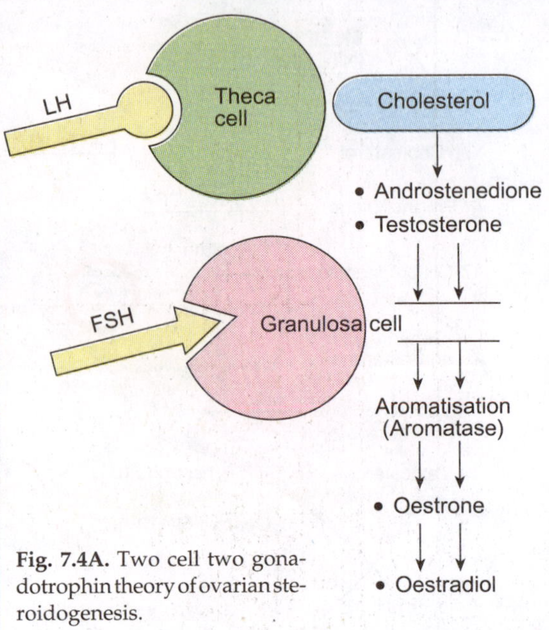

Fig. 7.4A. Two cell two gonadotrophin theory of ovarian steroidogenesis.

The blood level rises to about 300-600 pg/ml at ovulation. After a sharp fall, it rises again to about 150-200 pg/ml in the luteal phase (Fig. 7.5).

Total quantity of oestradiol production during a cycle from ovulatory ovary is estimated to be 10 mg.

Physiological action

Secondary sex characters — Oestrogen tends to induce feminine characteristics. The hormone is responsible for feminine body configuration and feminine mental make up including shyness. There is secretion in apocrine glands, change in voice and deposition of fat on the breasts, thighs and hips. **The growth of axillary and pubic hair is dependent predominantly on androgens of adrenal origin.**

Action on the genital organs — Under the action of oestrogen, the genital organs not only develop into maturity but induce cyclic changes for reproduction. After menopause, with the fall in the oestrogen level, atrophic changes of the organs occur.

Vulva and vagina — All the structures are influenced by the oestrogens. The vaginal vascularity and epithelial activity are related to oestrogen. Oestrogen induces thickening of the lining epithelium, cornification of the superficial cells and deposition of glycogen which is converted into lactic acid by the Doderlein's bacilli. **As such, the vaginal flora is maintained by oestrogen.**

Uterus — There is increased vascularity with hyperplasia of the muscles. It changes the uterus from the infantile to adult form. Cyclic changes in the endometrium includes regeneration and proliferation of the endometrium. **It produces receptors for progesterone.** Withdrawal of oestrogen causes shedding of the endometrium and menstruation.

Cervix — Oestrogen causes hypertrophy of the cervix and increases the cervical gland secretion. The secretion is more watery, alkaline with less protein and more electrolytes. These favour penetration of the sperm.

Fallopian tubes — There is increased vascularity with increased motility of the tubes.

Breasts — There is increased proliferation of the ducts and stromal tissues. There is also increased vascularity and pigmentation of the areola. Accumulation of fat also occurs. Breast secretion, however, cannot occur.

Blood — Oestrogen increases the coagulability of blood by increasing many procoagulants, chiefly fibrinogen. The platelets become more adhesive.

Locomotor system — Oestrogen conserves calcium and phosphorus and encourages bone formation.

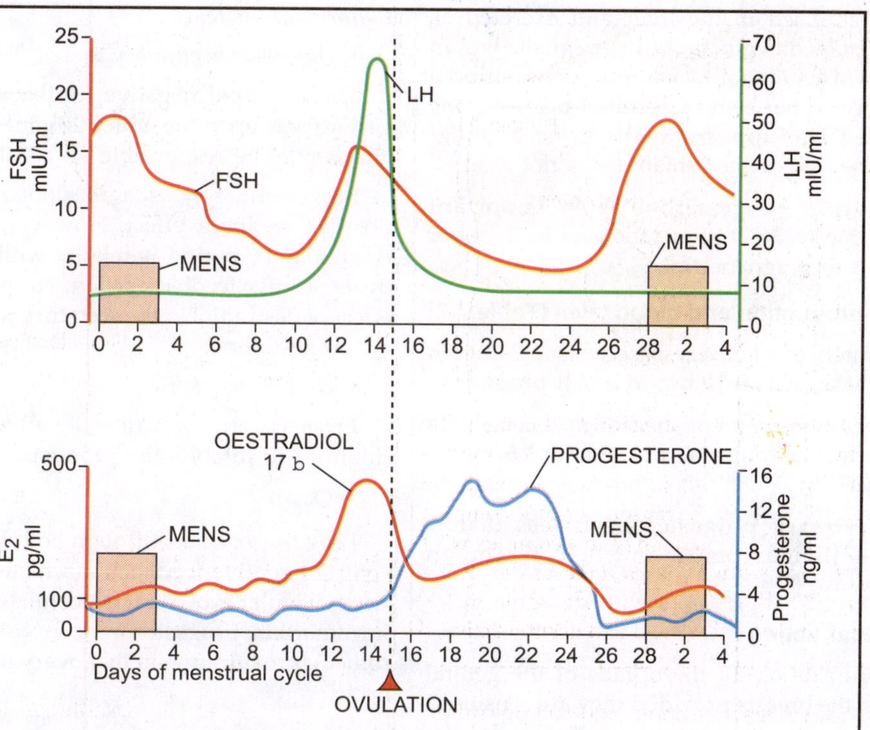

Fig. 7.5. Fluctuation of different hormone levels during menstrual cycle (ovulatory)

General — Oestrogen increases sodium, nitrogen and fluid retention of the body. It lowers the blood cholesterol and lowers the incidence of coronary heart disease in women prior to menopause. It has got widespread capillary vasodilatation effect.

Endocrine system

- *Hypothalamopituitary axis*

Negative feedback

Oestrogen exerts a negative feedback effect on the release of FSH. This is by :

(i) Direct action on pituitary, decreasing the sensitivity of the gonadotroph to GnRH.

(ii) Direct action on the hypothalamus with a decrease in GnRH secretion, possibly via increased inhibitory dopaminergic activity.

Positive feedback

High levels of oestrogen (> 200 pg/ml) exert a positive feedback effect on LH (mid cycle LH surge). Sustained (24-48 hours) elevated levels of oestrogen lead to sustained and elevated LH secretion. It may be due to :

(i) Increasing pituitary responsiveness to GnRH.

(ii) Stimulating the hypothalamus in secreting GnRH.

The positive feedback effect cannot occur in the postovulatory phase because of the presence of progesterone.

- *Ovary* : The presence of E_2 and FSH in the antral fluid is essential for sustained proliferation of granulosa cells and continued follicular growth.

- It increases the binding globulin in circulation and raises the blood levels of protein bound iodine and protein bound cortisol.

Progesterone

Site of secretion

The progesterone is secreted from the luteinised theca-granulosa cells of the corpus luteum. A trace amount is however, secreted from the theca-granulosa cells of the follicle and also from the ovarian stroma.

Metabolism

Progesterone is bound mainly to albumin (79%) and corticosteroid binding globulin (17.7%).

It is metabolised in the liver and excreted as sodium pregnanediol glucuronide (pregnanediol) in the urine. This metabolite has no progestational activity. Only 20 per cent of secreted progesterone is conjugated and appears in the urine as pregnanediol. The fate of the remainder is not clear.

17-α-hydroxy progesterone is an important product of the ovary. It is metabolised in the liver and reduced to pregnanetriol.

Amount of production and blood level (Table 7.2)

Daily production of progesterone is 2-3 mg in follicular phase and 20-30 mg in luteal phase.

Daily excretion of pregnanediol in the urine is less than 1 mg in follicular phase and 3-6 mg in luteal phase.

Serum value of progesterone is less than 1 ng/ml in follicular phase and 5-15 ng/ml in midluteal phase (Fig. 7.5).

Physiological action

Progesterone acts on all the organs of the genital tract and on the breasts provided they are sensitised by oestrogen.

Uterus — Progesterone produces myohyperplasia and diminishes the contractility of the myometrium. It however, increases the tone of the circular muscle fibres at the isthmus. It produces secretory activity in the endometrium; enhances secretion of the glands rich in glycogen. The character of the cervical mucus is changed and become more thick and viscid preventing sperm penetration.

Vagina — The maturation of the vaginal epithelium is hindered. There is more shedding of the intermediate cells with folded edges and a tendency to clump.

Fallopian tubes — The epithelial cells are stimulated to secrete clear mucus which helps in migration of the ovum. Tubal motility is however, decreased which may predispose to tubal pregnancy.

Breasts — Along with oestrogen, it produces hypertrophy and growth of the acinar structures.

General — Progesterone is thermogenic, raises the basal body temperature by 0.2°C – 0.5°C. There may be enhanced deposition of fat in the tissues. It relaxes smooth muscles and ligaments — specially during pregnancy. It promotes the secretion of sebum by the skin. Like other steroids, it causes fluid retention.

Endocrinal system

- *Hypothalamopituitary axis*

The principal negative feedback action of progesterone is upon the midcycle gonadotrophin surge and it may be responsible for its short duration.

Progesterone by itself does not appear to exert a positive feedback effect. However, its rise during preovulatory period is related with the FSH surge by its positive feedback action. The positive feedback effect of oestradiol in the secretory phase is inhibited by progesterone.

- *GnRH secretion*

Progesterone first (low level) stimulates, then (high level) inhibits the production of GnRH.

- *Ovary*

Progesterone acts through both intraovarian and central negative feedback mechanisms to suppress new follicular growth. It is postulated that increased intraovarian progesterone concentration prevents follicular maturation in that ovary in the subsequent cycle.

Androgens

The androgens are produced in the ovary by all three types of cells — stroma, theca and granulosa, but mainly by the theca interna of the follicles. The production of androgens is primarily under the control of LH. **The principal androgens secreted are** — dehydroepiandrosterone, androstenedione and testosterone.

The principal site of metabolism is liver. The androgens are reduced to androsterone and etiocholanolone. These can be measured in the urine as 11 deoxy-17 ketosteroids.

Total daily production of androstenedione is 3 mg and of testosterone 0.2-0.3 mg.

Plasma level of androstenedione is 1.3-1.5 ng/ml, that of testosterone 0.3-0.6 ng/ml and of SHBG 38-103 nmol/L.

Peptides and their role

Inhibin, Activin and Follistatin are the peptides, secreted by the granulosa cells in response to FSH. Inhibin, inhibits FSH secretion and activin stimulates FSH release. Follistatin, suppresses FSH activity through activin.

Inhibin

Inhibin is produced by the granulosa cells of the

ovarian follicle. It has got a preferential negative feedback effect on FSH release. In premenopausal women with anovulatory cycles, high level of FSH with normal steroid levels may be due to depletion of inhibin. The same is probably true in resistant ovarian syndrome having elevated FSH despite adequate oestrogen.

Relaxin

Relaxin is secreted from the preovulatory follicle and corpus luteum. It probably facilitates follicular rupture during ovulation.

Growth factors are polypeptides and they act locally through paracrine and autocrine way. Important growth factors are : Insulin-like growth factors (IGF), Epidermal Growth Factor, Tumour Necrosis Factor α (TNFα) and Interleukin-1 system.

Insulin-like growth factors (IGF) — are most abundant. IGF-II is produced in theca cells, granulosa cells and luteinised granulosa cells. IGF-II enhances gonadotrophin (FSH and LH) actions to stimulate granulosa cell proliferation, aromatase activity and progesterone synthesis.

THYROID

The thyroid gland consists of numerous acini and follicles. Between the follicles, there are parafollicular or 'C' cells. The follicular cells synthesise iodine containing thyroxine (T_4) and triiodothyronine (T_3) under the influence of TSH of the anterior pituitary (Table 7.1). These hormones are related to body growth and metabolic needs. Ovarian function is markedly related to the thyroid activity. Normal enlargement of the gland occurs during puberty, pregnancy and menopause. Menstrual function may be significantly disturbed in thyroid dysfunction. Calcitonin is secreted from the parafollicular cells in response to elevated blood calcium.

Table 7.1

Normal serum values of thyroid profile

TSH	0.4-5 mmol/L	(3 μU/ml)
T_3	1.1-2.3 nmol/L	(70-190 ng/100 ml)
T_4	10-25 pmol/L	(5-12 μg/100 ml)

ADRENAL GLANDS

Adrenal gland consists of two zones — outer cortex and inner medulla. The medulla secretes adrenaline and noradrenaline.

Control of cortical secretions

Zona glomerulosa

Aldosterone is secreted from this zone. The secretion is principally controlled by the renin–angiotensin mechanism and is not markedly affected by ACTH. It produces retention of sodium and increased excretion of potassium through the renal tubules.

Zona reticularis and fasciculata

They act as a single unit. The principal hormones that are secreted are cortisol, corticosterone (glucocorticoids); androstenedione, androsterone and dehydroepiandrosterone (collectively called androgens) and to some extent oestrogen and progesterone. These constitute the extraovarian sources of steroids.

The control of cortisol synthesis through ACTH is regulated by the negative feedback, diurnal rhythm and stress. Stress can override the negative feedback mechanism and diurnal rhythm. A rise of plasma cortisol causes a rapid suppression of ACTH. A fall in cortisol level leads to increased production of ACTH probably through release of CRH from the hypothalamus.

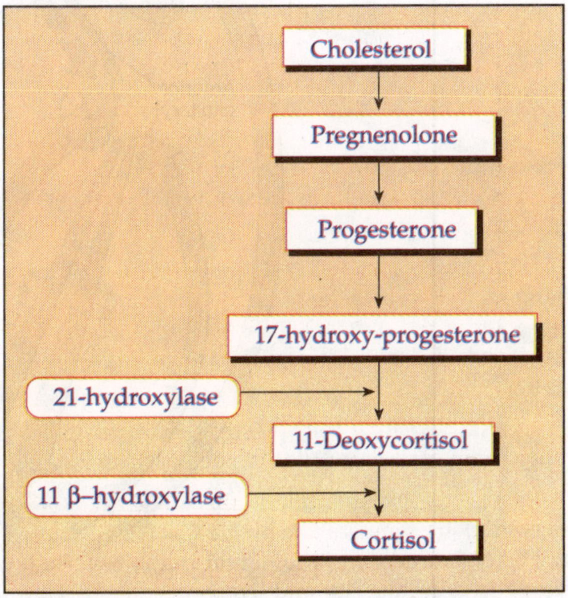

The biosynthetic pathway in the secretion of cortisol through series of enzymatic action (predominantly 21-hydroxylase) is as follows :

(a) **Action of glucocorticoids**

The main action of cortisol is anabolic.

(i) Antagonistic to insulin and tends to raise the blood sugar.

(ii) Suppression of inflammatory reaction.

(iii) Lipogenic effect.

(b) **The action of androgens and adrenal steroids** is anabolic to antagonise the catabolic effects of the glucocorticoids.

HYPOTHALAMO-PITUITARY OVARIAN AXIS

The hormones liberated from the hypothalamus, pituitary and ovary are dependent to one another. A well-coordinated axis is formed called hypothalamo-pituitary ovarian axis, (Fig. 7.6). The secretion of hormones from these glands is modified through feedback mechanism operating through this

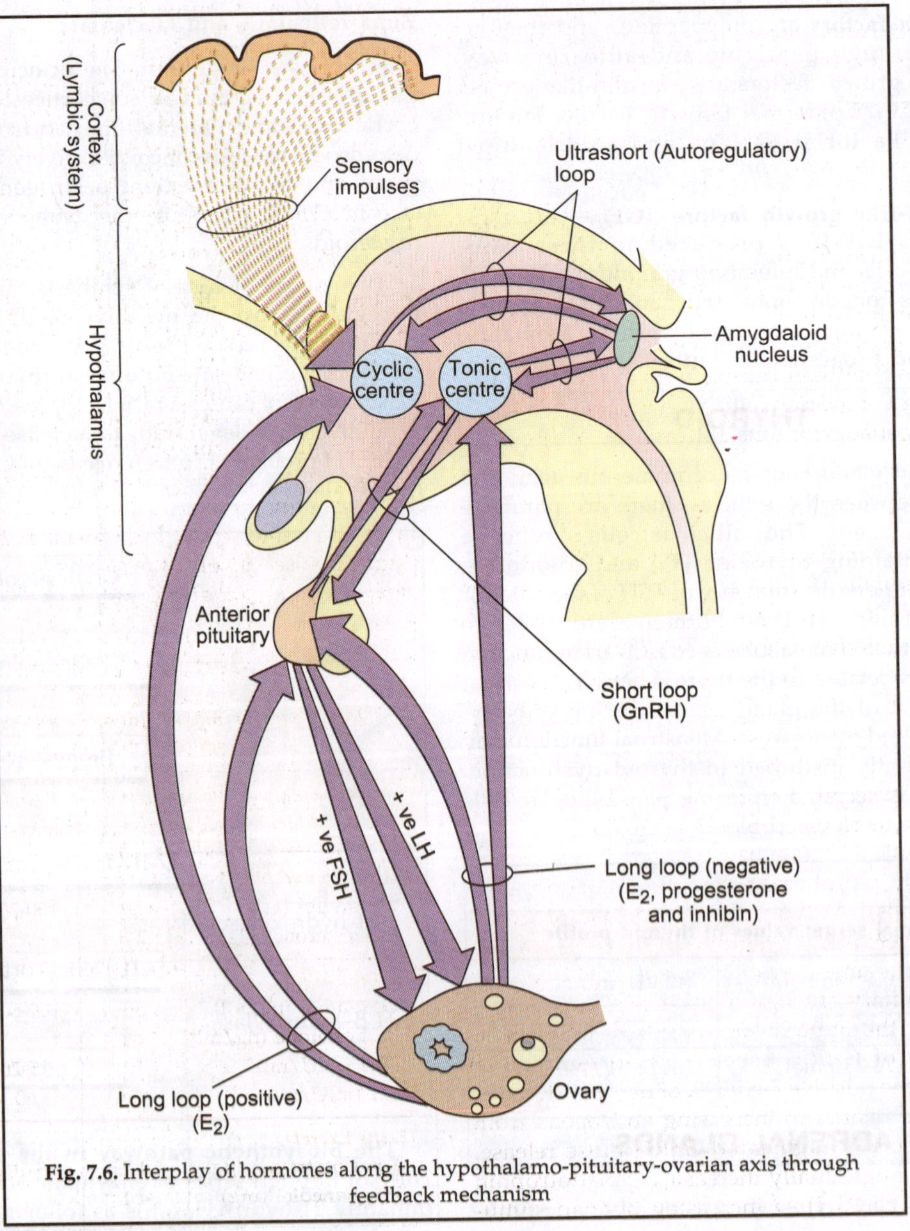

Fig. 7.6. Interplay of hormones along the hypothalamo-pituitary-ovarian axis through feedback mechanism

axis. The axis may also be modified by hormones liberated from the thyroid or adrenal glands.

Feedback loop

• The long feedback loop refers to the feedback effects of the ovarian steroids on both the hypothalamus and pituitary. It is usually inhibitory (negative) but may be stimulatory (positive-preovulatory).

• The short feedback loop relates the secretion of GnRH by gonadotrophins by interplay between the neurotransmitters and the pituitary gonadotrophins. FSH and LH exert negative feedback effect on the hypothalamic production of GnRH.

• Ultrashort feedback loop refers to auto-regulation of the releasing hormones of the hypothalamus on its own synthesis (Fig. 7.6).

Fetal life

In terms of hormone production, the hypothalamo-pituitary ovarian axis is active and functional from approximately 20 weeks of fetal life. In fact, the circulatory gonadotrophin levels remain at a higher level in fetal life than during neonatal period. The development of ovarian follicles in the fetus depends upon the gonadotrophins released from the fetal pituitary.

Infancy and childhood

The high level of FSH and to a lesser degree of LH at birth gradually decline and the minimum levels are achieved by two years of age. The FSH levels are highly sensitive to exogenous oestrogen.

Prepuberty and puberty

The hypothalamo-pituitary-gonadal feedback system is in operation for many years prior to puberty. Prior to puberty, the hypothalamus is very much sensitive to the negative feedback by even a small amount of extragonadal steroids (oestrogens produced by peripheral conversion of androgens from adrenals). As a result, the release of gonadotrophin releasing hormone (GnRH) from the hypothalamus and that of FSH and LH from the anterior pituitary are kept in abeyance. As puberty approaches, the hypothalamic centres involved in the release of GnRH becomes more and more sensitive to the positive feedback of ovarian steroids. This may be related to increasing androgens from adrenals. There is augmented GnRH pulse release. This results in gradually increasing gonadotrophin secretion (LH > FSH) → increasing ovarian stimulation → increasing oestrogen levels → tonic and pulsatile discharge of gonadotrophins.

This increasing level of oestrogen is responsible for the growth and initiation of thelarche and finally menarche. The development of the positive feedback response to oestrogen resulting in cyclic release of gonadotrophins occurs after a variable period following menarche. As such, the first few cycles are expected to be anovulatory. The growth of pubic and axillary hair is related to increase in the secretion of adrenal androgens. The onset of this increase is called adrenarche which occurs at age 8-10 years.

Ovarian and menstrual cycle (p. 81)

Pregnancy and during 'Pill' intake — As the oestrogen level is high in both the conditions, the pituitary gonadotrophins remain static at low levels by the negative feedback mechanism.

Following delivery

During pregnancy, there is hypofunction of the axis induced by high level of oestrogen. The hypothalamic hypofunction results in low levels of GnRH. In the immediate postpartum period, there is pituitary refractoriness to GnRH resulting in low FSH and LH levels. High prolactin levels render the ovary less sensitive to the already low gonadotrophin stimulation resulting in ovarian inactivity, low oestrogen status and anovulation. Even when ovarian activity resumes, raised levels of prolactin give rise to short luteal phase and reduced fertility.

Table 7.2
Daily production, serum values and urinary excretion of hormones

Hormones	Follicular phase	At ovulation	Luteal phase
Daily production			
Oestradiol (μg)	50	150-300	100
Progesterone (mg)	2-3		20-30
Serum values			
Oestradiol (pg/ml)	50	300-600	150-200
Progesterone (ng/ml)	< 1		> 5
FSH (mIU/ml)	10	15-20	10
LH (mIU/ml)	5	60	5
Daily Excretion			
Total oestrogen (μg)	10-25	35-100	25-75
Pregnanediol (mg)	< 1		3-6

Thus, the picture of the first three weeks postpartum is one of hypothalamo-pituitary-ovarian inactivity which is prolonged by lactation under the influence of prolactin secretion.

Perimenopausal period

Few years prior to menopause, the ovarian follicles become gradually resistant to the pituitary gonadotrophins. As a result of impaired folliculogenesis, less oestrogen is secreted. There is decrease in the negative feedback effect of oestrogen on the hypothalamo-pituitary axis, resulting in increase of FSH. The increase of FSH may also be due to diminished follicular inhibin (see p. 72).

When menopause sets in, the oestradiol level comes down to basal 20 pg/ml and cannot have any negative feedback effect on hypothalamo-pituitary axis (see p. 74).

As a result, GnRH release is enhanced resulting in increased synthesis and release of gonadotrophins. The pulsatile pattern is maintained and while the frequency remains unaltered, the amplitude is markedly increased.

Gradually with senescence, the GnRH secretion is diminished and so also the gonadotrophins and oestrogens, when the true menopause sets in.

KEY POINTS

- Hypothalamus has got neural connection with the cortex and through hypothalamo-portal system of vessels, connected with the anterior pituitary.
- Among the specific releasing hormones, the important ones are GnRH, TRH, CRH and the prolactin secretion is inhibited by PIF. Dopamine is a physiological inhibitor.
- GnRH is a decapeptide with a very short half-life (p. 64).
- GnRH is secreted in a pulsatile manner. The amplitude and frequency vary in the menstrual cycle. The frequency is rapid (one pulse/hr) in the follicular phase but slower (1 pulse/2-3 hours) in the luteal phase (p. 64).

  GnRH stimulates the release and synthesis of both LH and FSH from the same cells of the anterior pituitary in pulsatile manner.

  GnRH binds to the specific receptor on the surface membrane of the gonadotrophs. A second messenger is activated combining Ca^{++}, protein kinase C and cAMP together to stimulate the release of stored LH and FSH and their subsequent synthesis (Fig. 7.2).
- The neurohormonal control of GnRH secretion is very complex. A number of neurotransmitters and neuromodulators (see p. 65) are involved to play their inhibitory (endogenous opioids, dopamine, inhibin) and stimulatory (norepinephrine, prostaglandin, activin) roles (p. 65).
- Gonadotrophins are secreted from the beta cells of anterior pituitary. These are glycoproteins. The hormone specificity is ascertained by β subunits.

  Down regulation is the decrease in sensitivity of the gonadotroph (adenohypophysis) receptors, due to continued stimulation of GnRH. Upregulation is the increase in receptor sensitivity due to intermittent exposure to GnRH (p. 64).

  GnRH analogues are produced by substitution of amino acids in the parent molecule (p. 64) at the 6 and 10 positions. The agonists have greater potencies and longer half-lives than the parent GnRH.
- Ovarian hormones determine the cyclic pattern of FSH and LH release (Fig. 7.6).

KEY POINTS

- The half-life of LH is 30 minutes and that of FSH is 3.9 hours. LH acts primarily on the theca cells to produce androgens. Granulosa cells convert androgens to oestrogen by the enzyme aromatase.
- FSH is predominantly morphogenic but in conjunction with LH, it is involved in maturation of oocyte, ovulation and steroidogenesis. LH is predominantly steroidogenic. It also stimulates resumption of meiosis, helps in ovulation and formation and maintenance of corpus luteum (p. 67).
- LH acts primarily on theca cells to produce androgens, whereas FSH acts primarily on the granulosa cells to produce oestrogens by aromatisation of androgens (p. 67). The ovary secretes three principal steroid hormones : estradiol from the follicle, progesterone from the corpus luteum and androstenedione from the stroma (p. 68).
- Prolactin is secreted from the alpha cells and is a polypeptide. Thyrotrophic hormone is produced by the beta cells.
- The α subunits of LH, FSH, TSH and hCG are similar. It is due to the different β subunits which provide specific biologic activity for each hormone.
- A number of peptides like activin, inhibin and follistatin are produced by GnRH from pituitary cells as well as from the granulosa cells of the ovary. Follistatin inhibits GnRH secretion (p. 72).
- Two cell, two gonadotrophin concept of ovarian steroidogenesis states that LH stimulates the theca cells to produce androgens, which are subsequently aromatised in the granulosa cells by FSH to produce oestrogens (p. 68; Fig. 7.4A).
- LH acts upon the luteinised granulosa cells to produce progesterone. Oestrogen is also produced in luteal phase under the influence of FSH and LH.
- The midcycle LH surge initiates the resumption of meiosis-I. The primary oocyte under goes first meiotic division giving rise to secondary oocyte and first polar body (p. 80).
- The second meiotic division is completed only after fertilisation by a sperm. The ovum and second polar body is then developed (p. 80).
- The sites of production of oestrogens, predominantly the oestradiol, are granulosa cells, luteinised granulosa cells, theca cells and stroma of the ovary. The oestrogens are produced by two-cell two gonadotrophin concept (Fig. 7.4A, p. 68).
- Androstenedione is converted to oestrone in the adipose tissue. Oestradiol and oestrone are interconvertible. Oestrone sulphate is the major circulating oestrogen and has a long half-life.
- Oestradiol exerts a negative feedback effect on the hypothalamo-pituitary axis. However, when the level is raised to more than 200 pg/ml and sustained for 24-48 hours, it has got positive feedback effects. The positive feedback effect cannot occur in the luteal phase because of progesterone.
- Progesterone has 21 carbon atoms, Androgens have 19 Carbon atoms and oestrogens have 18 carbon atoms. The progesterone is secreted from the luteinised theca-granulosa cells of the corpus luteum, theca granulosa cells of the follicle and from the stroma. Trace amount of 17-α-hydroxy progesterone in the preovulatory period is essential for final maturation of the oocyte and involved in LH surge.
- Serum progesterone levels are < 1 ng/ml before ovulation and reach 10-20 ng/ml at the mid luteal phase.
- Progesterone has got negative feedback on the hypothalamo-pituitary axis; principally upon the midcycle gonadotrophin surge and is responsible for its short duration.

KEY POINTS

- Oestrogen stimulates the synthesis of both oestrogen and progesterone receptors in target tissues. Progestins inhibit the synthesis of both the receptors. Progesterone has antimitotic and antiproliferative action (p. 70).
- Normal enlargement of thyroid gland occurs during puberty, pregnancy and menopause.
- Menstrual function is significantly disturbed in thyroid dysfunction.
- The biosynthetic pathway in the secretion of cortisol is through series of enzymatic action from cholesterol via 17-α-hydroxy progesterone.
- The hypothalamo-pituitary axis is active and functional from 20 weeks of fetal life (p. 74).
- At puberty, increasing oestrogen levels result in pulsatile release of gonadotrophins. The development of positive feedback effect occurs 2-3 years following menarche (p. 75).
- During pregnancy and 'pill' taking period, gonadotrophins remain static at low levels (p. 75).
- During first three weeks postpartum, there is hypothalamo-pituitary-ovarian inactivity due to high level of prolactin. As menopause approaches, there is less production of oestrogens and the remaining ovarian follicles become resistant to gonadotrophins. There is decrease in follicular inhibin. The combined effects result in increase in FSH and later on LH also. When the oestradiol level falls below 20 pg/ml, menopause sets in (p. 55).

  GnRH release is also enhanced because of decrease in negative feedback effect of oestrogen. This results also in increased release and synthesis of gonadotrophins (p. 56).
- Dominant follicle is selected by days 5 and 7. The dominant follicle has a maximum diameter of about 20 mm and a volume of 3.8 ml. The dominant follicle secretes more oestradiol which in turn induces more FSH receptors (p. 83, Fig. 8.3A, 8.4)
- FSH induces LH receptors on granulosa cells.
- The actions of FSH and LH on the follicles are modulated by a group of peptides and growth factory by autocrine and paracrine nodes. Inhibin, secreted in the granulosa cells by FSH, directly suppresses FSH. Activin augments FSH secretion and action (p. 72).
- Successful development of a follicle depends on the FSH induced aromatase activity in the granulosa cells to convert the follicular microenvironment from androgen dominated to an oestrogen dominated one (see p. 67, 82).

Menstruation

8

Definition

Menstruation is the visible manifestation of cyclic physiologic uterine bleeding due to shedding of the endometrium following invisible interplay of hormones mainly through hypothalamo-pituitary-ovarian axis. **For the menstruation to occur**, the axis must be actively coordinated, endometrium must be responsive to the ovarian hormones (oestrogen and progesterone) and the outflow tract must be patent.

Anatomical aspect

The period extending from the beginning of a period (mens) to the beginning of the next one is called menstrual cycle. The first menstruation (menarche) occurs between 11-15 years **with a mean of 13 years.** It is more closely related to bone age than to chronological age. For the past couple of decades, the age of menarche is gradually declining with improvement of nutrition and environmental condition. Once the menstruation starts, it continues cyclically at intervals of 21-35 days with a mean of 28 days. Physiologically, it is kept in abeyance due to pregnancy and lactation. Ultimately, it ceases between the ages 45-50 when menopause sets in. **The duration of menstruation (mens) is about 4-5 days and the amount of blood loss is estimated to be 20 to 80 ml with an average of 35 ml. Nearly 70 per cent of total menstrual blood loss occurs in the first 2 days. The menstrual discharge consists** mainly of dark altered blood, mucus, vaginal epithelial cells, fragments of endometrium, prostaglandins, enzymes and bacteria.

FOLLICULAR GROWTH AND ATRESIA

- Germ cells
- Primordial follicle
- Cyclic maturation of the follicle (ovarian cycle)
  - Ovulation
  - Corpus luteum
- Follicular atresia.

GERM CELLS

Origin

The germ cells migrate from the endoderm of the yolk sac in the region of hindgut. From there, they migrate into the genital ridge passing through the dorsal mesentery of the hindgut. A peptide, called, telopheron directs this anatomic migration. The migration is probably through amoeboid activity or by chemotactic mechanism. In the gonadal ridge, the oogonia are surrounded by clumps of epithelial cells (Fig. 3.4.).

Multiplication

The germ cells undergo rapid mitotic division and by 20 weeks, the number reaches about 7 million. While majority of the oogonia continue to divide until 7th month of gestation, some enter into the prophase of first meiotic division and **are called primary oocytes.** These are surrounded by flat cells from the stroma (pregranulosa cells) and are called **primordial follicles.** The primary oocytes continue to grow through various stages of prophase (leptotene, zygotene, pachytene and diplotene) and ultimately reach to the stage of diplotene or else become atretic. Primary oocytes are then arrested in the diplotene stage of prophase of first meiotic division, until ovulation.

Total number of oocytes **at 20 weeks of intrauterine life is about 6-7 million. At birth**, the total number of primordial follicles is estimated to be about 2 million. The primary oocytes do not finish the first meiotic division until puberty is reached. **At puberty, some 400000 primary oocytes are left** behind, the rest become atretic. **During the entire reproductive period**, some 400 are likely to ovulate. Thus, the important feature is the tendency of the sex cells to undergo degeneration. **The degeneration starts in the intrauterine life** and continues throughout childhood and the child-bearing period. As a result, no more follicles with ova can be detected in menopausal women.

Maturation

The essence of maturation is reduction of the number of chromosomes to half. The primary oocyte remains in diplotene phase until shortly before ovulation unless it undergoes atresia. **It is the midcycle LH surge that initiates the resumption of meiosis-1.** The primary oocyte undergoes **first meiotic division** giving rise to secondary oocyte and **one polar body**. The two are of unequal size, the secondary oocyte contains haploid number of chromosomes (23, X) but nearly all the cytoplasm. The small polar body also contains haploid number of chromosome (23, X) but with scanty cytoplasm. **The formation of secondary oocyte occurs** with full maturation of Graafian follicle just prior to ovulation.

The secondary oocyte immediately begins the **second meiotic division** but stops at metaphase. **The secondary oocyte completes the second meiotic division (homotypical) only after fertilisation by a sperm in the fallopian tube**. The division results in the formation of the two unequal daughter cells each possessing 23 chromosomes (23, X). The larger one is called the ovum (female pronucleus) and the smaller one is the **second polar body. In the absence of fertilisation, the secondary oocyte, does not complete the second meiotic division and degenerates as such**. Thus, the first stage of maturation of the oocyte occurs within the follicle but the final stage is achieved only after fertilisation in the fallopian tube.

The arrested meiotic division of the oocyte prior to ovulation is probably due to oocyte maturation inhibition (OMI) factor present in the follicular fluid. OMI is secreted by the granulosa cells. The resumption of meiosis occurs due to the midcycle LH surge.

PRIMORDIAL FOLLICLE

The primordial follicle consists of an oocyte, which is surrounded by a single layer of flattened granulosa cells. The follicle measures about 0.03-0.05 mm. The oocyte (primitive ovum) measures about 18-24 μ in diameter, nucleus 12 μ and nucleolus 6 μ. Throughout childhood, the primordial follicles grow very slowly. Thin growth is not dependent on gonadotrophins.

MORPHOLOGY OF THE OOCYTE

With the maturation of the follicle, there is simultaneous enlargement of the oocyte although at a lesser pace. While the follicle continues to enlarge

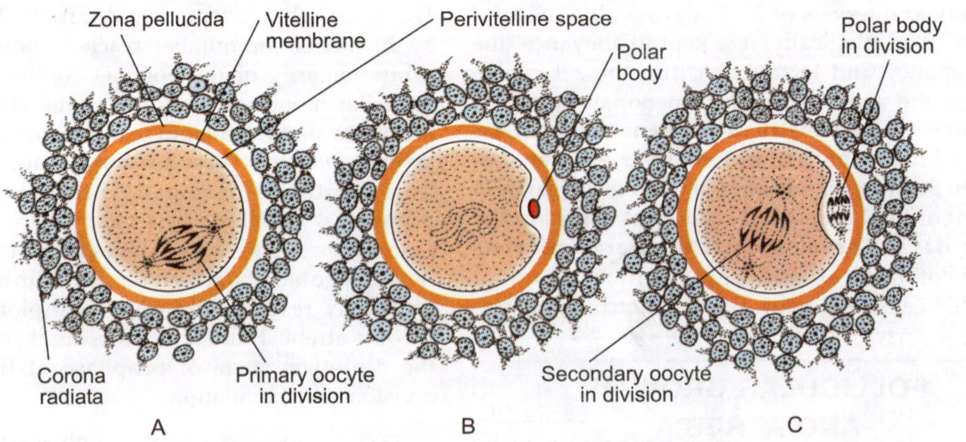

Fig. 8.1. Morphology of the oocyte

until just prior to ovulation, the oocyte ceases to enlarge around the time of antrum formation. **The morphological features of the primary oocyte just prior to ovulation (often erroneously called mature ovum) are as follows**:

It measures about 130 microns and the nucleus measures 20-25 microns. This is in contrast with 20 microns and 10 microns respectively in the primordial follicle. The radially arranged granulosa cells surrounding the oocyte is called **corona radiata.** The oocyte is surrounded by an outer envelope called **zona pellucida**, a glycoprotein layer, secreted by the growing oocyte. The cytoplasm, also called vitellus contains nutritive yolk granules and is limited by a definite membrane called **vitelline membrane**. The space between the vitelline membrane and the zona pellucida is called **perivitelline space**. The spherical nucleus is located near the centre of the cytoplasm. The nucleolus is large with sparsely distributed chromatin. Shortly before ovulation, meiosis is reinitiated. At the completion of the first and second meiotic division, the number of chromosomes in the oocyte is halved (23, X) and the two polar bodies which are formed are pushed to the perivitelline space. **The first polar body is formed just prior to ovulation and the second one just after fertilisation (Figs. 8.1 and 8.2).**

MENSTRUAL CYCLE

OVARIAN CYCLE

Definition

The development and maturation of a follicle, ovulation and formation of corpus luteum and its degeneration constitute an ovarian cycle. All these events occur within 4 weeks.

Thus, the ovarian cycle consists of:

- Recruitment of groups of follicles.
- Selection of dominant follicle and its maturation.
- Ovulation.
- Corpus luteum formation.
- Demise of the corpus luteum.

Recruitment of groups of follicles (Preantral phase)

The cohort of the growing follicles undergoes a process of development and differentiation which takes about **85 days and spreads over 3 ovarian cycles**.

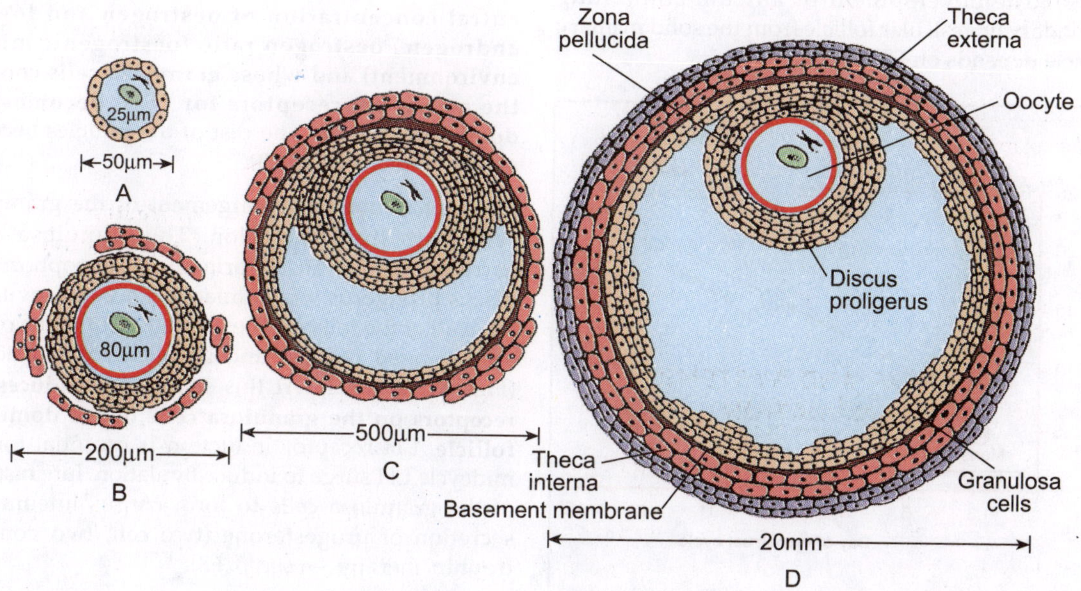

Fig. 8.2. Development of Graafian follicle

It is not clear as to how many and which of the primordial follicles amidst several thousands are recruited for a particular cycle. It is presumed that about 20 antral follicles (about 5-10 per ovary) proceed to develop in each cycle.

The initial recruitment and growth of primordial follicles are not under the control of any hormone. After a certain stage (2-5 mm in size) the growth and differentiation of primordial follicles are under the control of FSH. **Unless the follicles are rescued by FSH at this stage, they undergo atresia**.

There is predominant change is in the oocyte which is enlarged out of proportion to the size of the follicle. The oocyte is now surrounded by an acellular barrier of glycoprotein produced by the follicular cells and is called zona pellucida. The flattened outer single layer pregranulosa cells become cuboidal and multilayered — now called granulosa cells. There is appearance of channels (gap junctions) between the granulosa cells and the oocyte. Through these gap junctions nutrition to the oocyte is maintained. There is noticeable beginning of differentiation of the theca interna layer of ovarian stroma surrounding the follicle. The granulosa cells now acquire FSH receptors.

Selection of a dominant follicle and its maturation

The Graafian follicle is named after the Dutch physician and anatomist Reijnier de Graaf (1641-1673). The development of antrum containing secondary or vesicular follicle from the solid primary follicle depends on FSH.

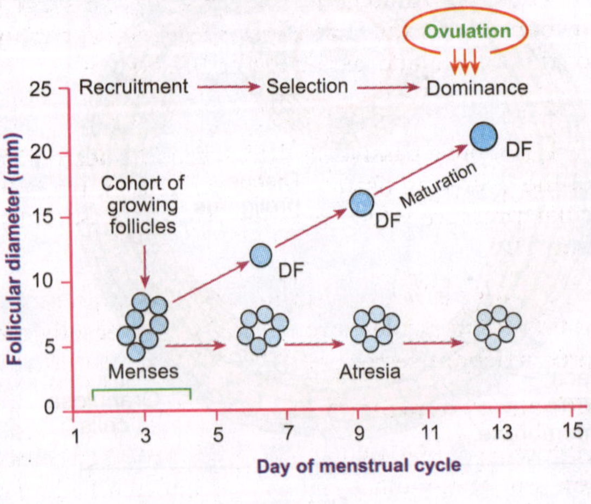

Fig. 8.3. Selection and maturation of the dominant follicle (DF) during a natural cycle

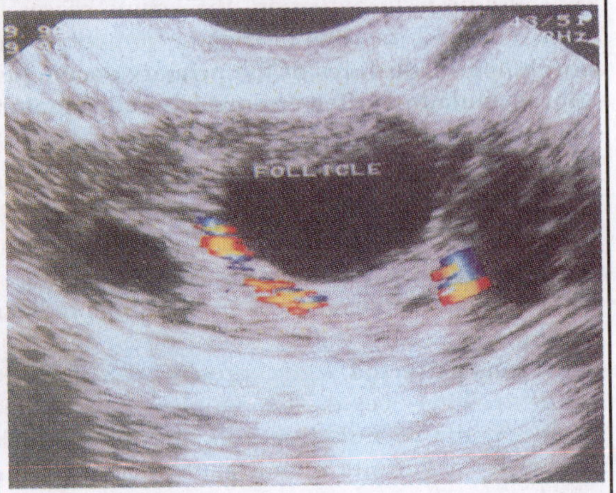

Fig. 8.3A. Colour Doppler (TV) sonogram showing a mature Graafian follicle prior to ovulation

There is accelerated growth of all the components of the follicles of the preantral phase. The granulosa cells grow faster than the theca cells. There is production of follicular fluid which is primarily an ultra filtrate of blood from the vessels within theca interna. The fluid-filled space is formed amidst the granulosa cells. The spaces coalesce to form an antrum.

Dominant follicle

As early as day 5-7, one of the follicles out of so many becomes dominant and undergoes further maturation. It seems probable that the **one with highest antral concentration of oestrogen and lowest androgen : oestrogen ratio (oestrogenic microenvironment) and whose granulosa cells contain the maximum receptors for FSH, becomes the dominant follicle**. The rest of the follicles become atretic by day 8 (Fig. 8.3).

There is marked enlargement of the granulosa cells with lipid inclusion. The granulosa cells surround the ovum to form cumulus oophorus or discus proligerus which infact anchors the ovum to the wall of the follicle. The cells adjacent to the ovum are arranged radially and is called corona radiata (Figs. 8.2 and 8.4). At this stage, **FSH induces LH receptors on the granulosa cells of the dominant follicle**. LH receptor induction is essential for the midcycle LH surge to induce ovulation, luteinisation of the granulosa cells to form corpus luteum and secretion of progesterone (two cell, two gonadotrophin therapy — see p. 68).

Theca cells becomes vacuolated and more vascular than those of other antral follicles. The theca cells are separated from the granulosa cells by a polymerised membrane called membrana granulosa. Just prior to ovulation, LH may act to depolymerise this membrane to facilitate vascularisation of the granulosa cells.

The follicular fluid is increased in amount. **The fluid contains** oestrogens, FSH, trace amount of androgen, prolactin, OMI (oocyte maturation inhibitor), LI (luteinisation inhibitor), inhibin-which acts centrally to inhibit FSH, proteolytic enzymes, plasmin, etc.

The fully mature Graafian follicle just prior to ovulation measures about 20 mm, and is composed of the following structures from outside inward (Fig. 8.4).

(a) Theca externa.

(b) Theca interna.

(c) Membrana granulosa (limitans).

(d) Granulosa cell layer.

(e) Discus proligerus in which the ovum is incorporated with cells arranged radially (corona radiata).

(f) Antrum containing vesicular fluid.

As previously mentioned, it takes 3 months for the follicle to grow and mature to ovulation — 2 months to reach an antral stage measuring 1 mm; 2 weeks to reach 5 mm and another 2 weeks to reach 20 mm before ovulation.

Ovulation

The dominant follicle, shortly before ovulation reaches the surface of the ovary. The cumulus becomes detached from the wall so that the ovum with the surrounding cells (corona radiata) floats freely in the liquor folliculi. The oocyte completes the first meiotic division with extrusion of the first polar body which is pushed to the perivitelline space. The follicular wall near the ovarian surface becomes thinner.The stigma develops as a conical projection which penetrates the outer surface layer of the ovary and persists for a while ($^1/_2$-2 minutes) as a thin membrane. The cumulus escapes out of the follicle by a slow oozing process, taking about 1-2 minutes along with varying amount of follicular fluid. The stigma is soon closed by a plug of plasma.

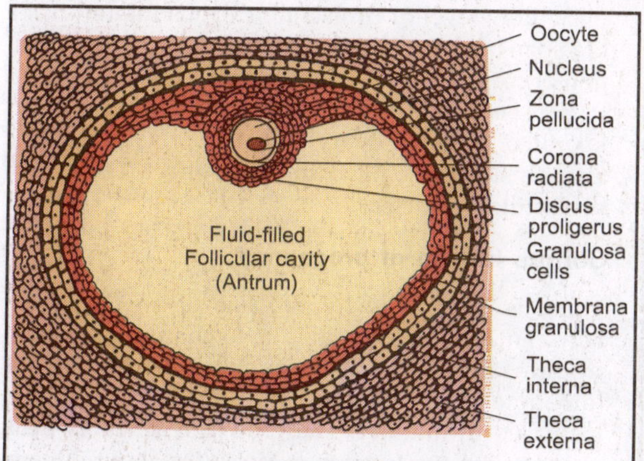

Fig. 8.4. A mature Graafian follicle

Causes

The following are the possible explanations which may operate singly or in combination.

1. ***Endocrinal***

• *LH surge*

Sustained peak level of oestrogen for 24-48 hours in the late follicular phase results in LH surge from the anterior pituitary (positive feedback effect). Effective LH surge persists for about 24 hours. The **LH surge stimulates** completion of reduction division of the oocyte and initiates luteinisation of the granulosa cells, synthesis of progesterone and prostaglandins.

• *FSH rise*

Preovulatory rise of 17-α-hydroxy progesterone facilitates the positive feedback action of oestrogen to induce FSH surge → increase in plasminogen activator → plasminogen → plasmin → helps lysis of the wall of the follicle.

Thus, the combined LH/FSH midcycle surge is responsible for the final stage of maturation, rupture of the follicle and expulsion of the oocyte.

2. ***Stretching factor***

It is more a passive stretching causing necrobiosis of the overlying tissue rather than rise in intrafollicular pressure which remains static at about 10-15 mm Hg.

3. ***Contraction of the micromuscles*** in the theca externa and ovular stroma due to increased local prostaglandin secretion.

Effects of ovulation

Following ovulation, the follicle is changed to corpus luteum. The ovum is picked up into the Fallopian tube and undergoes either degeneration or further maturation, if fertilisation occurs. **Menstruation is unrelated to ovulation and anovular menstruation**

is quite common during adolescence, following childbirth and in women approaching menopause.

Corpus luteum

After ovulation, the ruptured Graafian follicle develops into corpus luteum. The life cycle is divided into four stages :

- **Proliferation**
- **Vascularisation**
- **Maturation**
- **Regression**

Stage of proliferation

The collapsed walls of the empty follicle form convolutions. The opening through which the ovum escapes soon becomes plugged with fibrin. The granulosa cells undergo hypertrophy without multiplication. The cells become larger, polyhedral with pale vesicular nuclei and frothy cytoplasm. The cells are called granulosa lutein cells. The colour of the corpus luteum at this stage is greyish yellow due to presence of lipids (Fig. 8.5).

Stage of vascularisation

Within 24 hours of rupture of the follicle, small capillaries grow into granulosa layer towards the lumen accompanied by lymphatics and fibroblasts. The sprouting vessels may rupture and bleed in the cavity.

Stage of maturation

By 4th day, the luteal cells have attained the maximum size. Approximately about 7-8 days following ovulation, the corpus luteum attains a size of about 1-2 cm and reaches its secretory peak. There is hypertrophy of the theca interna cells. The cells persist in the periphery and in the septa and are called paralutein cells. Some theca lutein cells called 'K' cells invade the granulosa layer. The lutein cells become greatly enlarged and develop lipid inclusion, giving the cells a distinctive yellowish colour. **The colour is due to the pigment carotene.** The cavity may be small containing scanty fluid.

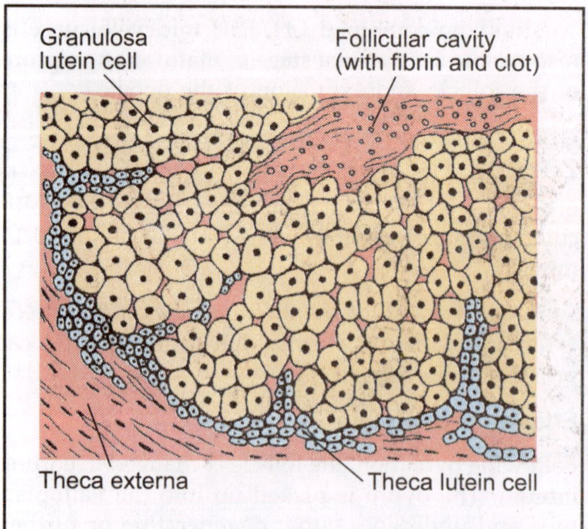

Fig. 8.5. Histologic appearance of a section of corpus luteum

Stage of regression

On the day 22-23 of cycle, retrogression starts. The first evidence of degeneration is appearance of vacuolation in the cells. There is deposition of fat in the lutein cells and appearance of hyaline tissue between them. The lutein cells atrophy and the corpus luteum becomes corpus albicans. Regression of corpus luteum is due to withdrawal of tonic LH support.

If, however, fertilisation occurs in the particular cycle, regression fails to occur, instead it is converted into corpus luteum of pregnancy.

Hormones in relation to formation and maintenance of corpus luteum

1. FSH in presence of high level of oestrogen induces LH receptors in the granulosa cells of the dominant follicle. There after midcycle LH surge causes luteinisation of the granulosa cells and progesterone secretion. LH secretion must be continued for the function of corpus luteum, failing which the corpus luteum will regress.

2. Adequate folliculogenesis in the preovulatory phase with increased secretion of oestradiol and of 17-α-hydroxy progesterone is a prerequisite for adequate corpus luteum formation.

3. Low level of prolactin : Corpus luteum has a life-span of about 12-14 days. The cause of degeneration of corpus luteum in an infertile cycle is not clear. It has been suggested that prostaglandin F2 α liberated from the ovary is luteolytic. Oestradiol is also considered to have luteolytic effect. The role of prolactin is not clear.

Corpus luteum of pregnancy

There is a surge of hyperplasia of all the layers between 23rd to 28th day due to chorionic gonadotrophin. hCG, like LH will stimulate the corpus luteum to secrete progesterone. The 'K' cells are also increased in number. The growth reaches its peak at about 8th week when it measures about 2-3 cm. It looks bright orange, later on becomes yellow and finally pale. Regression occurs following low levels of chorionic gonadotrophin and the degenerative changes take place most frequently at about 6 months of gestation.

Hormone secretion

Hormones—predominantly progesterone is secreted by the corpus luteum to support the endometrium of the luteal phase. There is also secretion of oestrogen, inhibin and relaxin. Progesterone along with oestrogen from corpus luteum maintain the growth of the fertilised ovum. This is essential till the luteal function is taken over by the placenta. **This turn over of function from corpus luteum of pregnancy to placenta is called luteal-placental shift. This transition period continues from seven weeks to ten weeks.** In the absence of pregnancy there is fall in the levels of serum oestradiol, progesterone and inhibin. This removes the inhibitory control of GnRH and FSH. Gradual increase in FSH is responsible for fresh recruitment of follicles for the next cycle.

FOLLICULAR ATRESIA

Atresia is a continued process which actually starts at 20th week of intrauterine life and ends at

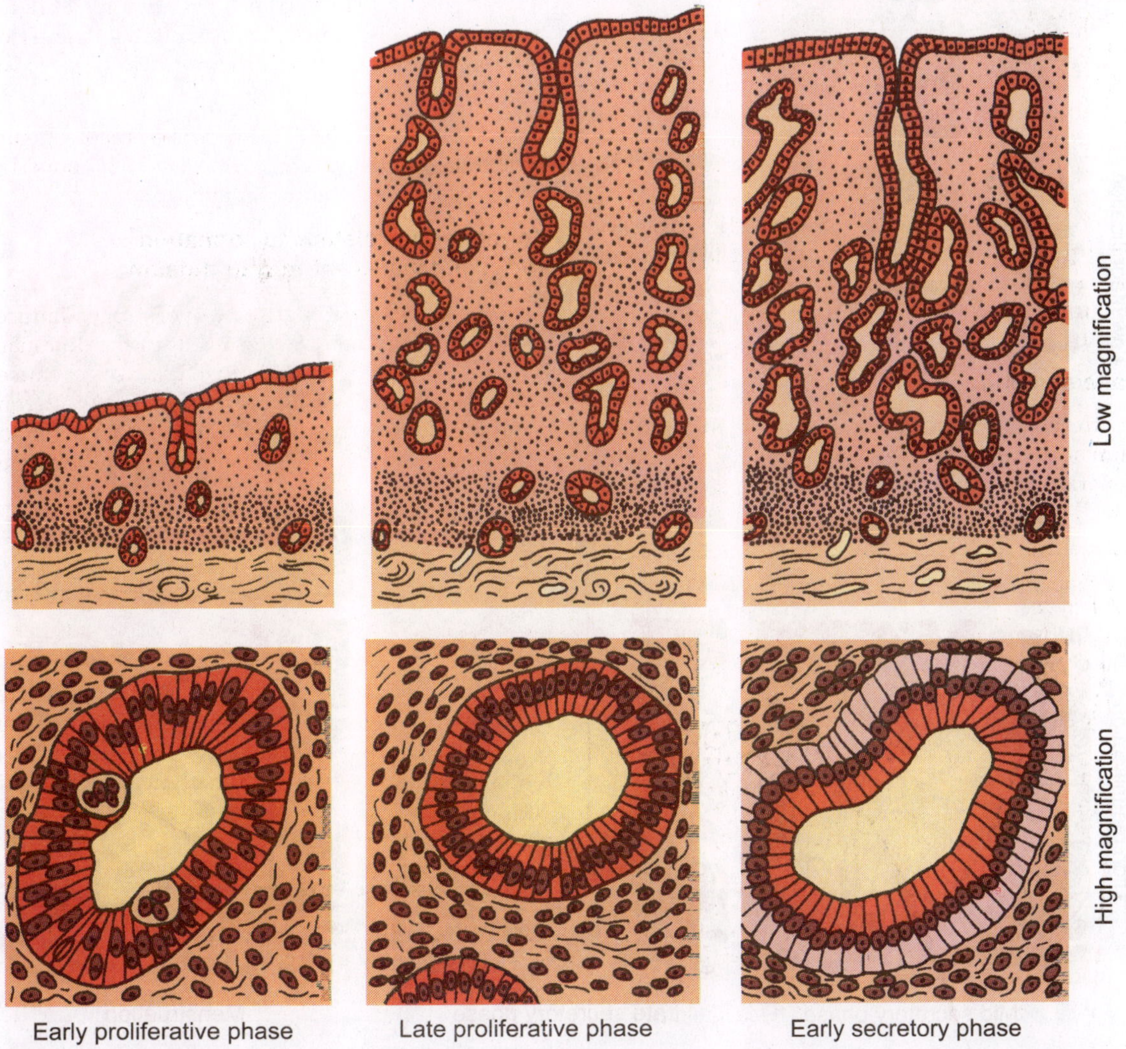

Fig. 8.6. Endometrium in proliferative and early secretory phase. Note the tendency of tortuosity of the glands and the characteristic subnuclear vacuolation in early secretory phase (cf compare with those of proliferative phase)

menopause. It may affect a follicle at any stage of development. However, the following descriptions are related to atretic changes of a maturing follicle which is ultimately left out in the race of a dominant follicle.

Changes in the ovum occur first. The ovum swells and undergoes hyaline and fatty degeneration. Granulosa cells then regress at a faster rate than the cells of theca interna. Hyaline tissue is deposited beneath the membrana granulosa to form the glass membrane which is the classic feature of follicular degeneration. Liquor folliculi is gradually absorbed with increasing formation of hyaline tissue in the glass membrane. Eventually, the follicle collapses; its cavity is obliterated when the opposing surfaces of the glass membranes come in contact. In the periphery, deep staining theca interna cells persist and are called interstitial cells of the ovary. These cells atrophy after menopause.

Causes of germ cell loss and follicular atresia

Exact factors are unknown. The following are the possible explanations for follicular degeneration and atresia :

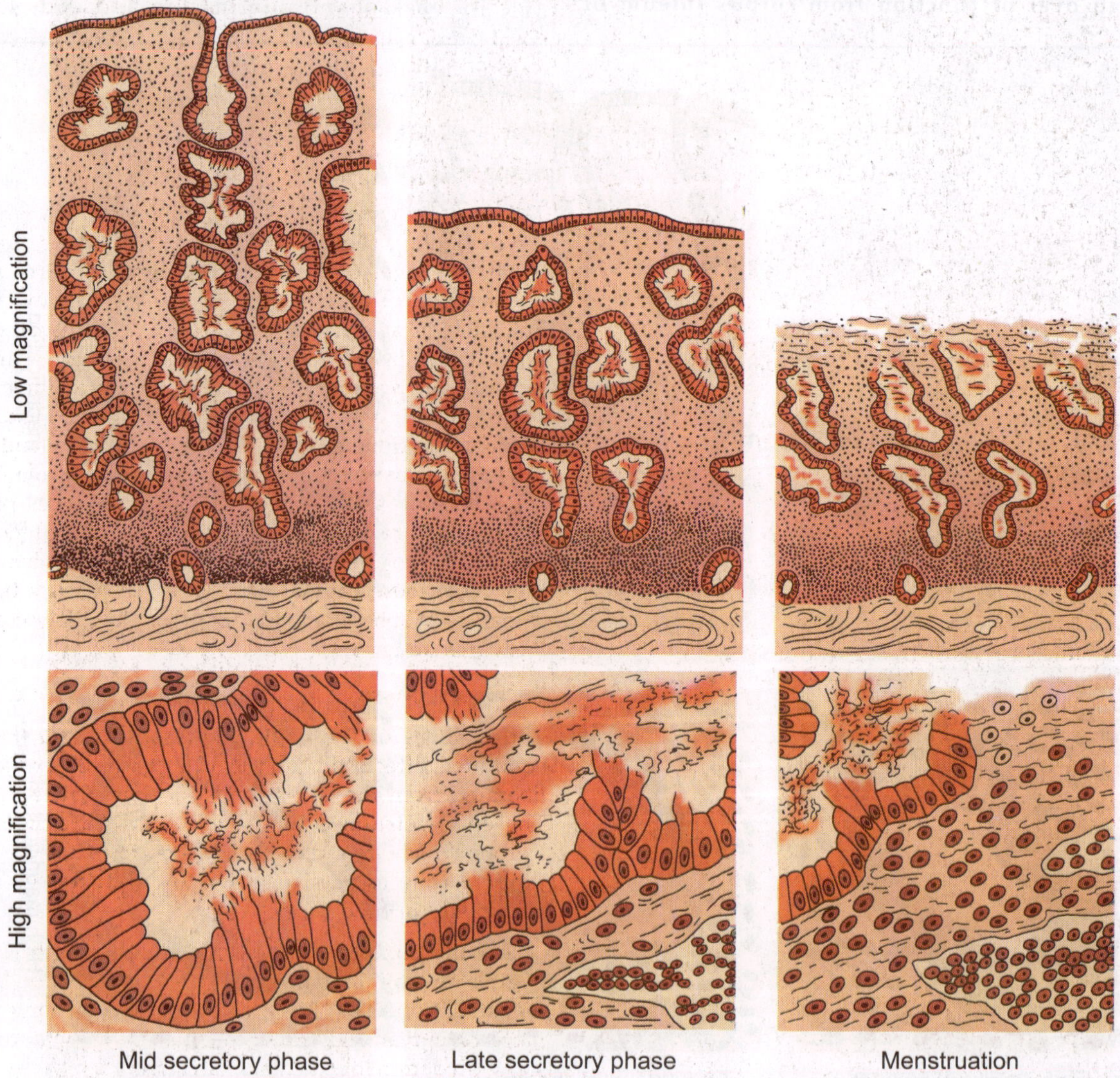

Fig. 8.7. Endometrium in secretory and menstrual phase. Note the marked tortuosity of the glands with secretion in the lumen in the midsecretory phase. The nucleus is pushed to the base.

- Oogonia having no granulosa cell layer envelope.
- Follicles that do not enter the germ cell meiotic division.
- Follicles not rescued by FSH.
- Follicles not having oestrogen induced FSH receptors.
- Follicles loosing FSH receptors due to negative feedback effect of oestrogen secreted by the dominant follicle.
- Follicles loosing FSH receptors due to high androgen : oestrogen ratio (androgenic follicular microenvironment).
- Genetic influence — as in 45, X individual.
- Apoptosis — programmed cell death.

Under the action of LH, more **androgens** are formed from these thecal cells which perhaps have got two functions : (i) **to enhance the process of atresia** of the small follicles and (ii) **to stimulate libido** specially noticed in midmenstrual period.

ENDOMETRIAL CYCLE

The endometrium is the lining epithelium of the uterine cavity above the level of internal os. It consists of **surface epithelium, glands, stroma and blood vessels**. Two distinct divisions are established — **basal zone (stratum basalis) and the superficial functional zone**.

Basal zone

It is about one-third of the total depth of the endometrium and lies in contact with the myometrium. It consists of stromal cells which stain deeply and are compactly placed. The base of the endometrial glands extends into the layer. The zone is supplied by the basal arteries. The zone is uninfluenced by hormone and as such, no cyclic changes are observed. After shedding of the superficial part during menstruation, the regeneration of all the components occurs from this zone. **It measures about 1 mm**.

Functional zone

This zone is under the influence of fluctuating cyclic ovarian hormones, oestrogen and progesterone. The changes in different components during an ovulatory cycle has been traditionally divided into four stages (Figs. 8.6, 8.7 and 8.9).

- Regenerative phase.
- Proliferative phase.
- Secretory phase.
- Menstruation.

Stage of regeneration

Regeneration of the endometrium starts even before the menstruation ceases and is completed 2-3 days after the end of menstruation. The cubical surface epithelium is derived from the gland lumina and stromal cells. New blood vessels grow from the stumps of the old one. The glands and the stromal cells are regenerated from the remnants left in the basal zone. The glands are lined by the cubical epithelium and lie parallel to the surface. The stromal ground substance re-expands. **The thickness averages 2 mm**.

Stage of proliferation

This stage extends from 5th or 6th day to 14th day (till ovulation). The proliferative changes occurs due to rise in level of ovarian oestrogens. There is proliferation of all the elements — at first slowly but later on at a rapid pace. **The glands** become tubular and lie perpendicular to the surface. **The epithelium** becomes columnar with the nuclei placed at the base. The epithelium of one gland becomes continuous with the neighbouring gland. Mitosis is evident in the epithelial cells. **The stromal cells** become spindle-shaped with evidences of mitosis and are compact. **The spiral vessels** extend unbranched to a region below the epithelium where they form loose capillary network. There may be evidences of subepithelial congestion. **The thickness measures about 3-4 mm**.

Secretory phase

The changes of the components are due to the combined effects of oestrogen and progesterone liberated from the corpus luteum after ovulation. The endometrium contains receptors for progesterone which are induced by oestrogen. **Thus, the progesterone can only act on the endometrium previously primed by oestrogen**.

All the components display their growth. It begins on day 15 and ceases 5-6 days prior to menstruation. **The surface epithelium** becomes more columnar and ciliated at places. The glands show predominant changes. **The glands** increase in size. The lining epithelium become taller. There is appearance of vacuoles due to secretion of glycogen between the nuclei and the basement membrane.

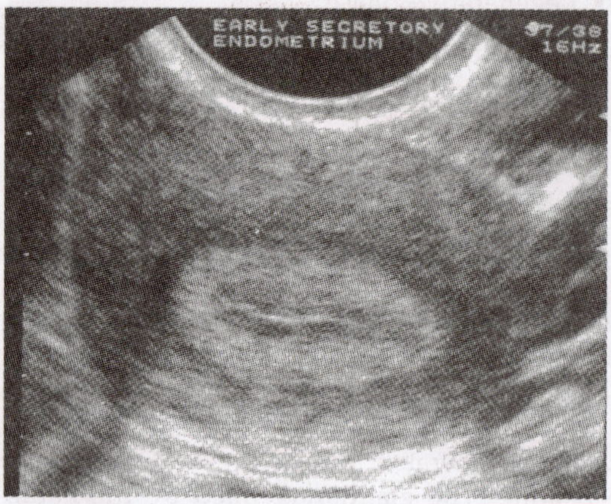

Fig. 8.8. Transvaginal scan demonstrating thickened, early secretory endometrium

This is called **subnuclear vacuolation**, which is the **earliest (36-48 hours) evidence of progesterone effect (ovulation). The subnuclear vacuolation persists until about 21st day of cycle.** The intracellular secretion then enters the gland lumina on the way to the uterine cavity pushing the nuclei back towards the basement membrane. The effect is a saw-toothed glandular epithelium. The fluid has got nutritive value for any fertilised ovum reaching the uterus during that time. **The glands become corkscrew-shaped. The blood vessels undergo marked spiralling.**

The stromal cells become swollen, large and polyhedral and after the 21st day tend to collect more superficially around the neck of the glands. The deeper spongy layer is composed of convoluted glands, coiled arterioles and comparatively few stromal cells in oedematous stroma. Histochemical studies show increase in glycogen and acid phosphatase. Histological staining is eosinophilic **The thickness of the endometrium reaches its highest (6-8 mm) (Fig. 8.8).**

The endometrial growth ceases 5-6 days prior to menstruation (22nd or 23rd day of cycle) in an infertile cycle. This is due to dehydration of the glands. The subepithelial capillaries and the spiral vessels are engorged. **The regressive changes in the endometrium are pronounced 24-48 hours prior to menstruation.** There is marked spiralling of the arteries and the withdrawal of hormones oestrogen and progesterone causes intense spasm of the spiral arterioles at the basal part. These two lead to stasis and tissue anoxaemia. There are evidences of infiltration of leucocytes and monocytes in the stroma.

Menstrual phase

It is essentially degeneration and casting off of an endometrium prepared for a pregnancy. **Regression of corpus luteum with fall in the level of oestrogen and progesterone is an invariable preceding feature.** As a result of withdrawal of hormone support, there is retrogressive changes in the endometrium as mentioned earlier.

Mechanism of menstrual bleeding

The degenerative changes are predominantly of vascular origin. Stasis of blood and spasm of the arterioles lead to damage of the arteriolar walls. Phase of relaxation leads to escape of blood out of the vessels through the damaged walls. The degenerative process is rapid and involves all the components of the functional damaged layer. There is local tissue destruction by release of proteolytic enzymes from the breakdown of lysosomes. **So there is enzymatic autodigestion of the functional zone. The bleeding occurs** from the broken arteries, veins and capillaries and also from the stromal haematoma. The blood along with the superficial functional layer is shed into the uterine cavity. The blood coagulates in the uterine cavity but soon liquefies by plasmin unless the bleeding is very brisk and rapid. **The menstrual flow** stops as a result of combined effect of prolonged vasoconstriction, myometrial contraction and local aggregation of platelets with deposition of fibrin around them. Endothelin and platelet activating factor present in the endometrium are potent vasoconstrictors. Resumption of oestrogen secretion leads to clot formation over the decapitated stumps of endometrial vessels. There is simultaneous repair of endometrium. This is under control of oestrogen and different growth factors.

Role of prostaglandins

It is likely that the arteriolar constriction and endometrial necrosis are caused by prostaglandins. The endometrium and partly the myometrium, synthesize the prostaglandins from arachidonic acid by the enzyme cyclo-oxygenase. Different prostaglandins have got different action. $PGF_2\alpha$ causes myometrial contraction and vasoconstriction. It seems to play a dominant role in normal cycle. PGE_2 produces myometrial contraction but causes vasodilatation. PGI_2 (Prostacyclin) causes myometrial relaxation and vasodilatation. It also inhibits platelet activity. Thus, the menstrual pain and blood flow are probably related to the relative proportion of different prostaglandins present in the endometrium.

Hormones in relation to ovarian and menstrual cycle

The outcome in relation to hormonal interplay in normally menstruating women includes :

- Growth and development of the Graafian follicle.
- Ovulation.
- Maintenance and demise of corpus luteum.
- Endometrial growth and shedding.

Growth and development of the follicle (Fig. 8.9)

At the beginning of a menstrual cycle, a low level of oestrogen and inhibin secreted from the previous weaning corpus luteum maintains a high FSH level through release of negative feedback of oestrogen. The FSH increases not only its own receptors in the granulosa cells but also LH receptors in theca cells. Initial sustained low level of LH stimulates the production of oestrogen. Under the synergistic effect of FSH and oestrogen, multiplication of the granulosa cells, formation of the follicular fluid and synthesis of more LH receptors in the theca cells occur.

With increased secretion of oestrogen, the FSH level is lowered through a negative feedback mechanism. Thus, the initial high level of FSH comes down to a static base level by day 5. Paradoxically, the increasing LH level with the rising oestrogen level stimulates androgen production in the theca cells. Granulosa cells now utilise the increased androgen produced from the theca cells for the synthesis of oestrogen.

The falling FSH level with peak rise of oestrogen in the late follicular phase increases the LH receptors in the granulosa cells. Final maturation of the follicle is thus achieved by the combined effect of FSH and LH.

Role of peptides and growth factors (p. 72)

Peptides — FSH stimulates the granulosa cells to produce a number of peptides like inhibin, activin and follistatin. Activin is also secreted by the pituitary gland. Inhibin directly inhibits FSH, where as activin stimulates FSH.

Growth factors — Insulin like growth factors (IGF), epidermal growth factors and others, modulate the action of FSH, LH and the peptides. IGF-11, is produced in the theca cells. It stimulates aromatase activity and progesterone synthesis in the granulosa cells.

OVULATION

LH surge initiates luteinisation acting through its receptors about 24-48 hrs. prior to ovulation. A trace amount of 17-α-hydroxy progesterone is formed which is probably responsible for completion of the first meiotic division of the oocyte and compounds the effect of oestrogen for LH surge. Progesterone also facilitates the positive feedback action to induce FSH surge → increase in plasminogen activator → plasminogen → plasmin → helps lysis of the follicular wall.

After the oestradiol reaches beyond the critical level of 200 pg/ml and is sustained for about 48 hours, it exerts a positive feedback action to LH from the anterior pituitary (LH surge). **Ovulation occurs approximately 10-12 hours after the LH peak or 32-36 hours after the onset of LH surge.** A threshold of LH surge generally persists for 24 hours. **Ovulation coincides approximately 24-36 hours after the peak oestradiol level. LH surge stimulates** completion of the reduction division of the oocyte and initiates luteinisation of the granulosa cells and synthesis of progesterone and prostaglandins.

Thus, the **combined LH/FSH midcycle surge** is responsible for the final stage of maturation of the follicle, completion of the first meiotic division of the oocyte with extrusion of the first polar body and expulsion of the oocyte (ovulation).

The drop in LH level following its peak may be due to desensitisation of LH receptors or due to negative feedback effect of progesterone. This down regulation results in a refractory state during which there is diminished steroidogenesis.

Table 8.1
APPROXIMATE TIME INTERVAL OF EVENTS IN MENSTRUAL CYCLE PRIOR TO OVULATION

Events	Hours
Oestradiol rise	83
Onset of LH surge	34-36
Oestradiol peak	24-36
LH peak	10-12
Progesterone rise	8

Maintenance and demise of corpus luteum

Soon following the LH surge, the level of oestrogen drops down within an hour and the LH peak after 24 hours. LH initiates and maintains the corpus luteum from which both progesterone and oestrogen are secreted. The oestrogen attains a lower level and maintains a plateau curve as against a peak rise in follicular phase. 17-α-hydroxy progesterone parallels with the oestradiol level in the luteal phase. **Progesterone attains its highest peak about 8 days after the LH peak**. Through intraovarian and central negative feedback mechanisms, **progesterone acts to suppress new follicular growth**. As the oestrogen and progesterone attain their highest peak, they exert a negative feedback effect on LH and FSH in an infertile cycle and the level of LH and FSH drops down to a minimum. The lysis of the corpus luteum occurs and so the secretion of progesterone and oestrogen falls. **The life span of corpus luteum is about 12-14 days**. With the fall of oestrogen and progesterone, FSH level again rises under the influence of GnRH to exert its effect on follicular growth and maturation for the next cycle (Figs. 8.9 and 8.10).

Endometrial growth and shedding

Oestrogen secreted in the follicular phase produces proliferative changes in the endometrium and induces receptors for progesterone. In the luteal phase, progesterone acts on the oestrogen primed endometrium having sufficient number of receptors and produces secretory changes. In the infertile cycle, with the fall of oestrogen and progesterone, the endometrium becomes unsupported to the hormones and degeneration occurs → menstruation (Fig. 8.10).

Endometrial sample biopsy and histology can precisely determine the date of menstrual cycle. Any discrepancy of **more than two days** when examined in the post ovulatory phase is called **luteal phase defect**. This method of endometrial examination is called **dating of endometrium**.

LUTEAL-FOLLICULAR SHIFT

This period extends from the demise of corpus luteum (fall of serum oestradiol, inhibin and progesterone level) to the selection of a dominant follicle for the next cycle. The recruitment of follicles is done by FSH. The decrease in inhibin level removes its suppressive effect of FSH secretion in the pituitary. FSH level starts rising about 2 days before the onset of menses. Fall in the level of oestradiol and progesterone allows pulsatile secretion of GnRH. Rising FSH level rescues the follicles from atresia and selects the dominant follicle.

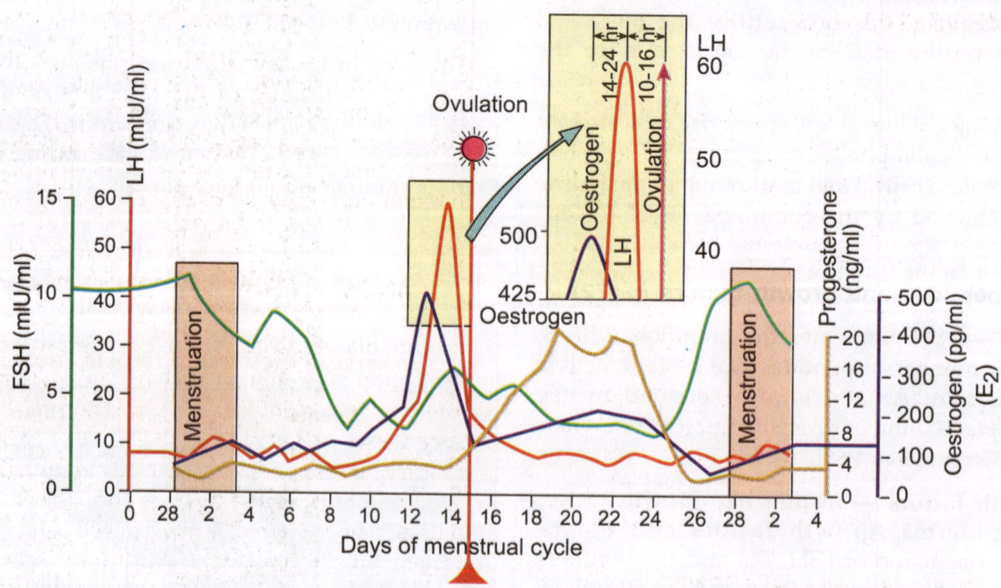

Fig. 8.9. Fluctuation of serum levels of ovarian steroids and gonadotrophins in a normal ovulatory cycle

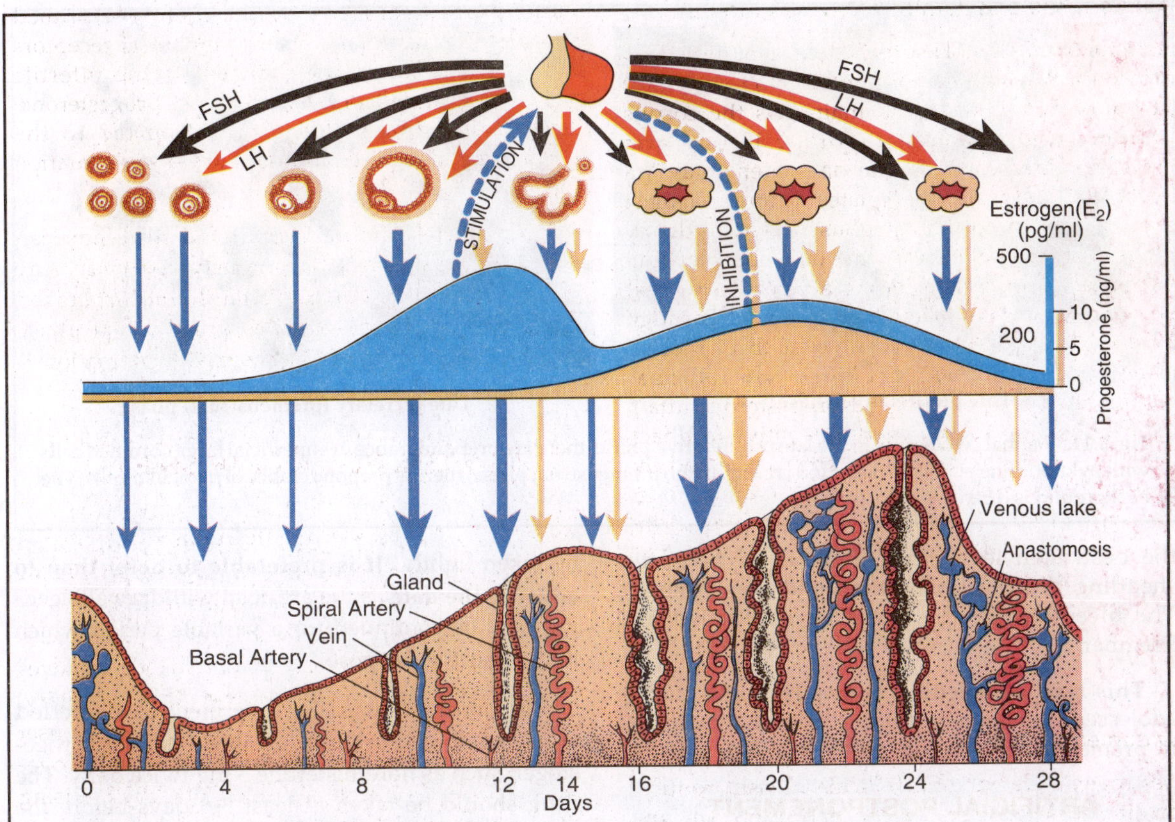

Fig. 8.10. Hormones controlling the ovarian and endometrial cycles

MENSTRUAL SYMPTOMS

In majority, apart from bleeding per vaginam there is no symptom. Initially, it begins as pink discharge but on day 2 and 3 it becomes dark red. In teenagers or nulliparous, there may be associated tolerable colicky pain at the beginning due to uterine contraction. If the pain is of sufficient magnitude so as to incapacitate the day-to-day activities, it is called dysmenorrhoea (see chapter 14). There may be premonitory symptoms such as pelvic discomfort, backache, fullness of the breasts or mastalgia just prior to menstruation. Headache or depression may be present. If these premonitory symptoms are predominant, these are grouped into a syndrome called "premenstrual syndrome" and is dealt separately in a later chapter.

MENSTRUAL HYGIENE

Sympathetic and careful handling of the young girls experiencing first menstruation is of paramount importance. This should be done by the mother explaining the physiological and other associated changes during period. The girls should continue with their normal activities. The daily bath should not be suspended. During initial few periods, the girl may use sanitary pads comfortably but with experience may be changed to tampon, if so desired.

ANOVULAR MENSTRUATION

In an anovulatory cycle, the follicles grow without any selection of dominant follicle. The oestrogen is secreted in increasing amount. There may be imbalance between oestrogen and FSH or because of temporary unresponsiveness of the hypothalamus to the rising oestrogen, GnRH is suppressed → no ovulation. The net effect is unopposed secretion of oestrogen till the follicles exist. The endometrium remains in either proliferative or at times hyperplastic state. There is inadequate structural stromal support and the endometrium remains fragile. When

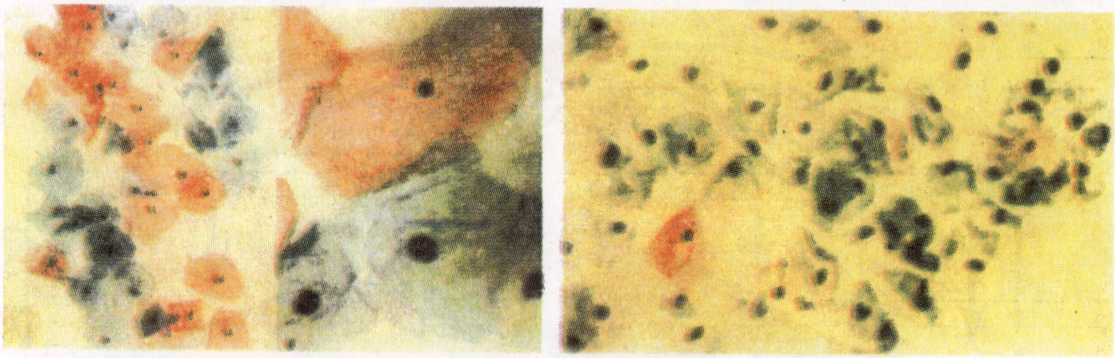

Late proliferative phase | Late secretary (premenstrual) phase

Fig. 8.11. Vaginal cytology — In the late proliferative phase, there are preponderance of superficial large cornified cells with pyknotic nuclei. The background is clear. In the premenstrual phase, there is preponderance of navicular cells. The background is dirty.

the oestrogen level falls, there is asynchronus shedding of the endometrium and menstruation. The bleeding may be heavy or prolonged and irregular.

This type of bleeding is mostly found during adolescence, following childbirth and abortion and in premenopausal period.

ARTIFICIAL POSTPONEMENT

Artificial alteration of the date of menstrual flow should be judiciously comply with. It should not be taken lightly. **It is preferable to defer than to advance the date** as the artificial withdrawal bleeding may be continued for a variable period which may spoil the purpose.

The hormones used for deferment of the period are — combined oral pill, 2 tablets daily or progestogen such as norethisterone 5 mg twice daily. The drug should be taken at least 3-6 days before the expected date of the period and continued until the crisis is over. The period is expected 2-3 days after the drug is suspended.

Table 8.2

Cervical cycle, Vaginal cycle and General changes in follicular and luteal phase

Cervical Cycle	
Follicular phase	**Luteal phase**
• Internal os — funnel-shaped	• Tightly closed
• Mucus — thin and watery	• Thick and viscid
• Stretchability — increased to beyond 10 cm	• Lost
• Fern tree pattern present	• Lost
• Glycoprotein network — parallel, thus facilitating sperm penetration	• Interlacing bridges, preventing sperm penetration
• Glandular epithelium — taller	• Glands — more branched
Vaginal Cycle (Fig. 8.11)	
Follicular phase	**Luteal phase**
• Cytology — showing preponderance of superficial large cornified cells with pyknotic nuclei	• Preponderance of intermediate cells with folded edges (navicular cells)
• Background of the smear — clear	• Dirty due to presence of leucocytes and bacilli

General changes		
Preovulatory	**Ovulatory**	**Premenstrual**
• No symptom	• Pain abdomen on either iliac fossa • Slight vaginal bleeding • Mucoid vaginal discharge	• Irritability, lethargy, constipation • Acne • Pelvic discomfort • Abnormal gain in weight • Mastalgia

KEY POINTS

➤ Menstruation is the visible manifestation of cyclical physiologic uterine bleeding due to shedding of the endometrium as a result of invisible interplay of hormones mainly through hypothalamo-pituitary-ovarian axis.

➤ Average age of menarche is 13 years. The average menstrual blood loss is 35 ml (may be upto 80 ml). Average loss of iron in each menses is 13 mg. and about 70 per cent of total menstrual blood loss (MBL) occurs in the first 2 days (p. 79). Alkali haematin method is most precise to measure the MBL.

➤ The primordial follicle measures 0.03-0.05 mm. Primitive ovum measures 18-24 microns in diameter.

➤ The primary oocyte undergoes first meiotic division giving rise to secondary oocyte and one polar body just prior to ovulation. The measurement of a primary oocyte just prior to ovulation (mature ovum) is 130 microns.

➤ The secondary oocyte completes the second meiotic division only after fertilisation by a sperm in the fallopian tube.

➤ It is presumed that those follicles which are less exposed to progesterone environment are likely to run in the race for dominance in the next cycle.

➤ One follicle with highest antral concentration of oestrogen and lowest androgen : oestrogen ratio and the granulosa cells containing the maximum receptors for FSH becomes the dominant follicle. The fully mature Graafian follicle measures about 20 mm with a volume of 3.5 ml.

➤ LH surge stimulates the completion of first meiotic division, luteinisation of granulosa cells, synthesis of progesterone and prostaglandins.

Preovulatory FSH surge (which is progesterone dependent) enhances conversion of plasminogen to plasmin for the lysis of follicular wall.

Oestradiol (E_2) exerts negative feedback effect to FSH but bears a positive feedback effect to LH.

Both FSH and LH regulates follicular development through a number of growth factors and peptides by autocrine and paracrine mechanism (see p. 81).

Insulin growth factor II (IGF-II) is produced by theca and granulosa cells. IGF-II stimulates granulosa cell proliferation and aromatase activity.

Inhibin is a peptide, secreted by the granulosa cells in response to FSH. Inhibin is a potent inhibitor of FSH. Activin, another peptide secreted by the granulosa cells and by the pituitary, stimulates FSH.

➤ Sustained peak level of oestradiol for about 24 hours beyond 200 pg/ml in late follicular phase results in LH surge (positive feedback effect). Ovulation occurs about 32-36 hours after the onset of LH surge. The mean duration of LH surge is about 24 hours. The peak LH levels plateau for about 14 hours. The cause of LH decline is probably due to acute down regulation or due to negative feedback effect of progesterone (Table 8.1).

KEY POINTS

- After ovulation, the ruptured Graafian follicle becomes corpus luteum.

  The yellowish colour is due to lipid and pigment carotene. Regression starts on day 22-23 of infertile cycle.
- LH hormone, with adequate number of LH receptors in the granulosa cells, as induced during folliculogenesis with increased secretion of oestradiol, is the key factor of adequate corpus luteum formation (p. 84).
- The hormones — oestrogen and progesterone are secreted from the corpus luteum.
- The follicles containing high androgen : oestrogen ratio are destined to undergo atresia. Under the action of LH, more androgens are produced from the active thecal compartments (p. 85).
- The functional zone of the endometrium is under the influence of fluctuating cyclic ovarian hormones, oestrogen and progesterone. Progesterone can only act on the endometrium previously primed by oestrogen. Subnuclear vacuolation is the earliest evidence of ovulation and appears on 18th day and persists up to 21st day. The mechanism of menstrual bleeding is due to degenerative changes predominantly of vascular origin. The menstrual flow stops as a result of combined effect of prolonged vasoconstriction, myometrial contraction and local aggregation of platelets.
- $PGF_{2}\alpha$ causes myometrial contraction and vasoconstriction, PGE_2 produces myometrial contraction but causes vasodilatation, PGI_2 (prostacyclin) causes myometrial relaxation and vasodilatation.
- Under the synergistic effect of FSH and oestrogen, multiplication of the granulosa cells, formation of the follicular fluid and synthesis of more LH receptors in the theca cells occur. The falling FSH level with peak rise of oestrogen in the late follicular phase increases the LH receptors in the granulosa cells. Final maturation of the follicle is achieved by the combined effect of FSH and LH.
- Preovulatory FSH surge increases the plasmin which helps lysis of the follicular wall. LH surge stimulates completion of reduction division of the oocyte and initiates luteinisation of the granulosa cells and synthesis of progesterone and prostaglandins.
- Progesterone attains its highest peak about 8 days after the LH peak. Through intra-ovarian and central negative feedback mechanisms, progesterone acts to suppress new follicular growth.
- When the endometrium becomes unsupported by the fall of oestrogen and progesterone, degeneration occurs resulting in menstruation. The regressive changes in the endometrium are pronounced 24-48 hours prior to menstruation (p. 88).
- LH stimulates granulosa cell proliferation and luteinisation and production of progesterone.
- The theca cells and the stroma of atretic follicles produce more androgens in the midcycle. This raised androgen level enhances further atresia of the small follicles. This also increases libido.
- Demise of corpus luteum is due to the luteolytic action of oestrogen, prostaglandin $F_{2\alpha}$, nitric oxide, endotheline, TNFα and the proteolytic enzymes. hCG rescues the corpus luteum.
- **Luteal-Placental shift** is the turnover of function from corpus luteum of pregnancy to placenta. This transition period continues from seven weeks to ten weeks. This is essential for the growth of the fertilized ovum (p. 85).
- **Luteal-Follicular shift** is the period that extends from the demise of corpus lutcum to the selection of a new dominant follicle for the next cycle. It is due to fall in the levels of oestradiol, progesterone and inhibin. There is simultaneous rise in the levels of GnRH and FSH (p. 90).
- Rising in FSH level rescues follices from apoptosis and selects the dominant follicle (p. 82, 85).
- Menstrual cycle is associated with other changes like cervical, vaginal and general (see Table 8.2). The cervical cycle includes changes in the cervix and cervical mucus. Vaginal cytology varies with the phases of menstruation. General changes includes the different symptoms (Table 8.2).

Examination of a Gynaecological Patient

9

The clinical examination should be thorough and meticulous. These include in-depth history taking and examinations — general, abdominal and internal. It should be emphasised that a meticulous history taking alone can give a positive diagnosis in majority of cases without any physical examination. The examination should, in fact, proceed with the provisional diagnosis in mind. On occasion, ancillary aids are required to confirm the diagnosis. For a careful history taking, the following outlines are of help :

Name	Age ....
Marital status	Parity ....
Social status	Address ....
Chief complaint	

A patient hearing should be given about the complaints made by the patient in her own words. In order to substantiate the guess made out of her complaints, some leading questions may have to be asked tactfully and judiciously.

HISTORY

This should be taken in details. If multiple symptoms are present, their chronologic appearances are to be noted. Integration of the symptomatology to one pathology is to be tried first before embarking on the diagnosis of multiple pathology. Enquiry should be made about the bowel habits and urinary trouble, if any.

Menstrual History

Enquiry should be made about :

- Age of onset of the first period (menarche).
- Regularity of the cycle.
- Duration of period.
- Length of the cycle.
- Amount of bleeding — Excess is indicated by the passage of clots or number of pads used.
- First day of the last menstrual period (LMP).

The menstrual history can be reproduced as 13/4/28, representing that the period began at the age of 13, lasts for 4 days and occurs every 28 days.

Obstetric History

If the patient had been previously pregnant, details are to be enquired as per tabulation below. Many a times, the complaints may be related to the pregnancy complications or lactation.

No. date	Year and events	Pregnancy events	Labour delivery	Method of	Puerpe-rium	Baby wt. and sex. Birth asphyxia. Duration of breast feeding
1.						
2.						

The obstetric history is to be summed up as —

No. of living children ....Boys.........Girls..........	
Health status of the baby	
Immunisation	
Last issue..	

Past Medical History

Relevant medical disorders — systemic, metabolic or endocrinal should be enquired. Their presence requires care during operative procedure, if it deems necessary. Through tactful and intelligent interrogation, exposure to sexually transmitted disease is to be enquired.

Past Surgical History

This includes general, obstetrical or gynaecological surgery. The nature of the operation, anaesthetic complication if any, postoperative convalescence are to be enquired. Any histopathological report or relevant investigation related to the previous surgery is most often helpful.

Family History

It is of occasional value. Malignancy in the breast, colon, ovary or other genital organs is often related. Tubercular affection of any family member can give a clue in diagnosis of pelvic tuberculosis.

Personal History

Occupation, marital status — married, widow, divorced or separated should be enquired. If married — details of sexual life should be noted, specially in case of infertility. Contraceptive practice, if any should be enquired — specially relevant in pill users or cases having IUCD, as these methods often produce some adverse symptoms. History of taking drugs for a long time or allergy to certain drugs is to be noted.

EXAMINATION

The examination includes :

- General and systemic examination
- Gynaecological examination
  - Breast examination.
  - Abdominal examination.
  - Pelvic examination.

GENERAL AND SYSTEMIC EXAMINATION

The general and systemic examination should be thorough and meticulous.

Built — Too obese or too thin — May be the result of endocrinopathy and related to menstrual abnormalities.

Nutrition — Average/Poor.

Stature — including development of secondary sex characters.

Pallor Jaundice

Teeth, gums and tonsils — for any septic foci.

Neck — Palpation of thyroid gland and lymph nodes, specially the left supraclavicular glands.

Oedema of legs

Cardiovascular and respiratory systems — Any abnormality may modify the surgical procedure, if it deems necessary.

Pulse Blood pressure

GYNAECOLOGICAL EXAMINATION

Breast examination (Fig. 9.1)

This should be a routine specially in women above the age of 30, to detect any breast pathology, the important being carcinoma. In India, breast carcinoma is the second most common site of malignancy in female, next to carcinoma cervix.

Abdominal Examination

Prerequisites

- **Bladder should be empty.** The only exception to the procedure is the presence of history suggestive of stress incontinence. If history is suggestive of chronic retention of urine, catheterisation should be done taking aseptic precautions, using sterile simple rubber catheter.
- The patient is to lie flat on the table with the thighs slightly flexed and abducted to make the abdominal muscles relaxed.
- The physician usually prefers to stand on the right side.

Actual steps :

- **Inspection**
- **Palpation**
- **Percussion**
- **Auscultation**

Inspection

The skin condition of the abdomen — presence of old scar, striae, prominent veins or eversion of the umbilicus is to be noted. By asking the patient to strain, one can elicit either incisional hernia or divarication of the rectus abdominis muscles. In intestinal obstruction, the abdomen is uniformly distended and the respiration is of thoracic type. In pelvic peritonitis, the lower abdomen is only distended with diminished inspiratory movements. In ascites, one can find fullness only in the flanks with the centre remaining flat. A huge pelvic tumour

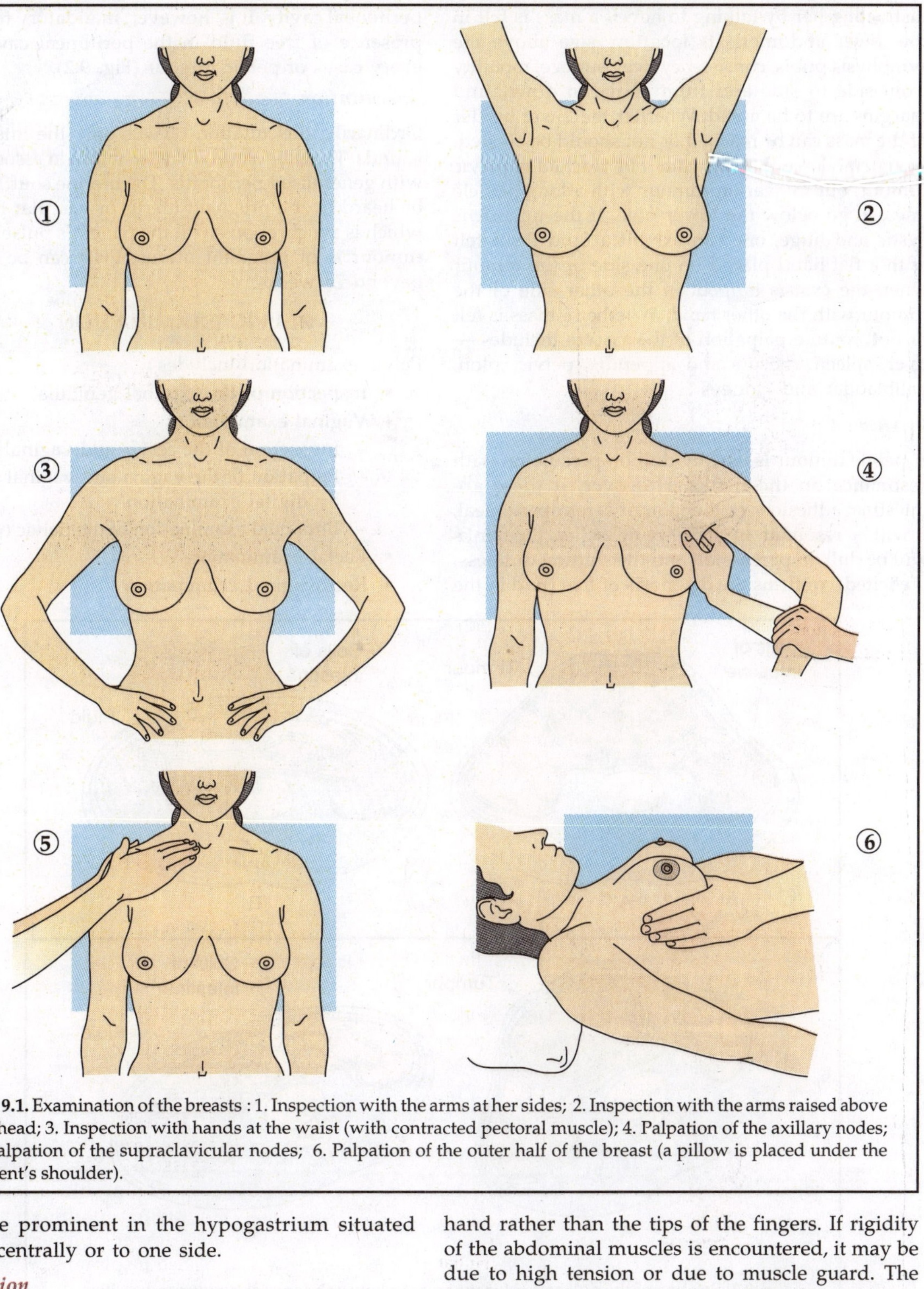

Fig. 9.1. Examination of the breasts : 1. Inspection with the arms at her sides; 2. Inspection with the arms raised above the head; 3. Inspection with hands at the waist (with contracted pectoral muscle); 4. Palpation of the axillary nodes; 5. Palpation of the supraclavicular nodes; 6. Palpation of the outer half of the breast (a pillow is placed under the patient's shoulder).

is more prominent in the hypogastrium situated either centrally or to one side.

Palpation

The palpation should be done with the flat of the hand rather than the tips of the fingers. If rigidity of the abdominal muscles is encountered, it may be due to high tension or due to muscle guard. The former may be overcome by asking the patient to take deep breaths with the mouth open or by distracting her by talking to her. If a mass is felt in the lower abdomen, its location, size above the symphysis pubis, consistency, feel, surface, mobility from side to side and from above to down, and margins are to be noted. Whether the lower border of the mass can be reached or not should be elicited. In general, lower border cannot be reached in pelvic tumour, but in ovarian tumour with a long pedicle one can go below the lower pole. If the tumour is cystic and huge, one can exhibit a fluid thrill–felt with a flat hand placed on one side of the tumour when the cyst is tapped on the other side of the tumour with the other hand. Whether a mass is felt or not, routine palpation of the viscera includes — liver, spleen, caecum and appendix, pelvic colon, gallbladder and kidneys.

Percussion

A pelvic tumour is usually dull on percussion with resonance on the flanks. However, if there are intestinal adhesions or the tumour is retroperitoneal, it will be resonant. In presence of ascites, the flanks will be dull on percussion and the shifting dullness, if elicited, confirms the diagnosis of free fluid in the peritoneal cavity. It is, however, mandatory to elicit presence of free fluid in the peritoneal cavity in every cases of pelvic tumour (Fig. 9.2).

Auscultation

Ordinarily, auscultation reveals only the intestinal sounds. These however, may be absent in association with generalised peritonitis. The uterine souffle may be heard over a pregnant uterus or vascular fibroid which is synchronous with the patient's pulse. If the tumour is of pregnant uterus, FHR can be heard beyond 24 weeks.

PELVIC EXAMINATION

Pelvic examination includes :

- Inspection of the external genitalia
- Vaginal examination
  - Inspection of the cervix and vaginal walls.
  - Palpation of the vagina and vaginal cervix by digital examination.
  - Bimanual examination of the pelvic organs.
- Rectal examination
- Rectovaginal examination

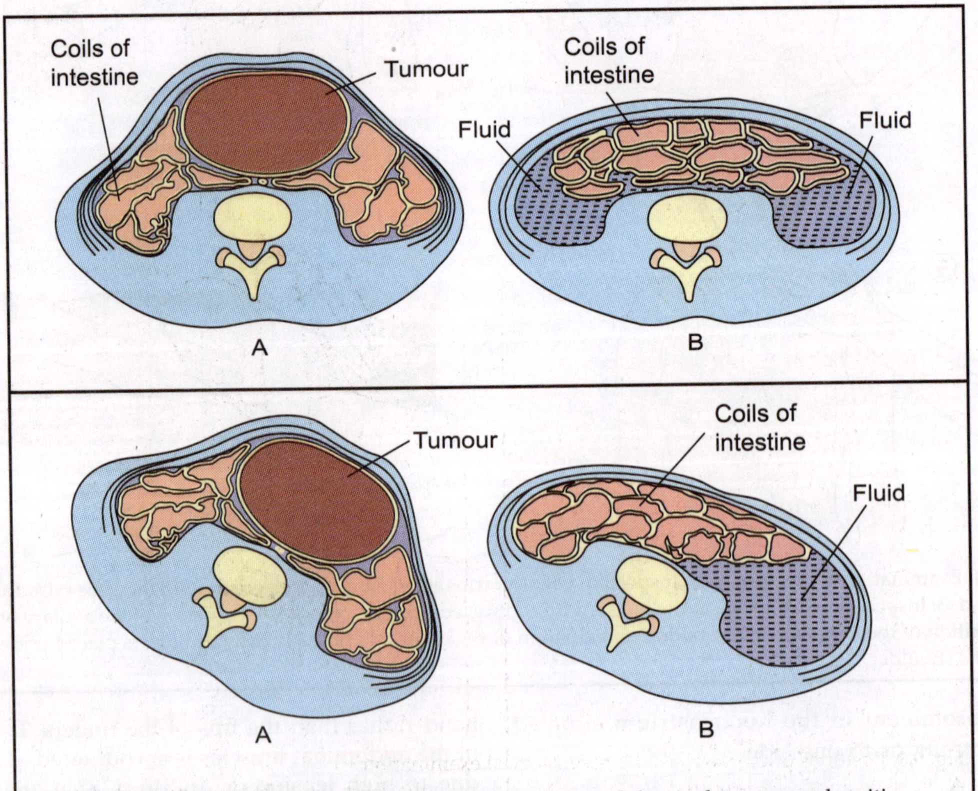

Fig. 9.2. Relation of the dull and resonant areas in lower abdominal tumour and ascities. **Upper figure** in dorsal position. **Lower figure** with patient in turned position.

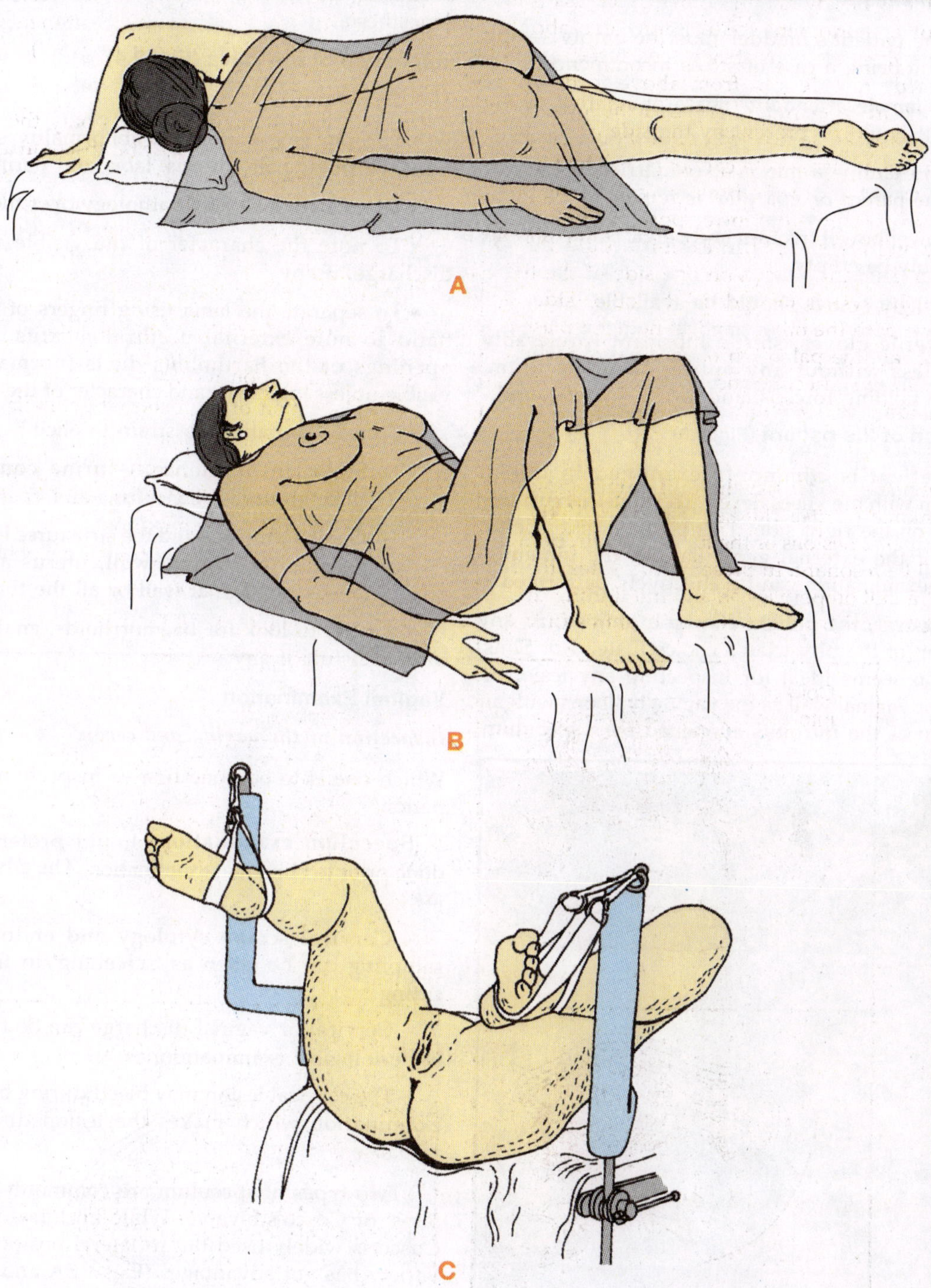

Fig. 9.3. Positions of the patient for gynaecological examination :
A. Sims' position — The patient lies on her left side with the chest, the right knee and thigh drawn up, the left arm along the back. B. Dorsal position. C. Lithotomy position.

Prerequisites

• The patient's bladder must be empty — the exception being a case of stress incontinence.

• A female attendant (nurse or relative of the patient) should be present by the side.

• To examine a minor or unmarried, a consent from the parent or guardian is required.

• Lower bowel (rectum and pelvic colon) should preferably be empty.

• A light source should be available.

• Sterile gloves, sterile lubricant (preferably colourless without any antiseptics), speculum, sponge holding forceps, and swabs, are required.

Position of the patient (Fig. 9.3)

The patient is commonly examined in dorsal position with the knees flexed. The physician usually stands on the right side. This position gives better view of the external genitalia and the bimanual pelvic examination can be effectively performed.

However, the patient can be examined, in any position of the physician's choice. Lateral or Sims' position seems ideal for inspecting any lesion in anterior vaginal wall as the vagina balloons with air as soon as the introitus is opened by a speculum.

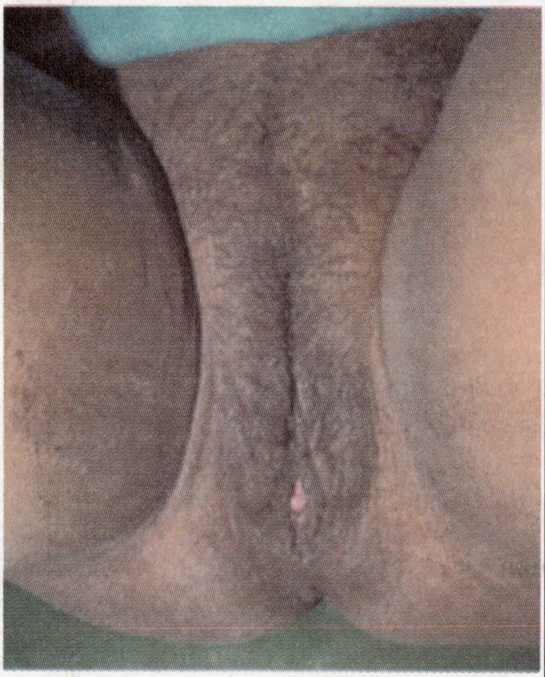

Fig. 9.4. Inspection of vulva in dorsal position

Lithotomy position is ideal for examination under anaesthesia.

Inspection of the vulva (Fig. 9.4)

This includes:

• To note any anatomical abnormality starting from the pubic hair, clitoris, labia and perineum.

• To note any palpable pathology over the areas.

• To note the character of the visible vaginal discharge, if any.

• To separate the labia using fingers of the left hand to note external urethral meatus, visible openings of the Bartholin's ducts (normally not visible unless inflamed) and character of the hymen.

• To ask the patient to strain to elicit :

- Stress incontinence — urine comes out through urethral meatus.
- Genital prolapse and the structures involved — anterior vaginal wall, uterus alone or posterior vaginal wall or all the three.

• Lastly, to look for haemorrhoids, anal fissure or anal fistula if any.

Vaginal Examination

Inspection of the vagina and cervix

Which one is to be done first — inspection or palpation?

Speculum examination should preferably be done prior to bimanual examination. **The advantages are :**

– Cervical scrape cytology and endocervical sampling can be taken as 'screening' in the same sitting.

– Cervical or vaginal discharge can be taken for bacteriological examination.

– The cervical lesion may bleed during bimanual examination which makes the lesion difficult to visualise.

Two types of speculum are commonly used — Sims' or Cusco's bivalve. While in dorsal position, Cusco is widely used but in lateral position, Sims' variety has got advantages (Figs 9.5A and B).

The cervix is best visualised with the Cusco's variety. But while the vaginal fornices are only visualised by Cusco, **the anterior vaginal wall is to be visualised by Sims' variety**. Sims' speculum is advantageous in cases of genital prolapse.

Apart from inspection, collection of the discharge from the cervix or from the vaginal fornices or from the external urethral meatus is taken for bacteriological examination.

It is a routine practice to take cervical scrape cytology and endocervical sampling for cytological examination in all patients in the advanced countries, and selected centres in the developing one as a screening procedure.

Digital examination

Digital examination is done using a gloved index finger lubricated with sterile lubricant. In virgins with intact hymen, this examination is withheld but can be employed under anaesthesia.

Palpation of any labial swelling (commonly Bartholin's cyst or abscess) is made with the finger placed internally and thumb placed externally (Fig. 9.6). The urethra is now pressed from above down for any discharge escaping out through the meatus.

Palpation of the vaginal walls is to be done from below upwards to detect any abnormality either in the wall or in the adjacent structures.

The vaginal cervix is next palpated to note :

- Direction — In anteverted uterus, the anterior lip is felt first and in retroverted position either the external os or the posterior lip is felt first.
- Station — Normally the external os is at the level of ischial spines.
- Texture — In nonpregnant state, it feels firm like tip of the nose.
- Shape — It is conical with smooth surface in nulliparae but cylindrical in parous.
- External os — It is smooth and round in nulliparous but may be dilated with evidence of tear in parous women.
- Movement — painful or not.
- Whether it bleeds to touch.

Integrity and tone of the perineal body are to be elicited by flexing the internal finger posteriorly and palpating the perineal body between the internal finger and the thumb placed externally. The finger is now turned laterally above the level of levator

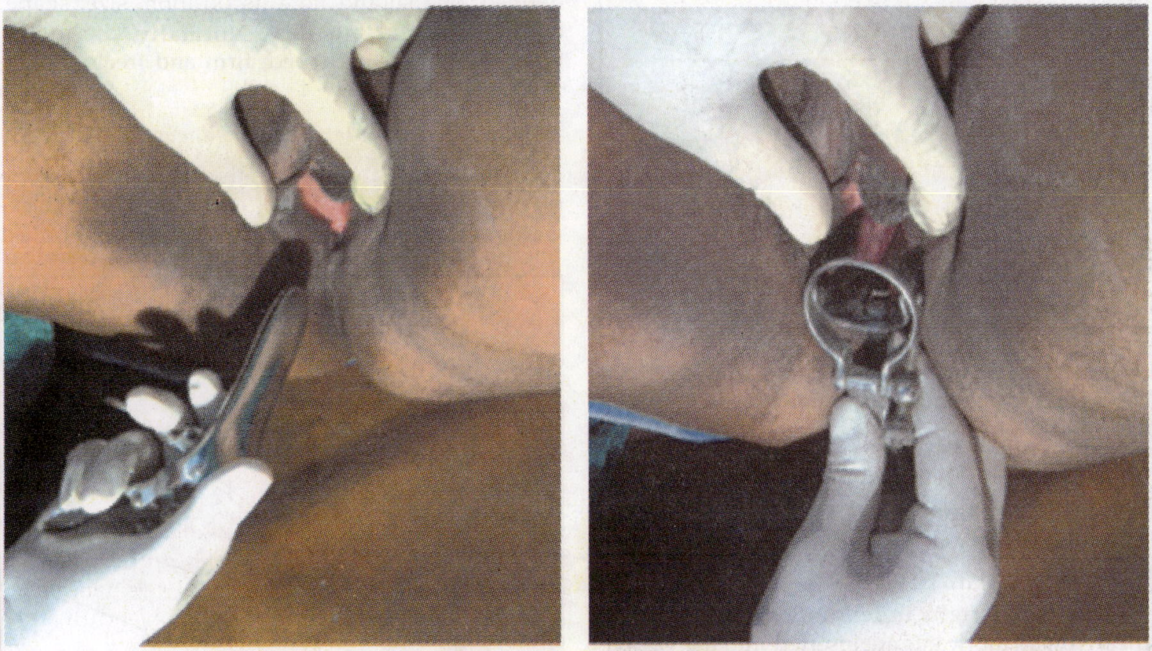

A B

Figs. 9.5A and B. Introduction of Cusco's speculum : A – Vertical with blades closed and slightly oblique to minimise pressure on the urethra. B – Rotate to 90° and then open up the blades

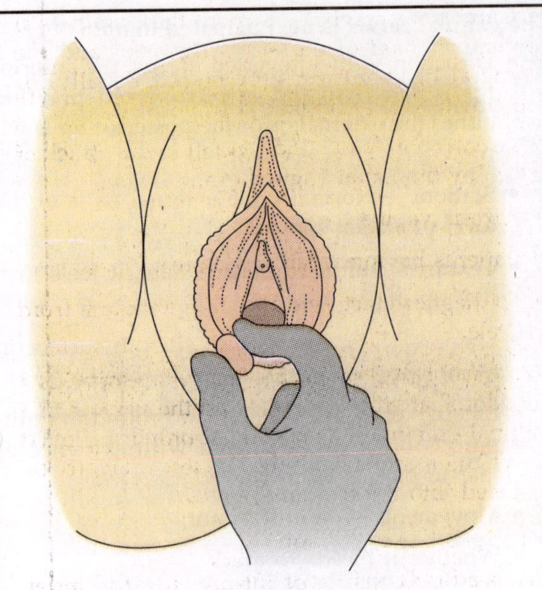

Fig. 9.6. Palpation of a labial swelling *(Bartholin's gland)*

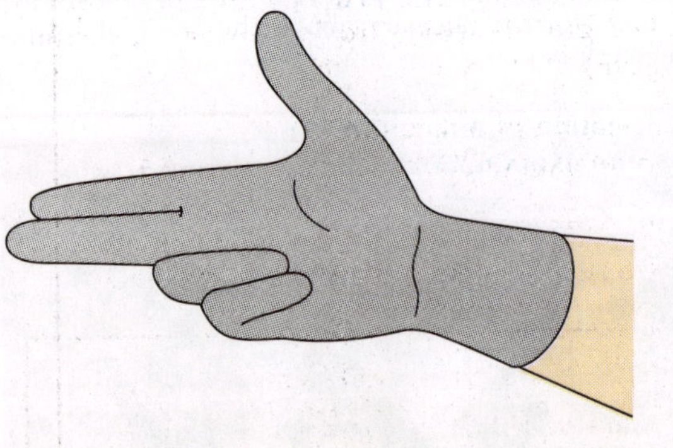

Fig. 9.7. Position of the fingers during bimanual examination

ani muscles. The muscles can be palpated between the vaginal finger and the thumb placed externally over the labium majus.

Bimanual Examination

The techniques are difficult to describe in words but perfectness will be achieved only through experience.

The gloved right index and middle fingers smeared with lubricants are inserted into the vagina. If the introitus is narrow or tender, one finger may be used. The relative position of the fingers during introduction is shown in Figure 9.7. The left hand is placed on the hypogastrium well above the symphysis pubis so that the pelvic organs can be palpated between them. **The examination should be methodical, gentle but purposeful**. To be more informative, abdominal hand is to be used more than the vaginal fingers and the patient is asked to breathe through the mouth for better relaxation of the abdominal muscles.

The information obtained by bimanual examination includes :

- Palpation of the uterus
- Palpation of the uterine appendages
- Pouch of Douglas.

Palpation of the uterus

The two internal fingers which are placed in the anterior fornix exert a pushing force at the uterocervical junction in an upward direction towards the lumbar vertebrae and not towards the symphysis pubis. The pressure exerted by the left hand should be not only downwards but from behind forwards (Fig. 9.8). The uterine outline between the two hands can thus be palpated clearly as anteverted. If the uterus is retroverted, it will not be so felt but can be felt if the internal fingers push up the uterus through the posterior fornix. After the uterine outline is defined, one should note its position, size, shape, consistency and mobility. **Normally**, the uterus is anteverted, pear-shaped, firm and freely mobile in all directions.

Palpation of the uterine appendages

For palpation of the adnexa, the vaginal fingers are placed in the lateral fornix and are pushed backwards and upwards. The counter pressure is applied

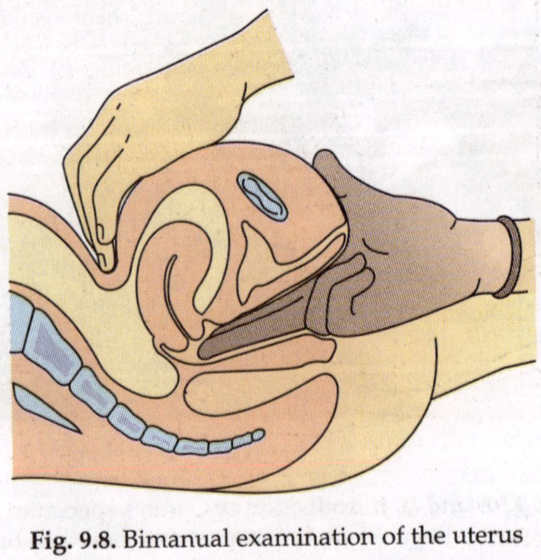

Fig. 9.8. Bimanual examination of the uterus

by the abdominal hand placed to one side of the uterus in a backward direction. **The normal uterine tube cannot be palpated.** A normal ovary may not be felt. If it is palpable, it is mobile and sensitive to manual pressure.

The pouch of Douglas

The pouch of Douglas can be examined effectively through the posterior fornix. Normally, the faecal mass in the rectosigmoid or else the body of a retroverted uterus is only felt. Some pathology detected in the pouch of Douglas should be supplemented by rectal examination.

Rectal or Rectoabdominal Examination

Rectal examination can be done in isolation or as an adjunct to vaginal examination.

It is indicated in :

- Children or in adult virgins.
- Painful vaginal examination.

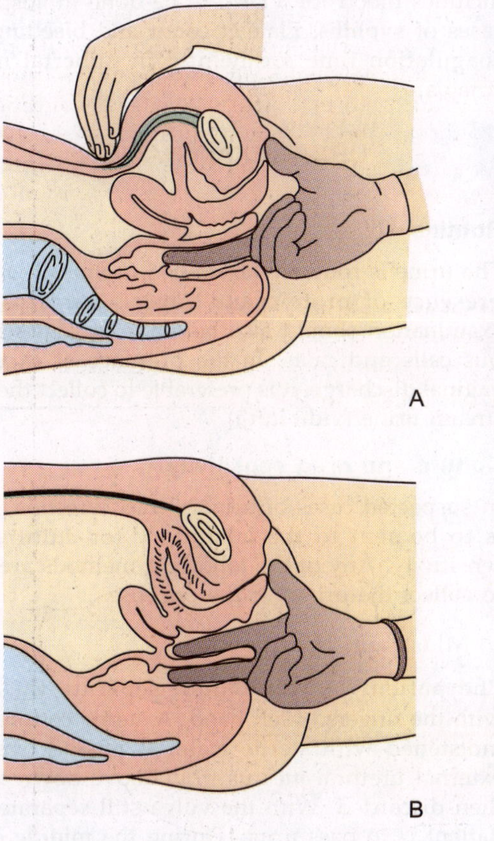

Figs. 9.9A and B. Rectoabdominal (A) and Rectovaginal examination (B)

- Carcinoma cervix — to note the parametrial involvement (base of the broad ligament and the uterosacral ligament can only be felt rectally) or involvement of the rectum.
- To corroborate the findings felt in the pouch of Douglas by bimanual vaginal examination.
- Atresia vagina.
- Patients having rectal symptoms.
- To diagnose rectocele and differentiate it from enterocele.

The lower bowel should preferably be empty. The rectoabdominal procedure is almost the same as that of vaginal examination except that only the gloved index finger smeared with vaseline is to be introduced into the rectum (Fig. 9.9A).

Rectovaginal examination

The procedure consists of introducing the index finger in the vagina and the middle finger in the rectum. This examination may help to determine whether the lesion is in the bowel or between the rectum and vagina. **This is of special help** to differentiate a growth arising from the ovary or rectum (Fig. 9.9B).

Identification of a mass felt on bimanual examination

Uterine tumour **(Fig. 9.10)**

- Uterus is not separated from the mass.

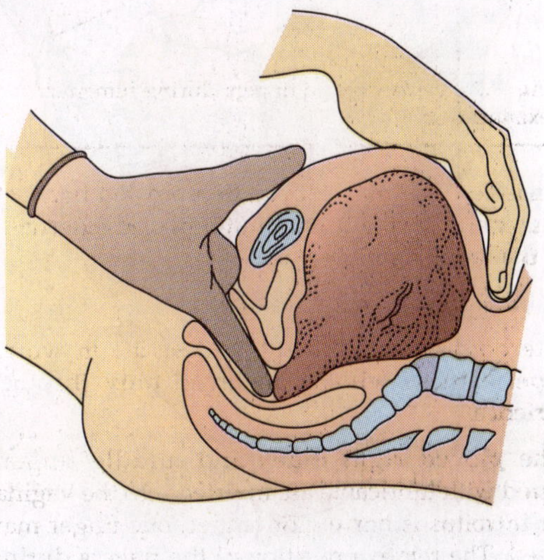

Fig. 9.10. Identification of an uterine tumour in bimanual examination

• Movements of the mass felt per abdomen are transmitted to the cervix and *vice versa,* the exception being one of subserous pedunculated fibroid.

Adnexal mass

• The uterus is separated from the mass (Figs. 9.11 and 9.12).

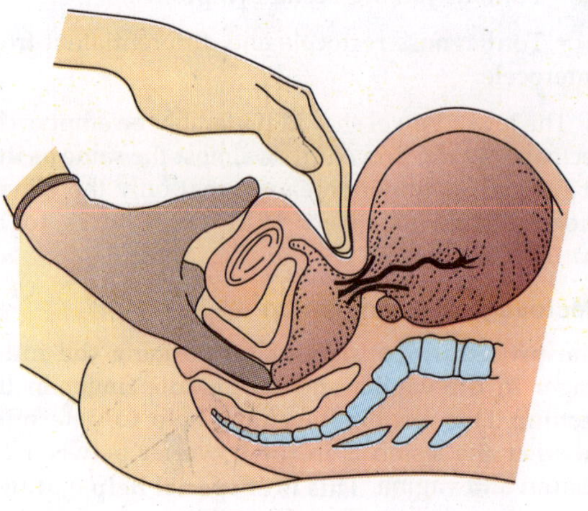

Fig. 9.11. Identification of ovarian tumour in bimanual examination

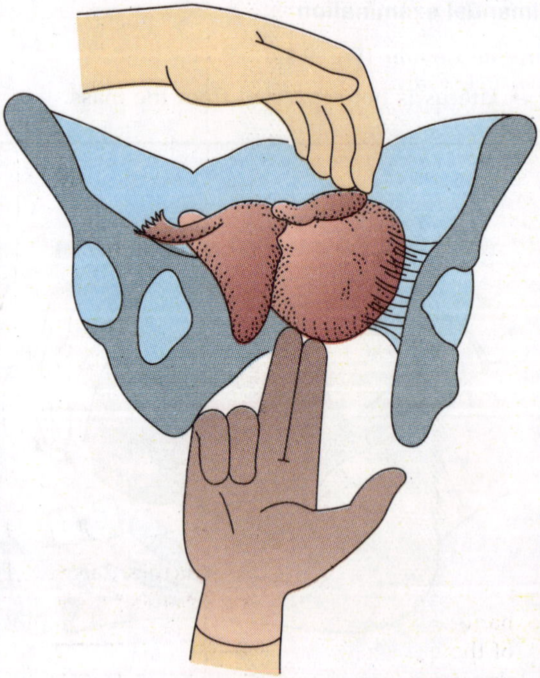

Fig. 9.12. Identification of an adnexal mass in bimanual examination

• Movements of the mass (tumour) are not transmitted to the cervix, the exception being one if the mass is fixed with uterus.

ANCILLARY AIDS TO CLINICAL DIAGNOSIS

A meticulous history and methodical examinations as mentioned earlier in the chapter most often help the clinician to arrive at a diagnosis. For confirmation of diagnosis or rarely in cases with confused diagnosis, ancillary aids are required. Their application should be judiciously executed considering the surrounding the patients are placed in.

BLOOD VALUES

Haemoglobin estimation should be done in all cases of excessive bleeding. Total and differential count of white cells and ESR are helpful in diagnosis of pelvic inflammation. Serological investigation includes blood for VDRL to be done in suspected cases of syphilis. Platelet count and bleeding and coagulation time are helpful in pubertal menorrhagia.

URINE EXAMINATION

Routine

The urine is routinely examined chemically for the presence of protein and sugar. A microscopic examination should also be made for detection of pus cells and casts. In the presence of excessive vaginal discharge, it is preferable to collect the midstream urine (vide infra).

Culture and drug sensitivity

In suspected cases of urinary tract infection, urine is to be sent to the laboratory for culture and sensitivity. Any of the following methods are used to collect the urine for the purpose.

(i) Midstream collection

The patient herself should separate the labia with the fingers of left hand. A sterile cotton swab moistened with sterile water is passed over the external urethral meatus from above down and is then discarded. With the vulva still separated the patient is to pass urine. During the middle of the act of micturition, a part of urine is collected in a sterile wide mouth container.

(ii) Catheter collection

This should be collected by a doctor or a nurse. This is specially indicated when the patient is not ambulant or having chronic retention. **Meticulous washing of the hands with soap and wearing sterile gloves are mandatory.** The patient is in dorsal position with the thighs apart. The labia are separated using the fingers of left hand. A sterile cotton swab moistened with sterile water is passed from above down over the external urethral meatus. The sterile autoclaved rubber catheter or a disposable plastic catheter is to be introduced with the proximal 4 cm remaining untouched by the fingers. With meticulous asepsis, the technique does not increase urinary tract infection (Figs. 9.13A and B).

(iii) Suprapubic bladder puncture

In many centres, it is now done in preference to other methods of collection of urine. The result is more reliable and bladder infection is minimum. The patient is asked not to void urine to make the bladder full. A fine needle fitted with a syringe is passed through the abdominal wall just above the symphysis pubis into the bladder. About 5-10 ml of urine is collected. **The patient is asked to void the urine immediately**.

Whatever method employed in the collection of urine, **the sample should be sent immediately to the laboratory.** There may be multiplication of the organisms with time.

URETHRAL DISCHARGE

With a sterile gloved finger, the urethra is squeezed against the symphysis pubis from behind forwards. The discharge through the external urethral meatus is collected with sterile swabs. One swab may be sent for culture and the other to be spread on to a slide, stained and examined under microscope.

VAGINAL OR CERVICAL DISCHARGE

The patient is advised not to have vaginal douche at least in previous 24 hours. **Cusco's bivalve**

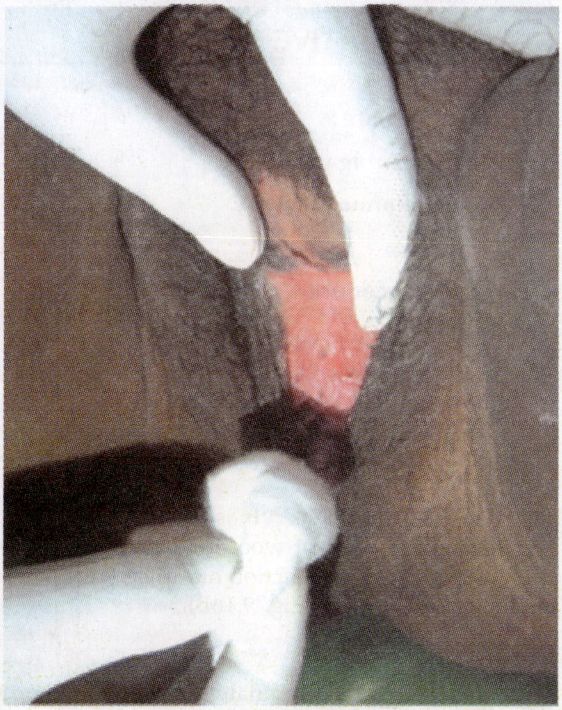

Fig. 9.13(A). Methods of catheterisation by rubber catheter. Cleansing of the vestibule from above down by a moist swab

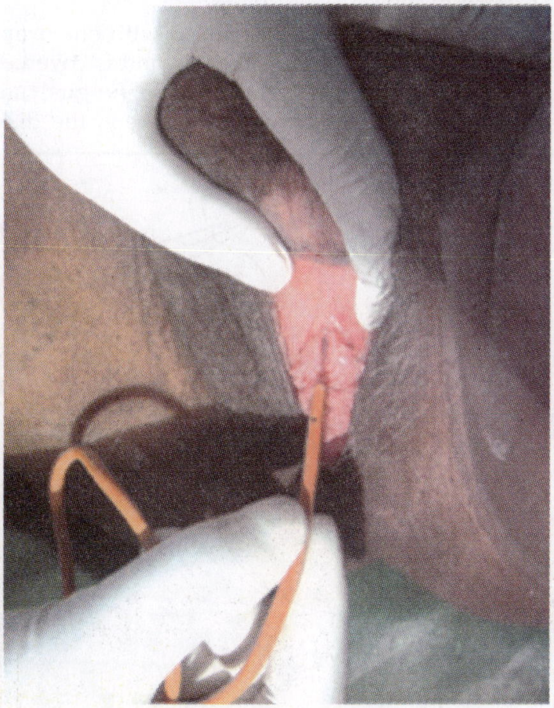

Fig. 9.13(B). Note the use of left fingers for disposition of the external urethral meatus and holding the catheter well away from the tip by the right hand

speculum is introduced without lubricant and prior to internal examination. The material collected in the posterior blade or from the cervical canal as the case may be, is taken either by a platinum loop or swab stick.

For culture

The cotton swab stick is put in a sterile container with a stopper and to be sent immediately to the laboratory. The culture is usually unnecessary in vaginal infection. For trichomoniasis, Kupferberg's media or Feinberg Whittington media; for *Candida albicans* — Nickerson's or Sabouraud's media is used.

Identification of organism in slide

(a) Trichomonas vaginalis

The material is dropped over a slide and then mixed with one drop of normal saline. It is then covered with a coverslip. Actively motile trichomonads can be seen under microscope easily (Fig. 9.14). It can be effectively visualised after staining with 1 per cent brilliant cresyl violet; leucocytes and other bacteria will not take up the dye.

(b) Monilia

One drop of the discharge is mixed with one drop of 10 per cent potassium hydroxide and is covered with a coverslip. The mycelia of the fungus can be seen under microscope. Alternatively, the discharge is spread over a slide, dried and stained with methylene blue to demonstrate the mycelia (Fig. 9.15).

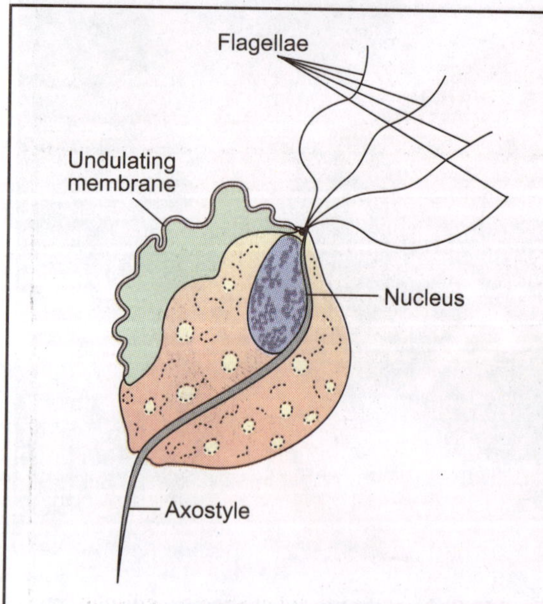

Fig. 9.14. Identification of organism in slide — Trichomonas vaginalis

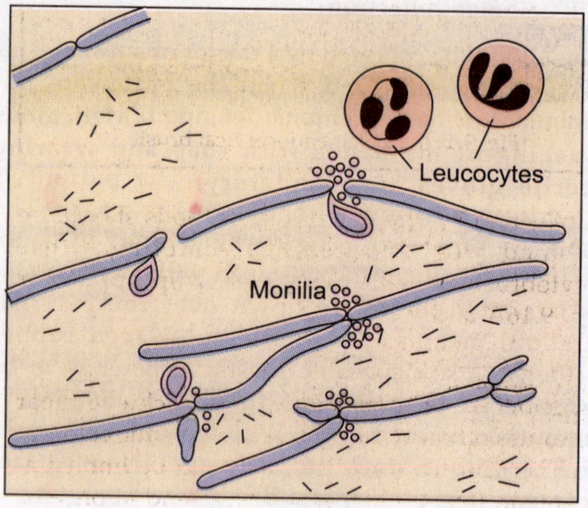

Fig. 9.15. Identification of organism in slide — Monilia

CERVICAL AND VAGINAL SMEAR FOR EXFOLIATIVE CYTOLOGY

The indications are :

- **As a screening procedure**
- **For cytohormonal study**
- **Others**

Screening procedure

Collection of material

The cervix is exposed with a vaginal speculum without lubricant and prior to bimanual examination. Lubricants tend to distort cell morphology.

Cervical scraping

The material from the cervix is best collected using Ayre's spatula made of wood or plastic. Whole of the squamocolumnar junction has to be scrapped to obtain good material (Fig. 9.16B).

Vaginal pool aspiration

The exfoliated cells accumulated in the vaginal pool in the posterior fornix is collected either using a glass pipette about 15 cm long and 0.5 cm in diameter with a strong rubber bulb at one end or by a swab stick. This is not much reliable.

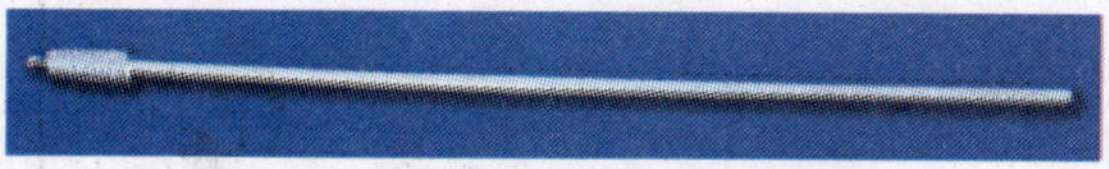

Fig. 9.16A. Rocket endocervical brush

Collection by any one of the methods should be combined with endocervical sampling either by cytobrush or with moist cotton tip applicator (Figs. 9.16A and 9.16B).

Fixation and staining

The principle of the staining is to achieve clear nuclear definition and to define cytoplasmic colouration. The material so collected should be immediately spread over a microscopic slide and at once be put into the fixative ethyl alcohol (95%) before drying. After fixing for about 30 minutes, the slide is taken out, air dried and sent to the laboratory with proper identification. The slide so sent is stained either with Papanicolaou's or Sorr's method and examined by a trained cytologist. Indeed, **trained cytopathologist and cytotechnologist are vital for the success of any screening programme**.

Benefits : The objective of screening is to reduce the incidence and mortality from cervical cancer. Even a single smear in a life time, if appropriately timed, will produce some benefits. If extended only to high-risk group, the mortality from the cancer deaths will still be reduced to 60 per cent.

Pap smear test has been effective reducing the incidence of cervical cancer by 80% and the mortality by 70%. As a result of Pap test, more and more

Table 9.1

Women subjected to cervical cancer screening programme

	Screening schedule
• ***Low risk***	
– Women who had never been sexually active. – Women aged 70, who had three negative smears in the past 10 years. – Women who had hysterectomy for benign lesion.	Nil
• ***At risk***	
– Women aged 21 years or having sex for last 3 years upto the age of 70 who are or have been sexually active.	Every 2-3 years after 3 negative yearly smears
• ***High risk***	
– Early marriage – Early intercourse – Early pregnancy – Smoking habits – Oral pill users – Multiple sexual partners – Human papilloma virus (p. 312) infection – Women who are immuno-suppressed (HIV positive).	Every 2-3 years after 3 negative yearly smears

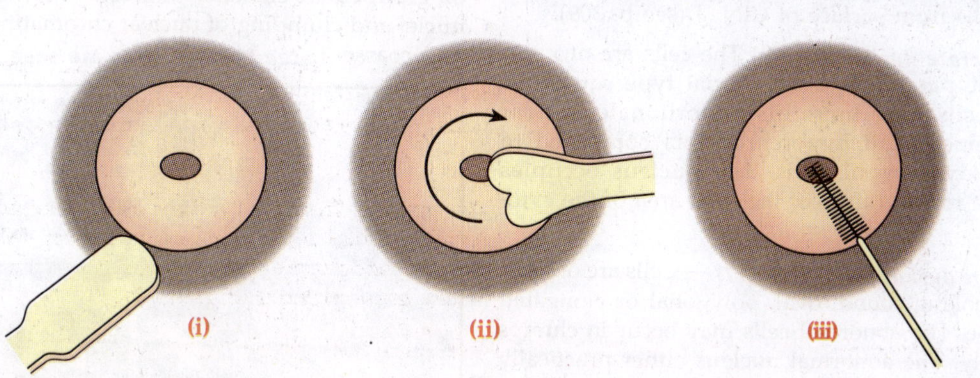

Fig. 9.16B. Collection of smear — (i) : By wooden spatula from the lateral vaginal fornix for cytohormonal study. (ii) : By Ayre's spatula from the squamocolumnar junction for screening. (iii) : By cytobrush taking endocervical sampling for screening

preinvasive carcinoma is detected. Opportunistic screening done by a trained staff is effective when follow up (call and recall) is maintained. Pap testing after total hysterectomy, done for benign lesion is not recommended.

Intervals : All sexually active women should be screened starting from the age of 21 years or after 3 years of vaginal sex upto the age of 70. Screening should be yearly till the age of 30. Thereafter, it should be at the interval of every 2-3 years after three consecutive yearly negative smears (ACOG 2003). The high risk group should be screened with **HPV DNA testing combined with cytology (p. 311)**. **The negative predictive value of one negative HPV DNA test and two negative cytology tests are almost 100%**. When both the tests are negative, the screening interval may be increased to 6 years.

Morphological abnormalities of the nucleus (Dyskaryosis)

- Disproportionate nuclear enlargement.
- Irregularity of the nuclear outline.
- Abnormalities of the nucleus — in number, size and shape.
- Hyperchromasia.
- Condensation of chromatin material.
- Multinucleation.

Abnormal cells are :

Mild dyskaryosis — Cells are of superficial or intermediate type squamous cells. Cells have angular borders with translucent cytoplasm. The nucleus occupies less than half of the total area of cytoplasm. Binucleation is common. Mild dyskaryosis correlates with cells from surface of CIN I (see p. 309).

Moderate dyskaryosis — The cells are of intermediate, parabasal or superficial type squamous cells. Cells have more disproportionate nuclear enlargement and hyperchromasia compared to mildly dyskaryotic cells. The nucleus occupies one half to two-thirds of the total area of the cytoplasm.

***Severe dyskaryosis* (Fig. 9.17)** — Cells are of basal type, looking round, oval, polygonal or elongated in shape. The abnormal cells may occur in clumps or singly. The abnormal nucleus either practically fills the cell or there may be a thick, dense and narrow rim of cytoplasm around it. The nucleus is irregular with coarse chromatin pattern. The cells may be different in size and shape. Severely dyskaryotic cells when elongated, are sometimes called **fibre cells**. A severely dyskaryotic cell with an elongated tail of cytoplasm is described as a **tadpole cell**. Severely dyskaryotic cells correlate with CIN 3.

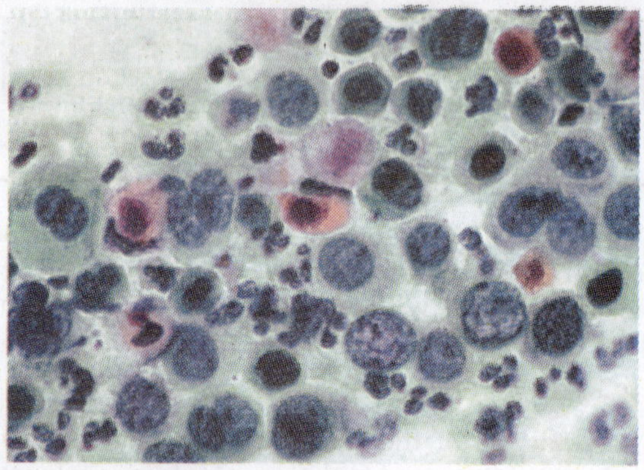

Fig. 9.17. Severe dyskaryosis

Koilocytosis is the nuclear abnormalities associated with human papilloma virus infection. Cells show typical central clearing (perinuclear halo) with peripheral condensation of cytoplasm. The nucleus is irregulary enlarged and shows hyperchromasia with multinucleation. Patients with koilocytosis on repeated smear, need colposcopic evaluation (see p. 112).

***Carcinoma in situ* (Fig. 9.18)** — Cells are parabasal type with increased nuclear cytoplasmic ratio. The nucleus may be irregular sometimes multiple. The chromatin pattern is granular. Cytoplasm is scanty.

***Invasive carcinoma* (Fig. 9.19)** — Cells are single or grouped in clusters. The cells show irregular nuclei and clumping of nuclear chromatin which is also coarse. **Large tadpole cells are seen.**

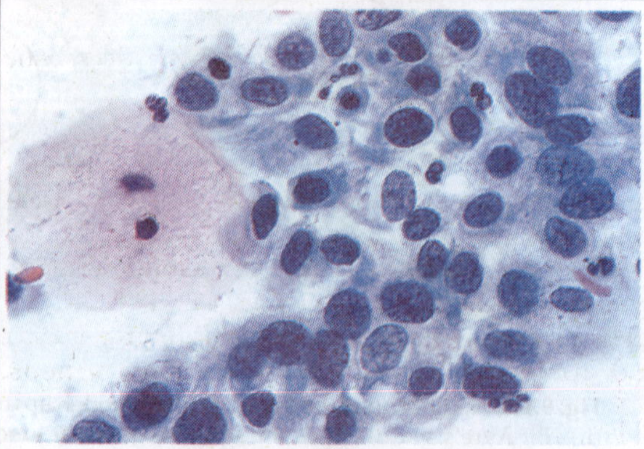

Fig. 9.18. Carcinoma *in situ*

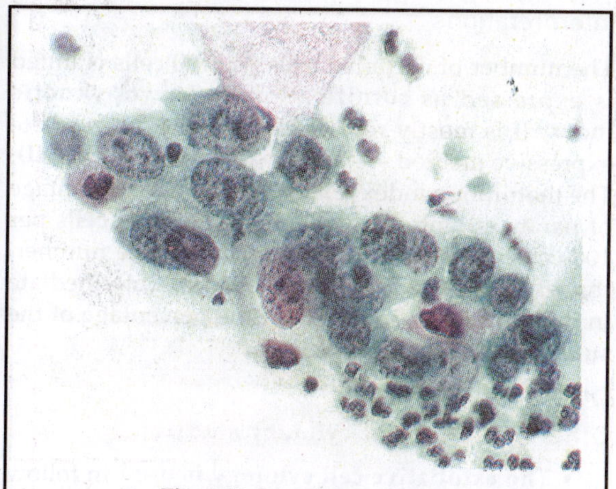

Fig. 9.19. Invasive carcinoma

Reporting system : Reporting system on the grading basis (Papanicolaou's) is replaced by some with two remarks only — normal or abnormal (Table 9.2). An abnormal smear indicates the presence of lesion either CIN and/or papilloma virus infection or invasive malignancy. A doubtful or inconclusive smear dictates repeat smear.

Table 9.2
Papanicolaou's grading

Group – I	—	Normal
Group – II	—	Presence of borderline atypical cells — probably due to infection. No evidence of malignancy.
Group – III	—	Cells suspicious of malignancy.
Group – IV	—	Presence of few malignant cells.
Group – V	—	Presence of large number of malignant cells.

Accuracy : A single Pap smear has a diagnostic sensitivity of about 60 per cent. **False-negative rate of Pap smear after three consecutive negative tests is less than 1 per cent.** There are several reasons for false-negative smear. This may be due to technical error where smear is too scanty, too thick, too bloody, poorly stained or due to misinterpretation by the cytologist. Error in cytology could be reduced further by liquid-based thin layer slide preparation and automated (computer) screening methods. **Abnormal cytology is an indication of colposcopic evaluation and directed biopsy.** If colposcopy is not available, biopsy is to be taken from the unstained areas following **application of Schiller's or Lugol's iodine** (see Ch. 22). In the presence of infection, repeat cytology has to be done after the infection is controlled.

Liquid-based Cytology (LBC)

Cervical smear is taken using a plastic spatula. The spatula is rinsed in a buffered methanol solution. Cells are separated by centrifugation. Thin layer smears are made. National Institute of Clinical Excellence (NICE) has recommended to replace the conventional smear with LBC. LBC avoids the risk of false-positive, false-negative or unsatisfactory smears.

Comparison of different classification system

Papanicolaou (1943)	CIN (WHO 1975)	SIL (Bethesda 1988)
I	Normal	Normal
II	Inflammatory	Infection • HPV • ASCOUS
III	CIN I	Low SIL
	CIN II	
	CIN III	High SIL
IV	CIS	
V	SCC	SCC

CIN = Cervical intraepithelial neoplasia (see p. 309)
SIL = Squamous intraepithelial lesion (see p. 309)
SCC = Squamous cell carcinoma
ASCOUS = Atypical squamous cell of undetermined significance.

Cytohormonal study

The vaginal epithelium is highly sensitive to the hormones oestrogen and progesterone. The non-invasive study of the epithelium for hormonal status is steadily increasing owing to the speed, cheapness and accuracy.

Instructions to the patient

- To avoid intercourse for about 48 hours.
- Not to use vaginal douche for 24 hours.
- To withhold use of hormonal drugs.

Procedures

The lateral wall of the upper-third of the vagina (most sensitive to hormonal influence) is lightly scraped with a wooden spatula after taking due precautions mentioned earlier. The material so collected is to be fixed and stained as mentioned earlier. **The physician should mention the following information** such as age, first day of the last period, menstrual pattern and any hormone therapy.

Inferences

The exfoliated vaginal epithelial cells normally include parabasal, intermediate and superficial cells. The parabasal cells are small, round and basophilic; the intermediate cells are transparent and basophilic while the superficial cells are large, thin acidophilic with pyknotic nuclei. The oestrogen produces superficial cell maturation; progesterone, androgen, corticosteroids, 'pill' and pregnancy produce intermediate cell maturation, whereas lack of any hormonal activity produces parabasal cell dominance (Table 9.3).

The oestrogenic smear is suggested by preponderance of large eosinophilic cells with pyknotic nuclei (cornified cells). The background remains clear (Fig. 8.11).

The progesterone smear is of predominantly basophilic cells with vesicular nuclei. The background looks dirty (Fig. 8.11).

Interpretations

The number of cornified cells per 100 cells counted is expressed as **cornification or karyopyknotic index**. It is mostly replaced by a more appropriate expressive method — called **maturation index (MI)**. The maturation index relates the relative percentage of parabasal, intermediate and superficial cells per 100 cells counted. It is expressed in three number, the left one parabasal percentage, the intermediate in the centre and on the right, the percentage of the superficial cells (Table 9.3).

Others

Other indications of cytology study are :

- **The exfoliative cell cytology is used** in follow up cases of carcinoma cervix treated either by surgery or radiotherapy.
- **Sex chromatin study** — The materials are from scraping of buccal mucosa and to be stained with Papanicolaou stain. The presence of Barr body in more than 25 per cent cells is diagnostic of female sex.
- **Aspirated** ascitic, cystic or pleural fluid is subjected to Papanicolaou stain for evidences of malignant cells.

Table 9.3

Maturation index from birth to menopause

	MI	Smear features	Inference
At birth	0/95/5	—	Combined effect of circulating maternal hormones — oestrogen, progesterone and corticoids.
Childhood	80/20/0	—	MI shifting to left because of diminished steroid hormones.
Reproductive period :			
– Preovulatory	0/40/60	Smear clear, cells are discrete.	Oestrogen ++
– Mid secretory	0/70/30	Smear dirty, cells in clusters.	Oestrogen + Progesterone ++
– During pregnancy	0/95/5	Marked folding of the intermediate cells–'navicular cells'.	Oestrogen ++ Progesterone ++ Corticosteroids +
– Postpartum	100/0/0	—	Parabasal maturation
Postmenopausal	0/100/0 or 100/0/0	—	Lack of oestrogen

EXAMINATION OF CERVICAL MUCUS

- **Bacteriological study** • **Hormonal status**
- **Infertility investigation**

Bacteriological study

Cusco's bivalve speculum is introduced without lubricant. With the help of a sterile cotton swab, the cervical canal is swabbed. The material is either sent for culture or spread over a microscopic slide for Gram staining.

Hormonal status

The physical, chemical and cellular components of the cervical secretion are dependent on hormones — oestrogen and progesterone. Oestrogen increases the water and electrolyte content with decrease in protein. As such, the mucus becomes copious, clear and thin. Progesterone, on the other hand, decreases the water and electrolytes but increases the protein. As a result, the mucus becomes scanty, thick and tenacious. The influence of the hormones on the cervical mucus is utilised in detection of ovulation in clinical practice.

- pH around the time of ovulation is about 6.8–7.4.

- **Spinnbarkeit** (stretchability or elasticity) — During the midcycle, the cervical secretion is collected with a pipette and placed over a glass slide. Another glass slide is placed over it. Because of increased elasticity due to high oestrogen level during this period, the mucus placed between the slides **can withstand stretching upto a distance of over 10 cm.** After ovulation when corpus luteum forms, progesterone is secreted. Under its action, the cervical mucus looses its property of elasticity and while attempting the above procedure, the mucus fractures when put under tension much earlier. **This loss of elasticity after its presence in the midcycle is the indirect evidence of ovulation.**

- **Fern test** — During the midcycle, the cervical mucus is obtained by a platinum loop or pipette and spread on a clean glass slide and dried. When seen under low power microscope, it shows characteristic pattern of fern formation. **It is due to high sodium chloride** and low protein content in the mucus due to high oestrogen in the midmenstrual phase prior to ovulation. After ovulation with increasing progesterone, the ferning disappears completely after 21st day. **Thus, the presence of ferning even after 21st day suggests anovulation and its disappearance is presumptive evidence of ovulation (Fig. 9.20).**

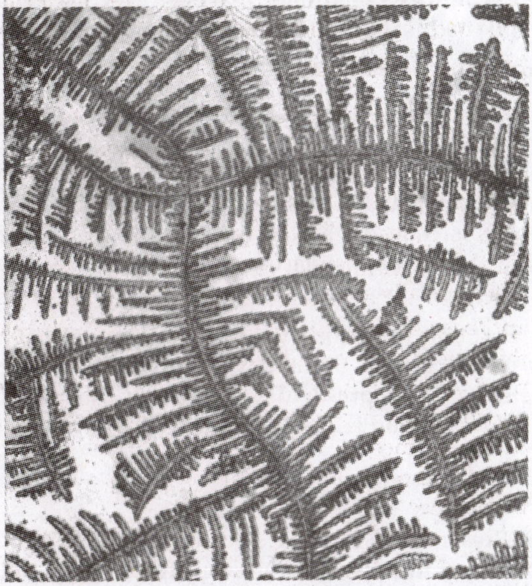

Fig. 9.20. Fern tree appearance of cervical mucus

The cervical scoring system of Insler (1979) takes into the account of amount, spinnbarkeit, ferning of the mucus along with state of the external os of the cervix. A score of 10-12 indicates complete follicular maturation.

Infertility investigations

Postcoital test (PCT) — Marion Sims (1866) and Max Huhner (1913)

Cervical mucous is a glycoprotein gel with interstitial channel between mucin strands. These strands expand and contract in response to steroid hormones. This helps sperm transport upwards (see Fig. 16.4).

Principle

Spermatozoa are able to penetrate the cervical mucus during the late proliferative and early secretory phase of menstrual cycles — a span of about 6 days. Best time to perform the test is on day 12 or 13 in a regular 28 day cycle (1-2 days before ovulation).

Prerequisites

- To avoid intercourse for 2 days.
- To avoid intravaginal medication or douching on the day preceding the test.

- The material should preferably be examined within 8-12 hours of intercourse.

Collection of material

The patient should report to the clinic preferably within 8-12 hours following intercourse. The cervix is exposed with a Cusco's speculum. Using a polythelene catheter attached to syringe, the endocervical mucus is collected and placed over a warm glass slide. A coverslip is placed over it and is examined microscopically under high power.

Best time to perform the test is on the day before or on the day of the midcycle urinary LH surge. Detection of a pre-ovulatory follicle by transvaginal ultrasound is also helpful for proper timing of PCT.

Inferences

(1) **Presence of at least 10 progressively motile sperm per high power field signifies the test to be normal.** The count, however, decreases with passing of time. It signifies adequate sperm count with good quality, good coital technique without any evidence of cervical hostility.

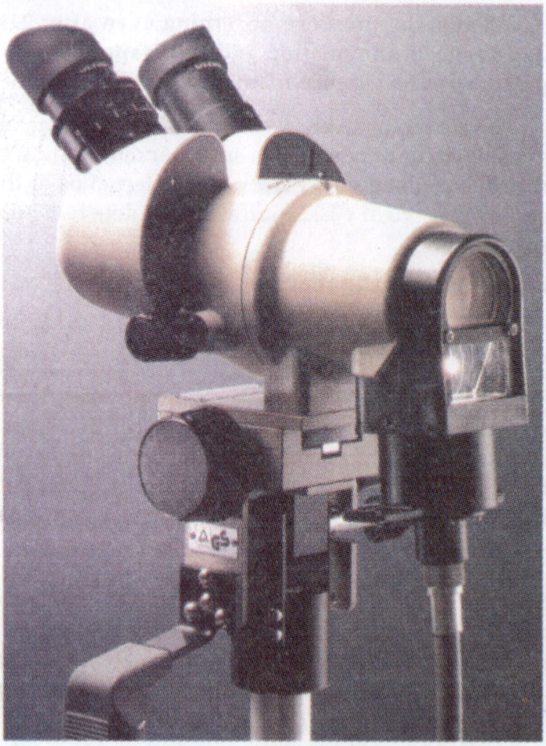

Fig. 9.21. Colposcope

Technique of colposcopy needs ease of maneuver (frontal distance of 225 to 250 mm), magnification (6-16 times), adequate light source (30,000 lux), the stand to permit mobility and the examination table for patient's comfort.

(2) Absence of any sperm signifies either aspermia or imperfect coital techniques and the test should be repeated and examined within 2-4 hours of intercourse **(early PCT)**.

(3) Presence of immotile sperm with a normal sperm count in a good quality of cervical mucus signifies presence of immunological factors (sperm antibodies). This requires confirmation by either detection of antisperm antibody in the serum or by sperm penetration test, known as, Sperm Cervical Mucus Contact Test (SCMCT) — see p. 232.

Limitations of Postcoital Test

PCT has got poor predictive value. It has neither improved the treatment of infertility nor the outcome in terms of conception. The test procedure is inconvenient and embarrassing also. Routine postcoital test is not recommended.

COLPOSCOPY

The instrument was devised by Hinselmann in 1925. Colposcope and colpomicroscope are sophisticated and complicated instruments. It is designed to magnify the surface epithelium of the vaginal part of the cervix including entire transformation zone. The magnification is to the extent of 15-40 times in colposcopy and about 100-300 times in colpomicroscopy (Fig. 9.21).

Procedure : The patient is placed in lithotomy position. The cervix is visualised using a Cusco's speculum (Fig. 9.5). Colposcopic examination of the cervix and vagina is done using low power magnification (6-16 fold). Cervix is then cleared of any mucous discharge using a swab soaked with normal saline. Green filter and high magnification can be used now. Next, the cervix is wiped gently with 3 per cent acetic acid and examination repeated. Acetic acid causes coagulation of nuclear protein which is high in CIN. This prevents transmission of light through the epithelium which is visible as white (acetowhite) areas. **The important selective groups to be examined are** :

1. Women with abnormal smears.

2. Women with clinically suspicious cervices specially with history of contact bleeding despite the presence of negative smear.

Where the lesion is not clinically detected,

colposcopic directed biopsy offers maximum reliability.

Conservative methods of treatment in CIN can be effectively performed colposcopically as an OPD procedure.

Table 9.4
Colposcopic terminology

I.	Normal colposcopic findings
	A – Normal squamous epithelium
	B – Columnar epithelium
	C – Transformation zone
II.	Abnormal colposcopic findings (see p. 314)
	A – Atypical transformation zone
	(a) Mosaic (b) Punctate
	(c) White epithelium
	(d) Keratosis
	(e) Atypical vessels
	B – Suspected frank invasive cancer— The cancer is evident only colposcopically.
III.	Unsatisfactory — Transformation zone not seen (p. 310)
IV.	Other findings — Condyloma and papilloma are of importance.

IMAGING TECHNIQUES IN GYNAECOLOGY

• X-ray • Ultrasound • CT Scan • MRI • PET

X-RAY

A chest X-ray and intravenous urogram are essential for investigation in pelvic malignancy, cervical cancer in particular, prior to staging. Plain X-ray of the pelvis is helpful to locate an IUCD or to look for shadows of teeth or bone in benign cystic teratoma. Special X-ray using contrast media are :

- HSG (details in p. 559).
- Lymphangiography — to locate the lymph glands involved in pelvic malignancy.
- Pelvic pneumography — It has been replaced absolutely by sonar and laparoscopy.

ULTRASOUND

There is rapid and continuing evolution of ultrasound, since its first introduction by Ian Donald (Glasgow – 1950) in the field of medicine. Sonography is used widely in Gynaecology either with the transabdominal (TAS) or with the transvaginal (TVS) probe. Because of safety, high patient acceptance and relatively low cost, ultrasonography has become a common diagnostic modality in gynaecology, these days.

Transabdominal Sonography (TAS) is done with a linear or curvilinear array transducer operating at 2.5–3.5 MHz. TAS requires full bladder to displace the bowel out of pelvis. Otherwise gas in the bowel acts as a complete barrier to ultrasound waves. TAS is best used for large masses like fibroid or ovarian tumour. Higher is the frequency of ultrasound wave, better is the image resolution but lesser is the depth of tissue penetration.

Transvaginal Sonography (TVS) is done with a probe which is placed close to the target organ. There is no need of a full bladder. It also avoids the difficulties due to obesity, faced in TAS. TVS operates at a high frequency (5-8 MHz). Therefore, detailed evaluation of the pelvic organs (within 10 cm of the field) is possible with TVS. But the drawbacks of TVS are mainly due to narrow vagina as in virgins, postmenopausal women or post radiation vaginal stenosis.

Transvaginal Colour Doppler Sonography (TV–CDS) — Provides additional information of blood flow to, from or within an organ (uterus or adnexae). This flow can be measured by analysis of the waveform using the pulsatility index.

Use of ultrasound in gynaecology

- **Use in infertility workup**

– Serial measurement of ovarian follicular diameter (folliculometry) and endometrial thickness are done using TVS. **Mature follicle** should measure between 18 and 20 mm in diameter. The favourable peri-ovulatory endometrium should be between 7 and 11 mm thick (see Chapter 16).

– Ultrasound can provide presumptive evidence of ovulation. **Following ovulation**, internal echoes appear and free fluid is observed in pouch of Douglas.

– To detect **correct timing of ovulation** by folliculometry in conjunction with plasma oestradiol.

This helps in induction of ovulation, artificial insemination and ovum retrieval in IVF.

– Sonographic guided **oocyte retrieval** in IVF and GIFT programmes, is now accepted as the best method.

• **Ectopic pregnancy** can be detected on TVS as a **"tubal ring"**, separate from the ovary in a patient with empty uterine cavity. **TV–CDS** is of more help to detect the vascularity of "tubal ring" when it is unruptured.

• **Pelvic mass** can be evaluated as regard to its location and consistency. Uterine fibroid, ovarian mass, endometrioma, tubo-ovarian mass, etc. can be delineated when there is confusion in clinical diagnosis. However, major limitation is due to its lack of specificity.

• **Oncology** : TV-CDS can assess the vascularity of the mass. Low flow impedance with high flow velocity raises the suspicion of a malignant tumour.

Presence of papillary excrescences, mural nodules, septations, cystic lesion with solid components and ascites are the other sonographic features of malignancy.

• **Endometrial disease** : Women with unexplained uterine bleeding, or postmenopausal bleeding are better studies with TVS. An endometrial thickness of less than 5 mm is considered atrophic. Endometrial biopsy is needed for postmenopausal women with thicker endometrium.

• **Sonohysterography** involves instillation of saline in the uterine cavity and study with TVS. Submucous fibroid or polyp is better diagnosed with this method.

• **To locate missing IUD (see ch. 29).**

• **Sonohysterosalpingography (see p. 231).**

• **Sonographically guided procedures.**

A needle guide is attached to the shaft of the vaginal probe. With the use of real time, TVS can guide the needle course in a safe path. This technique can be utilised for many diagnostic and therapeutic purposes :

– Aspiration of cystic masses, e.g. Chocolate cyst (see p. 301).

– Follicular aspiration, e.g. Ovum retrieval in IVF (see p. 244).

– Aspiration of tubo-ovarian abscess.

– Biopsies.

• **Transrectal sonography** can be used where TVS cannot be used due to vaginal narrowing.

• **Saline Infusion Sonography (SIS)**

Infusion of normal saline into the uterine cavity and doing transvaginal (high resolution) sonography is helpful for the diagnosis of many uterine pathology. SIS catheter is inserted through the cervical os. Normal saline is infused slowly (5-10 ml) when the uterus is imaged with vaginal ultrasound.

Common indications of SIS are :

• Postmenopausal bleeding.

• Abnormal uterine bleeding.

• Recurrent miscarriage.

• Infertility.

COMPUTED TOMOGRAPHY(CT SCAN)

CT scan provides high resolution two dimensional images. Cross sectional images of the body are taken at very close intervals in the form of multiple slices. CT scan differentiate tissue densities and this greyscale pictures can be read on an X-ray film or a television monitor. Pelvic organs could be differentiated from gastrointestinal and urinary systems using contrast media. Contrast media can be given orally, IV or rectally. CT is most useful in the diagnosis of lymph node metastases, depth of myometrial invasion in endometrial cancer, ovarian mass and myomas. **However, lymph nodes must be enlarged at least by 2 cm to be detected by CT. Cerebral metastases of choriocarcinoma or microadenoma of the pituitary** can best be detected by CT procedure. CT scan also facilitates the percutaneous needle biopsy of suspicious lymph nodes. In obese or

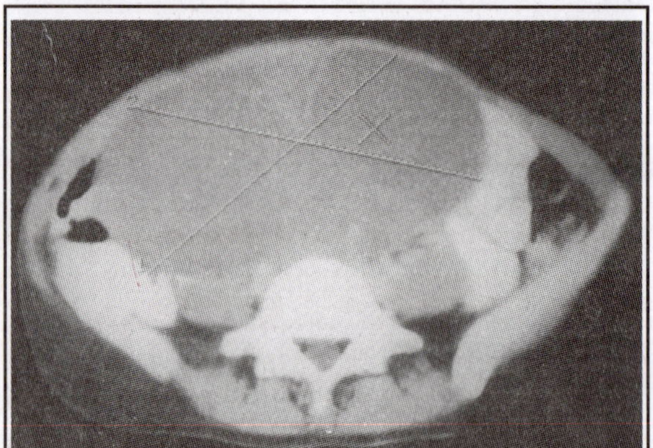

Fig. 9.22. CT scan of the pelvis showing an ovarian mass

in cases of distended stomach or gut, it is an ideal alternative to sonar (Fig. 36.81). CT is useful in assessing tumour extent and detecting metastases (Fig. 9.22). CT has its role in staging of ovarian cancer as it can detect pertoneal, omental and serosal deposits in addition to liver and nodal metastasis (p. 624). However, it is more costly and there is chance of surface radiation. Surface radiation dose of CT scan of the abdomen and pelvis is between-2 and 10 CGY. Value of CT in the assessment of pelvic organs is limited. MRI is preferred where available.

MAGNETIC RESONANCE IMAGING (MRI)

The phenomenon of nuclear magnetic resonance was first described by Felix Bloch and Edward Purcell in 1946. MR as a basis for an imaging technique was employed in practice about 30 years later by Lauterbur.

MRI creates cross-sectional images of the body using a combination of radiowaves (non-ionising radiation) and magnetic fields. Biologic tissue nuclei with protons or neutrons have got magnetic properties. When a pulse of radiowaves is imposed on the nuclei a strong resonance will occur and the energy is absorbed by the nuclei. A signal is detected in a receiver coil, situated close to the tissue, when the energy is emitted by the nuclei. The strength of the emitted signal varies directly with the proton density. In gynaecology, MRI is found superior to CT, in the delineation of pelvic organs in multiple planes. Respiratory movements have got little effect on the pelvic organs. Sagittal and coronal views can be obtained without moving the patient. Patients with implants (pacemakers) cannot undergo MRI. Gadolium is used as IV contrast for better visualisation of organs and their abnormalities.

Use of MRI

• MRI can differentiate the different zones (endometrium, inner and outer myometrium) of the uterus clearly (see Fig. 36.82). It can measure the depth of myometrial penetration of endometrial cancer preoperatively.

• MRI can detect accurately the parametrial invasion of cervical cancer but cannot identify lymphatic metastases reliably. It is more reliable in distinguishing post-treatment fibrosis and recurrence.

• Endovaginal or endorectal coils produce high resolution images of the cervix and parametrium. Tumour volume can be measured with 3D imaging system. Coronal and axial planes are used to determine the invasion of the bladder, rectum, parametrium and uterine body.

• Leiomyomas are better diagnosed with MRI.

• MRI is a non-invasive tool in the diagnosis of endometriosis. It can measure the depth of penetration which is responsible for pelvic pain.

• MRI is superior to CT in the evaluation of metastatic lymph nodes or recurrent pelvic tumour. However, neither CT nor MRI can detect microscopic malignant disease (p. 625).

MRI is twice more expensive than CT.

Hazards : **Main hazards** are electroconvulsions and atrial fibrillation. This is due to rapidly changing magnetic field. Hence, caution should be exercised with epileptic patients and who had recent myocardial infarction.

POSITRON EMISSION TOMOGRAPHY (PET)

PET is based on the tissue uptake of 18F-fluro-2 deoxyglucose. FDG-PET can measure the difference between the normal tissue and cancerous tissue. Cancer tissues process this glucose analog differently compared to that of normal tissues. This glucose analog is given IV. FDG-PET scan is then done and the images are interpreted.

FDG-PET scan is more sensitive for detection of metastatic disease and recurrence of ovarian malignancy. It is also useful to assess the response following tumour therapy. FDG-PET scan is found to be more sensitive and specific compared to CT or MRI.

CONCLUSIONS

All the imaging systems have got their role in gynaecological practice.

X-ray, either plain or using contrast media have got its place. It is cheaper and quite informative with minimal risks of irradiation.

Sonar establishes a definite place in diagnostic evaluation. Ultrasound guided procedures are used for both the diagnostic and therapeutic purposes.

CT is costly and should be employed in selected cases to detect microadenoma of pituitary or metastatic lesions in the brain or liver.

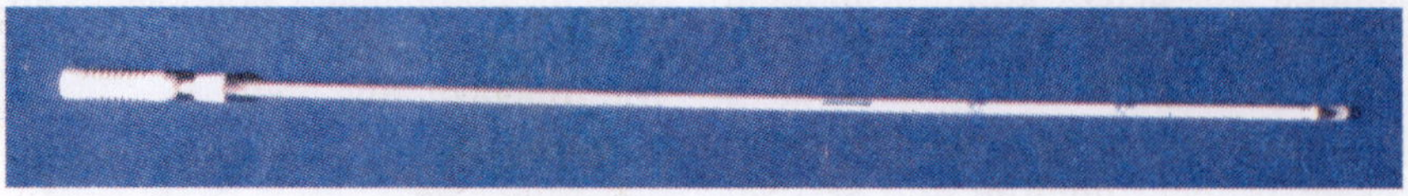

Fig. 9.23. Endometrial sampler

MRI may be employed in cases where sonar or CT fails to detect the lesion and specially to differentiate post-treatment fibrosis or tumour. It is very costly with limited availability.

• PET is helpful to differentiate normal tissues from cancerous one.

ENDOMETRIAL SAMPLING

Endometrial sampling is one of the diagnostic tests, most frequently performed as an outdoor procedure. This rapid, safe and inexpensive test is employed in the clinical work up of women with infertility or abnormal uterine bleeding or for periodic screening during HRT. The instrument commonly used is either a Vabra aspirator or a Sharman curette. **Currently endometrial sampler (Pipelle) is used as an out-patient procedure** (Fig. 9.23). A thin plastic cannula, with a plunger within, is negotiated within the uterus. **It is done as an out-patient procedure.** When the plunger is withdrawn, adequate endometrium is obtained due to suction action. This procedure is reliable and is accepted by the patient. To study the hormonal effect, material from the fundus and upper part of the body is to be taken. However, when a large tissue mass is needed for histological studies, a thorough endometrial curettage is to be done under anaesthesia as in endometrial tuberculosis or postmenopausal bleeding.

ENDOMETRIAL BIOPSY

The most reliable method to study the endometrium is by obtaining the material by curettage after dilatation of the cervix usually under general anaesthesia. Its clinical application is described in appropriate chapters (see p. 533).

TESTS FOR TUBAL PATENCY

These are described in the Chapter 16 (p. 233).

CERVICAL BIOPSY

To confirm the clinical diagnosis of the cervical pathology, biopsy is mandatory. It can be done in the out-patient or in indoor. Biopsy can be taken safely at the out-patient, if the pathology is detectable, but for wider tissue excision as in cone biopsy, it should be done as an in-patient. The details are described in page 560.

CULDOCENTESIS

Definition

Culdocentesis is the transvaginal aspiration of peritoneal fluid from the cul-de-sac or pouch of Douglas.

Indications

- In suspected disturbed ectopic pregnancy or other causes producing haemoperitoneum.
- In suspected cases of pelvic abscess.

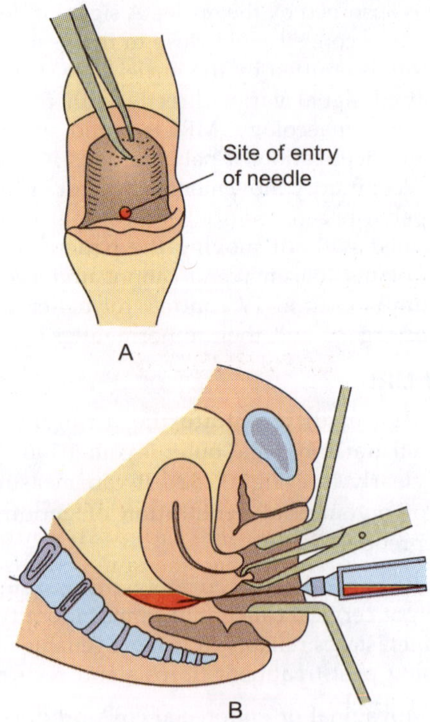

Fig. 9.24. Culdocentesis

Steps

- The procedure is done under sedation.
- The patient is put in lithotomy position.
- Vagina is cleaned with Betadine.
- A posterior vaginal speculum is inserted.
- A 18 gauge spinal needle fitted with a syringe is inserted at a point 1 cm below the cervico-vaginal junction in the posterior fornix (Fig. 9.24).
- After inserting the needle to a depth of about 2 cm, suction is applied as the needle is withdrawn.
- **If unclotted blood is obtained, the diagnosis of intraperitoneal bleeding is established.** If no blood or fluid is obtained, the needle is withdrawn slowly while intermittent suction should be maintained. If the tap is found dry, another attempt is to be made.

ENDOSCOPY IN GYNAECOLOGY (see ch. 35)

Endoscopy has become an essential armamentarium in the diagnostic evaluation of gynaecologic lesions as well as for operative procedures. Gynaecological endoscopy includes the procedures as mentioned in the Table 9.5.

Table 9.5
Gynaecological Endoscopy

• Laparoscopy	• Hysteroscopy	• Salpingoscopy
• Falloposcopy	• Cystoscopy	• Culdoscopy
• Sigmoidoscopy and proctoscopy		

LAPAROSCOPY

Laparoscopy is a technique of visualisation of peritoneal cavity by means of a fibre optic endoscope introduced through the abdominal wall. Prior pneumoperitoneum is achieved by introduction of carbon dioxide or air. For diagnostic purposes, either local or general anaesthesia may be used. Its use is gradually widening both in diagnostic and therapeutic field in gynaecology. The details are in Chapter 35 (Fig. 9.25).

Indications

- **Diagnostic**
- **Operative (chaper 35)**

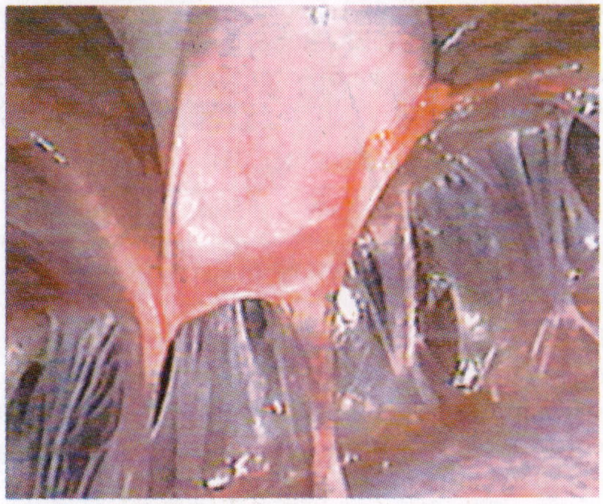

Fig. 9.25. Chlamydial infection causing perihepatic adhesions (Fitz-Hugh-Curtis Syndrome) diagnosed by Laparoscopy

Diagnostic

- Infertility work up (chapter 16)
  - Peritubal adhesions.
  - Chromopertubation (p. 231).
  - Minimal endometriosis (p. 298).
  - Ovulation stigma of the ovary.
  - Before reversal of sterilisation operation (p. 239).
- Chronic pelvic pain (see p. 530)
- Nature of a pelvic mass : Fibroid, Ovarian cyst
- To diagnose an acute pelvic lesion
  - Ectopic pregnancy (p. 529).
  - Acute appendicitis.
  - Acute salpingitis — diagnosis and collection of pus for culture.
- Follow up of pelvic surgery (second look)
  - Tuboplasty.
  - Ovarian malignancy.
  - Evaluation of therapy in endometriosis.
- Investigation protocol of amenorrhoea.
- Diagnosis of suspected Müllerian abnormalities (p. 43).
- Uterine perforation.

Timing of Laparoscopy

In infertility work up, it may be done in the peri-ovulatory period to facilitate chromopertubation and also diagnosis of ovulation. However, in endometriosis, it is preferably done in the premenstrual period when the ectopic endometrial implants increase in size.

Operative — (see chapter 35).

Complications — (see p. 586).

HYSTEROSCOPY (see p. 587)

Hysteroscopy is an operative procedure whereby the endometrial cavity can be visualised with the aid of fibre optic telescope. **The uterine distension is achieved by** carbon dioxide, normal saline or glycine. The instrument is to pass transcervically, usually without dilatation of the cervix or local anaesthetic. However, for operative hysteroscopy, either paracervical block or general anaesthesia is required. **Diagnostic hysteroscopy should be performed in the postmenstrual period** for better view without bleeding. The chance of conception disturbance is absent (Fig. 9.26).

Recently, contact hysteroscopy has become more popular since a distending medium is not needed. The interpretation of endometrial pathology is similar to colposcopy in that it depends on colour, contour and vascular pattern.

Indications

- **Diagnostic** • **Operative**

The technical details and operative hysteroscopy are dealt in Chapter 35.

Diagnostic

- Unresponsive irregular uterine bleeding to exclude uterine polyp, submucous fibroid or products of conception.

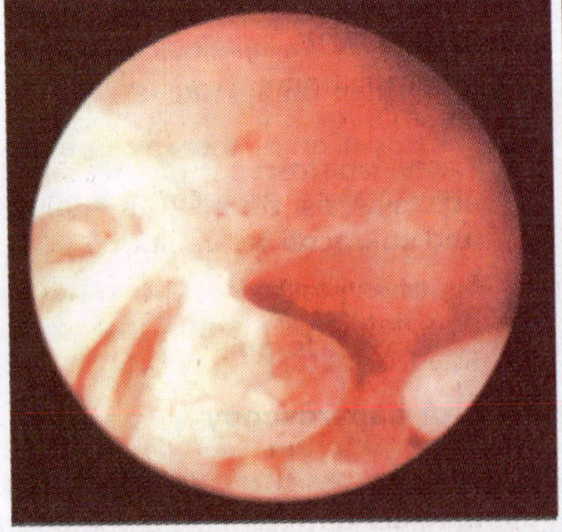

Fig. 9.26. Hysteroscopic view of a submucous fibroid polyp

- Congenital uterine septum in recurrent abortion.
- Missing threads of IUD.
- Intrauterine adhesions (uterine synechiae).
- To visualise transformation zone with colpomicrohysteroscopy when colposcopic finding is unsatisfactory.

Operative — (see p. 589).

Complications — (see p. 590).

Conclusion

The instruments for endoscopic procedures are costly and require a great deal of expertise for diagnostic and specially for operative procedures.

SALPINGOSCOPY

In salpingoscopy, a firm telescope is inserted through the abdominal ostium of the uterine tube so that the tubal mucosa can be visualised by distending the lumen with saline infusion. The telescope is to be introduced through laparoscope.

Salpingoscopy allows study of the physiology and anatomy of the tubal epithelium and **permits more accurate selection of patients for IVF rather than the tubal surgery.**

Falloposcopy — see p. 232.

CYSTOSCOPY

The main use of cystoscopy in gynaecology is to evaluate cervical cancer prior to staging and, to investigate the urinary symptoms including haematuria, incontinence and fistulae.

CULDOSCOPY

Culdoscopy is an optical instrument designed to visualise the pelvic structures through an incision in the pouch of Douglas. Its use has almost been replaced by laparoscopy.

PROCTOSCOPY AND SIGMOIDOSCOPY

For rectal involvement of genital malignancy, a digital examination or at best proctoscopy is usually adequate.

Table 9.6
Common laser systems used in gynaecology

Laser type	Wavelength	Tissue penetration
Carbon dioxide	10.6 μm	0.1 mm
Neodymium : yttrium-aluminium gernate (Nd : YAG)	1.06 μm	0.6-4.2 mm
Potassium titanyl-phosphate (KTP 532)	0.532 μm	0.4-0.8 mm
Argon	0.5 μm	0.2 mm

EXAMINATION UNDER ANAESTHESIA (EUA)

EUA is indicated where bimanual examination cannot be conducted properly either because of extreme tenderness or inadequate relaxation of abdominopelvic muscles or non-cooperative patient. It should be done routinely in all cases of uterine malignancy for clinical staging. It is extended freely to examine virgins or in cases with paediatric gynaecological problems.

LASER IN GYNAECOLOGY

The word 'Laser' is an acronym for ***light amplification by stimulated emission of radiation*** :

Physics of laser

The important physical properties of laser are :

(i) Monochromacity — Light beams of a particular laser have got the same wavelength.

(ii) Coherent — The light waves are all perfectly aligned and uni-directional.

(iii) Collimated — The light beams run parallel and do not diverge.

(iv) The laser beam can be converged by a convex lens to a sharp focus, called spot size.

(v) Power density is the measure of laser effects upon tissue. It is expressed as watts/cm^2.

(vi) Smaller the spot size, greater is the power density.

(vii) Laser – tissue interaction — The water in the cells (80% by volume) boils instantly at the temperature of 100°C. The cell explodes and vaporises. The cell protein and minerals are incinerated and look charred.

(viii) The depth of tissue destruction is very precise and there is very little lateral effect.

(ix) Laser effect depends on power (watts), spot size, power density, and laser-tissue contact time.

(x) Beams of CO_2 and Nd : YAG laser are invisible. There is preferential absorption of laser by one tissue from another.

Common laser systems used in gynaecology are carbon dioxide, Nd : YAG, KTP and Argon (Table 9.6).

Fiber-optic laser laproscopy (KTP 532 and Argon) has the following advantages : Accurate targetting, better haemostasis, contact modes of cutting, vaporisation, coagulation and less laser plume production.

Use of laser in gynaecology

Principal use of laser in gynaecology is for the purpose of tissue cutting, coagulation or vaporisation. It is used widely in genital tract surgery and with endoscopic surgery. It is commonly used in the management of :

(i) Cervical intra-epithelial neoplasia (CIN) (see p. 309).

(ii) Conisation of the cervix (see p. 560).

(iii) Vulvar intra-epithelial neoplasia (VIN) (see p. 307).

(iv) Vaginal intra-epithelial neoplasia (VAIN) (see p. 308).

(v) Vaporisation of pelvic endometriosis (see p. 301).

(vi) Laser laparoscopy for ovarian cystectomy, adhesiolysis, removal of ectopic pregnancy and presacral neurectomy.

(vii) Laser laparoscopy assisted hysteroscopy, for dividing large pedicles that have been coagulated or suture ligated.

(viii) Hysteroscopic surgery — Laser ablation of endometrium (see p. 189), resection of uterine septum (metroplasty) and submucous fibroids (see p. 272).

Limitations of Laser

- The equipment is expensive.
- Technical complexity — requires sufficient training.

HAZARDS OF LASER SYSTEMS

Laser must be used by a trained person. Laser protection guidelines must be strictly followed to protect the operator, assistant, the theatre staff and the patient from the accidental hazards. A laser controlled area (LCA) must have warning signs when laser is in use. Special spectacles are used to protect the eyes. Common hazards are :

A. (i) Eyes — visual loss due to corneal or retinal damage.

(ii) Skin damage.

(iii) Damage from laser smoke.

B. General

(i) Burn injury (use of spirit and paper drapes must be avoided in theatre).

(ii) Inflammable anaesthetic gases are to use with great care.

(iii) Reflections of laser beam is dangerous. Shining instruments are not to be used.

KEY POINTS

- The clinical examination should be thorough and meticulous. The examination should in fact proceed with the provisional diagnosis in mind. A patient hearing should be given about the complaints made by the patient in her own words.
- Menstrual history includes age of menarche, cycle length, regularity, duration of period, amount of flow and the first day of the last menstrual period.
- Integration of the symptomatology to a single pathology is to be tried first before embarking on the diagnosis of multiple pathology.
- The general and systemic examination should be thorough and meticulous.
- Breast examination should be a routine specially in women above the age of 30 years.
- Bladder should be empty prior to examination.
- Abdominal palpation should be done with the flat of the hand rather than the tips of the fingers. Whether a mass is felt or not, routine palpation of the viscera includes liver, spleen, caecum, pelvic colon, gallbladder and kidneys.
- It is mandatory to elicit presence of free fluid in the peritoneal cavity in all cases of pelvic tumours.
- Pelvic examination includes inspection of external genitalia, vaginal examination (inspection with a speculum, palpation and bimanual examination), rectal examination and rectovaginal examination.
- Rectovaginal examination is of special help to differentiate a growth arising from the ovary or rectum.
- Dyskaryosis in the morphological abnormalities of the nucleus. It may be mild, moderate or severe. Koilocytosis is associated with human papilloma virus infection.
- As a screening procedure, the material from the cervix is best collected using Ayre's spatula. About 5 cases of cervical intra-epithelial neoplasia are diagnosed per 1000 patients and invasive carcinoma of the cervix in order of 1 in 1000. The Pap smear screening should best be done at interval of 3 years after 2 yearly negative smear from 18 years to 60 years. However, screening interval depends on patient's risk level (Table 9.1).
- Diagnostic accuracy of Pap smear after three consecutive negative test is about 99 per cent.
- For cytohormonal study, the smear is taken from the lateral wall of the upper-third of the vagina. The oestrogenic smear is suggested by preponderance of large eosinophilic cells with pyknotic nuclei. The progesterone smear is predominantly basophilic with vesicular nuclei. The background is dirty.

KEY POINTS

- Maturation index (M1), is expressed by three numbers as the percentage of parabasal, intermediate and superficial cells written from left to the right. There is significant shift in maturation index from birth to menopause.
- Examination of cervical mucus is done for bacteriological study, to know the hormonal status and in infertility investigation.

  Oestrogenic mucus is clear, abundant and has got the power of elasticity and shows pattern of fern tree formation. Progesterone smears is thick and viscid, losses its property of elasticity and ferning disappears.
- Postcoital test (PCT) is done on day 12 or 13. The reporting time is within 8-12 hours following intercourse. Presence of at least 10 progressively motile sperm per high power field signifies the test to be normal.
- Menstrual cycles after puberty and before menopause are frequently anovulatory and irregular.
- Pap smears should be performed every 1-3 years depending upon patients risk factors.
- Ultrasonography (TAS, TVS or TV-CDS) has become a common diagnostic modality in gynaecology. It is widely used in infertility work up (sonohysterosalpingography, folliculometry, detection of ovulation and oocyte retrieval in IVF programme), evaluation of pelvic mass, ectopic pregnancy and endometrial disease. Sonographically guided procedures provide added information.

  CT is useful in detection of enlarged pelvic lymph nodes and microadenoma of pituitary. Considering its limitations MRI is preferred where available.
- MRI uses radiowaves (nonionising) and magnetic fields. It accurately shows parametrial invasion of cervical cancer but cannot reliably identify the lymph node metastases. It can measure the depth of myometrial penetration in endometrial carcinoma preoperatively. High resolution images in multiple planes are obtained. Tumour volume can be measured with 3D imaging system.
- Endometrial sampling is useful in the clinical work up of women with infertility or abnormal perimenopausal bleeding. It can be performed in the OPD using a narrow plastic cannula (pipette).
- Culdocentesis is indicated in suspected cases of haemoperitoneum or pelvic abscess.
- Colposcope is a valuable adjunct in the screening procedure. It is employed in cases with abnormal cervical smear and with clinically suspicious cervices specially with history of contact bleeding even if the smear is negative. Colposcopic directed biopsy is the best one when the lesion is not clinically detected.
- The use of laparoscopy is gradually widening. The major diagnostic uses are infertility, chronic pelvic pain and to exclude pelvic lesion (see Ch. 35).
- Hysteroscopy is gaining popularity as a diagnostic aid in unresponsive uterine bleeding, uterine synechiae, congenital uterine septum or missing threads of IUD (see ch. 35).
- **Salpingoscopy** — is the evaluation of tubal mucosa with a telescope, introduced through the abdominal ostium of the tube.
- Principal use of laser in gynaecology is for tissue cutting, coagulation or vaporisation. Laser effects depend on power (watts), spot size, power density and laser-tissue contact time. Commonly used laser system in gynaecology are CO_2, Nd:YAG, KTP 532 or Argon (Table 9.6).

Pelvic Infection

10

Defence of the genital tract

As there is free anastomosis between the lymphatics and blood vessels, the infection of one pelvic organ usually spreads to the other more frequently. There is direct communication of the peritoneal cavity to the exterior through the vagina. In spite of these, the frequency and intensity of pelvic infection is kept lowered by the defence mechanism.

Vulval defence

Anatomic — (i) Apposition of the cleft by labia. (ii) Compound racemose type of Bartholin's glands.

Physiologic — (i) Fungicidal action of the secretion (undecylenic acid) of the apocrine glands (ii) Natural high resistance to infection of the vulval and perineal skin.

Vaginal defence

Anatomic — (i) Apposition of the anterior and posterior walls with its transverse rugae (ii) Stratified epithelium devoid of glands.

Physiologic — This is maintained by the hormone oestrogen (see Table 10.1).

At birth, under the influence of maternal oestrogen circulating into the newborn, the vaginal epithelium become multilayered. The desquamated epithelium containing glycogen is converted into lactic acid probably by enzymatic action for the first 48 hours. Subsequently, the Doderlein's bacilli appear probably from the gut and convert the glycogen into lactic acid. As a result, **for about 10-12 days following birth, the vaginal defence is good and infection is unlikely**.

Thereafter and upto puberty, there is no circulatory oestrogen. The vaginal epithelium is reduced to few layers; glycogen is absent and so also the Doderlein's bacillus. The vaginal pH becomes neutral or alkaline. **During the reproductive period** with high oestrogen, the vaginal defence is fully restored. But again in **postmenopause**, after the withdrawal of oestrogen, the vaginal defence is lost.

It should be emphasised that only the **Doderlein's bacilli can grow in the acid media with pH 4–4.5.** But when the pH increases, the other organisms normally present in the vagina will grow.

Table : 10.1
Defence of the vagina in relation to age

	Newborn (0-10 days)	*Up to puberty*	*Childbearing period*	*Postmenopause*
Epithelium	Multilayered	Thin	Multilayered	Thin
Glycogen	++	(–)	++	(–)
Doderlein's bacillus	+	(–)	++	(–)
pH	Acidic (4-5)	Neutral or alkaline (6-8)	Acidic (4-5)	Neutral (6-7)

The vaginal defence is lost :

(i) Following 10 days of birth till puberty is reached.

(ii) During reproductive period — in the following situation :

- *During menstruation* — The vaginal pH becomes increased due to contaminated blood and fall of oestrogen. The protective cervical mucus disappears and the endometrium sheds.
- *Following abortion and childbirth* — The contaminated lochia increases the pH. The raw placental site, inevitable tear of the cervix, bruising of the vagina and presence of blood clots or remnants of decidua favour nidation of the bacterial growth. The general resistance is also lowered somehow.

(iii) During menopause.

Cervical defence

Anatomic — (i) Racemose type of glands, (ii) mucus plug.

Physiologic — Bactericidal effect of the mucus.

Uterine defence

(i) Cyclic shedding of the endometrium (ii) Closure of the uterine ostium of the fallopian tube with slightest inflammatory reaction in the endometrium.

Tubal defence

Anatomic — Integrated mucus plicae and epithelial cilia.

Physiologic — Peristalsis of the tube and also the movement of the cilia are towards the uterus.

Causative organisms

The bacterial pathogens involved in upper genital tract infections are principally derived from the normal flora of the vagina and endocervix. Exogenous sources are sexually transmitted or following induced criminal abortion or during delivery in unhygienic surroundings. The factors responsible for alteration leading to development of pelvic infections are :

- Impairment of local blood supply.
- Presence of foreign bodies.
- Destruction of tissue by trauma or infection.
- Growth of aerobic infection.

Aerobes produce tissue destruction and alteration of the local environment that paves the way for lower genital tract flora, especially anaerobes, to gain access to the upper genital tract.

Organisms

1. **Pyogenic (50 %)** — This is the commonest type – the organisms responsible are:

Aerobes

The gram-positive organisms are *staphylococcus*. **The gram-negatives are** *E. coli, pseudomonas, klebsiella, N. gonorrhoeae*, etc.

Anaerobes

The gram-positives are anaerobic streptococcus. *Clostridium welchii, Cl. tetani*, etc. **The gram-negatives** are mainly bacteroides group of which *Bacteroides fragilis* is the commonest.

2. **Sexually transmitted disease (STD)** — The organisms are *N. gonorrhoeae, Chlamydia trachomatis, Treponema pallidum, Herpes simplex virus type II, Human papilloma virus, Gardnerella vaginalis (Haemophilus vaginalis), Haemophilus ducreyi, Donovan bodies, HIV I or II*, etc.

3. **Parasitic** — *Trichomonas vaginalis*

4. **Fungal** — *Candida albicans*

5. **Viral** — *Herpes simplex virus type II, Human papilloma virus, HIV, Condylomata accuminata*, etc.

6. **Tubercular** — *Mycobacterium tuberculosis.*

Modes of spread of infections

The route of infection is most commonly ascending in nature. However, the classic modes of infection of some specific organisms are —

- **Through continuity and contiguity** — gonococcal infection (Fig. 10.1).
- **Through lymphatics and pelvic veins** — post-abortal and puerperal infection — by pyogenic organisms other than gonococcus (Fig. 10.2).
- **Through blood stream** — tubercular
- **From adjacent infected extra-genital organs** like intestine.

ACUTE PELVIC INFECTION

- Pelvic inflammatory disease (PID).
- Following delivery and abortion.
- Following gynaecological procedures.
- Following IUD.
- Secondary to other infections — appendicitis.

PELVIC INFLAMMATORY DISEASE (PID)

Definition

PID is a disease of the upper genital tract. **It is a spectrum of infection and inflammation of the upper genital tract organs typically involving the endometrium, fallopian tubes, ovaries, pelvic peritoneum and surrounding structures**. It is attributed to the ascending spread of microorganisms from the cervicovaginal canal to the contiguous pelvic structures. The clinical syndrome is not related to pregnancy and surgery.

But, as the terminology fails to pinpoint the precise organ or organisms involved, it is better to use the anatomical terminology in relation to which organ is involved in the infectious process. Thus, **the better terminology should be** either endometritis, salpingitis, pelvic peritonitis or tubo-ovarian abscess. **The cervicitis is not included in the list.**

Many, however, prefer the term salpingitis as because it ultimately bears the brunt of acute infection.

From a clinical perspective, it is more pragmatic to describe acute salpingitis as sexually transmitted or not.

Epidemiology

Despite better understanding of the aetiology, pathogenesis, improved diagnostic tools such as sonar or laparoscopy and advent of wide range of antimicrobials, it still constitutes a health hazard both in the developed and more so in the developing countries. The incidence of pelvic infection is on the rise due to the rise in sexually transmitted diseases.

The ready availability of contraception together with increased permissive sexual attitude has resulted in increased incidence of sexually transmitted diseases and, correspondingly, acute PID (more in p. 142).

The incidence varies from 1-2 per cent per year among sexually active women. About 85 per cent are spontaneous infection in sexually active females of reproductive age. The remaining 15 per cent follow procedures, which favours the organisms to ascend up. Such iatrogenic procedures include endometrial biopsy, uterine curettage, insertion of

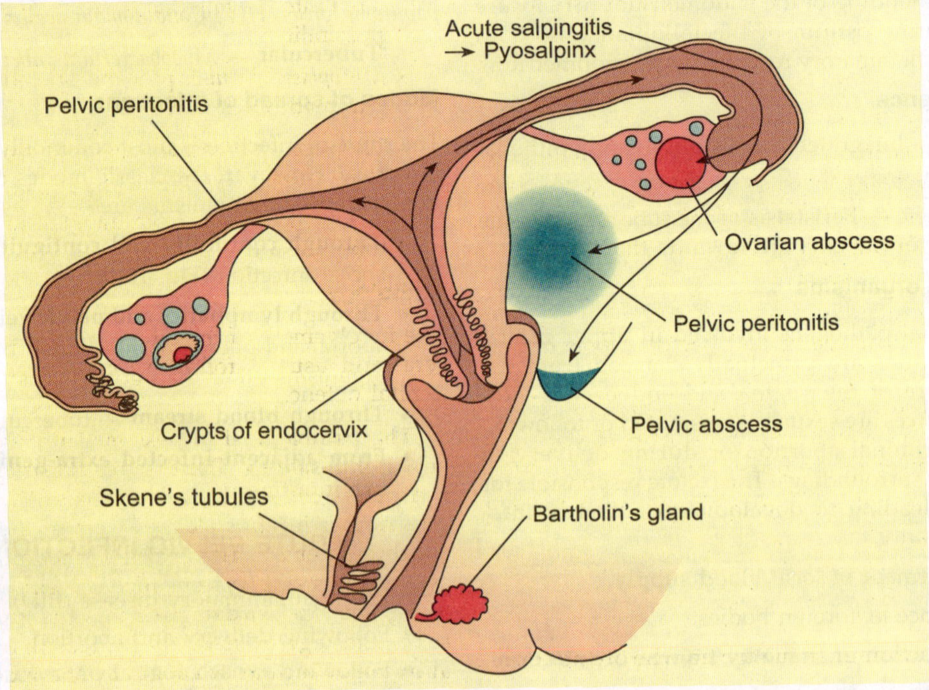

Fig. 10.1. Mode of spread in gonococcal infection

IUD and hysterosalpingography. Two-thirds are restricted to young women of less than 25 years and the remaining one-third limited among 30 years or older.

Pelvic inflammatory disease is a major problem to the reproductive health of young women. PID may be asymptomatic or subclinical. Currently there is **certain changes in the epidemiology of PID.** (A) Shift from *in-patient PID to out-patient PID.* (B) Change in clinical presentation. Less severe disease is commonly seen. (C) Shift in the microbial aetiology of more *Chlamydia trachomatis* than gonococcus and others.

Risk factors

- Menstruating teenagers.
- Multiple sexual partners.
- Absence of contraceptive pill use.
- Previous history of acute PID.
- IUD users.
- Area with high prevalence of sexually transmitted diseases.

Teenagers have got low hormonal and cell mediated immune defence in response to genital tract infection. Wider area of cervical epithelium allows colonisation of *Chlamydia trachomatis* and *N. gonorrhoeae*. (See p. 143).

Protective

Contraceptive practice

- Barrier methods, specially condom along with spermicidal chemicals containing Nonoxynol-9 which is both bactericidal and virucidal.
- Oral steroidal contraceptives have got two preventive aspects.
  - Produce thick mucus plug preventing ascent of sperm and bacterial penetration (see p. 465).
  - Decrease in duration of menstruation, creates a shorter interval of bacterial colonisation of the upper tract.
- Woman with monogamous partner who had vasectomy.
- Pregnancy.
- Menopause.
- PID is uncommon in women who are not menstruating.
- Husband who is azoospermic.

Microbiology

Acute PID is usually a **polymicrobial** infection caused by organisms ascending upstairs from downstairs.

The primary organisms are sexually transmitted and limited approximately to *N. gonorrhoeae* in 30 per cent, *Chlamydia trachomatis* in 30 per cent and *Mycoplasma hominis* in 10 per cent.

The secondary organisms normally found in the vagina are almost always associated sooner or later. These are :

Aerobic organisms — non-haemolytic streptococcus.

E. coli, group B *streptococcus* and *staphylococcus*.

Anaerobic organisms — *Bacteroides* species – *fragilis* and *bivius*, *peptostreptococcus* and *peptococcus*.

Mode of affection

- The classic concept is that the gonococcus ascends up to affect the tubes through mucosal continuity and contiguity. However, ascent of the bacteria from lower to upper genital tract is facilitated by the sexually transmitted vectors such as sperm and trichomonads.
- Reflux of menstrual blood along with gonococci into the fallopian tubes may be the other possibility.
- *Mycoplasma hominis* probably spreads across the parametrium to affect the tube.
- The secondary organisms probably affect the tube through lymphatics.
- Rarely, organisms from the gut may affect the tube directly.

Pathology

The involvement of the tube is almost always bilateral and usually following mens due to loss of genital defence.

The pathological process is initiated primarily in the endosalpinx. There is gross destruction of the epithelial cells, cilia and microvilli. In severe infection, it invades all the layers of the tube and produces acute inflammatory reaction; becomes oedematous and hyperaemic. The exfoliated cells along with the exudate pour into the lumen of the tube and agglutinate the mucosal folds. **The abdominal ostium is closed** by the indrawing of the oedematous fimbriae and by inflammatory adhesions. The uterine end is closed by congestion.

The closure of both the ostia results in pent up of the exudate inside the tube. **Depending upon the virulence, the exudate may be watery producing hydrosalpinx or purulent producing pyosalpinx.** The purulent exudate then changes the microenvironment of the tube which favours growth of other pyogenic and anaerobic organisms resulting in deeper penetration and more tissue destruction. The organisms spontaneously die within 2-3 weeks. As the serous coat is not much affected, **the resulting adhesions of the tube with the surrounding structures are not so dense,** in fact flimsy, unlike pyogenic or tubercular infection.

On occasions, the exudate pours through the abdominal ostium to produce pelvic peritonitis and pelvic abscess or may affect the ovary (the organisms gain access through the ovulation rent) producing ovarian abscess. A tubo-ovarian abscess is thus formed (Fig. 10.1).

CLINICAL FEATURES

Symptoms

Patients with acute PID present with a wide range of non-specific clinical symptoms. Symptoms usually appear at and immediately following the mens.

- Bilateral lower abdominal and pelvic pain which is dull in nature. The onset of pain is more rapid and acute in gonococcal infection (3 days) than in chlamydial infection (5-7 days).
- There is fever, lassitude and headache.
- Irregular and excessive vaginal bleeding is usually due to associated endometritis.
- Abnormal vaginal discharge which becomes purulent and or copious.
- Nausea and vomiting.
- Dyspareunia.
- Pain and discomfort in the right hypochondrium due to concomitant perihepatitis **(Fitz-Hugh-Curtis syndrome)** may occur in 5-10 per cent of cases of acute salpingitis. **The liver is involved** due to transperitoneal or vascular dissemination of either gonococcal or chlamydial infection.

Signs

- The temperature is elevated to beyond 38.3°C.
- Abdominal palpation reveals tenderness on both the quadrants of lower abdomen. The liver may be enlarged and tender.
- Vaginal examination reveals — (1) Abnormal vaginal discharge which may be of purulent. (2) Congested external urethral meatus or openings of Bartholin's ducts through which pus may be seen escaping out on pressure. (3) Speculum examination shows congested cervix with purulent discharge from the canal. (4) Bimanual examination reveals bilateral tenderness on fornix palpation, which increases more with movement of the cervix. There may be thickening or a definite mass felt through the fornices.

CLINICAL DIAGNOSTIC CRITERIA OF PID (CDC-2001)

Minimum criteria

- Lower abdominal pain.
- Adnexal tenderness.
- Cervical motion tenderness.

Additional criteria

- Oral temperature > 38.3°C.
- Abnormal cervical or vaginal discharge.
- Raised C-reactive protein and/or ESR.
- Laboratory documentation of positive cervical infection with Gonorrhoea or C. trachomatis.
- Histopathologic evidence of endometritis on biopsy.
- Sonographic evidence of tubo-ovarian complex.
- Laparoscopic evidence of PID (p. 127).

Investigations

Identification of organisms

For identification of organisms, the materials are collected from the following available sources :

(i) Discharge from the urethra or Bartholin's gland.

(ii) Cervical canal.

(iii) Collected pus from the fallopian tubes during laparoscopy or laparotomy.

The material so collected is subjected to Gram stain and culture (aerobic and anaerobic). The findings of gram-negative diplococci is very much suggestive of gonococcal infection. Except in highly sophisticated centres, the detection of *Cl. trachomatis* is difficult (for diagnosis see p. 146). As the process of investigation is not specific and is time consuming, treatment for *Cl. trachomatis* should be started from the clinical diagnosis. A positive Gram stain smear from endocervical mucus is non-specific and a negative smear does not rule out upper genital tract infection.

Blood : Leucocyte count shows leucocytosis to more than 10,000 per cu mm and an elevated ESR value of more than 15 mm per hour. The results correlate with the severity of the inflammatory reactions of the fallopian tubes as seen on laparoscopy. **Serological test for syphilis should be carried out for both the partners in all cases.**

Laparoscopy : Laparoscopy is considered the "**gold standard**". While it is the **most reliable aid** to support the clinical diagnosis but it may not be feasible to do in all cases. It is reserved only in those cases in which differential diagnosis includes salpingitis, appendicitis or ectopic pregnancy. Non-responding pelvic mass needs laparoscopic clarification (also see p. 138).

Laparoscopic findings and severity of PID are :

- Hyperaemia and oedema of the tubes.
- Purulent exudates from the fimbrial ends.
- Tubes not freely movable.
- Pyosalpinx, pus in the POD.
- **'Violin string'** like adhesions in the pelvis and around the liver suggests chlamydial infection.

Laparoscopy helps to aspirate fluid or pus for microbiological study from the fallopian tube, ovary or pouch of Douglas.

Sonography : It is of limited value. Dilated and fluid-filled tubes, fluid in the pouch of Douglas or adnexal mass are suggestive of PID. It may be employed where clinical examination is difficult or is not informative because of acute tenderness or obesity.

Table 10.2
Clinical Features of Acute PID

- Rise of temperature > 38°C
- Lower abdominal tenderness
- Tenderness on movement of the cervix
- Adnexal mass
- The supportive diagnostic aids are :
  - Blood :– Leucocytosis > 10,000 per cu mm
    – ESR raised > 15 mm per hour
  - Laparoscopic evidences of tubal affection
  - Culdocentesis with purulent fluid having white cell count > 30,000/ml.

Culdocentesis : Aspiration of peritoneal fluid and its white cell count, if exceeds 30,000 per ml. is

Table 10.3 : Clinical features of acute salpingitis, acute appendicitis and disturbed ectopic

Symptoms and signs	*Acute salpingitis (Table 12.3)*	*Acute appendicitis*	*Disturbed ectopic*
• Pain	Acute lower abdominal on both sides	Starts near umbilicus but settles to right iliac fossa	Acute lower abdomen on one side
• Amenorrhoea and bleeding PV	Unrelated	Unrelated	Usually present
• GI symptoms such as nausea, vomiting	Inconsistantly present	Usual	Absent
• General look	Face-flushed	Toxic	Pale
• Tongue	No significant change	Furred	Pale
• Pulse	Rapid but proportionate with temperature	Rapid, out of proportion to temperature	Persistent rise even with normal temperature
• Temperature	More raised	Slightly raised	Not raised
• Tenderness	Lower abdomen on both sides	On McBurney's point may have muscle guard	Lower abdomen more on one side
• Per vaginam	Tenderness on both fornices. A mass may be felt	Tenderness on right fornix and high up	Mass may be felt through one fornix extending to pouch of Douglas.

significant in acute PID. Bacterial culture from the fluid is not informative because of vaginal contamination.

Investigations are also to be extended to male partner and smear and culture are made from urethral secretion.

Diagnosis

The anatomic diagnosis of infection to the upper genital tract is made from the following clinical features (Table 10.2).

Microbial diagnosis is difficult. But as already emphasised, one should not wait for the report, instead treatment should be started empirically. **The materials for identification of organisms are** from the cervical and urethral discharge and secretion from the Bartholin's gland, and laparoscopic or laparotomy collection of pus from the fallopian tubes. The materials are to be subjected to Gram stain and culture (aerobic and anaerobic).

Gram stain of the discharge may be positive for gram-negative intracellular diplococci of *N. gonorrhoeae*. Bacteriologic diagnosis of *Chlamydia trachomatis* is difficult. However, the status of the sexual partner is the single most important clue to the diagnosis of chlamydial infection. **If the woman has a stable sexual relationship with asymptomatic man, the clinical manifestations are unlikely to be due to chlamydial infection.**

Differential diagnosis

The clinical condition may be confused with —

(1) appendicitis, (2) disturbed ectopic pregnancy, (3) torsion of ovarian pedicle, haemorrhage or rupture of ovarian cyst, (4) endometriosis, (5) diverticulitis and (6) urinary tract infection (Table 10.3).

The two conditions — acute appendicitis and disturbed ectopic pregnancy must be ruled out, because both the conditions require urgent laparotomy where as acute salpingitis is to be treated conservatively.

Complications

Immediate : (1) Pelvic peritonitis or even generalised peritonitis. (2) Septicaemia — producing arthritis or myocarditis.

Late : (1) Dyspareunia. (2) Infertility rate is 12 per cent, after two episodes increases to 25 per cent and after three raises to 50 per cent. It is due to tubal damage or tubo-ovarian mass. (3) Chronic pelvic inflammation is due to recurrent or associated pyogenic infection. (4) Formation of adhesions or hydrosalpinx or pyosalpinx and tubo-ovarian abscess. (5) Chronic pelvic pain and ill health. (6) Increased risk of ectopic pregnancy (6-10 fold).

Treatment

Essential steps in the prevention are :

- Community based approach to increase public health awareness.
- Prevention of sexually transmitted diseases with the knowledge of healthy and safer sex.
- Liberal use of contraceptives.
- Routine screening of high-risk population.

The principles of therapy are :

- To control the infection energetically.
- To prevent infertility and late sequelae.
- To prevent reinfection.

Out-patient therapy : Apart from adequate rest and analgesic, antibiotics are to be prescribed even before the microbiological report is available. As because the infection is polymicrobial in nature, instead of single, combination of antibiotics should be prescribed. Out-patients antibiotic therapy for acute PID is given in the Table 10.4.

Table 10.4
Out-patient antibiotic therapy

- **Patient should receive oral therapy for 7-14 days (any one) :**
  - Doxycycline 100 mg two times a day
  - Erythromycin 500 mg four times a day
  - Tetracycline 500 mg four times a day

For anaerobic coverage metronidazole, 400 mg orally two times a day.

Antibiotic therapy should be modified depending on the culture and sensitivity report when ever available.

Specific antibiotic therapy (any one) for gonococcal and chlamydial infections.

- ***Chlamydia trachomatis* infection :**
  - Doxycycline 100 mg orally, two times a day for 7 days.
  - Azithromycin 1 gm orally single dose.
  - Ofloxacin 400 mg orally two times a day for 7 days.
- ***N. gonorrhoeae* infection :**
  - Ceftriaxone 250 mg deep IM single dose.
  - Ciprofloxacin 500 mg orally single dose.

All patients treated in the out-patients are **evaluated after 48 hours and if no response, are to be hospitalised.**

In-patient therapy : The patients are to be hospitalised for antibiotic therapy in the conditions as mentioned in Table 10.5.

Table 10.5
Indications of in-patient antibiotic therapy

- Suspected pelvic abscess
- Severe illness, temperature > 38°C
- Uncertain diagnosis — where surgical emergencies, e.g. ectopic pregnancy cannot be excluded
- Unresponsive to out-patient therapy for 48 hours
- Intolerance to oral antibiotics
- Co-existing pregnancy
- Patient is known to have HIV infection

Bed rest is imposed. Oral feeding is restricted. Dehydration and acidosis are to be corrected by intravenous fluid.

Intravenous antibiotic therapy is recommended for at least 48 hours but may be extended to 4 days, if necessary (Table 10.6).

Table 10.6
In-patient antibiotic therapy

- Cefoxitin 2 gm IV 4 times a day for 2-4 days

Or

- Gentamicin 2 mg/kg IV (loading dose), followed by 1.5 mg/kg IV (maintenance dose) every 8 hours

and

- Metronidazole 500 mg IV every 8 hours.

Improvement of the patient is evidenced by remission of temperature, improvement of pelvic tenderness, normal white blood cell count and negative report on bacteriological study.

Indications of surgery

The indications of surgery is comparatively less. The unequivocal indications are :

- Generalised peritonitis.
- Pelvic abscess.
- Tubo-ovarian abscess which does not respond (48-72 hours) to antimicrobial therapy.

To prevent reinfection

The following formalities are to be rigidly followed to prevent reinfection :

- Educating the patient to avoid reinfection and the potential hazards of it.
- The patient should be warned against multiple sexual partners.
- To use condom.
- The sexual partner or partners are to be traced and properly investigated to find out the organism(s) and treated effectively. If they have got non-gonococcal urethritis, they should be treated with tetracycline 500 mg 6 hourly or doxycycline 100 mg twice daily for 7 days.

Follow up

Repeat smears and cultures from the discharge are to be done after 7 days following the full course of treatment. The tests are to be repeated following each menstrual period until it becomes **negative for three consecutive reports when the patient is declared cured.** Until she is cured and her sexual partner(s) have been treated and cured, the patient must be prohibited from intercourse.

The only unequivocal proof of successful treatment after salpingitis is an intrauterine pregnancy.

FOLLOWING DELIVERY AND ABORTION

The common organisms producing acute infection following delivery are anaerobic *streptococcus, staphylococcus pyogenes*, non-haemolytic *streptococcus, E. coli* and *bacteroides group*. Too often, multiple organisms are present and it is difficult to pinpoint a particular organism responsible for a particular type of infection.

As previously mentioned, the defence is lost following childbirth and abortion. Malnutrition, unhygienic environment during delivery, dehydration and ketoacidosis during labour are the additional factors in underprivileged women. Infections are common following caesarean section. Following abortion, specially when induced criminally, exogenous infection is quite likely and potentially virulent.

Pathology

The infection is either localised to the cervix, producing acute cervicitis or may affect the placental

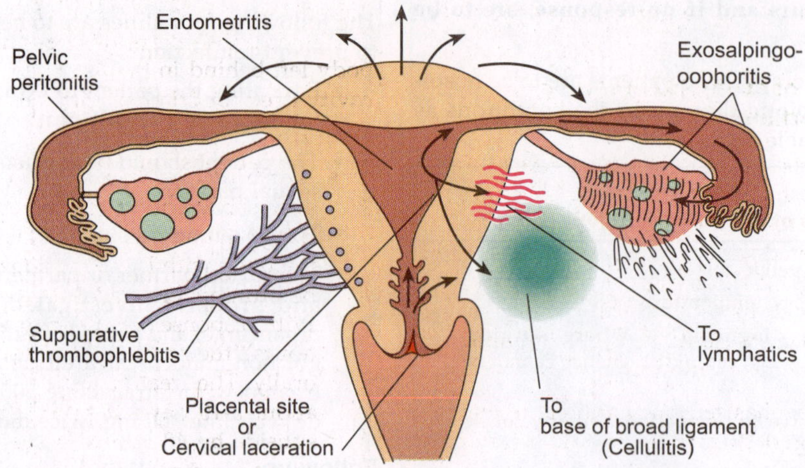

Fig. 10.2. Mode of spread in postabortal or puerperal infection

site producing endometritis. The infection may spread to the myometrium producing endomyometritis which is limited by a leucocytic barrier. On occasion, the infection spreads to the parametrium, usually to one side, through lymphatics or directly through the tear of the cervix; thereby gaining access to the base of the broad ligament. The infection may also spread upwards through the tubal openings into the tubal lumen producing endosalpingitis. **Thus, the fallopian tube is affected** either from outside following parametritis, through lymphatics producing perisalpingitis or through endosalpingitis. The ovary may be affected through involvement of the tube or following pelvic peritonitis. Thus, an acute tubo-ovarian mass is formed (Fig. 10.2).

Spread of infection

Depending upon the virulence of the organisms and resistance of the host, the following events may occur.

The infection is localised principally to the cervix and subsequently develops into chronic cervicitis. **The parametrial exudate** may resolute completely leaving behind scarring or fibrosis or may undergo suppuration. The abscess so formed usually points above the inguinal ligament. **The tubal affection results in cornual block,** hydrosalpinx or pyosalpinx following blockage of the fimbrial end. **There may be peritonitis** either localised or at times generalised. In others, the tube may be adherent with the ovary, intestine and omentum producing tubo-ovarian mass, the abdominal ostium usually remaining patent. **The pelvic veins may be involved producing thrombophlebitis,** which is either confined to the pelvis or spreads upwards along the ovarian veins or downwards along the iliofemoral veins. The systemic effect varies from minimal to a fatal one, specially with gram-negative organisms following criminal abortion. **The serious complications include** septic shock, acute renal failure and disseminated intravascular coagulopathy.

Clinical features

The onset may be acute or insidious and the clinical picture varies widely depending upon the severity and spread of infection. But the **chief complaints** of varying magnitude are fever, lower abdominal and pelvic pain and offensive vaginal discharge following delivery or abortion.

On examination, the patient looks ill and may be restless. She likes to lie on her back with the legs flexed. Pulse rate is rapid and is out of proportion to the temperature. Abdominal examination reveals tenderness or even rigidity on lower abdomen.

Vaginal examination is painful. The discharge is offensive. The uterus is tender, more with movement of the cervix. The fornices are tender. Depending upon the spread, there may be unilateral or bilateral mass (tubo-ovarian), an unilateral tender indurated mass pushing the uterus to the contralateral side (parametritis) or a bulging fluctuating mass felt through the posterior fornix (pelvic abscess). Rectal examination is useful to corroborate the pelvic findings.

Complications of acute PID following delivery or abortion

(1) Endotoxic shock. (2) Oliguria or anuria. (3) Disseminated intravascular coagulopathy. These are predominantly due to gram-negative organisms and are too often associated with criminal abortion. (4) Tubo-ovarian abscess. (5) Peritonitis. (6) Parametritis. (7) Thrombophlebitis — Features usually appear 7-10 days following the initial events. (8) Pulmonary embolism.

It must be emphasised that the fatal outcome is due to prolonged duration of shock, failure to remove surgically accessible sepsis, including retained products, and inappropriate antibiotic therapy.

Treatment

Preventive : The pyogenic infection following delivery is prevented by the following :

(1) To maintain asepsis and antiseptic measures during labour. (2) To avoid traumatic and difficult vaginal deliveries. (3) To use prophylactic antibiotic when labour is delayed following rupture of the membranes or when there are intrauterine manipulations like forceps or manual removal of placenta. (4) To boost up family planning acceptance to prevent the unwanted pregnancies.

Curative

- Hospitalisation — The patient may be admitted if clinically indicated (p. 129).
- **Triple swabs** are to be taken — one from high vagina, one from the endocervix and the third from the urethra. These are to be sent for aerobic and anaerobic culture, drug sensitivity test and Gram stain. **The swabs are to be taken prior to bimanual examination.**
- Vaginal and rectal examinations are then made to note the extent of pelvic infection.
- Investigations.

Routine

(a) **Triple swabs** — already mentioned (b) **Blood** is sent for haemoglobin estimation, total and differential count of white cells, depending on severity of infection blood culture and serum electrolytes are done. (c) **Urine** analysis including culture.

Special investigations are to be done as required : (a) **Ultrasonography** of abdomen and pelvis to detect physometra or presence of any foreign body left behind in the uterus or in the abdominal cavity used for criminal interference.

Definitive treatment

- **Antibiotics** — Pending sensitivity report, potent bactericidal drugs such as gentamicin 2 mg/kg body weight and clindamycin IV 600 mg daily with IV metronidazole 500 mg are to be administered at every 6-8 hours interval. With response (usually noticeable within 24-36 hours), the route of administration is changed orally. The treatment should be continued for about 8-10 days. If the temperature does not subside by 48 hours, the antibiotic should be changed according to microbiology and sensitivity report.

Supportive therapy

- **Blood transfusion** — to improve anaemia.
- **Appropriate therapy** is directed to treat generalised peritonitis, endotoxic shock, renal failure or disseminated intravascular coagulopathy.

Active surgery

It includes :

- Evacuation of uterus • Posterior colpotomy
- Laparotomy — A suspected case of acute appendicitis or rupture tubo-ovarian abscess.

Indications of surgery in septic abortion are :

(1) Injury to the uterus. (2) Suspected injury to the gut. (3) Presence of foreign body in the abdomen as evidenced by the USG or felt through the fornix on bimanual examination. (4) Unresponsive peritonitis suggestive of collection of pus. (5) Patient's clinical condition not responding to the conservative treatment.

Late sequelae

These include :

- Infertility either due to cornual block, or damage to the wall of the tube.
- Residual infection with periodic acute exacerbation.
- Intestinal obstruction.
- Chronic ill health.
- Chronic pelvic pain.
- Dyspareunia and marital disharmony.

FOLLOWING GYNAECOLOGICAL PROCEDURES

Infection of the residual pelvic organs or cellular tissues is frequent following hysterectomy, more in vaginal than abdominal one. It is more common in infected or potentially infected cases than in 'elective' non-infective cases.

Organisms

Escherichia coli and *Bacteroides fragilis* are the predominant organisms.

Pathology

The vaginal cuff may be indurated due to infected haematoma → cellulitis → abscess. The infection may spread to produce pelvic cellulitis, thrombophlebitis or tubo-ovarian mass.

Clinical features

Fever and lower abdominal or pelvic pain of varying degrees appear few days (3-4) following surgery.

Per vaginam

Discharge is offensive and the vaginal vault is indurated and tender. Speculum examination may reveal exposed vaginal cuff with purulent discharge coming through the gaping vault. Rectal examination reveals induration on the vault or its extension to one side (parametritis). Rarely, a fluctuant mass may be felt (pelvic abscess).

Treatment

Prophylactic

Pre-operative cleaning of the vagina with antiseptic lotion, perfect haemostasis during surgery and leaving behind the vault open in infected cases could reduce the postoperative infection. **Chemoprophylaxis** in potentially or actually infected cases using **intravenous metronidazole 500 mg 8 hourly for 3 such and intravenous ceftriaxone 1 gm, given during the operation and 1-2 doses after the operation is quite effective to lower the risk of infection.**

Definitive treatment

Appropriate antibiotic and drainage of pus through the vault are enough to arrest the infection. However, in parametritis and thrombophlebitis, the response is poor. Adnexal abscess requires urgent exploration and removal of the infected mass.

IUD AND PELVIC INFECTION

IUD is one of the iatrogenic causes of pelvic infection in gynaecology (see ch. 29). All types of IUDs are responsible. The incidence ranges from 2-10 per cent. **The chance is, however, more in nulliparae.** It may flare up pre-existing pelvic infection. IUD tail may be implicated in ascent of the organisms from the vagina in infections long after insertion. The bacteria may be carried from the cervix into the endometrium during insertion. Actinomycosis has been found rarely in association with the use of copper devices. Risk of PID is highest in the first month after insertion. Again risk of PID is highest when the patient has multiple sexual partners.

As a preventive measure, **it is better not to insert in nulliparae or in cases with previous history of pelvic inflammatory disease.** Insertion should be carried out under strict aseptic condition. Once the pelvic infection occurs, the device should be removed in addition to antibiotic and supportive therapy. Actinomycosis responds well with penicillin.

CHRONIC PELVIC INFECTION

Chronic pelvic infection is a distressing clinical entity not only to the patients but also to the physicians. It results :

- Following acute pelvic infection — the initial treatment have either been delayed or otherwise inadequate.
- Following low grade recurrent infection.
- Tubercular infection.

The first two types are predominantly due to pyogenic organisms including those responsible for acute PID. There is often history of previous acute pelvic infection. Tubercular infection is chronic from the beginning and is described as a separate entity.

PYOGENIC

Pathology

The pathology in the uterus is most often spared because of periodic shedding of the endometrium. The tubal changes are secondary to the changes induced by previous acute salpingitis. The tubal epithelium is usually lost, specially in gonococcal infection; the wall gets thickened with plasma cell infiltration and the openings are blocked. These result in hydrosalpinx, with loss of the lining mucosa with its plicae. The peritoneal surface is involved in recurrent infection producing **either flimsy (gonococcal) or dense (non-gonococcal pyogenic) adhesions.** The tubes are thus kinked and may get adherent to the ovaries, uterus, intestine, omentum and pelvic peritoneum. A tubo-ovarian mass or a frozen pelvis results. The serum and lymph exudate in the parametrium of acute infection coagulates, which later either completely resolutes or becomes fibrotic. The fibrosis pulls the uterus, the cervix in particular, to the same side.

Clinical features

- There may be previous history of acute pelvic infection following childbirth or abortion. Recurrent episodes of reinfection is often present. The recent presence of IUCD is highly corroborative.
- The entity may remain asymptomatic and reveals on laparoscopy or hysterosalpingography for investigation of infertility.

Symptoms

- Chronic pelvic pain of varying magnitude is present in almost all cases. The pain aggravates prior to menstruation due to congestion.
- Dyspareunia, which is deep and may be located unilaterally or bilaterally.
- Congestive dysmenorrhoea.
- Lower abdominal pain.
- Menorrhagia due to congestion and at times polymenorrhagia due to ovarian involvement.
- Vaginal discharge is almost a constant manifestation and may be mucoid or mucopurulent.
- Infertility, which may be primary or more commonly secondary.

Important factors for infertility are — cornual block (Fig. 36.68), loss of cilia, loss of peristalsis due to thickening of the tubal wall, closure of the abdominal ostium and distortion of the tube due to peritubal adhesions.

- Deteriorating general health status is due to presence of septic foci, pelvic pain and agony. Marital disharmony arises out of dyspareunia.

On examination

Per abdomen : There may be tenderness on one or both iliac fossa. An irregular tender pelvic mass may be felt.

Per vaginam : The findings are as mentioned in page 126.

Rectal examination corroborates the findings of vaginal examination and should not be omitted, specially when the vaginal examination is painful. The involvement of the parametrium and uterosacral ligaments are better assessed rectally.

It should be once more emphasised that there may not be any palpable clinical findings to establish the diagnosis of chronic pelvic infection.

Investigations

The investigations include :

- Blood examination for evidences of leucocytosis, Hb estimation and ESR. Urine examination — routine and, if necessary, culture sensitivity. This may be of help if there is history of recent re-infection.

Laparoscopy : This is helpful to confirm the diagnosis and to know the extent of the lesion specially in cases of infertility. However, in cases where too much adhesions are anticipated, diagnostic laparotomy is a safer substitute.

Differential diagnosis

- Endometriosis — Chronic pelvic pain, dyspareunia, and parametrial thickening too often are confused with endometriosis.
- Disturbed ectopic pregnancy.
- Chronic appendicitis.
- Chronic colitis.
- Intracystic haemorrhage or twisted ovarian cyst.
- Chronic cystourethritis.

Management

• General • Specific • Surgery

General

- Improvement of general health, specially to correct anaemia, is imperative.
- Analgesics as required, may be prescribed for temporary palliation. Pelvic heat application by short wave diathermy is comforting to the patient.

Specific

- The IUCD is to be removed, if it is still inside.
- Antibiotic therapy has got little benefit unless there is recent acute exacerbation. The long-

term broad spectrum antibiotics to be administered include doxycycline or tetracycline or cephalosporin for three weeks. In proved cases of gonococcal infection, specific therapy is directed as outlined in acute infection (p. 144).

Surgery : ***Indications*** — It is indeed difficult to categorise the indications of surgery, but the following are unequivocal indications :

- Persistence of symptoms in spite of adequate conservative treatment.
- Recurrence of acute attacks.
- Increase in size of the pelvic mass despite treatment.
- General deterioration in health despite intensive conservative treatment.
- Persistence of menorrhagia that is incapacitating and/or causing anaemia.
- Infertility — Restorative tubal surgery even with asymptomatic minimal lesion detected by laparoscopy.

Precautions prior to surgery

The surgery should be done when the acute symptoms are controlled.

Broad spectrum antibiotic should be given prior to and following surgery.

Nature of surgery

Due consideration should be given to age, parity and extent of the lesion.

In women with infertility, restorative tubal plastic operations such as salpingolysis, salpingostomy or tubal anastomosis may be done with varying degree of success (see p. 239). Chance of ectopic pregnancy is however more. An alternative is IVF and ET.

In general, the ideal surgery should be total hysterectomy with bilateral salpingo-oophorectomy for women that they have completed their family.

GENITAL TUBERCULOSIS

Incidence

The incidence of genital tuberculosis varies widely with the social status of the patient and her environment. The incidence is about 1 per cent amongst the gynaecological patients attending the out-patient department in the developing countries. Incidence is high (5-10 %) amongst the patients with infertility. With the prevalence of HIV infection incidence of genital tuberculosis is rising.

Pathogenesis

The causative organism is *Mycobacterium tuberculosis* of human type. Very rarely the bovine type may affect the vulva. **Genital tuberculosis is almost always secondary to primary infection** elsewhere in the extragenital sites such as lungs (50%), lymph nodes, urinary tract, bones and joints. **The fallopian tubes are invariably the primary sites** of pelvic tuberculosis from where secondary spread occurs to other genital organs.

Mode of spread

Bloodstream

From any of the primary sites, the pelvic organs are involved by haematogenous spread in about 90 per cent cases. If the post-primary haematogenous spread coincides with the growth spurt of the pelvic vessels, the genital organs, the tubes in particular, are likely to be affected. Thus, the pelvic organs are infected during puberty. If the spread precedes the growth phase, the genital organs are spared. The infection remains dormant for a variable period of time (4-6 years) until clinical manifestations appear (Fig. 10.3).

Lymphatic or direct

The pelvic organs are involved directly or by lymphatics from the infected organs such as peritoneum, bowel or mesenteric nodes.

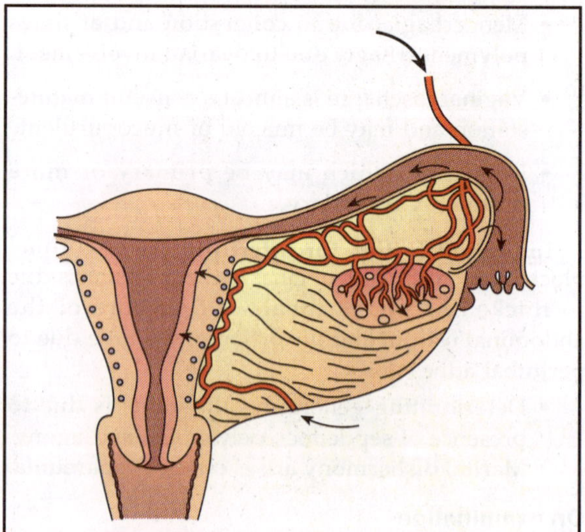

Fig. 10.3. Mode of spread in tubercular infection through blood-stream

Ascending

Although difficult to prove but sexual transmission from a male with urogenital tuberculosis is possible in vulval, vaginal or cervical lesion.

Pathology of Pelvic Organs

Fallopian tube : **The commonest site of affection is the fallopian tubes (100%). Both the tubes are affected simultaneously. The initial site of infection** is in the submucosal layer (interstitial salpingitis) of the ampullary part of the tube.

The infection may spread medially along the wall causing destruction of the muscles which are replaced by fibrous tissue. The walls get thickened, become calcified or even ossified. The thickening may at time become segmented. The infection may spread inwards; the mucosa gets swollen and destroyed. The fimbrial are everted and **the abdominal ostium usually remains patent**. The elongated and distended distal tube with the patent abdominal ostium gives the appearance of **"tobacco-pouch"**. Occlusion of the ostium may however occur due to adhesions. The tubercles burst pouring the caseous material inside the lumen producing tubercular pyosalpinx, which may adhere to the ovaries and the surrounding structures. Often the infection spreads outwards producing perisalpingitis with exudation, causing dense adhesions with the surrounding structures — tubercular tubo-ovarian mass. Rarely, miliary tubercles may be found on the serosal surface of the tubes, uterus, peritoneum or intestines. These are often associated with tubercular peritonitis (Fig. 10.4).

However, not infrequently the tubes may look absolutely normal or nodular at places. If the nodules happen to be present in the isthmus near the uterine cornu, it constitutes salpingitis isthmica nodosa. **Salpingitis isthmica nodosa** is the nodular thickening of the tube due to proliferation of tubal epithelium within the hypertrophied myosalpinx (muscle layer). Exact aetiology is unknown. It is diagnosed radiologically as a small diverticulum (Fig. 10.7). It is however not specific to tubercular infection only (see p. 168). It is also observed in pelvic endometriosis.

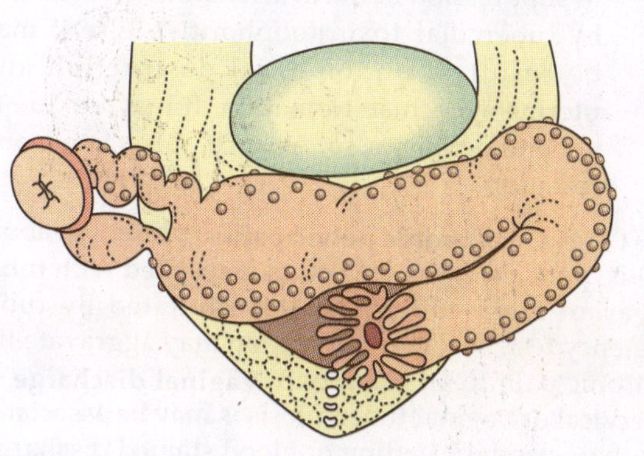

Fig. 10.4. Miliary tubercle on the tubes and uterus. Note the patent abdominal ostium of the left tube (tobacco-pouch appearance)

Uterus

The endometrium is involved in 60 per cent of cases. The infection is from the tubes either by lymphatics or by direct spread through continuity. Cornual ends are commonly affected due to their dual blood supply, as well as their anatomical proximity to tubes. The tubercle is situated in the basal layer of the endometrium only to come to the surface premenstrually. After the endometrium is shed at each menstruation, reinfection occurs from the lesions in the basal layer or from the tubes. Endometrial ulceration may lead to **adhesion or synechiae formation (Asherman's syndrome)**. This may cause infertility, secondary amenorrhoea or recurrent abortion (p. 438). Rarely, the infection spreads to the myometrium (2.5%) and if caseation occurs, a pyometra results, specially in postmenopausal women.

Cervix : **The cervical affection is not so uncommon (5-15%).** Primary infection of the cervix by sexual intercourse though rare, has been recorded. It may be ulcerative or may be bright nodular in type. Both may bleed to touch, thereby causing confusion with carcinoma. Histologically genital tuberculosis is associated with marked epithelial hyperplasia with some degree of atypia. This may lead to erroneous diagnosis of carcinoma (see Fig. 10.8).

Vulva and vagina : The affection of these sites is **very rare (1%)**. The lesion may be ulcerative with undermined edges. Rarely the lesions may be of hypertrophic variety. The diagnosis is made only by histology.

Ovary : The ovaries are involved in **about 30 per cent of tubercular salpingitis**. The manifestation may be surface tubercles, adhesions, thickening of the capsule or even caseating abscess in the substance of the ovary.

Pelvic peritoneum

Pelvic peritonitis is present in about 40-50 per cent

of cases. Tuberculous peritonitis may be 'wet' (exudative type) or 'dry' (adhesive type).

In the **'wet' variety** there is ascites with straw coloured fluid in the peritoneal cavity. The parietal and visceral peritoneum are covered with numerous small tubercles (Fig. 10.4).

In the **'dry' variety** there is dense adhesion with bowel loops. The adhesion is due to fibrosis when the 'wet' variety heals.

Microscopic appearance of the lesion

Microscopic picture of the lesion is very characteristic irrespective of the organ involved. **Typical granuloma consists of infiltration of multinucleated giant cells (Langhans), chronic inflammatory cells and epithelioid cells, surrounding a central area of caseation necrosis (Fig. 10.5).** Caseation may not be a constant feature.

Clinical features

Patient profile : The infection is restricted mostly (80%) to childbearing period (20-40 years). There may be past history of tubercular affection of the lungs or lymph glands. **Genital tuberculosis occurs in 10-20 per cent of patients who have pulmonary tuberculosis in adolescence.** A family history of contact may be available. Onset is mostly insidious.

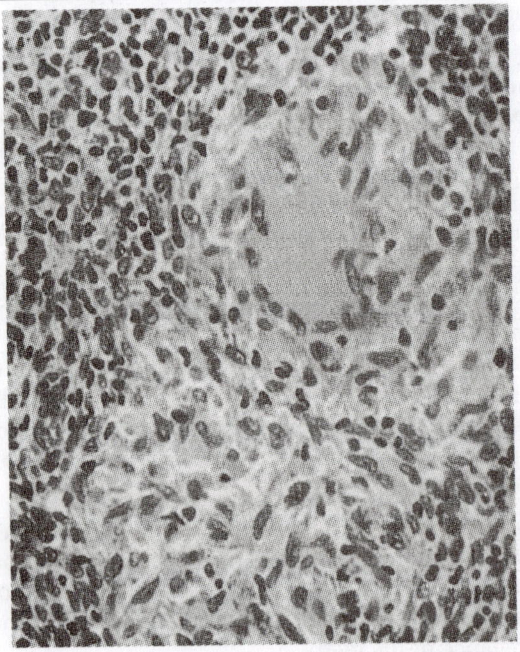

Fig. 10.5. A typical tubercular granuloma formed by lymphocytes, epithelioid cells and Langhans giant cells. Central area of caseation necrosis is seen

A flare up of the infection may occur acutely either spontaneously or following diagnostic endometrial curettage or hysterosalpingography.

Symptoms : Symptoms vary considerably with the severity and stage of the disease. At one extreme, there is neither any symptom nor any palpable pelvic pathology. **Sometimes symptoms like** weakness, low grade fever, anorexia, anaemia or night sweats may be present. The lesion is accidentally diagnosed during investigation for infertility or dysfunctional uterine bleeding. These cases are often designated as "silent tuberculosis". **In others, the clinical manifestations appear.** These are :

Infertility — It may be primary or secondary and is present in about 70-80 per cent cases of pelvic tuberculosis. In India, about 10 per cent infertile women have got genital tuberculosis. The causes are predominantly due to tubal blockage, adhesions in the endometrial cavity (uterine synechiae) or associated ovulatory dysfunction.

Menstrual abnormality — In about 50 per cent, the menstrual function is normal.

The menstrual abnormalities include :

- Menorrhagia or irregular bleeding is probably due to ovarian involvement, pelvic congestion or endometrial proliferative lesion. It is the early manifestation. These patients fail to respond with hormone therapy. Endometrial tuberculosis is a rare cause of puberty menorrhagia and postmenopausal bleeding.
- Amenorrhoea or oligomenorrhoea — Secondary amenorrhoea is more common and may be the only presenting symptom that makes the patient seek for medical advice. It may be due to suppression of the ovarian function probably by tubercular toxin (oophoritis). Else it may be result of endometrial destruction and uterine synechiae formation. It may be due to general debility also. As such, it is a late manifestation.

Others — **Chronic pelvic pain** is present in about 20-30 per cent cases. It is often associated with tubo-ovarian mass and may be precipitated by tubal patency test. Secondary infection may aggravate the chronic pain to an acute one. **Vaginal discharge** — Cervical or vaginal tuberculosis is may be associated with postcoital bleeding or blood stained discharge. **Constitutional symptoms** such as loss of weight, malaise, anorexia, pyrexia and anaemia are present in the acute phase of the disease.

Signs

Health status — The general health usually remains unaffected. There may be constitutional symptoms like weakness, low grade fever, anorexia, anaemia and night sweats. There may be evidences of active or healed extra-genital tubercular lesion.

Per abdomen — Abdominal findings may be negative or rarely one may find an irregular tender mass in lower abdomen arising out of the pelvis. Abdomen may **feel doughy due to matted intestines.** Evidences of free peritoneal fluid are rare. **Tubercular ascites when encysted mimics an ovarian cyst.**

Per vaginam — The pelvic findings may be negative in 50 per cent cases. Vulval or vaginal ulcer presents with undermined edges. There may be thickening of the tubes which are felt through the lateral fornices or nodules, felt through posterior fornix. At times, there is bilateral pelvic mass of varying sizes quite indistinguishable from that due to pyogenic infection. Per rectum, one may confirm the vaginal findings.

Investigations

The investigations aim at :

- To identify the primary lesion.
- To confirm the genital lesion.

Blood — The leucocyte count and ESR values may be raised. Periodic examination is of value to evaluate the progress of the lesion.

Mantoux test — Positive test with high dilution is suggestive that the patient is sensitised to tuberculoprotein. A negative test excludes tuberculosis.

Chest X-ray is taken for evidence of healed or active pulmonary lesion.

Diagnostic uterine curettage — This is to be done during the week preceding menstruation. The tubercles are likely to come to the surface during this period. **The material should be sent to the laboratory in two portions.**

(a) One part in formal-saline for histopathological examination to detect the giant cell system. Histology could detect tuberculosis in about 10 per cent of cases only. False-positive histology may be due to the presence of chronic lesions (like talc or catgut granuloma) or sarcoidosis. False-negative result is due to improper timing of uterine curettage or due to less incidence of uterine infection.

(b) One part in normal saline for :

(i) Culture in Löwenstein-Jensen media.

(ii) Identification of the acid-fast bacilli by Ziehl-Neelsen's stain (AFB-Microscopy).

(iii) Nucleic acid amplification.

(iv) Guineapig inoculation.

A positive culture is suggestive while a positive guineapig inoculation test is diagnostic. Bacteriological test, if positive, should be able to type the bacilli and report on their drug sensitivity.

Nucleic acid amplification (16S ribosomal DNA) techniques with Polymerase Chain Reaction (PCR), **can identify *M. tuberculosis* from endometrium or menstrual blood (clinical specimens).** PCR is more sensitive (85-95%) than microscopy and bacteriological culture. **This method can detect fewer than 10 organisms in clinical specimens compared to 10,000 necessary for smear positivity. Genital TB is usually paucibacillary.**

First day menstrual discharge — This is to be collected by a pipette and the material subjected to micobacterial nucleic acid amplification, culture and guineapig inoculation. **It should be emphasised that while a positive report on AFB-microscopy, PCR, culture and histology gives the diagnosis, a negative report does not rule out tuberculosis.**

Sputum and urine is to be cultured for tubercle bacillus.

Lymph node biopsy is to be done, specially from the neck in lymphadenitis.

Biopsy from the lesion cervix, vagina or vulva.

Hysterosalpingography (HSG) — In a proved case, HSG is contraindicated for the risk of reactivation of the lesion. HSG done as a routine work up in the investigation of infertility may reveal the following suggestive features :

- Vascular or lymphatic extravasation of dye (Fig. 10.6).
- Rigid (lead-pipe) tubes with nodulations at places.
- 'Tobacco pouch' appearance with blocked fimbrial end (Fig. 10.4).
- Beaded appearance of the tube with variable filling density (Fig. 10.7).
- Distal tube obstruction.
- Coiling of the tubes or calcified shadow at places.

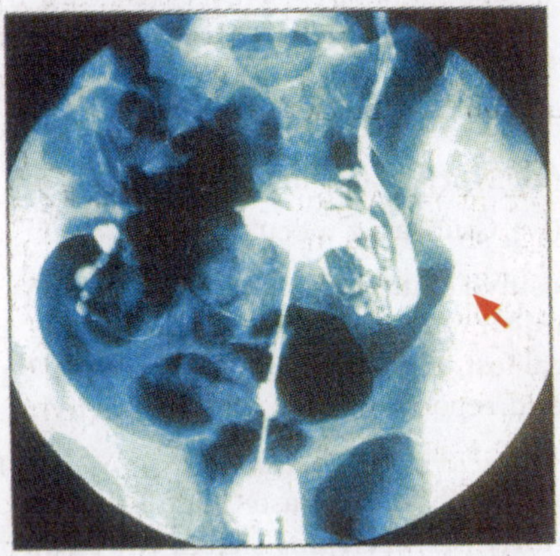

Fig. 10.6. Hysterosalpingogram showing marked extravasation of dye in venous and lymphatic channels. It was proved to be a case of tubercular endometritis.

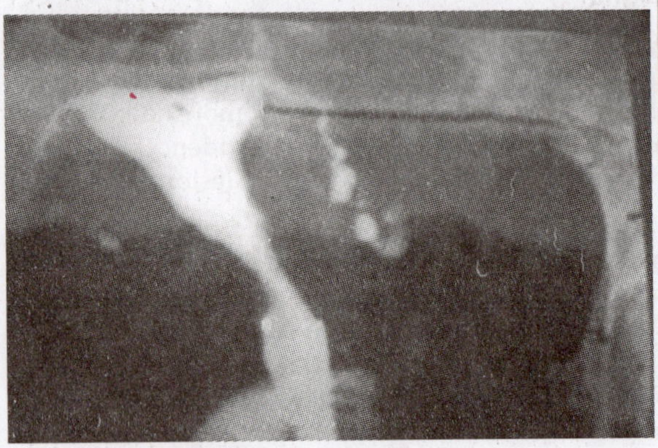

Fig. 10.7. Hysterosalpingogram showing beaded appearance of the tube with variable filling density. Pelvic tuberculosis was later confirmed.

[*By courtesy : Dr. P. Panigrahi, Consultant Gynaecologist, JLN Hospital, Bhilai*]

- Bilateral cornual block (Fig. 36.69).
- Tubal diverticula and/or fluffiness of tubal outline.
- Uterine cavity — irregular outline, honeycomb appearance or presence of uterine synechiae.

Imaging : Abdominal and pelvic ultrasound, CT or MRI is helpful where a mass and/or ascites is present. However, it cannot confirm the diagnosis.

Laparoscopy : In the absence of endometrial evidence, one may take the advantage of laparoscope for identification of tubercles in the pelvic organs or characteristic segmented nodular appearance of the tubes. Biopsy may be taken from peritoneal tubercles for histology. Aspiration of fluid is done for culture. This may be accidentally discovered during diagnostic laparoscopy for infertility work up or for chronic pelvic pain.

Diagnosis

Considering the high prevalence of extragenital tuberculosis, pulmonary in particular, the physicians of the Third World Countries should look out for the presence of genital tuberculosis. For this, **the following guidelines may be prescribed** :

(a) The physician should be conscious of the entity.

(b) One should suspect and exclude genital tuberculosis in the following conditions :

- Unexplained infertility or amenorrhoea.
- Recurrent episodes of pelvic infections, not responding with usual course of antibiotics.

(c) Presence of pelvic mass with nodules in the pouch of Douglas.

Differential diagnosis

The pelvic mass is often confused with : (i) Pyogenic tubo-ovarian mass. (ii) Pelvic endometriosis. (iii) Adherent ovarian cyst. (iv) Chronic disturbed ectopic pregnancy.

Treatment

- **General** • **Chemotherapy** • **Surgery**

General : In the presence of active pulmonary tuberculosis, hospital admission is preferred. Otherwise, pelvic tuberculosis *per se* need not require hospitalisation or bed rest except in acute exacerbation. To improve the body resistance, due attention is to be paid as regards diet and to correct anaemia. Until the infection is controlled, the husband should use condom during intercourse to prevent possibility of contracting urogenital tuberculosis.

Chemotherapy : Antituberculous chemotherapy is the treatment of first choice.

Initial phase : Four drugs are used for 2 months to reduce the bacterial population and to prevent emergence of drug-resistance. The drugs used are isoniazid, rifampicin, pyrazinamide and ethambutol. Ethambutol is essential to those who have been treated previously or are immunocompromised (HIV positive individual).

Continuation phase : Treatment is continued for a period of further 4 months with isoniazid and rifampicin.

This standard regimen may be used **during pregnancy and lactation (Table 10.7).**

After about a year of treatment, diagnostic endometrial curettage is to be done. If the histological and/or bacteriological examination becomes positive, the treatment must be continued further. If these are negative, the endometrium is examined at interval of six months. **A patient may be considered cured,** if at least two reports including histological and bacteriological examination become negative. Majority of the patients (90-95 %) respond well to chemotherapy.

Surgery — ***Indications*** : (i) Unresponsiveness of active disease in spite of adequate anti-tuberculous chemotherapy. (ii) Tubercular pyosalpinx, ovarian abscess or pyometra (iii) Persistent menorrhagia and/or chronic pelvic pain causing deteriorating health status.

Contraindications : (i) Presence of active tuberculosis in extragenital site. (ii) Favourable response to antimicrobial therapy with diminishing size of the pelvic mass. (iii) Accidental discovery of tubercular tubo-ovarian mass on laparotomy in young patient. The abdomen is to be closed after taking tissue for biopsy.

Precautions — Antitubercular drug therapy in full dosage should be instituted at least six weeks prior to surgery and similar treatment should be continued following surgery.

Type of surgery — The ideal surgery should be total hysterectomy with bilateral salpingo-oophorectomy. In young women at least one ovary, if found apparently healthy, should be preserved. Isolated excision of tubo-ovarian mass, drainage of pyometra or repair of fistula may be done in selected cases.

Results of treatment

In terms of future reproduction, the prognosis is most unfavourable. Pregnancy is rare (5-10 %), and if occurs, chance of ectopic pregnancy is more (40 %). In uterine pregnancy, abortion is likely and a pregnancy going upto term is a rare event.

With the help of assisted reproductive technology (ART) higher pregnancy rate is observed following successful chemotherapy.

Table 10.7 : Antituberculous Chemotherapy For Initial Treatment

Drug	*Daily oral dosage (adult)*	*Nature*	*Toxicity*	*Comments*
Isoniazid	5 mg/kg : max. 300 mg.	Bactericidal	Hepatitis, Peripheral neuropathy	• Check liver function • Combine pyridoxin 50 mg daily
Rifampicin	10 mg/kg : max. 600 mg.	Bactericidal	Hepatic dysfunction Orange discolouration of urine. Febrile reaction	• Drug interaction (p. 466) • Oral contraceptives to be avoided (p. 466) • Monitor Liver enzymes (AST)
Pyrazinamide	20-25 mg/kg : max. 2 gm.	Bactericidal	Hepatitis, Hyperuricaemia, GI upset and Arthralgia	• Active against intracellular dividing forms of mycobacterium. • Monitor (AST)
Ethambutol	15-20 mg/kg : max. 2.5 gm.	Bacteriostatic	Visual disturbances Optic neuritis, Loss of visual acuity.	• Ophthalmoscopic examination prior to therapy.

Intermittent dose schedule is also recommended. Treatment should be supervised by the DOTS provider.

Revised National TB Control Programme (RNTCP) 1993 and Directly Observed Treatment by Short Course Chemotherapy (DOTS).

- *Isoniazid* : 15 mg/kg, 3 times a week for 6 months.
- *Rifampicin* : 600 mg, 3 times a week for 6 months.
- *Pyrazinamide* : 30 mg/kg, 3 times a week for first 2 months only.
- *Ethambutol* : 30 mg/kg, 3 times a week for first 2 months only.

VULVAL TUBERCULOSIS

The patient complains of a painful and tender ulcer in the vulva. Confirmation is done by biopsy. The medical treatment is the same as that outlined in pelvic tuberculosis. In unresponsive cases, local vulvectomy is to be done.

CERVICAL TUBERCULOSIS

The presenting complaints are mucopurulent discharge and postcoital bleeding. Cervical tuberculosis on speculum examination (Fig. 10.8) appears as an ulcerated or hypertrophic growth which bleeds on touch.

Cervical cytology — may reveal multinucleated giant cells, epithelioid cells and dyskaryotic cells. **Biopsy** confirms the diagnosis. Antitubercular drug therapy as outlined in pelvic tuberculosis is prescribed (Table 10.7). In unresponsive cases, hysterectomy is justified.

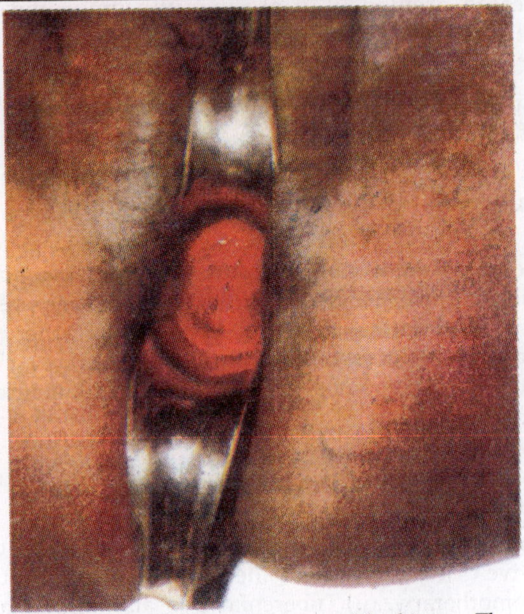

Fig. 10.8. Tubercular cervix proved by biopsy. The clinical diagnosis was confused with malignancy

CHRONIC PID

The term chronic pelvic inflammatory disease has largely been abandoned. The long-term sequelae of acute PID such as adhesions or hydrosalpinx are bacteriologically sterile.

True chronic PID such as **genital tuberculosis and actinomycosis** is rare although the former is not infrequent in the developing countries.

Actinomycosis is caused by *Actinomyces israelii*, a gram-positive anaerobe. It may be associated in IUCD users more with noncopper devices. It is sensitive to penicillin. The treatment should be continued for 6 weeks. Following the course of antibiotic treatment, Pap smear is repeated after 3 months. If infection is still present IUCD should be removed.

KEY POINTS

- The vaginal defence is lost following 10 days of birth till puberty, in reproductive period-during menstruation, following abortion and childbirth and following menopause.
- Pelvic inflammatory disease according to anatomic location may be in the endometrium (endometritis), the oviducts (salpingitis), the ovary (oophoritis), the myometrium (myometritis), uterine serosa and broad ligaments (parametritis) and the peritoneum (pelvic peritonitis).
- The primary organisms of PID are predominantly sexually transmitted. Acute PID is polymicrobial in nature. As the symptoms of PID are nonspecific, over treatment is preferred to missed diagnosis.
- Clinical diagnostic criteria for acute PID includes : Minimum and Additional (routine and definitive) criteria (see p. 126).
- Gonococcal affection of the tubes is by direct spread from downstairs to upstairs across the mucosal surface of the endometrium, reflux of the menstrual flow with gonococci into the tubes and carried along the spermatozoa or the trichomonads. The pathological process is initiated primarily in the endosalpinx.

  For detection of Gonococcus, the materials are collected from the urethra or Bartholin's duct, cervical smear and laparoscopic collection of pus from the uterine tube. Acute gonorrhoea is treated by drugs (Table 11.2 on p. 144) to both the partners.

KEY POINTS

In acute condition, the diagnosis is confused with acute appendicitis and disturbed ectopic pregnancy.

Immediate complications include pelvic peritonitis and septicaemia and late complications include infertility, chronic pelvic pain and chronic ill-health.

Repeat smears and cultures from the discharge are to be done following each menstrual period until it becomes negative for 3 consecutive reports when the patient is declared cured.

- *Chlamydia trachomatis* — a gram-negative obligatory intracellular bacteria, is now the commonest organism proved to be sexually transmitted from the non-gonococcal urethritis in male consort. The clinical picture is almost the same to that of gonococcal infection but is milder in nature. Perihepatic inflammation (Fitz-Hugh-Curtis syndrome) is observed in 5-10 per cent women with acute PID.

  The late sequelae include tubal obstruction, infertility, early abortion and ectopic pregnancy.

  Detection can be done by tissue culture. The specific antibody can be detected by immunofluorescent test or complement fixation test. Chlamydial DNA amplification and detection by PCR is a very sensitive test.

  The organism is sensitive to azithromycin, erythromycin or ofloxacin. The same treatment is to be given to the sexual partner.

- The commonest organisms producing acute infection following delivery and abortion are anaerobic Streptococcus, *Staphylococcus pyogenes, Esch. coli* and Bacteroides groups.

- The fallopian tube is affected either following parametritis through the lymphatics producing perisalpingitis or through endosalpingitis. Tubal affection to cause infertility depends on the severity and number of episodes of the disease.

- Triple swabs are to be taken prior to bimanual examination one from the high vagina, one from the endocervix and the third from the urethra. These are to be sent for aerobic and anaerobic culture, drug sensitivity and Gram stain. Culture from the endocervical materials does not give a reliable indicator of the microbiology of tubal infection.

- Clinical diagnostic criteria of PID (CDC-2001) include minimum and additional ones (p. 126). Diagnostic laparoscopy is considered the gold standard (p. 127). Women may have antibiotherapy either as an out-patient (Table 10.4) or as an in-patient (Table 10.6) depending on her evaluation (Table 10.5).

- IUD may produce pelvic infection (2-10 %). The chance is more in nulliparae. The highest risk is in the first month after insertion. Bacteria ascends along the nylon threads. Actinomycosis is often implicated.

- Combined oral contraceptive use offers some protection against PID. causing thick cervical mucous and decrease in duration of menstrual flow. Contact tracing and treatment of sexual partner should be a routine for effective treatment of PID.

- The incidence of genital tuberculosis is about 1 per cent amongst the gynaecological patient. The pelvic organs are affected secondarily, the primary site is predominantly in lung. The spread is by haematogenous route. fallopian tube is almost always affected by interstitial salpingitis, endometrium in 60 per cent and cervix in 15 per cent cases. Infertility is present in 70 per cent. About 10 per cent of the infertile couple have got genital tuberculosis.

  Although menorrhagia may be the early symptom but more commonly, the patient presents with oligomenorrhoea or amenorrhoea. The diagnosis is confirmed by histological examination, culture in Löwenstein-Jensen media and guineapig inoculation and identification of the bacteria by Ziehl-Neelsen's stain from the uterine curettage materials. PCR is more sensitive (p. 137).

- The suggestive features of HSG are extravasation of dye, rigid tubes with nodulation at places and tobacco-pouch appearance (p. 137). The result in terms of fertility following treatment (Table 10.7) is unsatisfactory. Pregnancy is rare and if occurs, risk of ectopic pregnancy is more. In uterine pregnancy, abortion is likely and a pregnancy upto term is a rarity.

Sexually Transmitted Infections

11

Introduction

Sexually transmitted infections (STIs) include those infections which are predominantly transmitted through sexual contact from an infected partner. Although the transmission of the infections is mostly due to sexual contact, other modes of transmission include placental (HIV, syphilis), by blood transfusion or infected needles (HIV, hepatitis B or syphilis) or by inoculation on to the infant's mucosa when it passes through the birth canal (gonococcal, chlamydial or herpes). Gynaecological morbidities associated with sexually transmitted

Table 11.1
Sexually transmitted infections (STIs)

Disease	Agent
	• **Bacterial**
Gonorrhoea	*Neisseria gonorrhoeae*
Non-gonococcal urethritis	*Chlamydia trachomatis* (D-K serotypes)
Syphilis	*Treponema pallidum*
Lymphogranuloma venereum	*Chlamydia trachomatis* (L serotypes)
Chancroid	*Haemophilus ducreyi*
Granuloma inguinale	*Donovania granulomatis*
Non-specific vaginitis	*Haemophilus vaginalis*
Mycoplasma infection	*Mycoplasma hominis*
	• **Viral**
AIDS	*Human immunodeficiency virus* (HIV 1 or HIV 2)
Genital herpes	*Herpes simplex virus* (HSV 2)
Condyloma acuminata	*Human papilloma virus* (HPV)
Molluscum contagiosum	*Pox virus*
Viral hepatitis	*Hepatitis B* and *C virus*
CIN	*HPV – 16, 18* or *31*
	• **Protozoal**
Bacterial vaginosis (BV)	*Gardnerella vaginalis*
Trichomonas vaginitis	*Trichomonas vaginalis*
	• **Fungal**
Monilial vaginitis	*Candida albicans*
	• **Ectoparasites**
Scabies	*Sarcoptes scabiei*
Pediculosis pubis	Crab louse (*Phthirus pubis*)

diseases (STDs) are high. Chronic pelvic infection, pain, infertility, ectopic pregnancy, vulval and cervical neoplasia are the long-term sequelae.

Transplacental infection (during pregnancy) to the fetus results in high perinatal morbidity and mortality. **There is rising trend of STD throughout the globe.** With the improvement of diagnostic methods and increased interest on STD, more and more diseases are included mostly of viral origin (HIV, Hepatitis B and C, HPV).

The reasons for increasing incidence are :

- Rising prevalence of viral infections like HIV, hepatitis B and C.
- Development of antibiotic resistance by gonococci and other microbial organisms.
- Increased promiscuity and permissiveness.
- Increased use of 'Pill' and IUCD which cannot prevent STI.
- Lack of sex education and inadequate practice of safer sex.
- Increased rate of overseas travel.
- Increased detection due to heightened awareness.
- Inclusion of more diseases mostly of viral origin.

Important sexually transmitted diseases are grouped in Table 11.1.

GONORRHOEA

Gonorrhoea still remains an important health problem. The causative organism is *Neisseria gonorrhoeae* — a gram-negative diplococcus. The incubation period is 3-7 days.

The principal site of invasion is the columnar and transitional epithelium of the genitourinary tract. As such, **the primary sites of infection are** endocervix, urethra, Skene's gland and Bartholin's gland. The organism may be localised in the lower genital tract to produce urethritis, bartholinitis or cervicitis. Other sites of infection are oropharynx anorectal region and conjunctiva. As squamous epithelium is resistant to gonococcal invasion, vaginitis in adult is not possible but vulvovaginitis is possible in childhood. In about 15 per cent of untreated cervicitis, gonococcal infection may ascend up to produce acute PID. Rarely, it may produce septicaemia with distant involvement to cause tenosynovitis and septic arthritis. Upper genital organs are involved as the infect ion is spread along the spermatozoa. Gonococci attach to the spermatozoa and are being carried up. Endometritis and salpingitis are common (see p. 125). **It should be remembered that *N. gonorrhoeae*** is often present with other sexually transmitted diseases and women with gonorrhoea are considered to be at risk for incubating syphilis. One-third is associated with chlamydial infection.

Clinical features in adult

About 50 per cent of patients with gonorrhoea are asymptomatic and even when the symptoms are present, they are non-specific. The clinical features of acute gonococcal infection is described as follows :

- Local.
- Distant or metastatic.
- PID (Chapter 10, p. 124).

Local

Symptoms

- Urinary symptoms such as dysuria or frequency of micturition.
- Excessive irritant vaginal discharge.
- Acute unilateral pain and swelling over the labia due to involvement of Bartholin's gland.
- There may be rectal discomfort due to associated proctitis from genital contamination.

Signs

- Labia may be swollen and look inflamed.
- The vaginal discharge is purulent.
- The external urethral meatus and the openings of the Bartholin's ducts look congested. On squeezing the urethra and giving pressure on the Bartholin's glands, purulent exudate escapes out through the openings. Bartholin's gland may be palpably enlarged, tender with fluctuation, suggestive of formation of abscess.
- Speculum examination reveals congested ectocervix with increased mucopurulent cervical secretions escaping out through the external os.

Distant or metastatic

There may be features of perihepatitis and septicaemia. Perihepatitis results from spread of infection to the liver capsule. There is formation of adhesions with the abdominal wall. This is not infrequently (5-10%) associated with acute PID.

Septicaemia is characterised by low grade fever, polyarthralgia, tenosynovitis, septic arthritis, perihepatitis, meningitis, endocarditis and skin rash.

Complications — Acute pelvic inflammation leads to chronic pelvic inflammatory disease unless adequately treated. Infertility, ectopic pregnancy (due to tubal damage), dyspareunia, chronic pelvic pain, tubo-ovarian mass and Bartholin's gland abscess are the commonly seen.

Diagnosis

In the acute phase, secretions from the urethra, Bartholin's gland and endocervix are collected for Gram stain and culture.

A presumptive diagnosis is made following detection of gram-negative intracellular diplococci on staining. DNA-based tests are used for screening.

Culture of the discharge in Thayer-Martin medium further confirms the diagnosis. Drug sensitivity test is also to be performed.

In all cases, serological test for syphilis and rapid diagnostic tests for *Cl. trachomatis* — monoclonal antibody and ELISA are to be employed. Gonococcal complement fixation test is only positive after some weeks of the disease and as such is of no use in acute cases.

Treatment

Preventive

- Adequate therapy for gonococcal infection and meticulous follow up are to be done till the patient is declared cure.
- To treat adequately the male sexual partner simultaneously.
- To avoid multiple sex partners.
- To use condom till both the sexual partners are free from disease.

Curative

The specific treatment for gonorrhoea is **single dose regimen** of any one of the following drugs (Table 11.2).

Table 11.2
Drugs used in acute gonorrhoea (CDC guidelines 2002)

• Ceftriaxone	—	125 mg IM
• Ciprofloxacin	—	500 mg orally
• Ofloxacin	—	400 mg orally
• Cefixime	—	400 mg orally
• Levofloxacin	—	250 mg orally

Conjunctivitis of the newborn should be treated with a single dose of ceftriaxone (20-30 mg/kg) IM and gentamicin eye ointment (1%).

It should be borne in mind that the patient with gonorrhoea must be suspected of having syphilis or chlamydial infection. As such, treatment should cover all the three.

Follow up

Cultures should be made 7 days after the therapy. Repeat cultures are made at monthly intervals following mens for three months. **If the reports are persistently negative, the patient is declared cure.**

SYPHILIS

Syphilis is caused by the spirochaeta *Treponema pallidum*. Syphilitic lesion of the genital tract is acquired by direct contact with another person who has open primary or secondary syphilitic lesion. Transmission occurs through the abraded skin or mucosal surface.

Clinical features

The incubation period ranges between 9-90 days.

The primary lesion (chancre) may be single or multiple and is usually located in the labia. Fourchette, anus, cervix and nipples are the other sites of lesion. A small papule is formed which is quickly eroded to form an ulcer. The margins are raised with smooth shiny floor. The ulcer is painless without any surrounding inflammatory reaction. The inguinal glands are enlarged, discrete and painless. The **primary chancre** heals spontaneously in 1-8 week leaving behind a scar.

The tubes are not affected and infertility does not occur unless associated with gonococcal infection.

Secondary syphilis — Within 6 weeks to 6 months from the onset of primary chancre, the secondary syphilis may be evidenced in the vulva in the form of **condyloma lata**. These are coarse, flat-topped, moist, necrotic lesions and teeming with treponemes. Patient may present with systemic symptoms like fever, headache and sore throat. Maculopapular skin rashes are seen on the palms and soles. Other features include generalised lymphadenopathy, mucosal ulcers and alopecia.

The primary and secondary stage can last upto two years and during the period, the woman is a source of infection.

Latent syphilis — It is the quiescence phase after the stage of secondary syphilis has resolved. It may be early (duration less than 2 years from the onset of disease) or late duration more than 2 years from the onset of disease.

Tertiary syphilis — About one-third of untreated patients progress from late latent stage to tertiary syphilis. The risks are the development of neurosyphilis and cardiovascular syphilis. The important pathology is endarteritis and periarteritis of small and medium sized vessels. Tertiary syphilis is characterised by **gumma**. A gummatous ulcer is a deep punched ulcer with rolled out margins. It is painless with a moist leather base. Serpiginous outline may also be produced.

The systemic manifestations of the secondary and tertiary syphilis are better dealt with in Textbook of Medicine.

Congenital syphilis — See author's Textbook of Obstetrics (Chapter 19).

Diagnosis

1. History of exposure to an infected person.

2. Identification of the organism — *Treponema pallidum*, an anaerobe.

A smear is taken from the exudate which is obtained after teasing the primary chancre (base and edge) with a swab dipped in normal saline. It is examined under dark ground illumination through a microscope. The treponemata appear as motile white cork-screw shaped organisms.

3. Serological test — (a) VDRL : This is the common flocculation test performed and is **positive after 6 weeks of initial infection**.

(b) The specific tests include *Treponema pallidum* haemagglutination (TPHA) test and *Treponema pallidum immobilisation (TPI) test*.

(c) Fluorescent treponemal antibody absorption test (FTA-abs). FTA-abs is expensive but a **confirmatory test**. FTA-IgM is produced only in active treponemal infection and it declines after adequate treatment.

(d) ELISA test for treponemal specific IgG or IgM is now routinely used.

(e) Currently immunoblotting and PCR tests are evaluated as more sensitive and confirmatory tests.

(f) VDRL and TPHA tests are used for screening and FTA-abs test is used for confirmation.

(g) Serological tests are invariably positive in secondary syphilis.

Treatment (CDC Recommendation – 1998)

Early syphilis (primary, secondary and early latent syphilis of less than 1 year duration)

Benzathine penicillin G 2.4 million units is given intramuscularly in a single dose half to each buttock.

In penicillin hypersensitive cases, tetracycline or erythromycin 500 mg, 4 times a day orally for 14 days is effective.

Late syphilis

Benzathine penicillin G 2.4 million units is given IM weekly for three weeks. This should be in consultation with the STD clinic.

Alternative regimen : Doxycycline 100 mg orally twice daily or Tetracycline 500 mg orally 4 times a day for 4 weeks.

Follow up

Serological test is to be performed 1,3,6 and 12 months after treatment of early syphilis. In late symptomatic cases, surveillance is for life; the serological test is to be done annually.

CHLAMYDIAL INFECTIONS

The causative organism is *Chlamydia trachomatis* (of D-K serotypes) an obligatory intracellular gram-negative bacteria. Its prevalence is more than *N. gonorrhoeae* as a causative agent for sexually transmitted disease in developed countries. Chlamydia has longer incubation period (6-14 days) compared to gonorrhoea (3-7 days).

The organisms affect the columnar and transitional epithelium of the genitourinary tract. The lesion is limited superficially. As there is no deeper penetration, the pathological changes to produce symptoms may not be apparent. **The infection is mostly localised** in the urethra, Bartholin's gland and cervix. It can ascend upstairs like gonococcal infection to produce acute PID. Too often (20-40%), it is associated with gonococcal infection.

Clinical features are non-specific and asymptomatic in most cases (75%). Dysuria, dyspareunia, postcoital bleeding and intermenstrual bleeding are the presenting symptoms.

Findings include mucopurulent cervical discharge, cervical oedema, cervical ectopy and cervical friability.

The clinical features of acute PID — has been mentioned in chapter 10 (p. 126).

Complications : Urethritis and bartholinitis are manifested by dysuria and purulent vaginal discharge. Chlamydial cervicitis spreads upwards to produce endometritis and salpingitis. Chlamydial salpingitis is asymptomatic in majority of the cases. It causes tubal scarring resulting in infertility and ectopic pregnancy. It is the more common cause of perihepatitis **(Fitz-Hugh-Curtis syndrome)** than in the gonococcus. The spread to the liver from the pelvic organs is via the lymphatics and the peritoneal cavity.

Diagnosis

In uncomplicated cases, the materials are to be collected from the urethra and endocervical canals.

- *C. trachomatis* elementary bodies are detected using fluorescein-conjugated monoclonal antibodies. It is a rapid, simple, sensitive (90%) and specific (95%) test. This slide test is performed with endocervical smears.
- Chlamydia antigen (lipopolysaccharide) can be detected by ELISA technique. Samples are taken from endocervix (endocervical swab). Sensitivity and specificity of this test is similar to fluorescent monoclonal antibody test.
- Chlamydial DNA amplification and detection by polymerase chain reaction (PCR) is a very sensitive test. First void urine specimen is most effective and specific.
- Chlamydia can be demonstrated in tissue culture. (McCoy cell monolayers). It is expensive, technically difficult and takes 3-7 days to obtain result.

Treatment (see Table 11.3)

Table 11.3
Drugs used in chlamydial infections (CDC Guidelines 2002)

Azithromycin	– 1 gm orally single dose or
Doxycycline	– 100 mg orally bid × 7 days or
Ofloxacin	– 200 mg orally bid × 7 days or
Erythromycin	– 500 mg orally bid × 7 days.

The sexual partner should also be treated with the same drug regimen.

Treatment failure with the above strict guidelines are indicative of either lack of patient compliance or reinfection.

CHANCROID (SOFT SORE)

The causative organism is a gram-negative streptobacillus — *Haemophilus ducreyi*. The incubation period is very short 3-5 days or less.

The lesion starts as multiple vesicopustules over the vulva, vagina or cervix. It then sloughs to form shallow ulcers circumscribed by inflammatory zone. The lesion is very tender with foul purulent and haemorrhagic discharge. There may be cluster of ulcers. Unilateral inguinal lymphadenitis may occur which may suppurate to form abscess (buboes).

Diagnosis

Syphilis must be ruled out first. Demonstration of *Ducreyi bacillus* in specialised culture media is confirmatory. Discharge from the ulcers or pus from the lymph glands is taken for culture. In the stained film (Gram stain) the organisms appear classically as 'Shoal of fish'. It is difficult to grow this organism in culture method.

Treatment (CDC recommendation)

- Ceftriaxone 250 mg IM single dose is effective. Sexual partner should also be treated.
- Azithromycin 1 gm by mouth single dose.
- Erythromycin 500 mg by month every 6 hours for 7 days can also be given.

Longer course of treatment is needed for patients who are positive with HIV.

LYMPHOGRANULOMA VENEREUM (LGV)

Lymphogranuloma venereum (LGV) is caused by one of the aggressive L serotypes of *Chlamydia trachomatis* usually acquired sexually. It is an obligatory intracellular organism. The incubation period is 2-21 days. It is more commonly found in the sea ports of the Far East, Malaysia, Africa and South America.

Initial lesion is a painless papule, pustule or ulcer in the vulva. The inguinal glands are involved and feel rubbery. There is acute lymphangitis and lymphadenitis. **The glands become necrosed and abscess (bubo) forms**. The healing occurs with intense fibrosis with lymphatic obstruction. **The secondary phase** is noted by painful adenopathy. **The classical clinical sign of LGV is the "groove**

sign" a depression between the groups of inflamed nodes. The lymphatic obstruction leads to vulval swelling where as lymphatic extension to the vulva, vagina or rectum leads to ulceration, fibrosis and stricture of the vagina or rectum.

Complications include — (i) vulval elephantiasis, (ii) perineal scarring and dyspareunia, (iii) rectal stricture and (iv) sinus and fistula formation.

Diagnosis

(a) Culture and isolation of LGV (chlamydia serotypes $L_{1,2,3}$) is confirmatory.

(b) Detection of LGV antigen in pus obtained from a bubo with specific monoclonal antibodies using immunofluorescence method.

(c) Detection of LGV antigen by ELISA method.

(d) LGV complement fixation test — when positive with rising titre.

(e) Intradermal Frei test is nonspecific and unreliable.

Treatment

Prevention — Use of condom or to avoid intercourse with a suspected infected partner.

Definitive treatment — CDC recommends Doxycycline 100 mg bid for at least 21 days. Alternatively erythromycin 500 mg orally every 6 hours for 21 days is given (indicated for pregnant women). Sexual partner should also be treated.

Surgical — (i) Abscess should be aspirated but not be excised. (ii) Manual dilatation of the stricture weekly. It is essential to use antibiotics during the perioperative period.

GRANULOMA INGUINALE (VENEREUM)

This is a chronic progressive granulomatous diseases of the vulva, vagina or cervix. It commonly found in some tropics and subtropics like South China, South India, Papua New Guinea and South America. **The causative organism is** gram-negative bacillus — *Calymmatobacterium granulomatis* (*Donovania granulomatis*).

Clinical features

The disease usually manifests itself 10-40 days after coitus with an infected partner. The lesion starts as pustules which breakdown and erode the adjacent tissues through continuity and contiguity. The ulcer looks hypertrophic due to indurated granulation tissue. The margins are rolled and elevated. Biopsy may be needed to exclude neoplasia. The lymph nodes do not undergo suppuration and abscess formation (cf. Lymphogranuloma venereum).

Diagnosis is confirmed by demonstrating the *Donovan bodies* within the mononuclear cells in material (scrapings) from the ulcer when stained by the Giemsa method. **The bipolar appearance (safety pin) is characteristic of Donovan bodies.**

Treatment

Usually, it does respond well to a broad spectrum antibiotic. However, CDC recommends Doxycycline 100 mg bid for at least 3 weeks. Alternatively ciprofloxacin 750 mg bid for at least 2 weeks is given. The residual destructive lesion in the vulva may require plastic surgery or vulvectomy.

BACTERIAL VAGINOSIS (BV) (Bacterial Vaginitis)

The causative organism was previously thought to be *Gardnerella vaginalis* (*Haemophilus vaginalis*). The present concept is that along with *G. vaginalis*, anaerobic organisms such as *Bacteroides* species, *Peptococcus* species, mobiluncus and *Mycoplasma* hominis act synergistically to cause vaginal infection.

Clinically characterised by creamy vaginal discharge with fishy smell without extensive evidence of inflammation.

Clinical features

Bacterial Vaginosis (BV) is characterised by malodorous vaginal discharge. The term vaginosis preferred as there is no vaginal inflammation. The discharge is homogeneous, greyish-white and adherent to the vaginal wall. Clinical implications of BV, in pregnancy are, preterm rupture of membranes, preterm labour and chorioamnionitis.

Complications

(i) Recurrent infection leading to PID. (ii) Development of PID following abortion or (iii) vaginal cuff infection following hysterectomy (iv) Pregnancy complications : second trimester miscarriage, PROM, preterm birth, endometritis.

Diagnosis

(a) Litmus paper test — vaginal pH is alkaline (pH > 4.7).

(b) **Whiff test** : Fishy (amine) odour when a drop of discharge is mixed with 10 per cent potassium hydroxide solution.

(c) A smear of vaginal discharge is prepared with drops of normal saline on a glass slide and is seen under a microscope. Vaginal epithelial cells are seen covered with these coccobacilli and the cells appear as stippled or granular. At times the cells are so heavily stippled that the cell borders are obscured. **These stippled epithelial cells are called "clue cells" (Fig. 11.1). Clue cells are diagnostic of BV.**

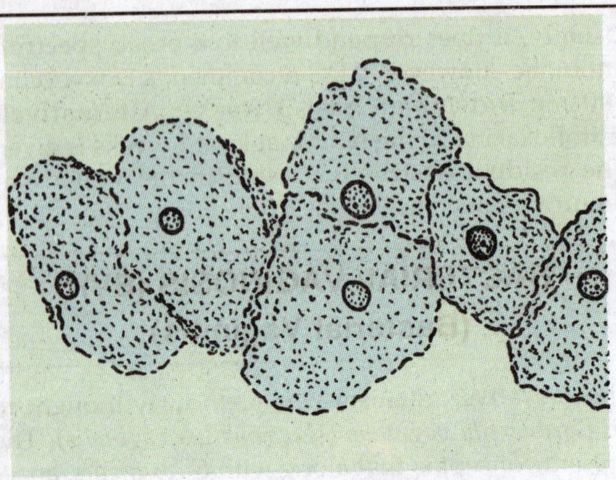

Fig. 11.1. Clue cells

Treatment is highly effective with metronidazole — 200 mg orally thrice daily for 7 days or Metronidazole 2 gm single dose orally can be used. Clindamycin cream (2%) and metronidazole gel are recommended for vaginal application to prevent obstetric complications. The patient's sexual partner should be treated simultaneously.

HERPES GENITALIS

The causative organism is herpes simplex virus (HSV) type 1 and 2. It is usually transmitted sexually by an infected partner but may possibly be transmitted by orogenital contact. The incubation period is 2-14 days.

Clinical features

Symptoms of the first attack usually appear less than 7 days after sexual contact. Initially, red painful inflammatory area appears commonly on the clitoris, labia, vestibule, vagina, perineum and cervix. Multiple vesicles appear which progress into multiple shallow ulcers and ultimately heal up spontaneously by crusting. It takes about three weeks to complete the process. Inguinal lymphadenopathy occurs. Constitutional symptoms include fever, malaise and headache. There may be vulvar burning, pruritus, dysuria or retention of urine.

First episodes are severe compared to the recurrent disease. Frequency of recurrent infection is high with HSV-2.

Diagnosis

(a) Virus tissue culture and isolation — confirmatory.

(b) Detection of virus antigen by ELISA or immunofluorescent method.

(c) PCR test to identify the HSV is the new and most accurate test.

Risks

(a) Physical and psychological trauma may precipitate recurrence.

(b) Possibly linked with cervical dysplasia and cancer.

(c) Adverse effects in primary infection during pregnancy.

- Increased chance of abortion and premature labour.
- Maternal transfer to neonates during vaginal delivery, if primary (50%) or recurrent (5%) attacks occur late in pregnancy.
- Baby may suffer from damage to central nervous system.
- **Delivery by caesarean section is indicated with primary genital herpes infection.**

Cautions

- Both the partners are warned that they are infectious whenever any lesions are evident.
- Women should have annual cervical smear.
- The women should inform the physician about the past history of herpes when becoming pregnant.

Treatment (CDC recommended regimens)

The specific treatment is yet to be explored. Rest and analgesics are helpful. **Acyclovir which inhibits the intracellular synthesis of DNA by the virus, has been found to be effective in acute attacks.** It is better to be given orally in doses of 200 mg 5 times a day for 7 days. Acyclovir is effective in reducing the symptoms, duration of viral shedding and helps rapid healing. Its prophylactic use can reduce the episodes of recurrence. Famciclovir 250 mg orally thrice daily for 7 days can be used alternatively. Saline bath may relieve local pain.

HUMAN IMMUNODEFICIENCY VIRUS (HIV) INFECTION AND ACQUIRED IMMUNODEFICIENCY SYNDROME (AIDS)

The virus

The causative agents are human immunodeficiency viruses (HIV) of strains HIV 1 and HIV 2. The first HIV virus was discovered in 1983 by Barre-Sinoussi and colleagues in Paris. HIV belongs to retrovirus (double stranded RNA) family. Retroviruses possess the enzyme **reverse transcriptase** which allows viral RNA to be transcribed into DNA. The viral DNA when gets incorporated into the host cell genome, **chronic infection begins**.The basic structure of this icosahedral HIV (RNA-retrovirus) consists of a core protein (P-24) with glycoprotein (GP 120; GP 41) envelope. Of the various core antigens, **P-24 is most widely used for investigation study**. Antibodies to envelope proteins (GP 120) have got some protective role. The virus is destroyed by heating at 56°C for 30 minutes or by disinfectants with glutaraldehyde.

Incidence

The incidence is difficult to work out but the fact remains that the disease is spreading alarmingly fast both in the developed and developing countries and now has become a global problem.

In India, an estimated 4 million (more than 50% of them are women and children) people are infected with HIV. In most Asian countries infection rates are less than 0.5 per cent.

Mode of transmission

- Sexual intercourse — Women are affected more than the men because in female, larger mucosal surface is exposed and semen contains high viral load. Transmission of virus from male to female is high.

  – Homosexual and bisexual – Heterosexual
- Intravenous drug abusers.
- Transfusion of contaminated blood or blood products.
- Use of contaminated needles, needle stick injuries.
- Breastfeeding—Infants who have been infected through one of infected blood or blood products or unsterile needles may infect their mothers during breastfeeding specially in presence of cracked nipples.
- Perinatal transmission—The vertical transmission to the neonates of the infected mothers is about 25–35%. The baby may be affected *in utero* (30%) through transplacental transfer, during delivery (70–75%) by contaminated secretions and blood of the birth canal and through breast milk in neonatal period (10–20%).

However, many health promoting benefits of breastfeeding may outweigh the risk of HIV transmission particularly in the developing world. For the other high risk factors for AIDS, see Table 11.4.

Immunopathogenesis

The target for HIV is the CD 4 receptor molecule. Cells within the immune system that have this molecule are : **CD 4 + T lymphocytes** (predominantly affected), monocytes, macrophages and other antigen presenting cells like fibroblasts, neurons, renal, hepatic and intestinal cells.

Following infection, there is profound cellular immunodeficiency as the CD 4^+ are progressively depleted by cytopathic effects of HIV.

Primary infection $\xrightarrow[\text{weeks}]{3\text{-}6}$ Acute syndrome $\xrightarrow[\text{3 months}]{\text{1 week to}}$ Immune response to HIV $\xrightarrow[\text{weeks}]{1\text{–}2}$ Clinical latency (7 - 10 years).

Immunological markers that are used to determine the **progression of the disease are** :

- CD 4 T lymphocyte count—patients with count from 200 to 500 cells/mm^3 are more likely to have HIV related symptoms and count < 200 cells/mm^3 is taken into AIDS defining criteria.
- Measurement of HIV RNA levels by RT-PCR and the b DNA assays. Effectiveness of therapy is evaluated by monitoring of HIV RNA every 3–4 months.
- Raised P-24 (core) antigen titre—reflects the viral load.
- Raised serum β_2 microglobulin—reflects the immune response.

Clinical presentation

Following exposure to HIV infection, a patient develops antibodies against HIV in about 8-12 weeks. The development of antibodies marks the stage of seroconversion and in some cases manifest clinically as a **'flu' like syndrome.**

Acute infection syndrome is characterised by fever, skin rash, arthralgia, lymphadenopathy and diarrhoea. This is called seroconversion illness. It lasts less than 2-3 weeks and resolves spontaneously.

After the initial exposure, the person remains asymptomatic for many years. The median time to develop AIDS is approximately 7-10 years. During this period, the patient shows progressive immune depletion. With increasing immunodeficiency, the person becomes susceptible to secondary infection by opportunistic organisms. Some individuals may just have persistent generalised lymphadenopathy during this period.

AIDs-related complex (ARC) refers to subjects having non-specific clinical features of weight loss, fever, diarrhoea, skin rash, lymphadenopathy, herpes simplex, oral candidiasis, oral or genital ulcers, PID, tubo-ovarian abscess, thrombocytopenia without full blown pictures of AIDS.

Any HIV infected individual with a CD4 + T cell count of < 200/µl, has AIDs by definition regardless of the presence of symptoms or opportunistic diseases.

Table 11.4 Risk factors for AIDS
• Multiple sex partners. • Prostitutes. • Homosexual males. • Intravenous drug abuser (IVDA). • Multiple transfusions of blood or blood products. • Sexually transmitted disease. • Mother to infant.

HIV related other diseases include :

- Common secondary infections are : atypical tuberculosis, pneumonia (Pneumocystis carinii pneumonia), systemic candidiasis and meningitis.
- Encephalitis, myelopathy and polyneuropathy are neurological manifestations.
- There is increased incidence of high-grade lymphoid neoplasms, Kaposi sarcoma and non-Hodgkin's lymphoma.
- Viral infections with herpes simplex, human papilloma virus (HPV) and cytomegalo virus (CMV) are common.

HIV related specific gynaecological problems are :

- **Infection of the genital tract** is high due to progressive immunodeficient state
  - Recurrent vaginal candidiasis.
  - Pelvic inflammatory diseases including sexually transmitted infections (STIs) (see p. 142).
  - Other viral infections HSV (p. 148), Genital Warts (p. 152) are commonly seen.
- **Neoplasms of the genital tract are increased**
  - Increased incidence of cervical intra-epithelial neoplasia (CIN) and carcinoma of the cervix.
  - Increased incidence of vulval intra-epithelial neoplasia (VIN).
- **Increased morbidity following gynaecological surgery**
  - Increased risk of wound infection and chest infection, an intensive antibiotic therapy is needed.
- **Menstrual abnormality** : Menorrhagia, amenorrhoea, may be due to associated weight loss, thrombocytopenia.
- **Pregnancy does not worsen the disease** neither the disease affect pregnancy adversely.

Diagnosis

The effect on cellular immunity is manifested by decrease in CD 4 cells. **An absolute CD 4 cell count below 200/mm^3 is considered as cut off point when there is risk of opportunistic infections.**

The organism can be detected from the blood, semen, vaginal secretions, breast milk or saliva (body fluids) of the infected persons.

Diagnostic tests for antibodies to HIV are :

- Detection of IgG antibody to Gp 120 (envelope glycoprotein component) is most commonly used. Antibody production may take upto 3 months (window period) from the time of infection. These antibodies are not protective.
- Viral P-24 antigen can be detected very soon after the infection and it usually disappears by 8-10 weeks time.
- **ELISA** (enzyme linked immunosorbent assay) is extremely sensitive (99.5%) but less specific. It is easy, cheap and less time consuming

(2-5 hours). As such, it can be employed as a screening procedure extended to 'at risk' persons.

- **Western blot or immunoblot** — It is highly specific but complicated and time consuming (1-2 days). It is expensive too.
- **Polymerase chain reaction (PCR)** is gold standard for diagnosis of HIV. Viral DNA is amplified following isolation of the virus from peripheral mononuclear cells.

Causes of death

- **Widespread infection** as it cannot be controlled effectively.
- **Profound immunodeficiency** leads to opportunistic infections and poor response to therapy.
- **Development** of unusual malignant lesions (lymphoma and Kaposi's sarcoma).

Treatment :

• **Preventive** • **Definitive**

Preventive measures include :

- 'Safer sex' practice by health education. Use of latext condoms and spermicides will prevent HIV.
- Use of blunt tipped needles to avoid needle stick injury during surgery.
- HIV negative blood transfusion (screening of donors).
- HIV negative frozen semen to use for artificial donor insemination.
- To maintain protocols for correct handling of all body fluids (p. 152).
- Postexposure prophylaxis with zidovudine and lamivudine is advisable (p. 152).
- Termination of pregnancy in HIV positive women.
- Avoiding breastfeeding — in the developing world, avoidance of breastfeeding may not be possible. Mother needs to be counselled as regard the risks and benefits of breastfeeding. **She is helped to make an informed choice.**
- Wide spread voluntary counselling and testing (VCT).

Definitive :

HIV treatment protocols change frequently.

Antiretroviral therapy : Antiretroviral drugs are grouped into — (A) **Nucleoside Reverse Transcriptase Inhibitors (NRTIs)** : Zidovudine, Zalcitabine, Lamivudine, Stavudine. (B) **Non-Nucleoside Reverse Transcriptase Inhibitors (NNRTIs)** : Delvirdine, Nevirapine, Efavirenz. (C) **Protease Inhibitors** (PI) : Indinavir, Saquinavir, Ritonavir, Amprenavir. (D) **Fusion inhibitor** : Enfuvirtide. The combinations of these drugs are effective in increasing CD4 counts and reducing viral load. Monotherapy is not used as it hastens drug resistance. Combination therapy is known by the acronym **HAART** (Highly Active Antiretroviral Therapy).

Drug combinations : Uptodate treatment recommendations available at : www.AIDSinfo.nih.gov.

- Two from Gr. A (NRTIs) plus one from Gr. B OR 2 from Gr. A (NRTIs) plus one from Gr. C (PI).

Plasma HIV RNA levels indicate the degree of viral replication and CD4 + T cell count indicate level of immune competence.

Important side effects of drugs are : lactic acidosis, anaemia, granulocytopenia, pancreatitis, peripheral neuropathy, hepatic dysfunction and carbohydrate intolerance.

When to start therapy :

- Acute HIV infection syndrome.
- Symptomatic HIV infection.
- Asymptomatic but CD 4 cell count < 350 cells/μl or with viral load — HIV RNA > 50,000 copies/ml.
- Post-exposure prophylaxis (see p. 152).
- Patients with CD 4 count < 200/μl should also receive trimethoprim and sulphamethoxazole combination (P. carinii prophylaxis).
- Opportunistic infections (mycobacterium) should be treated simultaneously with specific drugs when CD4 + T cells < 50/μl.
- Zidovudine is given in a dose of 200 mg every 8 hours. Nevirapine is found to reduce the viral transmission to breastfed infants.

With effective treatment viral load should reach 'undetectable' levels (< 50 copies/ml) and CD4 count should rise.

Colposcopy and cervical cytology screening should be routinely done.

When to change therapy : (i) Failure to reduce viral load. (ii) Persistently declining CD4 + T cell count. (iii) Clinical deterioration.

- **Post-exposure Prophylaxis** : A combination of two NRTIs is given for 4 weeks. Prophylactic use zidovudine (300 mg bid) and lamivudine (150 mg bid) for a period of 4 weeks immediately following an exposure may reduce the risk of seroconversion (CDC-2001).

Precautions to prevent occupational transmission of HIV (Universal Blood and Body Fluid Precautions) :

- All blood and body fluids should be considered potentially infectious for HIV.
- Non-surgical management whenever possible.
- Barrier precautions : Use of cap, mask, gown, double gloves, eye wear (goggles) and boots.
- Use of blunt tipped needles (risk of HIV infection following needle stick injury is 0.3%).
- Washing of any body fluid contamination off the skin immediately.
- Use of disposable syringes, needles and anaesthetic circuits.
- Resuscitation bags or mouthpieces should be available for emergency resuscitation.
- Thorough theatre disinfection after the operation.

GENITAL WARTS (CONDYLOMA ACUMINATA)

Condylomata are papillary lesions caused by **Human Papilloma Virus (HPV) usually type 6 and 11** (see p. 312). These are usually multiple and can be contaminated from other parts of the body. They can be transmitted sexually. Associated vaginal discharge favours their growth and so does pregnancy. Typically, they grow in clusters along a narrow stalk giving it a cauliflower appearance but at times the stalk may be broad and thick (Fig. 11.2). The condylomata may at times, spread to the vagina or even the cervix. **Anatomic distribution of anogenital HPV infection is : Cervix 70%, Vulva 25%, Vagina 10% and Anus 20%.** The lesion should be differentiated from syphilitic condylomata or vulval carcinoma. Very rarely, it becomes malignant. Conditions known to predispose women to infection with HPV are : Immunosuppression, diabetes, pregnancy and local trauma.

There may be an **association between HPV infection and malignant epithelial transformation of the cervix, vagina and vulva. It is usually associated with HPV types 16, 18, 45, 56 (see p. 312).**

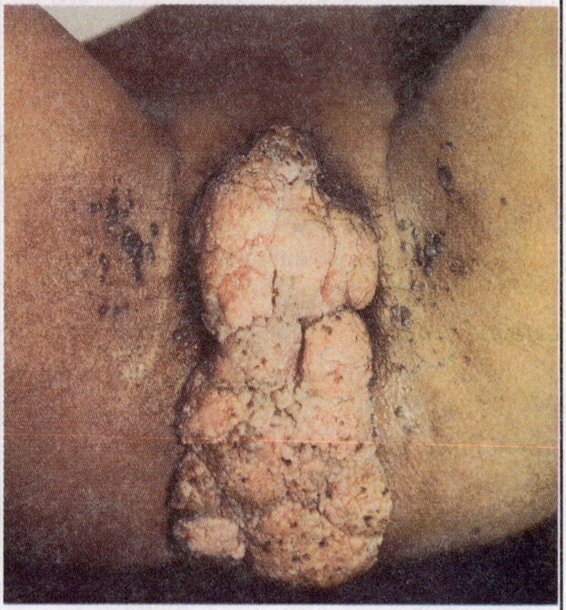

Fig. 11.2. Giant condyloma accuminata of vulva

Treatment

Podophyllotoxin is the main active ingredient of Podophyllin. Liquid and cream preparations are used locally two times daily for 3 days then repeated after a break of 4 days. **Its use is contraindicated during first trimester of pregnancy. Trichloroacetic** acid (90-100%) solution is used for isolated warts that respond poorly to podophyllin.

Other chemical agents : Interferon injection, 5 fluoracil, imiquimod (immunomodulator) 5 per cent cream have been used locally.

Destructive methods are used for resistant cases. These include cryotherapy, electrodiathermy, laser therapy or surgical removal.

MOLLUSCUM CONTAGIOSUM

Molluscum contagiosum is caused by a pox virus transmitted by body contact or towels or clothing. It is commonly seen in immunodeficient subject or with HIV infections. They vary in size upto 1 cm, dome-shaped, pearly-white in colour and often umbilicated. They are usually multiple and can occur anywhere in the skin and genitalia. Microscopic appearance reveals numerous inclusion bodies (molluscum bodies) in the cytoplasm of the cells.

Treatment is by application of tincture of iodine to the centre of each papule using a pointed stick. In unresponsive cases, diathermy or cryosurgery can be used.

PEDICULOSIS PUBIS

The infective agent is a crab louse (*Phthirus pubis*) which affects the coarse hair of the pubis. The louse alongwith its eggs are attached to the hair. It is transmitted by sexual contact or infected clothes encouraged by inadequate hygiene. It produces intense pruritis → scratching → secondary infection → suppuration.

Treatment

Permethrin cream (1%) is applied over the affected area and washed off after 10 minutes. Lindane 1% is used as a shampoo.

Treatment may also be done by application of 1 per cent gamma-benzene hexachloride or malathion (0.5%) cream. After rubbing the preparation, the area should not be washed for 24 hours. The application may be repeated after 4 days, if necessary. It is mandatory to treat the contact and sterilise the clothings by boiling.

SCABIES

This is caused by *Sarcoptes scabiei*. It produces intense itching and often excoriation of skin. It is often associated with poor local hygiene.

Treatment

Permethrin cream 5 per cent is applied to all areas of the body below the neck and washed off after 8-14 hours.

The treatment is also done by local application of 25 per cent benzyl benzoate emulsion for the entire body below the neck. Single application is often enough. The clothings should be boiled. The family members are also to be treated simultaneously to prevent reinfection.

KEY POINTS

- Sexually transmitted infections (STIs) includes those diseases which are predominantly transmitted through sexual contact from an infected partner. A patient with a STI is likely to have another one and as such, possible investigation is to be directed. *Chlamydia trachomatis* is now on the top in the list of the organisms causing STD, the other common diseases are bacterial vaginosis, gonorrhoea, syphilis, trichomonas vaginitis.
- Neisseria gonorrhoea commonly invades the columnar and transitional epithelium of the genito-urinary tract (endocervix, urethra, Bartholin's gland). Infertility, ectopic pregnancy, chronic pelvic pain are the long term complications (p. 144). Treatment should include Syphilis or Chlamydia infection also (p. 145).
- Herpes genitalis is caused by herpes simplex virus (HSV) type 1 and 2. Frequency of recurrent infection is high with HSV-2. It is possibly linked with cervical dysplasia and cancer. Acyclovir orally in doses of 200 mg 5 times a day for 7 days is effective in reducing the constitutional symptoms, duration of viral shedding and helps rapid healing.
- Syphilis is caused by *Treponema pallidum*. The hard chancre of primary syphilis is painless with an indurated base. About 33 per cent patients, who are not adequately treated during the primary, secondary or latent phases, develop tertiary syphilis. VDRL and TPHA tests are used for screening and FTA – ABS is used for confirmation. Treatment according to CDC recommendation includes Benzathine-penicillin IM (see p. 145).
- Chancroid (soft sore) is caused by a gram-negative *Haemophilus ducreyi*. Soft sore of chancroid is always painful. Unilateral inguinal lymphadenitis may occur which may suppurate to form abscess. Demonstration of Ducreyi bacillus from the discharge of the ulcer or aspirated pus from the lymph gland is confirmatory. Ceftriaxone 250 mg IM single dose is effective.

KEY- POINTS

- Granuloma inguinale (venerum) is caused by gram-negative *Donovania granulomatis*. There is localised ulcer formation without lymph node suppuration and abscess formation. Diagnosis is confirmed by demonstrating *Donovan bodies* within the mononuclear cells in materials from the ulcer when stained by Giemsa. Doxycycline 100 mg bid for at least 3 weeks is effective.
- Lymphogranuloma venerum is caused by L serotype *Chlamydia trachomatis*. The inguinal glands are involved early, become necrosed and abscess forms. Healing occurs with intense fibrosis and lymphatic obstruction. Diagnosis is made by detection of LGV antigen by ELISA method. Doxycycline 100 mg bid for at least 21 days is effective.
- AIDS is caused by human immunodeficiency virus (HIV). The methods of transmission are by sexual intercourse, transfusion of contaminated blood or blood products, use of contaminated needles and vertical transmission to the baby (25–35%) during pregnancy and childbirth. It is not spread by casual contact. Male condom is protective. It suppresses the immune system (depletion of CD 4 + T lymphocytes) so that the opportunistic organisms flare up.

  Plasma HIV-RNA levels indicate the degree of viral replication and CD 4 + T cell count indicate level of immune competence (p. 151). Screening test is by ELISA and confirmation is by Western blot. Viral DNA amplification and detection by PCR is gold standard (p. 151). Any HIV infected individual with CD4 + T cell count < 200/μL has AIDS.

  HIV related other diseases are : recurrent vaginal candidiasis, PID, CIN, VIN, atypical tuberculosis and others as observed in an immunocompromised patient. Preventive measures (see p. 151) and infection control during surgery (see p. 152) must be rigorous.

  HAART inhibits reverse transcriptase and slows down the progress of the disease. For HIV treatment protocols see p. 151. HAART increases CD4 count and reduces viral load. Monotherapy hastens development of drug resistance.
- Barrier contraception (condom) is effective to reduce the risk of HIV transmission and to prevent unwanted pregnancy. In addition, another contraceptive may be used to increase the contraceptive efficacy. There is no evidence that the use of the COCs (p. 464), IUCDs, LNG-IUS (p. 459) or Depo-Provera (p. 470), alters the risk of transmission.
- Condyloma accuminata is viral (HPV) in origin. Rarely, it may become malignant. The treatment is to paint with 20 per cent podophyllin resin in liquid paraffin. The drug is contraindicated during pregnancy. Electrodiathermy, Cryotherapy or Laser can also be used.
- Molluscum contagiosum is caused by pox virus. It is commonly seen with immunodeficient subject or with HIV infection. Treatment is by application of iodine or by cryotherapy.
- Pediculosis pubis is caused by crab louse. Treatment is by application of 1 per cent permethrin cream or 1 per cent gamma-benzene hexachloride cream.
- Scabies is caused by *Sarcoptes scabiei*. The treatment is by local application of 5 per cent permethrin cream or 25 per cent benzyl benzoate emulsion for the entire body below the neck.
- Bacterial vaginosis is caused by Gardnerella vaginalis. The vaginal discharge is homogeneous, adherent to vaginal wall with pH > 4.7 and has an amine odour when mixed with KOH solution (Whiff test). Presence of clue cells (stippled epithelial cells) on the wet smear of vaginal discharge is diagnostic. Oral metronidazole is highly effective.

Infections of the Individual Pelvic Organs

12

VULVAL INFECTION

The vulval and perineal skin is usually resistant to common infection. But the defence is lost following constant irritation by the vaginal discharge or urine (urinary incontinence). Furthermore, there may be atrophy or degenerative changes either in disease or following menopause when the infection is more likely. The vulval infection can thus occur *de novo* or may be affected secondarily, the primary site may be elsewhere in the adjacent structures. **In this section, only the lesions affecting primarily the vulva will be discussed.**

It is indeed difficult to classify the vulval infection but the following aetiological classification is of help.

I. Due to specific infection.

II. Due to sensitive reaction.

III. Due to vaginal discharge or urinary contamination.

I. VULVITIS DUE TO SPECIFIC INFECTION

Bacterial

- Pyogenic (non-gonococcal)
- Sexually transmitted diseases (p. 142)
  - Gonorrhoea (p. 143).
  - Syphilis (p. 144).
  - Chancroid (p. 146).
  - Lymphogranuloma venereum (p. 146).
  - Granuloma inguinale (p. 147).
- Tubercular (p. 134)

Viral

- Condylomata accuminata (p. 152).
- Herpes genitalis (p. 148).
- Molluscum contagiosum (p. 152).
- Herpes zoster (p. 156).

Fungal

- Moniliasis (160).
- Ringworm (156).

Parasitic

- Pediculosis pubis (p. 153).
- Scabies (p. 153).
- Threadworm (156).

Pyogenic infection (Non-gonococcal)

Vulval cellulitis

Unhygienic condition associated with even minor scratching on the vulva may cause intense cellulitis. The causative organism is predominantly *Staphylococcus aureus*. The vulva is swollen, red and tender. There may be profuse exudation. The inflammation is limited, in majority, upto the labiocrural fold.

The patient complains of intense pain, itching and problem in micturition. There may be excoriation of the skin due to scratching and laceration.

Treatment is effective by systemic antibiotics, local hot compress and analgesics.

Furunculosis

The infection affects the hair follicles of the mons and labia majora → folliculitis → furunculitis. The offending organism is *Staphylococcus aureus*. If it is recurrent, glycosuria should be excluded. Treatment is effective with systemic and local antibiotics and local cleanliness.

Infection of sebaceous and apocrine glands

Infection of an apocrine or sebaceous gland looks and presents the features of a boil. If it recurs, excision is to be done in the quiescent state.

Impetigo

Impetigo is a pustular infection caused by *Staphylococcus aureus* or *Streptococcus*. It may be localised to vulva or spread to other parts of the body, face or hands.

Blebs should be incised or the crusts be removed aseptically. Systemic and local antibiotics are to be prescribed.

Erysipelas

This rare spreading cellulitis is caused by invasion of the superficial lymphatics by beta haemolytic *Streptococcus*. There may be systemic constitutional symptoms. It responds well to systemic broad spectrum antibiotics.

Intertrigo

Intertrigo is due to irritation and infection of retained secretions in the skinfolds usually in an obese patient. It may also result from friction of the undergarments or sanitary towels.

Treatment with local hygiene and local antiseptic application is quite effective. At times, systemic antibiotics may have to be used. Maintenance of local hygiene and dusting with starch and zinc oxide powder are helpful.

Infection resulting from trauma

Infections may occur following childbirth trauma or gynaecological operation on the perineum. Apart from these, the commonest traumatic cause of vulval infection is scratching with nails. This when secondarily infected with pyogenic organisms may lead to localised pus formation or at times spreading cellulitis.

Depending upon the extent of infection, either local antiseptic dressings or systemic antibiotics should be prescribed.

Viral infection

Herpes zoster

The causative agent is varicella zoster virus (VZV). This is due to re-emergence of VZV from posterior nerve roots. It produces an inflammatory painful eruption of groups of vesicles distributed over the skin corresponding to the course of peripheral sensory nerves (dermatome). It is commonly unilateral but may extend to the thigh or buttock of the same side. The vesicles may rupture or become dry with scab formation. It resolves spontaneously in 3 weeks time.

Treatment is by analgesics to relieve pain and antibiotics to prevent secondary infection. Acyclovir 800 mg orally five times daily for 7 days is recommended. Acyclovir cream (5%) may be used locally for less severe infection.

Fungal infection

Moniliasis : See p. 160.

Ringworm : The causative organism is *Tinea cruris*. The lesions look bright red and circumscribed. The fungus can be detected microscopically from scraping of the lesion.

Treatment is very effective with imidazole (clotrimazole or miconazole) cream. Some fungi (*Trichophyton rubrum*) respond well to griseofulvin 500 mg twice daily by mouth for 4 weeks.

Parasitic infection

Threadworm : The causative organism is *Oxyuris vermicularis*. It is common in children. Nocturnal perineal itching with evidences of perianal excoriation is observed. The parasite is detected in the stool. Anthelmintic drugs such as mebendazole and local application of gentian violet cures the condition.

II. DUE TO SENSITIVE REACTION

The vulval skin is very much sensitive to many agents (mostly chemicals) which may produce contact dermatitis. Such agents include drugs used locally to cure pruritis — douche, soap, powder, detergent or deodorants, condoms, contraceptive creams or jelly or foam tablets, etc. The vulva is intensely inflamed and swollen. There may be vesicular or pustular eruption. Pruritus is the predominant symptom.

Treatment

There is no specific treatment. Careful enquiry is to be made to find out any correlation between the onset of the symptoms and the use of the offending agents mentioned earlier. If it is detected, it should be withheld forthwith. Innocuous zinc or calamine cream produces soothing effect. Hydrocortisone ointment is of help. Antihistaminic ointment should better be avoided as the skin may also be sensitive to it.

III. VAGINAL DISCHARGE OR URINARY CONTAMINATION

As previously mentioned, the perineal skin defence is lost in moisture and trauma. Constant vaginal discharge makes the area moist → irritation → scratching → trauma. This favours growth of the organisms like *Candida albicans* or *Trichomonas vaginalis*. The growth is favoured by glycosuria. The same condition occurs in true urinary incontinence. The area becomes moist and sodden with evidences of scratching.

Treatment is directed to cure the primary lesion. Soothing lotion or ointment may be of help to relieve the distress. Spontaneous healing occurs when the cause is removed.

ACUTE BARTHOLINITIS

Causative organisms

Although *Gonococcus* is always in mind but more commonly other pyogenic organisms such as *Esch. coli*, *Staphylococcus*, *Streptococcus* or *Chlamydia trachomatis* or mixed types are involved.

Pathology

Both the gland and the duct are involved. The epithelium of the gland or the duct gets swollen. The lumen of the duct may be blocked or remains open through which exudates escape out.

Fate

The infection may resolute completely or an abscess is formed. If left untreated, the abscess may burst through the lower vaginal wall. In others, the infection subsides only to recur in future. In such cases, the gland becomes fibrotic. Too often, the duct lumen heals by fibrosis with closure of the orifice → pent up secretion of the gland → formation of bartholin cyst. **Thus, the end results of acute Bartholinitis are :** (i) Complete resolution (ii) Recurrence (iii) Abscess (iv) Cyst formation.

Clinical features

Initially, there is local pain and discomfort even to the extent of difficulty in walking or sitting. Examination reveals tenderness and induration of the posterior half of the labia when palpated between thumb outside and the index finger inside the vagina (Fig. 9.6). The duct opening looks congested and secretion comes out through the opening when the gland is pressed by fingers. The secretion should be collected with a swab for bacteriological examination.

Treatment

Hot compress over the area and analgesics to relieve pain are instituted. Systemic antibiotic like ampicillin 500 mg orally 8 hourly is effective or else appropriate antibiotic according to the bacteriological sensitivity should be instituted.

RECURRENT BARTHOLINITIS

Periodic painful attacks cause problems and annoyance to the patient. Appropriate treatment as outlined in acute bartholinitis should be instituted in active phase. Excision of the gland with the duct may have to be done in the quiescent phase.

BARTHOLIN'S ABSCESS

Bartholin's abscess is the end result of acute bartholinitis. The duct gets blocked by fibrosis and the exudates pent up inside to produce abscess. If left uncared for, the abscess may burst through the lower vaginal wall. A sinus tract may remain with periodic discharge through it.

Clinical features

The local pain and discomfort become intense. The patient cannot walk or even sit. Fever is often associated.

On examination, there is an unilateral tender swelling beneath the posterior half of the labium majus expanding medially to the posterior part of the labium minus. The overlying skin appears red and oedematous.

Treatment

Rest is imposed. Pain is relieved by analgesics and daily sitz bath. Systemic antibiotic — ampicillin 500 mg orally 8 hourly or tetracycline in chlamydial infection is effective. Abscess should be drained at the earliest opportunity before it bursts spontaneously.

Marsupialisation (p. 158)

By making an elliptical opening on the medial aspect of the labium minus not only helps in drainage of pus but prevents recurrence of abscess and future cyst formation. It should be done under general anaesthesia (vide infra).

In case of recurrent Bartholin's abscess, excision should be done in the quiescent phase after the infection is controlled.

BARTHOLIN'S CYST

There is closure of the duct or the opening of an acinus. The cause may be infection or trauma followed by fibrosis and occlusion of the lumen. Lateral or illdirected mediolateral episiotomy may cause trauma to the duct.

Pathology

It may develop in the duct (common) or in the gland. **Commonly, it involves the duct;** the gland is adherent to it posterolaterally. Cyst of the duct or gland can be differentiated by the lining epithelium. The content is glairy colourless fluid — secretion of the Bartholin's gland.

Clinical features

A small size often remains unnoticed to the patient or escapes attention to the physician even following internal examination. If it becomes large (size of hen's egg), there is local discomfort and dyspareunia. Examination reveals an unilateral swelling on the posterior half of the labium majus which opens up the posterior end of the labium minus. Its medial projection makes the vulval cleft 'S'-shaped. The overlying skin is thin and shiny. The cyst is fluctuant and not tender (Fig. 12.1).

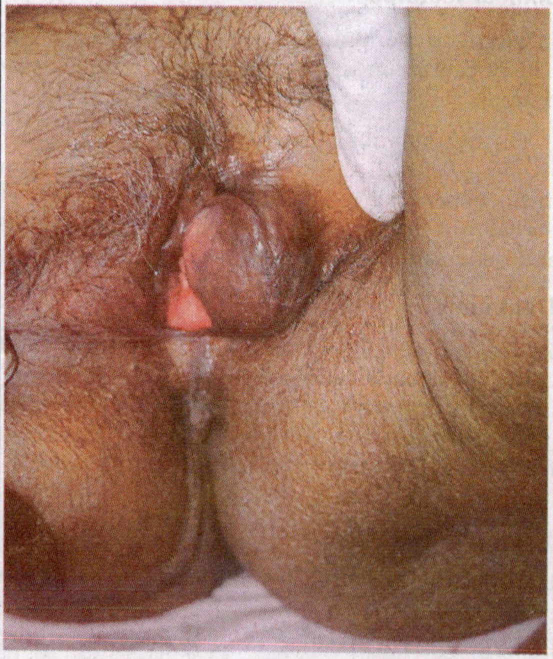

Fig. 12.1. Bartholin's cyst (*left*)

Treatment

Marsupialisation is the gratifying surgery for Bartholin's cyst. An incision is made on the inner aspect of the labium minus just outside the hymenal ring. The incision includes the vaginal wall and the cyst wall. The cut margins of the either side are to be trimmed off to make the opening an elliptical shape and of about 1 cm in diameter. The edges of the vaginal and cyst wall are sutured by interrupted catgut, thus leaving behind a clean circular opening.

The advantages of marsupialisation over the traditional excision operation are : (i) Simple. (ii) Can be done even under local anaesthesia. (iii) Shorter hospital stay (24 hours). (iv) Postoperative complication is almost nil. (v) Gland function (lubricant) remains intact.

VAGINAL INFECTION (VAGINITIS)

- Vulvovaginitis in childhood.
- Trichomoniasis.
- Moniliasis.
- Vaginitis due to *Chlamydia trachomatis*.
- Atrophic vaginitis.
- Non-specific vaginitis.
- Toxic shock syndrome.

VULVOVAGINITIS IN CHILDHOOD

Inflammatory conditions of the vulva and vagina are the commonest disorders during childhood. Due to lack of oestrogen, the vaginal defence is lost and the infection occurs easily, once introduced inside the vagina.

Aetiology

- Non-specific vulvovaginitis.
- Presence of foreign body in the vagina.
- Associated intestinal infestations — threadworm being the commonest.
- Rarely, more specific infection caused by *Candida albicans* or *Gonococcus* may be implicated.

Clinical features

The chief complaints are pruritus of varying degree and vaginal discharge. There may be painful micturition.

Inspection reveals soreness of the vulva. The labia minora may be swollen and red. The vaginal discharge varies from scanty to copious, at times offensive. If a foreign body is suspected, a vaginal examination with an aural or nasal speculum may help in diagnosis.

Investigations

The vaginal discharge is collected with a platinum loop and two smears are taken, one for direct examination and the other for Gram stain.

A small amount may be taken with a pipette for culture in Stuart's media. To exclude intestinal infestation, stool examination is of help.

Vaginoscopy is needed to exclude foreign body or tumour in a case with recurrent infection.

Treatment

In most cases, the cause remains unknown. Simple perineal hygiene will relieve the symptoms. In cases of soreness or after removal of foreign body, oestrogen ointment is to be applied locally every night for two weeks. Alternatively, ethinyl oestradiol vaginal cream is used for three weeks to improve the local vaginal defence. When the specific organisms are detected, therapy should be directed to cure the condition.

TRICHOMONAS VAGINITIS

Vaginal trichomoniasis is the most common and important cause of vaginitis in the childbearing period.

Causative organism

It is caused by Trichomonas vaginalis, a pear-shaped unicellular flagellate protozoa. It measures 20 μ long and 10 μ wide. It has got four anterior flagellae and a spear-like protrusion at the other end with an undulating membrane surrounding its anterior two-third. It is actively motile (Fig. 12.2).

Mode of transmission

The organism is predominantly transmitted by sexual contact, the male harbours the infection in the urethra and prostate. The transmission may also be possible by the toilet articles from one woman to the other or through examining gloves. The incubation period is 3-28 days.

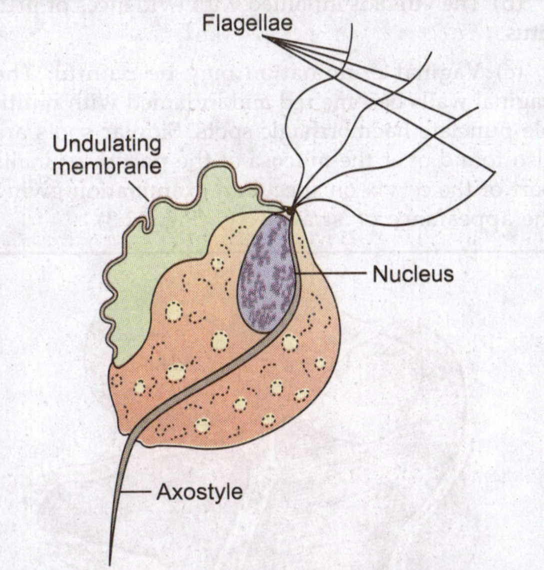

Fig. 12.2. Physical appearance of *Trichomonas vaginalis*

Pathology

In about 25 per cent of women in the reproductive period, the parasites harbour in the vagina in asymptomatic state. When the local defence is impaired — during and after menstruation, after sexual stimulation and following illness, the pH of the vagina is raised to 5.5-6.5. At this level of pH, the trichomonads thrive. The organisms usually lie in between the rugae and produce surface inflammatory reaction when the defence is lost. In about 75 per cent cases, the organism can be isolated from the urethra, Skene's tubules or even from the Bartholin's glands.

Clinical features

(a) There is sudden profuse and offensive vaginal discharge often dating from the last menstruation.

(b) Irritation and itching of varying degrees within and around the introitus are common.

(c) There is presence of urinary symptoms such as dysuria and frequency of micturition.

(d) There may be history of previous similar attacks.

Women with trichomoniasis should be evaluated for other STDs including *N. gonorrhoea, C. trachomatis* and HIV.

On examination

(a) There is thin, greenish yellow and frothy offensive discharge per vaginam.

(b) The vulva is inflamed with evidences of pruritus.

(c) Vaginal examination may be painful. The vaginal walls become red and inflamed with multiple punctate haemorrhagic spots. Similar spots are also found over the mucosa of the portio vaginalis part of the cervix on speculum examination giving the appearance of 'strawberry' (Fig. 12.3).

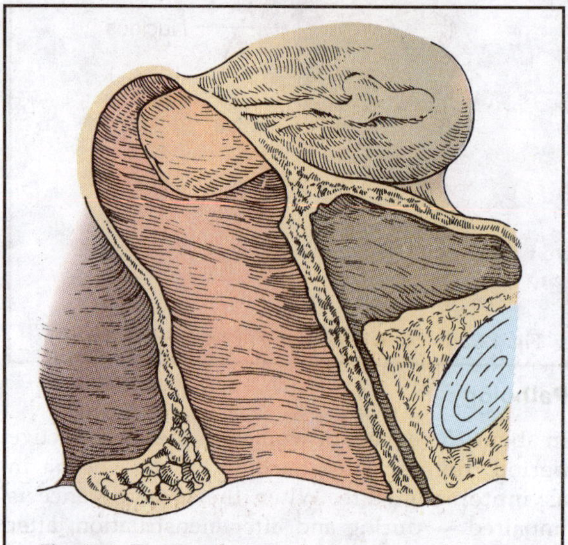

Fig. 12.3. Punctate haemorrhagic spots and 'strawberry' appearance on cervix

Diagnosis

(a) Identification of the trichomonads is done by hanging drop preparation (p. 106). If found negative even on repeat examination, the confirmation may be done by culture.

(b) Culture of the discharge collected by swabs in Kupferberg's or Feinberg Whittington medium.

In suspected cases, gonococcal or monilial infection should be excluded.

Treatment

The treatment is very much effective with metronidazole. Metronidazole 200 mg thrice daily by mouth is to be given for 1 week. A single dose regimen of 2 gm is an alternative. The husband should be given the same treatment schedule for 1 week. Resistance to metronidazole is extremely rare. The husband should use condom during coitus irrespective of contraceptive practice until the wife is cured.

If the symptoms persist, a second course of treatment is given after an interval of 7 days. To prevent recurrence, it is a sound policy to institute the treatment schedule to both the husband and wife for 7 days following menstruation for three consecutive cycles. During the three months period, the husband should use condom during intercourse.

CANDIDA VAGINITIS (MONILIASIS)

Causative organism

Moniliasis is caused by *Candida albicans*, a gram-positive yeast-like fungus (see Fig. 12.4).

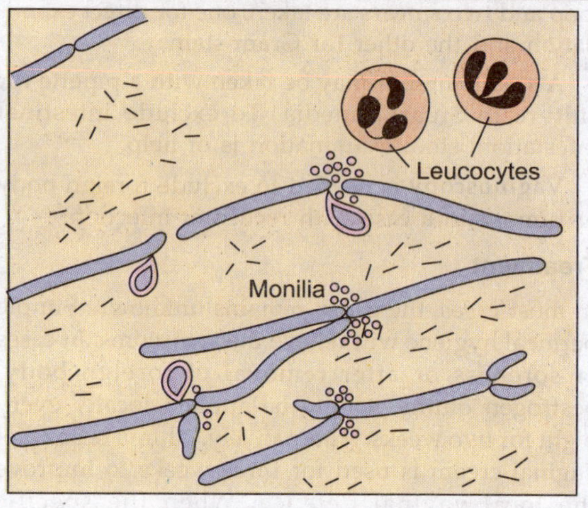

Fig. 12.4. Physical appearance of *Candida albicans*

Pathology

Predisposing factors for *Candida vaginitis*

- Diabetes : ↑ glycogen in the cells, glycosuria
- Pregnancy : ↑ Vaginal acidity, glycosuria
  ↑ Glycogen in the cells
- Broad spectrum antibiotics : ↓ Acid forming lactobacillus
- Combined oral pills
- Immunosuppression – HIV • Drugs–steroids
- Thyroid, Parathyroid disease

Clinical features

The patient complains of vaginal discharge with intense vulvovaginal pruritus. **The pruritis is out of proportion to the discharge.** There may be dyspareunia due to local soreness.

On examination

(a) The discharge is thick, curdy white and in flakes, often adherent to the vaginal wall (Fig. 12.5).

(b) Vulva may be red and swollen with evidences of pruritus.

(c) Vaginal examination may be tender. Removal of the white flakes reveals multiple oozing spots.

Diagnosis is confirmed by direct smear of the discharge or the flakes (Fig. 12.5) or by culture in Nickerson's or Sabouraud's media (Chapter 9).

Treatment

Corrections of the **predisposing factors** should be done, if possible. Local fungicidal preparations commonly used are of the polyene or imidazole group. Nystatin, clotrimazole, miconazole, econazole are used in the form of **either vaginal cream** or **pessary**.

One pessary is to be introduced high in the vagina at bedtime for consecutive 2 weeks. In severe cases, additional use of pessary in the morning is advocated. The treatment should be continued even during menstruation. *Single dose oral therapy* with fluconazole or itraconazole is also found effective.

Associated intestinal moniliasis should be treated by fluconazole 50 mg daily orally for 7 days. Husband should be treated with nystatin ointment locally for few days following each act of coitus. The use of condom is preferred.

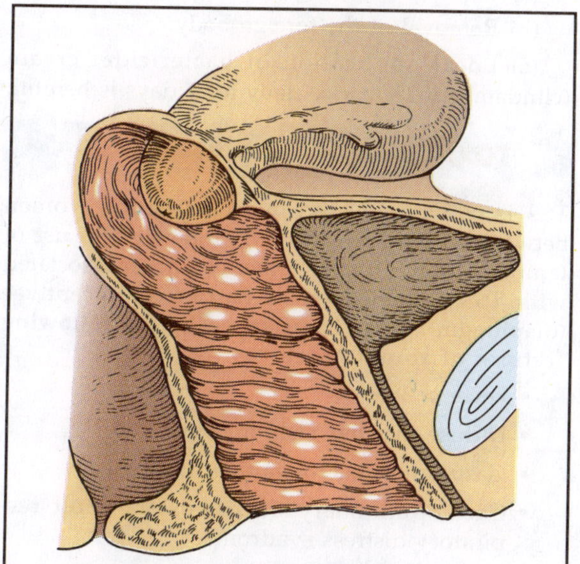

Fig. 12.5. Curdy white flakes adherent to the vaginal wall

Resistance to these drugs is not known. The systemic antifungal drugs fluconazole and itraconazole are effective in a single dose oral therapy.

CHLAMYDIAL VAGINITIS

The causative organism is *Chlamydia trachomatis*, a gram-negative obligate intracellular bacterium. This is a common sexually transmitted disease and causes vaginitis and urethritis. It is found in about 25-40 per cent of the female partners of men suffering for non-gonococcal urethritis.

The patient complains of dysuria and irritant mucopurulent vaginal discharge.

The **diagnosis** is confirmed by tissue culture and serological tests (see p. 146). Gonococcal infection must be excluded. **Complications include:** Pelvic pain, tubal damage causing infertility, ectopic pregnancy (see p. 146). **Treatment** with azithromycin 1 gm orally single dose to both the partners is very effective (see p. 146).

ATROPHIC VAGINITIS (SENILE VAGINITIS)

Vaginitis in postmenopausal women is called atrophic vaginitis. The term is preferable to senile vaginitis.

There is atrophy of the vulvovaginal structures due to oestrogen deficiency. The vaginal defence is lost. Vaginal mucosa is thin and is more susceptible to infection and trauma. There may be desquamation of the vaginal epithelium which may lead to formation of adhesions and bands between the walls.

Clinical features

(a) Postmenopausal yellowish or blood stained vaginal discharge.

(b) Discomfort, dryness, soreness in the vulva.

(c) Dyspareunia.

On examination

(a) Evidences of pruritus vulvae.

(b) The character of the discharge is yellowish or blood stained.

(c) Vaginal examination is often painful and the walls are found inflamed.

Table 12.1 : Differential diagnosis of vaginal discharge

Characteristics	Trichomoniasis	Candidiasis	Bacterial Vaginosis	Chlamydia	Normal vaginal discharge
Colour	Greenish yellow	Curdy white	Grey white to green	Mucopurulent yellow white	White
Consistency	Thin, Frothy	Thick	Thin	Thick	Thin
Whiff test : (see p. 148)	Negative	Negative	Positive (Fishy amine)	Negative	Negative
pH	5	< 4.5	5	< 4.5	< 4.5
Pruritus	+++	++	Non-irritating	—	—
Diagnosis : (Saline wet mount microscopy)	Motile trichomona (see p. 160)	Hyphae (see p. 160)	Clue cells (see p. 148)	Chlamydia DNA by PCR (see p. 146)	—
Treatment	Metronidazole 2 gm single dose or 200 mg. TID × 7 days (p. 160)	Imidazoles Fluconazole 150 mg P.O. weekly for 6 weeks (see p. 161)	Metronidazole 200 mg. TID × 7 days (p. 148)	Azithromycin 1 gm orally single dose (p. 146)	—

Diagnosis

Senile endometritis may co-exist and **carcinoma body or the cervix should be excluded prior to therapy (p. 532).** This can be achieved by examination under anaesthesia, diagnostic curettage, cervical cytology or biopsy (p. 331). These procedures are urgently indicated, if improvement does not rapidly follow the treatment of atrophic vaginitis.

Treatment

Improvement of general health and treatment of infection if present should be done. Systemic oestrogen therapy may be considered if there is no contraindications. This improves the vaginal epithelium, raises glycogen content and lowers vaginal pH.

Intravaginal application of oestrogen cream by an applicator is also effective. About one-third of the vaginal oestrogen is systemically absorbed.

NON-SPECIFIC VAGINITIS

During the reproductive period, when the vaginal defence is lost, the local pathogens-like *Staphylococcus, Streptococcus* (haemolytic and anaerobic), *Esch. coli*, etc. gain footing and produce acute symptoms. Foreign bodies-like pessary, tampon, IUCD or childbirth trauma or vaginal operations predispose to such infection.

Treatment

There is no specific treatment.

(a) Improvement of general health.

(b) Removal of the foreign body.

(c) Local application of bactericidal cream (clindamycin 2%) twice daily for 7 days is helpful.

TOXIC SHOCK SYNDROME (TSS)

TSS is commonly seen in menstruating women between 15 and 30 years of age following the use of tampons (polyacrylate). Other condition associated with TSS is use of female barrier contraceptives (diaphragm). **It is characterised by the following features of abrupt onset** :

- Fever > 38.9°C.
- Diffuse macular rash, myalgia.
- Gastrointestinal : Vomiting, diarrhoea.
- Cardiopulmonary : Hypotension, adult respiratory distress syndrome.
- Platelets : ≤ 100,000/mm^3.
- Renal : ↑ BUN ≥ twice normal.

- Hepatic : ↑ Bilirubin, ↑ SGOT; ↑ SGPT.
- Mucous membrane (vaginal, oropharyngeal) : Hyperaemia.

The pathological features are due to liberation of exotoxin by *Staphylococcus aureus*. It may lead to multiorgan system failure. Blood cultures are negative.

Treatment is supportive. Correction of hypovolemia and hypotension with intravenous fluids and dopamine infusion is done. Parenteral corticosteroids may be used. Blood coagulation parameters and serum electrolytes are checked and corrected. Infection is controlled by beta lactamase resistant anti-staphylococcal penicillin (cloxacillin, methicillin) for 10-14 days. The tampon should be removed. Mortality following TSS is 6-10 per cent.

CERVICITIS

The term cervicitis is reserved to infection of the endocervix including the glands and the stroma. The infection may be acute or chronic.

ACUTE CERVICITIS

The **endocervical infection** usually follows childbirth, abortion or any operation on cervix. The responsible organisms are usually pyogenic *Streptococcus, Staphylococcus, Esch. coli*, etc. Infection with STDs like *Gonococcus* or *Chlamydia trachomatis* may occur, the former being less common nowadays.

The organisms gain entry into the glands of the endocervix and produce acute inflammatory changes. The infection may be localised or spread upwards to involve the tube or sidewards involving the parametrium.

Clinical features

The vaginal examination is painful. The cervix is tender on touch or movements. Cervix looks oedematous and congested. **Mucopurulent discharge** is seen escaping out through the external os.

Prognosis

(a) It may resolute completely. (b) The infection may spread to involve the adjacent structures or even beyond that. (c) Becomes chronic.

Treatment

High vaginal and endocervical swabs are taken for bacteriological identification and drug sensitivity test. Appropriate antibiotics should be prescribed. General measures are to be taken as outlined in acute pelvic infection (ch. 10).

CHRONIC CERVICITIS

Chronic cervicitis is the commonest lesion found in women attending gynaecologic out-patient. It may follow an acute attack or usually chronic from the beginning. The infection usually occurs following childbirth or abortion by the pyogenic organisms — *Staphylococcus, Streptococcus* or *Esch. coli*. *Chlamydia trachomatis* is more and more implicated with *Gonococcus* being a rarity.

Pathology

The mucosa and the deeper tissues are congested, fibrosed and infiltrated with leucocytes and plasma cells. The glands are also hypertrophied with increased secretory activity. Some of the gland mouths are closed by fibrosis or plugs of desquamated epithelial cells to cause retention cyst — **nabothian follicles** (Fig. 18.4). Thus, in fact, it should be called chronic endocervicitis as the ectocervix is protected by the overlying stratified squamous epithelium. There is associated lacerated and everted endocervix, the so-called **eversion or ectropion.**

Clinical features

There may not be any symptom as it may be accidentally discovered during examination. Excessive mucoid discharge at times **mucopurulent** is the predominant symptom. History of contact bleeding or associated infertility may be present.

On examination : (a) The cervix may be tender to touch or on movement. (b) Speculum examination reveals — mucoid or mucopurulent discharge escaping out through the cervical os. There may be

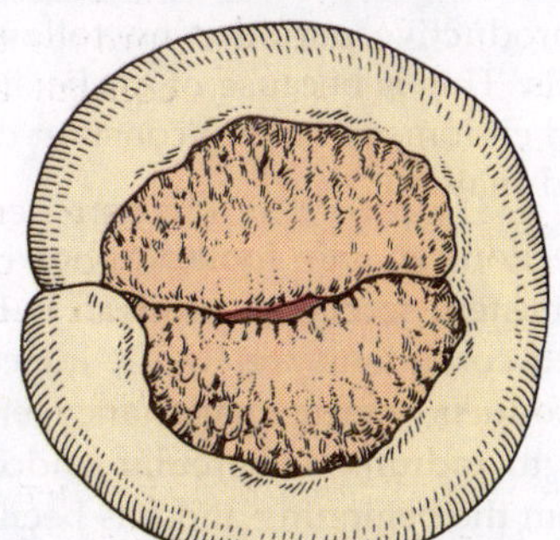

Fig. 12.6. Ectropion with unilateral tear of the cervix

enlargement, congestion or ectropion of the cervix. Associated ectopy may be present (Fig. 12.6).

Treatment

Cervical scrape cytology to exclude malignancy is mandatory prior to any therapy.

(i) There is no place of antibiotic therapy except in gonococcal or proved cases of chlamydial infection.

(ii) The diseased tissue may be destroyed by electro or diathermy cauterisation or laser or cryosurgery. The ectropion is corrected by deep linear burns and the coincidental erosion may be coagulated. (See p. 562).

(iii) Associated cervical tear may be reconstructed by trachelorrhaphy.

ENDOMETRITIS

During childbearing period, infection hardly occurs in the endometrium except in septic abortion or puerperal sepsis and acute gonococcal infection.

The bacterial invasion from the lower genital tract is prevented by the vaginal and cervical defence. Moreover, periodic shedding of the endometrium prevents the organisms to gain foothold.

ACUTE ENDOMETRITIS

Acute endometritis almost always occurs after abortion or childbirth. The details of such infection has been dealt in page 129. For details see author's Textbook of Obstetrics Chapter 29.

CHRONIC ENDOMETRITIS

It is indeed rare for chronic endometritis to occur during reproductive period even following acute endometritis. This is because of cyclic shedding of the infected endometrium and constant drainage of the infected material.

The infection can gain foothold, however, when there is persistent source of infection in the uterine cavity. Such conditions are IUCD, infected polyp, retained products, uterine malignancy, endometrial burns due to radium. Tubercular endometritis is chronic from the beginning and has been described in p. 135.

Women often presents with purulent or seropurulent vaginal discharge. **Diagnosis** is made by cervical smear, culture of the discharge and histology, of the endometrium.

Treatment

The offending cause is to be removed or eradicated. In unresponsive cases without any detectable source of infection and the patient approaching menopause, hysterectomy is justified.

ATROPHIC ENDOMETRITIS (SENILE ENDOMETRITIS)

Following menopause, due to deficiency of oestrogen, the defence of the uterocervicovaginal canal is lost. There is no periodic shedding of the endometrium. As a result, organisms of low virulence can ascend up to infect the atrophic endometrium. There is intense infiltration of the endometrium with polymorphonuclear leucocytes and plasma cells. The endometrium becomes ulcerated at places and replaced by granulation tissues. The purulent discharge either escapes out of the uterine cavity or may be pent up inside producing pyometra.

Clinical features

The postmenopausal women complain of vaginal discharge, at times offensive or even blood stained. Pelvic examination reveals features of atrophic vaginitis. Purulent discharge may be seen escaping out through the cervix. In presence of pyometra, the uterus is enlarged; feels soft and tender.

Diagnosis

The diagnosis is confused with carcinoma of the endometrium which must be excluded prior to treatment (see p. 344). In fact, pyometra may be present both in atrophic endometritis and endometrial carcinoma. Diagnostic curettage should be done and the endometrium is subjected to histological examination.

If however, pyometra is present, drainage of pus by simple dilatation should be done first. After 1-2 weeks, diagnostic curettage is to be done under cover of antibiotics.

Treatment

Oestrogen supplement — ethinyl oestradiol vaginal cream is helpful. In unresponsive cases or with recurrent attacks, hysterectomy should be done and **the specimen should be subjected to histological examination.**

PYOMETRA

Collection of pus in the uterine cavity is called pyometra. **The prerequisites for pyometra formation are** :

- Occlusion of the cervical canal.
- Enough sources of pus formation inside the uterine cavity.
- Presence of low grade infection.

Causes

- **Obstetrical** — The only condition is following infection of lochiometra.
- **Gynaecological** — The conditions which are associated with pyometra are : (a) Carcinoma in the lower part of the body of uterus (b) Endocervical carcinoma (c) Senile endometritis (d) Infected haematometra following amputation, conisation or deep cauterisation of cervix (e) Tubercular endometritis.

Pathology

There is abundant secretion of pus from the offending sites. The cervical canal gets blocked due to senile narrowing by fibrosis or due to debris. The accumulated pus distends the uterine cavity. The postmenopausal atrophic myometrium fails to expel the collected pus. Thus, the uterus gets enlarged more and more with thinning of its wall. The lining epithelium is lost at places and replaced by granulation tissue.

The organisms responsible are coliforms, *Streptococci* or *Staphylococci*. Rarely, it may be tubercular. Except in tubercular (caseous), the fluid is thin, offensive, at times purulent or blood stained. The pus may be sterile on culture or the offending organism can be detected.

Clinical features

The patient complains of intermittent blood stained purulent offensive discharge per vaginam. There may be occasional pain in lower abdomen. Systemic manifestation is usually absent.

Per abdomen

An uniform suprapubic swelling may be felt of varying size. It is cystic with well-defined margins but lower pole is not felt. It may be tender.

Internal examination reveals

The swelling is uterine in origin. The offensive discharge is seen escaping out through the cervix. **Pelvic ultrasonography** reveals distended uterine cavity with accumulation of fluid within.

Diagnosis is confirmed by dilatation of the cervix when pus escapes. In every case, **all types of investigation are to be made to exclude malignancy of the body of the uterus and endocervix.** Diagnostic curettage should be withheld for about 7-14 days following dilatation and drainage of pus. This will minimise such complications such as perforation of the uterus and spreading peritonitis. During the interval period, antibiotics should be prescribed.

Treatment

Once malignancy is excluded, the pyometra is drained by simple dilatation of the cervix. Even in non-malignant cases or in cases of recurrence, hysterectomy may be indicated. Definite surgery for malignancy is to be done following drainage of pus.

SALPINGITIS

Infection of the fallopian tube is called salpingitis. The details of salpingitis has already been described in the chapter of pelvic infection (ch. 10). The pathogenesis of salpingitis (acute and chronic) will be described in this section. **The following facts are to be borne in mind while dealing with salpingitis.**

- The infection is usually polymicrobial in nature (Table 12.2).
- Both the tubes are usually affected.
- Ovaries are usually involved in the inflammatory process and as such, the terminology of salpingo-oophoritis is preferred.
- Tubal infection almost always affects adversely the future reproductive function.

Table 12.2
The organisms responsible for salpingitis

Sexually transmitted :		
• Gonococcus	• Chlamydia trachomatis	
• Mycoplasma (rarely)		
Pyogenic :		
• Aerobes	—	*Streptococcus, Staphylococcus, Esch. coli.*
• Anaerobes	—	*Bacteroides fragilis, Actinomycosis* (rarely) *Peptococcus.*
Tubercular :		
• *Mycobacterium tuberculosis*		

Aetiology

I. Ascending infection from the uterus, cervix and vagina

• *Pyogenic* — The infection usually occurs following delivery and induced abortion. Minor operations like D + C, hysterosalpingography or presence of IUCD may be the responsible factors.

• *Sexually transmitted disease* — Salpingitis is the major complication following infections with *N. gonorrhoea* and *Chlamydia trachomatis*. Both the infections may remain asymptomatic but cause tubal damage (see p. 143, 145).

II. Direct spread from the adjacent infection

One or both the tubes are affected in appendicitis, diverticulitis or following pelvic peritonitis. The organisms are usually *Esch. coli* or *Streptococcus faecalis*. *Bacteroides fragilis* is too often involved whenever abscess is formed.

III. Tubercular (see p. 134)

The infection is usually chronic except in miliary form, when it manifests acutely.

Modes of spread to the tubes — See p. 123.

ACUTE SALPINGITIS

Pathology

• **Pyogenic** • **Gonococcal**

Acute pyogenic

The pathological changes in the tubes depend on the virulence of the organisms and the resistance of the host.

There is intense hyperaemia with dilated vessels visible under the peritoneal coat. The enlargement of the tube is greater than gonococcal infection because of interstitial involvement. The wall is enormously thickened and oedematous. The seropurulent or purulent exudate can be expressed out through the abdominal ostium.

Microscopically, the epithelium looks normal or the mucosa slightly oedematous. The muscularis shows marked oedema and acute inflammatory reaction. **As the outer coat is involved, adhesions are likely and are dense.**

There is simultaneous inflammatory reaction of the pelvic peritoneum to the extent of even pus formation. The pus collects in the pouch of Douglas forming pelvic abscess.

If the infection is very severe, the endosalpinx is destroyed in part or whole and pus is formed. If the fimbrial end is open, the pus escapes out. But if the fimbriae are adherent to each other and occlude the opening, the pus is pent up inside producing pyosalpinx. The organisms may be present for even a year and as such chances of repeated infections are more.

Acute gonococcal

Like pyogenic infection, there is hyperaemia and the tube is swollen and oedematous. The abdominal ostium initially remains open, through which the exudate can be expressed out. As the pathology is principally endosalpingitis, **adhesions are less and flimsy.**

The purulent exudate may escape in the peritoneal cavity and produces pelvic peritonitis and pelvic abscess. The ovaries may be involved in the process either directly or through lymphatics.

More often, the fimbriae get oedematous, phymotic and indrawn by cicatrical contraction of the serosa with closure of the abdominal ostium. The uterine opening is closed by congestion. The exudate is pent up inside the lumen producing **pyosalpinx.** The pus becomes sterile by 6 weeks.

Table 12.3
Clinical Diagnostic Criteria for Acute Salpingitis

- Abdominal tenderness.
- Rebound tenderness (±).
- Cervical and uterine motion tenderness.
- Adnexal tenderness.
- Temperature (> 38°C).
- Leucocytosis (> 10,000/mm^3).
- Purulent material from peritoneal cavity by laparoscopy or by culdocentesis (p.127).
- Pelvic abscess or tubo-ovarian mass on bimanual examination or on sonography.

Complication of acute salpingitis: (i) Pelvic or generalised peritonitis (ii) Pelvis cellulitis (iii) Pelvic thrombophlebitis (iv) Pelvic abscess (v) Tubo-ovarian abscess.

Fate of acute salpingitis

Complete resolution: Provided the tissue destruction is not appreciable, the tubes return to its normal structure and function.

But endosalpingitis too often produces loss of cilia which is responsible for **infertility** or delay in transport of the fertilised ovum, resulting in **ectopic pregnancy**.

Chronic : The infection may be chronic due to reinfection or flaring up of the infection at the site.

CHRONIC SALPINGITIS

Pathology

- Hydrosalpinx.
- Pyosalpinx.
- Chronic interstitial salpingitis.
- Salpingitis isthmica nodosa.

Hydrosalpinx

Collection of mucus secretion into the fallopian tube is called hydrosalpinx.

Pathogenesis : It is usually due to the end result of repeated attacks of mild endosalpingitis by pyogenic organisms of low virulence but highly irritant. The organisms involved are *Staphylococcus, Esch. coli, Gonococcus, Chlamydia trachomatis,* etc.

During initial infection, the fimbriae are oedematous and indrawn with the serous surface adhere together to produce closure of the abdominal ostium. The uterine ostium gets closed by congestion. The secretion is pent up to make the tube distended. The distension is marked on the ampullary region than the more rigid isthmus. As the mesosalpinx is fixed, the resultant distension makes the tube curled and **looks 'retort' shaped.** The wall is smooth and shiny containing clear fluid inside which is usually sterile (Figs. 12.7 and 36.55).

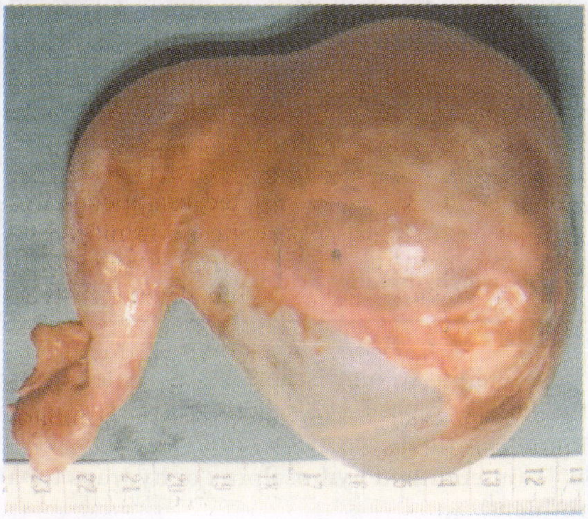

Fig. 12.7. Hydrosalpinx. Note the retort shape of the tube. Depending on tubal diameter **hydrosalpinx** may be **mild** < 15 mm; **moderate** 15-30 mm; **severe** > 30 mm.

Table 12.4
Comparative Features of Gonococcal and Pyogenic Salpingitis

Gonococcal	*Pyogenic*
• Sexually transmitted.	Endogenous organisms.
• Infection occurs usually during and following menstruation.	Following abortion and childbirth.
• **Mode of infection** — by continuity and contiguity (Fig. 10.1).	Through lymphatics and veins → pelvic cellulitis → tubal affection (Fig. 10.2).
• Always bilateral affection.	May be unilateral.
• Pathology :	
(i) Endosalpingitis.	(i) Perisalpingitis (predominantly).
(ii) Intraluminal exudation ++.	(ii) Less.
(iii) Closure of the abdominal ostium by phymotic and indrawn fimbriae.	(iii) Closure by adhesions. May remain patent.
(iv) Peritoneal coat is less involved, adhesions — scanty and flimsy.	(iv) More involvement and as such adhesions are more and dense.
• Pus becomes sterile by 6 weeks.	Takes longer time even a year.
• Restoration of reproductive function is unlikely.	May be possible.

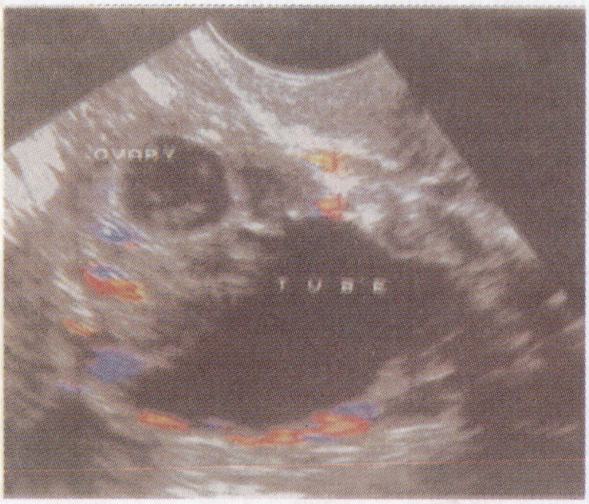

Fig. 12.8. Colour Doppler scan (TV) showing ovary and the tube with hydrosalpinx change

The uterine ostium is not closed anatomically, thus favours repeated infection. At times, there is intermittent discharge of the fluid into the uterine cavity **(intermittent hydrosalpinx or hydrops tubal profluens)**.

Hydrosalpinx is also considered as the end stage of pyosalpinx when the pus becomes liquefied to make the fluid clear. But the fact that there is intact but compressed epithelium with absence of chronic inflammatory reaction exclude its possibility.

Ultrasound and Colour Doppler (TVS)

Sausage-shaped complex cystic structure with reduced resistance index (RI) in the adnexal region is suggestive of the diagnosis (Fig. 12.8).

Complications

The following may happen : (i) Formation of tubo-ovarian cyst. (ii) Torsion. (iii) Infection from the gut. (iv) Rupture.

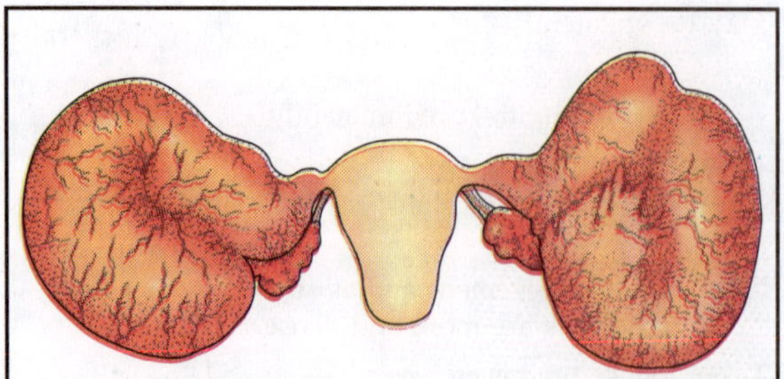

Fig. 12.9. Bilateral pyosalpinx

Pyosalpinx

The pyogenic organisms, if become virulent, produce intense inflammatory reaction with secretion of pus. The tube becomes closed at both ends; the abdominal ostium by adhesions of the fimbriae and the uterine end by exudate. Because of intense inflammatory reaction and or escape of pus into the peritoneal cavity, there is dense adhesions with the surrounding structures like ovaries, intestines, omentum and pelvic peritoneum. Thus, a tubo-ovarian mass is formed. The inner wall of the tube is replaced in part by granulation tissue (Figs. 12.9 and 12.11).

Chronic interstitial salpingitis

The tube enlarges mainly due to great thickness of the wall. The distension of the tube by the exudate is unusual. The abdominal ostium may be closed or partially open. The adjacent organs are adherent to the tube. Microscopically, there is extensive infiltration of plasma cells and histiocytes in all the layers. The epithelium is usually intact. There is intense fibrosis of the muscle coat along with inflammatory changes. This hinders the tubal motility and favours ectopic pregnancy.

Salpingitis isthmica nodosa

Pathogenesis : The exact nature still remains unclear.

The following are the probabilities :

(i) It is related to tubercular infection, although it may be the residue of any form of chronic interstitial salpingitis.

(ii) There is infiltration of the tubal mucosa directly into the muscularis resembling adenomyosis of the uterus.

(iii) It is one form of endometriosis of the tube. Absence of endometrial stroma, however, points against it.

Naked eye examination reveals one or two nodules in the isthmus of the tube, often involving the uterine cornu. The nodule is small but may be as large as 2 cm.

Microscopically, there is thickening of the muscularis in which the tubal epithelium lined spaces are scattered, giving an adenomatous picture. There may be inconsistent mild inflammatory reaction (Fig. 12.10).

The clinical features and investigations of **salpingitis have already been described in the chapter p. 166 (Table 12.3).**

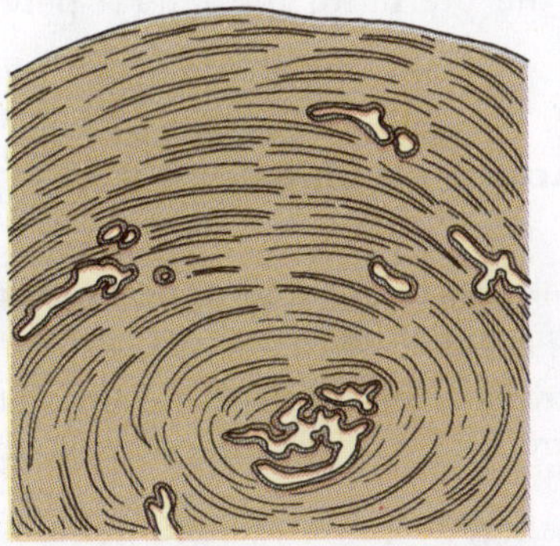

Fig. 12.10. Histology of salpingitis isthmica nodosa. Note the tubal epithelial lined spaces inside the muscularis

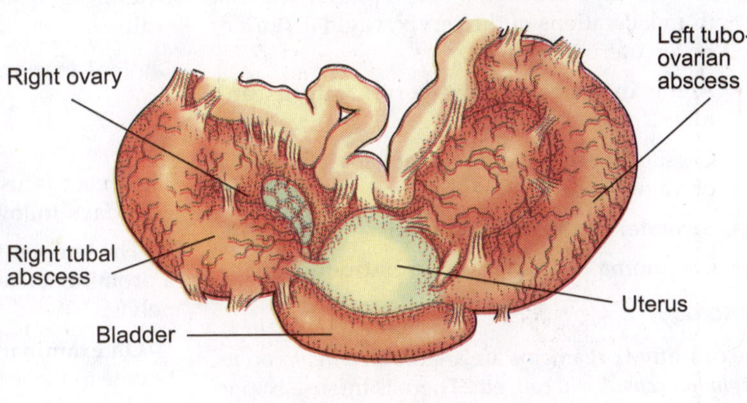

Fig. 12.11. Bilateral tubo-ovarian mass (TO mass)

Treatment of acute Salpingitis — Peritonitis (Regimens recommended by CDC)

- **Out-patient therapy** : (i) Ofloxacin 400 mg PO twice daily for 14 days plus metronidazole 500 mg PO twice daily for 14 days (see Table 10.4) are given. Patient is admitted for in-patient therapy if there is no response by 72 hours.

- **In-patient therapy** (Temp > 39°C, toxic look, lower abdominal guarding and rebound tenderness). Clindamycin 900 mg IV 8 hourly, plus gentamicin 2 mg/kg IV, then 1.5 mg/kg IV every 8 hours are given. This is followed by doxycycline 100 mg twice daily orally for 14 days. IV fluids to correct dehydration and nasogastric suction in the presence of abdominal distension or ileus are maintained. Laparotomy is done if there is clinical suggestion of abscess rupture.

Prognosis of salpingitis

With early diagnosis and therapy with potent antibiotics, the immediate risk is markedly reduced. With effective therapy, the prospect of future reproductive function of the tube is not so gloomy. But once the cilia is damaged, commonly with gonococcal infection or when involvement of the wall in pyogenic infection impairs the motility, the prospect of future fertility is very much poor even with reconstructive surgery. Even if pregnancy occurs, chance of ectopic is more.

OOPHORITIS

Isolated infection to the ovaries is a rarity. The ovaries are almost always affected during salpingitis and as such the nomenclature of salpingo-oophoritis is preferred. **The affection of the ovary from tubal infection occurs by the following routes** :

- Directly from the exudates contaminating the ovarian surface producing perioophoritis.
- Through lymphatics of the mesosalpinx and mesovarium producing interstitial oophoritis.
- Blood borne — mumps.
- Through the rent of the ovulation producing interstitial oophoritis.

If the organisms are severe, an abscess is formed and a tubo-ovarian abscess results. In others, the ovaries may be adherent to the tubes, intestine, omentum and pelvic peritoneum producing tubo-ovarian mass (TO mass). Such a mass is usually bilateral (Fig. 12.11).

Direct affection of the ovaries without tubal involvement may be due to mumps or influenza. In mumps, there is no sterilising effects on the ovaries unlike testes. This is because the capsule of the ovary is elastic and as such, ischaemic injury to the graafian follicles is not likely. Even if some follicles are damaged, many are left behind to carry on the reproductive function.

The symptomatology and treatment are like those of salpingitis.

PARAMETRITIS

Inflammation of the pelvic cellular tissue is called parametritis.

Aetiology

The infection gains access following :

- Delivery and abortion through placental site or from lacerations of the cervix, vaginal vault or lower uterine segment.
- Acute infections of the cervix, uterus and tubes.
- Caesarean section or hysterectomy-abdominal or vaginal (cuff cellulitis).
- Secondary to pelvic peritonitis.
- Carcinoma cervix or radium introduction.

Pathology

The causative organisms are anaerobic *Streptococcus, Staphylococcus, Esch. coli,* etc. There is intense hyperaemia with exudation of serous fluid, lymph and polymorphonuclear leucocytes. The exudate may resolute completely or an abscess is formed. The purulent exudate may be localised or may have extrapelvic extension along the tract of blood vessels and ureter. The abscess thus points towards the perinephric region along the ureter, to the buttock along the gluteal vessels, to the thigh along the external iliac vessels and to the groin above the inguinal ligament.

Rarely, the abscess may burst into the pelvic organs, or into the peritoneal cavity. There may be associated pelvic thrombophlebitis with chance of 'white leg' and pyaemia.

The cellulitis usually confined to one side but may extent to the other side either anteriorly or posteriorly. The infection affecting the posterior parametrium may spread on either side of the uterosacral ligaments.

The acute cellulitis usually subsides without any evidence. There may be variable degrees of scarring or fibrosis which is felt as a stony hard mass extending from the uterus to the lateral pelvic wall.

Clinical features

- **Acute**
- **Chronic**

Acute

The onset is usually insidious and appears about 7-10 days following initial infection.

The temperature rises to about 102°F. Pain is not a prominent feature, may be dull aching deep in the pelvis.

On examination, the pulse rate is raised proportionate to the temperature. There is generalised deep tenderness on lower abdomen. Rigidity is absent because the lesion is extra peritoneal. Pelvic examination reveals hot and tender vagina. There is an indurated tender mass usually unilateral which extends to the lateral pelvic wall and to which the uterus is firmly fixed. The uterus is pushed to the contralateral side (Fig. 12.12).

Rectal examination confirms the indurated tender mass or horse shoe-shaped induration of the uterosacral ligaments surrounding the rectum.

An abscess formation is featured by spiky rise of temperature, toxic look and fluctuant swelling in the regions mentioned earlier.

Chronic

The clinical features vary, as it is often associated with chronic salpingo-oophoritis and as such, the symptoms and signs are overshadowed by the latter condition. It may, however, be present without salpingitis.

The chief complaint is chronic deep seated pelvic pain, may be localised to one side. There is deep dyspareunia.

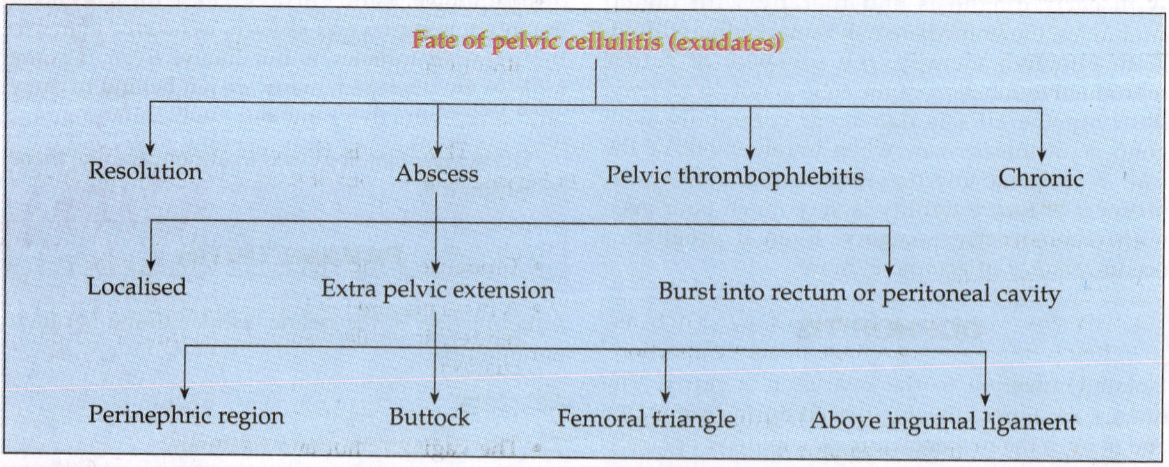

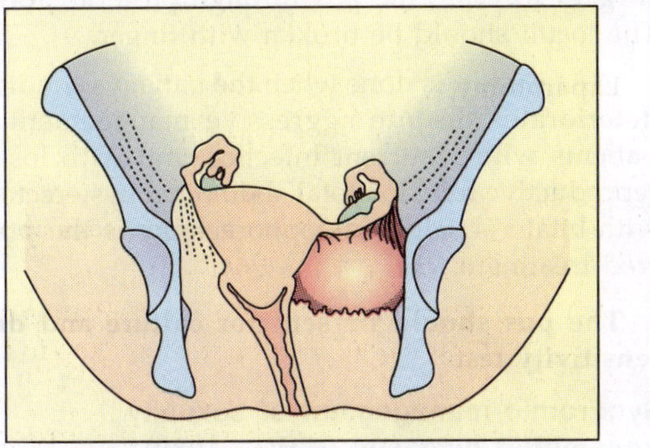

Fig. 12.12. Acute parametritis pushing the uterus to contralateral side

Pelvic examination reveals the uterus fixed to an indurated and tender mass. The uterus is also drawn to the affected side because of scarring. Movement of the cervix produces pain.

Treatment

Acute

The outline of management protocol is the same like that of acute salpingitis of pyogenic origin.

Only when an abscess is pointing and easily accessible that it should be drained surgically.

Chronic

The treatment is the same as for chronic salpingo-oophoritis. Deep pelvic short wave diathermy may be tried to relieve pain and dyspareunia. Too often, all the measures fail and considering the prolonged illness, debilitating condition and marital dysharmony, hysterectomy decision may have to be considered even at an early age specially in women whose family is completed.

PELVIC ABSCESS

Encysted pus in the pouch of Douglas is called pelvic abscess.

Aetiology

Pelvic causes (common)

- Postabortal and puerperal sepsis.
- Acute salpingitis.
- Perforation of an infected uterus such as attempted uterine curettage in septic abortion or pyometra.
- Infection of pelvic haematocele usually following disturbed tubal pregnancy.
- Postoperative pelvic peritonitis following abdominal or vaginal operation.
- Irritant peritonitis following contamination of urine, bile, vernix caseosa, meconium (spilled during Caesarean section), iodine containing dye used in hysterosalpingography or contents of ruptured ovarian cyst (sebum in dermoid cyst), etc.

Extrapelvic causes (rare)

Appendicitis, diverticulitis, ruptured gallbladder, perforated peptic ulcer usually produce generalised peritonitis. The condition may ultimately settle to the dependent pouch of Douglas and produces pelvic abscess.

The irritant peritoneal exudate (pus) either produced locally or settle down from the general peritoneal cavity is localised by coils of intestine and omentum on the top. The pus so localised may be loculated.

Fate : Complete resolution is unlikely. If left uncared for, the adhesions on the top may be disturbed producing generalised peritonitis. In others, the abscess may burst into the rectum but rarely through the vagina because of tough endopelvic fascial sheath.

Clinical features : Patient is ill from any of the causative factors mentioned earlier. **But the localisation of pus in the pouch of Douglas is evidenced by** :

Symptoms

- Spiky rise of high temperature with chills and rigor.
- Rectal tenesmus — frequent passage of loose mucoid stool.
- Pain lower abdomen — variable degrees.
- Urinary symptoms — difficulty or even retention of urine.

Signs

General : The face is flushed with anxious look. Pulse rate is raised out of proportion to temperature.

Per abdomen :

- Tenderness and rigidity in lower abdomen.
- A mass may be felt in the suprapubic region — tender, irregular, soft and resonant on percussion.

Per vaginam :

- The vagina is hot and tender.

- The uterus is pushed anteriorly; the movement of the cervix is painful.
- A boggy, fluctuant and tender mass is felt in the pouch of Douglas.
- A separate mass may be felt through the lateral fornix.

Rectal examination defines precisely the mass in the pouch of Douglas.

Investigations

Blood : There is high leucocytosis with increased polymorphs.

Bacteriological study : Swabs are taken from high vagina, endocervical canal and from the pus. Culture is done for both aerobic and anaerobic micro-organisms. Sensitivity of the micro-organisms to antibiotics is also to be detected.

Confirmation of diagnosis

The diagnosis is easy in most of the cases but at times confusion arises between pelvic haematocele and pelvic abscess. **Pelvic ultrasonography** reveals accumulation of fluid in the pouch of Douglas. **Examination under anaesthesia (EUA) and puncture of pouch of Douglas (culdocentesis)** give the correct diagnosis. Old blood comes out in the former and pus in the latter.

Treatment

General : Systemic antibiotics should cover anaerobic as well as aerobic micro-organisms (broad spectrum) : Cefoxitin 1-2 gm IV every 6-8 hours and gentamicin 5 mg/kg IV per 24 hours and metronidazole 500 mg IV 8 hourly are started. Antibiotic regimen may have to be changed depending upon the sensitivity report.

Surgery : **Posterior calpotomy** is the definitive surgery to drain the pus through posterior fornix. The loculi should be broken with finger.

Laparotomy is done when the patient's condition deteriorates despite aggressive management. In patients with recurrent infection and with loss of reproductive function total abdominal hysterectomy with bilateral salpingo-oophorectomy is the preferred treatment.

The pus should be sent for culture and drug sensitivity test.

Syndromic management of sexually transmitted diseases (WHO – 1988)

Principle : Treatment of STDs should be initiated at the patient's first visit to a clinic. At the same time the couple is counselled about the importance of condom use and prevention of STD transmission.

Method : Management is done by criteria for syndrome diagnosis of PID. These include detection of vaginal discharge, abdominal pain, cervical motion tenderness, bilateral adnexal tenderness and negative pregnancy test. Health care providers are trained up to follow a standardised protocol (flow charts) to treat such a patient. This is particularly suitable in a health care setting of developing countries.

Advantages :

- It avoids delay of treatment, where laboratory facilities are limited.
- It avoids loss of patient follow up, where referral system is not well-structured.
- Continued transmission of infection is prevented.
- It is a simple, inexpensive and rapid management for STDs.

KEY POINTS

- In recurrent vulvitis due to fungal infection, diabetes is to be excluded.
- Bartholin's cyst usually develops in the duct. The gratifying treatment is marsupialisation under local anaesthesia. A normal Bartholin's gland cannot be palpated.

  Excision of Bartholin's duct and gland is indicated for persistent and/or recurrent infections specially when it occurs beyond the age of 40.
- During childbearing period, vaginal trichomoniasis is the commonest STD caused by *Trichomonas vaginalis* — a flagellated parasite. Hanging drop preparation with identification of trichomonads is diagnostic.

KEY POINTS

Treatment is specific with metronidazole to both partners. The husband is to use condom during treatment. Vaginitis may be due to other causes also (p. 158).

- A vaginal discharge with pH > 5.0 indicate atrophic vaginitis, bacterial vaginosis or trichomonas infection whereas a vaginal discharge with pH < 4.5 may be either physiologic or due to fungal infection. Vaginal discharge needs to be differentiated before treatment (Table 12.1)
- Moniliasis is caused by *Candida albicans* — a gram-positive fungus. The infection is more likely related to diabetes, pregnancy or amongst 'pill' users (p. 160). Diagnosis is by identification of the mycelia by direct smear and stained by methylene blue or culture is Sabouraud's media.
- Toxic shock syndrome is due to improper use of vaginal tampon. The causative organism is *Staphylococcus aureus*. Dysfunction of multiple organ system is due to the bacterial exotoxin (p. 162). Treatment is supportive. Beta-lactamase resistant anti-staphylococcal penicillin (cloxacillin, methicillin) should be the choice.
- The feature of senile endometritis may simulate endometrial carcinoma which should be ruled out prior to treatment.
- Common causes of pyometra are endometrial carcinoma, endocervical carcinoma, senile endometritis, infected haematometra and tubercular endometritis.
- Pyogenic non-gonococcal organisms affect the tubes by producing perisalpingitis; gonococcal produces endosalpingitis and tubercular infection produces interstitial salpingitis.
- The organisms producing hydrosalpinx are *Staphylococcus, Streptococcus, Esch. coli, Gonococcus, Cl. trachomatis*, etc. Hydrosalpinx is the end result of repeated attacks of mild endosalpingitis. It may also be the end stage of pyosalpinx when the pus becomes liquefied. Prognosis of salpingitis in terms of reproductive function depends on the type of infection, severity and number of episodes. When the cilia is damaged and or motility is impaired (adhesion) prospect is very poor.
- Salpingitis isthmica nodosa may be one variety of endometriosis or related to tubercular infection. Tube is nodular and thickened. There is proliferation of tubal epithelium within the muscle layer (myosalpinx).
- Pelvic abscess is the encysted pus in the pouch of Douglas. The common causes are following acute salpingitis, postabortal sepsis, infected pelvic haematocele and postoperative pelvic peritonitis, etc.

  Confirmation of diagnosis is by culdocentesis and the definitive surgery is drainage of pus through posterior colpotomy.
- Most common site of chlamydia infection in the female genital tract is the columnar cells of the endocervix.
- **Mode of spread of infection to the tubes are : Pyogenic infection** spreads through veins and lymphatics causing perisalpingitis and endosalpingitis. Cornual block following postabortal or puerperal sepsis may occur.

  Gonococcal infection ascends through continuity and contiguity causing endosalpingitis.

  Tubercular infection spreads through blood stream causing interstitial salpingitis.
- **Clinical diagnostic criteria for acute salpingitis include** : Abdominal tenderness, cervical or uterine motion tenderness, adnexal tenderness plus one or more other features (see p. 166).
- Indication of surgery for PID are restricted to life-threatening infection, not responding to medical therapy (e.g. tubo-ovarian abscess, pelvic abscess or any clinical suggestion of abscess rupture).

Dysmenorrhoea and Other Disorders of Menstrual Cycles

13

DYSMENORRHOEA

Definition

Dysmenorrhoea literally means painful menstruation. But a more realistic and practical definition includes cases of **painful menstruation of sufficient magnitude so as to incapacitate day-to-day activities.**

Types

- **Primary**
- **Secondary**

PRIMARY DYSMENORRHOEA (Spasmodic)

The primary dysmenorrhoea is one where there is no identifiable pelvic pathology.

Incidence

The incidence of primary dysmenorrhoea of sufficient magnitude with incapacitation is about 5-10 per cent. With the advent of oral contraceptives and non-steroidal anti-inflammatory drugs, there is marked relief of the symptom.

Causes of pain

The mechanism of initiation of uterine pain in primary dysmenorrhoea is difficult to establish. **But the following are too often related.**

- Mostly confined to adolescents.
- Almost always confined to ovulatory cycles.
- The pain is usually cured following pregnancy and vaginal delivery.
- The pain is related to dysrhythmic uterine contractions and uterine hypoxia.

1. **Psychosomatic factor** due to tension and anxiety during adolescence; lower pain threshold is often attributed as an aggravating factor in pain perception. This may explain, in part, the disappearance of pain with advancing age.

2. **Abnormal anatomical and functional aspect of uterus**

Uterine myometrial hyperactivity has been observed in cases with primary dysmenorrhoea.

- Stenosis at the internal os or narrowing of the cervical canal → difficult for the menstrual blood to escape → strong uterine contractions → pain. This may explain relief of pain following dilatation of the cervix.
- Unequal development of Müllerian ducts, such as septate or bicornuate uterus. The pain is due to unequal muscular contractions.
- Uterine hypoplasia → inadequate expulsive force.
- Imbalance in the autonomic nervous control of uterine muscle.

There is overactivity of the sympathetic → hypertonicity of the circular fibres of the isthmus and internal os. The relief of pain following dilatation of the cervix or following vaginal delivery may be explained by the damage of the adrenergic neurons which fail to regenerate.

However, there is no sound basis to presume that these factors contribute to the pain of dysmenorrhoea.

3. **Role of vasopressin**

There is increased vasopressin release during menstruation in women with primary dysmenorrhoea. This explains the persistence of pain in cases even treated with antiprostaglandin drugs. The mechanism of action is yet to be explored. Vasopressin increases prostaglandin synthesis and also increases myometrial activity directly. It causes uterine hyperactivity and dysrhythmic contractions → ischaemia and hypoxia → pain.

4. Role of prostaglandins

In ovulatory cycles, under the action of progesterone, prostaglandins ($PGF_2\alpha$, PGE_2) are synthesized from the secretory endometrium. Prostaglandins are released with maximum production during shedding of the endometrium. $PGF_2\alpha$ is a strong vasoconstrictor, which causes ischaemia (angina) of the myometrium.

Either due to increased production of the prostaglandins or increased sensitivity of the myometrium to the normal production of prostaglandins, there is increased myometrial contraction with or without dysrhythmia. The possible cause of pain is shown schematically below.

5. Others

Endothelins and leukotrienes are vasoconstrictors and stimulate myometrial contractions. **Platelet activating factor (PAF)** is also associated with the aetiology of dysmenorrhoea as its concentration is found high.

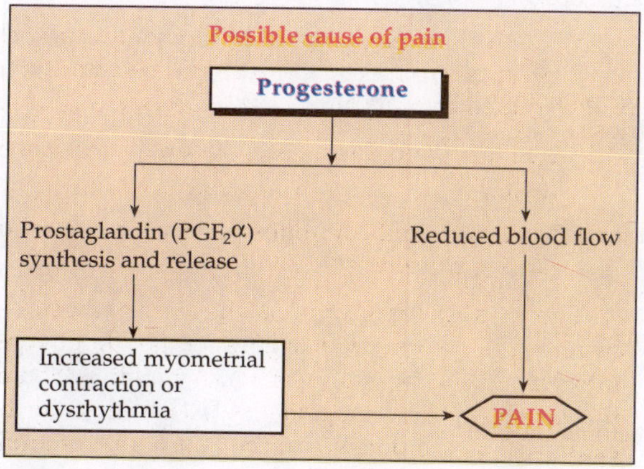

Patient profile

Primary dysmenorrhoea is predominantly confined to adolescent girls. It usually appears within 2 years of menarche. The mother or her sister may be dysmenorrhoeic. It is more common amongst girls from affluent society.

Clinical features

The pain begins a few hours before or just with the onset of menstruation. The severity of pain usually lasts for few hours, may extend to 24 hours but seldom persists beyond 48 hours. The pain is spasmodic and confined to lower abdomen; may radiate to the back and medial aspect of thighs. Systemic discomforts like nausea, vomiting, fatigue, diarrhoea and headache may be associated. It may be accompanied by vasomotor changes causing pallor, cold sweats and occasional fainting. Rarely, syncope and collapse in severe cases may be associated.

Abdominal or pelvic examination does not reveal any abnormal findings.

For detection of any pelvic abnormalities, **ultrasound** is very useful and it is not invasive.

Treatment

General measures include improvement of general health and simple psychotherapy in terms of explanation and assurance. Usual activities including sports are to be continued.

During menses, bowel should be kept empty; mild analgesics and antispasmodics may be prescribed. **Habit forming drugs such as pethidine or morphine must not be prescribed.** With these simple measures, the pain is relieved in majority.

In refractory or severe cases :

- **Drugs**
- **Surgery**

Drugs

The drugs used are :

- Prostaglandin synthetase inhibitors (Table 13.1).
- Oral contraceptives (combined oestrogen and progestogen).

Prostaglandin synthetase inhibitors (PSI)

These not only reduce the prostaglandin synthesis (by inhibition of cyclo-oxygenase enzyme) but also have a direct analgesic effect. Intrauterine pressure is reduced significantly. Any of the preparations listed in the table can be used orally for 2-3 days starting with the onset of period. The drug should be continued for 3-6 cycles.

Table 13.1

- **Fenamate group** — Mefanamic acid 250-500 mg 8 hourly or Flufenamic acid 100-200 mg 8 hourly.
- **Propionic acid derivatives** — Ibuprofen 400 mg 8 hourly or Naproxen 250 mg 6 hourly.
- **Indomethacin** 25 mg 8 hourly.

Management protocol of primary dysmenorrhoea

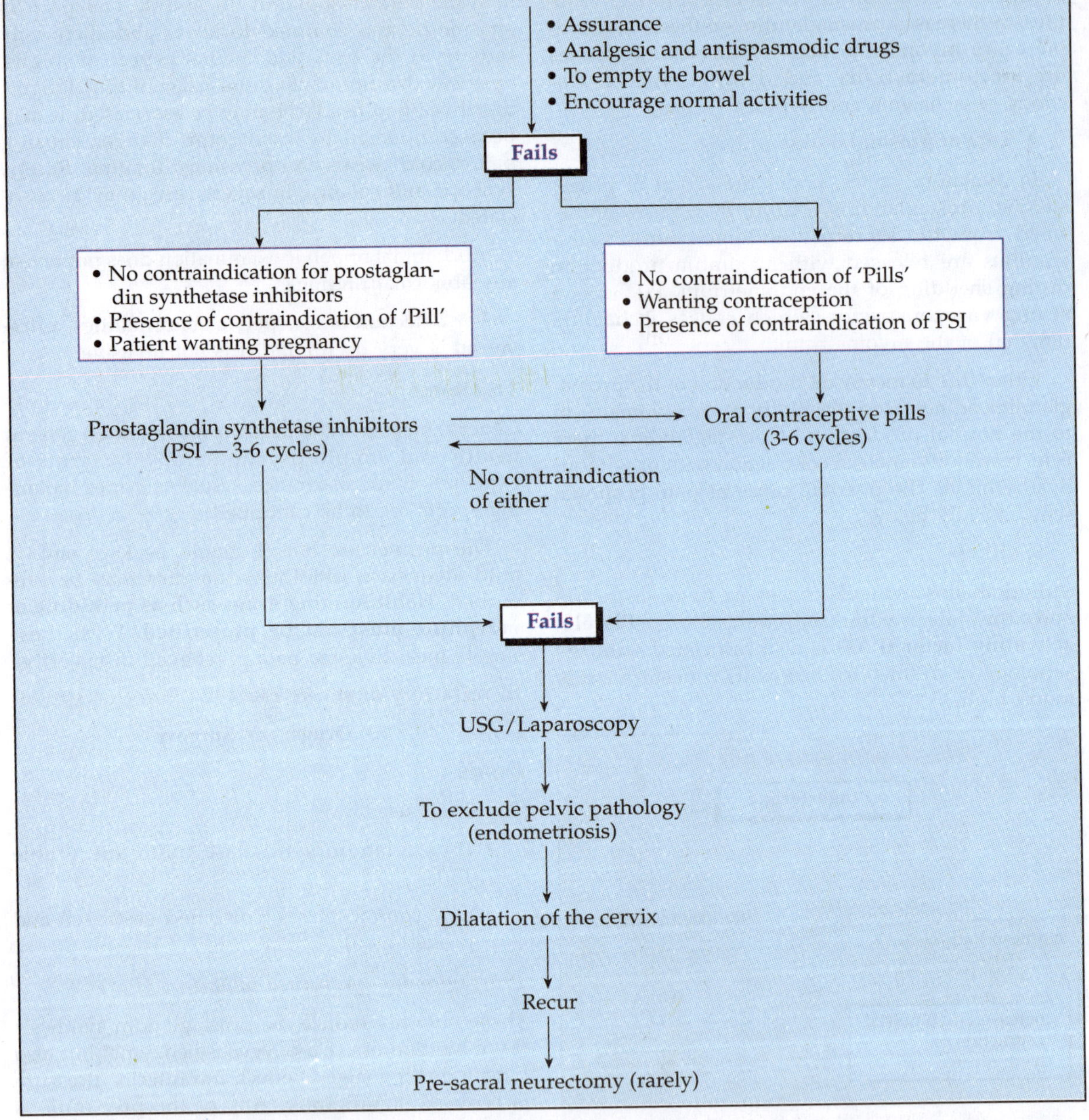

Newer drugs NSAIDS (Table 13.1) inhibit two different isoforms of the enzyme cyclo-oxygenase : COX–1 and COX–2. Selective inhibitors of the enzyme COX-2 may have similar analgesic efficacy but fewer side effects.

Transdermal use of smooth muscle relaxant glyceryl trinitrate is also used currently.

The suitable cases are — comparatively young age and having contraindications to 'pill'. The contraindications of its use include allergy to aspirin, gastric ulceration and history of asthma.

Oral contraceptive pills **:** The suitable candidates are patients — (i) wanting contraceptive precaution, (ii) with heavy periods and (iii) unresponsive or contraindications to anti-prostaglandin drugs. The pill should be used for 3-6 cycles.

Dydrogesterone — It does not inhibit ovulation but probably interferes with ovarian steroidogenesis.

The drug should be taken from day 5 of a cycle for 20 days. It should be continued for 3-6 cycles.

If the above protocol fails, laparoscopy is indicated to find out any pelvic pathology to account for pain, the important one being endometriosis.

Surgery

Dilatation of the cervical canal — Dilatation should be slow and gradual until the resistance of the internal os is overcome. It should be done under general anaesthesia. Sufficient dilatation with 6/9 Hegar is required. Curettage is unnecessary; may be of help if associated with menstrual abnormality or in membranous dysmenorrhoea (later in the chapter). **Late sequela may be cervical incompetence.**

Cervical dilatation relieves pain by — (i) stretching of the fibromuscular tissues at the level of internal os → loss of tone and (ii) by causing injury to the sensory nerve endings → cut down the pain pathway.

Bilateral block of the pelvic plexus — Paracervical block with alcohol may be carried out along with dilatation of the cervix to improve the result. It may be employed as a therapeutic test before a major operation like presacral neurectomy is undertaken.

Presacral neurectomy (Laparoscopic) — The objective is to cut down the sensory pathway (via T_{11}-L_2) from the uterus. It also increases the uterine blood supply. Presacral neurectomy is not helpful for adnexal pain (T_9-T_{10}) that is carried by the thoracic autonomic nerves along the ovarian vessels. On theoretical basis, it can only be done in a patient when all the measures fail. As such, its indication in true dysmenorrhoea is questionable.

SECONDARY DYSMENORRHOEA (Congestive)

Secondary dysmenorrhoea is normally considered to be menstruation — associated pain occurring in the presence of pelvic pathology.

Causes of pain

The pain may be related to increasing tension in the pelvic tissues due to premenstrual pelvic congestion or increased vascularity in the pelvic organs.

Common causes of secondary dysmenorrhoea: Chronic pelvic infection, pelvic endometriosis, pelvic adhesions, adenomyosis, uterine fibroid, endometrial polyp, IUCD *in utero* and pelvic congestion.

Patient profile

The patients are usually in thirties; more often parous and unrelated to any social status.

Clinical features

The pain is dull, situated in the back and in front without any radiation. It usually appears 3-5 days prior to the period and relieves with the start of bleeding. The onset and duration of pain depends on the pathology producing the pain. There is no systemic discomfort unlike primary dysmenorrhoea. The patients may have got some discomfort even in between periods. There are symptoms of associated pelvic pathology.

Abdominal and vaginal examinations usually reveal the offending lesion. At times, the lesion is revealed by laparotomy or laparoscopy.

Treatment

The treatment aims at the cause rather than the symptom. The type of treatment depends on the severity, age and parity of the patient.

MEMBRANOUS DYSMENORRHOEA

This is one variety of primary dysmenorrhoea but is rare. There is shedding of big endometrial casts during period. **It is probably due** to the deficiency in the tryptic ferment normally secreted in the endometrium. The treatment is the same as that for primary dysmenorrhoea. But the success rate is very low. It is not relieved even following pregnancy.

OVARIAN DYSMENORRHOEA

This clinical entity was first described by O'Donel Browne. The pain usually appears 2-3 days before menstruation. The pain is continuous and dull and is distributed to either one or both quadrants innervated by T_{10} to L_1 segments. The pain is ascribed to ovarian nerve degeneration or sclerocystic condition of the ovary. In obstinate cases, division of the infundibulopelvic ligament carrying ovarian sympathetic nerves is prescribed.

Right ovarian vein syndrome

Right ovarian vein crosses the ureter at right angle. During premenstrual period, due to pelvic congestion or increased blood flow, there may be marked engorgement in the vein → pressure on ureter → stasis → infection → pyelonephritis → pain.

Table 13.2
Causes of unilateral pain during period (Dysmenorrhoea)

- Ovarian dysmenorrhoea
- Bicornuate uterus
- Unilateral location of pelvic endometriosis
- Small fibroid polyp near one cornu
- Right ovarian vein syndrome
- Colonic or caecal spasm

MITTELSCHMERZ'S SYNDROME (Ovular pain)

Ovular pain is not an infrequent complaint. It appears in the midmenstrual period. The pain usually situated in the hypogastrium or to one iliac fossa. The pain is usually located on one side and does not change from side to side according to which ovary is ovulating. Nausea or vomiting is conspicuously absent. It rarely lasts more than 12 hours. It may be associated with slight vaginal bleeding or excessive mucoid vaginal discharge.

The exact cause is not known. **The probable factors are** — (i) increased tension of the Graafian follicle just prior to rupture, (ii) peritoneal irritation by the follicular fluid following ovulation and (iii) contraction of the tubes and uterus.

Treatment is effective with assurance and analgesics. In obstinate cases, the cure is absolute by making the cycle anovular with contraceptive pills.

PELVIC CONGESTION SYNDROME

There is disturbance in the autonomic nervous system which may lead to gross vascular congestion with pelvic varicosities. The patient has a congestive type of dysmenorrhoea without any demonstrable pelvic pathology.

The patient complains of vague disorders with backache and pelvic pain, at times with dyspareunia. There may be menorrhagia or epimenorrhoea. The uterus may feel bulky and boggy.

The treatment in unsatisfactory. Medroxy progesterone acetate (MPA) 50 mg daily for 4 months was found effective. In parous women with advancing age, hysterectomy may relieve the symptoms.

PREMENSTRUAL SYNDROME (PMS) (Syn : Premenstrual tension)

Premenstrual syndrome (PMS) is a psychoneuroendocrine disorder of unknown aetiology, often noticed just prior to menstruation. There is cyclic appearance of a large number of symptoms during the last 7-10 days of the menstrual cycle. **It should fulfil the following criteria :**

- Not related to any organic lesion.
- Regularly occurs during the luteal phase of each ovulatory menstrual cycle.
- Symptoms must be severe enough to disturb the life style of the woman or she requires medical help.
- Symptom-free period during rest of the cycle.

When these symptoms disrupt daily functioning they are grouped under the name **premenstrual dysphoric disorder (PMDD).**

Pathophysiology

The exact cause is not known but the **following hypotheses are postulated** :

(a) Alteration in the level of oestrogen and progesterone starting from the midluteal phase. Either there is altered oestrogen : progesterone ratio or diminished progesterone level.

(b) Neuroendocrine factors :

- **Serotonin** is an important neurotransmitter in the CNS. During the luteal phase, decreased synthesis of serotonin is observed in women suffering from PMS.
- **Endorphins** — The symptom complex of PMS is thought to be due to the withdrawal of endorphins (neurotransmitters) from CNS (see ch. 7) during the luteal phase.
- **γ-aminobutyric acid (GABA)** suppresses the anxiety level in the brain. Medications that are GABA agonist, are effective.

(c) Psychological and psychosocial factors may be involved to produce behavioural changes.

(d) Others — Variety of factors have been mentioned to explain the symptom complex of PMS. These are thyrotrophin releasing hormone (TRH) prolactin, renin, aldosterone, prostaglandins and others. Unfortunately nothing is conclusive.

Clinical features

PMS is more common in women aged 30-45. It may be related to childbirth or a disturbing life event.

Table 13.3
Symptomatology of PMS and PMDD

Related to water retention	• Abdominal bloating • Breast tenderness • Swelling of the extremities • Weight gain	
Neuropsychiatric symptoms	• Irritability • Depression • Mood swings • Forgetfulness • Restlessness • Increased appetite	• Tearfulness • Anxiety • Tension • Confusion • Headache
Behavioural symptoms	• Fatigue • Dyspareunia	• Tiredness

There is no abnormal pelvic findings excepting features of pelvic congestion.

CONFIRMATION OF DIAGNOSIS

If, by administering GnRH analogue, goserelin 3.6 mg in the form of depot at monthly intervals for 3 such, the symptoms are relieved along with amenorrhoea, the case is considered to be PMS.

TREATMENT

As the aetiology is multifactorial and too often obscure, various drugs are used either on speculation or empirically with varying degrees of success.

General

Nonpharmacological : (a) Assurance, Yoga, Stress management, Diet manipulation. (b) Avoidance of salt, caffeine and alcohol specially in second half of cycle improves the symptoms.

Nonhormonal :

(a) Tranquillizers or antidepressant drugs, may be of help logically.

(b) Pyridoxine – 100 mg twice daily is helpful by correcting tryptophan metabolism specially following 'pill' associated depression.

(c) Diuretics in the second half of the cycle – Frusemide 20 mg daily for consecutive 5 days a week reduces fluid retention.

(d) Alprazolam – 0.25 mg twice daily during the luteal phase improves the anxiety and depression symptoms.

(e) **Selective Serotonin Reuptake Inhibitors (SSRI)** are found to be very effective.

Fluoxetine is an antidepressant that inhibits neuronal uptake of serotonin. A single oral dose of 20 mg was found to improve the psychiatric and behavioural symptoms significantly.

The drugs are usually prescribed at least two days prior to the onset of symptoms and to be continued till menstruation starts.

Hormones

Any one of the following drugs is to be prescribed:

Oral contraceptive pills — The idea is to suppress ovulation and to maintain an uniform hormonal milieu. The therapy is to be continued for 3-6 cycles.

Progestogen — Dydrogesterone 10 mg daily or twice daily from 5th day of cycle for 20 days is of help on the presumption that progesterone deficiency is the cause. The therapy is to be repeated for 3-6 cycles. Levonorgestrel intrauterine system (IUS) is also used to suppress ovarian cycle.

Bromocriptine — 2.5 mg daily or twice daily may be helpful, at least to relieve the breast complaints.

Suppression of ovarian cycle — Suppression of the endogenous ovarian cycle can be achieved by :

- Danazol 200-400 mg daily is to be adjusted so as to produce amenorrhoea. Barrier method of contraception should be advised during the treatment.
- **GnRH analogues** **(p. 500)** — The gonadal steroids are suppressed by administration of GnRH agonist for 6 months (medical oophorectomy). GnRH analogues in PMS are used (i) to assess the role of ovarian steroids in the aetiology of PMS. (ii) This can also predict whether bilateral oophorectomy would be of any help or not. The preparations and doses used are as given :
  – Goserelin (Zoladex) 3.6 mg is given subcutaneously at every 4 weeks.
  – Leuprorelin acetate (Prostap) : 3.75 mg is given by SC or IM at every 4 weeks.
  – Triptorelin (Decapeptyl):3 mg is given IM every four weeks.

– Buserelin (Suprefact) : 200-500 μg daily SC or intranasally 300 μg (150 μg spray in each nostril) 3 times daily for 6 months.

Results of GnRH agonist therapy are dramatic.

GnRH agonist therapy is combined with oestrogen progestin "add-back" (see p. 502) to combat the hypoestrogenic symptoms.

- Oophorectomy.

In established cases of primary PMS with recurrence of symptoms and approaching to menopause, hysterectomy with bilateral oophorectomy is a last resort.

KEY POINTS

- Dysmenorrhoea is painful menstruation of sufficient magnitude so as to incapacitate the day-to-day activities. The incidence of primary dysmenorrhoea is about 10-15 per cent.

  Primary dysmenorrhoea is almost always confined to ovulatory cycle and relieved following pregnancy and vaginal delivery. The pain usually appears following painless periods after menarche.

  While primary dysmenorrhoea occurs before the age of 20, secondary dysmenorrhoea may occur at any age.

  Prostaglandin synthetase inhibitors (NSAIDs) or oral contraceptives or dydrogesterone are usually effective to minimise pain. Only cervical dilatation is required in obstinate cases. Secondary dysmenorrhoea is almost always secondary to other pelvic pathology such as PID, endometriosis or uterine polyps.

- Combined oral contraceptives reduce the severity of dysmenorrhoea. It is the drug of choice when contraception is required.

- In ovarian dysmenorrhoea, the pain is referred to the area innervated by T_{10} to L_1 segments.

- Right ovarian vein syndrome is due to engorgement of right ovarian vein premenstrually so as to compress the right ureter with resultant pyelonephritis and pain.

  Pain due to pelvic venous congestion is relieved by continuous high dose MPA.

- Mittelschmerz's syndrome (ovular pain) — is an indirect evidence of ovulation — occurring in the midmenstrual period.

- Premenstrual syndrome (PMS) regularly occurs in the luteal phase of each ovulatory menstrual cycle.

  There is no impairment of corpus luteal function for a woman who suffers from PMS.

  Exact aetiology is unknown. Altered oestrogen : progesterone ratio; reduced circulatory level of neurotransmitters (serotonin, GABA or endorphins) in the CNS may be responsible for the symptom complex.

  The symptoms are not specific (Table 13.3) and there is usually no abnormal pelvic finding.

  The most useful diagnostic tool for PMS is patient's symptom diary (Table 13.3).

  Treatment is supportive. In obstinate cases, hormones — 'pill', dydrogesterone, danazol are found helpful. Results of GnRH agonist therapy are dramatic. Tranquillizers (alprazolam – 0.25 mg) and/or antidepressants (fluoxetine 20 mg daily) significantly improve the symptoms.

  In proved cases — relief of symptoms with amenorrhoea either by danazol or GnRH analogues for 3 months; hysterectomy with bilateral salpingo-oophorectomy in patients approaching menopause is justified.

  Of the measures used in the management of PMS beneficial effects are observed with selective serotonin reuptake inhibitors (SSRI). Oral contraceptive pills suppressing ovulation. Bromocriptine (breast symptoms only) Vitamin B6 and GnRh analogues.

Abnormal Uterine Bleeding

14

MENORRHAGIA
(Syn : Hypermenorrhoea)

Definition

Menorrhagia is defined as cyclic bleeding at normal intervals; the bleeding is either excessive in amount (> 80 ml) or duration or both. The term menotaxis is often used to denote prolonged bleeding.

Causes

Menorrhagia is a symptom of some underlying pathology — organic or functional.

- **Organic**

Pelvic : The causes are tabulated in Table 14.1& 14.2.

Table 14.1
Pelvic pathology

Due to congestion, increased surface area or hyperplasia of the endometrium.

- Fibroid uterus
- Adenomyosis
- Pelvic endometriosis
- IUCD *inutero*
- Chronic tubo-ovarian mass
- Tubercular endometritis (early cases)
- Retroverted uterus — due to congestion
- Granulosa cell tumour of the ovary

Systemic — Liver dysfunction — failure to conjugate and thereby inactivates the oestrogens.

- Congestive cardiac failure
- Severe hypertension

Endocrinal

- Hypothyroidism • Hyperthyroidism

Blood dyscrasias

- Idiopathic thrombocytopenic purpura
- Leukaemia • von Willebrand's disease

Emotional upset

- **Functional**

Due to disturbed hypothalamo-pituitary-ovarian-endometrial axis.

Table 14.2
Common causes of menorrhagia

- Dysfunctional uterine bleeding • Fibroid uterus
- Adenomyosis
- Chronic tubo-ovarian mass

Diagnosis

Long duration of flow, passage of big clots, use of increased number of thick sanitary pads, pallor and low level of haemoglobin give an idea about the correct diagnosis and magnitude of menorrhagia.

Treatment

The definitive treatment is appropriate to the cause for menorrhagia.

POLYMENORRHOEA
(Syn : Epimenorrhoea)

Definition

Polymenorrhoea is defined as cyclic bleeding where the cycle is reduced to an arbitrary limit of less than 21 days and remains constant at that frequency. If the frequent cycle is associated with excessive and or prolonged bleeding, it is called epimenorrhagia.

Causes

Dysfunctional — It is seen predominantly during adolescence, preceding menopause and following delivery and abortion. Hyperstimulation of the ovary by the pituitary hormones may be the responsible factor.

Ovarian hyperaemia as in PID or ovarian endometriosis.

Treatment

Persistent dysfunctional type is to be treated by hormone as outlined in DUB (later in chapter).

METRORRHAGIA

Definition

Metrorrhagia is defined as irregular, acyclic bleeding from the uterus. Amount of bleeding is variable. While metrorrhagia strictly concerns uterine bleeding but in clinical practice, the bleeding from any part of the genital tract is included under the heading. Then again, irregular bleeding in the form of contact bleeding (Table 14.4) or intermenstrual bleeding (Tables 14.3 and 14.5) in an otherwise normal cycle is also included in metrorrhagia. In fact, it is mostly related to surface lesion in the uterus (Fig. 14.1).

Menometrorrhagia is the term applied when the bleeding is so irregular and excessive that the menses (periods) cannot be identified at all.

Table 14.3
Causes of acyclic bleeding

- DUB — usually during adolescence, following childbirth and abortion and preceding menopause
- Submucous fibroid
- Uterine polyp
- Carcinoma cervix and endometrial carcinoma

Table 14.4
Causes of contact bleeding

- Carcinoma cervix
- Mucous polyp of cervix
- Vascular ectopy of the cervix specially during pregnancy, pill use cervix
- Infections — chlamydial or tubercular cervicitis.
- Cervical endometriosis

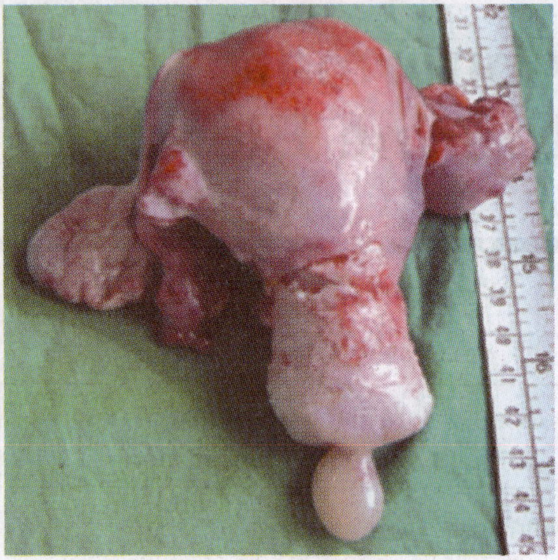

Fig. 14.1. Metrorrhagia due to cervical polyp

Table 14.5
Causes of intermenstrual bleeding

Apart from the causes of contact bleeding, other causes are :

- Urethral caruncle
- Ovular bleeding
- Breakthrough bleeding in pill use
- IUCD *in utero*
- Decubitus ulcer

Treatment

Treatment is directed to the underlying pathology.

Malignancy is to be excluded prior to any definitive treatment.

OLIGOMENORRHOEA

Definition : Menstrual bleeding occurring **more than 35 days** apart and which remains constant at that frequency is called oligomenorrhoea. Causes are mentioned in Table 14.6.

Table 14.6
Common causes of oligomenorrhoea

- Age-related—during adolescence and preceeding menopause

Table 14.6 contd. from previous page

- Weight-related – obesity (see p. 546)
- Stress and exercise related – (see p. 444)
- Endocrine disorders — PCOS (commonest), hyperprolactinaemia, hyperthyroidism (see p.440)
- Androgen producing tumours — ovarian, adrenal (see p. 371)
- Tubercular endometritis – late cases (see p. 136)

HYPOMENORRHOEA

Definition

When the menstrual bleeding is unduly scanty and lasts for less than 2 days, it is called hypomenorrhoea.

Causes

The causes may be local (uterine synechiae or endometrial tuberculosis), endocrinal (use of oral contraceptives, thyroid dysfunction and premenopausal period) or systemic (malnutrition).

DYSFUNCTIONAL UTERINE BLEEDING (DUB)

Definition

DUB is defined as **a state of abnormal uterine bleeding without any clinically detectable organic, systemic and iatrogenic cause. [Pelvic pathology e.g. tumour, inflammation or pregnancy is excluded.]**

Incidence

The prevalence varies widely but an incidence of 10 per cent amongst new patients attending the out-patient seems logical. The bleeding may be abnormal in frequency, amount or duration or combination of any three. As the diagnosis is based with the exclusion of 'organic lesion', so with the care and facilities to exclude such a lesion, the incidence varies. *Currently many authors define DUB as a state of abnormal uterine bleeding following anovulation due to dysfunction of hypothalamo-pituitary-ovarian axis.*

Pathophysiology

The current concept concludes that the abnormal bleeding is most likely due to local causes in the endometrium. There is some disturbance of the endometrial blood vessels and capillaries and coagulation of blood in and around these vessels. These are probably related to alteration in the ratio of endometrial prostaglandins which are delicately balanced in haemostasis of menstruation.

The endometrial abnormalities may be *primary or secondary* to **incoordination in the hypothalamo-pituitary-ovarian axis**. It is thus *more prevalent in extremes of reproductive period* — adolescence and premenopause or following childbirth and abortion.

Emotional influences, worries, anxieties or sexual problems sometimes are enough to disturb the normal hormonal balance.

The abnormal bleeding may be associated with or without ovulation and accordingly grouped into :

- **Ovular bleeding**
- **Anovular bleeding**

Ovular bleeding

Polymenorrhoea or polymenorrhagia

The condition usually occurs following childbirth and abortion, during adolescence and premenopausal period and in pelvic inflammatory disease.

The follicular development is speeded up with resulting shortening of the follicular phase. This is probably due to hyperstimulation of the follicular growth by FSH. Rarely, the luteal phase may be shortened due to premature lysis of the corpus luteum. Sometimes, it is related to stress induced stimulation.

Endometrial study prior to or within few hours of menstruation reveals secretory changes.

Oligomenorrhoea

Primary ovular oligomenorrhoea is rare. It may be met in adolescence and preceding menopause.

The disturbance may be due to ovarian unresponsiveness to FSH or secondary to pituitary dysfunction. There is undue prolongation of the proliferative phase with normal secretory phase.

Endometrial study prior to or within few hours of menstruation reveals secretory changes.

Functional menorrhagia

Ovular menorrhagia is quite uncommon. Two varieties are found :

- Irregular shedding of the endometrium.
- Irregular ripening of the endometrium.

Irregular shedding of the endometrium

The abnormality is usually met in extremes of reproductive period.

Normally, regeneration of the endometrium is completed by the end of third day of menstruation. In irregular shedding, desquamation is continued for a variable period with simultaneous failure of regeneration of the endometrium. **The possible explanations are**:

(i) Incomplete withdrawal of LH even on 26th day of cycle → incomplete atrophy of the corpus luteum → persistent secretion of progesterone.

(ii) Persistent LH → inhibition of FSH → suppresses ripening of the follicle in the next cycle → less oestrogen → less regeneration.

(iii) Variation of the endometrial receptors which are sensitive to the influence of oestrogen and progesterone.

Endometrial sampling performed after 5th or 6th day of the onset of menstruation reveals a mixture of secretory and proliferative endometrium. There is total absence of any surface epithelium.

Pregnanediol is found in the urine during menstrual phase.

Irregular ripening of the endometrium

There is poor formation and inadequate function of the corpus luteum. Secretion of both oestrogen and progesterone is inadequate to support the endometrial growth. As such, slight bleeding occurs and continues prior to the start of proper flow.

The endocrine profile in the luteal phase shows persistent low level of urinary pregnanediol level of less than 3 mg or plasma progesterone level less than 5 ng/ml.

Endometrial study prior to or soon after spotting reveals patchy area of secretory changes amidst proliferative endometrium.

Anovular bleeding

Menorrhagia

Anovular bleeding is usually excessive. In the absence of growth limiting progesterone due to anovulation, the endometrial growth is under the influence of oestrogen throughout the cycle. There is inadequate structural stromal support and the endometrium remains fragile.

Thus, with the withdrawal of oestrogen due to negative feedback action of FSH, the endometrial shedding continues for a longer period in asynchronous sequences because of lack of compactness.

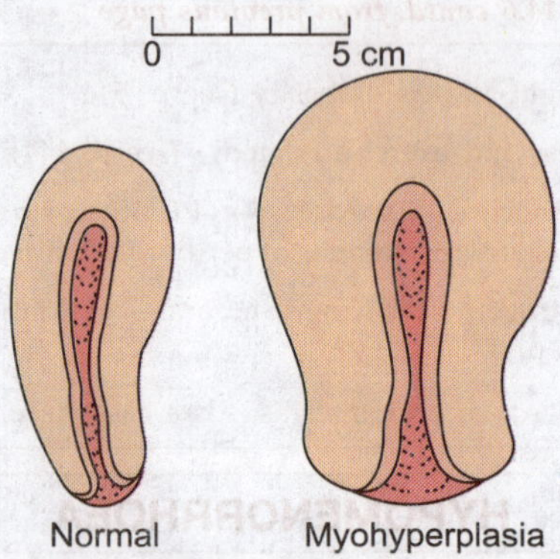

Fig. 14.2. Increased uterine size with myohyperplasia

Cystic glandular hyperplasia (*Syn : Metropathia haemorrhagica, Schroeder's disease*)

This type of abnormal bleeding is usually met in premenopausal women.

The basic fault may lie in the ovaries or may be due to disturbance of the rhythmic secretion of the gonadotrophins. There is slow increase in secretion of oestrogen but no negative feedback inhibition of FSH. The net effect is gradual rise in the level of oestrogen with concomittant phase of amenorrhoea for about 6-8 weeks. As there is no ovulation, the endometrium is under the influence of oestrogen without being opposed by growth limiting progesterone for a prolonged period. After a variable period, however, the oestrogen level falls resulting in endometrial shedding with heavy bleeding. Bleeding also occurs when the endometrial growth have outgrown their blood supply. Due to increased endometrial thickness, tissue breakdown continues for a long time. Bleeding is heavy as there is no vasoconstrictor effect of $PGF_2\alpha$. Bleeding is prolonged until the endometrium and blood vessels regenerate to control it.

Changes in the uterus

There is variable degree of myohyperplasia with symmetrical enlargement of the uterus to a size of about 8-10 weeks due to simultaneous hypertrophy of muscles (Fig. 14.2). The endometrial changes are classical. On naked eye examination, the endometrium looks thick, congested and often polypoidal (multiple polyposis).

Microscopically

(a) There is marked hyperplasia of all the endome-

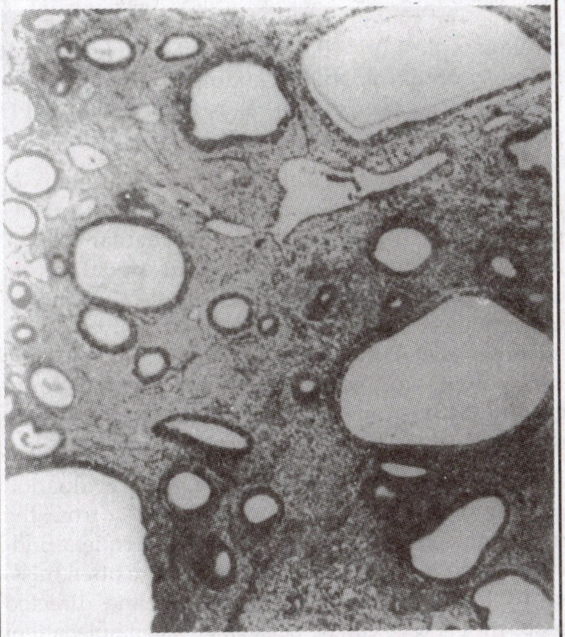

Fig. 14.3. Endometrium showing 'Swiss cheese' appearance

trial components. There is however, intense cystic glandular hypertrophy rather than hyperplasia with marked disparity in sizes. Some of the glands are small, others are large giving the appearance of "Swiss cheese" pattern (small and large holes of Swiss cheese made in Switzerland). The glands are empty and lined by columnar epithelium.

(b) Absence of secretory changes.

(c) Areas of necrosis in the superficial layers with small haemorrhages and leucocytic infiltration (Fig. 14.3).

Changes in the ovary

Cystic changes may be observed involving one or both the ovaries. The cyst may be single or multiple and the fluid contains oestrogen. The cyst is of follicular type. There is no evidence of corpus luteum.

Confusion in diagnosis

Phase of amenorrhoea followed by continued bleeding per vaginam with bulky uterus is too often confused with disturbed uterine pregnancy or ectopic gestation. **DUB of this type is absolutely painless.**

Atrophy of the endometrium

This type of abnormality is commonly met in postmenopausal women but may occur in reproductive period as final involutionary state of a previous metropathia.

The bleeding occurs from the rupture of the dilated capillaries beneath the atrophic surface epithelium. **The cause of endometrial atrophy** may be due to total absence of oestrogen or failure of uterine receptors to become responsive to oestrogen.

Endometrial pattern in DUB

The following are the histological patterns found in DUB. In majority (60 %), the endometrium is normal secretory in every aspect. In about 30 per cent, the endometrium is hyperplastic and in the remaining, there are evidences of irregular shedding, irregular ripening or atrophic pattern.

Investigations

The investigation aims at:

- To confirm the menstrual abnormality as stated by the patient.
- To exclude the 'organic' pelvic pathology.
- To identify the possible aetiology of DUB.
- To work out the definite therapy protocol.

History

Firstly, it is to be confirmed that the bleeding is through the vagina and not from the urethra or rectum. **The statement of excessive bleeding is assessed by** number of pads used, passage of clots (size and number) and duration of bleeding. If ambiguity is found from the estimated haemoglobin percentage, it is better to assess the blood loss by admitting the patient during period. Among the patients presenting with menorrhagia, only about 50 per cent have got excess blood loss (> 80 ml).

Nature of menstrual abnormality is then to be enquired — cyclic or acyclic, its relation to puberty, pregnancy events and last normal cycle. If there is wrong interpretation of the cycle duration and there is no urgency of any therapy, it is better to explain her to keep the menstrual records for 2-3 cycles. Not only does it help in diagnosis but spontaneous cure may occur on occasion.

Any emotional upset or psychosexual problem should be elicited tactfully. Use of steroidal contraceptives or IUCD insertion should be enquired. History of abnormal bleeding from the injury site, epistaxis, gum bleeding or that suggestive of PID should be enquired.

A thorough general and relevant systemic examination is to be made in an effort to find out the cause or effect of abnormal bleeding. In a suspected case of thrombocytopenic purpura, tourniquet test is performed.

Internal examination

Bimanual examination including speculum examination should be done in all cases except in virgins where rectal examination is to be done to exclude palpable pelvic pathology. If vaginal examination is required in virgins, it should be done under general anaesthesia and along with endometrial curettage.

Special investigations

• **Blood values** — Haemoglobin estimation is done in every case. In pubertal menorrhagia not responding to usual therapy, platelet count, prothrombin time, bleeding time, partial thromboplastin time are to be estimated. In suspected cases of thyroid dysfunction, serum TSH, T_3, T_4 estimation is to be done.

• ***Diagnostic uterine curettage (D & C)***

Diagnostic uterine curettage is indicated in DUB — (1) To exclude the **organic lesions in the endometrium** (incomplete abortion, endometrial polyp, tubercular endometritis or endometrial carcinoma). (2) To determine the functional state of the endometrium. (3) To have incidental therapeutic benefit.

In adolescent DUB, it should be done if bleeding fails to stop or is severe in nature (see p. 52).

During childbearing period (20-40 years), it should be done, **if the bleeding is acyclic. Risk of endometrial carcinoma in this age group is very low. During premenopausal period,** diagnostic curettage is **mandatory** prior to any therapy to exclude endometrial malignancy. **During postmenopausal period,** it is **mandatory** to exclude endometrial malignancy. Thin plastic endometrial tissue samplers (pipellae) are available (Fig. 9.23). It helps to obtain adequate endometrial sample for histological examination. It is done as an OPD procedure without any anaesthetic.

• **Ultrasound and colour Doppler** findings of endometrial hyperplasia are : (i) Endometrial thickness > 12 mm. (ii) Hyperechoic and regular outline. (iii) Angiogenesis and neovascular signal study. **Transvaginal sonography (TVS)** is also very sensitive to detect any anatomical abnormality (fibroid, adenomyosis) of the uterus, endometrium (endometrial polyps) and adnexae. **Saline Infusion Sonography (SIS)** is found very sensitive (p. 114) for the diagnosis of uterine pathology (polyps).

• **Hysteroscopy** — is done for better evaluation of endometrial lesion and to take biopsy from the offending site under direct vision. The frequent findings of polyp and submucous fibroid are often missed by blind curettage. Hysteroscopy and directed biopsy (H and B) can be performed as an out-patient basis. In many centres (H and B) has replaced conventional D and C (for details see p. 118).

• **Laparoscopy** — to exclude unsuspected pelvic pathology such as endometriosis, PID or ovarian tumour (granulosa cell tumour). The indication is urgent, if associated with pelvic pain.

• **Hysterography** — to exclude fibroid polyp or congenital malformation of uterus. Because of reduced specificity, HSG is mostly replaced by hysteroscopy (where facilities available).

Plan of special investigations

Blood values ⟶ ultrasonography ⟶ diagnostic uterine curettage/endometrial sampling (pipelle) ⟶ hysteroscopy/hysterography ⟶ laparoscopy.

MANAGEMENT

Because of diverse aetiopathology of DUB in

Time schedule for uterine curettage

Cyclic	• Menorrhagia • Irregular shedding • Irregular ripening	5-6 days prior to period 5-6 days after the period starts Soon after the period starts
Acyclic	—	Soon after the period starts
Continuous	—	Any time

different phases of woman's life, the management protocols have been grouped accordingly.

- Pubertal and adolescent menorrhagia < 20 years (see p. 52).
- Reproductive period (20-40 years).
- Premenopausal (> 40 years).
- Postmenopausal (see p. 532).

Reproductive period

- **General** • **Medical** • **Surgery**

General

Rest is advised during bleeding phase. Assurance and sympathetic handling are helpful particularly in adolescents. Anaemia should be corrected energetically by diet, haematinics and even by blood transfusion. Clinically evident systemic or endocrinal abnormalities should be investigated and treated accordingly.

MEDICAL MANAGEMENT OF DUB

Dysfunctional uterine bleeding (DUB), in majority responds well to conservative treatment during adolescence and early reproductive period. The derivatives of drugs used are listed in the Table 14.7.

Hormones : With the introduction of potent **orally active progestins, they became the mainstay in the management of DUB in all age groups** and practically replaced the isolated use of oestrogens and androgens.

Progestins : The common preparations used are norethisterone acetate and medroxyprogesterone acetate (Table 14.7). The latter one is better than the former as it does not alter the serum lipids. **Mechanism of antioestrogenic action of progestins are** : (i) It stimulates the enzyme (17-β-hydroxy steroid dehydrogenase) that converts oestradiol to oestrone (less potent). (ii) Inhibits induction of oestrogen receptor. (iii) It has antimitotic effect on the endometrium. While isolated progestins therapy is highly effective in anovular DUB in ovular DUB, combined preparations of progestogen and oestrogen (combined oral pills) are effective.

The preparations are used :

- Cyclic therapy • Continuous therapy

To stop bleeding and regulate the cycle :

Norethisterone preparations (5 mg tab) are used thrice daily till bleeding stops which it usually does by 3-7 days.

Table 14.7
Medical management of DUB

(A) Hormones (see p. 499)
• Norethisterone acetate (p. 509)
• Medroxyprogesterone acetate
• Dydrogesterone
• Equine conjugated oestrogen
• Combined oestrogens and progestogens (Contraceptive pills)
• 19 Norsteroid derivative (Gestrinone)
• Danazol (17 α-ethinyl testosterone)
• Progestin releasing IUCD LNG – IUS (p. 459)
• Mifepristone (RU 486) (p. 511)
• GnRH analogues (p. 500)
• Desmopressin
(B) Prostaglandin synthetase inhibitors (PSI)
• Fenamates (Mefenamic acid)
(C) Antifibrinolytic agents
• Tranexamic acid (TA)
• Ethamsylate
• Epsilon amino caproic acid (EACA)
For side effects of each drug used — see chapter 31

Cyclic therapy

- 5th to 25th day course.
- 15th to 25th day course.

5th to 25th day course :

In ovular bleeding — **Any low dose combined oral pills are effective** when given from 5th to 25th day of cycle for 3 consecutive cycles. It causes endometrial atrophy. Normal menstruation is expected to resume with restoration of normally functionating pituitary–ovarian-endometrial axis. It reduces menstrual blood loss by 50 per cent. It serves as a contraceptive as well.

In anovular bleeding — Cyclic progestogen preparation of medroxyprogesterone acetate (MPA) 10 mg or norethisterone 5 mg is used from 5th to 25th day of cycle for 3 cycles.

15th to 25th day course :

In ovular bleeding, where the patient wants pregnancy or in cases of irregular shedding or irregular ripening of the endometrium, dydrogesterone 1 tab (10 mg) daily or twice a day from 15th to 25th day may cure the state. This regimen is however, less effective than 5th to 25th day course. However, it does not suppress ovulation.

Continuous progestins : Synthetic progestins are widely used to treat menorrhagia. They counteract the effect of oestrogen, suppress the endometrium and the stroma is decidualised. Progestins also inhibit pituitary gonadotropin secretion and ovarian hormone production. Medroxyprogesterone acetate 10 mg thrice daily is given and treatment is usually continued for at least for 90 days.

Various continuous preparations may be used. Oral (Table 14.7), long-acting intramuscular injections, implants (p. 470), Progestogen only pill (p. 470) are effective to reduce menstrual blood loss. They may also result in oligomenorrhoea or amenorrhoea.

Oestrogen : In situations where the bleeding is acute and severe, conjugated oestrogen 25 mg is given IV. It may be repeated every four hours till the bleeding is controlled, when oral therapy is started. Haemostasis is achieved by conjugated equine oestrogen 2.5 mg tablet given 4 times a day. The bleeding usually stops within 2-3 days. In this situation oestrogen stimulates regeneration of the denuded endometrium and controls bleeding by process of healing. Proliferation of endometrium, increase in the level of fibrinogen, factors – V, X and platelet aggregation are the other mechanisms of action for oestrogen therapy. If bleeding continues further, D and C is indicated.

Intrauterine progestogen — Levonorgestrel intrauterine system (LNG IUS) induce endometrial glandular atrophy, stromal decidualisation and endometrial cell inactivation (see p. 459). It is effective for 5 years. It has minimal systemic absorption. Reduction of blood loss is upto 97 per cent. Results are comparable to TCRE (p. 189). It is considered as medical hysterectomy. In addition to its many other health benefits it is an effective contraceptive measure (p. 463).

Depot progestin preparations — have also been used to control excess menstrual blood loss. Depot medroxyprogesterone acetate (DMPA) may cause amenorrhoea (see p. 470).

Danazol : Danazol is suitable in cases with recurrent symptoms and in patients waiting for hysterectomy. The dose varies from 200-400 mg daily in 4 divided doses continuously for 3 months. A smaller dose tends to minimise the blood loss and a higher dose produces amenorrhoea (see p. 504).

Gestrinone : Gestrinone 2.5 mg orally twice a week for 3 months has been found useful (see p. 504).

Mifepristone (RU 486) : It is an anti-progesterone (19 nor steroid). It inhibits ovulation and induces amenorrhoea and reduces myoma size (p. 511).

GnRH agonists (see p. 500) : The subtherapeutic doses reduce the blood loss whereas in therapeutic doses produce amenorrhoea. It is valuable as short-term use in severe DUB, particularly if the woman is infertile and wants pregnancy. The drugs are used subcutaneously or intranasally. It improves anaemia, and is helpful when used before endometrial ablation (see below). A varying degree of hypo-oestrogenic features may appear.

NON-HORMONAL MANAGEMENT

Anti-fibrinolytic agents (Tranexamic acid) reduces menstrual blood loss by 50 per cent. It counteracts the endometrial fibrinolytic system. It is particularly helpful in IUCD induced menorrhagia. Gastrointestinal side effects are common. Antifibrinolytic agents can be used as a first line therapy.

Ethamsylate reduces endometrial capillary fragility. Results are often inconsistant.

Prostaglandin synthetase inhibitors : Mefenamic acid is much effective in women aged more than 35 years and in cases of ovulatory DUB. The dose is 150-600 mg orally in divided doses during the bleeding phase. The fenamates inhibit the synthesis of prostaglandins and interfere with the binding of PGE_2 to its receptor. NSAIDS can reduce menstrual blood loss by 25-40 per cent. Improvement of dysmenorrhoea headache, or nausea are the added benefits. Side effects (p. 176) are often mild. NSAIDS may be used as first line medical treatment.

Desmopressin — is a synthetic analogue of arginine — vasopressin. It is specially indicated in cases with von Willebrand's disease and factor VIII deficiency. It is given IV (0.3 μg/kg) or intranasally.

SURGICAL MANAGEMENT OF DUB

- Uterine curettage.
- Endometrial ablation/resection.
- Hysterectomy.

Uterine curettage

It is done predominantly as a **diagnostic tool but at times, it has got haemostatic and therapeutic effect by removing the necrosed and unhealthy endometrium.** It is hopefully expected that the normal relation of hypothalamo-pituitary-ovarian-endometrial axis is re-established by the time the regeneration of the endometrium occurs. **The indication is an urgent one, if the bleeding is acyclic and where endometrial pathology is suspected.**

Endometrial ablation/resection (see p. 589)

Indications are : (i) Women who have failed to respond to medical treatment (ii) Where hysterectomy is risky or the patient is unfit for longer duration surgery or because of obesity or adhesion (iii) When the patient prefers to preserve her uterus.

• **Laser ablation** of the endometrium using the Nd : YAG laser through hysteroscope is an alternative to hysterectomy. It is employed as an elective alternative to hysterectomy or when hysterectomy has been medically contraindicated. Tissue destruction (coagulation, vaporisation and carbonisation) to a **depth of 4-5 mm produces a therapeutic Asherman's syndrome and amenorrhoea**. The method should be employed in cases who have completed their families.

• **Transcervical resection** of the endometrium (TCRE) through continuous flow resectoscope is quicker and less costlier than laser ablation. It can be carried out even under paracervical block. Resectoscope loop must remove the basal layer of endometrium along with superficial layer of myometrium otherwise regeneration of endometrium causes failure of operation (Fig. 14.4).

• **Roller ball ablation** of endometrium is also effective. It coagulates endometrium up to a depth of about 4 mm.

Complications : Uterine perforations, fluid absorption (p. 590) may occur during hysteroscopic procedure.

• **Uterine thermal balloon** for destruction of endometrium is currently used with satisfactory result. Endometrium is destroyed using a thermal balloon with hot normal saline (85°C) for 10-15 minutes. No dilatation of the cervical canal is needed. This procedure is suitable for women who are not suitable for general anaesthetic or long duration surgery. The success rate is similar to TCRE. No pretreatment GnRH analogue is required. This is commonly done as a day care basis.

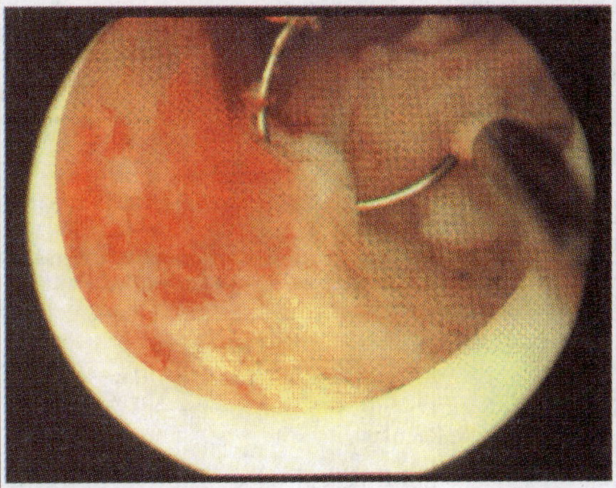

Fig. 14.4. Endometrial resection with the cutting loop

• **Microwave endometrial ablation** is simple and carried out as an out-patient procedure. Microwave electromagnetic heat energy causes ablation of the endometrium Endometrial tissue upto a depth of 6 mm is ablated. Temperature in the region is 75-80°C. Treat time (2-3 minutes) is less compared to TCRE.

• **Novasure :** Endometrial ablation is done using a bipolar electrode array mounted on an expandable frame. This creates a confluent lesion on the entire endometrial surface. Time required for global endometrial ablation is 90 seconds approximately. Radio frequency energy vaporises or coagulates the endometrium upto the myometrium. **Women with uterine cavity < 4 cm, PID, caesarean delivery are contraindicated.**

Table 14.8 : Common causes of abnormal vaginal bleeding

Abnormal menstrual bleeding	Non-menstrual bleeding
• Menorrhagia • Polymenorrhoea • Metrorrhagia • Oligomenorrhoea • Inappropriate (by age) – Precocious (see p. 49) – Delayed menopause (see p. 61) – Postmenopausal (see p. 532)	• Foreign body • Urethral caruncles (p. 398) • Genital malignancy (ch. 23) • Postcoital • Intermenstrual • Abortion • Breakthrough bleeding (see p. 468)

Methods of endometrial Ablation/Resection
Ablation • Laser • Rollerball • Thermal balloon • Microwave • Novasure **Resection** Transcervical resection (TCRE)

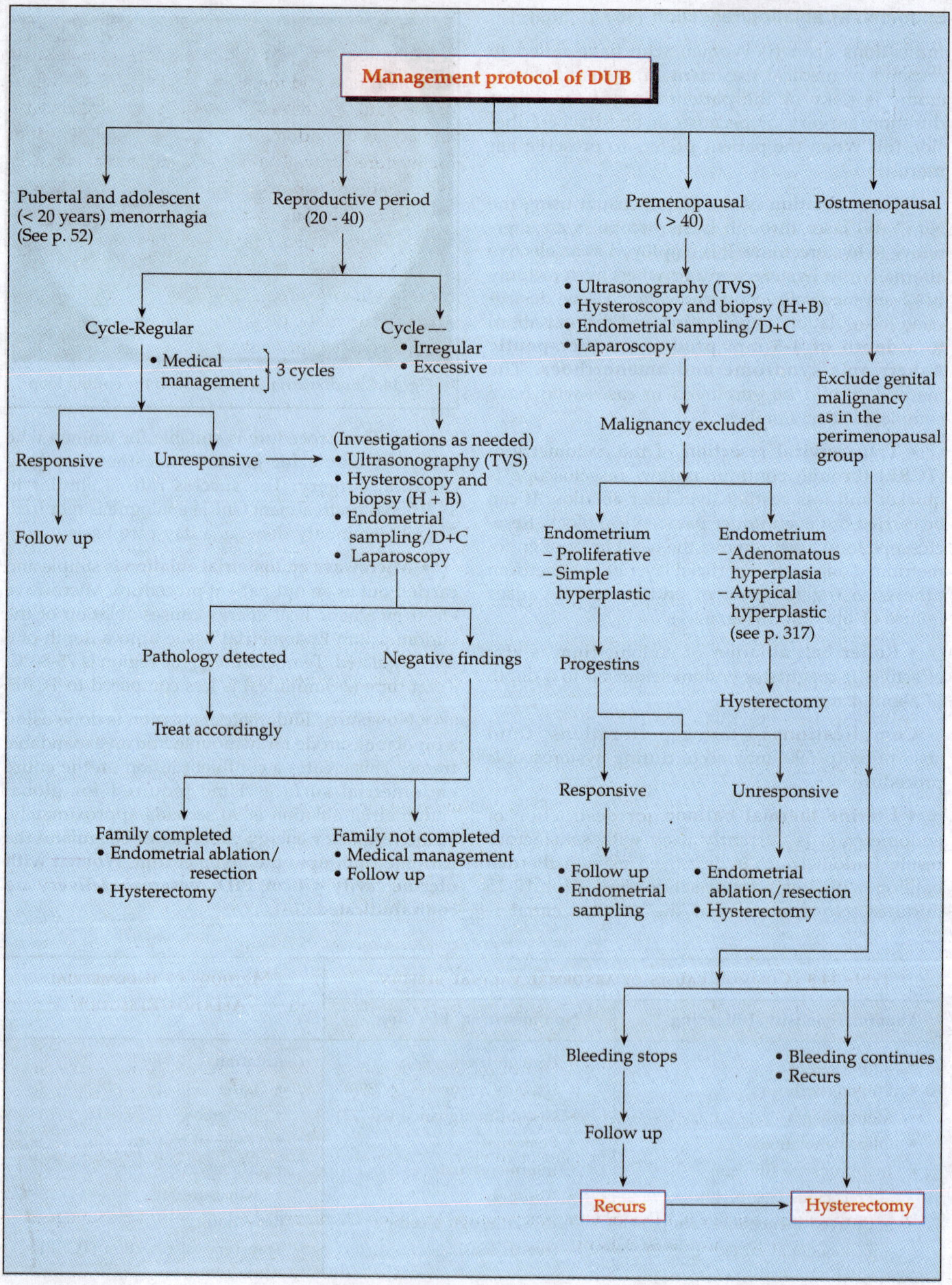

Management protocol of DUB
Pubertal and adolescent (< 20 years) menorrhagia (See p. 52)
Reproductive period (20 - 40)
Premenopausal (> 40)
Postmenopausal
Cycle-Regular
Cycle —
• Irregular
• Excessive
• Medical management
3 cycles
Responsive
Unresponsive
Follow up
(Investigations as needed)
• Ultrasonography (TVS)
• Hysteroscopy and biopsy (H + B)
• Endometrial sampling/D+C
• Laparoscopy
Pathology detected
Negative findings
Treat accordingly
Family completed
• Endometrial ablation/resection
• Hysterectomy
Family not completed
• Medical management
• Follow up
• Ultrasonography (TVS)
• Hysteroscopy and biopsy (H+B)
• Endometrial sampling/D+C
• Laparoscopy
Malignancy excluded
Exclude genital malignancy as in the perimenopausal group
Endometrium
– Proliferative
– Simple hyperplastic
Endometrium
– Adenomatous hyperplasia
– Atypical hyperplastic (see p. 317)
Progestins
Hysterectomy
Responsive
Unresponsive
• Follow up
• Endometrial sampling
• Endometrial ablation/resection
• Hysterectomy
Bleeding stops
• Bleeding continues
• Recurs
Follow up
Recurs
Hysterectomy

Pretreatment with danazol or GnRH agonists for 3 weeks prior to endometrial ablation is helpful to make the endometrium atrophic. The limitations and the effectiveness of endometrial ablation should be carefully evaluated before its wider application.

Results of Endometrial Ablation or Resection

Overall success with these methods is 70-80 per cent. About 40-50 per cent women become amenorrhoeic and another 40 per cent will have significant improvement of heavy blood loss. But 10 per cent of women may need repeat procedure or hysterectomy. For case selection, side effects, contraindications and complication (see p. 589).

Hysterectomy (p. 564)

Hysterectomy is justified when the conservative treatment fails and the blood loss impairs the health of the patient. Presence of endometrial hyperplasia and atypia on endometrial histology is an indication for hysterectomy. The decision can be taken easily as the patient is approaching 40. But even in women of thirties, prolonged procrastination with persistence of symptoms in spite of hormone therapy is often an indication of hysterectomy specially in those having desired number of children. Ovaries however, are to be preserved. The alternative in this group is endometrial ablation.

KEY POINTS

- Common causes of menorrhagia are DUB, fibroid, adenomyosis or chronic pelvic infection.
- Common causes of contact bleeding are carcinoma cervix, cervical mucous polyp and vascular erosion.
- The endometrial pattern in DUB is secretory in 60 per cent and hyperplastic in about 30 per cent.
- In late secretory phase the level of both PGE_2 and $PGF_{2\alpha}$ in the endometrium increases and during menses $PGF_{2\alpha}$ level rises over the PGE_2. The menstrual blood loss is inversely related to the level of endometrial $PGF_{2\alpha}/PGE_2$ ratio.
- In acyclic type of bleeding, diagnostic D + C should be done within 24 hours of mens.
- DUB is a state of abnormal uterine bleeding due to anovulation predominantly.
- D + C misses the diagnosis of uterine lesions in 10-20 per cent of women as it is a blind procedure. D + C can stop the acute episode of excess uterine bleeding but not the subsequent episodes.
- Diagnostic tests in women with menorrhagia include measurement of haemoglobin, serum iron, serum ferritin, TSH, endometrial biopsy and hysteroscopy.
- Hysteroscopy and biopsy is the best to evaluate the endometrial stature in DUB and to detect lesions such as submucous fibroid or polyp.
- To arrest acute episode of bleeding, potent progestogens are suitable in all periods of life, however, natural oestrogen administered parenterally (conjugated oestrogen 25 mg IV) is more effective in haemostasis during early reproductive period.
- For cycle regulation, either progestogens or combined preparations of oestrogen and progestogen (pill) may be used.
- In refractory cases or in cases of temporary contraindication of surgery, danazol or GnRH analogues may be used for short-term therapy.

KEY POINTS

- Prostaglandin synthetase inhibitors are effective in ovulatory DUB above the age of 35.
- Antifibrinolytic agents are suitable in case of DUB — following IUD.
- In cases of completed family, endometrial ablation/resection or hysterectomy is justified (p. 189).
- Endometrial ablation or resection (TCRE) is done in a woman who is over 35 years, has completed her family and without any significant endometrial pathology (e.g. cancer, submucous fibroid > 10 cm in diameter).
- Ablation of endometrium upto a depth of 4-5 mm using laser, roller ball, thermal balloon, microwave, is an effective method. Resection of endometrium upto the basal layer is also a quicker and less costlier method. Overall, amenorrhoea occurs in 50 per cent of women, about 40 per cent have decreased bleeding and 10 per cent may need repeat procedure or hysterectomy.
- In perimenopausal period, genital malignancy should be ruled out prior to any therapy.

Displacement of the Uterus

15

The uterus is not a fixed organ. Minor variations in position in any direction occur constantly with changes in posture, with straining, with full bladder or loaded rectum. Only when the uterus rests habitually in a position beyond the limit of normal variation, should it be called displacement.

RETROVERSION

Definition

Retroversion (RV) is the term used when the long axes of the corpus and cervix are in line and the whole organ turns backwards in relation to the long axis of the birth canal.

Retroflexion signifies a bending backwards of the corpus on the cervix at the level of internal os. **The two conditions are usually present together and are loosely called retroversion or retrodisplacement (Fig. 15.1).**

Degrees

Conventionally, three degrees are described.

First degree — The fundus is vertical and pointing towards the sacral promontory.

Second degree — The fundus lies in the sacral hollow but not below the internal os.

Third degree — The fundus lies below the level of the internal os.

Causes

- **Developmental**
- **Acquired**

Developmental

Retrodisplacement is quite common in fetuses and

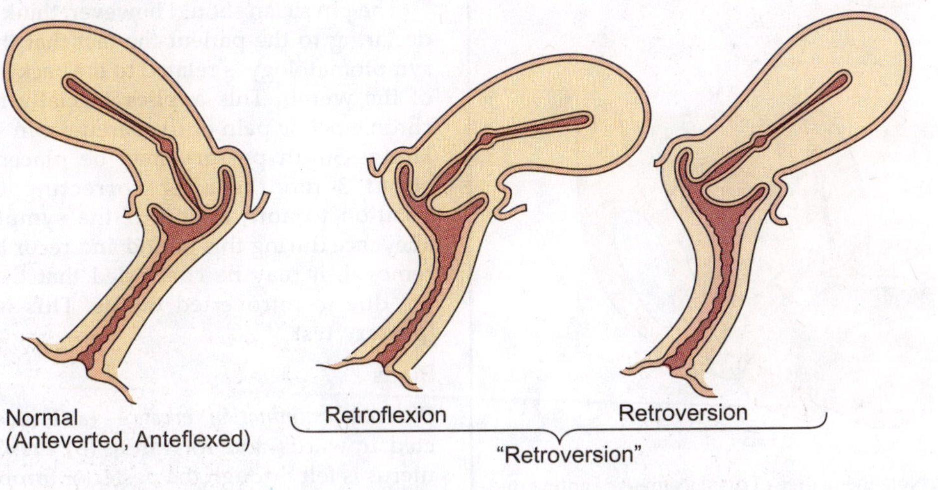

Fig. 15.1. Normal and retroverted uterus

young children. Due to developmental defect, there is lack of tone of the uterine muscles. The infantile position is retained. This is often associated with short vagina with shallow anterior vaginal fornix.

Acquired

Puerperal : The stretched ligaments caused by childbirth fail to keep the uterus in its normal position. A subinvoluted bulky uterus aggravates the condition.

Prolapse : Retroversion is usually implicated in the pathophysiology of prolapse which is mechanically caused by traction following cystocele.

Tumour : Fibroid, either in the anterior or posterior wall produces heaviness of the uterus and hence it falls behind.

Pelvic adhesions : Adhesions either inflammatory, operative or due to pelvic endometriosis pull the uterus posteriorly.

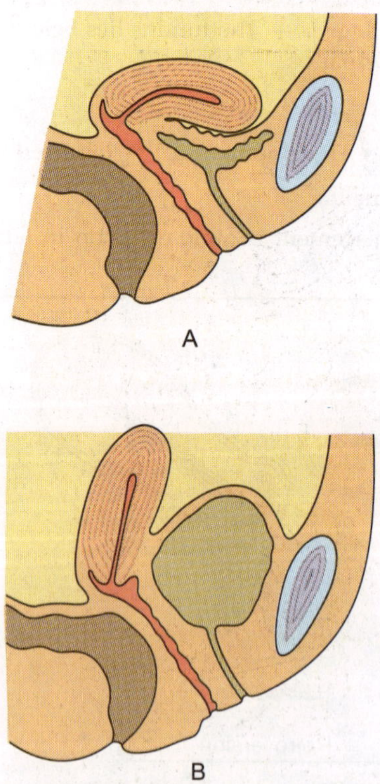

Fig. 15.2. Note the degree of displacement of anteverted uterus (B) due to full bladder (A) Reason to empty the bladder prior to examination

Incidence

Retroversion is present in about 15-20 per cent of normal women.

Clinical presentation

The condition is classified either as mobile and fixed or uncomplicated and complicated by pelvic diseases.

Mobile retroverted uterus

Symptoms

Mobile retroverted uterus is quite common and almost always remains asymptomatic. **However, the following symptoms may be attributed to it.**

- *Chronic premenstrual pelvic pain* — is due to varicosities in broad ligament produced by the kinks. The manifestations are those of 'pelvic congestion syndrome' (see p. 178, 530).
- *Backache.*
- *Dyspareunia* — Deep dyspareunia may be due to direct thrust by the penis against the retroflexed uterus or the prolapsed ovaries lying in the pouch of Douglas. Similar pain, if reproduced by pressing with examining fingers, may confirm its reality.
- *Infertility* — In third degree retroversion, the external os is away from the seminal pool at the posterior fornix during coitus or it may be occluded by the anterior vaginal wall. Associated underdevelopment of the uterus may also be a contributing factor.

The physician should however, think twice before declaring to the patient the fact that the particular symptomatology is related to the backward position of the womb. This applies specially to backache, chronic pelvic pain or dyspareunia. In such cases, a Hodge-Smith pessary may be placed inside for about 3 months after correcting the uterine position to anteversion. If the symptoms are in abeyance during this period and recur back after its removal, it may be concluded that the symptoms are due to retroverted uterus. **This is known as 'pessary test'.**

Signs

Bimanual examination reveals — (a) The cervix is directed upwards and forwards. (b) The body of the uterus is felt through the posterior fornix. It is found continuous with the cervix and it moves when the cervix is pressed up. The size of the uterus is difficult to assess at times.

Speculum examination reveals — the cervix comes in view much easily and the external os points forwards.

Rectal examination is of help to confirm the diagnosis.

Fixed retroversion

The symptoms are related to the associated pelvic pathology. Menstrual abnormalities (menorrhagia), congestive dysmenorrhoea, chronic pelvic pain or dyspareunia are usually associated.

Whether the uterus is fixed or mobile can be elicited by attempting to replace it by moving the cervix backwards and by pushing the fundus upwards. Rectal examination may be more effective to elicit the findings.

It is indeed of paramount importance to identify the position of the uterus as it is often necessary to identify prior to minor intrauterine manipulations such as insertion of IUCD or introduction of uterine sound. **Emptying the bladder prior to internal examination is mandatory (Fig. 15.2).**

Differential diagnosis

The retrodisplacement may be confused with hard faecal mass in the rectum, small fibroid on the posterior wall of the uterus and small ovarian cyst in the pouch of Douglas.

Pregnancy in retroverted uterus

Retroversion *per se* has got practically no adverse effect either on fertility or on early pregnancy wastage. In pregnancy, spontaneous correction usually occurs by 12-14 weeks. While the cause of infertility is mainly mechanical as mentioned earlier, repeated pregnancy wastage may be due to disturbance in uterine vascularity or due to thrust during intercourse specially in abortion prone women.

Prevention

The following guidelines are of help during the weeks after abortion or childbirth.

- To empty the bladder regularly.
- To increase the tone of the pelvic muscles by regular exercise.

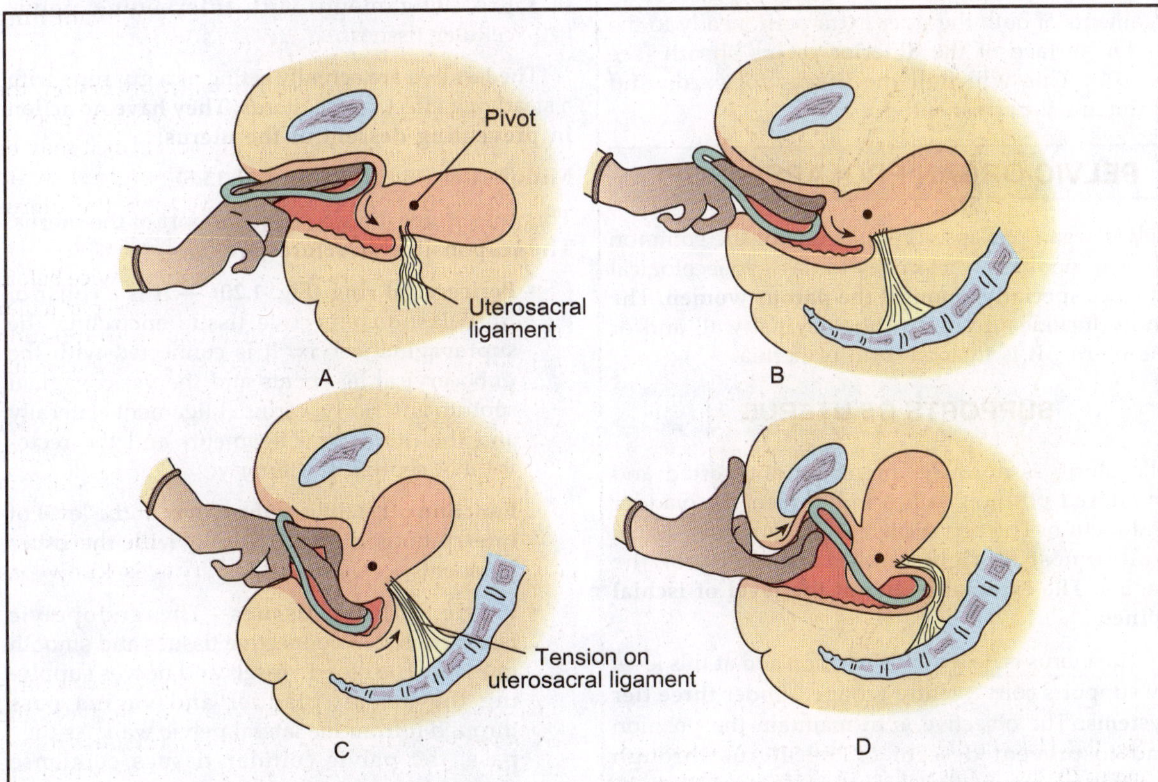

Fig. 15.3. Methods of introduction of pessary to correct the position of a RV uterus

- To encourage lying in prone position for half to one hour once or twice daily between 2 to 4 weeks postpartum.

Corrective treatment

- **Pessary** • **Surgical**

Pessary

Pessary is less commonly used in present day gynaecologic practice. However, it may be indicated : (1) for pessary test, (2) in subinvolution of uterus (see p. 194), (3) in pregnancy when spontaneous correction to anteversion fails by 12th week.

Usually Hodge-Smith pessary is used. The pessary acts by stretching the uterosacral ligaments so as to pull the cervix backwards (Fig. 15.3).

Surgical treatment

Surgical correction is indicated in : (1) Cases where the 'pessary test' is positive indicating that the symptoms are due to retroversion. (2) Fixed retroverted uterus producing symptoms like backache or dyspareunia.

The principle of surgical correction is ventrosuspension of the uterus by plicating the round ligaments of both the sides extra peritoneally to the under surface of the anterior rectus sheath (see p. 574). This will pull the uterus forwards and maintains it permanently.

PELVIC ORGAN PROLAPSE (POP)

Pelvic organ prolapse (POP) is one of the common clinical conditions met in day-to-day gynaecological practice **specially amongst the parous women**. The entity includes descent of the vaginal wall and or the uterus. It is infact a form of hernia.

SUPPORTS OF UTERUS

The uterus is normally placed in anteverted and anteflexed position. It lies in between the bladder and rectum. The cervix pierces the anterior vaginal wall almost at right angle to the axis of the vagina. **The external os lies at the level of ischial spines.**

The uterus is held in this position and at this level by supports conveniently grouped under **three tier systems.** The objective is to maintain the position and to prevent descent of the uterus through the natural urogenital hiatus in the pelvic floor (Fig. 15.4).

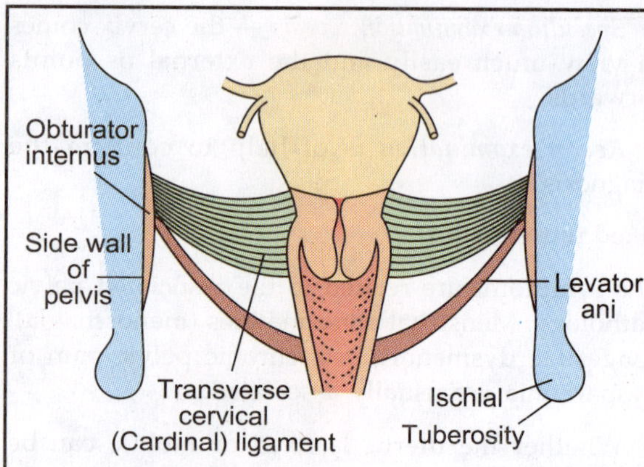

Fig. 15.4. Supports of uterus

Upper tier

The upper most supports of the uterus primarily maintain the uterus in anteverted position. **The responsible structures are** :

- Endopelvic fascia covering the uterus.
- Round ligaments.
- Broad ligaments with intervening pelvic cellular tissues.

The last two are actually acting as a guyrope with a steadying effect on the uterus. **They have no action in preventing descent of the uterus.**

Middle tier (Figures 15.5 and 15.6)

This constitutes the strongest support of the uterus. **The responsible structures are :**

- **Pericervical ring (Fig. 1.20)** — It is a collar of fibroelastic connective tissue encircling the supravaginal cervix. It is connected with the pubocervical ligaments and the vesicovaginal septum anteriorly, cardinal ligaments laterally and the uterosacral ligaments and the rectovaginal septum posteriorly.

  Function : It stabilises the cervix at the level of interspinous diameter along with the other ligaments.

- **Pelvic cellular tissues**—The endopelvic fascia consist of connective tissues and smooth muscles. The blood vessels and nerves supplying the uterus, bladder and vagina pass through it from the lateral pelvic wall. As they pass, the pelvic cellular tissues condense surrounding them and give good direct support to the viscera.

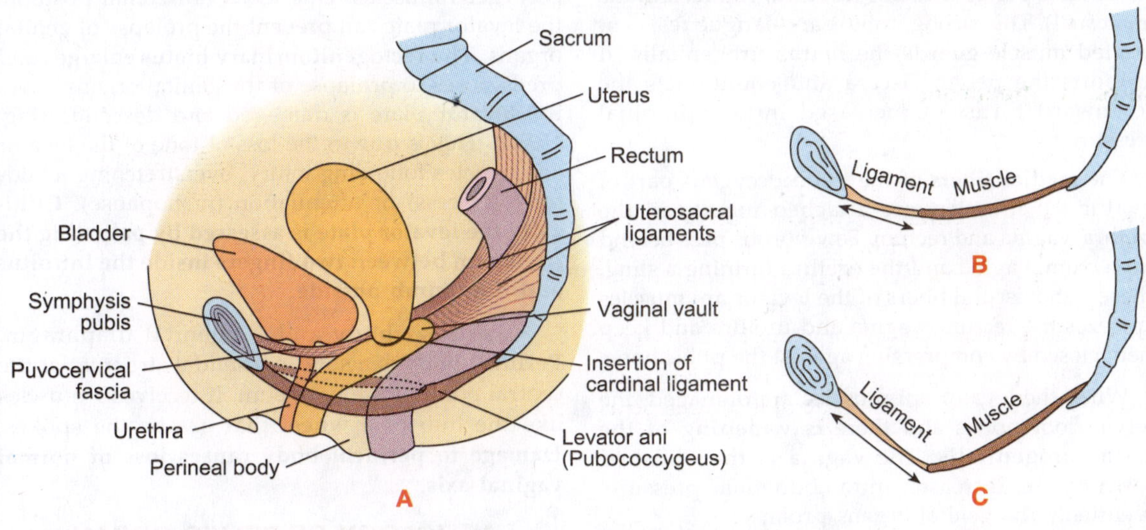

Fig. 15.5. Supports of uterus

The endopelvic fascia at places is condensed and reinforced by plain muscles to form ligaments — **Mackenrodt's, uterosacral and pubocervical. On the medial side, these are attached to the pericervical ring covering the cervicovaginal junction and on the other end are attached to the lateral, posterior and anterior walls of the pelvis (Figs. 15.5 and 15.6).** These are anatomically, morphologically and functionally the same unit. **This hammock like arrangement of condensed pelvic cellular tissues is the cardinal support of the uterus.**

Inferior tier

This gives the indirect support to the uterus. The support is principally given by the *pelvic floor muscles (Levator ani). Endopelvic fascia, Levator plate, Perineal body and the urogenital diaphragm.*

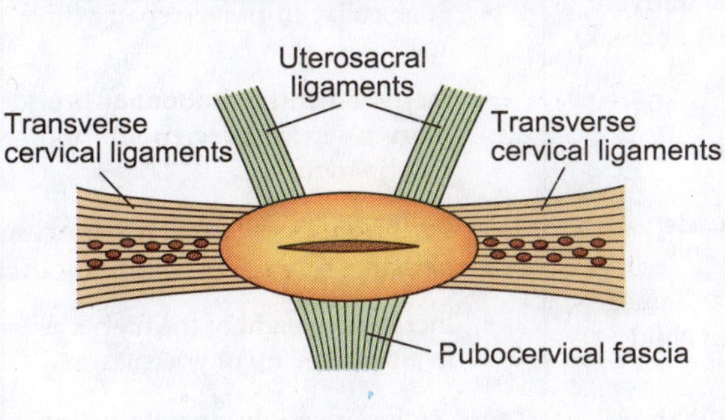

Fig. 15.6. Ligamentous supports of uterus

SUPPORTS OF VAGINA

Supports of the anterior vaginal wall

- ***Positional support*** — In the erect posture, the vagina makes an angle of 45° to the horizontal. Normal vaginal axis is horizontal in the upper two-third and vertical in the lower-third (see Fig. 15.5A). A well-supported vagina lies on the rectum and the levator plate (Figs.15.5A and 15.5B). Any raised intra-abdominal pressure is transmitted exclusively to the anterior vaginal wall which is apposed to the posterior vaginal wall.

- ***Pelvic cellular tissue*** — The vagina is ensheathed by strong condensation of pelvic cellular tissue called **endopelvic fascia.**

Traced below, this fascia form the posterior urethral ligament which is anchored to the pubic bones giving strong support to the urethra. Traced laterally, this fascia form the pubocervical fascia or ligament which is the anterior extension of the Mackenrodt's ligaments.

Supports of the posterior vaginal wall (Fig. 15.5)

- Endopelvic fascial sheath covering the vagina and rectum.

- Attachment of the uterosacral ligament to the lateral wall of the vault.

The levator ani muscles with its fascial coverings : This muscle is slug like a hammock around the midline pelvic effluents (urethra, vagina and the anal canal). This strong, robust and fatigue resistant striated muscle guards the hiatus urogenitalis. It supports the pelvic viscera and counteracts the downward thrust of increased intra-abdominal pressure.

The **medial fibers** of the pubococcygeus part of levator ani muscles, are attached mainly to the urethra, vagina and rectum. Few fibrous pass behind the rectum, vagina and the urethra forming a sling. These pubovisceral fibers of the levator ani muscles squeezes the rectum, vagina and urethra and keep them closed by compressing against the pubic bone.

When the levator ani muscles are damaged, the pelvic floor opens and there is **widening of the hiatus urogenitalis**. The vagina is then pushed down by the increased intra-abdominal pressure. Eventually the genital organs prolapse.

- **The levator plate (Figs. 15.5 A to C)** : Clinically it is a thick band of connective tissue formed by the medial fibers of the two levator ani muscles. Anatomically it is the anococcygeal raphe that extends between the anorectal junction and the coccyx. Some of the fibers extend anteriorly encircling the anorectal junction and are inserted into the **perineal body**.

The levator plate forms a horizontal supportive shelf upon which the rectum, upper vagina and the uterus rest (Figs. 15.5A and B). The horizontal position of this shelf is maintained by the anterior traction of the fibers of pubococcygeus and the iliococcygeus muscles. Due to its horizontal position, the levator plate can prevent the prolapse of genital organs. **The rectogenitourinary hiatus** enlarges and predisposes to prolapse of the genital organs when the levator plate is damaged and descends (Fig. 15.5C). This is due to the loss of tone of the levator ani muscles following injury, overstretching (childbirth process) or attenuation (menopause). **Clinically the levator plate is assessed by palpating the perineum between two fingers inside the introitus and the thumb outside.**

- **Perineal body** and urogenital diaphragm. **Perineal body** is a solid pyramidal structure at the central point of the perineum. It receives 9 muscles like the hub of a wheel that grasps the spokes. **Damage to perineal body causes loss of normal vaginal axis.**

AETIOLOGY OF PELVIC ORGAN PROLAPSE (POP)

The genital prolapse occurs due to weakness of the structures supporting the organs in position. These factors may be anatomical or clinical. **The clinical factors** are grouped as :

- **Predisposing** • **Aggravating**

Predisposing factors

- **Acquired** • **Congenital**

Acquired

Vaginal delivery with consequent injury to the

Table 15.1 : AETIOLOGY OF PELVIC ORGAN PROLAPSE (POP)

ANATOMICAL FACTORS	CLINICAL FACTORS	
	Predisposing factors	**Aggravating factors**
• Gravitational stress due to human bipedal posture. • Anterior inclination of pelvis directing the force more anteriorly. • Stress of parturiation (Internal rotation) causing damage maximum on puborectal fibers of levator ani. • Pelvic floor weakness due to urogenital hiatus and the direction of obstetric axis through the hiatus. • Inherent weakness of the supporting structures (Genetic).	A. Acquired **Trauma of vaginal delivery** causing injury (tear or break) to : (1) Ligaments (see p. 196) (2) Endopelvic fascia (see p. 196) (3) Levator ani muscle (4) Perineal body. (5) Neuromuscular damage due to repeated childbirth. B. Congenital (see p. 199) Inborn weakness of supporting structures.	• Postmenopausal atrophy. • Poor collagen tissue repair with age. • Increased intra-abdominal pressure as in chronic cough and constipation. • Asthenia and undernutrition. • Obesity. • Increased weight of the uterus as in fibroid or myohyperplasia. These factors possibly operate where the supports of the genital organs are already weak.

supporting structures is the single most important acquired predisposing factor in producing prolapse. The prolapse is unusual in cases delivered by caesarean section.

The injury is caused by :

(1) Overstretching of the Mackenrodt's and uterosacral ligaments : (i) Premature bear down efforts prior to full dilatation of the cervix. (ii) Delivery with forceps or ventouse with forceful traction. (iii) Prolonged second stage of labour. (iv) Downward pressure on the uterine fundus in an attempt to deliver the placenta. (v) Precipitate labour.

In all these conditions the uterus tends to be pushed down into the flabby distended vagina.

(2) Overstretching and breaks in the endopelvic fascial sheath.

(3) Overstretching of the perineum.

(4) Imperfect repair of the perineal injuries. Poor repair of collagen tissue.

(5) Loss of levator function.

(6) Neuromuscular damage of levator ani during childbirth.

(7) Subinvolution of the supporting structures. This is particularly noticeable in : (i) Ill-nourished and asthenic women. (ii) Early resumption of activities which greatly increase intra-abdominal pressure before the tissues regain their tone. (iii) Repeated childbirths at frequent intervals.

Congenital

Congenital weakness of the supporting structures is responsible for **nulliparous prolapse or prolapse following an easy vaginal delivery. One should be on the look out for an occult spina bifida** and associated neurological abnormalities.

CLINICAL TYPES OF PELVIC ORGAN PROLAPSE

The genital prolapse is broadly grouped into :

- **Vaginal prolapse** • **Uterine prolapse**

While vaginal prolapse can occur independently without uterine descent, the uterine prolapse is usually associated with variable degrees of vaginal descent.

Vaginal prolapse

Anterior wall

- *Cystocele* — The cystocele is **formed by laxity and descent of the upper two-thirds of the anterior vaginal wall.** As the bladder base is closely related to this area, there is herniation of the bladder through the lax anterior wall.

- *Urethrocele* — When there is laxity of the **lower-third of the anterior vaginal wall,** the urethra herniates through it. This may appear independently or usually along with cystocele and is called cysto-urethrocele.

Posterior wall

- *Relaxed perineum* — Torn perineal body produces gaping introitus with bulge of the lower part of the posterior vaginal wall.

- *Rectocele* — There is laxity of the middle-third of the posterior vaginal wall and the adjacent rectovaginal septum. As a result, there is herniation of the rectum through the lax area.

Vault prolapse

- *Enterocele* — Laxity of the upper-third of the posterior vaginal wall results in herniation of the pouch of Douglas. It may contain omentum or even loop of small bowel and hence called enterocele. **Traction enterocele** is secondary to uterovaginal prolapse. Pulsion enterocele is secondary to chronically raised intra-abdominal pressure.

- *Secondary vault prolapse* — This may occur following either vaginal or abdominal hysterectomy. Undetected enterocele during initial operation or inadequate primary repair usually results in secondary vault prolapse (Fig. 15.20).

Uterine prolapse

There are two types :

- *Uterovaginal prolapse* is the prolapse of the uterus, cervix and upper vagina.

This is the commonest type. Cystocele occurs first followed by traction effect on the cervix causing retroversion of the uterus. Intra-abdominal pressure has got piston like action on the uterus thereby pushing it down into the vagina.

- *Congenital*

There is usually no cystocele. The uterus herniates down along with inverted upper vagina. This is often met in nulliparous women and hence called **nulliparous prolapse**. The cause is congenital weakness of the supporting structures holding the uterus in position.

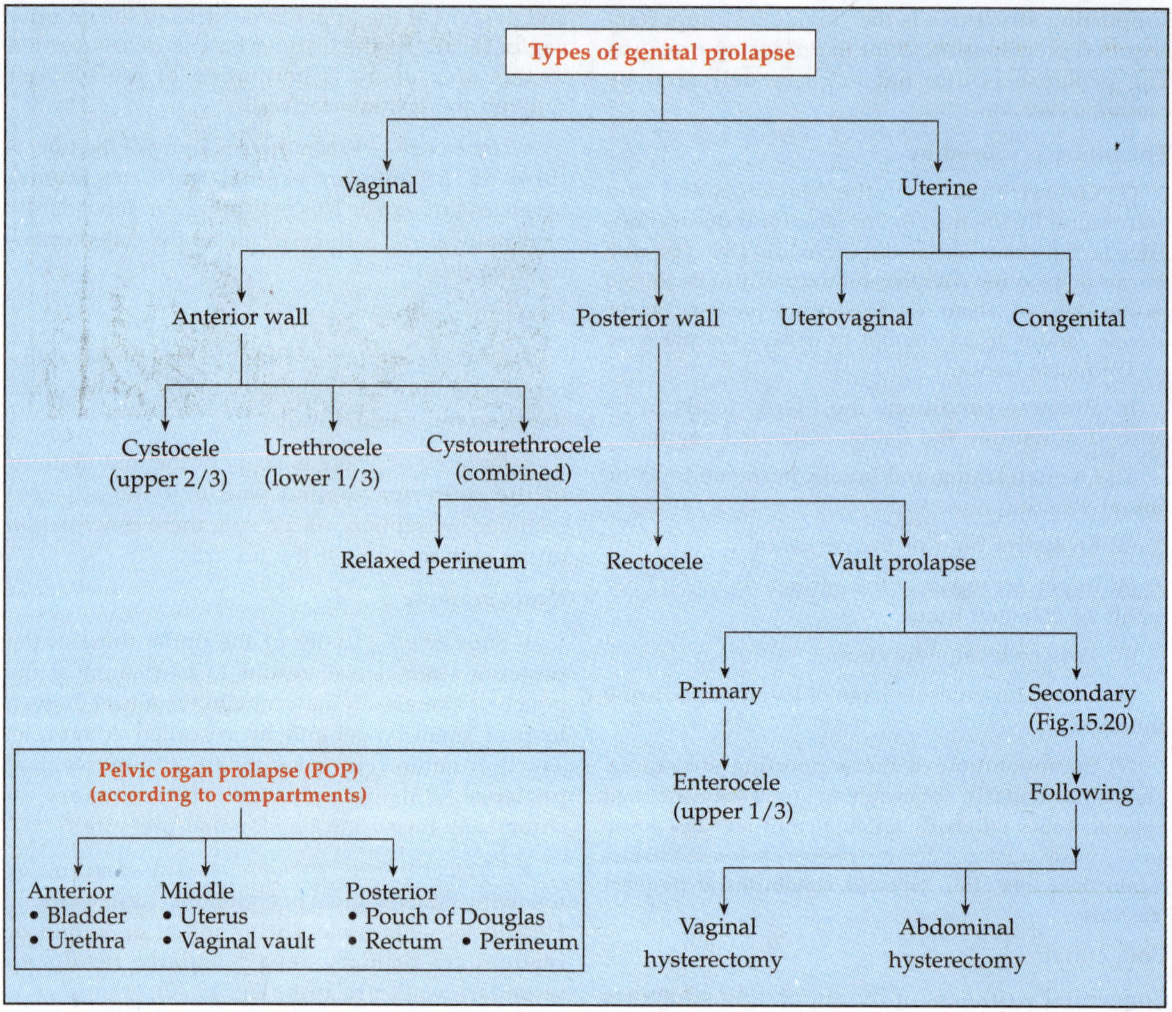

DEGREES OF UTERINE PROLAPSE (CLINICAL)

Three degrees are described :

First degree — The uterus descends down from its normal anatomical position (external os at the level of ischial spines) but the external os still remains inside the vagina.

Second degree — The external os protrudes outside the vaginal introitus but the uterine body still remains inside the vagina (Fig. 15.8).

Third degree (*Syn : Procidentia, Complete prolapse*) — The uterine body descends to lie outside the introitus (Fig. 15.9).

More recent grading system of prolapse considers the individual pelvic organ (according to compartment – see above) and its distance in relation to the hymen (Table 15.2). Pelvic Organ Prolapse Qualification (POP-Q) identifies several points (total 9) within and around the vagina and measures the distance of each point from the hymen. Staging is done according to the measurement (Fig. 15.10).

Table 15.2
Pelvic Organ Prolapse (POP) Quantitative Scoring (International Continence Society Terminology, American Urogynecologic Society, Society of Gynecologic Surgeons – 1996) Fig. 15.7 (Right hand side)

Stage	Description
0	No descent of pelvic organs.
I	Leading edge of the prolapse does not descend below 1 cm. above the hymenal ring.

Table 15.2 contd. from previous page

Stage	Description
II	Leading edge of the prolapse extends from 1 cm. above to 1 cm. below the hymenal ring.
III	From 1 cm. beyond the hymenal ring but without complete vaginal eversion.
IV	Essentially complete eversion of vagina.

Procidentia involves prolapse of the uterus with eversion of the entire vagina.

Complex prolapse is one when prolapse is associated with some other specific defects. **Complex prolapse** includes the following : Prolapse with urinary or faecal incontinence, nulliparous prolapse, recurrent prolapse, vaginal and rectal prolapse or prolapse in a frail woman.

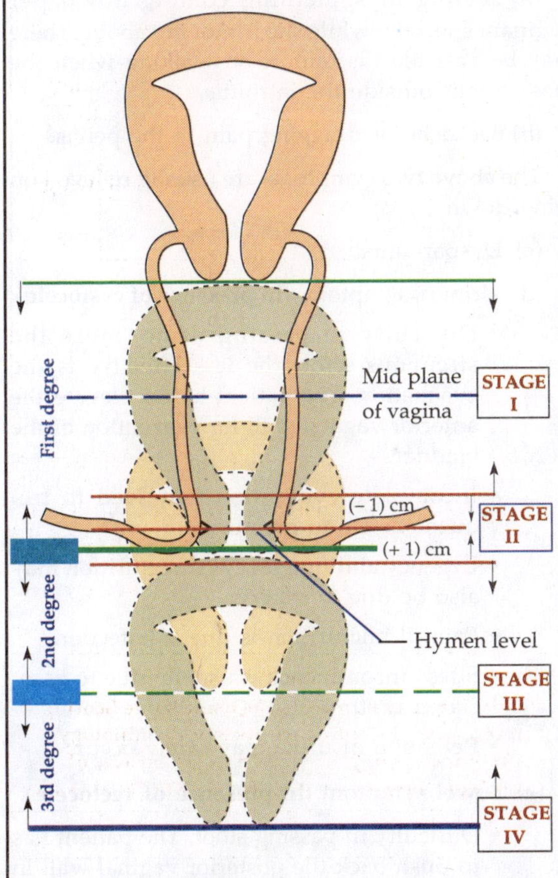

Fig. 15.7. Quantitative gradings of Pelvic Organ Prolapse [*ICS, AUGS, SGS – 1996*] stages–on the right hand side. Clinical degrees are shown on the left

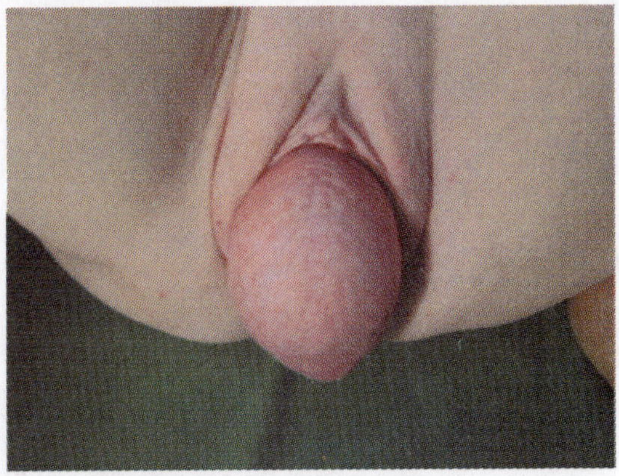

Fig. 15.8. Second degree uterine prolapse. Marked cystocele and there is decubitus ulcer

Morbid changes

Vaginal mucosa

The mucosa becomes stretched and if exposed to air, becomes thickened and dry with surface keratinisation. There may be pigmentation.

Decubitus ulcer (Fig. 15.8)

It is a trophic ulcer, always found at the dependent part of the prolapsed mass lying outside the introitus. There is initial surface keratinisation → cracks → infection → sloughing → ulceration. There is complete denudation of the surface epithelium. The diminished circulation is due to constriction of the prolapsed mass by the vaginal opening and narrowing of the uterine vessels by the stretching effect.

Cervix

Vaginal part — There is chronic congestion which may lead to hyperplasia and hypertrophy of the fibromusculoglandular components. These lead to vaginal part becoming bulky and congested. Addition of infection leads to purulent or at times blood stained discharge from ulceration.

Supravaginal part — The supravaginal part becomes elongated due to the strain imposed by the pull of the cardinal ligaments to keep the cervix in position, whereas the weight of the uterus makes it fall through the vaginal axis. Chronic interference of venous and lymphatic drainage favours elongation.

Urinary system

Bladder — There is incomplete emptying of the

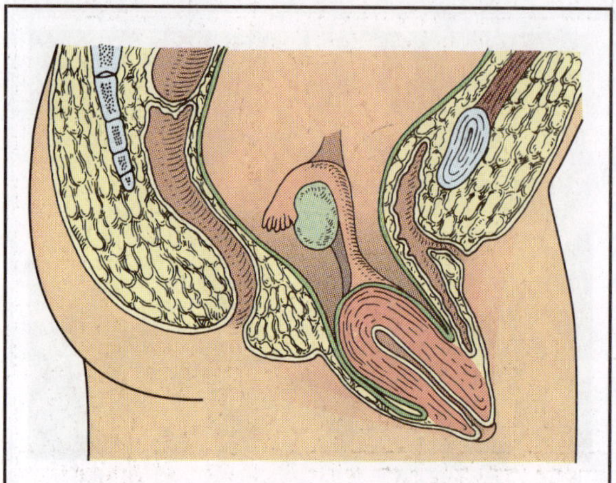

Fig. 15.9. Third degree uterine prolapse

bladder due to sharp angulation of the urethra against the pubourethral ligament during straining. As a result, there is hypertrophy of the bladder wall and trabeculation. Incomplete evacuation also favours cystitis.

Ureters — The ureters are carried downwards along with elongated Mackenrodt's ligaments and thus, mechanically obstructed by the hiatus of the pelvic floor. They may be compressed even by the uterine arteries at their crossing. As a result, hydroureteric changes may occur.

Infection of the bladder may thus ascend up to produce pyelitis or pyelonephritis. On rare occasions, uraemia may occur specially in long-standing cases of procidentia.

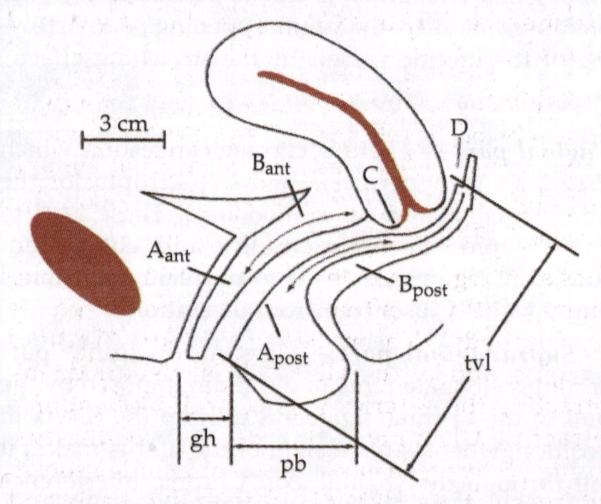

Fig. 15.10. Nine specific sites (points A_{ant}, B_{ant}, C, D, B_{post} and A_{post}), genital hiatus (gh), perineal body (pb), and total vaginal length (tvl) used for pelvic organ prolapse quantification system (p. 200). (Bump, Mattiason, Bo K, *et al* 1996)

Incarceration : At times, infection of the paravaginal and cervical tissues makes the entire prolapsed mass oedematous and congested. As a result, the mass may be irreducible.

Peritonitis : Rarely, the peritoneal infection (pelvic peritonitis) may occur through the posterior vaginal wall.

Carcinoma : Carcinoma rarely develops on decubitus ulcer.

Symptoms

The symptoms are variable. Even with minor degree, the symptoms may be pronounced, paradoxically there may not be any appreciable symptom even in severe degree. However, **the following symptoms are usually associated.**

(a) Feeling of something coming down per vaginam specially while she is moving about. There may be variable discomfort on walking when the mass comes outside the introitus.

(b) Backache or dragging pain in the pelvis.

The above two symptoms are usually relieved on lying down.

(c) Dyspareunia.

(d) Urinary symptoms (**in presence of cystocele**).

- Difficulty in passing urine, more the strenuous effort the less effective is the evacuation. The patient has to elevate the anterior vaginal wall for evacuation of the bladder.
- Incomplete evacuation may lead to frequent desire to pass urine.
- Urgency and frequency of micturition may also be due to cystitis.
- Painful micturition is due to infection.
- Stress incontinence is usually due to associated urethrocele.
- Retention of urine may rarely occur.

(e) Bowel symptom (**in presence of rectocele**).

- Difficulty in passing stool. The patient has to push back the posterior vaginal wall in position to complete the evacuation of faeces. Faecal incontinence may be associated.

(f) Excessive white or blood stained discharge per vaginam is due to associated vaginitis or decubitus ulcer.

Clinical examination and diagnosis of pelvic organ prolapse

- A composite examination — inspection and palpation : Vaginal, rectal, rectovaginal or even under anaesthesia may be required to arrive at a correct diagnosis.
- Pelvic Organ Prolapse (POP) is evaluated by pelvic examination in both dorsal and standing positions. The patient is asked to strain as to perform a Valsalva maneuver during examination. This often helps to demonstrate a prolapse which may not be seen at rest.
- A negative finding on inspection in dorsal position should be reconfirmed by asking the patient to strain on squatting position.
- Prolapse of one organ (uterus) is usually associated with prolapse of the adjacent organs (bladder, rectum).
- Aetiological aspect of prolapse should be evaluated.

Cystocele (Fig. 15.11) : There is a bulge of varying degree of the anterior vaginal wall which increases when the patient is asked to strain. This may be seen on inspection. In others, to elicit this, one may have to separate the labia or depress the posterior vaginal wall with fingers or using Sims' speculum, placing the patient in lateral position (see p. 99).

The mucosa over the bulge has got transverse rugosities. The bulge has got impulse on coughing, with diffuse margins and is reducible (Fig. 15.11).

Cystourethrocele : The bulging of the anterior vaginal wall involves the lower-third also. One may

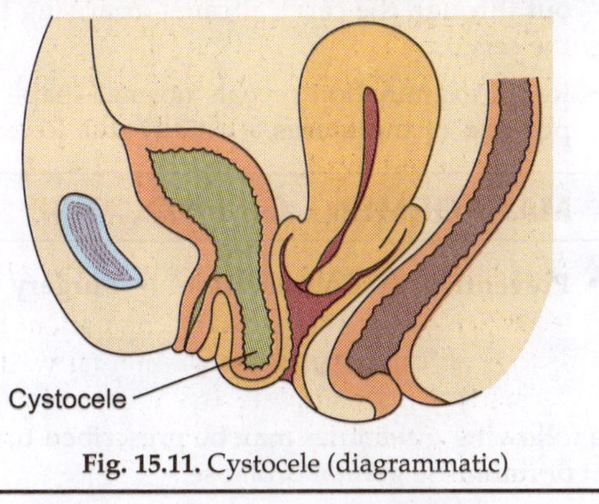

Fig. 15.11. Cystocele (diagrammatic)

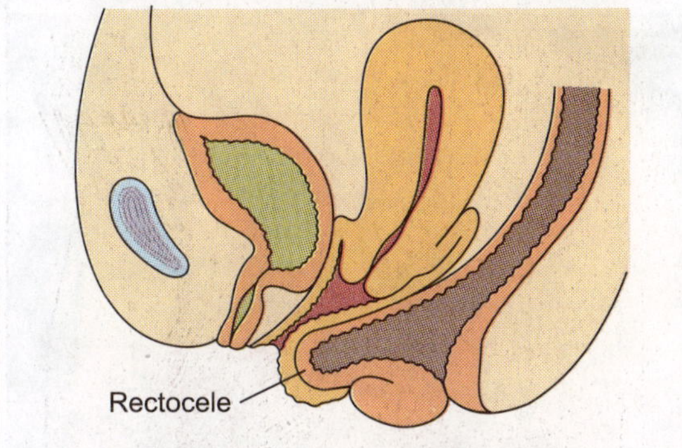

Fig. 15.12. Rectocele (diagrammatic)

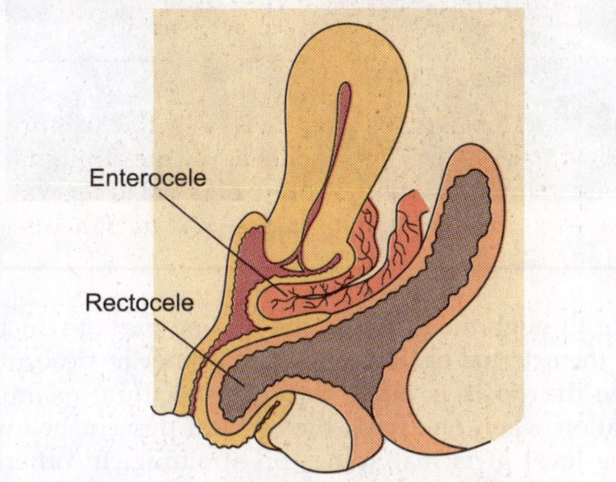

Fig. 15.13. Enterocele and rectocele (diagrammatic)

find the urine to escape out through the urethral meatus when the patient is asked to cough — stress incontinence. **To elicit the test, the bladder should be full.**

Relaxed perineum : There is gaping introitus with old scar of incomplete perineal tear. The lower part of the posterior vaginal wall is visible with or without straining.

Rectocele and enterocele : When the two conditions exist together, there is bulging of the posterior vaginal wall with a transverse sulcus between the two. The midvaginal one being rectocele with diffuse margins and reducible. This is visualised by retracting the anterior vaginal wall by Landon's retractor. **Ultimate differentiation of the two entities is by rectal or rectovaginal examination.** In enterocele, the bulging is close to the cervix and cannot be reached by the finger inside the rectum (Figs. 15.12 and 15.13).

Uterine prolapse : In second or third degree of prolapse, inspection can reveal a mass protruding

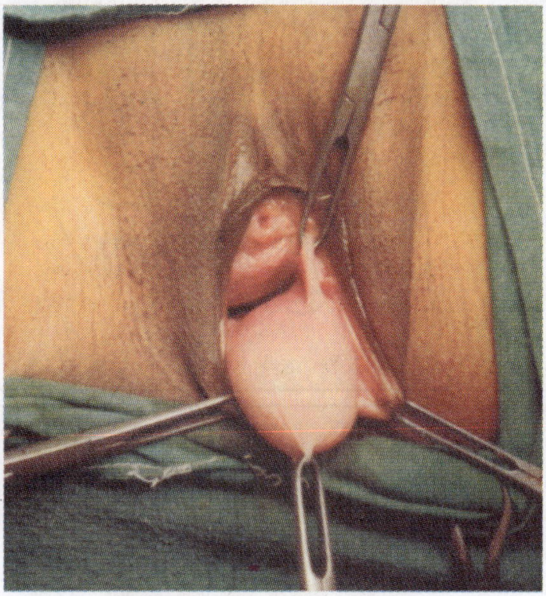

Fig. 15.14. Gartner's cyst

out through the introitus, the leading part of which is the external os. In first degree of uterine descent, the diagnosis is made through speculum examination when one finds the cervical descent below the level of ischial spines on straining. In others however, the external os is visible on separating the labia (Fig. 15.8).

To diagnose a third degree prolapse, palpation is essential. If the thumb placed anteriorly and the fingers posteriorly above the mass outside the introitus are apposed, it is a third degree (Fig. 15.9).

There may be evidences of decubitus ulceration or dark pigmented areas.

Bimanual examination reveals shallow vaginal fornices and normal length of the vaginal cervix with normal size uterine body. The introduction of a sound reveals marked increase in length of the uterine cavity. This signifies elongation of the supravaginal part of the cervix.

Differential diagnosis

Cystocele : The cystocele is often confused with a cyst in the anterior vaginal wall, the commonest being Gartner's cyst (retention cyst in remnants of Wolffian duct).

Features of Gartner's cyst are (Fig. 15.14)

- Situated anteriorly or anterolaterally and of variable sizes.
- Rugosities of the overlying vaginal mucosa are lost.
- Vaginal mucosa over it becomes tense and shiny.
- Margins are well-defined.
- It is not reducible.
- There is no impulse on coughing.
- The metal catheter tip introduced per urethra fails to come underneath the vaginal mucosa.

Uterine prolapse

(a) ***Congenital elongation of the cervix*** **(Fig. 18.6, p. 261)**

- It is unassociated with prolapse (usually).
- Vaginal part of the cervix is elongated.
- External os lies below the level of ischial spines.
- Vaginal fornices are narrow and deep.
- Cervix looks conical.
- Uterine body is normal size and in position.

(b) ***Chronic inversion*** **(Fig. 15.22)**

- Leading protruding mass is broad.
- There is no opening visible on the leading part.
- It looks shaggy.
- Internal examination reveals — cervical rim is on the top around the mass.
- Rectal examination confirms the absence of the uterine body and a cup-like depression is felt.

(c) ***Fibroid polyp*** **(Fig. 15.23)**

- The mass is saggy with a broad leading part.
- No opening is visible on the leading part.
- Internal examination reveals the pedicle coming out through the cervical canal or arising from the cervix.
- Rectal examination reveals normal shape and position of the uterus.

MANAGEMENT OF PROLAPSE

- **Preventive** • **Conservative** • **Surgery**

PREVENTIVE

The following guidelines may be prescribed to prevent or minimise genital prolapse.

Adequate antenatal and intranatal care

- To avoid injury to the supporting structures during the time of vaginal delivery either spontaneous or instrumental (see p.199).

Adequate postnatal care

- To encourage early ambulance.
- To encourage pelvic floor exercises by squeezing the pelvic floor muscles in the puerperium.

General measures

- To avoid strenuous activities, chronic cough, constipation and heavy weight lifting.
- To avoid future pregnancy too soon and too many by contraceptive practice.

CONSERVATIVE

As the genital prolapse is a sort of hernia, there is practically no scope of conservative treatment.

However, mild subjective symptoms of something coming down per vaginam may be tackled by palliative treatment :

- Improvement of general measures (see above).
- Oestrogen replacement therapy may improve minor degree prolapse in postmenopausal women.
- Pelvic floor exercises in an attempt to strengthen the muscles (Kegel exercises).

PESSARY TREATMENT

It should be emphasised that the pessary cannot cure prolapse but relieves the symptoms by stretching the hiatus urogenitalis, thus preventing vaginal and uterine descent. It may be used with advantages in selected cases such as :

- *Early pregnancy* — The pessary should be placed inside upto 18 weeks when the uterus becomes sufficiently enlarged to sit on the brim of the pelvis.
- *Puerperium* — to facilitate involution.
- *Patients absolutely unfit for surgery* specially with short life expectancy.
- *Patient's unwillingness* for operation.
- *While waiting for operation.* One disadvantage is, the patient may feel so comfortable that she may refuse operation in future.

Table 15.3 : Type of prolapse and the common surgical repair procedures

Organ descent	Clinical condition	Type of operation
VAGINAL WALL		
Anterior (Upper 2/3) or whole	Cystocele/cystourethrocele	Anterior colporrhaphy (p. 206), Paravaginal repair (p. 207).
Posterior (Lower 2/3)	Rectocele	Colpoperineorrhaphy (p. 207)
Posterior (Upper 1/3)	Enterocele	Vaginal repair of enterocele with PFR (p. 210) McCall culdoplasty (p. 210)
Combined anterior and Posterior	Cystocele and rectocele	Pelvic floor repair (PFR) (p. 210)
UTEROVAGINAL Uterus along with vaginal walls	Uterovaginal prolapse	Vaginal hysterectomy with PFR (p. 211) Fothergill's operation (preservation of uterus) (p. 210).
VAGINAL WALL **FOLLOWING HYSTERECTOMY** (Vaginal or abdominal)	Vault prolapse (secondary)	**Vaginal** : (i) Repair of vaginal vault along with PFR (p. 209) (ii) Sacrospinous colpopexy (p. 215) (iii) Colpoclesis (Le Fort) (p. 215) **Abdominal** : (i) Sacral colpopexy (p. 215)
Uterus (without vaginal walls)	Congenital or nulliparous prolapse	Cervicopexy or Sling (Purandare's) operation (p. 215).

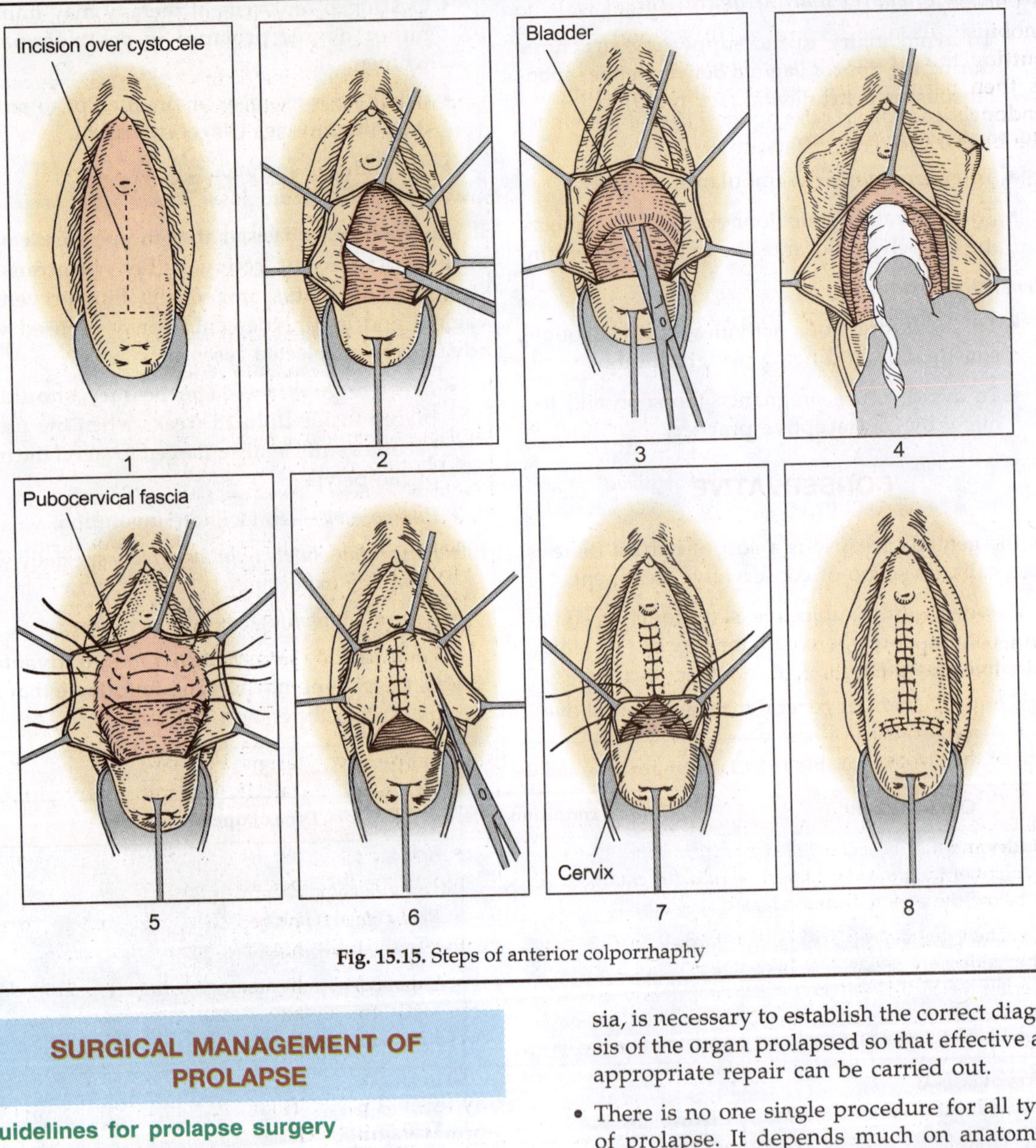

Fig. 15.15. Steps of anterior colporrhaphy

SURGICAL MANAGEMENT OF PROLAPSE

Guidelines for prolapse surgery

- Surgery is the treatment of symptomatic prolapse where conservative management has failed or is not indicated.
- Surgical procedures may be : (A) Restorative — (i) correcting her own support tissues (Table 15.3) or (ii) compensatory — using permanent graft material (p. 215). (B) Extirpative — removing the uterus and correcting the support tissues. (C) Obliterative — closing the vagina (colpocleisis p. 215).
- Meticulous examination, even under anaesthesia, is necessary to establish the correct diagnosis of the organ prolapsed so that effective and appropriate repair can be carried out.
- There is no one single procedure for all types of prolapse. It depends much on anatomical alteration of structures and the degree of prolapse (see p. 200).
- Due consideration is to be given about the age, reproductive and sexual function of the woman before any specific surgery.

Types of operation : See Table 15.3.

Anterior colporrhaphy (Fig. 15.15)

This operation is designed to correct cystocele and urethrocele. The underlying principles are to excise a portion of the relaxed anterior vaginal wall, to mobilise the bladder and push it upwards after cutting the vesicocervical ligament. The bladder is then permanently supported by plicating the endopelvic fascia and the pubocervical fascia under the bladder neck in the midline.

Steps of operation (Fig. 15.15)

Preliminaries

- The operation is done under general or epidural anaesthesia.
- The patient is placed in lithotomy position.
- Vulva and vagina are to be swabbed with antiseptic solution.
- The perineum is to be draped with sterile towel and legs with leggings.
- Bladder is to be emptied by metal catheter.
- Vaginal examination is done to assess the type and degree of prolapse.

Actual steps (Fig. 15.15)

- Sims' posterior vaginal speculum is introduced and the anterior lip of the cervix is held by multiple teethed vulsellum and firmly brought down by assistant (Fig. 15.15.1).
- A metal catheter is introduced to know the lower limit of the bladder.
- An inverted 'T' incision is made on the anterior vaginal wall. The horizontal incision is made below the bladder and the vertical incision is made starting from the midpoint of the transverse incision upto a point about 1.5 cm below the external urethral meatus (Fig. 15.15.1).
- The triangular vaginal flaps including the fascia on either sides are separated from the endopelvic fascia covering the bladder by knife and gauze dissection. The line of cleavage is vesicovaginal space and if properly negotiated, the dissection is easy with minimal blood loss (Fig. 15.15.2).
- The bladder with the covering endopelvic fascia (pubocervical) is now exposed as the edges of the vaginal wall are retracted laterally.
- The vesicocervical ligament is held up with Allis tissue or toothed dissecting forceps and divided. The bladder is then pushed up by gauze covered finger till the peritoneum of the uterovesical pouch is visible. The vesico-cervical space is now exposed (Figs. 15.15.3 and 15.15.4).
- The pubocervical fascia is plicated by interrupted sutures with No 'O' chromic catgut using round body needle. The lower one or two stitches include a bite on the cervix, thus closing the hiatus through which the bladder herniates (Fig. 15.15.5).
- The redundant portion of the vaginal mucosa is cut on either side (Fig. 15.15.6).
- The cut margins of the vagina are apposed by interrupted sutures with No. 'O' chromic catgut using cutting needle (Figs. 15.15.7 and 15.15.8).
- The catheter is reintroduced once more to be sure that the bladder is not injured.
- Toileting of the vagina is done.
- Vagina is tightly packed with roller gauze smeared with antiseptic cream.
- A self retaining catheter is introduced.

The last two formalities are optional.

Paravaginal defect repair : Anterior vaginal wall prolapse (cystocele) is repaired by anterior colporrhaphy and plicating the endopelvic fascia in the midline under the bladder neck. But anterior vaginal prolapse may be due to the detachment of the endopelvic fascia from the lateral pelvic side wall. In that case repair should be done by fixing (reattaching) the endopelvic fascia to the arcus tendineus fascia (white line) of the pelvis. This may be done retropubically through the space of Retzius or vaginally. This is indicated in cases with recurrent cystocele following repair.

Perineorrhaphy/Colpoperineorrhaphy

It is an operation designed to repair the prolapse of posterior vaginal wall. Its uses and extent of repair are employed in :

- *Relaxed perineum* — The operation is extended to repair the torn perineal body.
- *Rectocele* — The repair is extended to correct rectocele by tightening the pararectal fascia.
- *Enterocele* — High perineorrhaphy is to be done right upto the cervicovaginal junction along with correction of enterocele.

Restoration of perineal body is essential with any form of pelvic floor repair. This maintains the normal vaginal axis.

Steps of operation (Fig. 15.16)

Preliminaries : The preliminaries are to be followed as in anterior colporrhaphy.

Actual steps

- A pair of Allis tissue forceps is placed on each side at the lower end of labium minus and a third pair of Allis is placed on the posterior vaginal wall in the midline well above the rectocele bulge (Fig.15.16.1).
- A horizontal incision is made on the mucocutaneous junction joining the two Allis tissue forceps (Fig. 15.16.1).

• Through this incision, with the help of perineorrhaphy scissors, the posterior vaginal wall is dissected off from the perineal body and rectum upto the third Allis forceps placed on the posterior vaginal wall (Fig. 15.16.1).

• A vertical incision is made from the apex to the middle of the horizontal incision (inverted 'T' shaped incision) (Fig. 15.16.1).

• The two triangular flaps are now dissected laterally to expose the rectum and musculofascial structures levator ani muscle (Fig. 15.16.2).

• The lax vaginal flaps are excised.

• The rectocele is corrected by suturing the pararectal fascia with interrupted sutures.

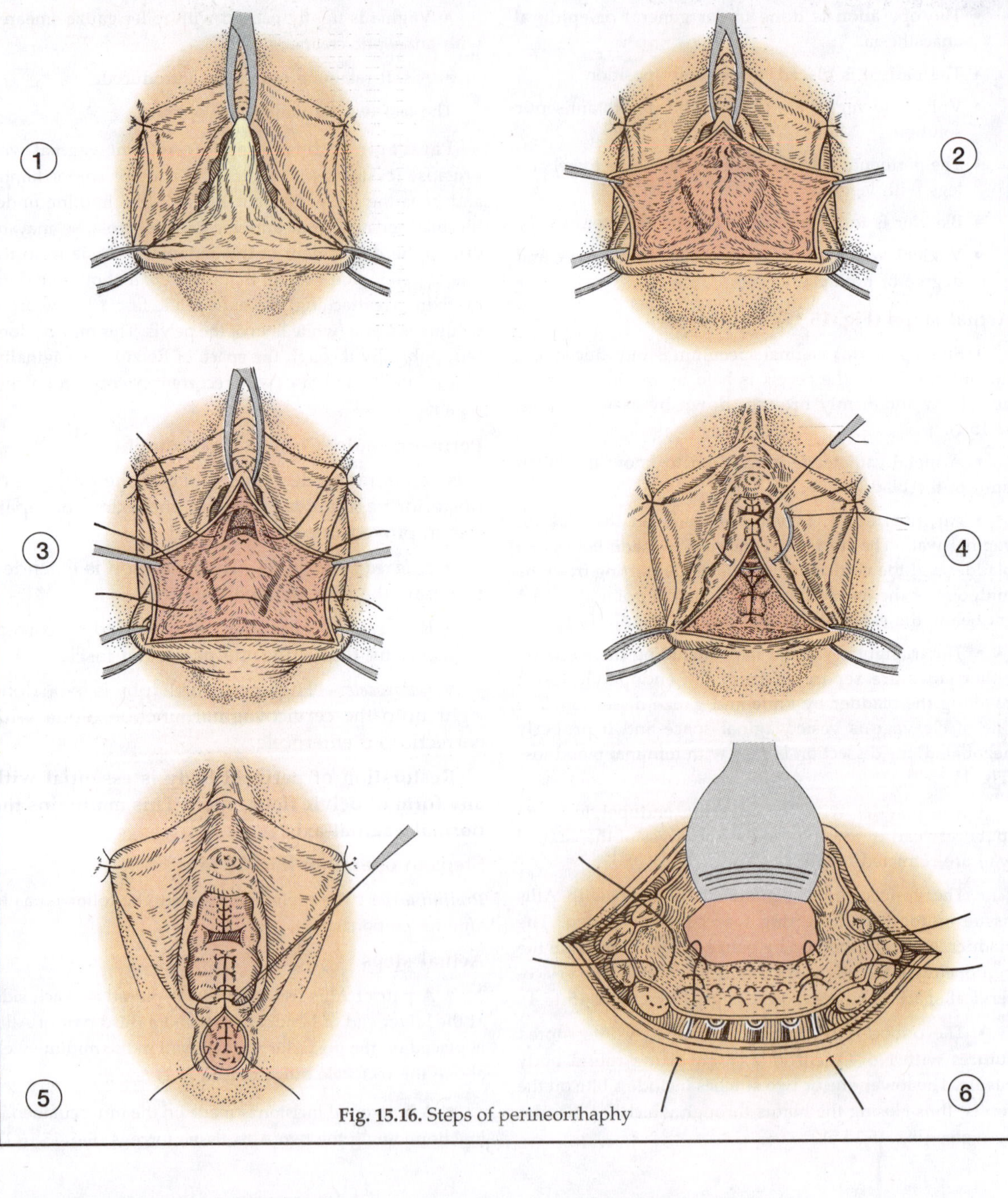

Fig. 15.16. Steps of perineorrhaphy

- Two or three interrupted sutures are placed through the levator ani and fibromuscular tissues of the perineal body using No. 'I' catgut. The rectum should be pressed back by finger while the sutures are placed. The knots are to be placed at a later stage (Fig. 15.16.3).
- The cut margins of the posterior vaginal wall are approximated, starting from the apex using No. 'O' catgut until it reaches upto the perineal body (Fig. 15.16.4).
- The knots are now placed to the sutures passed through the perineal body.
- The rest of the posterior vaginal wall and the skin margins are apposed by interrupted catgut sutures (Fig. 15.16.5).
- Toileting of the vagina is done.
- Tight vaginal pack is optional.

REPAIR OF ENTEROCELE AND VAULT PROLAPSE (FIG. 15.17)

Enterocele is almost always associated with genital prolapse. Along with repair operation, enterocele is to be corrected **transvaginally**. The principles of correction are to obliterate the neck of the enterocele sac as high as possible by purse string suture, to excise the excess peritoneal sac and approximation of the uterosacral ligaments (Fig. 15.17).

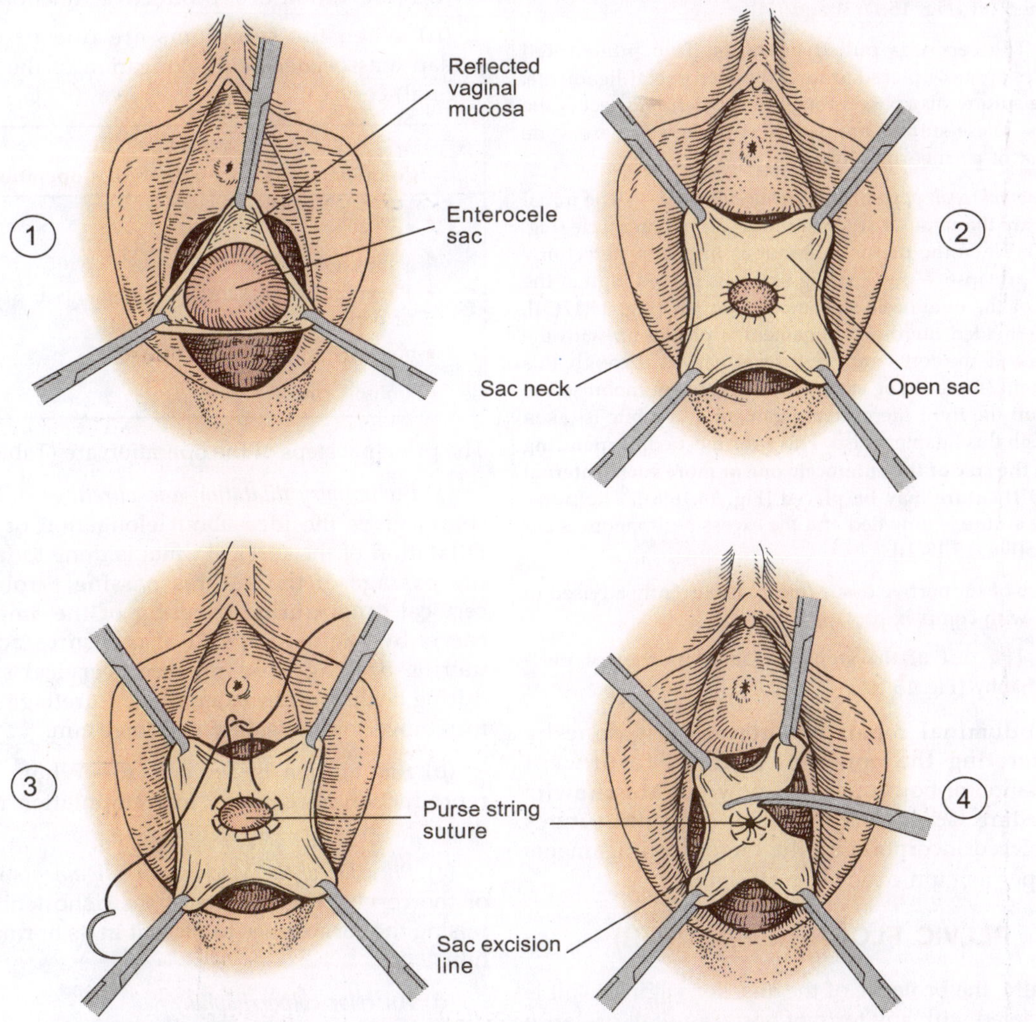

Fig. 15.17. Steps of enterocele repair operation with cervix still present — 1. Dissection to expose the enterocele. 2. To open the sac and reduce the contents if any. 3. A purse string suture is placed at the neck of the sac and tied. 4. The excess peritoneum is resected.

Actual steps

• An inverted 'T' shaped incision is made with the vertical arm of the 'T' extending up to the apex of the vaginal vault and the horizontal arm, along the mucocutaneous border (Fig. 15.16.1).

• Dissection is carried out to expose the enterocele sac [see Fig. 15.17(1)].

• The sac is opened, the contents (bowel, omentum) are pushed away [Fig. 15.17(2)].

• The peritoneum of the posterior *cul-de-sac* is dissected off the anterior surface of the rectum and lower sigmoid and excised.

• A purse string suture (2-0 vicryl) is placed high at the neck of the sac and tied. The excess peritoneum is resected off [Fig. 15.17(3) and (4)].

• The cervix is pulled upwards. Two interrupted sutures are now placed around the uterosacral ligaments. These sutures also pass through the posterior aspect of the cervix. These sutures are tied. Rest of the steps are same as that of perineorrhaphy.

Vaginal repair of posthysterectomy enterocele — The initial steps are the same as described in repair of enterocele (Fig. 15.17). When the uterus is absent as in posthysterectomy vault prolapse, a purse string suture is passed high at the neck of the enterocele sac and left untied [Fig. 15.17(3)]. The left sided uterosacral ligament is picked up with the fingers of the left hand. Suture is passed through this ligament (ureter to be excluded). Fingers are mobilised to pick up the right uterosacral ligament and a bite is taken through this ligament also. This suture is tied. **Depending upon the size of the enterocele one or more such (internal McCall) suture may be placed [Fig. 15.16(6)].** The purse string suture is now tied and the excess peritoneum is cut away [Fig. 15.17(4)].

Use of supportive tissue (mesh) is currently advised in cases with complex prolapse.

• The rest of the steps are same as that of perineorrhaphy (Fig. 15.16).

Abdominal repair of enterocele is done by obliterating the pouch of Douglas to prevent herniation of bowel. This is known as **Moschowitz procedure**. Generally three to four concentric sutures are placed incorporating the uterosacral ligaments and peritoneum over the rectosigmoid.

PELVIC FLOOR REPAIR (PFR)

Usually, the prolapse of the anterior vaginal wall is associated with any form of posterior wall prolapse and relaxed perineum. As such, the corrective operation is known as pelvic floor repair. **This includes anterior colporrhaphy and colpoperineorrhaphy.** It should be emphasized that the pelvic floor repair is not the operation for uterine descent. But as the uterine descent is most frequently associated with prolapse of the vaginal wall, pelvic floor repair has to be done along with operation for uterine descent.

FOTHERGILL'S OR MANCHESTER OPERATION

The operation is designed to correct uterine descent associated with cystocele and rectocele where **preservation of the uterus** is desirable.

The indications are :

(i) Preservation of reproductive function.

(ii) When the symptoms are due to vaginal prolapse associated with elongation of the (supravaginal) cervix.

Table 15.4
Composite steps of Forthergill's operation

- Preliminary D + C.
- Amputation of cervix.
- Plication of Mackenrodt's ligaments in front of cervix.
- Anterior colporrhaphy.
- Colpoperineorrhaphy.

The principal steps of the operation are (Table 15.4) :

(a) *Preliminary dilatation and curettage* — Uterine sound gives the idea about elongation of cervix. **Dilatation** of the cervical canal is done to facilitate the passage of the sutures passing through the cervical canal during covering of the amputated cervix by vaginal flaps. It also ensures adequate uterine drainage and prevents cervical stenosis during healing of the external os. **Curettage** is done to remove the unhealthy endometrium.

(b) *Amputation of the cervix* — Where future reproduction is required, low amputation is to be done.

(c) *Plication of the Mackenrodt's ligaments* in front of the cervix. This facilitates their shortening and raising the cervix so as to place it in its normal position.

(d) *Anterior colporrhaphy.*

(e) *Colpoperineorrhaphy.*

If the family is completed, vaginal sterilisation is to be done.

STEPS OF OPERATION

Preliminaries

The preliminaries are the same as those followed in anterior colporrhaphy.

Actual steps

- Preliminary D + C.
- The next step is like that of anterior colporrhaphy upto the pushing up the bladder.
- The posterior lip of the cervix is to be held with vulsellum and the cervix is drawn upwards.
- A pair of Allis forceps is placed in the midpoint of the posterior cervicovaginal junction.
- The anterior transverse incision is now extended posteriorly across the posterior cervicovaginal junction. The lateral and posterior vaginal wall is dissected off from the cervix by scissors and finger dissection.
- The Mackenrodt's ligament with descending cervical artery of either side is clamped at a higher level of amputation, cut and replaced by ligature (chromic catgut No. '1').
- The presence of enterocele should be searched for and if detected, to be repaired (Fig. 15.17).
- The cervix is now amputated at the calculated level.
- Anterior lip of the amputated cervix is now held with single-toothed vulsellum.
- The posterior lip of the amputated cervix is covered by the vaginal flap using a **Sturmdorff suture** (vide Figs. 15.18A and B) or by Bonney's method.

In **Bonney's method**, a catgut stitch is fixed at the apex of the posterior vaginal flap. The ends of the ligature are passed through the cervical canal and are taken out laterally on either side of new posterior fornix. The ends of the ligature are tied in the midline.

- The cut ends of the Mackenrodt's ligament are sutured to the anterior surface of the cervix (Fig. 15.18C). Alternatively, the ligaments are fixed using **Fothergill's stitch** (Fig. 15.18D). Fothergill's stitch is used to make the uterus anteverted. The stitch passes through the following tissues in sequence. Vaginal skin at the level of the Fothergill's lateral point → Mackenrodt's ligament → through the cervical tissue from outside inwards → cervical tissue from inside outwards → Mackenrodt's liga-ment of the other side → vaginal skin (Fothergill's lateral point) of the other side.
- Pubocervical fascia is approximated as in anterior colporrhaphy.
- Redundant portion of the vaginal mucosa is excised.
- The cut margins of the vagina are apposed by interrupted sutures.
- Posterior colpoperineorrhaphy is performed.
- Toileting the vagina is done.
- Vaginal pack is given.
- Self retaining catheter is introduced.

Complications : See Table 15.5 (p. 216).

VAGINAL HYSTERECTOMY WITH PELVIC FLOOR REPAIR

The operation is often designated as Ward Mayo's operation named after Mayo (1915) and Ward (1919) both from United States.

Removal of the uterus per vaginam (vaginal hysterectomy) is mostly done in cases of uterine prolapse. It should be emphasised that hysterectomy is not the surgery for the prolapse. It is the associated repair of the pelvic floor (PFR) which is the corrective surgery for prolapse.

Indications

- Uterovaginal prolapse in postmenopausal women.
- Genital prolapse in perimenopausal age group along with diseased uterus like DUB, unhealthy cervix or small submucous fibroid requiring hysterectomy.
- As an alternative to Fothergill's operation where family is completed.
- As an alternative to abdominal hysterectomy in undescended uterus either as a routine or in selected cases where abdominal approach is unsafe. PFR is not done in such cases.
- As an alternative to laparoscopic assisted vaginal hysterectomy (LAVH) in selected cases of undescended uterus. Compared to LAVH, vaginal hysterectomy is less expensive and the perioperative morbidity is no different (see p. 569).

Principles of the operation in prolapse

- Removal of the uterus through vaginal route.
- Correction of enterocele, if any.
- Approximation of the pedicles in the midline to have a good buttress.
- Fixation of the uterosacral ligaments to the vault to prevent vault prolapse.

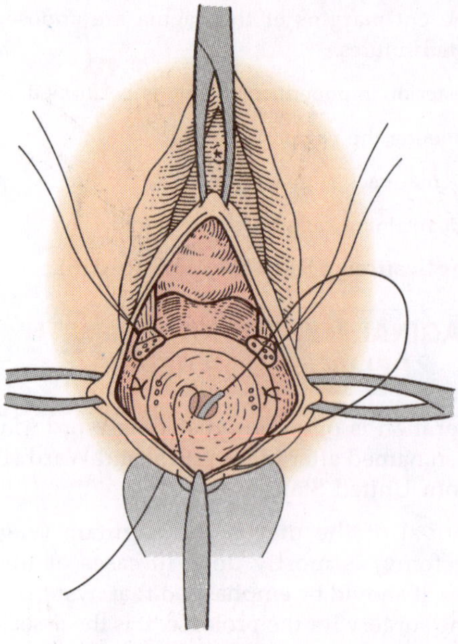

Fig.15.18(A). After amputation of the cervix, the raw posterior lip of the cervix is covered by the posterior vaginal mucosa using Sturmdorff suture

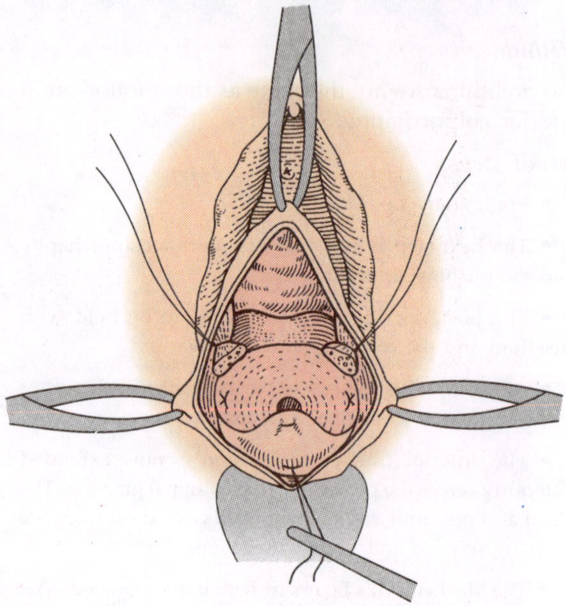

Fig.15.18(B). The knot is tied in the new posterior fornix

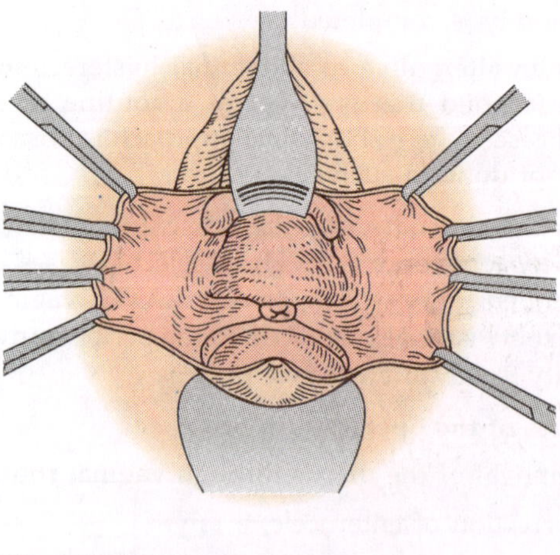

Fig.15.18(C). Approximation of the cut ends of the Mackenrodt's ligament and fixing them in front of the cervix

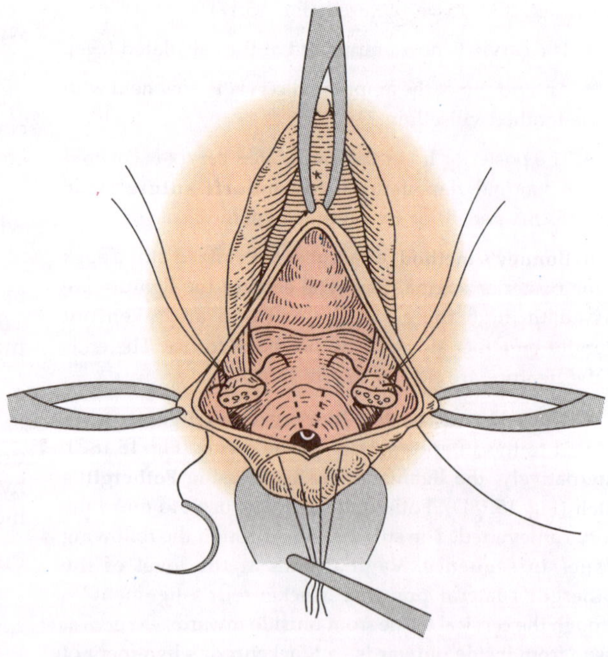

Fig.15.18(D). Approximation of the cut ends of the Mackenrodt's ligaments in front of the cervix using Fothergill's stitch

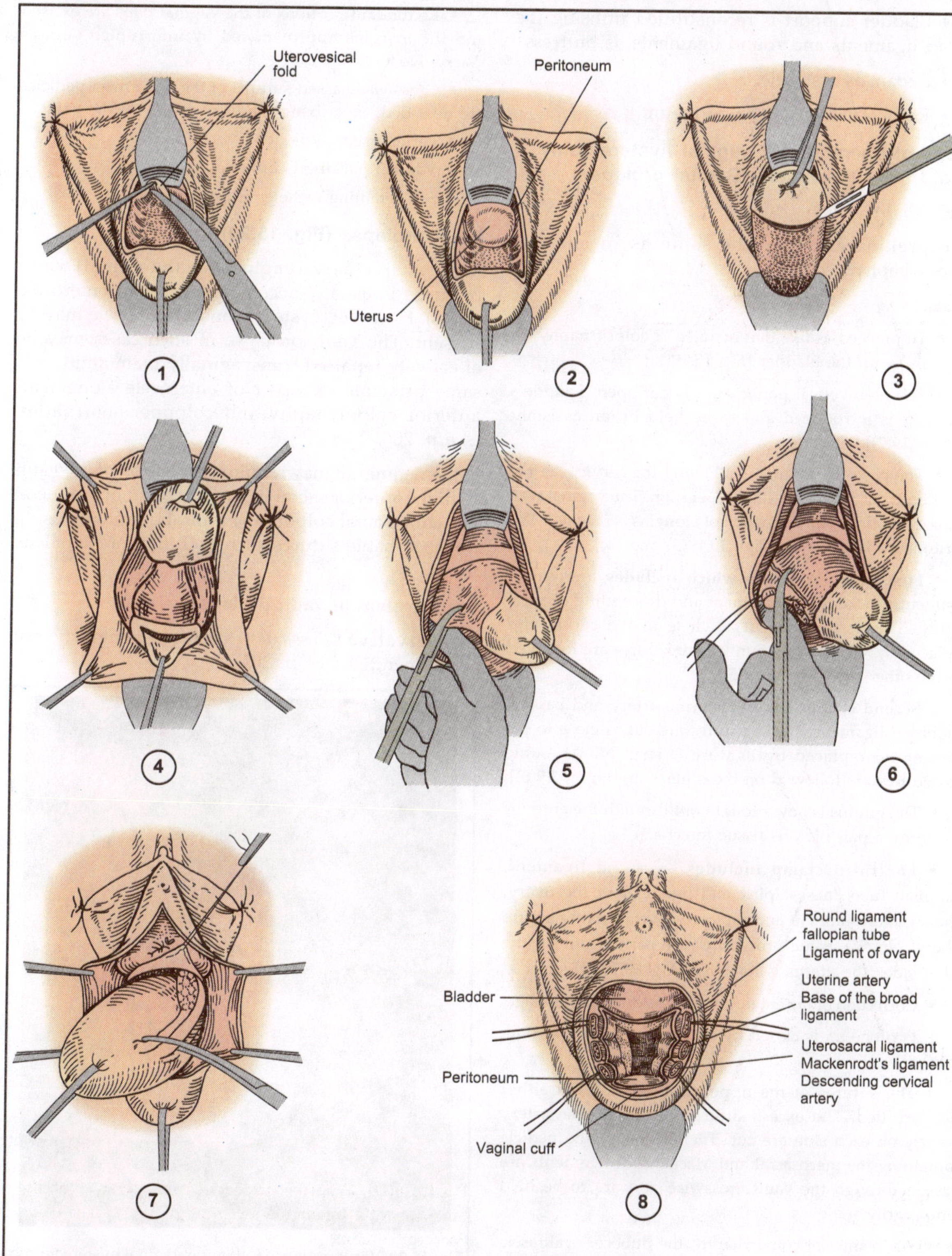

Fig.15.19. Principal steps of vaginal hysterectomy

- Bladder support is reconstituted utilising the broad ligaments and round ligaments as buttress.
- Repair of cystocele.
- Reconstruction of the perineum.

Steps of operation for vaginal hysterectomy (Fig. 15.19) (Indication—Genital prolapse)

Preliminaries

The preliminaries are the same as in anterior colporrhaphy.

Actual steps

- To proceed as like that of anterior colporrhaphy up to pushing up the bladder [Fig. 15.19(1)].
- The uterovesical peritoneum is cut open. Landon's retractor is introduced and to be held by an assistant [Fig. 15.19(2)].
- The posterior vaginal wall along the cervicovaginal junction is cut as in Fothergill's operation. The vaginal wall is dissected down till the pouch of Douglas is reached. The peritoneum is cut open [Figs. 15.19(3) and (4)].
- **First clamp is placed which includes** uterosacral ligament, Mackenrodt's ligament and descending cervical artery. The tissues are cut as close to the cervix and replaced by Vicryl No. 1. Similar procedures are followed on the other side [Fig. 15.19(5)].
- **Second clamp includes** uterine artery and base of the broad ligament. The structures are cut as close to the uterus and replaced by ligature (Vicryl No. 1). Same procedures are followed on the other side [Fig. 15.19(6)].
- The fundus is now brought out through the anterior pouch by a pair of Allis tissue forceps.
- **The third clamp includes** — round ligament, fallopian tube, mesosalpinx and ligament of the ovary. The structures are cut and replaced by transfixing suture (Vicryl No. '1'). Same procedures are carried out on the other side. The uterus is removed [Fig. 15.19(7)].
- Correction of the enterocele is to be done at this stage.
- Peritoneum is closed by a purse string suture [Fig. 15.19(8)].
- The sutures of the uppermost pedicles on either side are tied. The excess sutures of the uterine artery pedicle on each side are cut. The sutures of the pedicle containing the uterosacral and Mackenrodt ligaments are passed through the vault crosswise and are to be held temporarily.
- As in anterior colporrhaphy, the pubocervical fascia is approximated and fixed to the uppermost tied broad ligament pedicles to close the hiatus.
- Redundant portions of the vaginal flaps are excised and the margins approximated by interrupted sutures (Vicryl No.'O').
- Crosswise passed sutures of the lowermost pedicles are now tied, thus fixing the ligaments with the vault.
- Perineorrhaphy is done.
- Vaginal packing is optional.
- Self retaining catheter is introduced.

Vault prolapse (Fig. 15.20)

Posthysterectomy (vaginal or abdominal) vault prolapse is usually accompanied by an enterocele (70 %). However, cystocele and or rectocele may be present. The vault prolapse in such cases may be effectively repaired transvaginally maintaining the same principle of repair of enterocele along with anterior colporrhaphy and colpoperineorrhaphy (see p. 206, 207).

Sometimes, it may require suspension of the vault with the anterior sacral ligament infront of 3rd sacral vertebra (sacral colpopexy) transabdominally using nonabsorbable sutures such as Teflon or Mersilene mesh.

Management of vault prolapse

Conservative : *Pessary treatment*—generally not recommended (see p. 205).

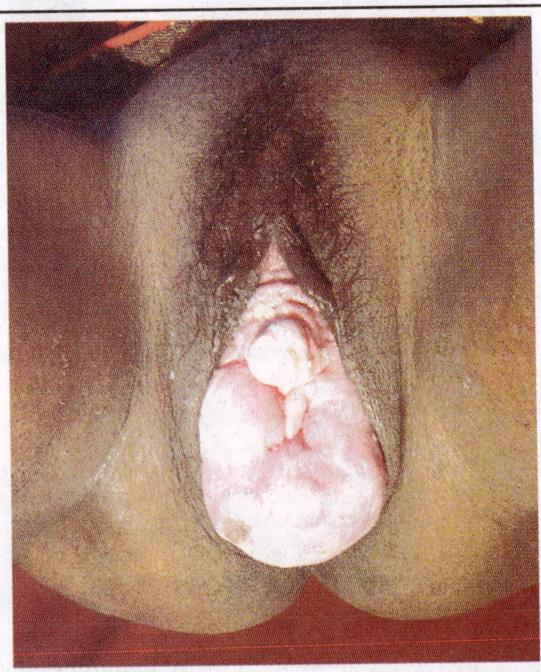

Fig. 15.20. Vault prolapse following vaginal hysterectomy. Scar is seen anteriorly.

Surgical :

Transvaginal approach

- Repair of enterocele along with pelvic floor repair (see p. 209).
- Le Fort operation.
- Colpocleisis (cases following hysterectomy).
- Sacrospinous colpopexy.

Abdominal approach

- Vault suspension (sacral colpopexy).

Le Fort operation

The procedure is almost obsolete. It may be done in old age with procidentia when the patient is unfit for longer duration of surgery as vaginal hysterectomy with PFR. There should not be any uterine or pelvic pathology. Cervical cytology (pap smear) should be normal. The operation can be done under local anaesthesia.

The principle steps of the operation are :

- Denudation of rectangular vaginal flap from the anterior and posterior vaginal walls.
- Apposition of the denuded anterior and posterior vaginal walls by chromic catgut. Two small channels are thus left in the vagina one on either side for drainage.

The complications include — pyometra and urinary stress incontinence.

Colpocleisis (after hysterectomy)

Denudation of vaginal mucosa is done all round. Successive purse string absorbable sutures are placed from above downwards to appose the vaginal walls. It is a simple, safe and effective operation for a woman who is no longer interested in coital function.

Sacrospinous colpopexy is done by fixing the vaginal vault to the sacrospinous ligament on the right side. This procedure may cause damage to bowel, ureter or the pudendal vessels. It has higher failure rates.

Abdominal approach

Vault suspension (Sacral colpopexy) : Principle of the operation is to suspense the vaginal vault to be anterior longitudinal ligament in front of the 3rd sacral vertebra. Non-absorbable suture material (Mersilene or Gore-Tex mesh) is used.

Actual steps

- Abdomen is opened by vertical or transverse incision.
- A vertical incision is made on the posterior peritoneum over the sacral hollow while the rectosigmoid is pulled up laterally.
- Lateral angles of the vagina are identified and grasped with Allis tissue forceps.
- Two strips or Mersilene or Gore-Tex mesh (1.5 cm wide) are fixed to the vaginal angles and are pulled up in the midline. The other ends are fixed to the anterior longitudinal ligament in front of 3rd sacral vertebra with proper tension.
- Posterior peritoneum is sewn over the strips to make them retroperitoneal.

Complications : Stress urinary incontinence is an important one.

Laparoscopic sacrocolpopexy is found to be effective with similar result to open sacrocolpopexy.

Effectiveness of "total mesh" (sheet of synthetic material) surgery to act as a new pelvic floor is not established. Complications are : mesh erosion, infection and fistula formation.

CERVICOPEXY OR SLING OPERATION (PURANDARE'S OPERATION)

The operation is indicated in **congenital** or **nulliparous prolapse** without cystocele where the cervix is pulled up mechanically through abdominal route. Strips of rectus sheath of either side passed extraperitoneally are stitched to the anterior surface of the cervix by silk.

Principle steps of the operation

- A transverse abdominal incision is made through the skin and fat.
- Two facial strips (rectus sheath) of 1.5 cm wide are dissected off, keeping its lateral attachment at the lateral border of the rectus muscle intact.
- The peritoneal cavity is opened in the midline. Bladder peritoneum is dissected off and the uterine isthmus is exposed mobilising the bladder.
- The medial ends of the facial strips are now brought down between the leaves of the broad ligament to this site of uterine isthmus. (This procedure is technically similar as described in Gilliam operation p. 574).
- The free edges of the facial strips are now fixed at the uterine isthmus with a sturdy bite using silk. This is done after adjusting the correct position of the uterus.
- Bladder peritoneum is repaired and abdomen is closed in layers. This operation may be combined with **Moschcowitz procedure**. Instead of fascial strips, currently non-absorbable (Marlex or Gore-Tex) tape is used for this purpose.

To know much details and variations of all the operations, the readers are requested to consult books of operative gynaecology.

COMPLICATIONS OF VAGINAL REPAIR OPERATIONS

Complications of PFR

Operative

- Haemorrhage — The haemorrhage may at times be brisk. The hypovolaemic state can be tackled by infusion and blood transfusion.
- Trauma — The bladder in anterior colporrhaphy or rectum in perineorrhaphy may be injured. The injury should be effectively repaired else, either VVF or RVF may develop later on.

Postoperative : **Urinary**

- Retention of urine is a common complication.

This is due to:

(i) Spasm, oedema and tenderness of pubococcygeus muscle.
(ii) Oedema of the urethral wall.
(iii) Reflex from the wounds.

- Infection leading to cystitis.

Haemorrhage

Primary haemorrhage occurs within 24 hours. **It is due to** imperfect haemostasis at operation or due to slipping of the ligature.

Along with the resuscitative procedures, the patient is to be brought to the operation theatre. Under anaesthesia, the suture sites in the vagina, both anterior and posterior are explored and haemostatic sutures are given. The vagina should be packed tightly with dry roller gauze which should be removed after 24 hours without anaesthesia.

Secondary haemorrhage occurs usually between 5-10th day but may occur even in the 3rd week. **It is due to sepsis of the wound.** If the haemorrhage is brisk, along with resuscitative procedures, the patient is to be brought to the operation theatre and under general anaesthesia, the vagina is explored. The clots are removed to find any bleeding point. **If only generalised oozing is found**, tight intravaginal pack using dry roller gauze is enough. **If bleeding point is visible**, haemostatic sutures should be given followed by vaginal packing. The plug should be removed after 24 hours. Antibiotics are to be started again.

Sepsis: Infection occurs on the vaginal or perineal wounds. Rarely, disruption of the perineal wound occurs.

Late:

- Dyspareunia.
- Recurrence of prolapse.
- VVF following bladder injury.
- RVF following rectal injury.

COMPLICATIONS OF VAGINAL HYSTERECTOMY WITH PFR

All the complications mentioned in PFR operation may occur, at times with increased intensity. Additional complications include:

Immediate

- Vault cellulitis
- Pelvic abscess
- Thrombophlebitis (see p. 569)
- Pulmonary embolism (see p. 569)

Late: • Vault prolapse (see p. 214)

Table 15.5
COMPLICATIONS OF FOTHERGILL'S OPERATION

During operation	• Haemorrhage • Injury to the bladder and rectum
Postoperative	• Retention of urine or cystitis • Haemorrhage—primary or secondary • Infection
Late	• Dyspareunia • Cervical stenosis–haematometra • Infertility • Cervical incompetency • Cervical dystocia in labour

CHRONIC INVERSION

Definition

Inversion is a condition where the uterus becomes turned inside out; the fundus prolapsing through the cervix.

Causes

- Incomplete obstetric inversion unnoticed or left uncared following failure to reduce for a variable period of 4 weeks or more.
- Submucous myomatous polyp arising from the fundus → traction effect (Fig. 15.21).

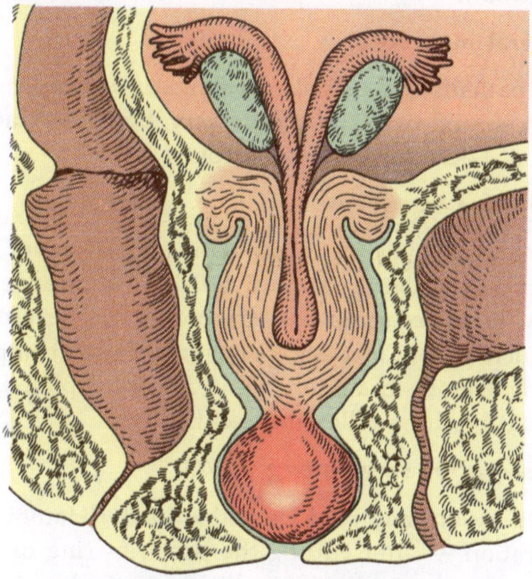

Fig. 15.21. Chronic incomplete inversion due to fundal fibroid (diagrammatic)

- Sarcomatous changes of fundal fibroma → infiltration of malignancy into the myometrium → softening of the wall.
- Senile inversion following high amputation of the cervix. It is probably due to cervical atony and incompetence.

Types

Two types are described in chronic inversion.

- **Incomplete** — The fundus protrudes through the cervix and lying inside the vagina.
- **Complete** — Whole of the uterus including the cervix are inverted. The vagina may also be involved in the process.

Symptoms

- Sensation of something coming down per vaginam.
- Irregular vaginal bleeding.
- Offensive vaginal discharge.

Signs

Inspection (Fig. 15.22)

The protruding mass has got the following features :

(i) Globular, (ii) No opening in the leading part, (iii) Shaggy look, (iv) Tumour may be present at the bottom.

Per vaginam : (a) The cervical rim is felt high up in incomplete variety but not felt in complete one. (b) Cup-shaped depression at the fundus is felt or the uterus is not felt in position.

Rectal examination : Rectoabdominal examination is more informative to note the fundal depression or displacement of the uterus.

Sound test : Demonstration of shortness or absence of uterine cavity using an uterine sound is reasonably confirmative.

EUA : At times, it is needed to confirm the diagnosis.

The diagnostic difficulty is much when inversion is secondary to a fibroid polyp or sarcoma and the inversion is incomplete, filling the vagina. A portion is to be removed from the tumour mass for histological examination to differentiate between a simple fibroid or sarcoma.

Differential diagnosis

Chronic inversion has to be differentiated from:

(i) Fibroid polyp.

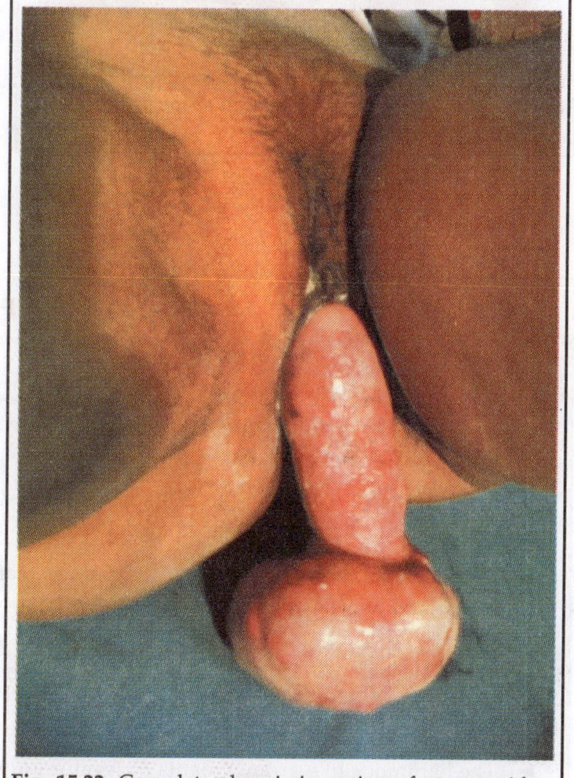

Fig. 15.22. Complete chronic inversion of uterus with a fundal fibroid [*By courtesy* : Dept. of Obst & Gynae., Govt. Maternity Hospital, Osmania Medical College, Hyderabad]

(ii) Uterine prolapse.

(iii) Prolapsed hypertrophied ulcerated cervix.

(iv) Fungating cervical malignancy.

In fibroid polyp — The uterus is in normal position and the uterine sound can be passed into the uterine cavity. In difficulty, examination under anaesthesia may be required (Fig. 15.23).

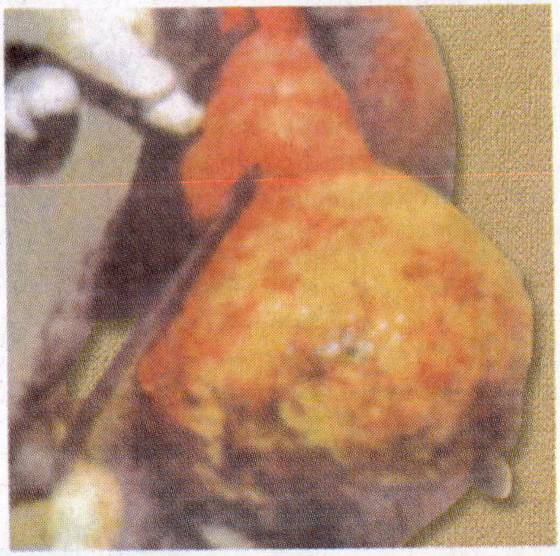

Fig. 15.23. Cervical fibroid polyp confusing diagnosis with chronic inversion. Note the uterine sound into the cervical canal

Treatment

General measures

The patients are usually anaemic. Prior improvement should be made if necessary, by blood transfusion. Local sepsis is to be controlled.

Definitive treatment

There is no place of manipulative replacement by taxis. Rectification should be done by surgery. Preservation or removal of the uterus is determined by such factors like age, parity, associated complicating factors. If hysterectomy is contemplated, it should be done following rectification.

Conservative surgery (see p. 573)

Rectification may be done abdominally (Haultain's operation — after cutting the posterior ring of the cervix) or vaginally (Spinelli's operation — after cutting the anterior ring of the cervix). Following Haultain's operation, some form of suspension operation has to be done to prevent posterior adhesions.

Contemplating polypectomy in suspected inversion, prior confirmation by 'sound test' is mandatory. **It is a sound policy to remove the tumour by shelling from its capsule rather than dividing the pedicle in such cases.**

KEY POINTS

- Retroversion of the uterus is quite common and is present in about 15-20 per cent of normal women. Emptying the bladder prior to its diagnosis is mandatory. Retroversion *per se* has got no adverse effect on fertility or early pregnancy.
- Pelvic Organ Prolapse is the prolapse of the pelvic organs into the vaginal canal. The important risk factors for prolapse is history of vaginal birth and age of the woman.
- Important support structures of uterus are the cardinal, uterosacral, pubocervical ligaments, endopelvic fascia, levator ani muscle (pubococcygeus, iliococcygeus, levator plate) and the perineal body.

  Prolapse is due to a combination of injury to the neuromuscular as well as supporting structures.
- Aetiology of genital prolapse includes the anatomical factors as well as the different clinical factors (p. 198).
- The hammock like arrangements of levator ani muscle, the condensed endopelvic fascia specially the Mackenrodt's ligaments are the cardinal support of the uterus. The levator plate and the perineal body maintains the normal vaginal axis (p. 196-198).

KEY POINTS

- Cystocele and urethrocele are more common with a gynaecoid pelvis than with android or anthropoid types. In cases of congenital prolapse, occult spina bifida should be looked for. Secondary vault prolapse is more following vaginal hysterectomy than abdominal one. Decubitus ulcer is a trophic ulcer. Malignancy is a rare association. Predominant urinary complaints in genital prolapse are difficulty in passing urine, incomplete evacuation, frequency, stress incontinence and rarely retention. To diagnose a third degree uterine prolapse, digital palpation is mandatory. Cystocele may be confused with Gartner's cyst. Uterine prolapse may be confused with congenital elongation of the cervix, chronic uterine inversion and fibroid polyp.
- The examination for prolapse should be done with the patient in dorsal position then standing and using Valsalva's manoeuvre for correct assessment.
- **Degree of urine prolapse** : ***1st degree*** : Uterus descends from its anatomical position but external uterine os remains in the vagina; ***2nd degree*** : External os protrudes outside the vaging but uterine body remains inside; ***3rd degree*** : Uterine body descends outside the vaginal introitus (procidentia). (Fig. 15.7, left hand side).
- **Newer classifications** of pelvic organ prolapse (POP) have been introduced for more objective quantification and to avoid confusion about the type and degree of prolapse. Prolapse must be documented in terms of anterior or posterior vaginal wall and the uterine descent (Table 15.2). In this regard fixed anatomic reference points are used (Fig. 15.10).
- Pessary treatment may be indicated in early pregnancy, puerperium, patient unfit for surgery or while the patients are waiting for operation.
- The surgical procedures for the management of prolapse are different. The type of surgery for an individual woman depends on her age, reproductive and sexual function as the type and degree of prolapse (p. 205).
- The component parts of Fothergill's operation are D + C, amputation of the cervix, plication of Mackenrodt's ligaments in front of the cervix, anterior colporrhaphy and colpoperineorrhaphy (p. 210).
- Posthysterectomy vault prolapse (0.1 – 10%) is usually accompanied by an enterocele (70%). Valut prolapse can be repaired either by vaginal or by abdominal route. Colpocleisis is an easy, safe and effective method for a woman who is no longer interested in coital function.
- When an enterocele is present, the sac should be dissected high up and ligated at its neck to prevent recurrence. McCall culdoplasty (p. 210) is done. External McCall suture is placed at a higher level than the internal McCall (p. 210). Vicryl (1-0) suture is passed through the left posterior vaginal wall, peritoneum, pararectal fascia (utero sacral ligament) and it is then carried over in front of the sigmoid colon to include the similar points on the right hand side. One or more such sutures may be placed. It is tied after the closure of the peritoneal purse string suture [Fig. 15.16(6)].
- Cervicopexy (sling operation) is the method of repair for a patient with congenital or nulliparous prolapse (p. 215).
- After pelvic floor repair, bladder drainage (transurethral catheter) for 3-5 days is generally necessary before normal voiding starts.
- The gynaecologic inversion is usually incomplete. Rectal examination is more informative in the diagnosis of chronic inversion. Chronic inversion may be confused with fibroid polyp, uterine prolapse, fungating cervical malignancy or prolapsed hypertrophied ulcerated cervix. There is no place of manipulative replacement of chronic inversion. Surgical rectification is done either abdominally (Haultain's) or vaginally (Spinelli's) (see p. 573).

Infertility

16

Definition

Infertility is defined as a failure to conceive within one or more years of regular unprotected coitus.

Primary infertility denotes those patients who have never conceived. **Secondary infertility** indicates previous pregnancy but failure to conceive subsequently.

Fecundability is defined as the probability of achieving a pregnancy within one menstrual cycle. In a healthy young couple it is 20 per cent. **Fecundity** is the probability of achieving a livebirth within a single cycle.

Incidence

Eighty per cent of the couples achieve conception if they so desire, within one year of having regular intercourse with adequate frequency (4-5 times a week). Another 10 per cent will achieve the objective by the end of second year. As such, 10 per cent remain infertile by the end of second year.

Factors responsible for fertility are :

- **Healthy spermatozoa** should be deposited high in the vagina at or near the cervix (male factor).
- The spermatozoa should undergo changes **(capacitation, acrosome reaction)** and acquire motility (cervical factor).
- The **motile spermatozoa** should ascend through the cervix into the uterine cavity and the fallopian tubes.
- There should be **ovulation** (ovarian factor).
- The fallopian tubes should be patent and the oocyte should be picked up by the fimbriated end of the tube (**tubal factor**).
- The spermatozoa should **fertilise** the oocyte at the ampulla of the tube.
- The embryo should reach the **uterine cavity** after 3-4 days of fertilisation.
- The **endometrium** should be receptive (by oestrogen, progesterone, IGF-1, cytokines, integrins) for **implantation** and the **corpus luteum** should function adequately.

Physiological consideration

Due to anovulation infertility is the rule prior to puberty and after menopause. But it should be remembered that the girl may be pregnant even before menarche and pregnancy is possible within few months of menopause. Conception is not possible during pregnancy as the pituitary gonadal axis is suppressed by hCG and hence no ovulation. During lactation, infertility is said to be relative. Despite the fact that the patient is amenorrhoeic during lactation, ovulation and conception can occur. However, in fully lactating women (breastfeeding 5-6 times a day and spending 60 minutes in 24 hours), pregnancy is unlikely up to 10 weeks postpartum.

CAUSES OF INFERTILITY

Conception depends on the fertility potential of both the male and female partner. **The male is directly responsible in about 30-40 per cent, the female in about 40-55 per cent and both are responsible in about 10 per cent cases.** The remaining 10 per cent, is **unexplained** in spite of thorough investigations with modern technical knowhow. It is also strange that 4 out of 10 patients of unexplained category become pregnant within 3 years without having any specific treatment.

It is also emphasised that the relative subfertility of one partner may sometimes be counterbalanced by the high fertility of the other.

Faults in the male (Table 16.1)

- Defective spermatogenesis

- Obstruction of the efferent duct system
- Failure to deposit sperm high in the vagina
- Errors in the seminal fluid.

Defective spermatogenesis

FSH stimulates spermatogenesis from basal cells of the seminiferous tubules. Sertoli cells envelope the germ cells and support spermatogenesis. Sertoli cell function is controlled by FSH and testosterone. Scrotal temperature should be 1°–2°F less than the body temperature. LH is required for the synthesis of testosterone from the Leydig cells. FSH also stimulates the Sertoli cells to produce androgen binding proteins (ABP) and inhibin B. ABP binds to testosterone and dihydrotestosterone to maintain the local high concentration of androgens. Spermatogenesis and sperm maturation need a high androgenic environment. Inhibin B inhibits FSH secretion. Spermatogenesis is controlled predominantly by the genes on Y chromosome. **Approximately 74 days are required to complete the process of spermatogenesis.** Additional 12-20 days are needed for spermatozoa to travel the epididymis. **The causes of defective spermatogenesis are :**

- **Congenital**
  - **Undescended testes** — the hormone secretion remains unaffected, but the spermatogenesis is depressed. Vas deferens is absent (bilateral) in about 1-2 per cent of infertile males.
  - **Kartagener syndrome** (autosomal disease) there is loss of ciliary function and sperm motility.
  - **Hypospadias** causes failure to deposit sperm high in vagina.
- **Thermal factor** — The scrotal temperature is raised in conditions such as varicocele, big hydrocele or filariasis. Varicocele probably interferes with the cooling mechanism or increases catecholamine concentration. Other causes are using tight undergarment or working in hot atmosphere. In all these conditions, the depressed spermatogenesis may be temporary and reversible.
- **Infection** — (a) Mumps orchitis after puberty may permanently damage spermatogenesis. (b) The quality of the sperm is adversely affected by chronic systemic illness like bronchiectasis. Bacterial or viral infection of the seminal vesicle or prostate depresses the sperm count. (c) *T. mycoplasma* or *Chlamydia trachomatis* infection is also implicated.
- **General factors** — Chronic debilitating diseases, malnutrition or heavy smoking reduce spermatogenesis. Alcohol inhibits spermatogenesis either by suppressing Leydig cell synthesis of testosterone or possibly by suppressing gonadotrophin levels.
- **Endocrine** — Testicular failure due to gonadotrophin deficiency (**Kallmann's syndrome**) is rare. FSH level is raised in idiopathic testicular failure with germ cell hypoplasia (**Sertoli-cell-only-syndrome**). Hyperprolactinaemia is associated with impotence.

Table 16.1
Common causes of male infertility

Pre-testicular	Testicular	Post-testicular
Endocrine • Gonadotrophin deficiency • Thyroid dysfunction • Hyperprolactinaemia **Psychosexual** – Erectile dysfunction – Impotence **Drugs** – Antihypertensives – Antipsychotics **Genetic** – 47 XXY (p. 222) – Y chromosome deletions	• Immotile cilia (Kartagener) syndrome • Cryptorchidism • Infection (mumps orchitis) • Toxins : Drugs, Radiation (p. 222) • Varicocele • Immunologic (p. 232) • Sertoli-cell-only syndrome (p. 221) • Primary testicular failure • Oligoastheno-teratozoospermia	**Obstruction of efferent duct** • Congenital – Absence of Vas deferens (Cystic fibrosis) – Young's syndrome (p. 222) • Acquired Infection : Tuberculosis, Gonorrhoea • *Surgical* – Herneorrhaphy, – Vasectomy. **Others** • Ejaculatory failure • Retrograde ejaculation • Hypospadius • Bladder neck surgery

• **Genetic** — Common chromosomal abnormality in azoospermic male is Klinefelter's syndrome (47 XXY). Gene deletion have been detected in the long arm of Y chromosome (Yq) for patients with severe oligospermia.

• **Iatrogenic** — Radiation, cytotoxic drugs, nitrofurantoin, cimetidine, β blockers, antihypertensive, anticonvulsant and antidepressant drugs are likely to hinder spermatogenesis.

• **Immunological factor** — Antibodies against spermatozoal surface antigens may be the cause of infertility. This results in clumping of the spermatozoa after ejaculation.

Obstruction of the efferent ducts — The efferent ducts may be obstructed by infection like tubercular, gonococcal or by surgical trauma (herniorrhaphy) following vasectomy. In **Young's syndrome** there is epididymal obstruction and bronchiectasis.

Failure to deposit sperm high in the vagina (coital problems)

- Erectile dysfunction
- Ejaculatory defect — premature, retrograde or absence of ejaculation
- Hypospadias.

Sperm abnormality — Loss of sperm motility (asthenozoospermia), abnormal sperm morphology (round headed sperm, teratozoospermia) are the important factors.

Errors in the seminal fluid

- Unusually high or low volume of ejaculate
- Low fructose content
- High prostaglandin content
- Undue viscosity.

CAUSES OF FEMALE INFERTILITY

According to FIGO manual (1990) causes are — tubal and peritoneal factors (25-35%), ovulatory factor (30-40%) and endometriosis (1-10%).

Ovarian factors — The ovulatory dysfunctions (dysovulatory) encompass :

- Anovulation or oligo-ovulation
- Decreased ovarian reserve (p. 503)
- Luteal phase defect (LPD)
- Luteinised unruptured follicle (LUF)

Anovulation or oligo-ovulation

The ovarian activity is totally dependant on the gonadotrophins and the normal secretion of gonadotrophins depends on the pulsatile release of GnRH from hypothalamus. As such, **ovarian dysfunction is likely to be linked with disturbed hypothalamo-pituitary-ovarian axis either primary or secondary from thyroid or adrenal dysfunction.**

Thus, the disturbance may result not only in anovulation but may also produce oligomenorrhoea or even amenorrhoea. Anovulatory cycles usually represent a lesser degree of disturbance with these normal pathways than does amenorrhoea. **Possible causes of anovulation** are given schematically.

As there is no ovulation, there is no corpus luteum formation. In the absence of progesterone, there is no secretory endometrium in the second half of the cycle. The other features of ovulation (later in the chapter) are absent.

Luteal phase defect (LPD)

In this condition there is inadequate growth and function of the corpus luteum. There is inadequate progesterone secretion. The life span of corpus luteum is shortened to less than 10 days. As a result, there is inadequate secretory changes in the endometrium which hinder implantation. LPD is due to defective folliculogenesis which again may be due to varied reasons. Drug induced ovulation, decreased level of FSH and/or LH, elevated prolactin, subclinical hypothyroidism, older women, pelvic endometriosis, dysfunctional uterine bleeding are the important causes.

Luteinised unruptured follicular syndrome (trapped ovum)

In this condition, the ovum is trapped inside the follicle which gets luteinised. The cause is obscure but may be associated with **pelvic endometriosis or with hyperprolactinaemia.**

Tubal and peritoneal factors are responsible for about 30-40 per cent cases of female infertility.

The obstruction of the tubes may be due to — (a) **Pelvic infections causing** : (i) Peritubal adhesions (ii) Endosalpingeal damage. (b) Previous tubal surgery or sterilisation. (c) Salpingitis isthmica nodosa (p. 168). (d) Tubal endometriosis (p. 168) and others. (e) Polyps or mucous debris within the tubal lumen, or tubal spasm.

Peritoneal factors — In addition to peritubal adhesions, even minimal endometriosis may produce infertility. Deep dyspareunia too often troubles the patient. The possible multifactorial mechanisms which operate in minimal endometriosis are depicted schematically below (Table 16.2).

Uterine factors — The endometrium must be sufficiently receptive enough for effective nidation and growth of the fertilised ovum. **The possible factors that hinder nidation are** uterine hypoplasia, inadequate secretory endometrium, fibroid uterus, endometritis (tubercular in particular), uterine synechiae or congenital malformation of uterus.

Cervical factors

Anatomic — Anatomic defects preventing sperm ascent may be due to congenital elongation of the cervix, second degree uterine prolapse and acute retroverted uterus. These conditions prevent the external os to bathe in the seminal pool. Pinhole os may at times be implicated, or the cervical canal may be occluded by a polyp.

Physiologic — The fault lies in the composition of the cervical mucus, so much that the spermatozoa fail to penetrate the mucus. The mucus may be scanty following amputation, conisation or deep cauterisation of the cervix. The abnormal constituents include excessive, viscous or purulent discharge as in chronic cervicitis. Presence of antisperm or sperm immobilising antibodies may be implicated as immunological factor of infertility.

Vaginal factors — Atresia vagina (partial or complete), transverse vaginal septum, septate vagina or narrow introitus causing dyspareunia are included in the congenital group.

Vaginitis and purulent discharge may at times be implicated but pregnancy too often occurs in presence of vaginitis, specific or nonspecific. However, dyspareunia may be the real problem in such cases.

Combined factors

- These include the presence of factors both in the male and female partners causing infertility.
- General factors : Advanced age of the wife beyond 35 is related but spermatogenesis continues throughout life although ageing reduces the fertility in male also.
- Infrequent intercourse, lack of knowledge of coital technique and timing of coitus to utilise the fertile period are very much common even amongst the literate couples.
- Apareunia and dyspareunia (see p. 541).
- Anxiety and apprehension.
- Use of lubricants during intercourse — which may be spermicidal.
- Immunological factors.

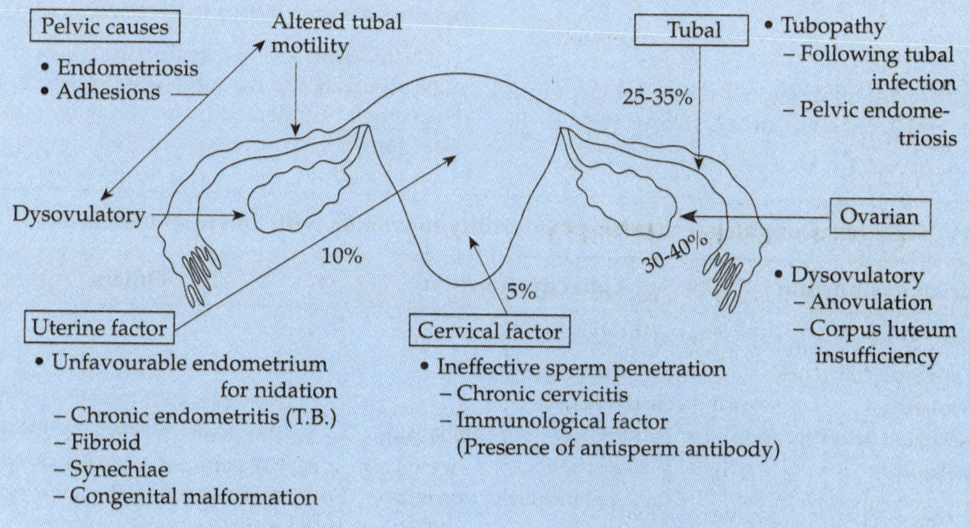

Scheme – 1 : Showing common causes of female infertility

INVESTIGATIONS OF INFERTILITY

Objectives of investigation

- To detect the aetiological factor(s).
- To rectify the abnormality in an attempt to improve the fertility.
- To give assurance with explanation to the couple if no abnormality is detected.

When to investigate? As per the definition, the infertile couple should be investigated after one year of regular unprotected exposure with adequate frequency. The interval is however, shortened to 6 months after the age of 35 of the woman and 40 years of man.

What to investigate? The basic investigations to be carried out are : (i) Semen analysis. (ii) Confirmation of ovulation and (iii) Confirmation of tubal patency.

It is important that both partners should come at the first visit. Detailed general and reproductive history should be taken in presence of both. However, the clinical examination of each partner is carried out separately. No one is to be blamed.

Clinical approach to investigation

- **Male** • **Female**

MALE

History

Age, duration of marriage, history of previous marriage and proven fertility if any, are to be noted.

A general medical history should be taken with special reference to sexually transmitted diseases, mumps orchitis after puberty, diabetes, recurrent chest infection or bronchiectasis. Relevant surgery such as herniorrhaphy, operation on testes or other surgery in the genital area are to be enquired. Occupational history should be directed towards exposure to excessive heat or radiation. Enquiry about the sexual history includes frequency of intercourse, full penetration of penis inside the vagina or orgasm in right time, whether either partner experiencing discomfort or lack of satisfaction. Social habits, particularly heavy smoking and alcohol are of importance.

Examination

A full physical examination is performed to determine the general state of health. Examination of the reproductive system includes — inspection and palpation of the genitalia. Attention should be paid to the size and consistency of the testicles. **Testicular volume** (measured by an orchidometer) should be at least 20 cm^3. Presence of varicocele should be elicited in the upright position.

Investigations

(a) **Routine investigations** include urine and blood examination including postprandial sugar.

(b) **Seminal fluid analysis — This should be the first step in investigation** because, if some gross abnormalities are detected (example being absence of sperm), the couple should be counselled for the need of assisted reproductive technology.

Collection — The collection is best done by masturbation failing which by coitus interruptus. The semen is collected in a clean wide mouthed dry glass jar. The sample so collected should be sent to

Table 16.2 : Possible mechanism of infertility in women with pelvic endometriosis

Ovarian dysfunction	Tubal dysfunction	Others
• Endocrinopathies (see p. 298) – Defective folliculogenesis – Anovulation – Luteal phase defect (p. 230) – LUFS (p. 230) – Hyperprolactinaemia (p. 548) • Oocyte maturation defect	• Altered tubal motility • Pelvic adhesions, tubal obstruction. • Distortion of normal tube and ovarian relationship. • Impaired pick up of oocyte by the fimbria.	• Dyspareunia (poor coital function, see p. 296, 541). • Abnormal peritoneal fluid (see p. 295). • Abnormal systemic immune response. • Increased sperm phagocytosis by macrophages. • Fertilisation and implantation failure. • Early miscarriage.

the laboratory as early as possible so that the examination can be performed within two hours. The coitus should be avoided for 2-3 days prior to the test (abstinence).

Normal values (Table 16.3) — The figures given are an average. Considerable variation occurs from person to person and at different times in any one individual.

It should be borne in mind that the sperm count gives reflection of the man's health status 74 days back, when actually the spermatozoa were produced.

As previously mentioned, there is wide range of normalcy and it is not wise to interpret the analysis as abnormal, if the values are found lower than mentioned. However, one should repeat the test at least twice at about two and half months interval, if the report is abnormal.

Table 16.3
Normal semen values as suggested by WHO (2002)

Volume	2.0 ml or more
pH	7.2-7.8
Sperm concentration	20 million/ml or more
Total sperm count	≥ 40 million per ejaculate
Motility	50 per cent or more progressive forward motility
Morphology	15 per cent or more normal form
Viability	75% or more living
Leucocytes	Less than 1 million/ml
Sperm agglutination	< 2 (scale 0-3)

In selected cases, biochemical tests of creatine phosphokinase and reactive oxygen species are done as sperm function tests. Creatinine phosphokinase helps sperm transport while reactive oxygen specis and the peroxides interfere with sperm function.

Normal male fertility requires a count of over 20 million spermatozoa per ml and a progressive motility of over 25 per cent. However, it is not rare to have pregnancy with a sperm count of 5 million per ml. If the semen analysis is normal and the wife confirms that ejaculation takes place in her vagina, no further investigations are needed in the male. Semen values normally vary widely. Two properly performed semen analysis at least 4 weeks apart should be done when one report is abnormal.

Nomenclature

- ***Aspermia*** : Failure of emission of semen (no ejaculate).
- ***Oligospermia/Oligozoospermia*** : Sperm count is less than 20 million per ml.
- ***Polyzoospermia*** : Count is more than 350 million/ml.
- ***Azoospermia*** : No spermatozoon in the semen.
- ***Asthenozoospermia*** : Reduced sperm motility. Leucocytospermia : Increased white cells in semen.
- ***Necrozoospermia*** : Spermatozoa are dead or motionless.
- ***Teratozoospermia*** : > 70% spermatozoa with abnormal morphology.
- ***Oligoasthenoteratozoospermia*** : Disturbance of all 3 variables.

In-depth evaluation

These are needed in cases of — (a) Azoospermia (b) Oligospermia (c) Low volume ejaculate (d) Problems of sexual potency. Further diagnostic protocols has been appropriately designed (Scheme 2).

- **Serum FSH, LH, testosterone, prolactin, and TSH** : Testicular dysfunction causes rise in FSH and LH. Low level of FSH and LH suggest hypogonadotrophic hypogonadism (see Scheme 2). Leydig cell dysfunction causes low testosterone and high LH level. Elevated prolactin due to pituitary adenoma may cause impotency.

- **Fructose content in the seminal fluid** — Its absence suggests congenital absence of seminal vesicle or portion of the ductal system or both.

- **Testicular biopsy** — is done to differentiate primary testicular failure from obstruction as a cause of azoospermia or severe oligospermia. **The biopsy material is to be sent in Bouin's solution and not in formol saline.**

Transrectal Ultrasound (TRUS) — is done to visualise the seminal vesicles, prostate and ejaculatory ducts obstruction. Indications of TRUS are : (i) Azoospermia or severe oligospermia with a normal testicular volume. (ii) Abnormal digital rectal examination. (iii) Ejaculatory duct abnormality (cysts, dilatation or calcification). (iv) Genital abnormality (hypospadius).

Vasogram is a radiographic study done to evaluate the ejaculatory duct obstruction. It is mostly replaced by TRUS.

- **Karyotype analysis** — This is to be done in cases with azoospermia or severe oligospermia and raised FSH. Klinefelter's syndrome (XXY) is the commonest. Micro

Scheme – 2 **Abnormal semen analysis (apparently unexplained)**

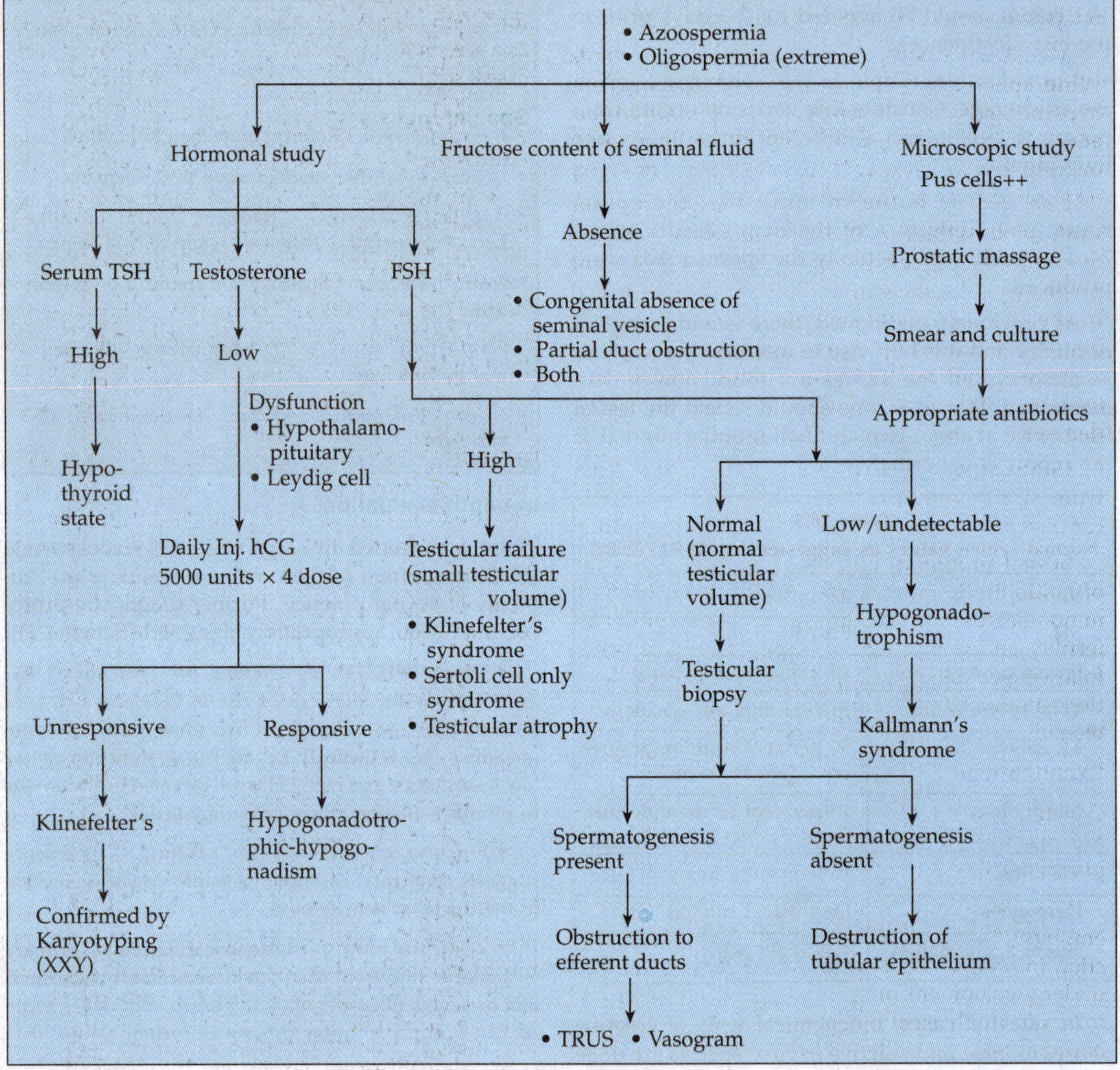

deletions of the long arm of Y chromosome can also cause severe seminal abnormalities.

• **Immunological tests** — Two types of antibodies have been described — sperm agglutinating and sperm immobilising; the latter is probably related to infertility. The antibodies are produced following infection (orchitis), trauma or vasectomy. These antibodies can be detected from the serum by the sperm immobilising test. Presence of sperm antibodies in the cervical mucous is demonstrated by **post-coital test** (see p. 111, 232).

• **Presence of plenty of pus cells** requires prostatic massage. The collected fluid is to be examined by staining and culture to detect the organisms and appropriate antibiotic sensitivity.

FEMALE

History

Age, duration of marriage, history of previous marriage with proven fertility if any, are to be noted.

A general medical history should be taken with special reference to tuberculosis, sexually transmitted disease, features suggestive of pelvic inflammation or diabetes.

The surgical history should be directed specially towards abdominal or pelvic surgery. This may be related to peritubal adhesions.

Menstrual history should be taken in details. Wide spectrum of abnormalities ranging from hypomenorrhoea – oligomenorrhoea to amenorrhoea are associated with disturbed hypothalamopituitary ovarian axis which may be either primary or secondary to adrenal or thyroid dysfunction.

Previous obstetric history — including number of pregnancies, the interval between them and pregnancy related complications are to be enquired. In the case of secondary infertility, the obstetric history is important. The history of premature rupture of the membranes or puerperal sepsis may be responsible for ascending infection and tubal damage.

Contraceptive practice should be elicited. Apart from IUCD which may produce PID, no other contraceptives have any adverse effect on fertility.

Sexual problems such as dyspareunia, and loss of libido are to be enquired. It should be borne in mind that the female orgasm is not essential for fertility and loss of semen from the vaginal orifice following coitus is normal. A psychosomatic evaluation should focus on general and infertility problems.

Examinations

General, systemic and gynaecological examinations are made to detect any abnormality which may hinder fertility.

General examination must be thorough – special emphasis being given to obesity or marked reduction in weight. Abnormal distribution of hairs or underdevelopment of secondary sex characters are to be noted. Physical features pertaining to endocrinopathies are carefully evaluated to detect features of PCOS, hirsutism and inappropriate galactorrhoea.

Systemic examination may accidentally detect such abnormalities like hypertension, organic heart disease, chronic renal lesion, endocrinopathies and alike.

Gynaecological examination includes adequacy of hymenal opening, evidences of vaginal infections, cervical tear or chronic infection, undue elongation of the cervix, uterine size, position and mobility, presence of unilateral or bilateral adnexal masses – fixed or mobile with or without tenderness and presence of nodules in the pouch of Douglas.

Speculum examination may reveal abnormal cervical discharge. The discharge is to be collected for Gram stain and culture. Cervical smear is taken as a screening procedure as a routine or in suspected cases.

Special Investigations

Guidelines

- In the presence of major fault in male such as azoospermia due to testicular destruction or intersex, there is very little scope to proceed for investigation for the female partner. However, considering the place of Assisted Reproductive Technology (ART) female investigation may not be withheld (p. 243).
- Similarly, when a major defect is detected in female such as müllerian agenesis or intersex, infertility investigations should be suspended. However, correctable abnormality should be rectified first prior to investigation, e.g. narrow vaginal introitus, overt hypothyroidism or diabetes mellitus.
- Noninvasive or minimal invasive methods are to be employed prior to major invasive one. However, it is not uncommon to have pregnancy soon after the first visit.
- Detection of abnormality of one factor does not negate investigation for another defect elsewhere. Multiple defects may be present in the same case, e.g. tubal defects may be associated with anovulation.
- Pregnancy following laparoscopy and dye test or hysterosalpingography is not uncommon. It is presumed that small flimsy adhesions or any mucus plug obstructing the tubal lumen is removed during such procedures. The cervical spasm may be relieved during dilatation.
- Genital tuberculosis as a cause of infertility is to be kept in mind specially in the developing countries. The association is as high as 10-15 per cent in contrast to a low figure of 0.5 per cent in the developed countries.

Ovarian factors

Ovarian dysfunctions (dysovulatory) commonly associated with infertility are :

- Anovulation or oligo-ovulation (infrequent ovulation).
- Luteal phase defect (LPD).
- Luteinised unruptured follicle (LUF).

DIAGNOSIS OF OVULATION

The various methods used in practice to detect ovulation are grouped as follows (see Table 16.4) :

- **Indirect** • **Direct** • **Conclusive**

Table 16.4 : Diagnosis of ovulation

Indirect
Menstrual history
Evaluation of peripheral or endorgan changes
• BBT
• Cervical mucus study
• Vaginal cytology
• Hormone estimation
– Serum progesterone
– Serum LH
– Serum oestradiol
– Urine LH
• Endometrial biopsy
Sonography
Direct
Laparoscopy
Conclusive
Pregnancy

INDIRECT

The indirect or presumptive evidences of ovulation are commonly used in clinical practice. **These are inferred from** :

- Menstrual history.
- Evaluation of peripheral or endorgan changes due to oestrogen and progesterone.
- Direct assays of gonadotrophins or steroid hormones preceeding, coinciding or succeeding the ovulatory process.

Menstrual history

The following features in relation to menstruation are strong evidences of ovulation.

- Regular normal menstrual loss between the age of 20-35.
- Midmenstrual bleeding (spotting) or pain or excessive mucoid vaginal discharge (Mittelschmerz syndrome).
- Features suggestive of premenstrual syndrome or primary dysmenorrhoea.

Evaluation of peripheral or endorgan changes (Table 16.4)

Basal body temperature (BBT)

Observation — **There is "biphasic pattern" of temperature variation in ovulatory cycle.** If pregnancy occurs, the rise of temperature sustains along with absence of the period. In anovulatory cycle, there is no rise of temperature throughout the cycle.

Principle — The rise of temperature is secondary to rise in progesterone output following ovulation. Progesterone is thermogenic. The primary reason for the rise is the increase in the production and secretion of norepinephrine which is also thermogenic.

Procedures — The patient is instructed to take her oral temperature **daily on waking in the morning before rising out of the bed.** The temperature is recorded on a special chart. Days when intercourse takes place should also be noted on the chart for better evaluation of coital frequency.

Interpretation — The body temperature maintaining throughout the first half of the cycle is raised to 0.5° to 1°F (0.2°-0.5°C) following ovulation. The rise sustains throughout the second half of the cycle and falls about 2 days prior to the next period – called "biphasic pattern" (Fig. 16.1). There may be a drop in the temperature to about 0.5°F before the rise and almost coincides with either LH surge or ovulation. The demonstrable rise actually occurs about 2 days after the LH peak and with a peripheral level of progesterone to greater than 5 ng/ml.

Clinical importance — Maintenance of BBT chart during investigation is of help in determining ovulation and timing of post-coital test, endometrial biopsy, cervical mucus or vaginal cytology study for ovulation. It also helps the couple to determine the most fertile period, if the cycle is irregular.

Limitations of BBT

- BBT indicates ovulation retrospectively.
- It cannot predict ovulation precisely with time.
- Rarely ovulation has been observed though BBT is monophasic.

How long to keep the record?

It should not be continued for more than 3-4 months for investigation purpose. However, it has to be maintained for longer periods during management of ovulation induction.

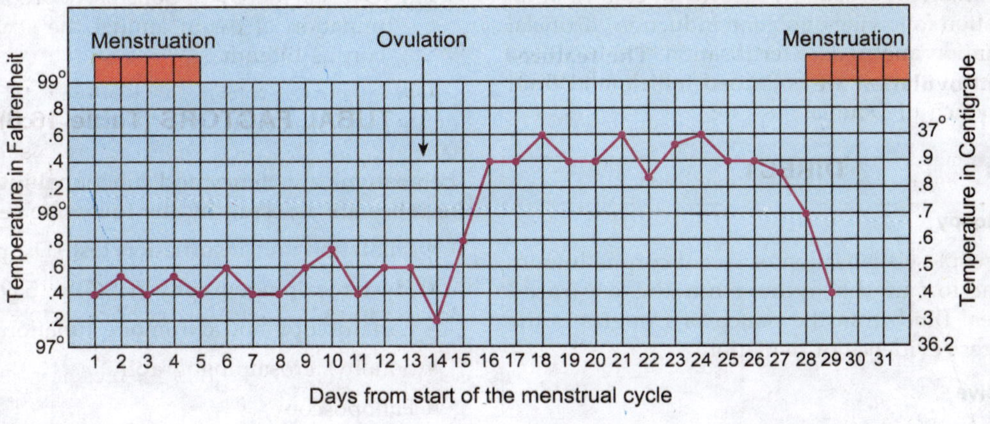

Fig. 16.1. Biphasic BBT Chart

Cervical mucus study

Alteration of the physicochemical properties of the cervical mucus occurs due to the effect of oestrogen and progesterone.

Disappearance of fern pattern beyond 22nd day of the cycle which was present in the midcycle is suggestive of ovulation. Persistence of fern pattern even beyond 22nd day suggests anovulation. Progesterone causes dissolution of the sodium chloride crystals. Following ovulation, there is loss of stretchability (spinbarkeit) which was present in the midcycle (see p.111).

Vaginal cytology

Maturation index shifts to the left from the midcycle to the mid second half of cycle due to the effect of progesterone (see p.111). However, a single smear on day 25 or 26 of the cycle reveals features of progesterone effect, if ovulation occurs.

Hormone estimation

- **Serum progesterone** — Estimation of serum progesterone is done on day 8 and 21 of a cycle. An increase in value from less than 1 ng/ml to greater than 6 ng/ml suggests ovulation.

- **Serum LH** — Daily estimation of serum LH at midcycle can detect the LH surge. Ovulation occurs about 34-36 hours after beginning of the LH surge. It coincides about 10-12 hours after the LH peak.

- **Serum oestradiol** attains the peak rise approximately 24 hours prior to LH surge and about 24-36 hours prior to ovulation.

The serum LH and oestradiol estimation is used for *in vitro* fertilisation.

Urinary LH

LH kits are available to detect midcycle LH surge. Ovulation usually occurs within 14-26 hours of detection of urine LH surge and almost always within 48 hours. (The test should be done on a daily basis. It is started 2 to 3 days before the expected surge depending upon the cycle length).

Endometrial biopsy

Endometrial tissues to detect ovulation (endometrial sampling) can easily be obtained as an out patient procedure using instruments such as Sharman curette or Pipelle endometrial sampler. Dilatation and curettage is however reserved in cases where bulk endometrial study is required as in endometrial tuberculosis.

***When to do?* Biopsy is to be done on 21st–23rd day of the cycle.** Barrier contraceptive should be prescribed during the cycle to prevent accidental conception. However, if the cycle is irregular, it is done within 24 hours of the period.

Findings — Evidences of secretory activity of the endometrial glands in the second half of the cycle give not only the diagnosis of ovulation but can predict the functional integrity of the corpus luteum.

Subnuclear vacuolation is the earliest evidence appearing 36-48 hours following ovulation.

Cause — The secretory changes are due to the action of progesterone on the oestrogen primed endometrium.

Sonography

Serial sonography during midcycle can precisely measure the Graafian follicle just prior to ovulation

(18-20 mm). It is particularly helpful for confirmation of ovulation following ovulation induction , artificial insemination and *in vitro* fertilisation. **The features of recent ovulation are** collapsed follicle and fluid in the pouch of Douglas.

DIRECT

Laparoscopy

Laparoscopic visualisation of recent corpus luteum or detection of the ovum from the aspirated peritoneal fluid from the pouch of Douglas is the only direct evidence of ovulation.

Conclusive

Pregnancy is the surest evidence of ovulation.

LUTEAL PHASE DEFECT (LPD)

Diagnosis of LPD is difficult. However, it is based on the following :

- BBT chart — (a) Slow rise of temperature taking 4-5 days following the fall in the midcycle. (b) Rise of temperature sustains less than 10 days.
- Endometrial biopsy — Biopsy done on 25-27th day of the period reveals the endometrium at least 2 days out of phase (***Example*** : If the biopsy is done on 25th day of cycle, the endometrial changes observed correspond to the day 23). This lag phase endometrium must be proved in more than one cycle (see p. 90). However, it is not conclusive.
- Serum progesterone estimated on 8th day following ovulation is less than 10 ng/ml.

LUTEINISED UNRUPTURED FOLLICLE (LUF)

Luteinised unruptured follicle (LUF) syndrome refers to an infertile woman with regular menses and presumptive evidences of ovulation without release of the ovum from the follicle (trapped ovum). The features of ovulation — formation of corpus luteum and its stigma are absent. It is often associated with pelvic endometriosis.

Diagnosis — In the presence of biologic effects of progesterone in the early luteal phase :

(i) Sonography — Persistence of echo-free dominant follicle beyond 36 hours after LH peak.

(ii) Laparoscopy — Failure to observe a stigma of ovulation.

(iii) Ovarian biopsy — Conclusive proof is determination of ovum amidst the structure of corpus luteum.

TUBAL FACTORS (Table 16.6)

The anatomical patency and functional integrity of the tubes are assessed by the following tests :

- Dilatation and insufflation test (DI) p. 558
- Hysterosalpingography (HSG) p. 559
- Laparoscopy and chromopertubation p. 231
- Sonohysterosalpingography
- Falloposcopy
- Salpingoscopy.

Insufflation test (Rubin's test)

Principle — The underlying principle lies with the fact that the cervical canal is in continuity with the peritoneal cavity through the tubes. As such, entry of air or CO_2 into the peritoneal cavity when pushed transcervically under pressure, gives evidence of tubal patency.

When to be done? It should be done in the post-menstrual phase at least 2 days after stoppage of menstrual bleeding.

Limitation — It should not be done in the presence of pelvic infection.

Observations — The patency of the tube is confirmed by : (1) fall in the pressure when raised beyond 120 mm Hg, (2) hissing sound heard on auscultation on either iliac fossa and (3) shoulder pain experienced by the patient (irritation of the diaphragm by the air).

Drawbacks — In about one-third of cases, it gives a false-negative findings due to cornual spasm. It also cannot identify the side and site of the block in the tube. As such, it is inferior to other methods of tubal study. This test is not commonly done these days.

Hysterosalpingography (HSG)

Principle — The principle is the same like that of insufflation test. Instead of air or CO_2, dye is instilled transcervically.

When to be done? As in D + I.

Limitation — As in D + I.

Advantages — It has got distinct advantages over insufflation test. It can precisely detect the side and site of block in the tube. It can reveal any abnormality in the uterus (congenital or acquired like synechiae, fibroid). As such insufflation of the tubes has largely been replaced by HSG (Fig. 16.2).

Disadvantages — It involves radiation risk.

LAPAROSCOPY AND CHROMOPERTUBATION (Fig16.3)

The scope of diagnostic laparoscopy in the investigation of infertility has been widened. It is an invasive investigation, **so this is done after male factor and ovulatory functions have been found normal or corrected. The indications of its use are** :

- Abnormal HSG findings.
- Failure to conceive after reasonable period (6 months) even with normal HSG.
- Unexplained infertility.
- Women who have comorbid pelvic pathology (PID, endometriosis).

Table 16.5
Indications of laparoscopy in infertility

Diagnostic	• Age > 35 years • Abnormal HSG • Failure to conceive after reasonable period (6 months) with normal HSG • Unexplained infertility
Operative	• GIFT and ZIFT procedures • Ovarian diathermy (p. 239) • Reconstructive tubal surgery • Fulguration of endometriotic implants

Protocols — A double puncture technique is to be applied. All the pelvic organs are to be properly visualised, of particular importance is to note the fimbrial end of the fallopian tubes and their relation with the ovaries. Proper documentation with the aid of diagram is mandatory.

Advantages over HSG — It can precisely diagnose peritubal adhesions, pelvic endometriosis or evidences of ovulation. **Chromopertubation with methylene blue** cannot only reveal patency of the tube but the nature of tubal motility.

Drawbacks — It is more invasive than HSG. It cannot detect abnormality in the uterine cavity or tubal lumen. Thus, the two procedures should be regarded as complementary to each other and should not be used as a substitute to the other procedure.

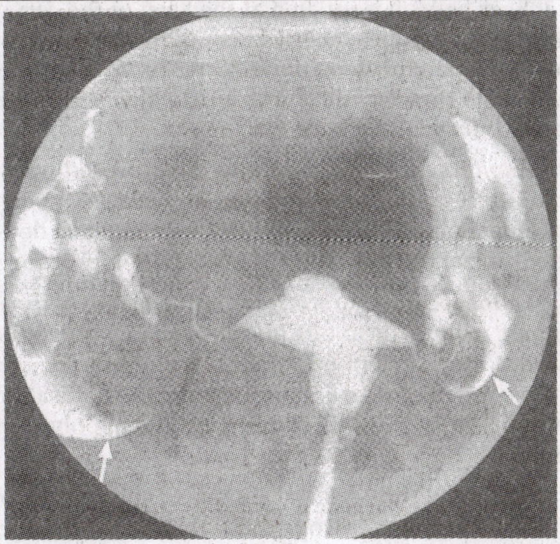

Fig. 16.2. Hysterosalpingogram showing bilateral peritoneal spillage

When to be done? It is preferably done in the secretory phase. Recent corpus luteum may be visualised and endometrial biopsy can be taken in the same sitting.

Sonohysterosalpingography

Principle — Normal saline is pushed within the uterine cavity with a paediatric Foley Catheter. The

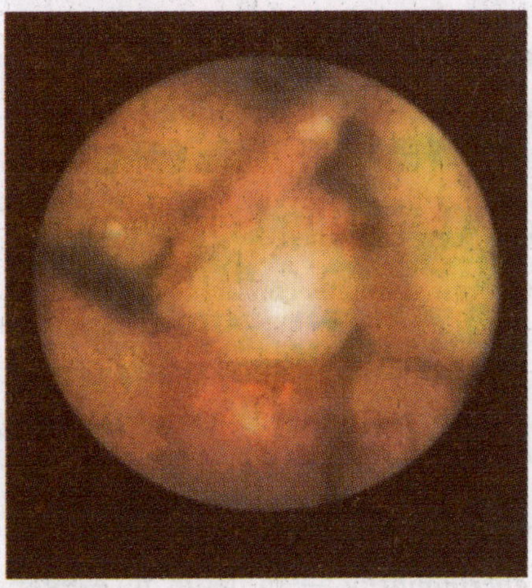

Fig. 16.3. Chromopertubation shows the patency of the tubes *(Courtesy : Dr. Manoj Samanta)*

catheter balloon is inflated at the level of the cervix to prevent fluid leak. Ultrasonography of the uterus and fallopian tubes are done. Ultrasound can follow the fluid through the tubes up to the peritoneal cavity and in the pouch of Douglas.

Advantages—It is a non-invasive procedure. It can detect uterine malformations, synechiae or polyps (superior to HSG). Tubal pathology could be detected as that of HSG. There is no radiation exposure.

Falloposcopy is to study the entire length of tubal lumen with the help of a fine and flexible fibreoptic device. It is performed through the uterine cavity, using a hysteroscope. It helps direct visualisation of tubal ostia, mucosal pattern, intratubal polyps or debris.

Salpingoscopy—Tubal lumen is studied introducing a rigid endoscope through the fimbrial end of the tube. It is performed through the operating channel of a laparoscope.

Uterine factor—Uterine factors commonly associated with subfertility are submucous fibroids, (see p. 267), congenital malformations (see ch. 4) and intrauterine adhesions (Asherman's syndrome). They are more likely to cause recurrent pregnancy loss rather than primary infertility.

Ultrasonography, HSG, hysteroscopy and laparoscopy are needed in the evaluation of uterine factor for subfertility.

Cervical factor (Table 16.6)—The cervix functions as a biological valve. This is in the sense that, in the proliferative phase, it permits the entry of sperm and in the secretory phase, hinders their penetration (Fig. 16.4). As such, dysfunction at this level should be carefully evaluated. This is done by :

Postcoital test (PCT) (Sims-Huhner test)

Principle — PCT is to assess the quality of cervical mucous and the ability of sperm to survive in it. This has been described in Chap. 9, p. 111.

Sperm cervical mucus contact test (SCMCT)

This *in vitro* cross over test is performed using midcycle cervical mucus of the wife and semen of the husband under question and compare with donor sperm and donor cervical mucus (see p. 112). **Routine postcoital test is not recommended** (see p. 112).

Endocrinopathy — In-depth investigations in suspected or overt endocrinopathy with or without menstrual abnormality or ovarian dysfunction include estimation of serum TSH, prolactin, FSH, LH, dehydroepiandrosterone sulphate, testosterone and progesterone in midluteal phase. In cases with family history of diabetes, postprandial blood sugar is to be estimated.

Immunological factor—Human sperm has immunologic potential. In susceptible women, it can elicit antibodies against the antigens producing a cervical immune response and infertility. The antibodies against sperm may affect fertility by immobilising sperm or causing agglutination.

Male may also produce autoantibodies against seminal or sperm components. Sperm coated with these antibodies fail to migrate through the cervix.

Most common variety of antisperm antibodies are IgG, IgM and IgA isotypes. IgG may be found in cervical mucous, serum and semen. Agglutinating antibodies of IgA class are found in cervical mucous and seminal plasma. The IgM (Larger) molecules are found exclusively in the serum. **These immunoglobulins can bind to different parts of the sperm (e.g. head, body or tail) and make them immobile.**

Detection of antisperm antibody has not been found to be helpful in the management of infertility. Treatment of antisperm antibodies has not improved the pregnancy outcome. Therefore antisperm antibody testing is rarely done these days specially with the advent of IUI, IVF or ICSI (see p. 243).

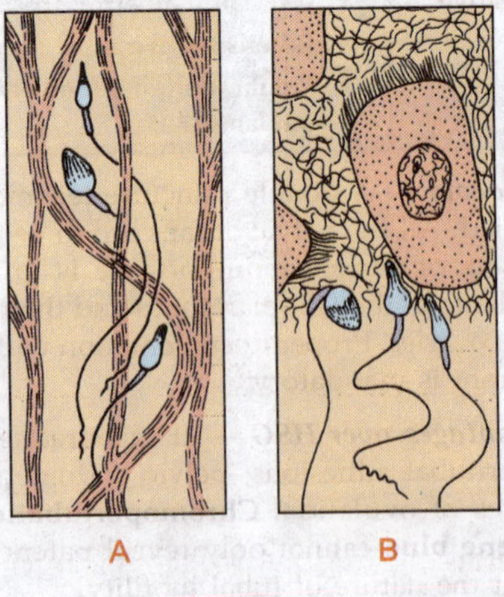

Fig. 16.4. (A) Oestrogenic effect on cervical mucus facilitates sperm penetration. (B) Progesterone effect hinders the penetration

Table 16.6
Infertility work up calendar

Identification of factor	Methods employed	Day of cycle	Observation
OVULATION	• BBT	Throughout cycle	Biphasic pattern
	• Endometrial biopsy	D 21-23	Secretory endometrium
	• Cervical mucus Nature Threadability Fern pattern	D 12-14 and D 21-23	D 12-14 / D 21-23 Clear, watery / Thick, viscid + / – + / –
	• Vaginal cytology	D 12-14 and D 21-23	D 12-14: Discrete cells, Pyknotic nuclei, background clear D 21-23: Folded edges. In clumps background dirty
	• Serum progesterone	D 8 and D 21	D-8 < 1 ng/ml D-21 > 6ng/ml
	• Serum LH	Midcycle daily (D 12-14)	Ovulation : About 10-12 hrs. after LH surge
	• Serial sonography	D 12-14	Follicular measurements — approaching 20 mm
	• Laparoscopy	Secretory phase	Recent corpus luteum
TUBAL FACTOR	• Insufflation test	Proliferative phase – 2 days after the bleeding stops	(i) Drop in pressure when raised to 120 mm Hg (ii) Hissing sound on iliac fossa (iii) Shoulder pain
	• Hysterosalpingography	As above	Spillage of dye into the peritoneal cavity
	• Laparoscopy and dye test	Proliferative phase	• Peritubal pathology • Pelvic pathology (Endometriosis) • Ovulation • Tubal patency by dye spillage from both the tubes
	• Sonohysterosalpingography	Proliferative phase	As HSG
	• Falloposcopy	Proliferative phase	Tubal luminal pathology
CERVICAL	• Postcoital test (PCT)	Around ovulation (D 12-14)	Presence of progressive motile sperm (10 per high power field)
	• Sperm cervical mucus contact test (SCMCT)	As above	Sperm antibodies (see p. 111, 232)

Unexplained infertility is defined when no obvious cause for infertility has been detected following all standard investigations. These include semen analysis, ovulation detection, tubal and peritoneal factors, endocrinopathy and PCT. Overall incidence is 10-20 per cent. With expectant management about 60 per cent of couples with unexplained infertility will conceive within a period of three years. IVF and ET (see p. 243) may be an option for those who fail to respond.

TREATMENT OF INFERTILITY

Couple instructions

Assurance

The infertile couple remains psychologically disturbed right from the beginning, more so as the investigation progresses. The couple in such cases should be tactfully handled to minimise psychologic upset.

When minor defects are detected in both the husband and the wife, each of which alone could not cause infertility but in combination, they significantly decrease the fertility potential. As such, **the faults should be treated simultaneously and not one after the other.** Even when a gross abnormality is detected and the prospect of pregnancy is bleak, an optimistic discussion is worth rewarding.

Body weight

Overweight or underweight of any partner should be adequately dealt with to obtain an optimum weight. Body mass index of 20-24 is optimum.

Smoking and alcohol

Excess smoking or alcohol consumption is to be avoided.

Coital problems

The coital problems should be carefully evaluated by intelligent interrogation. Advice to have intercourse during the midcycle too often gives the result early enough even prior to investigation. Using LH test kit, one can detect LH surge in urine by getting a deep blue colour of dipstick. The test should be performed daily between day 12 to day 16 of a regular cycle. Timed intercourse over 24-36 hours after the colour change reasonably succeeds in conception. Minor psychosexual problems should be corrected accordingly.

- **Male**
- **Female**
- **Combined**

Scheme — 3 **Initial investigation protocol of an infertile couple**

- **Husband semen analysis — normal (Table 16.3)**
- **Female partner**

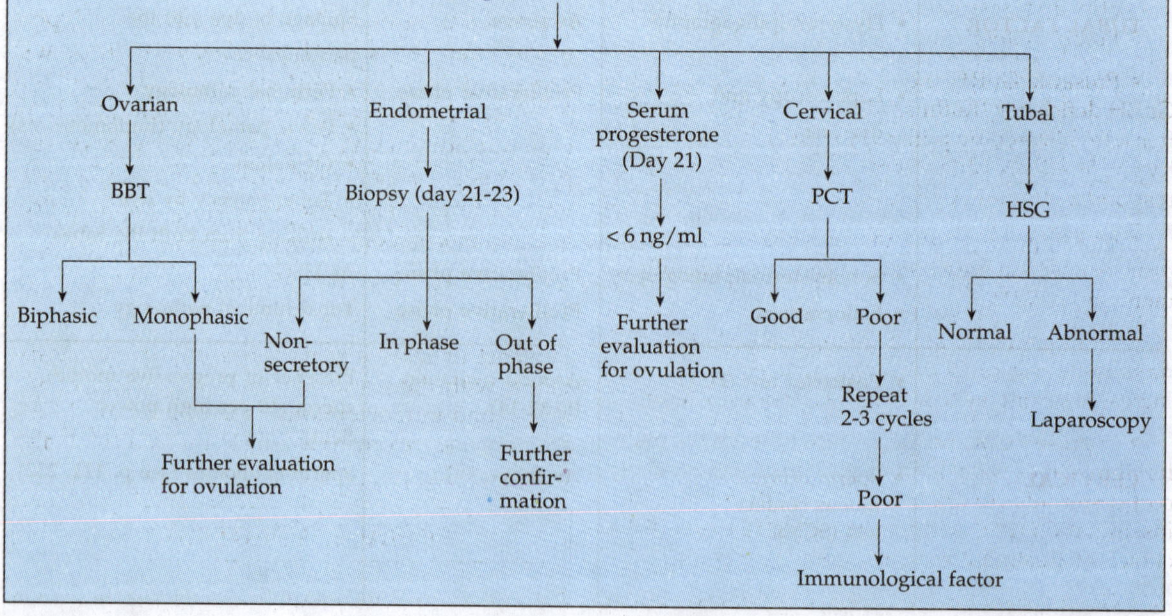

MALE INFERTILITY

The treatment of male is indicated in (i) extreme oligospermia, (ii) azoospermia, (iii) low volume ejaculate and (iv) impotency. Management is often difficult and unsatisfactory.

To improve spermatogenesis the following measures may be helpful.

General care : Improvement of general health, reduction of weight in obese, avoidance of alcohol and heavy smoking are of help. Avoidance of tight and warm undergarments or occupation that may elevate testicular temperature is helpful.

- Use of vitamins E, C, D, B_{12} and folic acid as antioxidants to improve spermatogenesis is of doubtful value.
- Medications that interfere spermatogenesis (p. 222) should be avoided.
- In **hypogonadotrophic-hypogonadism**, the disorders of spermatogenesis can be treated with the following therapy with varying success.
  - hCG 5000 IU intramuscularly once or twice a week is given to stimulate endogenous testosterone production.
  - hMG is added to hCG when there is no sperm in the ejaculate with hCG alone.
  - Dopamine agonist (cabergoline) is given in hyperprolactinaemia to restore normal prolactin and testosterone level. This improves libido, potency and fertility.
- Pulsatile GnRH therapy in infertile male with GnRH deficiency (Kallmann's syndrome) is effective. It is administered by minipump infusion. Cases with hypogonadotrophic hypogonadism may also respond with GnRH therapy.
- In **hypergonadotrophic-hypogonadism**, no form of medical treatment can improve fertility in men (see p. 221).
- Clomiphene citrate 25-50 mg orally daily for 25 days with rest for 5 days for 3 cycles is given. It increases serum level of FSH, LH and testosterone.
- In presence of antisperm antibodies in the male, its significance is uncler and the benefits of systemic corticosteroids are uncertain. Currently intrauterine insemination (IUI) with washed spermatozoa is the choice of treatment for such cases (see p. 242).
- Genital tract infection needs prolonged course of antibiotics. Generally doxycycline or erythromycin is given for a period of 4-6 weeks depending on the response.
- In retrograde ejaculation — phenylephrine (α-adrenergic agonist) is used to improve the tone of internal urethral sphincter. Sperm may be recovered from the neutralised urine. Processed spermatozoa could be used for IUI (see p. 242).
- In teratospermia, asthenospermia specific causes are unknown. No treatment is available. Donor insemination (AID) is the option (see p. 242).
- In genetic abnormality — artificial insemination with donor sperm (AID) is the option as no other treatment is available.

Surgical

- When the patient is found to be azoospermic and yet testicular biopsy shows normal spermatogenesis, obstruction of vas must be suspected. This should be corrected by microsurgery — vasoepididymostomy or vasovasostomy. After vasovasostomy patency is obtained in about 80 per cent of cases and pregnancy rate is about 50 per cent.
- Surgery for vericocele for improvement of fertility is not helpful. Hydrocele is corrected by surgery.
- Orchidopexy in undescended testes should be done between 2-3 years of age to have adequate spermatogenesis in later life.

Impotency

Psychosexual treatment may be of help. Hyperprolactinaemia needs further investigation and treatment (see p. 445). For erectile dysfunction sildenafil (25-100 mg) or tadalafil (10-20 mg) is currently advised. A single dose (depending on response) is given orally one hour before sexual activity. In unresponsive cases, artificial insemination is to be thought of (see p. 242).

Assisted reproductive technology (ART) for male infertility

Prospect of male infertility has improved significantly with the advent of ART. IUI, TESE, PESA, MESA and intracytoplasmic sperm injection (ICSI) are now the treatment available for infertile males (see p. 245).

FEMALE INFERTILITY

For convenience, the treatment modalities in female

infertility are grouped as follows according to the disorders identified :

- Ovulatory.
- Tubal.
- Associated disorders like endometriosis, infections or endocrinopathy.
- Cervical.
- Immunological.
- Unexplained infertility.
- Uterovaginal canal.
- Assisted reproductive technology (ART).

Ovulatory dysfunction

- **Anovulation** • **LPD** • **LUF**

For WHO classification — see p. 249.

Anovulation

Anovulation is a common factor for female infertility. It may be present in otherwise normal menstrual cycle or may be associated with oligomenorrhoea or amenorrhoea.

Induction of ovulation

To facilitate effective folliculogenesis and ovulation, the following may be prescribed :

- **General** • **Drugs** • **Surgery**

General

- Psychotherapy to improve the emotional causes, if any.
- Reduction of weight in obesity as in PCOS cases (see p. 450) is essential to have a good response of drug therapy for induction. This facilitates spontaneous ovulation.

Drugs : The following drugs are of use either singly or in combination (see Table 16.7).

Monitoring during ovulation induction (Table 16.8)

For diagnosis of ovulation, BBT recording is enough. With some therapies, diagnosis of ovulation is obtained from BBT chart supplemented by cervical mucus study (clear, watery, stretchable type). But when a complicated regimen is followed to achieve pregnancy by time intercourse or by ART, a detailed monitoring is a must which is only possible in selected centres. Not only the drugs are costly, the regimens are complicated and time consuming.

Table 16.7
Drugs used in induction of ovulation

Stimulation of ovulation
- Clomiphene citrate (CC)
- Letrozole (p. 508)
- hMG (Humegon, Pergonal) (FSH 75 IU + LH 75 IU)
- FSH
  - purified urinary FSH
  - highly purified urinary FSH (Metrodin HP)
  - recombinant FSH (Gonal-F, Recagon)
- hCG (Profasi, Pregnyl)
  - recombinant hCG
- GnRH (see p. 239)
- GnRH analogues (see p. 244)

Correction of Biochemical Abnormality

• Hyper-insulinaemia (insulin resistance)	– Metformin (see p.450)
• Androgen excess	– Dexamethasone (see p.450)
• Prolactin raised	– Bromocriptine (see p. 450)

Substitution therapy

• Hypothyroidism	– Thyroxin
• Diabetes mellitus	– Antidiabetic drugs

Table 16.8
Objectives of monitoring for induction of ovulation

- To select time for preovulatory administration of hCG.
- To prevent ovarian hyperstimulation syndrome.
- To select time for intercourse or artificial insemination.
- To select time for ovum retrieval in IVF.

Apart from BBT chart and cervical mucus study which are noninvasive, simple and quite informative, other parameters used are serial estimation of plasma E_2 and ultrasonic measurement of growing follicles (folliculometry). These last two are obligatory in ART.

Clomiphene citrate

Patient selection

- Normogonadotrophic–normoprolactinaemic patients who are having normal cycles with absent or infrequent ovulation.

- PCOS cases with oligomenorrhoea or amenorrhoea. The oestradiol level should be > 40 pg per ml.
- Hypothalamic amenorrhoea following stress or 'pill' use.

Dose : Clomiphene therapy is simple, safe and at the same time cost-effective. Most centres use an initial dose of 50 mg daily. Dose is increased in 50 mg steps to a maximum 250 mg daily, if ovulation is not induced by the lower dose. The actual starting day of its administration in the follicular phase varies between day 2 and day 5 and therapy is given for 5 days. Ovulation is expected to occur about 5-7 days after the last day of therapy. Therapy for six cycle is generally given.

Mechanism of action of clomiphene : Clomiphene citrate is anti-oestrogenic as well as weakly oestrogenic. It blocks the oestrogen receptors in the hypothalamus. This results in increased GnRH pulse amplitude causing increased gonadotrophin secretion from the pituitary. Anti-oestrogenic effects are seen on the endometrium and on the cervical mucus.

Side effects are : hot flushes, nausea, vomiting, headache, visual symptoms and ovarian hyperstimulation (rare). Incidence of abortion and congenital fetal malformations are not increased.

Couple instruction — The couple is advised to have sexual intercourse as per following guidelines :

- Daily or on alternate days beginning 5-7 days after the last dose of clomiphene therapy.
- Several times for 24-48 hours after the colour change in urine when tested by LH kit.
- Number of times over 24-36 hours following hCG administration.

Result : Successful induction rate is as high as 90 per cent but pregnancy rate is about 50 per cent. **The discrepancy is due to** premature luteinisation, LPD, cervical mucus hostility and other non-ovulatory factors. The incidence of multiple pregnancy is about 5 per cent.

Adjuvant therapy

Despite the high success rate of clomiphene, some adjuvant therapy is often needed.

(a) **Hyperinsulinaemia and Insulin sensitiser** — Patients with polycystic ovarian disease with BMI > 25 (see p. 440) are often found insulin resistant. Correction of their metabolic abnormality (see p. 450) along with weight reduction gives satisfactory result. Treatment with **metformin** (insulin sensitiser) is found to reduce hyperinsulinaemia and hyperandrogenaemia. Combination treatment with metformin and clomiphene increases ovulation rate significantly.

(b) Pre-existing or induced **elevated androgens** may be suppressed by dexamethasone 0.5 mg daily for 10 days, starting from 1st day of cycle. The drug should be stopped soon after ovulation.

(c) Eltroxin 0.1 mg may be administered daily during the therapy in obese patients with **subclinical hypothyroidism**.

(d) **Elevated prolactin level** with or without galactorrhoea indicates abnormal GnRH pulse secretion. This causes ovulatory dysfunction, LPD or amenorrhoea. **Bromocriptine or cabergoline (dopamine agonist)** therapy (see p. 450) increases the ovarian responsiveness to clomiphene. Patients with normal or minimally elevated prolactin when treated with bromocriptine and clomiphene are found to have increased pregnancy.

Results : Dopamine agonist treatment normalises prolactin level (80%), restores cyclic menses (80%) and ovulation in majority (70%) of women.

Side effects : Nausea, diziness, vomiting and orthostatic hypotension are common. Side effects of cabergoline are less. Specially when it is used by the vaginal route.

(e) **hCG** — In cases of anovulation due to failure of LH surge, hCG 5000 IU is administered usually 7 days after the last dose of clomiphene therapy. Prior monitoring of serum oestradiol level and ultrasonic measurement of follicular diameter (18-20 mm) is preferred to get a good result.

(f) Growth hormone — is combined to the poor responders specially, in the elderly group.

(g) Because of the anti-oestrogenic effect of clomiphene citrate, the cervical mucus becomes thick and viscid and it hinders sperm penetration. Conjugated oestrogen 1.25 mg given daily for 10 days starting on first day of cycle may be helpful.

Letrozole : See p. 508.

Gonadotrophins

Prerequisites for gonadotrophin therapy

- **Ovarian reserve** must be present (p. 503). Decline in fertility status due to oocyte depletion is known as **decreased ovarian reserve. Age of the woman is the strongest determinant of ovarian reserve. Value of serum FSH more than 10 IU/L, measured on D3, is suggestive poor ovarian reserve.**

• Other (non-ovulatory) factors for infertility must be ruled out. hMG (human menopausal gonadotrophin) is a mixture of FSH and LH [Pergonal = FSH (75 IU) + LH (75 IU)].

INDICATIONS OF GONADOTROPHIN USE

- Hypogonadotrophic hypogonadism (WHO Group I). See p. 249.
- Clomiphene failed or resistant cases (WHO Group II). See p. 249.
- Unexplained infertility.

Dose schedule

• hMG stimulates follicular growth with a variable dose schedule starting with a low dose (75 IU IM/day)

• Stimulation is started any time from D_2 to D_5 of the cycle and is continued for 7-10 days depending on the response.

• Follicular growth is monitored with serum oestradiol estimation and follicular number and size are measured by transvaginal sonography (TVS).

• Serum oestradiol level of 500-1500 pg/ml (150-300 pg/mature follicle) and maximum follicular diameter of 18-20 mm are optimum.

• When this optimum levels are obtained 5000-10000 IU of hCG is administered IM to induce ovulation.

• Endometrial thickness of 8-10 mm (as measured by TVS) on the day of hCG administration favours successful implantation.

• Ovulation is expected to occur, approximately 36 hours after the hCG administration.

Couple instruction

Couple is advised for the timing of intercourse or insemination (ART) accordingly (see above).

Patients with PCOS are more sensitive to hMG stimulation. Purified FSH (metrodin) or highly purified FSH (metrodin HP) or recombinant FSH (Gonal F, Recegon) have been used successfully with minimal side effects.

In cases of hypergonadotrophic hypogonadism, high gonadotrophin levels are lowered with the use of combined oestrogen and progestogen preparations (oral pill). Use of long-acting GnRH agonist also suppresses high endogenous gonadotrophin levels (see p. 500). When the levels reach normal, gonadotrophin therapy may be employed to achieve ovulation. The success rate is poor.

Side effects of Gonadotrophin therapy (see p. 503)

Contraindications of Gonadotrophin therapy

(1) Primary ovarian failure with raised serum FSH and (2) Uncontrolled thyroid and adrenal dysfunction. (3) Sex hormone dependent tumour in the body.

Results : Pregnancy rate after six courses of treatments is 90 per cent. Incidence of multiple pregnancy (10-30%), overall incidence of miscarriage (20-25%) and ectopic pregnancy are high. Risks of congenital anomalies are not increased.

GnRH

Exogenous GnRH — Pulsatile GnRH treatment stimulates physiologic levels of pituitary gonadotrophin secretion. So development of follicular growth, selection, recruitment and ovulation occurs as in normal menstrual cycle.

Patient selection

When ovulatory dysfunction is due to :

- Hypothalamic amenorrhoea
- Hypogonadotrophic hypogonadism
- Women with hyperprolactinaemia.

GnRH is administered intravenously or subcutaneously with an infusion pump in a pulsatile fashion.

A pulse of 5 μg is used IV at every 90 minutes. Follicular growth is similar to a normal menstrual cycle. Follicular growth monitoring, hCG administration and couple instructions are same as in hMG therapy.

Results : Pregnancy rate is 80 per cent following six course of treatment. Multiple pregnancy rate is 5 per cent. Overall risk of miscarriage is 30 per cent. The risk of ovarian hyperstimulation is low (see p. 503).

GnRH analogues (p. 500)

Patient selection

- Patients refractory to gonadotrophins.
- Patients having elevated LH.
- Patients with normal gonadotrophins.
- Patients with premature follicular luteinisation or premature ovulation due to premature LH surge.

GnRH agonist (buserelin, nafarelin) is given subcutaneously or intranasally either maintaining a short or long protocol. GnRH agonist is used for down regulation of pituitary gland by desensitisation of pituitary GnRH receptors (see p. 64). GnRH agonist initially produce stimulation of gonadotrophin secretion known as *'flare'* effect. Generally this flare effect lasts for about 2-3 weeks. Adequate pituitary suppression is achieved when serum oestradiol level is less than 10 pg/ml and FSH level is less than 10 mIU/ml. Follicular stimulation is achieved with highly purified or recombinant FSH. Follicular number and growth monitoring is similar as in hMG therapy. hCG is also administered when criteria is fulfilled as discussed with hMG therapy (see p. 238).

Results — ovulation rate is about 75 per cent and pregnancy rate is about 25 per cent.

GnRH antagonists — can block pituitary GnRH receptors completely without any initial stimulation (flare effect). Cetrorelix is currently being tried to prevent premature LH surge. As with GnRH analogue gonadotrophin stimulation is done (see above).

When pregnancy occurs following superovulation with GnRH agonist therapy, luteal phase support should be maintained either by giving hCG or progesterone.

It should be emphasised that the gonadotrophins, GnRH and GnRH analogues are costly drugs. **Their uses have to be monitored carefully with sophisticated gadgets** not only to control the regimen but also to minimise the hazards (Table 16.7). Thus, its use is restricted in selected centres and is commonly used in ART.

LUTEAL PHASE DEFECT (LPD)

Treatment : The following treatment may be of help in the idiopathic groups :

• Natural progesterone as vaginal suppositories 100 mg thrice daily starting from the day of ovulation is effective. It should be continued until mens begins. If mens fails to appear after 14 days, pregnancy test is to be done. If the test is positive, it should be continued upto 10th week of pregnancy.

• hCG is a potent luteotropic hormone, however, the response of LPD to hCG is unpredictable.

• In unresponsive cases, clomiphene citrate may be tried. It increases FSH which may improve folliculogenesis and normal corpus luteum formation with adequate production of progesterone. In refractory cases, IVF may be tried.

Luteinised unruptured follicle (LUF)

Defective folliculogenesis or inadequate LH surge may be corrected with :

• Optimally timed intramuscular injection of hCG 5000-10,000 IU.

• Administration of ovulation inducing drugs in the follicular phase followed by ovulatory hCG (5000-10000 IU).

• Bromocriptine therapy, if associated with hyperprolactinaemia (see p. 445).

SURGERY

• **Laparoscopic ovarian drilling (LOD) or laser vaporisation** : This is done by multiple puncture of the cysts in polycystic ovarian syndrome by diathermy or laser. It reduces systemic and intraovarian androgen levels. This procedure is helpful in clomiphene resistant, hyperandrogenic anovulatory women. The woman ovulates spontaneously following LOD (p. 450).

• **Wedge resection** — This is not commonly done these days. Bilateral wedge resection of the ovaries is done in PCOS cases where clomiphene citrate fails to induce ovulation. It produces adhesions.

• **Surgery** for pituitary prolactinomas (see p. 450).

• **Surgical removal** of virilising or other functioning ovarian or adrenal tumour (see p. 547).

Tubal and peritoneal factors

Tubal factors for infertility are corrected only by surgery. The different surgical methods are :

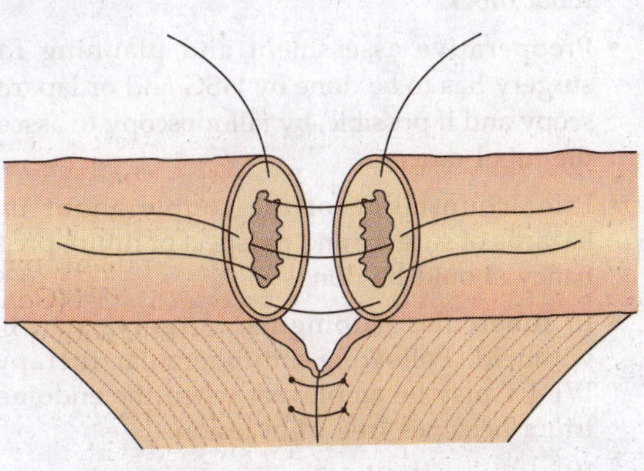

Fig. 16.5. Tubotubal anastomosis. Placement of four to five interrupted sutures using 8-0 polyglactin (under × 10 magnification)

(i) **Peritubal adhesions :** Correction is done by salpingo-ovariolysis either by laparoscopy or by laparotomy.

(ii) **Proximal tubal block :** Salpingography under fluroscopy may be helpful to remove any block due to mucous plugging. Otherwise proximal tubal cannulation with a guide wire under hysteroscopic guidance is done. In about 85 per cent cases tubal patency can be restored and over all pregnancy rate of about 45-50 per cent is reported. **Cannulation and balloon tuboplasty can avoid the need of ART which are expensive.**

(iii) **Distal tubal block :** (a) *Fimbrioplasty* — release of fimbrial adhesions and/or dilatation of fimbrial phimosis. (b) *Neosalpingostomy* — to create a new tubal opening in an occluded tube. Success rate in terms of pregnancy following fimbrioplasty is more compared to neosalpingostomy.

(iv) **Mid tubal block** : Reversal of tubal ligation — pregnancy rates after this procedure varies between 50-75 per cent. Success rate depends on — (a) age, (b) the method of sterilisation (Pomeroy's, Fallope rings, Diathermy, etc.), (c) site of anastomosis (isthmic-isthmic or isthmic-cornual), (d) final length of reconstructed tube. Risk of ectopic pregnancy following tubal reanastomosis is 3-7 per cent.

GUIDELINES FOR TUBAL SURGERY

- Tubal surgery may be considered in young women after previous tubal sterilisation or in women with mild disease at the distal tubal segment.
- Tubal surgery may be tried for mild proximal tubal block.
- Preoperative assessment and planning for surgery has to be done by HSG and or laparoscopy and if possible, by falloposcopy to assess the tubal mucosa.
- Prior counselling of the couple about the hazards of surgery and prospect of future pregnancy should be done.
- In tubercular salpingitis, surgery is to be withheld. Following antitubercular therapy, IVF-ET may be employed, when the endometrium becomes free from lesion.
- IVF is considered as the best treatment option for any complicated tubal occlusive disease.
- Salpingectomy should be done before IVF when hydrosalpinges are present (p. 620).

METHODS OF TUBAL SURGERY

Tuboplasty is the name given to the finer surgery on the tubes to restore the anatomy and physiology as far as practicable (see Table 16.9).

- The **operation** can be done by conventional methods, or by microsurgical techniques which may be employed following laparotomy or by laparoscopy (Fig. 35.5).
- **Microsurgical techniques give better result** due to minimal tissue handling and damage, perfect haemostasis and minimal adhesion formation. **Laparoscopic surgery gives the best result.**
- Nylon may be used as a temporary splint to facilitate suturing the ends. It should be removed following anastomosis and if kept inside, should be removed after 48 hours to minimise mucosal damage.
- Intraoperative instillation of Ringer lactate mixed with heparin or hydrocortisone may be employed to minimise adhesion formation.

Table 16.9 : Tuboplasty operation

Adhesiolysis (Salpingo-ovariolysis)	Separation or division of adhesions.
Fimbrioplasty	Separation of the fimbrial adhesions to open up the abdominal ostium.
Salpingostomy	That creates a new opening in a completely occluded tube. It is called **terminal or 'cuff'** at the abdominal ostium. The eversion of the neo-ostium is maintained by few stitches of 6-0 Vicryl.
Tubotubal anastomosis	When the segment of the diseased tube or following tubectomy operation is resected and end to end anastomosis is done (Fig. 16.5).
Tubocornual anastomosis	When there is cornual block, the remaining healthy tube is anastomosed to the patent interstitial part of the tube.

Adjuvant therapy

Adjunctive procedures to improve the result of tubal surgery include prophylactic antibiotics, use of adhesion prevention devices (interceed, seprafilm) and postoperative hydrotubation.

Hydrotubation — Hydrotubation is a procedure to flush the tubal lumen by medicated fluids passed transcervically through a cannula. The fluid contains antibiotic and hydrocortisone (Gentamicin 80 mg and dexamethasone 4 mg in 10 ml distilled water). It should be done in postmenstrual phase.

Results of tuboplasty — The result depends upon the nature of pathology, type of surgery and techniques employed — macro or microsurgery. **Overall pregnancy rate (following laparoscopic surgery) is as follows :** Salpingo-ovariolysis 65%; Fimbrioplasty 32%; Tubotubal anastomosis 75%; Tubocornual anastomosis 55%. The result is better in microsurgical techniques when done laparoscopically. **The result is best in reversal tubal sterilisation by tubotubal anastomosis using microsurgical techniques.**

Factors for poor outcome following tuboplasty :

- Dense pelvic adhesions.
- Loss of fimbriae.
- Bilateral hydrosalpinx > 3 cm (see p. 167).
- Length of the reconstructed tube < 4 cm.
- Reversal done after 5 years of sterilisation operation.
- Presence of other factors for infertility.

Endometriosis

Minimal asymptomatic pelvic endometriosis may be an incidental finding and intensive medical or surgical therapy does not improve the fertility status. However, the therapy should be instituted in minimal endometriosis with otherwise unexplained infertility. Mild endometriosis with involvement of the ovary or moderate endometriosis should be treated with drugs or surgery or both. For details see Chapter 21.

Cervical factor

Cervical mucus protects sperm from the hostile environment of the vagina and also from phagocytosis. The cervical mucus quality can be improved by conjugated oestrogen 1.25 mg orally daily starting on day eight for 5 days.

In proved cases of *Cl. trachomatis* or *M. hominis*, doxycycline 100 mg twice daily for 14 days is to be given to both the partners. **Cervical factor when cannot be treated, is overcome by ART procedures like IUI, IVF or GIFT (see p. 243).**

Immunological factor

In the presence of antisperm antibodies in the cervical mucus, dexamethasone 0.5 mg at bed time in the follicular phase may be given. As there is no distinct benefit of such treatment in antisperm antibody positive patients, COH and IUI (p. 242) or IVF (p. 243) or ICSI (p. 245) is recommended.

Uterovaginal surgery

The operations in the uterus to improve the fertility includes :

- Myomectomy (see p. 271) specially in submucous fibroid. Care should be taken to prevent or to minimise adhesions causing tubopathy.
- Metroplasty (see Ch. 4) either removal of septum or unification operation may be tried when no other cause is detected. This abnormality seldom causes infertility.
- Adhesiolysis with insertion of IUCD in uterine synechiae (see p. 451).
- Enlargement of the vaginal introitus (Fenton's operation p. 562) or removal of vaginal septum causing dyspareunia results in improvement of fertility.
- Apart from cauterisation, amputation of the cervix may have to be done for congenital elongation of the cervix (p. 561).
- Gilliam's type of operation to correct third degree retroversion in unexplained infertility (see p. 574).

Table 16.10
Attempt for pregnancy after infertility surgery

Type of surgery	Interval
Microsurgical tubal anastomosis	6 weeks
Uterotubal implantation	6 months
Salpingostomy	6-12 months
Surgery for endometriosis	Soon following surgery
Myomectomy/metroplasty	3-6 months
Adhesiolysis	Soon following surgery

Unexplained infertility

Unexplained infertility is earmarked to those couples who have undergone complete basic infertility work up and in whom no abnormality has been detected and still remains infertile. The incidence is extremely variable and largely dependent on the magnitude of the in-depth investigation protocol extended to the couple. **The reported incidence varies from 10-20 per cent.**

About 60-80 per cent of these couples become pregnant within 3 years without having any specific treatment.

Therapy : The prospect of spontaneous conception decreases with increasing age of the woman and the duration of infertility. The recommended treatment for unexplained infertility are induction of ovulation, IUI, Superovulation combined with IUI and Assisted Reproductive Technology (see below).

Combined factor : The faults detected in both the partners **should be treated simultaneously and not one after the other.**

ARTIFICIAL INSEMINATION (AI)

Different methods are :

- IUI — Intrauterine insemination
- Fallopian tube sperm perfusion.

INTRAUTERINE INSEMINATION (IUI)

IUI may be either AIH (artificial insemination husband) or AID (artificial insemination donor). Husband's semen is commonly used. **The purpose of IUI** is to bypass the endocervical canal which is abnormal and to place increased concentration of motile sperm as close to the fallopian tubes. The indications are tabulated in the Table 16.11.

Table 16.11 : Indications of IUI

- Hostile cervical mucus
- Cervical stenosis
- Oligospermia or asthenospermia
- Immune factor (male and female)
- Male factor – impotency or anatomical defect (hypospadias) but normal ejaculate can be obtained
- Unexplained infertility.

Technique

Washing, centrifugation and swim-up methods are commonly used. About 0.3 ml of washed and concentrated sperm is injected through a flexible polyethylene catheter within the uterine cavity around the time of ovulation (see Table 16.12). Washing in culture media removes the proteins and prostaglandins from semen that may cause uterine cramps or anaphylactoid reactions. Swim-up method selects the motile spermatozoa. Density Gradient Centrifugation may also be used. **The processed motile sperm for insemination should be at least 1 million.** Best results are obtained when the motile sperm count exceeds 10 million. Fertilising capacity for spermatozoa is for 24-48 hours. The procedure may be repeated 2-3 times over a period of 2-3 days. To increase sperm motility, pentoxyphylline (phosphodiesterase inhibitor) have been used. Generally 4-6 cycles of insemination with superovulation is advised (see Table 16.6).

Timing of IUI : In cervical insemination, timing is not so much vital because the sperm can survive in the cervical canal for a day or two. As the reservoir function is not available in IUI, some form of **controlled ovarian hyperstimulation (COH)** is required (see Table 16.12).

Table 16.12 : Timing of IUI

- Spontaneous cycles
  Cervical mucus study and BBT chart
  IUI × 2, likely on day 12 and 14
- Clomiphene induced cycles
  IUI – 5 and 7 days after completion of CC
- Urinary LH detection
  IUI – 24 hours after colour change
- Use of hCG and sonography
  – hCG at 18 mm diameter of the follicle
  IUI × 2, following 34-40 hours of hCG administration.

Results

The result varies widely in different centres, ranging 20-40 per cent. The best results are obtained in the treatment of cervical factor and unexplained infertility and in stimulated cycle. IUI along with superovulation (induction of ovulation with hMG/hCG) gives higher result.

ARTIFICIAL (THERAPEUTIC) INSEMINATION DONOR (AID)

When the semen of a donor is used for insemination it is called therapeutic insemination donor. **The indications are :**

- Untreatable azoospermia, asthenospermia.
- Genetic disease.

- Rh-negative donor insemination — for woman with Rh-sensitisation.

The donor should be healthy and of the same ethnic group as husband. He should be serologically and bacteriologically free from venereal diseases including AIDS and hepatitis. The recipient and donor must be matched for blood grouping and Rh typing. Either fresh or frozen semen is used. Sperm specimen should only be used when it is kept sequestered for at least 180 days and thereafter it has been found negative for HIV. The legal, psychological and religious aspects should be counselled before its application.

Results : A total of 3-6 cycles may have to be utilised to get a success. The success rate is about 50-60 per cent. Insemination when combined with superovulation, enhances success rate.

FALLOPIAN TUBE SPERM PERFUSION

Indications are same as that of IUI.

Technique : Large volume of washed and processed sperm is injected within the uterine cavity around the time of ovulation (see Table 16.12). This causes perfusion of the fallopian tubes with spermatozoa. In conjunction with ovulation induction pregnancy rate is 25-30 per cent per cycle.

ASSISTED REPRODUCTIVE TECHNOLOGY (ART)

ART encompasses all the procedures that involve manipulation of gametes and embryos outside the body for the treatment of infertility (see Table 16.13).

Table 16.13 : Different methods of ART

IVF-ET	: *In vitro* fertilisation and embryo transfer
GIFT	: Gamete intra-fallopian transfer
ZIFT	: Zygote intra-fallopian transfer
POST	: Peritoneal oocyte and sperm transfer
SUZI	: Subzonal insemination
ICSI	: Intracytoplasmic sperm injection
Methods of sperm recovery	
TESE	: Testicular sperm extraction
MESA	: Microsurgical epididymal sperm aspiration
PESA	: Percutaneous epididymal sperm aspiration

IN VITRO FERTILISATION AND EMBRYO TRANSFER (IVF-ET)

The field of reproductive medicine has changed for ever with the birth of Louise Brown in 1978 by IVF-ET. **Patrick Steptoe and Robert Edwards of England are remembered for their revolutionary work.**

The past decade has witnessed two more dramatic changes in the technique protocol of IVF-ET. One such change was from natural cycle to superovulation protocol and the other one was replacement of laparoscopy by vaginal sonography for ovum retrieval.

Indications of IVF–ET — See Table 16.14.

Table 16.14 : Indications of IVF

- Tubal disease (see p. 620).
- Unexplained infertility.
- Endometriosis.
- Male factor infertility.
- Cervical hostility.
- Failed ovulation induction.
- Ovarian failure (Donor oocyte IVF).
- Women with normal ovaries but no functional uterus (müllerian agenesis).
- Women with genetic risk (IVF and PGD).

Patient selection (ideal)

- Age < 35 years
- Presence of ovarian reserve (D-3, serum FSH <10 IU/L).
- Husband — normal seminogram.
- Couple must be screen negative for HIV and hepatitis.
- Normal uterine cavity as evaluated by hysteroscopy/sonohysterography.

Principal steps of an ART cycle

1. Down regulation using GnRH agonist.
2. Controlled ovarian hyperstimulation (COH).
3. Monitoring of follicular growth.
4. Oocyte retrieval.
5. Fertilisation *in vitro* (IVF, ICSI, GIFT).
6. Transfer of gametes or embryos.
7. Luteal support with progesterone.

GnRH analogues for down regulation

Currently most ART procedures involve the use of GnRH agonists (see p. 502).

- GnRH agonist therapy used for down regulation of pituitary, gives higher pregnancy rates.
- GnRH agonist therapy is continued either subcutaneously or intranasally during the gonadotrophin treatment phase (see p. 502).
- GnRH antagonists are currently tried along with gonadotrophin stimulation to prevent premature LH surge or premature ovulation. Cetrorelix and Ganirelix are the available drugs (see p. 502).

Different schedules for GnRH agonist are available :

- *Long follicular down regulation* — When therapy is started in the follicular phase of previous cycle.
- *Long luteal down regulation* (most commonly used) therapy is begun on D-21 of the previous cycle. Gonadotrophin stimulation is started following the menses (see p. 500).
- *Short protocol* — therapy is started in the follicular phase (D-1) along with gonadotrophin stimulation. This is also called 'flare' protocol, as gonadotrophin can work over the stimulatory effect of GnRH agonist.

Controlled ovarian hyperstimulation (COH)

In the first case, Steptoe and Edwards (1978) achieved the success from collecting the oocyte from a **natural cycle,** 36 hours after the onset of LH surge. But subsequently, it has been found that the success rate is much higher when more embryos are transferred which is only possible by COH. The other advantages of induction of superovulation are improved quality of the oocyte, timing of ovulation can be controlled, suited to the personnel involved and extended to all cases of ovulatory dysfunction (Fig. 16.6).The drug regimens used differ in each centre. Following drugs or combination of drugs are commonly used (Table 16.15).

Monitoring of follicular growth

The follicular growth response is monitored by cervical mucus study, sonographic measurement of the follicles and serum oestradiol estimation, commencing on the 8th day of treatment cycle. When three or more follicles are greater than 18 mm in diameter and serum E_2 levels > 250 pg/ml/per follicle, 5,000-10,000 IU of hCG (250 µg of recombinant hCG) is given intramuscularly. Oocyte is retrieved 36 hours after the hCG is given. hCG induces oocyte maturation. The individual woman may be a **high responder** or a **poor responder** (see p. 503). Depending upon the response management is done (see p. 503).

Table 16.15 : Drugs commonly used

- Clomiphene citrate (CC)
- CC + human menopausal gonadotrophin (hMG)
- CC + pure FSH
- CC + Recombinant FSH
- hMG
- FSH (see Table 16.7)
- GnRH analogues + hMG or pure FSH.

hCG is administered in each regimen (see Table 16.7)

Oocyte retrieval

Oocyte retrieval is done aseptically through vaginal route under ultrasound guidance. With the development of vaginal transducers, vaginal needle aspiration is done about 36 hours after hCG administration but before ovulation occurs (Fig. 16.6). Intravenous analgesia and sedation is adequate in most of the cases. The oocyte is readily recognisable as a single cell surrounded by a mass of cumulus cells. After recovery, the oocytes are maintained in culture *in vitro* for 4-6 hours.

Fertilisation (*in vitro*)

The sperm used for insemination *in vitro* is prepared by the wash and swim-up or density gradient centrifugation technique. Approximately 50,000 to 100,000 capacitated sperm are placed into the culture media containing the oocyte within 4-6 hours of retrieval. The eggs may demonstrate signs of fertilisation when examined 16-18 hours after insemination (presence of two pronuclei in the presence of a second polar body). **Sperm density and motility are the two most important criteria for successful IVF.** The semen is collected just prior to ovum retrieval.

Embryo transfer

The fertilised ova at the 4-8 cell stage are placed into the uterine cavity close to the fundus about 3 days after fertilisation through a fine flexible soft catheter transcervically. **Not more than three embryos are transferred** per cycle to minimise multiple pregnancy.

The process of transfer should be accurate, atraumatic and aseptic. Trial transfer is beneficial. The number of embryos to be transferred depends mainly on maternal age and the embryo quality.

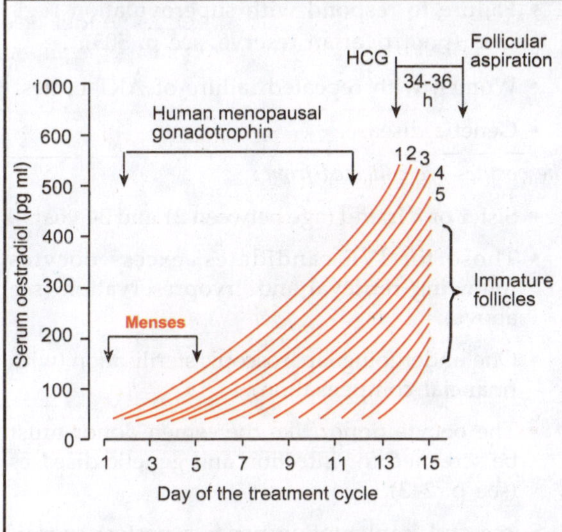

Fig. 16.6. Example of stimulated cycle in ART

Excess oocytes and embryos can be **cryopreserved** for future use. This will reduce the cost of ovulation stimulation as well as the risk of ovarian hyperstimulation (see p. 503).

- **Luteal phase support** is maintained with progesterone. It is started on the day after oocyte retrieval. hCG is given in supplemental doses (1,500-2,500 IU). Micronised progesterone 200 mg twice a day oral or as vaginal suppository or progesterone in oil injection 50 mg IM daily is continued for about 14 days. By this time diagnosis of pregnancy by estimation of β-hCG (quantitative value) is possible.

Result : The overall **delivery rate varies from 25-35 per cent per oocyte retrieval.**

There is increased risk of abortion (18%), multiple pregnancy (30%), ectopic (0.9%), low birth weight baby and prematurity. The risk of congenital malformation of the baby remains similar to general population.

GAMETE INTRAFALLOPIAN TRANSFER (GIFT)

GIFT was first described by Asch and colleagues in 1984. It is a more invasive and expensive procedure than IVF but the result seems better than IVF. In this procedure, both the sperm and the unfertilised oocytes are transferred into the fallopian tubes. Fertilisation is then achieved *in vivo*.

The prerequisite for GIFT procedure is to have normal uterine tubes. The indications are the same as that of IVF except the tubal factor. Best result is obtained in unexplained infertility and the result is poor in male factor abnormality.

The superovulation is done as in IVF. Two collected oocytes along with approximately 200,000-500,000 motile sperm for each fallopian tube are placed in a plastic tube container. It is then passed through laparoscope and inserted 4 cm. into the distal end of the fallopian tube where the combination is injected.

Result : The overall delivered pregnancy rate is as high as 27-30 per cent.

ZYGOTE INTRAFALLOPIAN TRANSFER (ZIFT)

Zygote intra-fallopian transfer was first described by Devroey *et al.* (1986).

The placement of the zygote (following one day of *in vitro* fertilisation) into the fallopian tube can be done either through the abdominal ostium by laparoscope or through the uterine ostium under ultrasonic guidance.

This technique is a suitable alternative of GIFT when defect lies in the male factor or in cases of failed GIFT. *Results* are similar to that of IVF. GIFT or ZIFT is avoided when tubal factors for infertility are present.

MICROMANIPULATION

Intracytoplasmic sperm injection (ICSI)

ICSI was first described by van Steirteghem and colleagues in Belgium (1992).

Indications :

- Severe oligospermia (< 5 million sperm/ml)
- Asthenospermia, Teratospermia
- Presence of sperm antibodies
- Obstruction of efferent duct system (male)
- Congenital absence of vas (bilateral)
- Failure of fertilisation in IVF
- Fertilisation of cryopreserved oocytes (with hardened zona pellucida)
- Unexplained infertility.

Sperm is recovered from the ejaculate. Otherwise sperm is retrieved by TESE (testicular sperm

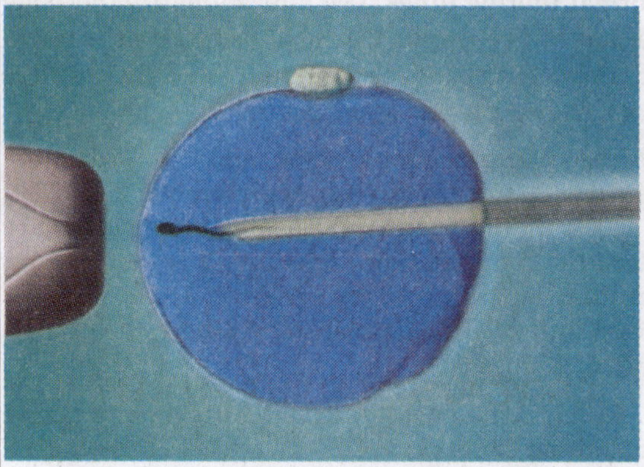

Fig. 16.7. Technique of intracytoplasmic sperm injection (ICSI)

extraction) or by MESA (microsurgical epididymal sperm aspiration) procedures.

Technique

One single spermatozoon or even a spermatid is injected directly into the cytoplasm of an oocyte by micropuncture of the zona pellucida. This procedure is carried out under a high quality inverted operating microscope. Micropipette is used to hold the oocyte while the spermatozoon is deposited inside the ooplasm by an injecting pipette (see Fig. 16.7).

ICSI is found to be very effective compared to other micromanipulation methods like subzonal insemination (SUZI). ICSI is very effective to reduce the need of AID.

Results : Fertilisation rate is about 60-70 per cent. Pregnancy rate is 20-40 per cent per embryo transfer.

EMBRYO OR OOCYTE DONATION

Ovum donation and IVF can help women with successful pregnancy. The essential requirements for successful outcome are : (i) successful ovum donation and IVF. (ii) Embryoendometrial synchronisation and (iii) Exogenous hormonal support until luteal–placental shift (see p. 245).

Indications

- Women with premature ovarian failure.
- Women with removed ovaries.
- Older women (poor oocyte quality).
- Failure to respond with superovulation regimen (poor ovarian reserve, see p. 503).
- Women with repeated failure of ART cycles.
- Genetic disease.

The oocytes are collected from :

- Sister or a friend (age between 21 and 34 years).
- Those for IVF candidates, excess oocytes following retrieval and cryopreservation (see above).
- One undergoing laparoscopic sterilisation (with financial compensation).
- The oocyte donor like the semen donor must be screened for infection and genetic diseases (see p. 243).

Successful implantation needs a perfect coordination of embryo and the endometrium. Oestrogen therapy (in the recipient) is started at the same time when the donor gets cycle stimulation. Progesterone treatment in the recipient generally begins on the day the donor undergoes ovum retrieval. Generally D3 embryos are transferred on the fourh day of progesterone therapy.

Luteal support : As the recipient has no corpus luteum, exogenous luteal support is needed. Exogenous oestrogen and progesterone treatment should therefore be continued until 10 weeks of gestation. Oocytes and embryos can be cryopreserved (at –196° under liquid nitrogen) for restoration of fertility in future. Survival of cryopreserved embryo is more than that of oocytes.

Results : Livebirth rate is approximately 47 per cent.

GESTATIONAL SURROGACY

A woman without a functional uterus, can have her genetic offspring with the help of ART. Embryos are transferred to the uterus of an another woman who is willing to carry the pregnancy on behalf of the infertile couple.

Cryopreservation of ovarian tissue

Restoration of reproductive function of a woman undergoing chemotherapy or radiotherapy is possible these days with the help of cryobiology. Cryopreservation of ovarian tissue or autotransplantation may allow natural pregnancy later on. With this method, ovulation using exogenous gonadotrophins can be achieved.

Oocyte cryopreservation by freezing is an alternative method. Vertification, using high concentration of cryoprotectant can solidify cells without ice formation. Human pregnancies and deliveries from vertified mature oocytes have been recorded.

Health hazards of ART

- **Most of the ART procedures are not associated with any increased risk of fetal congenital malformations or birth defects.** ICSI is often done due to male factors for infertility and it eliminates the natural process of sperm selection. It is not yet certain whether ICSI is associated with increased chromosomal abnormalities of the offspring.
- **Peri-implantation genetic diagnosis (PGD)** is done by blastomere biopsy. Genetic screening can avoid transferring embryos with aneuploidy and autosomal recessive or autosomal dominant gene mutation.
- Increased number of pregnancy loss, multiple pregnancy and ectopic pregnancy have been observed.
- Perinatal mortality and morbidity are high.
- Ovarian hyperstimulation syndrome (see p. 503) though rare but is a known health risk.
- Fertility drugs and cancer — no association have been found between ovulation induction drugs and ovarian cancer.
- Psychological stress and anxiety of the couple are severe. It is specially so when there is failure in the treatment or with a pregnancy loss.

PROGNOSIS OF INFERTILITY

The pregnancy rate within two years after the start of investigation, ranges between 30-40 per cent. The rate is however, increased to about 50-60 per cent, if AID cases are included.

Adoption

In spite of excellent advances in the field of infertility management, expectations are not always fulfilled. Couple must understand the infertility factors, cost and risk of management. End point of management must be realistically understood. Adoption is an alternative for many couples.

KEY POINTS

- Infertility is defined as a failure to conceive within 1 year of regular unprotected coitus.
- 10 per cent remain infertile by the end of 2nd year. The incidence increases further after the age of 30.
- In fully lactating women, pregnancy is unlikely up to 10 weeks postpartum.
- Male factor is responsible in 30-40 per cent, the female in 40-50 per cent, both in 10 per cent and unexplained in 10 per cent.
- Common causes of male infertility include defective spermatogenesis, obstruction of efferent duct, failure to deposit sperm high in vagina and error in seminal fluid (Table 16.1).
- Important causes of female infertility are tubal factor (25-35%), ovulatory factor (20-25%) and endometriosis (1-10%) (Scheme–1).
- Ovulatory dysfunction is likely to be linked with disturbed hypothalamo-pituitary-ovarian axis either primary or secondary from thyroid or adrenal dysfunction.
- Luteal phase defect is observed with older women, drug induced ovulation, elevated prolactin, patients with repeated pregnancy wastage, pelvic endometriosis, DUB and subclinical hypothyroidism.
- Serum progesterone more than 10 ng/ml on 8th postovulatory day indicates adequate luteal function.
- Luteinised unruptured follicle is often associated with pelvic endometriosis or with hyperprolactinaemia.
- Tubal factors are related to tubal infection, peritubal adhesions or endometriosis. The commonest peritoneal factor is endometriosis.
- Investigation of the infertile couple should be started after 1 year. The initial investigations of an infertile couple include : semen analysis (Male factor), hysterosalpingography (tubal factor), BBT and/or serum progesterone (evidence of ovulation) (see Scheme–3).

  BBT increases when circulating levels of progesterone is increased following ovulation.

KEY POINTS

- Diagnosis of ovulation is from indirect, direct and conclusive evidences (see Table 16.4).

  Subnuclear vacuolation of the endometrial glandular epithelium is the earliest evidence of ovulation (36-48 hours).

  A persistent rise in BBT and/or a serum progesterone more than 5 ng/ml is the presumptive evidence of ovulation. Sonographic evidences of ovulation are collapsed follicle and fluid in the pouch of Douglas. Pregnancy is the surest evidence of ovulation.

- A thorough investigation following an abnormal semen analysis, is needed to find out the specific cause of male infertility (Scheme–2).

- Tubal factor is assessed by HSG and laparoscopy; the two are complimentary. Sonohysterosalpingography has got no radiation exposure. Falloposcopy and salpingoscopy are used to study the tubal mucosa (Table 16.6).

- Postcoital test (PCT) is done in late proliferative phase. The examination is done 8-12 hours after coitus. The presence of active motile sperm numbering at least 10 per HPF is satisfactory. Routine PCT is not recommended.

  Presence of antisperm antibodies may not be the cause of infertility.

- Of all the aetiological factors, best result is obtained following treatment of anovulation.

- For induction of ovulation, the commonly used drugs are clomiphene citrate, hMG, FSH, hCG, GnRH analogues, bromocriptine (see Table 16.7).

  The suitable patients for clomiphene citrate (CC) are — normogonadotropic-normoprolactinaemic, PCO with amenorrhoea or hypothalamic amenorrhoea (see p. 237).

  Following CC therapy, incidence of multiple gestation is about 5 per cent and all being twins. The incidence of miscarriage, ectopic pregnancy or congenital malformation is not increased.

  Gonadotrophin therapy is indicated in cases with hypogonadotrophic-hypogonadism and clomiphene failure (see p. 238).

- GnRH is used in a pulsatile manner for cases with hypothalamic amenorrhoea and hypogonadotrophic hypogonadism.

  GnRH analogues are used in patients refractory to gonadotrophins, with elevated LH, with normal gonadotrophins and in cases with premature LH surge (see p. 238).

  Gonadotrophins and GnRH analogues and hCG are mostly used in ART with careful monitoring.

  Bromocriptine is indicated in cases of hyperprolactinaemia with or without galactorrhoea.

- Corpus luteum insufficiency can be treated by progesterone as vaginal suppositories or by hCG.

- Unruptured luteinised follicle is treated by intramuscular injection of hCG 5000-10,000 IU or ovulation inducing drugs or bromocriptine, if associated with hyperprolactinaemia.

- Tuboplasty is the surgical procedure performed to restore the anatomy and physiology of the tube (Table 16.9). Endoscopic surgery gives the best result. Prognosis for fertility depends upon the extent and the site of damage to the tube.

  Tubal reconstructive surgery may be considered for mild proximal tubal block. For any complicated tubal occlusive disease, IVF is the best therapy (see p. 239).

- Proximal tubal obstruction is usually treated by cannulation through tubes with catheters under hysteroscopic visualisation.

  No tubal surgery should be attempted in women with pelvic tuberculosis. IVF may be considered once endometrium is free from the disease (see p. 240).

  Overall result in terms of pregnancy following tuboplasty ranges between 15-60 per cent. The pregnancy rate after salpingolysis and fimbrioplasty is about 65 per cent. The result is best in reversal of tubal sterilisation by tubo-tubal anastomosis (see p. 241).

KEY POINTS

- Any form of therapy for minimal endometriosis does not improve fertility status. Unexplained infertility is observed in about 10-15 per cent cases. ART is an option for those who fail to conceive with expectant management (see p. 241).
- Assisted reproductive technology (ART) includes different methods (see Table 16.13). These are expensive and need sophisticated laboratory facilities.
- The best results of IUI are obtained in the treatment of cervical factor and unexplained infertility (Table 16.11) and in stimulated cycle (controlled ovarian hyperstimulation). Overall pregnancy rate ranges between 20-40 per cent.
- Controlled ovarian hyperstimulation (COH) and IUI (Table 16.12) are the options for women with unexplained infertility and for women whose male partner (husband) suffers from oligospermia.
- Donor insemination (AID) should be performed with frozen sperm, stored at least for 6 months. The donor should be retested negative for antibodies to HIV during this time of insemination. This is because antibodies to HIV may take several months to develop after the infection (see p. 242).
- IVF-ET (Steptoe and Edwards – 1978) — overall pregnancy rate varies from 20 to 30 per oocyte retrieval. Take home baby rate is about 15-20 per cent per procedure.
- GIFT (Asch-1984) procedure needs normal fallopian tubes. In some centres the success rate of GIFT and IVF-ET is the same.
- ICSI (Van Steirteghem – 1992) is an effective method for male infertility (severe oligospermia or sperm dysfunction). It reduces the need of AID.
- Pregnancy following donor oocyte or embryo is the option for women with ovarian failure, removed ovaries or with genetic disease.
- The pregnancy rate within 2 years after the start of investigations for infertility is 30-40 per cent. The rate is however increased to 50-60 per cent, if AID cases are included. When the couple fails to conceive after 2 years of therapy, the chance of conception is remote.
- Health hazards of ART include psychological stress of the couple, increased number of pregnancy loss, multiple pregnancy and ectopic pregnancy. Risk of fetal congenital malformations is not increased. Ovarian hyperstimulation syndrome is rare but is a known health hazard.
- Ovarian hyperstimulation syndrome (see p. 503) is a complication of ovulation induction. Basic pathology is increased capillary permeability (VEGF) leading to ascites, hypovolaemia, oliguria and electrolyte imbalance. Management is conservative. Abdominal paracentesis, to relieve respiratory distress and human albumin (IV), to correct hypovolaemia may be needed.
- **According to WHO, Ovulatory disorders are grouped into :**

  Group I : **Hypothalamic-Pituitary failure :** women in this group have hypogonadotrophic hypogonadism, low gonadotrophin and oestrogen level, normal prolactin and negative progesterone challenge test. Included in this group are : stress related amenorrhoea, Kallmann's syndrome, anorexia nervosa (p. 444, 450). These women are treated with hMG or GnRH.

  Group II : **Hypothalamic Pituitary Dysfunction** — Women are normogonadotrophic, normoestrogenic, anovulatory and oligomenorrhoeic. Women with PCOS are in this group (p. 440). These women are treated with clomiphene citrate.

  Group III : **Ovarian failure** — Women are hypergonadotrophic and hypogonadal with low oestrogen level (p. 444). These women are treated with ovum donation.

Benign Lesions of the Vulva and Vagina

17

VULVAL EPITHELIAL DISORDERS

Terminology, definition and types

The term "dystrophy" was used to embrace several lesions in the vulva characterised by epithelial abnormalities which result in either red or white appearance of the skin of the region.

Within the spectrum, various patterns of epithelial changes may be found. The changes may be interchangeable in the same patient in different times or at different sites of the lesion at the same time. The process may be reversible or remain static.

There has been much confusion about the nomenclature of vulval 'dystrophies'. The latest terminology recommended by **International Society for the Study of Vulval Disease (1989)** are listed in the Table 17.1. **Only the non-neoplastic disorders will be discussed in this chapter.**

Aetiology

The precise mechanism of vulval epithelial disorder is not clear. Multiple factors such as traumatic (scratching), allergic, irritation, nutritional (deficiency of folic acid, vit. B_{12}, riboflavine, achlorhydria, etc.), infection (fungus), immunological or metabolic, etc. are possibly implicated. Autoimmune disorders like thyroid disease, pernicious anaemia and diabetes are often associated.

Lichen sclerosis

As because the epithelium is metabolically active, the justification of the term 'atrophicus' is inappropriate and the terminology of only lichen sclerosis is preferred.

It usually occurs following menopause; may occur even in childhood but in that case it resolves after menarche.

Table 17.1
Terminology of disorders of vulval skin and mucosa

Non-neoplastic

- Lichen sclerosus
- Squamous cell hyperplasia (Formerly hyperplastic dystrophy)
- Other dermatoses

Vulval intra-epithelial neoplasia (VIN)

- Squamous VIN
  VIN I — Mild dysplasia
  VIN II — Moderate dysplasia
  VIN III — Severe dysplasia
- Non-squamous VIN
  Paget's disease

Note 1 : When mixed epithelial disorders occur, they should be reported separately. For example, lichen sclerosus associated with squamous cell hyperplasia should be reported separately and not as mixed dystrophy.

Note 2 : When the squamous cell hyperplasia is secondary to specific dermatoses involving the vulva, the primary lesion should be mentioned. Such primary lesions are psoriasis, lichen planus, Candida infection, condyloma acuminatum.

Note 3 : Leukoplakia is a descriptive term used for irregular thickening and whitening of the vulval skin. It is seen in several pathological conditions of the vulva. It should not be used as a diagnostic term.

Distribution of lesion

The entire vulva is involved. It may even extend to the perineum and beyond the labiocrural folds to the thighs. It may also affect other parts of the body. The distribution of lesion is thus more wider.

Histology

The epithelium is thin, at times with hyperkeratosis. There is flattening of the rete ridges with evidence of hyalinisation. Fibroblasts are absent. There is presence of lymphocytes and plasma cells (Fig. 17.2).

Clinical features

Pruritus is more than soreness. There is dyspareunia (excluding childhood) and dysuria. This is due to stenosis of the vulval outlet. The skin is thin and looks white. On rubbing, the skin becomes thickened (Fig. 17.1).

Diagnosis

The diagnosis should be confirmed by biopsy having characteristic changes.

The risk of malignancy is about 1-4 per cent.

Squamous cell hyperplasia

The term squamous cell hyperplasia is applied to histological evidences of hyperplasia without any other clinical features to account for the lesion. As such, the associated local pathology to produce squamous cell hyperplasia must be excluded prior hand.

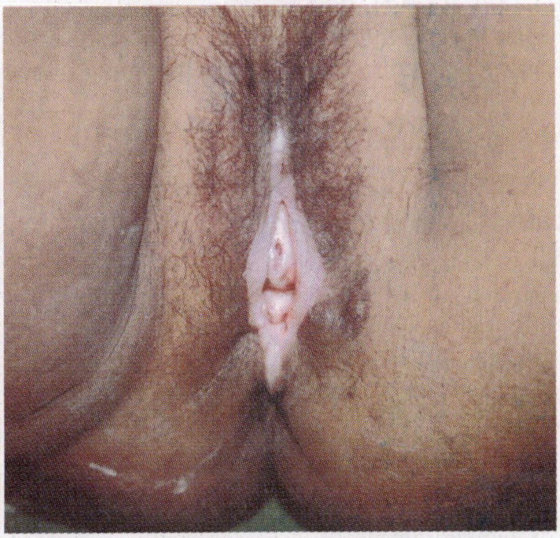

Fig. 17.1. Lichen sclerosis

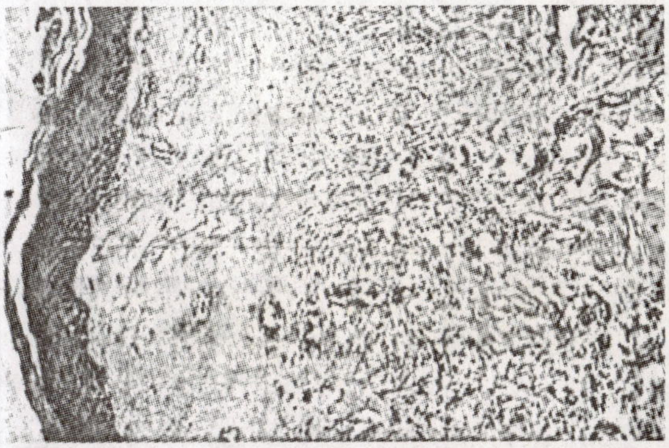

Fig. 17.2. Histologic picture of Lichen sclerosis showing atrophic and flat epithelium with loss of rete ridges. There is presence of hyalinised collagen tissue and chronic inflammatory cells.

The median age is younger, may be premenopausal but mostly postmenopausal.

Distribution of lesion : It is confined to the inner aspects of the labia majora, the labia minora, the introitus and the prepuce of clitoris.

Histology : The microscopic picture is nonspecific. The characteristic features are elongation of rete pegs, hyperkeratosis and the presence of dermal inflammation.

Biopsy is mandatory not only to clinch the diagnosis but to assess the presence or absence of atypia. Atypia is found in about 10 per cent of cases.

Clinical features : Pruritus is the chief complaint. There may be dysuria. When cracks develop, there may be increased soreness and pain.

The affected area of the vulva looks white with well-defined margins.

Prognosis : The cases with severe atypia are considered to be precancerous and chance of malignancy is much high.

Psoriasis : Psoriasis may occur exclusively on the vulva. But often, there are lesions elsewhere or have a positive family history.

Relation with malignancy

About 50 per cent of all invasive carcinomas of the vulva arise in an area of chronic vulval epithelial disorder. The malignant potential of vulval intraepithelial neoplastic (VIN) disorders is about 2-4 per cent and that for non-neoplastic epithelial disorders is very low. The chance is more with hyperplastic variety with cellular atypia (Fig. 17.3).

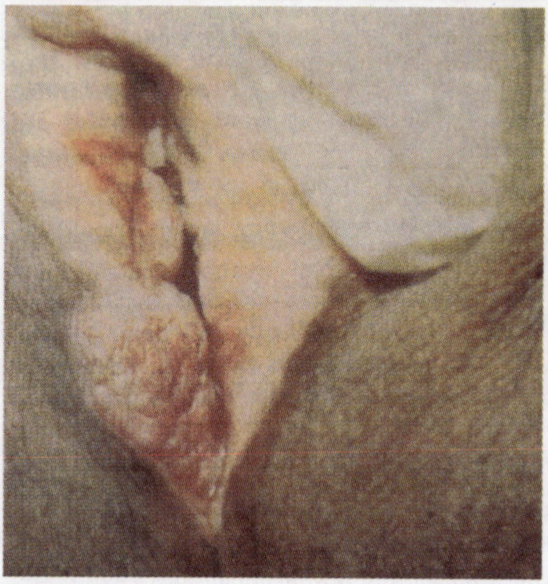

Fig. 17.3. Vulval dystrophy associated with malignancy

Confirmation of diagnosis of vulval epithelial disorders

Multiple punch biopsies are needed prior to therapy. The objectives of biopsy are to diagnose the type of disorder and to differentiate it from other skin lesions such as vitiligo or psoriasis.

The sites for biopsy are from the margins of cracks and fissures and the sky blue areas left behind after applying 1 per cent aqueous toluidine blue to the vulva and washing it off after 1 minute with 1 per cent acetic acid. Laboratory investigations as and where necessary are to be carried out as mentioned in the aetiology to determine the cause.

Treatment of vulval epithelial disorders

General

- The patient should avoid the use of deodorants or douches.
- A non-irritant soap should be used in the area and dried carefully without much rubbing.
- The patient should use either cotton underwear or nothing at all.
- Histopathological diagnosis has to be made by biopsy prior to institution of any therapy.
- All possible contributing factors should be dealt adequately.

Individual protocol

Lichen sclerosis

In asymptomatic cases, no treatment is required. In symptomatic cases, a 2 per cent of testosterone ointment gives good result when applied locally 2-3 times a day. This results in thickening and softening the skin — relieves the pruritus. Thereafter, testosterone cream should be applied locally once or twice a week indefinitely. The patient should be checked at interval of 3 months.

In prepubertal girls, local application of 1 per cent hydrocortisone cream is quite effective. Potent steroid cream like clobetasol propionate (0.05%) also gives good response.

There is no place of vulvectomy or laser vaporisation.

Squamous cell hyperplasia

- Without atypia — Local application with 2 per cent hydrocortisone cream is effective. The oedema and inflammation of the nerve endings subside → relief of pruritus. Alternatively, potent fluorinated corticosteroid cream, clobetasol propionate 0.05 per cent have been recommended three times daily for 8-10 weeks.

- With atypia — Considering the risk involved in development of malignancy, local vulvectomy is justified. Serial section should be done from the suspected areas to exclude malignancy. There is chance of recurrence.

Local therapy with antimitotic agent such as fluorouracil which inhibit an enzyme essential for pyrimidine synthesis is helpful when applied as 5 per cent cream twice daily for a minimum period of 6-8 weeks.

Psoriasis

Treatment is by topical corticosteroids.

White lesions of the vulva

The melanocytes loose their ability to manufacture melanin resulting in depigmentation and subsequent white lesions. **The lesions include** :

- Lichen sclerosis
- Squamous cell hyperplasia
- Vitiligo
- Albinism — enzyme deficiency preventing normal formation of melanin
- Leukoderma
- Intertrigo.

Table 17.2
Ulcers of the vulva

STD related (see chapter 11)	Idiopathic	Tuberculosis	Malignancy (see ch. 23)	Systemic disease related or dermatoses
• Syphilitic • Herpes genitalis • Chancroid • Granuloma inguinale • Lymphogranuloma venerum	Behçet's disease Aphthous ulcers Lipschutz ulcers	Tubercular	**Primay** • Squamous cell carcinoma • Malignant melanoma • Basal cell carcinoma **Secondary** • Leukaemia • Choriocarcinoma (p. 349)	• Lupus erythematosus • Crohn's disease • Lichen planus • Lichen sclerosis

Red lesions of the vulva are due to infection (candida), allergy, dermatitis and melanosis.

VULVAL ULCERS

Vulval ulcers are predominantly due to sexually transmitted diseases. Rarely, it may be due to non-specific causes. Malignant ulcer is also rare. The various aetiological factors related to vulval ulcers are given in the Table 17.2.

All are described in appropriate chapters (see p. 155, 307, 321). **Other systemic diseases with vulvar manifestation.**

Crohn's disease

Crohn's disease affecting the intestine may involve the vulva in late stage of the disease in about 25 per cent of cases. The ulcer looks like knife cuts in the skin.

Behçet's disease

This is a rare chronic inflammatory disease characterised by recurrent oral and genital ulcers with ocular ulcer (anterior uveitis). The exact aetiology is unknown. It may be the manifestation of an underlying autoimmune process. Monoarticular arthritis may also be associates. The vulval ulceration may be extensive and leaving behind dense scar after healing.

There is no specific treatment. Topical and systemic corticosteroids are used for relief of the symptoms. Oestrogen dominated oral contraceptives are often beneficial.

Lipschutz ulcer

The lesion affects mainly the labia minora and introitus. In acute state, there may be constitutional upset with lymphadenopathy. The causative agent may be Epstein-Barr virus. Treatment is with antiseptic lotions and ointment.

Vulval ulcer

Leukaemia — Rarely may cause nodular infiltration and ulceration of the vulva.

Dermatological disorders : Disseminated lupus erythematosus may cause recurrent ulcerations of the vulva and mucous membrane of the mouth and vagina.

Vulvar manifestations of systemic diseases

(1) **Dermatologic disorders** : (i) Contact dermatitis — due to agents that may be locally irritant. (ii) Psoriasis. (iii) Ulceration due to disseminated lupus erythematosus.

(2) Vulvar ulceration or deposits due to **leukaemia**.

(3) **Acanthosis nigricans** — hyperpigmented lesion of the vulva. It may be associated with glucose intolerance (insulin resistance), chronic anovulation and androgen excess (see p. 440).

(4) **Chronic vulvo vaginal candidiasis** : due to diabetes.

(5) **Behçet's syndrome.**

MISCELLANEOUS SWELLINGS

Vulval cysts

Bartholin's cyst — See p. 158.

Sebaceous cyst — These are usually multiple and are formed by accumulation of the sebaceous material due to occlusion of the ducts. These are located in the labia majora. If infected, treatment is done by antibiotics and surgical drainage.

Cyst of the canal of Nuck — Part of the processus vaginalis which accompanied the round ligament and obliterated prior to birth may persist to form a cyst. It invariably occupies the anterior part of the labium majus.

Inguinolabial hernia

When the entire processus vaginalis remains patent there may be herniation of the abdominal contents along the tract. The hernia may be limited to the inguinal canal or may extend upto the anterior part of the labium majus. The contents of the sac may be intestine or omentum. The swelling is reducible and impulse on straining can be elicited. **One should be conscious of the entity** as casual surgical incision on labial swelling may cause inadvertent injury to the gut.

Vulval varicosities

These are met predominantly during pregnancy and subside following delivery. Sometimes, they may produce intolerable aching on standing. Support pads and tights or T-bandage may be tried to relieve the symptoms. If fails, treatment by injecting sclerosing fluids or high ligature of the long saphenous vein may be of help.

Elephantiasis vulvae

It is mainly due to consequence of lymphatic obstruction by microfilaria (filariasis). Plastic surgery may be tried to restore the normal anatomy along with antifilarial treatment. There is chance of recurrence.

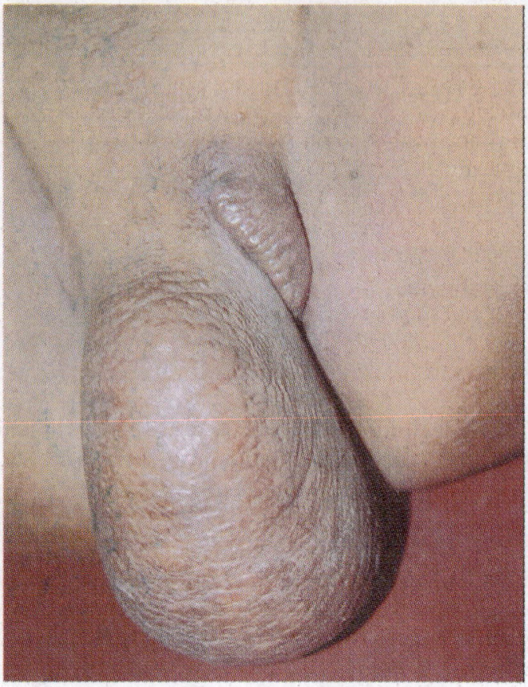

Fig. 17.4. Vulval fibroma
[*By courtesy* : Dr. (Ms.) C. Das, Associate Professor, Dept. of OB-Gynae., NRS Medical College, Kolkata

Benign Tumours of the Vulva

Fibroma, lipoma, neurofibroma

These are all benign tumours of varying sizes, Surgical removal is necessary if they produce discomfort (Figs 17.4 and 17.5).

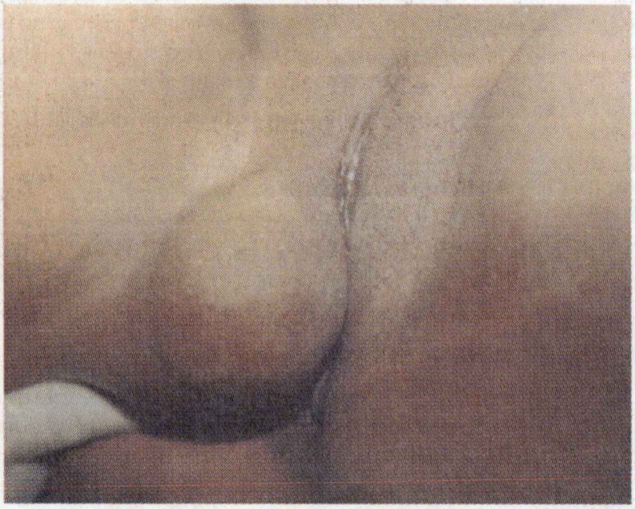

Fig. 17.5. Vulval lipoma

Hydradenoma : Hydradenoma arises from the sweat gland in the vulva, usually located in the anterior part of the labia majora. It rarely exceeds 1 cm. It is a benign lesion but its reddish look and complex adenomatous pattern on histology may be confused with malignancy. Simple excision is adequate.

Endometriosis

Endometriosis usually appears as a swelling near the insertion of the round ligaments in the anterior part of the labia majora. It may be associated with pelvic endometriosis. Its presence is limited only during reproductive period and becomes enlarged and tender during menstruation. Treatment is surgical excision and confirmation by biopsy (endometrial glands and stroma with haemosiderin – laden macrophages).

VAGINAL CYSTS

Vaginal cyst is rare as there is no gland in the mucous coat. Small cysts may remain unnoticed. The common cysts that are found include Gartner's duct cyst and epithelial inclusion cyst.

Gartner's cyst

The Gartner's duct cyst is usually situated in the anterolateral wall of the vagina. The epithelium is low columnar and secretes mucinous material which is pent up forming the cyst. The treatment is by surgical excision (Fig. 17.6).

Inclusion cyst

The epithelial inclusion cysts arise from the vaginal epithelium buried under the mucosa during healing from a traumatic injury following childbirth or surgery. They usually locate in the lower-third of the vagina on the posterior or posterolateral wall. The lining epithelium is stratified squamous. The content is a thick cheesy substance. The treatment in symptomatic cases is by surgical excision (Fig. 17.7).

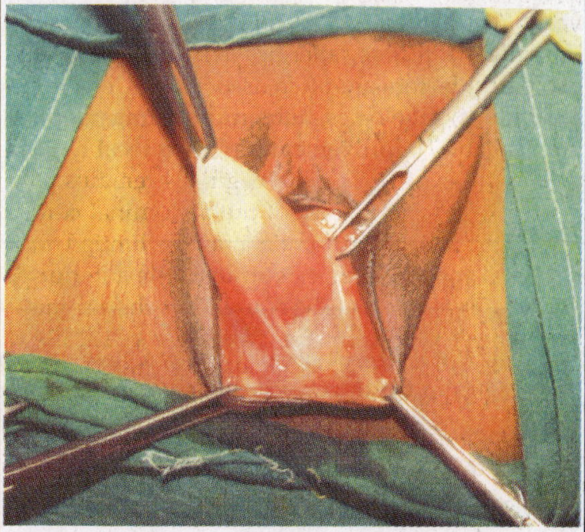

Fig. 17.6. Gartner's duct cyst

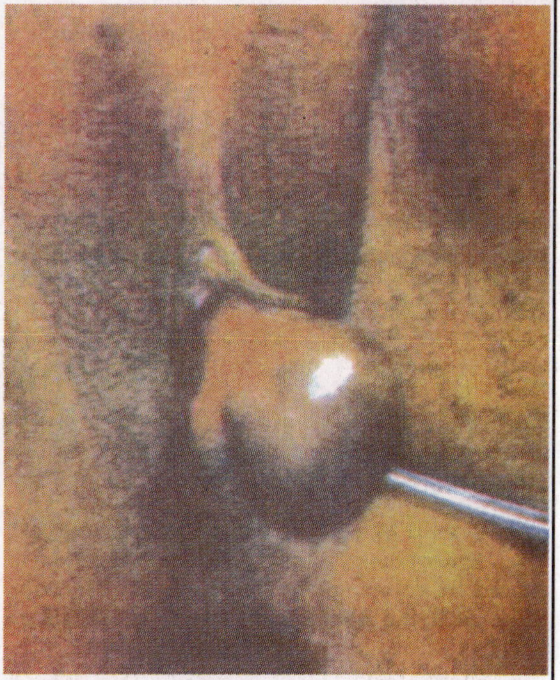

Fig. 17.7. Intracystic haemorrhage in inclusion cyst

VULVAL PAIN SYNDROME

Vulvar pain may be burning, stinging or irritation. It may be due to several reasons.

- Aphthous ulcer
- Vulval dermatoses
- Herpes genitalis
- Pudendal or genitofemoral nerve neuralgia
- Vulvodynia (burning vulva syndrome)
- Vulval vestibulitis syndrome
- Referred pain from urethral or vagina
- Psychological.

Vulvodynia is characterised by burning sensation over the vulva (burning vulva syndrome). It is often seen in perimenopausal or postmenopausal women. Exact aetiology is not known. Infective, allergic or psychological factors may be related. It is not associated with dyspareunia. Clinical examination does not reveal any abnormality in many cases. Colposcopic examination may show acetowhite or erythematous change of the epithelium. Treatment unsatisfactory. Tricyclic anti-depressant (amitriptyline) is found helpful. A dose of 60 mg/day for 3-6 months is given. Gabapentin is also beneficial. Psychosexual counselling and behaviour therapy are needed for some cases. Surgery is contraindicated.

Vulval vestibulitis syndrome is characterised by pain around the ducts of Bartholin gland and the introitus. There may be superficial dyspareunia and vestibular tenderness on touch. Exact aetiology is unknown. Infective, allergic, dermatologic or psychological factors are often associated. Considering the various, aetiologies, numerous treatment options are available. Improvement of vulvar local hygiene, control of infective agents and allergens, diet modification (low oxalate), psychological (tricyclic antidepressants), behavioural treatment and even surgery (vestibuloplasty, laser vaporisation) have been tried. Treatment results are often unsatisfactory.

KEY POINTS

- Lichen sclerosus usually occurs following menopause. The lesion can extend beyond the labiocrural folds to the thighs. Pruritus is more than soreness. The risk of malignancy is 1-4 per cent.
- Hyperplastic dystrophy is usually confined to inner aspects of labia majora, the labia minora and the introitus. Pruritus is the chief complaint.

  About 50 per cent of all invasive carcinomas of the vulva arise in an area of chronic vulval epithelial disorder. Only 2-4 per cent of VIN may develop malignancy. Multiple biopsies are to be taken from the sky blue areas left behind after applying 1 per cent aqueous toluidine blue and washed off with 1 per cent acetic acid. Cases with atypia have got increased chance of malignancy. Considering the risk, local vulvectomy is justified specially with atypia (see p. 308).
- Vulval cyst may be — Bartholin's cyst, sebaceous cyst or cyst of canal of Nuck.
- Vulval ulcers are predominantly STI related.
- Vulvodynia is a painful condition of the vulva of unknown aetiology. Psychosexual counselling, behavioural therapy, tricyclic antidepressants (amitriptyline) are helpful.
- Vulval vestibulitis syndrome — may be a generalised or focal painful condition of unknown aetiology. Topical agents (steroids, antifungal creams), vestibulectomy, behavioural therapy, have been tried.
- Vaginal ulcer is rare. Common vaginal cysts are Gartner's cyst and epithelial inclusion cyst.

Benign Lesions of the Cervix

18

CERVICAL ECTOPY (EROSION)

Definition

Cervical ectopy is a condition where the squamous epithelium of the ectocervix is replaced by columnar epithelium which is continuous with the endocervix. It is not an ulcer (Fig. 18.1).

Aetiology

- **Congenital**
- **Acquired**

Congenital

At birth, in about one-third of cases, the columnar epithelium of the endocervix extends beyond the external os. This condition persists only for a few days until the level of oestrogen derived from the mother falls. Thus, the congenital ectopy heals spontaneously.

But real congenital ectopy reappears at or soon after puberty under the influence of oestrogen in about one-third of cases.

Acquired

Hormonal

The squamocolumnar junction is not static and its movement, either inwards or outwards is dependent on oestrogen. When the oestrogen level is high, it moves, out so that the columnar epithelium extends onto the vaginal portion of the cervix replacing the squamous epithelium. This state is observed during pregnancy and amongst 'pill users'. The squamocolumnar junction returns back to its normal position after 3 months following delivery and little earlier following withdrawal of 'pill'.

Infection

The role of infection as the primary cause of ectopy has been discarded. However, chronic cervicitis may be associated or else the infection may supervene on an ectopy because of the delicate columnar epithelium which is more vulnerable to trauma and infection.

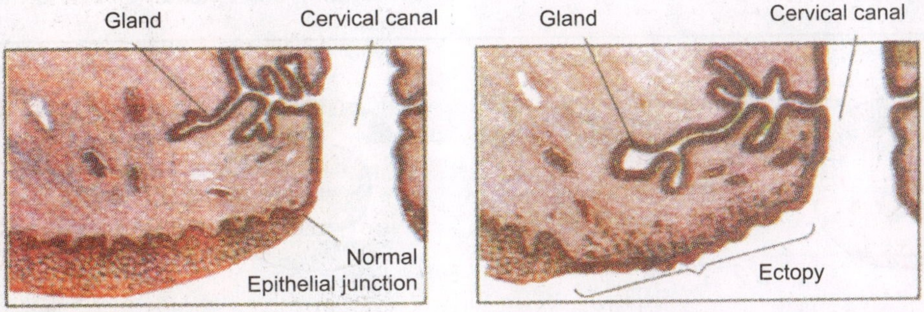

Fig. 18.1. (A) Normal squamocolumnar junction; (B) Ectopy

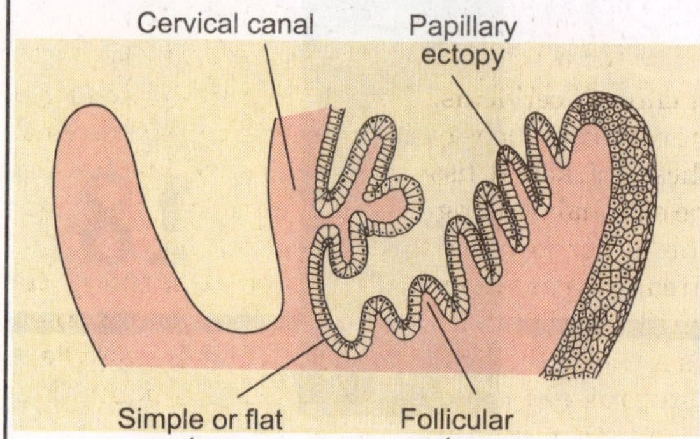

Fig. 18.2. Different types of erosion

Pathogenesis

In the active phase of ectopy, the squamocolumnar junction moves out from the os. The columnar epithelium of the endocervix maintains its continuity while covering the ectocervix replacing the squamous epithelium. The replaced epithelium is usually arranged in a single layer (**flat type**) or may be so hyperplastic as to fold inwards to accommodate in the increased area — **a follicular ectopy**. At times, it becomes heaped up to fold inwards and outwards — **a papillary ectopy** (Fig. 18.2). Underneath the epithelium, there are evidences of round cell infiltration and glandular proliferation. The features of infection are probably secondary rather than primary. The columnar epithelium is less resistant to infection than the squamous epithelium.

During the process of healing, the squamocolumnar junction gradually moves towards the external os. The squamous epithelium grows beneath the columnar epithelium until it reaches at or near to its original position at the external os. The columnar epithelium gradually disintegrates. Alternatively, the replacement is probably by squamous metaplasia of the columnar cells. The possibility of squamous metaplasia of the reserve cells is also likely (details in Chap. 22).

During the process, the squamous epithelium may obstruct the mouth of the underlying glands (normally not present in ectocervix) → pent up secretion → retention cyst → **Nabothian follicle**. Alternatively, the epithelium may burrow inside the gland lumina. In oblique cut-section, it may simulate the histologic picture of squamous cell carcinoma. **This process of replacement by the squamous epithelium is called epidermidisation.**

Ectopy is not to be considered as precancerous but the squamocolumnar junction is vulnerable to malignant changes.

Clinical features

Symptoms

The lesion may be asymptomatic. However, the following symptoms may be present.

- Vaginal discharge — The discharge may be excessively mucoid from the overgrowth or overactive cervical crypts. It may be mucopurulent, offensive and irritant in presence of infection; may be even blood-stained due to premenstrual congestion.
- Contact bleeding specially during pregnancy and 'pill use' either following coitus or defecation may be associated.
- Associated cervicitis may produce backache, pelvic pain and at times infertility.

Signs

Internal examination reveals (Fig. 18.3) :

- Per speculum — There is a bright red area surrounding and extending beyond the external os

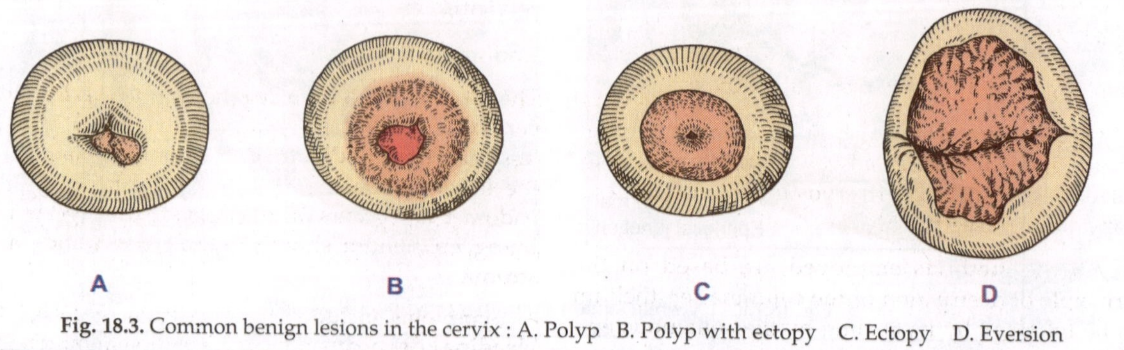

Fig. 18.3. Common benign lesions in the cervix : A. Polyp B. Polyp with ectopy C. Ectopy D. Eversion

in the ectocervix. The outer edge is clearly demarcated. The lesion may be smooth or having small papillary folds. It is neither tender nor bleeds to touch. On rubbing with a gauze piece, there may be multiple oozing spots (sharp bleeding in isolated spots in carcinoma).

The feel is soft and granular giving rise to a grating sensation.

Diagnosis

The diagnosis is confused with :

Ectropion : The lips of the cervix are curled back to expose the endocervix. This may be apparent when the lips of the cervix are stretched by the bivalve speculum.

Early carcinoma : It is indurated, friable and usually ulcerated which bleeds to touch. Confirmation is by biopsy, if necessary following Schiller's iodine application or colposcopy directed.

Primary sore : There is denudation of the epithelium without excavation of the cervical tissue. The ulcer has a punched-out appearance. Smear examination under dark ground illumination microscopy, identifies the treponemata.

Tubercular ulcer : There is indurated ulcer with caseation at the base. Biopsy confirms the diagnosis.

Management

Guidelines : **All cases should be subjected to cytological examination** from the cervical smear to exclude dysplasia or malignancy. In doubtful smear, colposcopy and or cervical biopsy should be done.

In asymptomatic cases discovered on routine examination, active treatment should be withheld.

Symptomatic cases

• Detected during pregnancy and early puerperium, the treatment should be withheld for at least 12 weeks postpartum. In pill users, the 'pill' should be stopped and barrier method is advised.

• Persistent ectopy with troublesome discharge should be treated surgically by — (i) thermal cauterisation (see Fig. 34.2), (ii) cryosurgery and (iii) laser vaporisation (see p. 561).

All the methods employed are based on the principle of destruction of the columnar epithelium to be followed by its healing by the squamous epithelium.

EVERSION (ECTROPION)

In chronic cervicitis, there is marked thickening of the cervical mucosa with underlying tissue oedema. These thickened tissues tend to push out through the external os along the direction of least resistance. The entity is most marked where the cervix has already been lacerated. In such conditions, the longitudinal muscle fibres are free to act unopposed. As a result, the lips of the cervix curl upwards and outwards to expose the red looking endocervix so as to be confused with ectopy (Fig. 18.3).

CERVICAL TEAR

Varying degrees of cervical tear is invariable during vaginal delivery. One or both the sides may be torn or the tear may be irregular (stellate type). If there is no superimposed infection and the tear is small, the torn surfaces may appose leaving behind only a small notch. However, if infection supervenes, eversion occurs confusing the diagnosis of ectopy (Fig. 18.3).

Non-obstetric causes of cervical lacerations are during operative procedures of dilatation of the cervix. Postmenopausal atrophy or chronic cervicitis predisposes to tear.

CERVICAL CYSTS

Nabothian cysts (Fig. 18.4)

These are usually multiple. They are formed due to blocking of the cervical gland mouths usually as a result of healing of ectopy (epidermidisation). The pent up secretion produces cysts of varying sizes from microscopic to pea. **The presence of the cysts furthest from the external os indicates the extent of transformation zone**. The lining epithelium is columnar. The treatment is directed towards chronic cervicitis.

Endometriotic cysts

These are situated in the portio vaginalis part of the cervix. The cyst is small and reddish and of less than 1 cm in diameter. It is more explained by the implantation theory. The implantation of the endometrium occurs during delivery or surgery. The lining epithelium shows endometrial glands and stroma.

Symptoms include intermenstrual or postcoital bleeding, deep dyspareunia and dysmenorrhoea.

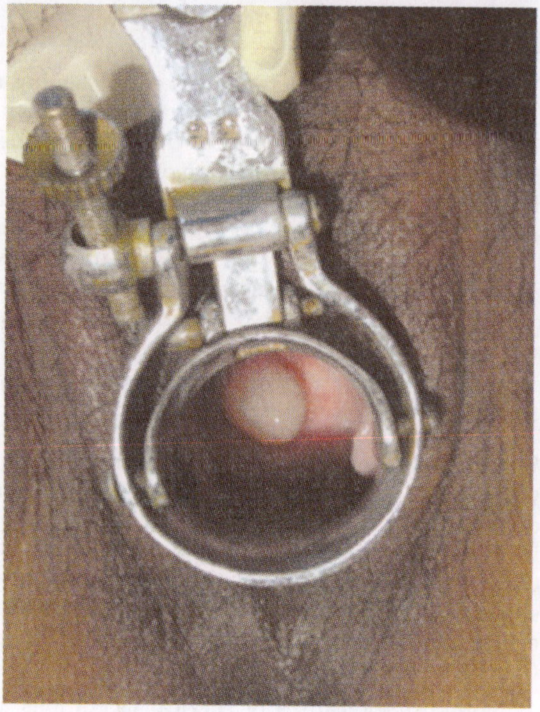

Fig. 18.4. Nabothian cyst of cervix

Speculum examination reveals a small reddish cyst. The treatment is destruction by cauterisation and rarely by excision.

Mesonephric cysts

These are usually situated on the outerside of the cervical stroma. They seldom exceed 2.5 cm. These are lined by cuboidal epithelium. They are asymptomatic. The existence of the cyst is discovered on speculum examination and confirmation by excision biopsy.

ELONGATION OF THE CERVIX

The normal length of the cervix is about 2.5 cm. The vaginal and the supravaginal parts are of equal length. The elongation may affect either part of the cervix.

Causes

Elongation of the supravaginal part is commonly associated with the uterine prolapse. The mechanism has been described in p. 201.

Vaginal part is always elongated congenitally. Chronic cervicitis may produce some hypertrophy and makes the cervix bulky.

Symptoms

There is no specific symptom for supravaginal elongation. However, congenital elongation of the vaginal part may present the following :

- Sensation of something coming down
- Dyspareunia
- Infertility

Pelvic examination

Supravaginal elongation is featured by (Fig. 18.5) :

- Associated uterine prolapse.
- Fornix — shallow.
- Vaginal cervix — normal length.
- Uterine body — normal in size.
- Uterocervical canal — increased in length evidenced by introduction of an uterine sound. This indirectly proves that the increase is in the supravaginal part.

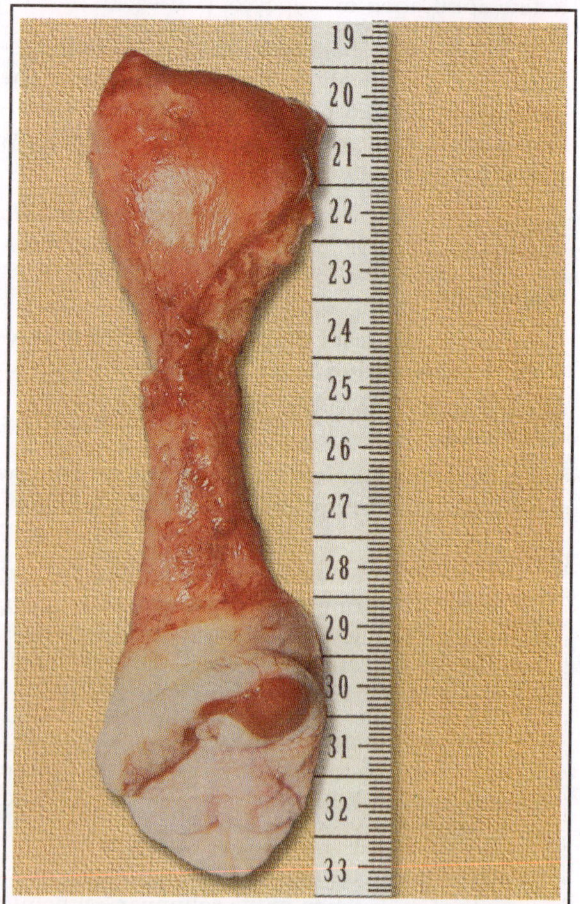

Fig. 18.5. Supravaginal elongation of cervix in prolapse

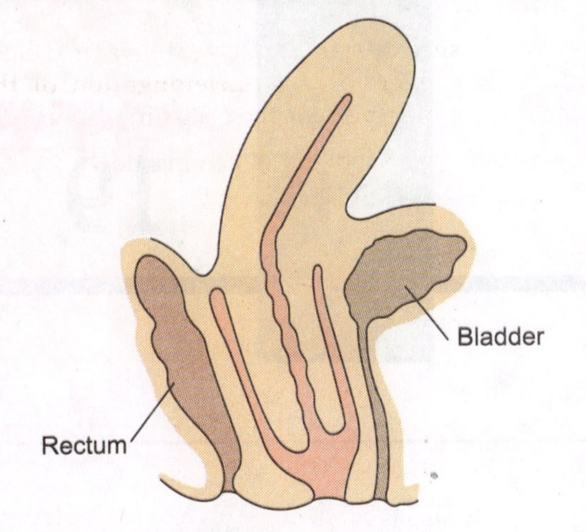

Fig. 18.6. Congenital elongation of cervix

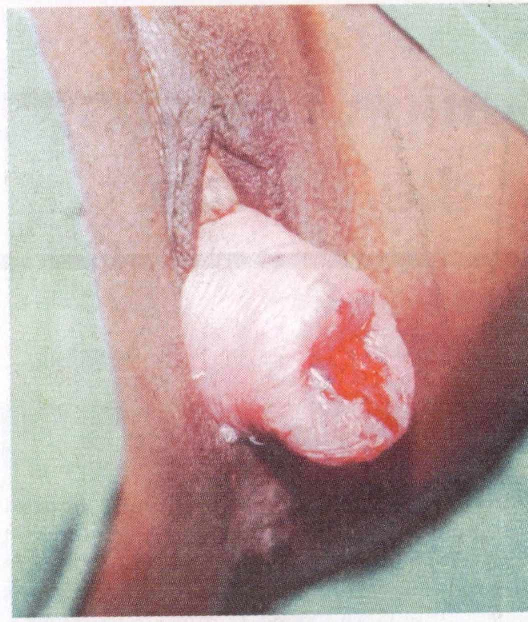

Fig. 18.7. Congenital elongation of cervix with prolapse

Congenital elongation is featured by (Fig. 18.6) :

- Fornix — deep.
- Vaginal cervix — elongated.
- Uterine body — normal in size.
- Uterocervical canal — increased in length, evidenced by uterine sound.

Treatment

Supravaginal elongation (Fig. 18.5)

As it is associated with uterine prolapse, its treatment protocol will be the same as that for prolapse.

Congenital elongation (Fig. 18.7)

The excess length of the cervix is amputated (cervical amputation). In presence of congenital prolapse, some form of cervicopexy has to be done (see p. 215).

KEY POINTS

- Chronic cervicitis and cervical erosion are the two most common cervical lesions encountered in gynaecological practice.
- Cervical ectopy (erosion) may be congenital (circumoral) or acquired due to hormonal effect as observed during pregnancy and 'pill users'. The role of infection as the primary cause has been discarded.
  Histologically, the erosion is either flat, papillary or of follicular variety.
  Healing of the erosion occurs through replacement of the columnar epithelium by downgrowth of the squamous epithelium or by squamous metaplasia of the columnar cells or the reserve cells. This process of replacement is called epidermidisation. Ectopy is not a precancerous state.
  Ectopy is not an ulcer as it is entirely lined by columnar epithelium.
  All cases should be subjected to cytological examination to exclude dysplasia or malignancy.
  In asymptomatic cases, treatment should be withheld.
  Detected during pregnancy, treatment should be withheld for at least 12 weeks postpartum.
  Persistent erosion with troublesome discharge should be treated surgically by thermal cauterisation, cryosurgery or best by laser vaporisation.
- Cervical cysts may be Nabothian, endometriotic or mesonephric. The confirmation of diagnosis is by histology.
- Supravaginal elongation of the cervix is associated with uterine prolapse and elongation of the vaginal part of the cervix is congenital in origin.

Benign Lesions of the Uterus

19

FIBROID

Fibroid is not only **the commonest benign tumour of the uterus** but is the commonest benign solid tumour in female. Histologically this tumour is composed of smooth muscle and fibrous connective tissue, so named as uterine leiomyoma, myoma or fibromyoma.

Incidence

It has been estimated that at least 20 per cent of women at the age of 30 have got fibroid in their wombs. Fortunately, most of them remain asymptomatic. The incidence of symptomatic fibroid in hospital outpatient is about 3 per cent. A high incidence of 10 per cent prevails in England. In coloured races (black women), the incidence is even higher.

These are more common in nulliparous (Fig. 19.2) or in those having one child infertility (Table 19.1). The prevalence is highest between 35-45 years.

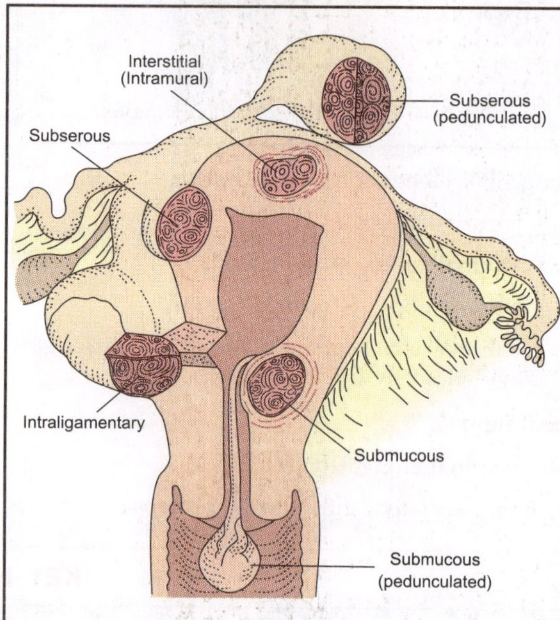

Fig. 19.1. Various types of uterine fibroids

Histogenesis

Origin

The aetiology still remains unclear. The prevailing hypothesis is that, it arises from the neoplastic single smooth muscle cell of the myometrium. The stimulus for initial neoplastic transformation is not known. The following are implicated :

- **Chromosomal abnormality** — In about 40 per cent of cases there is a varying type of chromosomal abnormality particularly the chromosome six or seven (rearrangements, deletions). Abnormal cellular proliferation may be due to this genetic potential.
- **Role of polypeptide growth factors** — Epidermal growth factor (EGF), insulin-like growth factor-1 (IGF-1), transforming growth factor (TGF), stimulate the growth of leiomyoma either directly or via oestrogen.
- A positive family history is often present.

Growth

It is predominantly an oestrogen-dependent tumour. Oestrogen and progesterone is incriminated as the cause. Oestrogen dependency is evidenced by :

- Growth potentiality is limited during child-bearing period.
- Increased growth during pregnancy.
- They do not occur before menarche.
- Following menopause, there is cessation of growth and there is no new growth at all.

- It seems to contain more oestrogen receptors than the adjacent myometrium.
- Frequent association of anovulation.

The growth potentiality is not squarely distributed amongst the fibroids which are usually multiple, some grow faster than the others. On the whole, the rate of growth is slow and it takes about 3-5 years for the fibroid to grow sufficiently to be felt per abdomen (c.f. — ovarian tumour grows in months).

Table 19.1 : Risk factors for fibroid

Increased risk	*Reduced risk*
• Nulliparity • Obesity • Hyperoestrogenic state • Black women	• Multiparity • Smoking

However, **the fibroid grows rapidly** during pregnancy or amongst pill users (high dose pills). Rapid growth may also be due to degeneration or due to malignant change.

The newer low dose oral contraceptives are not associated with increase in the growth of a fibroid.

Types

- **Body**
- **Cervical**

(See chart below)

Body : The fibroids are mostly located in the body of the uterus and are usually multiple (Figs. 19.1 and 19.2).

Interstitial or intramural (75%)

Initially, the fibroids are intramural in position but subsequently, some are pushed outwards or inwards. Eventually, in about 70 per cent they persist in that position.

Subperitoneal or subserous (15%)

In this condition, the intramural fibroid is pushed outwards towards the peritoneal cavity. The fibroids are either partially or completely covered by peritoneum. When completely covered by peritoneum, it usually attains a pedicle — called pedunculated subserous fibroid. On rare occasion, the pedicle may be torn through; the fibroid gets its nourishment from the omental or mesenteric adhesions and is called **'wandering'** or **'parasitic'** fibroid. Sometimes, the intramural fibroid may be pushed out in between the layers of broad ligament and is called broad ligament fibroid (false or pseudo).

Submucous (5%) (Fig. 19.3)

The intramural fibroid when pushed towards the uterine cavity, and is lying underneath the endometrium, it is called submucous fibroid. Submucous fibroid can make the uterine cavity irregular and distorted. Pedunculated submucous fibroid may come out through the cervix (Fig. 19.7). It may be

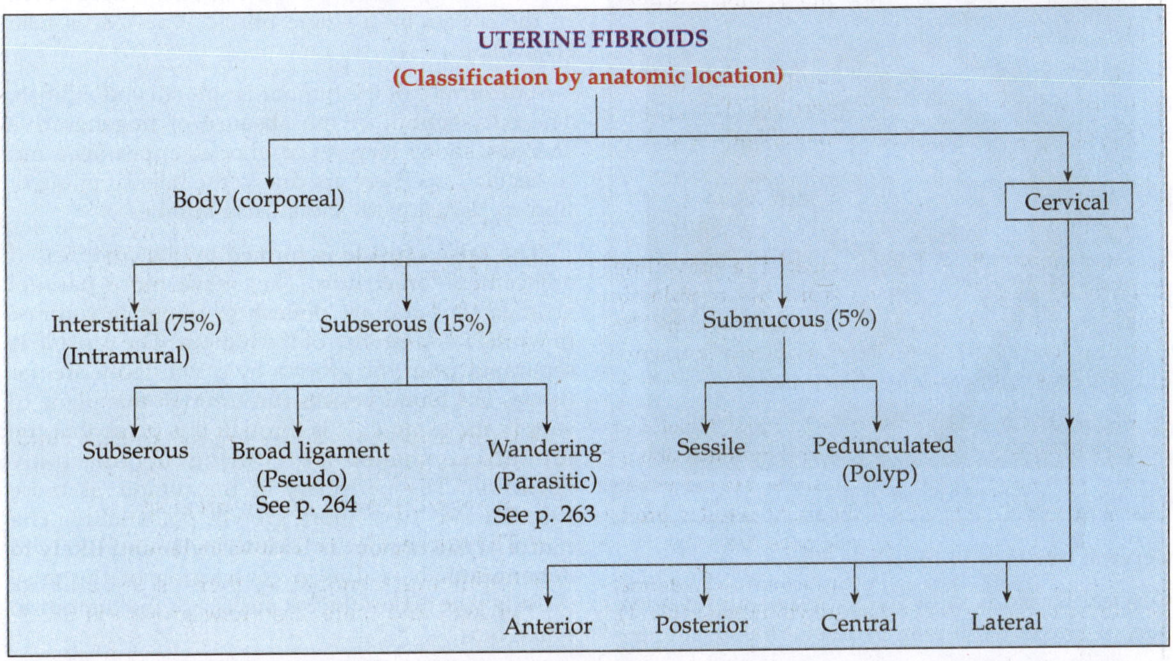

infected or ulcerated to cause metrorrhagia. Although, **this variety is least common (about 5 %)** but it produces maximum symptoms (Fig. 19.12).

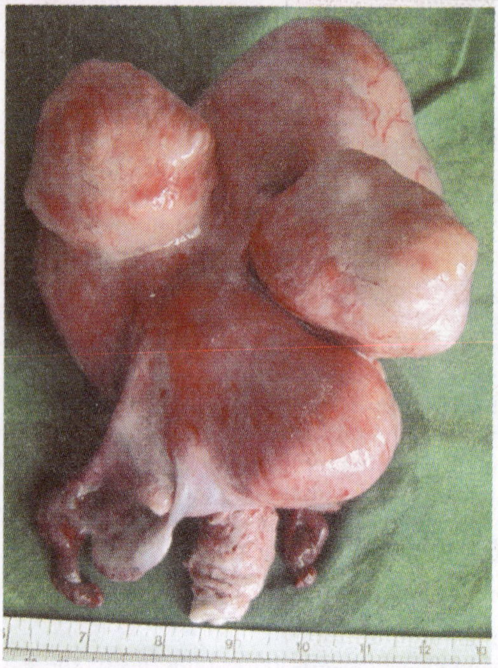

Fig. 19.2. Multiple fibroids causing marked distortion of the uterus. The uterine corpus is almost completely replaced by multile myomas in subserous, intramural and submucous positions.

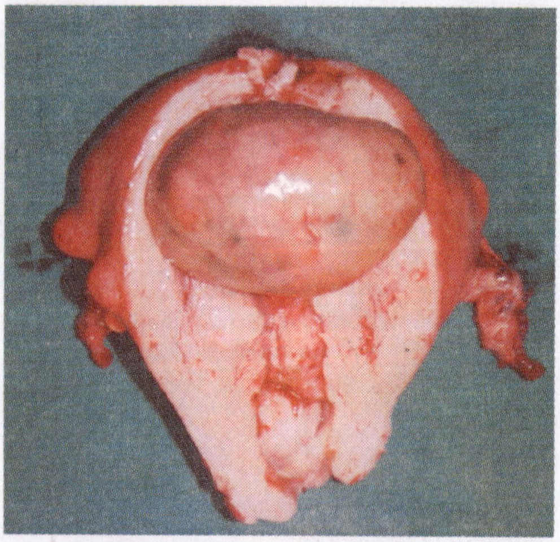

Fig. 19.3. Submucous fibroid

Cervical (see Figs 19.10 and 36.50)

Cervical fibroid is rare (1-2 %). In the supravaginal part of the cervix, it may be interstitial or subperitoneal variety and rarely polypoidal. Depending upon the position, it may be anterior, posterior, lateral or central. Interstitial growths may displace the cervix or expand it so much that the external os is difficult to recognise. **All these disturb the pelvic anatomy, specially the ureter.**

Table 19.2
The fate of a submucous fibroid

- Surface necrosis
- Polypoid change — following pedicle formation
- Infection
- Degenerations including sarcomatous change

In the vaginal cervix, the fibroid is usually pedunculated and rarely sessile.

Pseudocervical fibroid : A fibroid polyp arising from the uterine body when occupies and distends the cervical canal, it is called pseudocervical fibroid.

BODY OR CORPOREAL FIBROIDS

Pathology

Naked eye appearance

The uterus is enlarged; the shape is distorted by multiple nodular growth of varying sizes. Occasionally, there may be uniform enlargement of the uterus by a single fibroid. The feel is firm (Fig. 19.3).

Cut surface of the tumour is smooth and whitish. The cut section, in the absence of degenerative changes, shows features of whorled appearance and trabeculation. These are due to the intermingling of fibrous tissues with the muscle bundles.

The false capsule is formed by the compressed adjacent myometrium. They have more parallel arrangement and are pinkish in colour in contrast to whitish appearance of the tumour. The capsule is separated from the growth by a thin loose areolar tissue. The blood vessels run through this plane to supply the tumour. It is through this plane that the tumour is shelled out during myomectomy operation. The periphery of the tumour is more vascular and have more growth potentiality. **The centre of the tumour is least vascular and likely to degenerate.** It is due to contraction of the false capsule that makes the cut surface of the tumour to bulge out.

Microscopic appearance (Fig. 19.4)

The tumour consists of smooth muscles and fibrous connective tissues of varying proportion. Originally, it consists of only muscle element but later on, fibrous tissues intermingle with the muscle bundles. As such, the nomenclature of 'fibroids' although commonly used, is inappropriate and should better be called either 'myomata' or fibromyomata.

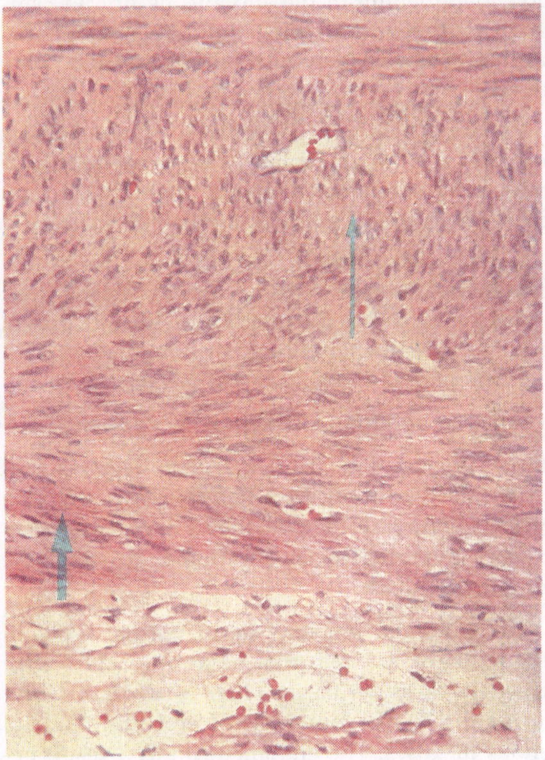

Fig. 19.4. Histological picture of fibroid

SECONDARY CHANGES IN FIBROIDS

Table 19.3
Secondary changes in fibroid

• Degenerations	• Infection
• Atrophy	• Vascular changes
• Necrosis	• Sarcomatous change

Degenerations

Hyaline degeneration is the most common (65%) type of degeneration affecting all sizes of fibroids except the tiny one. It is common specially in tumours having more connective tissues. The central part of the tumour which is least vascular is the common site. The feel becomes soft elastic in contrast to firm feel of the tumour.

Naked eye examination on the cut surface shows irregular homogenous areas with loss of whorl-like appearance.

Microscopic examination reveals hyaline changes of both the muscles and fibrous tissues.

Cystic degeneration usually occurs following menopause and is common in interstitial fibroids. It is formed by liquefaction of the areas with hyaline changes. The cystic spaces are lined by irregular ragged walls. The cystic changes of an isolated big fibroid may be confused with an ovarian cyst or pregnancy.

Fatty degeneration is usually found at or after menopause. Fat globules are deposited mainly in the muscle cells.

Calcific degeneration (10%) usually involves the subserous fibroids with small pedicle or myomas of postmenopausal women. It is usually preceded by fatty degeneration. There is precipitation of calcium carbonate or phosphate within the tumour. When whole of the tumour is converted into a calcified mass, it is called "**womb stone**".

Red degeneration (carneous degeneration) occurs in a large fibroid mainly during second half of pregnancy and puerperium. Partial recovery is possible and as such called necrobiosis. The cause is not known but is probably vascular in origin. Infection does not play any part.

Naked eye appearance of the tumour shows dark areas with cut section revealing raw-beef appearance often containing cystic spaces. The odour is often fishy due to fatty acids. Colour is due to the presence of haemolysed red cells and haemoglobin.

Microscopically, evidences of necrosis are present. Vessels are thrombosed but extravasation of blood is unlikely.

Atrophy : Atrophic changes occur following menopause due to loss of support from oestrogen. There is reduction in the size of the tumour. Similar reduction also occurs following pregnancy enlargement.

Necrosis : Circulatory inadequacy may lead to central necrosis of the tumour. This is present in submucous polyp or pedunculated subserous fibroid.

Infection : The infection gains access to the tumour core through the thinned and sloughed surface epithelium of the submucous fibroid. This usually happens following delivery or abortion. Intramural fibroid may also be infected following delivery.

Vascular changes : Dilatation of the vessels (telangiectasis) or dilatation of the lymphatic channels (lymphangiectasis) inside the myoma may occur. The cause is not known.

Sarcomatous changes : Sarcomatous change may occur **in less than 0.1 per cent cases**. The usual type is leiomyosarcoma. Recurrence of fibroid polyp, sudden enlargement of fibroid or fibroid along with postmenopausal bleeding raises the suspicion.

Associated changes in the pelvic organs

Uterus : The shape is distorted; usually asymmetrical but at times, uniform. Myohyperplasia is almost a constant finding. It may be due to hyperoestrinism or work hypertrophy in an attempt to expel the fibroid.

The endometrium may be of normal type. In others, there are features of anovulation with evidences of hyperplasia. There is dilatation and congestion of the myometrial and endometrial venous plexuses. The endometrium as a result becomes thick, congested and oedematous. The endometrium overlying the submucous fibroid may be thin and necrotic with evidences of infection.

The uterine cavity may be elongated and distorted in intramural and submucous varieties.

Table 19.4
Complications of fibroids

- Degenerations
- Necrosis
- Infection
- Sarcomatous change
- Torsion of subserous pedunculated fibroid
- Haemorrhage
  - Intracapsular
  - Rupture surface vein of subserous fibroid → intraperitoneal
- Polycythemia due to
  - Erythropoietic function by the tumour
  - Altered erythropoietic function of the kidney through ureteric pressure

Uterine tubes : The frequent tubal infection (about 15%) detected in association with fibroid seems coincidental.

Ovaries : The ovaries may be enlarged, congested and studded with multiple cysts. The cause may be due to hyperoestrinism.

Ureter : There may be displacement of the anatomy of the ureter in broad ligament fibroid. The compression effect results in hydroureter and or hydronephrosis.

Endometriosis : There is increased association of pelvic endometriosis and adenomyosis (30%).

Endometrial carcinoma : The incidence remains unaffected.

CLINICAL FEATURES

Patient profile

The patients are usually nulliparous or having long period of secondary infertility. However, early marriage and frequent childbirth make its frequency high even amongst the multiparous women. The incidence is at its peak between 35-45 years. There is a tendency of delayed menopause.

Symptoms : The majority of fibroids remain asymptomatic (75%). They are accidentally discovered by the physician during routine examination or at laparotomy or laparoscopy.

The symptoms are related to anatomic type and size of the tumour. **The site is more important than the size.** A small submucous fibroid may produce more symptoms than a big subserous fibroid.

Menstrual abnormalities

(a) **Menorrhagia (30%) is the classic symptom of symptomatic fibroid.**

The menstrual loss is progressively increased with successive cycles. It is conspicuous in submucous or interstitial fibroids. **The causes are** :

- Increased surface area of the endometrium (Normal is about 15 sq cm).
- Interference with normal uterine contractility due to interposition of fibroid.
- Congestion and dilatation of the subjacent endometrial venous plexuses caused by the obstruction of the tumour.
- Endometrial hyperplasia due to hyperoestrinism (anovulation).
- Pelvic congestion.
- Role of prostanoids — imbalance of thromboxane (TXA_2) and prostacyclin (PGI_2) with relative deficiency of TXA_2.

(b) **Metrorrhagia or irregular bleeding may be due to :**

- Ulceration of submucous fibroid or fibroid polyp
- Torn vessels from the sloughing base of a polyp
- Associated endometrial carcinoma.

SYMPTOMS OF FIBROID UTERUS

- Asymptomatic – majority (75%)
- Menstrual abnormality : Menorrhagia, metrorrhagia (p. 266).
- Dysmenorrhoea
- Dyspareunia
- Infertility
- Pressure symptoms
- Recurrent pregnancy loss (miscarriage, preterm labour)
- Lower abdominal or pelvic pain
- Abdominal enlargement.

Dysmenorrhoea : The congestive variety may be due to associated pelvic congestion or endometriosis. Spasmodic type is associated with extrusion of polyp and its expulsion from the uterine cavity.

Subserous, broad ligament or cervical fibroids are usually unassociated with menstrual abnormalities.

Infertility : Infertility (30%) may be a major complaint. **The probable known attributing factors are :**

Uterine

- Distortion and or elongation of the uterine cavity → difficult sperm ascent.
- Preventing rhythmic uterine contraction due to fibroids during intercourse → impaired sperm transport.
- Congestion and dilatation of the endometrial venous plexuses → defective nidation.
- Atrophy and ulceration of the endometrium over the submucous fibroids → defective nidation.
- Menorrhagia and dyspareunia.

Tubal

- Cornual block due to position of the fibroid.
- Marked elongation of the tube over a big fibroid.
- Associated salpingitis with tubal block.

Ovarian : • Anovulation

Peritoneal : • Endometriosis

Unknown — (majority)

Pregnancy related problems like abortion, preterm labour and intrauterine growth restriction are high. The reasons are defective implantation of the placenta, poorly developed endometrium, reduced space for the growing fetus and placenta. Red degeneration and torsion of subserous pedunculated fibroid is common in pregnancy. Postpartum haemorrhage is also more.

Pain lower abdomen

The fibroids are usually painless. Pain may be due to some complications of the tumour or due to associated pelvic pathology.

Due to tumour

- Degeneration
- Torsion subserous pedunculated fibroid
- Extrusion of polyp.

Associated pathology

- Endometriosis
- PID.

Abdominal swellings (lump)

The patient may have a sense of heaviness in lower abdomen. She may feel a lump in the lower abdomen even without any other symptom.

Pressure symptoms

Pressure symptoms are rare in body fibroids. The fibroids in the posterior wall may be impacted in the pelvis producing constipation, dysuria or even retention of urine. A broad ligament fibroid may produce ureteric compression → hydroureteric and hydronephrotic changes → infection → pyelitis.

Signs

General examination reveals varying degrees of pallor depending upon the magnitude and duration of menstrual loss.

Abdominal examination

The tumour may not be sufficiently enlarged to be felt per abdomen. But if enlarged to 14 weeks or more, the following features are noted.

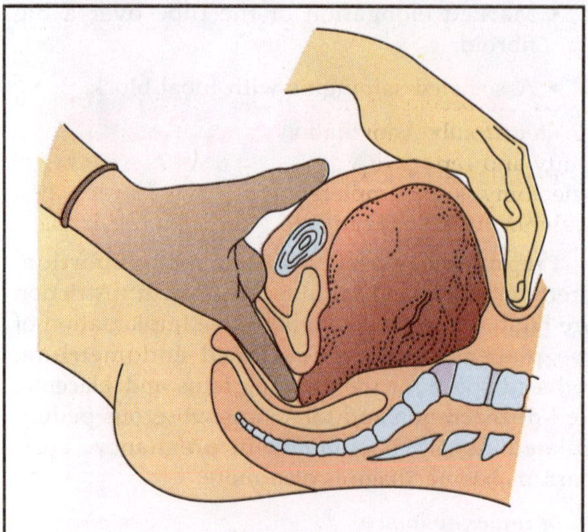

Fig. 19.5. Bimanual examination in a case of uterine fibroid

Palpation

- Feel is firm, more towards hard; may be cystic in cystic degeneration.
- Margins are well-defined except the lower pole which cannot be reached suggestive of pelvic in origin.
- Surface is nodular; may be uniformly enlarged in a single fibroid.
- Mobility is restricted from above downwards but can be moved from side to side.

Percussion

The swelling is dull on percussion.

Pelvic examination

Bimanual examination reveals the uterus irregularly enlarged by the swelling felt per abdomen. **That the swelling is uterine is evidenced by**:

- Uterus is not felt separated from the swelling and as such a groove is not felt between the uterus and the mass (Fig. 19.5).

- The cervix moves with the movement of the tumour felt per abdomen.

The only exception of these two findings is a subserous pedunculated fibroid. As such, such type is too often confused with an ovarian tumour. However, a submucous fibroid may produce symmetrical enlargement of the uterus and at times, it is difficult to diagnose accurately.

Table 19.5
Causes of symmetrical enlargement of uterus

• Pregnancy	• Haematometra
• Submucous or intramural (solitary)fibroid	• Lochiometra
• Adenomyosis	• Malignancy
• Myohyperplasia	– Carcinoma body
• Pyometra	– Choriocarcinoma
	– Sarcoma

Table 19.6
Life-threatening complications of fibroids

- Persistent menorrhagia, metrorrhagia or continued vaginal bleeding → severe anaemia.
- Severe intraperitoneal haemorrhage due to rupture of veins over subserous fibroid.
- Severe infection leading to peritonitis or septicaemia.
- Sarcoma.

INVESTIGATIONS

The investigations aim at :

- To confirm the diagnosis
- Preoperative assessment.

To confirm the diagnosis

Although, the majority of uterine fibroids can be diagnosed from the history and pelvic examination but at times pose problems in diagnosis.

Ultrasound and Colour Doppler (TVS) findings are : (i) Uterine contour is enlarged and distorted. (ii) Depending on the amount of connective tissue or smooth muscle proliferation, fibroids are of different echogenecity-hypoechoic or hyperechoic. (iii) Vascularisation is at the periphery of the fibroid. (iv) Central vascularisation indicates degenerative changes. Ultrasound is an useful diagnostic tool to confirm the diagnosis of fibroid and to differentiate it from ovarian mass or pregnancy. However, in pedunculated subserous fibroid, ultrasound cannot differentiate it from solid ovarian tumour specially when the ovaries are not visualised. Transvaginal ultrasound can accurately assess the myoma location, dimensions and also any adnexal pathology. Hydroureter or hydronephrotic changes can be diagnosed. **3-Dimensional** ultrasonography can locate fibroids accurately. Serial ultrasound exami-

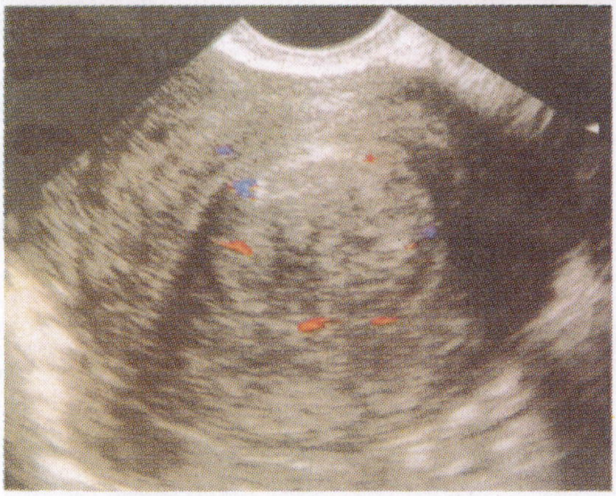

Fig. 19.6. Ultrasonographic view of a uterine fibroid

nation is needed during medical or conservative management (Figs. 19.6 , 19.7 and 19.13).

Saline Infusion Sonography (SIS) is helpful to detect any submucous fibroid or polyp (p. 114).

Magnetic resonance imaging (MRI) — is more accurate compared to ultrasound (p. 625). It helps to differentiate adenomyosis from fibroids. MRI is not used routinely for the diagnosis. It is expensive and not widely available.

Laparoscopy — Laparoscopy is helpful, if the uterine size is less than 12 weeks and associated with pelvic pain and infertility. Associated pelvic endometriosis and tubal pathology can be revealed. It can also differentiate a pedunculated fibroid from ovarian tumour not revealed by clinical examination and ultrasound.

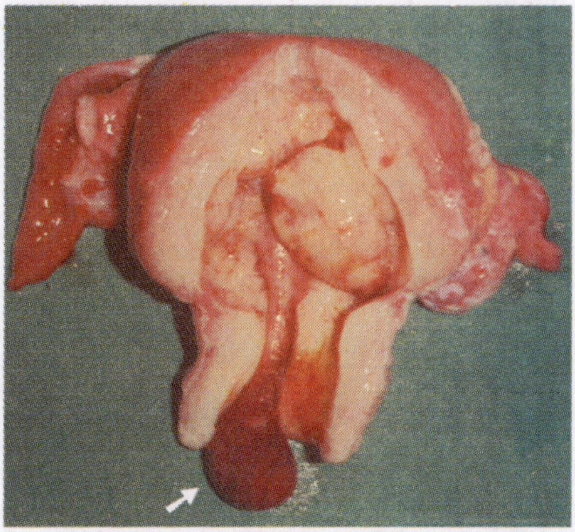

Fig. 19.7. Submucous fibroid polyps, sessile and pedunculated (see also Fig. 36.49)

Hysteroscopy or HSG — The methods are of help to detect submucous fibroid in unexplained infertility and repeated pregnancy wastage where myomectomy is contemplated. The presence and site of submucous fibroid can be diagnosed by direct visualisation during hysteroscopy (Fig. 19.8) or indirectly as a filling defect on hysterosalpingography.

Uterine curettage — In the presence of irregular bleeding, to detect any co-existing pathology and to study the endometrial pattern, curettage is helpful. It additionally helps to diagnose a submucous fibroid by feeling a bump. However, hysteroscopy and biopsy is a better alternative.

Preoperative assessment : Apart from routine preoperative investigations, intravenous pyelography to note the anatomic changes of the ureter may be helpful.

Differential diagnosis : The fibroid of varying sizes may be confused with : (1) Pregnancy (2) Full bladder (3) Adenomyosis (4) Myohyperplasia (5) Ovarian tumour (6) TO mass. The differentiating features are described in p. 287, ch. 20.

MANAGEMENT OF FIBROID UTERUS

- **Symptomatic** • **Asymptomatic**

Symptomatic fibroids

MEDICAL MANAGEMENT

Drug therapy has established a firm place in the management of symptomatic fibroids. The drugs are used either as a temporary palliation or may be used in rare cases, as an alternative to surgery. **Prior to drug therapy, one must be certain about the diagnosis. The objectives of medical treatment are :**

- To improve menorrhagia and to correct anaemia before surgery.
- To minimise the size and vascularity of the tumour in order to facilitate surgery.
- In selected cases of infertility to facilitate hysteroscopic or laparoscopic surgery (see chapter 35).
- As an alternative to surgery in perimenopausal women or women with high-risk factors for surgery.
- Where postponement of surgery is planned temporarily.

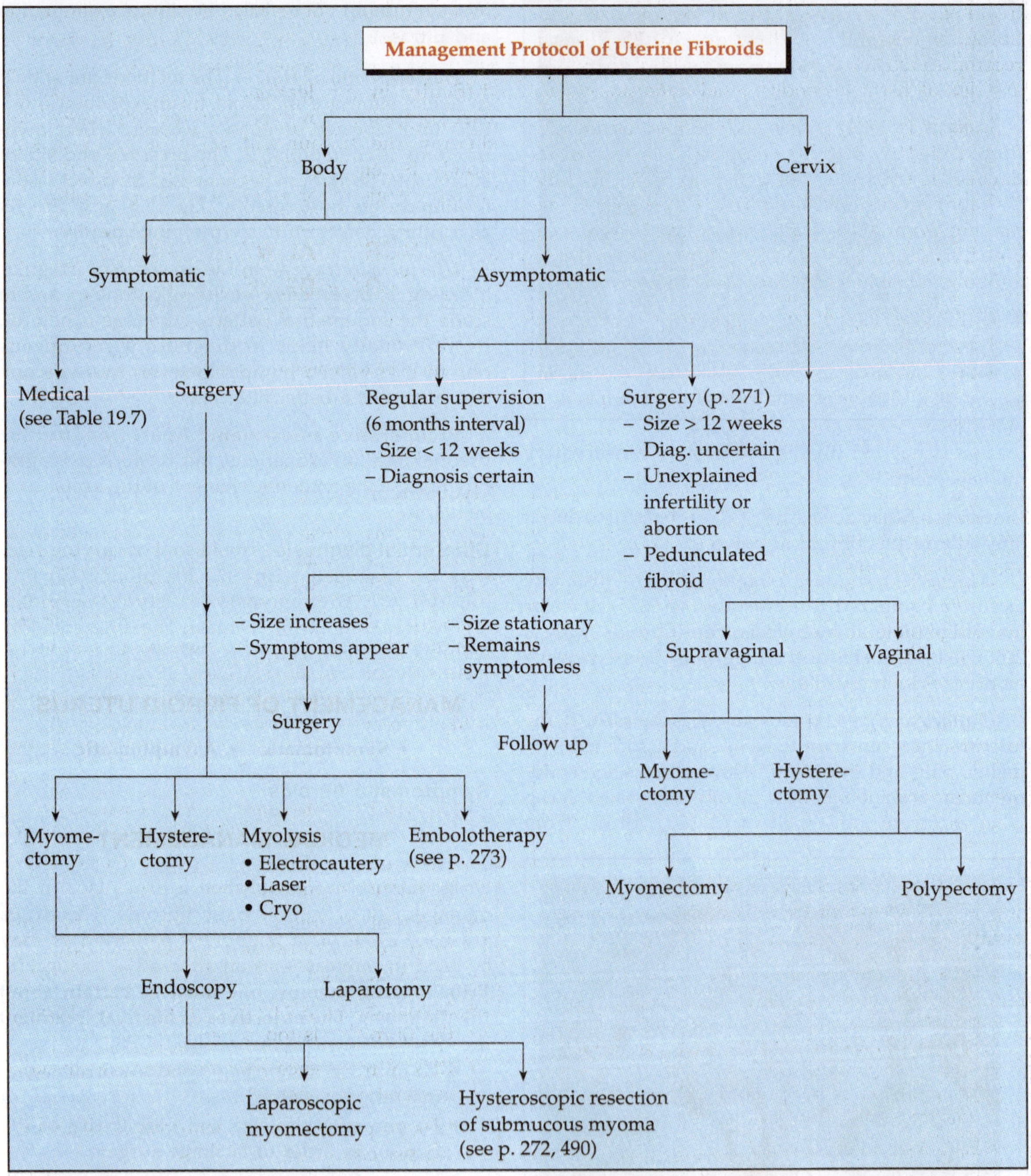

To minimise blood loss

As a temporary palliation, various drugs are used to minimise blood loss and to correct anaemia when a definite surgery cannot be undertaken for certain periods (Table 19.7).

Antiprogesterones (p. 511) — Mifepristone (RU 486) has been found to be very effective in the

Table 19.7 : Drugs used to minimise blood loss

Antifibrinolytics
Antiprogesterones
Danazol
GnRH analogues : • Agonists • Antagonists
Prostaglandin synthetase inhibitors

treatment of menorrhagia. It reduces the size of the fibroid significantly. A daily dose of 25-30 mg is recommended for 3 months. Long-term therapy is avoided as it causes endometrial hyperplasia.

Danazol (p. 504) — can reduce the volume of a fibroid slightly. Because of androgenic side effects, danazol is used only for a period of 3-6 months. Danazol administered daily in divided doses ranging from 200-400 mg for 3 months minimises blood loss or even produce amenorrhoea by its antigonadotrophin and androgen agonist actions.

GnRH agonists (p. 500) — Drugs commonly used are goserelin, luporelin, buserelin or nafarelin (see p. 500). Mechanism of action is sustained pituitary down regulation and suppression of ovarian function. There is initial transient pituitary stimulation.

GnRH antagonists (p. 502) — Cetrorelix or ganirelix causes immediate suppression of pituitary and the ovaries. They do not have the initial stimulatory effect. Benefits are same as that of agonists (see Table 19.8). Onset of amenorrhoea is rapid.

Antifibrinolytics have been found to reduce the amount of blood loss significantly. Tranexamic acid, 2-4 gm orally daily is useful for fibroid related menorrhagia.

Prostaglandin synthetase inhibitors —These are used to relieve pain due to associated endometriosis or degeneration of the fibroid. They cannot improve menorrhagia due to fibroids.

Levonorgestrel-releasing Intrauterine System (LNG-IUS) reduces blood loss and uterine size. However, this is not recommended when the uterine size is ≥ 12 weeks or there is distortion of uterine cavity.

Preoperative therapy : It is indeed advantageous to reduce the size and vascularity of fibroid prior to either myomectomy or hysterectomy. While operation will be technically easier in broad ligament or cervical fibroid, in myomectomy, there may be little difficulty in enucleation of the tumour from its pseudocapsule. However, with the stoppage of the therapy, the tumour will attain its previous size slowly. Benefits (see Table 19.8) are achieved when therapy is given for a period of three months.

Table 19.8 : Benefits of GnRH analogue therapy

- Improvement of menorrhagia and may produce amenorrhoea.
- Improvement of anaemia.
- Relief of pressure symptoms.
- Reduction in size (50%) when used for a period of 6 months.
- Reduction in vascularity of the tumour.
- Reduction in blood loss during myomectomy.
- May facilitate laparoscopic or hysteroscopic surgery.

SURGICAL MANAGEMENT OF FIBROID UTERUS

- **Myomectomy** (may be done by)
  - Laparotomy
  - Laparoscopy
  - Hysteroscopy
- **Embolotherapy**
- **Myolysis**
- **Hysterectomy**

Myomectomy (see p. 574, Tables 19.9 to 19.12)

Myomectomy is the enucleation of myomata from the uterus leaving behind a potentially functioning organ capable of future reproduction.

As such, the surgeon should be satisfied with the operation designed to serve the objective. It is indeed useless to perform a hectic surgery to remove such myomata only to leave behind an uterus which is unlikely to conceive in future.

Table 19.9
Important considerations prior to myomectomy

- It should be done mainly to preserve the reproductive function.
- The wish to preserve the menstrual function in parous women should be judiciously complied with.
- Myomectomy is a more risky operation when the fibroid(s) is too big and too many.
- Risk of recurrence and persistence of fibroid is about 30-50 per cent.
- Risk of persistence of menorrhagia is about 1-5 per cent.
- Risk of relaparotomy is about 20-25 per cent.
- Pregnancy rate following myomectomy is about 40-60 per cent.
- Pregnancy following myomectomy should have a mandatory hospital delivery, although the chance of scar rupture is rare (little more when the cavity is open).

TABLE 19.10 : INDICATIONS OF MYOMECTOMY

- Persistent uterine bleeding despite medical therapy.
- Excessive pain or pressure symptoms.
- Size > 12 weeks, woman desirous to have a baby.
- Unexplained infertility with distortion of the uterine cavity.
- Recurrent pregnancy wastage due to fibroid.
- Rapidly growing myoma during follow up.
- Subserous pedunculated fibroid.

TABLE 19.11 : PRE-REQUISITES TO MYOMECTOMY

- Hysteroscopy or hysterosalpingography — to exclude any submucous fibroid or a polyp or any tubal block.
- Diagnostic D + C — in cases of irregular cycles, not only to remove a polyp but also to exclude endometrial carcinoma.
- Examination of the husband from fertility point of view (semen analysis).

TABLE 19.12 : CONTRAINDICATIONS OF MYOMECTOMY

- Infected fibroid.
- Growth of myoma after menopause.
- Suspected malignant change (sarcoma).
- Parous women where hysterectomy is safer and is a definitive treatment (Table 19.9).
- Function less fallopian tubes (bilateral hydrosalpinx, tubo-ovarian mass) – decision must be judicious with the advent of microsurgery and ART (p. 243).
- Pelvic or Endometrial tuberculosis.
- During pregnancy or during caesarean section.

Among the contraindications few are relative rather than absolute. Restoration of anatomy and function of the uterus, tubes and ovaries following myomectomy are important, not only for future reproductive function but also to avoid the future hazards (see Table 19.9).

However, the final decision as to whether to perform myomectomy or hysterectomy is to be taken following laparotomy. As such, it is prudent on the part of surgeon to declare the operative decision as '**myomectomy to be tried**' and if the conditions arise so, it may end in hysterectomy.

Pre-treatment with GnRH analogues may be used to reduce the size and vascularity of the uterus. Steps of myomectomy and complications of myomectomy have been discussed (see p. 574).

Vaginal myomectomy : Submucous pedunculated myoma can be removed vaginally. **Morcellation** (removal by piecemeal) is needed if the tumour is large. A moderate size fibroid can be removed by twisting. In that case fibroid is grasped with a sponge forceps.

Endoscopic surgery

Hysteroscopy : Generally a fibroid of 3-4 cm in diameter or a polyp is resected with a hysteroscope. Pedicle or the base of the fibroid is coagulated using electrocautery (Fig. 19.8). Nd : YAG laser can also be used (p. 590).

Complications of hysteroscopic surgery are uterine perforation, fluid overload, haemorrhage and others (see p. 590).

Laparoscopy : Subserous and intramural fibroids could be removed laparoscopically. Electrocautery, laser and extra corporeal sutures are used for haemostasis. Laparoscopic surgery is not suitable when the fibroid is large, deep intramural, multiple or technically inaccessible. Leiomyomas can be desiccated **(myolysis)** using laser or bipolar diathermy. Complications of laparoscopic surgery,

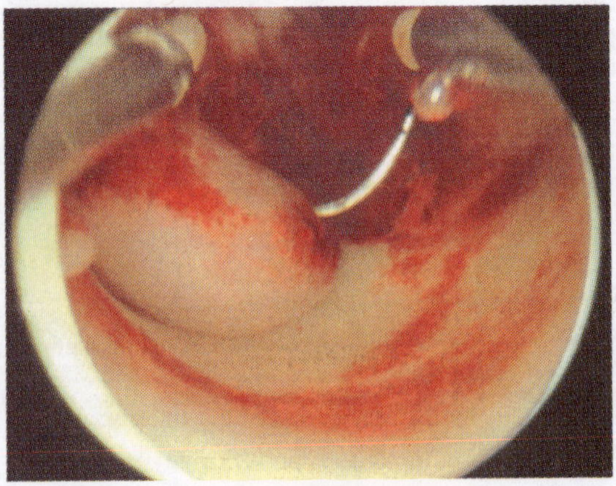

Fig. 19.8. Hysteroscopic view of a submucous fibroid. Endoscopic resection is possible

contraindications and others are discussed in Chapter 35 (p. 586).

Embolotherapy : Embolisation of uterine arteries causes avascular necrosis followed by shrinkage of fibroid. Uterine arteries are occluded by injecting polyvinyl alcohol particles through percutaneous femoral catheterisation. This may be an option to women with symptomatic fibroid where surgery is not preferred.

Result : Improvement of menorrhagia is observed in 80-90 per cent with 60 per cent reduction in size.

Contraindications : Active pelvic infection, desire for future pregnancy, drug allergy.

Levonorgestrel-Releasing IUS (see p. 459) can be used to control menorrhagia where the uterine size is ≤ 12 weeks and there is no distortion of the cavity.

High-Intensity Focussed Ultrasound has been used currently for its thermal and cavitational effects on tissues. It is a non-invasive procedure. Initial reports had shown its safety and efficacy.

Magnetic Resonance guided percutaneous laser ablation is found effective. Laser is used for thermal ablation of the fibroid.

Hysterectomy

Hysterectomy in fact, is the operation of choice in symptomatic fibroid. As such, in the absence of indication of myomectomy, hysterectomy is done. The patients over the age of 40 years and in those not desirous of further child are the classic indications.

Total hysterectomy is performed. However, **a subtotal hysterectomy may have to be done in conditions such as** :

- Sudden deterioration of the general condition of the patient during operation specially when the operation is done in anaemic state.
- Associated endometriosis specially involving the rectovaginal septum.

Removal of the ovary

It is preferable to remove the ovaries in postmenopausal women and to preserve the same in earlier age, if they are found healthy. (For details see p. 565).

Advantages of hysterectomy

- There is no chance of recurrence.
- Adnexal pathology and the unhealthy cervix if any are also removed.

Place of vaginal hysterectomy

Fibroids with size of 10-12 weeks of pregnancy associated with uterine prolapse are better dealt by the vaginal route. Vaginal hysterectomy with repair of pelvic floor is the operation of choice. Pretreatment with GnRH analogue may facilitate vaginal hysterectomy.

Table 19.13
Indications of emergency surgery in a fibroid

- Torsion of subserous pedunculated fibroid.
- Massive intraperitoneal haemorrhage following rupture of veins over subserous fibroid.
- Uncontrolled infected fibroid.
- Uncontrolled bleeding fibroid.

ASYMPTOMATIC FIBROID (75%)

Fibroids detected accidentally on routine examination for complaints other than fibroids are dealt with as follows :

• Observation • Surgery

Observation

A certain diagnosis of fibroid should be a must prior to contemplating expectant management. The risk of sarcomatous changes is so insignificant (0.1%) that prophylactic removal of fibroid is unjustified in asymptomatic cases.

The judicious observations may be instituted in cases :

- Size < 12 weeks (of pregnancy size).
- Diagnosis certain.
- Follow up possible.

Periodic examination at interval of 6 months is needed. If the symptoms of fibroid appear and or it grows and increases in size, surgery is indicated.

CERVICAL FIBROID (Figs. 19.9 and 19.10)

Symptoms

In nonpregnant state, the symptoms are predominantly due to pressure effect on the surrounding structures.

Anterior cervical : Bladder symptoms like frequency or even retention of urine are conspicuous. The retention is more due to pressure than elongation of urethra.

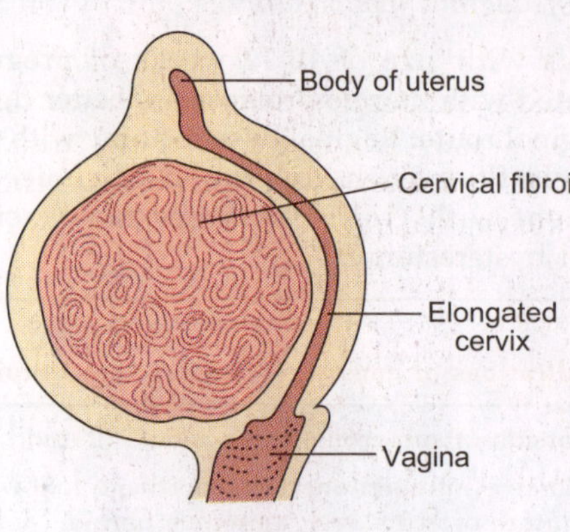

Fig. 19.9. Cervical fibroid

Posterior cervical : (Fig. 36.51) Rectal symptom is in the form of constipation.

Lateral cervical : Vascular obstruction may lead to haemorrhoids and oedema legs (rare). The ureter is pushed laterally and below the tumour.

Central cervical (Fig. 19.10) : Central fibroid produces predominantly bladder symptoms. The cervix is expanded on all sides. The uterus sits on the top of the expanded cervix (lantern on the dome of St. Paul's).

In pregnancy, it remains asymptomatic but produces insuperable obstruction during labour.

Fibroids arising from the vaginal part of the cervix may remain asymptomatic during nonpregnant state but produces obstruction during labour. If pedunculated, there may be a sensation of something coming down or if infected a foul smelling discharge per vaginam (Fig. 19.14).

Treatment

Supravaginal fibroids : Myomectomy may be tried if the patient is young and desirous of having a baby. But, it is not only technically difficult but the anatomic and functional restoration of the cervix cannot be adequate to achieve the objective of future reproduction.

As such, mostly it is dealt with by hysterectomy. **The principle to be followed is enucleation followed by hysterectomy** to minimise the injury to the ureter.

Preoperative GnRH analogues administration for 3 months facilitates surgery.

Vaginal part fibroids : If the tumour is sessile, myomectomy and if pedunculated, polypectomy is done.

POLYPS

Table 19.14 : Different types of polyp

Benign	*Malignant*
– Mucous	– *De novo*
– Fibroid	– Secondary changes
– Placental	of benign polyp

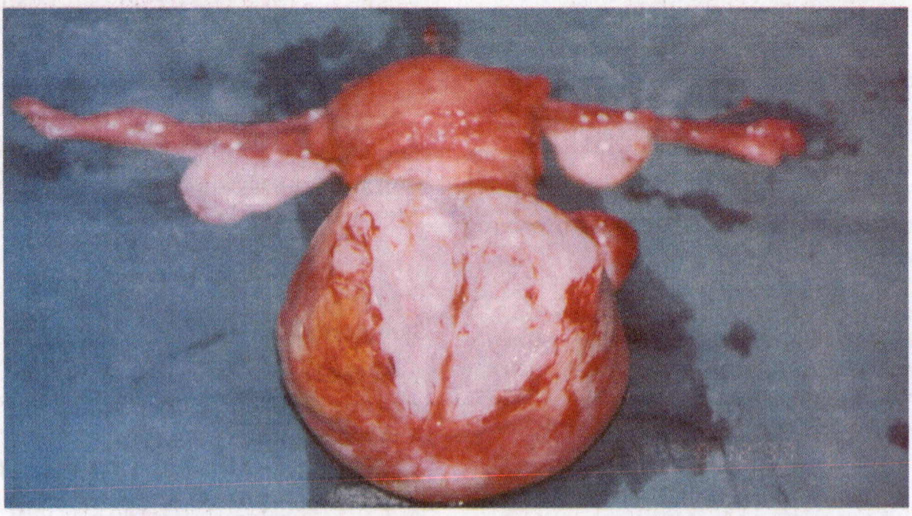

Fig. 19.10. Central cervical fibroid (huge) [*Courtesy : Dr. Biswajit Ghosh, Burnpur*]

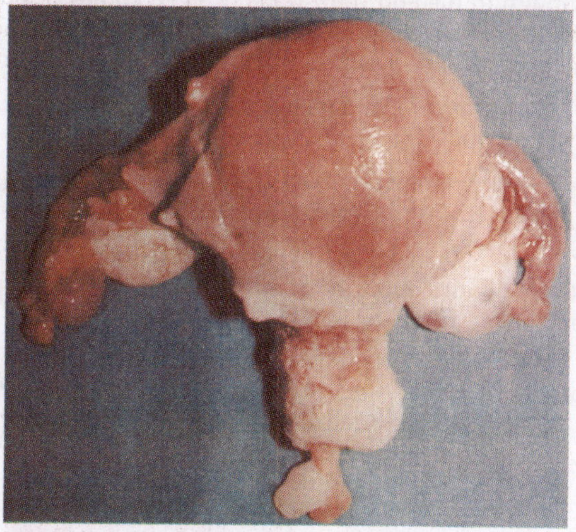

Fig. 19.11. Cervical mucous polyp

Benign : Polyp is a clinical entity referring a tumour attached by a pedicle.

Mucous : **The commonest type of benign uterine polyp is mucous one.** It may arise from the body of the uterus or from the cervix (Fig. 19.11).

Pathogenesis — ***Body*** : A part of the thick endometrium projects into the cavity and ultimately attains a pedicle. It seems to arise from the basal endometrium surrounded by the functional zone. This explains its unresponsiveness to hormones. Multiple polyposis as met in endometrial hyperplasia due to hyperoestrinism is excluded from such a discrete polyp..

Naked eye appearance shows a small polyp size of about 1-2 cm, looks reddish and feels soft. The pedicle may at times be long enough to make the polyp protruded from the cervix.

Microscopically — The core contains stromal cells, glands and large thick-walled vascular channels. The surface is lined by endometrium. The tip may undergo squamous metaplasia. Malignant change is rare but may coexist with endometrial carcinoma. The pedicle contains thin fibrous tissue with thin blood vessels. Rarely, smooth muscles invade the polyp and is then called adenomyomatous polyp. In such cases, the pedicle is usually broad. Such type is usually associated with adenomyosis.

Cervical : The polyp mainly arises from the endocervix and rarely from the ectocervix. The stimulus of epithelial overgrowth is probably due to hyperoestrinism, chronic irritation by infection or localised vascular congestion.

Naked eye appearance shows the polyp of usually small size rarely exceeding 1-2 cm, single and red in colour. The pedicle may at times be long enough to reach the vaginal introitus (Fig. 19.14).

Microscopically — The stroma consists of fibrous connective tissues with numerous small blood vessels and occasional cervical glands.The lining epithelium is tall columnar like that of endocervix. The tip may undergo squamous metaplasia. Sometimes, the stroma is more dense and fibrous and the term fibroadenomatous polyp is used. Malignant change is rare and usually of squamous cell carcinoma.

Symptoms : There may not be any symptom. The entity is accidentally discovered during speculum examination, following hysterosalpingography (filling defect), hysteroscopy or on opening the uterine cavity following hysterectomy.

However, the following symptoms are related :

- Irregular uterine bleeding, either pre-or-post menopausal
- Contact bleeding, if the polyp is situated at or outside the cervix
- Excessive vaginal discharge which may be offensive.

Signs : Unless the polyp is at or outside the external os, no positive finding is present.

However, if it protrudes out of the cervix, it feels small in size and slippery. Per speculum, it looks reddish in colour, attached usually by a slender pedicle.

FIBROID POLYP

The fibroid polyp may arise from the body of the uterus or from the cervix.

Pathogenesis

Body (Figs. 19.12 and 19.13)

Fibroid polyp is almost always due to extrusion of a submucous fibroid into the uterine cavity. During this process, it attains a pedicle which is often broad and usually attached to the posterior wall. The torn ends of the pseudocapsule are retracted in the base of the pedicle. The uterus contracts to expel the polyp out and as a result, the polyp may be pushed out through the cervix to lie even in the vagina.

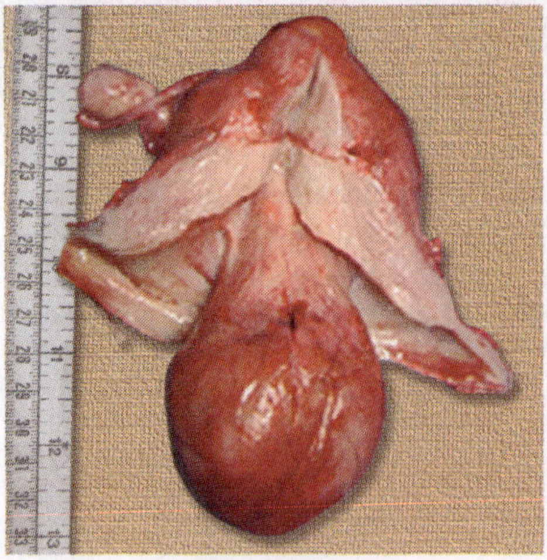

Fig. 19.12. Fibroid polyp. Note the wide pedicle and thinning out of the cervix

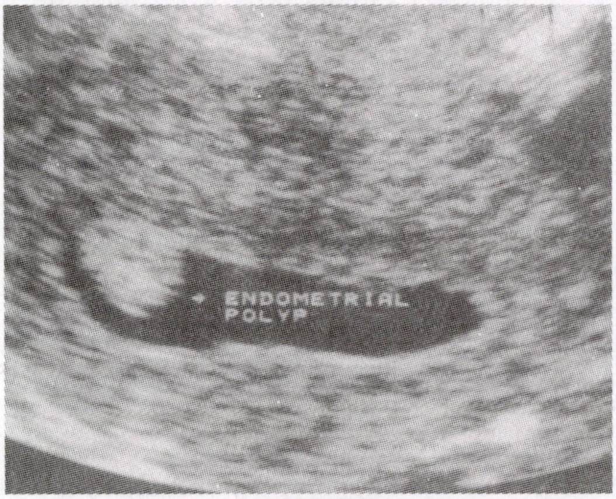

Fig. 19.13. Sonogram (TV) of the uterus showing an echogenic area within the endometrial cavity — submucous polyp

Naked eye — The polyp is usually single, of varying sizes. There may be evidences of necrosis, infection and haemorrhage specially at the tip. The pedicle is broad. There may be associated other varieties of fibroids in the uterus.

Microscopically, the polyp including the pedicle is covered by endometrium. In the tip, there may be squamous metaplasia. The core of the polyp is composed of fibromuscular structures. The pedicle is composed of fibrous tissues with slender blood vessels.

Cervical : Cervical fibroid polyp usually arises from the ectocervix and from its posterior lip. It may be small and usually single. At times, it is big enough to distend the vagina or even comes out of the introitus confusing the diagnosis of uterine inversion (Fig. 19.14).

Symptoms : The patients are usually in reproductive period. The chief complaints are :

• Intermenstrual bleeding, often continuous specially in fibroid polyp arising from the body.

• Colicky pain in the lower abdomen due to uterine contraction in an effort to expel the polyp out of the uterine cavity.

• Excessive vaginal discharge which may be offensive.

• Sensation of something coming down when the polyp becomes big distending the vagina.

Signs : General examination reveals varying degrees of anaemia.

Per vaginam

• The uterus may be bulky.

• The cervix may be patulous and the tip of the polyp is felt or else, the polyp is felt distinctly outside the external os.

Speculum examination — reveals the size and colour of the polyp which is usually pale; may be

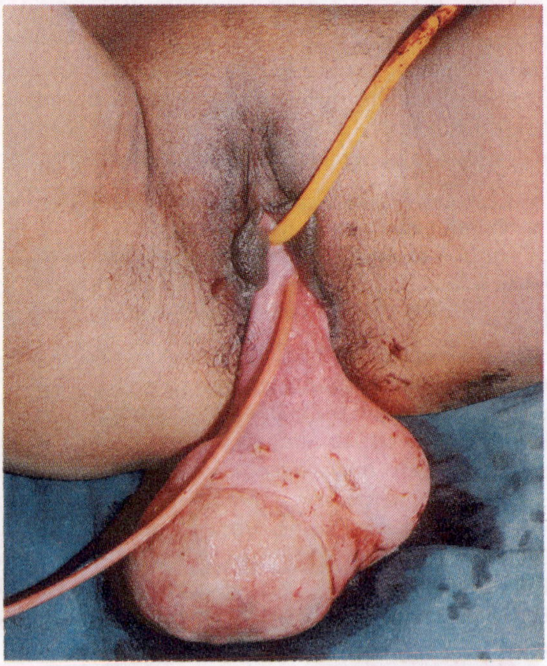

Fig. 19.14. Cervical fibroid polyp may be confused with inversion. ***Catheters*** : one in urethra and the other in the cervical canal — [*By courtesy : Prof. D. Banerjee, NRSMC&H*]

haemorrhagic. Whereas, the attachment of the pedicle to the cervix can be visualised but attachment higher up may be at times difficult to locate (Fig. 19.11).

Diagnostic aids

- Sound test — to differentiate a fibroid polyp from chronic inversion, sound test is done. If an uterine sound is passed all round between the pedicle and the dilating cervical canal, it is a polyp. In complete chronic inversion, the sound cannot be passed (see Fig. 15.21).
- Hysterosalpingography — to detect the filling defect in fibroid polyp.
- Hysteroscopy — to visualise the uterine polyp (Fig. 35.10).
- Examination under anaesthesia and exploration of the uterine cavity by curette or ovum or ring forceps can accidentally help in diagnosis of an uterine polyp.

PLACENTAL POLYP

A retained bit of placental tissue when adherent to the uterine wall gets organised with the surrounding blood clots. The mass, so formed, is infact not pedunculated and as such the term placental polyp is a misnomer.

Clinical features : There is history of recent childbirth or abortion. Irregular bleeding per vaginam and offensive vaginal discharge are present dated back to the pregnancy events.

Per vaginam, the uterus is bulky with the patulous cervical canal.

MANAGEMENT OF A POLYP

- **Mucous polyp**
- **Fibroid polyp**
- **Placental polyp**

Mucous polyp : Endometrial polyps are usually removed by uterine curettage or using ring or ovum forceps. In cases of recurrence and patients who have completed the family, hysterectomy is justified. **The causes of recurrence of polyps are** : (1) Incomplete removal, some left behind (2) Persistence of the cause leading to polyp formation (3) Malignancy.

Cervical polyps are removed by twisting of the pedicle. The base of the pedicle should be cauterised to prevent recurrence. Routine uterine curettage is done to remove the unhealthy endometrium and associated endometrial polyp, if any.

Fibroid polyp : The principle of tackling fibroid polyp depends on the age of the patient, family profile and associated uterine pathology — only fibroid or else and location of the polyp.

Diagnosed polyp confined to the cavity

- Uterus to be preserved — Removal of the polyp is done by cutting the anterior wall of the uterus (anterior hysterotomy like incision).
- Uterus to be removed — Hysterectomy is done with the fibroid polyp *in situ*.

Polyp lying in the cervical canal

Uterus to be preserved :

- Pedicle is thin — The polyp is removed by twisting after being caught by Allis or Lane's tissue forceps. The bleeding will be checked by crushing effect and contraction of the muscles at the base of the polyp.
- Pedicle is thick — If the pedicle is not accessible even by traction of the polyp, the anterior lip of the cervix is to be cut vertically so as to gain access to the pedicle. A transfixation suture is placed in the pedicle and the pedicle is cut distal to the ligature.

Uterus to be removed : Hysterectomy can be done with the fibroid polyp inside.

Big fibroid lying in the vagina : Be sure that it is a polyp and not uterine inversion or fibroid with inversion.

- Diagnosed polyp — Removal of polyp by **morcellement** (piecemeal) followed by transfixation suture on the pedicle and removal of the redundant pedicle distal to the ligature.
- Associated with chronic uterine inversion — The incision is made close to the fibroid and enucleate it.

When hysterectomy is indicated, the polyps of such type are expected to be infected and are to be removed first. Antibiotics are to be administered. The general condition of the patient is to be improved and hysterectomy should be done at a later date. This will minimise postoperative complications, the important one being infection.

It is once more to be emphasised that in all cases, the polyps should be sent for histological examination after its removal.

MALIGNANT POLYPS

Malignant polyps may arise *de novo* or may undergo secondary malignant changes on benign polyps.

It should be borne in mind that not infrequently, a benign endometrial polyp may co-exist with discrete endometrial carcinoma. As such, all possible investigations are to be done before declaring the absence of a malignant condition specially in postmenopausal women.

The following malignant changes occur in benign polyps — adenocarcinoma in endometrial polyp, sarcoma in fibroid polyp and choriocarcinoma in placental polyp.

To differentiate a malignant polyp or malignant changes in a benign polyp, the polyp including the pedicle is to be sent for histology. **In primary**, evidences of malignancy are present both in the pedicle and the core of the tumour. **In secondary** changes, the pedicle shows benign features but there are evidences of malignancy in the core of the polyp.

Treatment: Appropriate treatment is to be instituted depending upon the nature of malignancy (see p. 341).

KEY POINTS

- Fibroid is the most common pelvic tumour. The incidence of symptomatic fibroid varies from 3-10 per cent. It is common in nulliparous and the prevalence is highest between 35-45 years.

  Fibroid arises from the smooth muscle elements of the myometrium, could be genetically determined and the growth is dependent on the polypeptide growth factors (EGF, IGF-1, TGF) and oestrogen. It is slow growing compared to ovarian neoplasm.

  Fibroids may affect the reproductive outcome adversely by enlargement and distortion of the uterus, anovulation cervical or cornual black or poor endometrial vascularity.

  Corporeal fibroid is common and often multiple. All fibroids are interstitial but later on become submucous or subserous. Cervical fibroid is rare (1-2%).

  Fibroid has got a false capsule formed by the compressed myometrium. The centre is least vascular and degeneration is common.

  Hyaline degeneration is the commonest secondary change and sarcoma is rare 0.1 per cent. Red degeneration occurs mainly in pregnancy and puerperium.

  Associated endometriosis and adenomyosis is found in 30 per cent and pelvic infection in 15 per cent.

  Majority of fibroids remain asymptomatic (75%). Menorrhagia is the classic symptom of fibroid. Pelvic examination is supportive — the tumour of uterine origin. For confirmation of diagnosis, the help of sonar, laparoscopy, hysteroscopy or HSG may be useful in selected cases.

  Life-threatening complications include — severe anaemia, intraperitoneal haemorrhage from ruptured veins over the subserous fibroid, severe infection and sarcomatous changes.

  There is definite place of observation in asymptomatic fibroid provided one is certain of diagnosis and follow up is possible.

  Medical management aims mostly as palliative and the drugs used are progestogens, antiprogesterones, danazol, GnRH analogues (agonists and antagonists). Benefits of preoperative GnRH analogue therapy are many (see Table 19.8).

  The surgical treatment of fibroid concentrates to hysterectomy or myomectomy depending upon the age of the patient and need for preservation of reproductive function. Indications of myomectomy may be either due to a symptomatic or due to an asymptomatic fibroid (see Table 19.10).

  Myomectomy is a risky operation. There is chance of recurrence (30-50%), persistence of menorrhagia (1-5 %) and relaparotomy (20-25%). Pregnancy rate following myomectomy is about 40-60 per cent. Subserous and interstitial fibroids could be removed laparoscopically. Hysteroscopic resection of the submucous fibroid can be done in selected cases (Fig.19.8).

  Uterine Artery Embolisation (UAE) and myolysis are newer methods of treatment (P. 273). They need more clinical trials to establish their benefits on long-term basis.

- The commonest type of benign uterine polyp is a mucous one. It is associated with hyperoestrinism. Fibroid polyp is mostly due to extrusion of a submucous fibroid. A big polyp may be confused with chronic uterine inversion or may be associated with it.

Benign Lesions of the Ovary

20

OVARIAN ENLARGEMENT

- **Non-neoplastic** • **Neoplastic (Benign)**

NON-NEOPLASTIC

The non-neoplastic enlargement of the ovary is usually due to accumulation of fluid inside the functional unit of the ovary.

The causes are :

- Follicular cysts.
- Corpus luteum cyst.
- Theca lutein and granulosa lutein cysts.
- Polycystic ovarian syndrome (see p. 430).
- Endometrial cyst (chocolate cyst) — see p. 301.

Except the last one, all are functional cysts of the ovary and are loosely called cystic ovary.

The features of the functional cysts are :

(a) Related to temporary hormonal disorders.

(b) Rarely becomes complicated.

(c) Sometimes confused with neoplastic cyst but **can be distinguished by the following features.**

- Usually 6-8 cm in diameter.
- Usually asymptomatic.
- Spontaneous regression usually following correction of the functional disturbances to which it is related.
- Unilocular.
- Contains clear fluid inside unless haemorrhage occurs.
- Lining epithelium corresponds to the functional epithelium of the unit from which it arises.

Follicular cysts

Follicular cysts are the commonest functional cysts. They are usually multiple and small as seen in cases of cystic glandular hyperplasia of the endometrium or in association of fibroid. Hyperoestrinism is implicated as its cause. However, an isolated cyst may be formed in unruptured Graafian follicle which may be enlarged but usually not exceeding 5 cm. The cyst is lined by typical granulosa cells without lutein cells or the cells may be flattened due to pressure (Fig. 20.1).

In majority of cases, the detection is made accidentally on bimanual examination, sonography, laparoscopy or laparotomy. The cyst may remain asymptomatic or may produce vague pain.

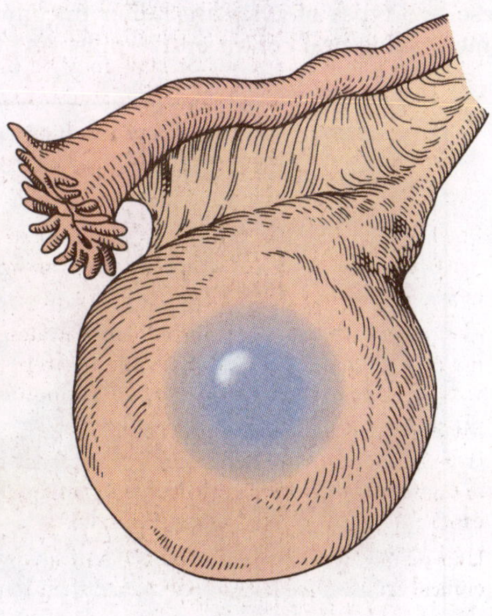

Fig. 20.1. Follicular cyst

In uncomplicated cases — it should be followed up for about 3-6 months with check up at monthly intervals. During this period, functional cysts are likely to retrogress. However, the period of expectancy should be curtailed with advancing ages (approaching menopause).

If, the size increases or there is doubt about its nature or intracystic haemorrhage and rupture occur causing acute abdomen, laparotomy is indicated.

Corpus luteum cysts

Corpus luteum cyst usually occurs due to overactivity of corpus luteum. There is excessive bleeding inside the corpus luteum. In spite of the blood filled cyst, the progesterone and oestrogen secretion continues. As a result, the menstrual cycle is prolonged followed by heavy and or continued bleeding. It is then confused with a case of threatened abortion or else, if the intracystic bleeding is much, it may rupture producing features of acute intraperitoneal haemorrhage with clinical picture simulating disturbed tubal pregnancy.

It may often be associated with pregnancy and persists for about 12 weeks. Unless complicated, spontaneous regression is expected.

If features of acute abdomen appears, laparotomy with enucleation of the cyst is to be done along with resuscitative measures as in disturbed tubal pregnancy.

These two types of cysts are rather uncommon in women taking oral contraceptive pills. As such, if the cyst persists after three months of pill therapy, it is more likely to be a neoplastic cyst.

Lutein cysts (Fig. 20.2)

Lutein cysts are usually bilateral and caused by excessive chorionic gonadotrophin secreted in cases of gestational trophoblastic tumours. These may also be formed with administration of gonadotrophins or even clomiphene to induce ovulation. These are usually lined either by theca lutein cells, called theca lutein cyst or by granulosa lutein cells, called granulosa lutein cyst.

Spontaneous regression is expected within few weeks following effective therapy of the tumours with the gonadotrophin level returning back to normal.

BENIGN OVARIAN NEOPLASMS

Incidence

The incidence of ovarian tumour amongst gynaecologic admission varies from 1-3 per cent. About 75 per cent of these are benign.

Classification

The classification of ovarian tumour is unsatisfactory and full of confusion. Classification based on morphological characteristics, histological features or clinical behaviours have been tried but none did last long.

A brief resume of the ovarian structures is

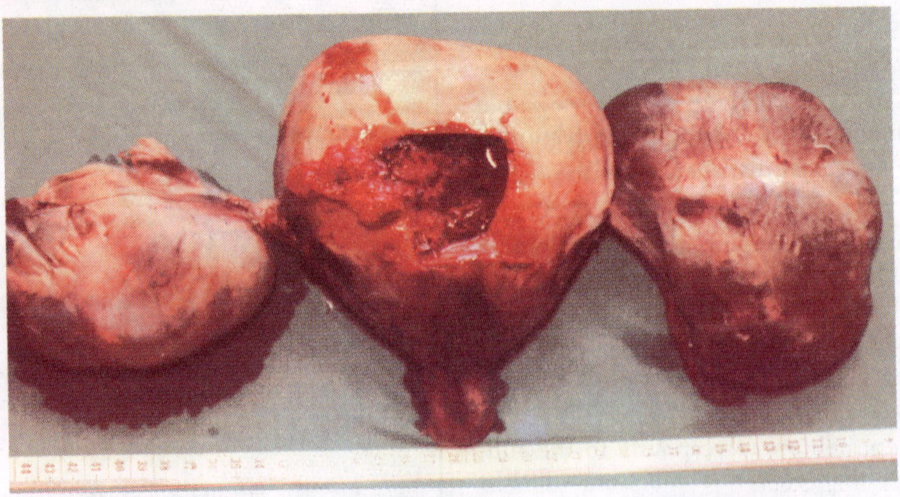

Fig. 20.2. Bilateral lutein cysts in association with hydatidiform mole

worthwhile to have an idea about the histogenesis of the ovarian neoplasms. **The ovarian tissues are constantly in a dynamic state.** Not only they are under the action of the gonadotrophins and have got steroidogenic potentialities, but even before puberty and after menopause, the ovarian tissues remain in a dynamic state.

The principal ovarian tissue components are :

- Epithelial cells derived from the **coelomic epithelium**.
- Oocytes derived from the primitive **germ cells**.
- Mesenchymal elements from the **gonadal stroma**.

For some reasons, not known, abnormal growth may occur from any of these elements and the classification is based on the structure from which the growth occurs. The classification given in the text is based more or less on WHO classification (Table 20.1).

Table 20.1
Classification of ovarian tumour

I. Epithelial tumour

These tumours may be benign, borderline malignant or malignant.

- Serous tumour
- Mucinous cyst adenoma
- Endometrioid tumours
- Mesonephroid
  or
  Clear cell tumours
- Brenner tumours
- Mixed epithelial tumours
- Undifferentiated carcinoma
- Unclassified epithelial tumours

II. Sex cord stromal tumours

a. Granulosa cell tumours
b. Tumours of thecoma-fibroma group
  - Thecoma
  - Fibroma
  - Unclassified
c. Androblastoma
  - Sertoli cell tumour
  - Sertoli Leydig cell tumour
  - Hilus cell tumour
d. Gynandroblastoma
e. Unclassified

Table contd.

III. Lipid cell tumour

IV. Germ cell tumours of the ovary

(15-20% of all primary ovarian neoplasms)

I. *Germ cell tumours*
  a. Dysgerminoma
  b. Endodermal sinus tumour
  c. Embryonal cell carcinoma
  d. Polyembryoma
  e. Choriocarcinoma
  f. Teratoma : (i) Immature;
    (ii) Mature (Dermoid cyst);
    (iii) Monodermal : • Struma ovarii • Carcinoid
  G. Mixed forms (combinations of types A to F)

II. *Tumours composed of germ cells and sex cord stromal derivatives* :
  a. Gonadoblastoma
  b. Mixed germ cell — sex cord stromal tumour

V. Gonadoblastoma

VI. Unclassified

VII. Secondary metastasis

Although full classification of the ovarian neoplasms has been presented but **only the benign ovarian tumours and that too, only the common varieties** will be presented in this chapter. These are :

- Mucinous cyst adenoma
- Serous cyst adenoma
- Brenner tumour
- Dermoid cyst

These cysts constitute about 80 per cent of the primary ovarian tumours and are called ovarian cysts as opposed to cystic ovaries in functional ones.

MUCINOUS CYST ADENOMA

Origin

The following diverse modes of origin of mucinous cyst adenoma are described :

- It arises from the totipotent surface epithelium of the ovary.
- Its association with Brenner tumour suggests its origin as mucinous metaplasia of the epithelioid cells.

Pathology

These are quite common and account for about 20-25 per cent of all ovarian tumours. The tumours

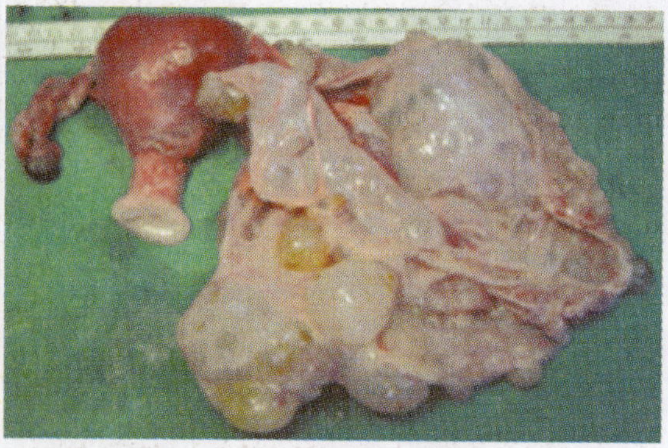

Fig. 20.3. Cut section showing mucinous cyst adenoma

are bilateral in about 10 per cent cases. The chance of malignancy is about 5-10 per cent.

Naked eye appearance

It may attain a huge size if left uncared for. In fact, **it is the largest benign ovarian tumour.**

The wall is smooth, lobulated with whitish or bluish white hue. At places, it is thin so as to be translucent.

On cut section

The content inside is thick, viscid, mucin — a glycoprotein with high content of neutral polysaccharides. It is colourless unless complicated by haemorrhage. The cyst is frequently multiloculated, sometimes with papillary growth arising from the septum (Fig. 20.3).

Microscopic examination

The cyst is lined by a single layer of tall columnar epithelium with dark staining basal nucleus but without any cilia. The epithelial characteristics are like those of endocervix (Figs. 20.4 and 20.5).

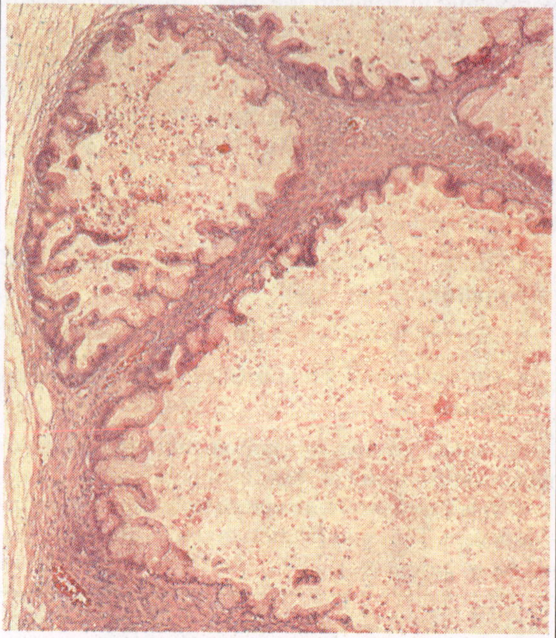

Fig. 20.4. Microphotograph showing the lining epithelium of mucinous cyst adenoma. The epithelium does not invade the wall and the serosa is intact

As the secretion is not abundant, there is more chance of proliferation of the lining epithelium to form papillary projection. As such, intracystic haemorrhage is more likely. Often, the papillary growth projects outwards perforating the cyst wall in about 15 per cent cases.

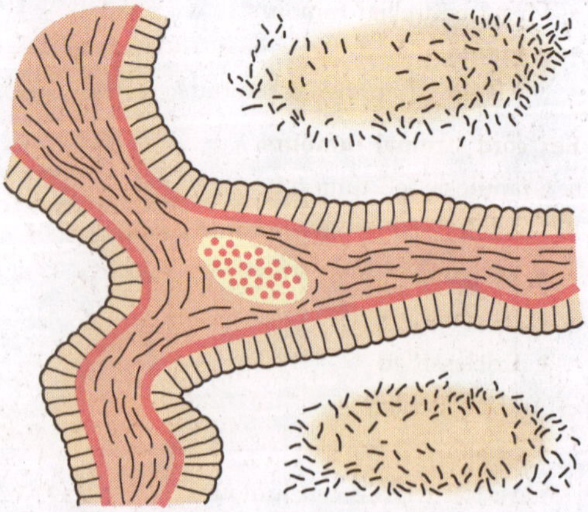

Fig. 20.5. Diagrammatic picture showing a single layer of tall columnar epithelial cells with basal nuclei. These cells secrete mucin — mucinous cyst adenoma

SEROUS CYST ADENOMA

Origin

Serous cyst arises from the totipotent surface epithelium of the ovary.

It is quite common and **accounts for about 40 per cent** of ovarian tumours. It is **bilateral in about 40 per cent** and **chance of malignancy is about 40 per cent.**

Pathology

The cysts are not so big as that of mucinous type.

Naked eye appearance

The wall is smooth, shiny and greyish white. At times, there are exuberant papillary projection. It may be multilobulated on cut section. The content fluid is clear, rich in serum proteins — albumin and globulin.

Microscopic examination

It is lined by a single layer of cubical epithelium.

The papillary structures consist of broad dense fibrous stroma covered by single or multiple layers of columnar epithelium. There may be presence of ciliated, secretory and peg cells resembling tubal epithelium (Fig. 20.6).

Psammoma bodies : These are tiny, spherical, laminated calcified structures which are most often found in areas of cellular degeneration (15%). Its presence *per se* does not denote malignancy. It is not present in slow growing tumour.

BRENNER TUMOUR

Brenner tumour account for 1-2 per cent of all ovarian tumours, 8-10 per cent are bilateral and usually seen in women above the age of 40. Majority are solid and are less than 2 cm in diameter. It usually arises from squamous metaplasia of surface epithelium. Gross picture of Brenner is similar to that of fibroma. Histologically islands of transitional epithelium (Walthard nests) in a compact fibrous stroma are seen. **The cells look like "coffee bean" as the nuclei have longitudinal grooves.** They are usually benign in nature. Oestrogen is secreted by the tumour and the woman may present with abnormal vaginal bleeding. Unilateral oophorectomy in a young woman and total hysterectomy and bilateral salpingo-oophorectomy in elderly women is the treatment choice.

DERMOID CYST

Origin : Dermoid cyst **arises from the germ cells** arrested after the first meiotic division.

Pathology : Dermoid cyst constitutes about 97 per cent of teratomata. Its incidence is about 15-20 per cent amongst ovarian tumours. The tumour is bilateral in about 15-20 per cent. It constitutes about 20-40 per cent of all ovarian tumours in pregnancy. **Torsion is the most common (15-20%) and rupture is an uncommon (1%) complication. The chance of malignancy is about 1-2 per cent.** Squamous cell carcinoma is the commonest.

Naked eye appearance (Fig. 20.7)

The cyst is of moderate size. The capsule is tense and smooth. On cut section, the content is a predominantly sebaceous material with hair. There may be clear fluid (cerebrospinal fluid) derived from the neural tissues (choroid plexus). There is one area of

Table 20.2 : Differentiation between benign and malignant ovarian tumours

Clinical examination: Benign	Clinical examination: Malignant	Laparotomy findings: Benign	Laparotomy findings: Malignant
• Unilateral	Bilateral	• **Ascites** — Absent	Present — often haemorrhagic
• Mobile	Fixed		
• **Feel** — Cystic	Solid/variegated	• **Exophytic growth on surface** — Absent	Present
• **Surface** — Smooth	Irregular	• **Adhesions** — Absent	Present
• **Ascites** — Absent	Present	• **Cut section** — Cystic	Solid and haemorrhagic areas
• **Growth** — Slow	Rapid		
• **Patient's Age** — Younger	Older		
• **Nodules in POD** — Absent	Present	• **Peritoneal nodules** — Absent	Present

Diagnostic criteria of a ovarian tumour on ultrasonography

Benign	Malignant
• Cystic areas with uniformly thin or thick multiple linear echoes (see Fig. 20.11).	• Cystic areas with irregular heterogenous solid part in more than 50% total tumour volume
• **Colour Doppler (TVS) evaluation of blood flow** : regular vascular branching and flow.	• Neovascularisation, low resistance flow with pulsatility index < 1.0.

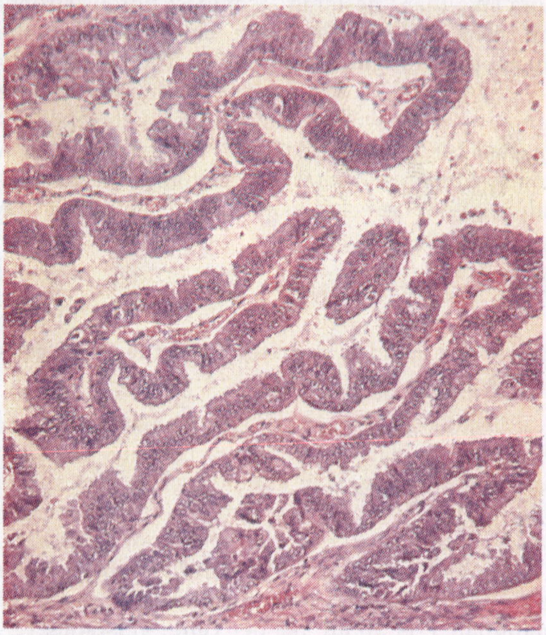

Fig. 20.6. Microphotograph showing the lining epithelium of papillary serous cyst adenoma. The cells form long papilliform processes

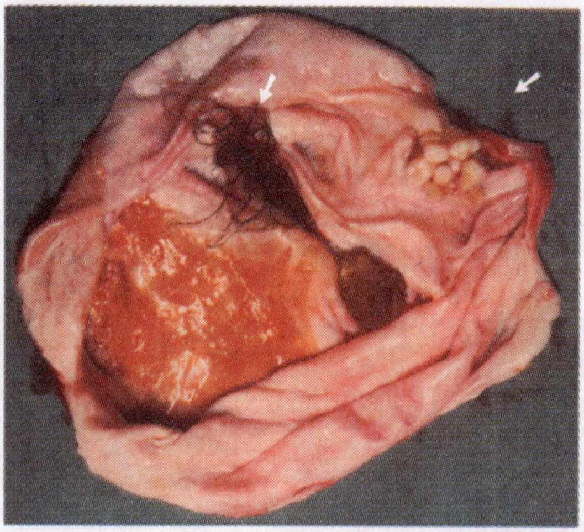

Fig. 20.7. Cut section of a dermoid cyst showing hair and teeth

solid projection called **Rokitansky's protuberance** which is covered by skin with sweat and sebaceous glands. It is here that teeth and bones are found. **Histological section should be made from this area.** A rare one consists predominantly of thyroid tissue — called **struma ovarii** which may be associated with hyperthyroidism.

Microscopic examination

The wall is lined by stratified squamous epithelium; and at places by granulation tissue. The epithelium may be transitional or columnar. **The most common tissue elements are ectodermal.**

The terminology of 'dermoid cyst' is misnomer, as apart from ectodermal element, there may be endodermal and mesodermal tissues as well. Besides dermal components bone, cartilage, neural tissue, thyroid and salivary gland tissues are often present.

Struma Ovarii and Strumal Carcinoids

Rarely ovarian teratomas contain a specialised tissue type. **Struma ovarii is composed of thyroid tissue.** This accounts for less than 3 per cent of **mature teratomas**. Malignant changes in a struma ovarii is extremely rare. **Strumal carcinoids** are also rare teratomas. Primary carcinoid tumours of the ovary account for less than 5 per cent of ovarian teratomas. These tumours may be **hormonally active with secretion of serotonin, bradykinin and other peptide hormones from the argentaffin cells** as found in gastrointestinal tract or bronchial tissues. **Carcinoid syndrome** is characterised by episodic facial flushing, abdominal pain, diarrhoea and bronchospasm. Metastatic carcinoid tumours are often bilateral. Carcinoid syndrome is more common in metastatic carcinoid than in ovarian primaries.

CLINICAL FEATURES OF BENIGN TUMOURS

Age : Benign tumours predominantly manifest in the late childbearing period. However, dermoid (90%) specially with mucinous cyst adenoma, is common in the reproductive period. As such, the dermoid is more common during pregnancy (10 per cent).

Parity : There is no correlation with parity of the patient (c.f. Fibroid — more related with nulliparity).

Symptoms : Most tumours are asymptomatic. These are detected accidentally by a general physician to find a lump in the lower abdomen during routine abdominal palpation or by a gynaecologist to find a tumour during pelvic examination, laparoscopy or laparotomy.

However, the patient may present the following symptoms :

- Heaviness in the lower abdomen.

• A gradually increasing mass in lower abdomen (ovarian tumour grows in months — c.f. fibroid).

• Dull aching pain in lower abdomen.

• In neglected cases, the tumour may be big enough to fill whole of the abdomen. It then produces cardiorespiratory embarrassment or gastrointestinal symptoms like nausea or indigestion.

• **Menstrual pattern remains unaffected unless associated with hormone producing tumours** — menorrhagia or postmenopausal bleeding or precocious puberty in feminising tumour-like granulosa cell tumour or amenorrhoea in masculinising tumour-like Sertoli-Leydig cell tumour (p. 371).

Signs

• General condition remains unaffected. However, in huge mucinous cyst adenoma, the patient may be cachetic due to protein loss (Fig. 20.8).

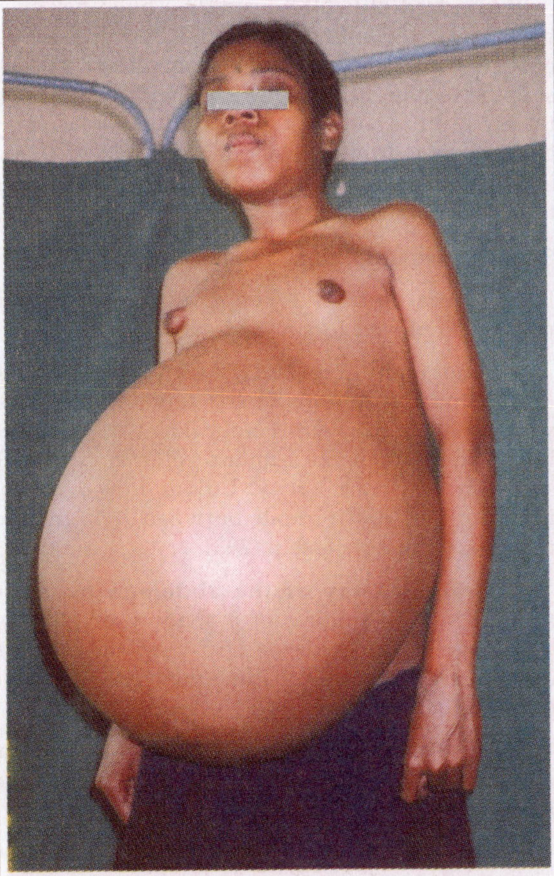

Fig. 20.8. Marked enlargement of the abdomen due to a huge mucinous cyst adenoma
[*Courtesy* : Dr. A. Halder, Asst. Professor, Obst.Gynae, N.B. Medical College, Sushrutnagar, Darjeeling].

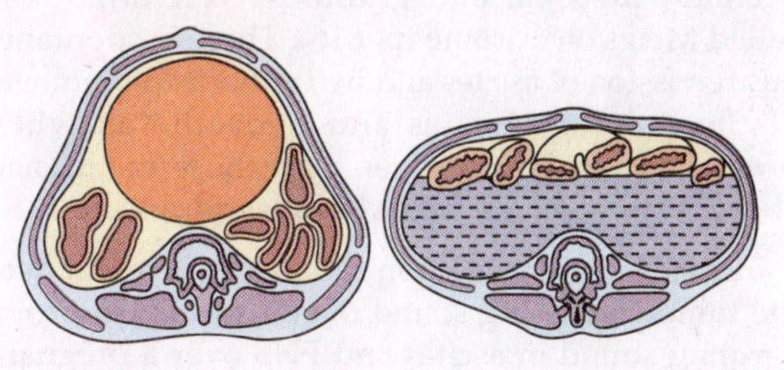

Fig. 20.9. Note the contour of the abdomen in ovarian tumour (left) and ascites (right)

• Pitting oedema of legs may be present when a huge tumour presses on the great veins.

Abdominal examination : An ovarian tumour which is enlarged sufficiently so as to occupy the lower abdomen presents with the following :

Inspection : There is bulging of the lower abdomen over which the abdominal wall moves freely with respiration. The mass may be placed centrally or in one side. At times, the mass fills the entire abdominal cavity everting the umbilicus with visible veins under the skin; the flanks remain flat (c.f. Flanks are full with ascites) (Fig. 20.9).

Palpation

• Feel is cystic or tense cystic. Benign solid tumours such as fibroma, thecoma, Brenner tumour are rare.

• Freely mobile from side to side but restricted from above down unless the pedicle is long. Too big a tumour or adhesions make its mobility restricted.

• Upper and lateral borders are well-defined but the lower pole is difficult to reach suggestive of pelvic origin. However, with long pedicle, the tumour may be displaced upwards so as to reach the lower pole.

• Surface over the tumour is smooth but often grooved in lobulated tumour.

• It is usually not tender.

***Percussion* (Fig. 20.9)** : Percussion note is dull in the centre and resonant in the flanks (c.f. In ascites — just the opposite). A fluid thrill may be elicited when the walls are thin and the content is watery. Co-existing ascites may be present even in a benign solid tumour (fibroma) and is called Meigs' syndrome.

Meigs' syndrome : Ascites and right side hydrothorax in association with fibroma of the ovary,

Brenner, thecoma and granulosa cell tumour is called Meigs' syndrome (p. 616). There is spontaneous remission of ascites and hydrothorax on removal of the tumour. Ascites and hydrothorax when present in conditions other than those mentioned above, are called pseudo-Meigs' syndrome.

Auscultation : A friction rub may be present over the tumour (Hissing sound over a vascular fibroid, gargling sound in ascites and FHS over a pregnant uterus).

Pelvic examination

***Bimanual examination reveals* (Fig. 9.10)**

- The uterus is separated from the mass.
- A groove is felt between the uterus and the mass.
- Movement of the mass per abdomen fails to move the cervix.
- On elevation of the mass per abdomen, the cervix remains in stationary position.
- The lower pole of the cyst can be felt through the fornix.
- Absence of pulsation of the uterine vessels through the fornices.

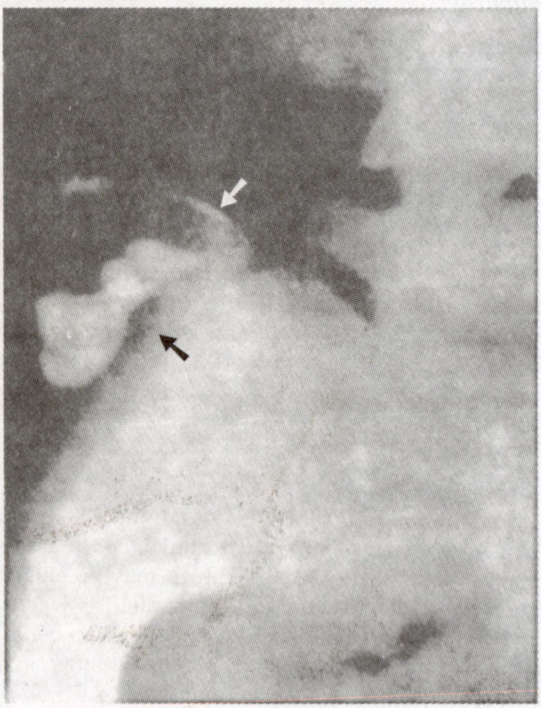

Fig. 20.10. Plain X-ray of the abdomen over a tumour showing shadow of a tooth in dermoid

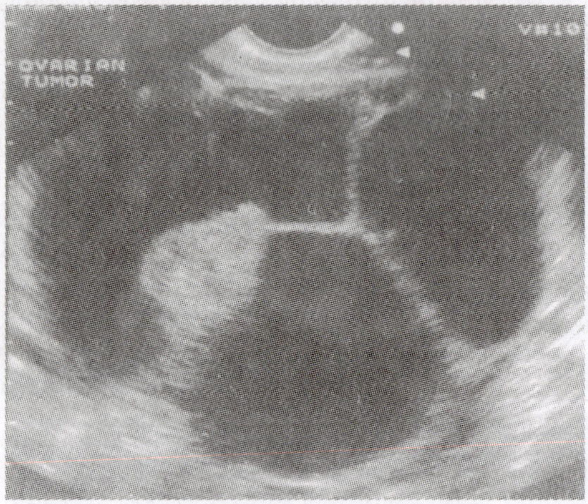

Fig. 20.11. Sonography (TV) of a benign ovarian cyst — multilocular with thin septum

It is indeed difficult to identify a huge cyst even by bimanual examination as the findings are all obscured. It is also difficult to foretell from which side the tumour arises. However, with elevation of the tumour per abdomen, the stretched pedicle may be felt through the corresponding fornix. **If a cyst is felt lying anterior to the uterus, it is more likely to be dermoid**.

Special investigations

If the clinical features are equivocal, the following may be employed to substantiate the diagnosis.

- **Sonography (Fig. 20.11)** — It can identify the uterus and the tumour in the same scan. Transvaginal sonography with colour flow Doppler gives information about the tumour volume, cyst wall, septa and the vascularity. Colour flow Doppler imaging can distinguish between benign and malignant tumours (see p. 283).
- **Straight X-ray of the abdomen over the tumour** — The finding of a shadow of teeth or bones is a direct evidence of a dermoid cyst. An outline of a soft tissue shadow may also be visible (Fig. 20.10).
- **CT** — (Fig. 20.12). The presence of an adnexal mass with mixed attenuation due to the presence of large amount of fat, calcification and tooth.
- **EUA** — In doubtful diagnosis specially in virgins, EUA is helpful.
- **Laparoscopy** — This is of help to differentiate a painful cystic mass with disturbed ectopic pregnancy.

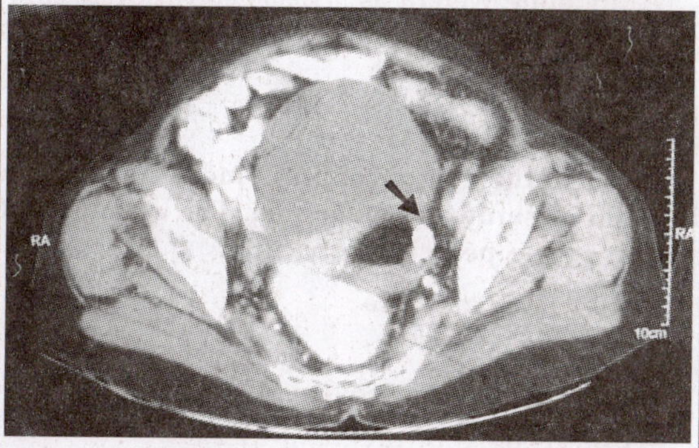

Fig. 20.12. CT scan shows a typical benign cystic teratoma containing fat, dental elements (arrow) and a fat-fluid level (p. 625)

• **Laparotomy** — If the clinical and ancillary aids fail to diagnose the mass, laparotomy is justified to arrive at a diagnosis. This is specially indicated when a suspected functional cyst fails to regress in follow up.

• **Cytology** — When the patient presents with ascites or pleural effusion, cytological examination of the aspirated fluid is done for malignant cells.

DIFFERENTIAL DIAGNOSIS OF A BENIGN OVARIAN TUMOUR

An ovarian tumour, apparently uncomplicated, may be confused (depending upon its size) with the following (see also p. 530) :

- Full bladder
- Pregnancy
- Fibroid
- Chocolate cyst of the ovary (see p. 301, 305)
- Encysted peritonitis
- Ascites
- Functional ovarian cyst
- Pregnancy with fibroid.

Full bladder

Always examine the patient with the bladder empty; if necessary following catheterisation. One should not be confused with overflow incontinence in chronic retention as normal urination, as stated by the patient.

Pregnancy : A pregnancy of 16-18 weeks is very much deceptive and one should be very much careful to exclude pregnancy during child-bearing period irrespective of the status of the women. If necessary, the help of X-ray or sonar may be taken. If none is available, it is a sound policy to re-examine the patient after 4 weeks when all the diagnostic features of pregnancy will be clinically evident.

Fibroid : Confusion arises specially in cases of pedunculated subserous fibroid more so, if degeneration occurs. Sonar or laparoscopy may be helpful. However, in either condition laparotomy is indicated when the diagnosis can be made.

Chocolate cyst of the ovary (see p. 301).

Encysted peritonitis : There may be features of tubercular affection elsewhere or in the abdomen. The encysted mass is usually irregular, not movable with ill-defined margins and usually situated high up. Pelvic examination usually gives a negative finding.

Ascites : There is fullness of the flanks. On percussion, flanks are dull with resonance in the centre. There may be presence of fluid thrill and positive shifting dullness. On auscultation, there is absence of any rub sound unlike in ovarian tumour.

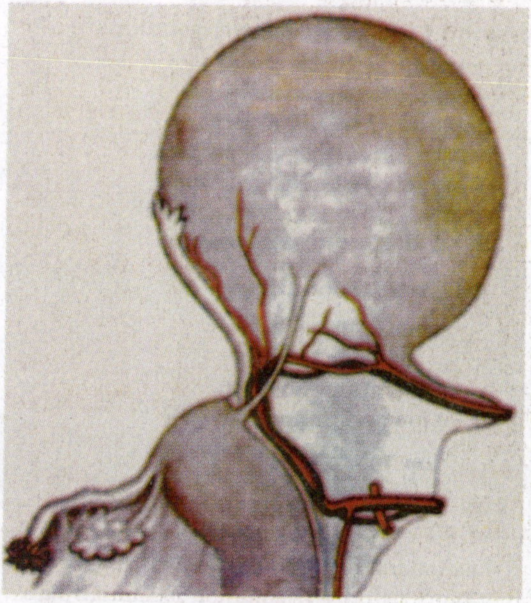

Fig. 20.13. Structures forming the ovarian pedicle

Sometimes, the ovarian tumour is so big as in mucinous cyst adenoma, that it is difficult to differentiate by clinical examination alone. In such cases, abdominal paracentesis and examination of the fluid can give a clue in the diagnosis.

Functional cyst : These cysts are small and re-examination after 12 weeks solves the diagnosis in most cases. The follicular or corpus luteum cyst usually regresses, while neoplastic cyst usually increases in size. Laparoscopy is of help.

Pregnancy with fibroid : In such condition, the pregnant uterus feels more soft and cystic but the fibroid feels little firm. As such, the former is confused as ovarian cyst and the latter one as uterus. Sonar can differentiate and prevent an unnecessary laparotomy with mistaken diagnosis of pregnancy with ovarian cyst.

COMPLICATIONS OF BENIGN OVARIAN TUMOURS

- Torsion of the pedicle (axial rotation)
- Intracystic haemorrhage
- Infection
- Rupture
- Pseudomyxoma peritonei
- Malignancy

Torsion of the pedicle (axial rotation)

Table 20.3
Structures forming the ovarian pedicle (Fig. 20.13)

Laterally

- Infundibulopelvic ligament containing structures therein, i.e. ovarian vessels, nerves and lymphatics.

Medially

- Ovarian ligament.
- Medial end of the Fallopian tube.
- Mesosalpinx containing utero-ovarian anastomotic vessels.

Middle

- Broad ligament.

The axial rotation is found in about 10-15 per cent cases at operation. It is common in tumour having :

- Moderate size, preferably with round contour.
- Moderate weight as *dermoid cyst* (due to high fat content).
- Free mobility.
- Long pedicle.

As such, **the complication is more common in dermoid or serous cystadenoma. The aetiology of torsion of the pedicle is obscure.**

***Predisposing factors* are** :

- Trauma.
- Violent physical movements.
- Contractions of pregnant uterus.
- Intestinal peristalsis.

These probably initiate axial rotation.

Precipitating factor : The haemodynamic theory is perhaps most satisfactory to explain the final onslaught of torsion. Slight axial rotation of the pedicle → venous occlusion and partial arterial compression → intermittent forcible arterial pulsation → further aggravating the axial rotation until it becomes complete. The rotation occurs usually towards midline. Torsion leads to ischaemia and tissue necrosis (Fig. 20.15).

Fate : The partial torsion may often untwist spontaneously but if complete torsion of few turns occur, there is obstruction of both the veins and arteries. As a result, there is intense venous congestion with extravasation of blood inside the cyst. The cyst becomes tense and may rupture or else, the intestine may adhere to the gangrenous cyst which may be infected; the organisms are derived from the gut or from the uterine tube. Rarely, the pedicle may be detached; the **tumour gets its nourishment from some other abdominal structures to which it is adherent (parasitic tumour)**.

Symptoms : The clinical presentation depends on the extent of interference with ovarian blood supply. With complete vascular occlusion, the pain will be severe.

The patient complains of sudden acute pain lower abdomen along with a lump. The lump may be present before or manifested with pain.

On examination, the general condition remains unaffected except that the patient is in agony with pain. Abdominal examination reveals a tender, tense cystic mass, with restricted mobility, situated in the hypogastrium and arising from the pelvis.

Pelvic examination reveals the mass felt per abdomen is separated from the uterus.

Table 20.4
Summary of Torsion of Ovarian Pedicle

- Common in dermoid or simple serous cyst.
- Partial axial rotation followed by complete torsion is explained by haemodynamic theory.
- Symptoms of acute pain lower abdomen with a lump.
- General condition remains unaffected.
- Abdominal examination reveals a tense cystic tender mass in the hypogastrium arising from the pelvis.
- Pelvic examination reveals the mass separated from the uterus.
- Treatment is laparotomy and ovariotomy.

Differential diagnosis

The diagnosis is often confused with — (1) disturbed ectopic pregnancy, (2) acute hydramnios, (3) perforating hydatidiform mole and (4) torsion of subserous pedunculated fibroid.

Treatment : To suppress pain, morphine 15 mg IM is given. Laparotomy is to be done at the earliest. The definitive surgery is usually ovariotomy (salpingo-oophorectomy) as the structures usually become gangrenous. The clamps are placed prior untwisting the pedicle to minimise dislodgement of the thrombi. However, for better grip, clamps may be placed after untwisting the pedicle (Table 20.3).

Intracystic haemorrhage : It is more common in serous cyst adenoma with papillary varieties. Intracystic haemorrhage also occurs following venous congestion due to axial torsion of the pedicle and also in malignant changes.

Infection : Infection is common following torsion. The organisms are derived from the intestines or uterine tubes when they are adherent to the cyst.

Rupture : Rupture of the cyst usually follows in big and tense cysts with degeneration of a part of cyst wall. The rupture also occurs following intracystic haemorrhage or direct trauma, in papillary variety or in malignancy.

Pseudomyxoma peritonei : It is a condition of mucinous ascites usually secondary to mucinous tumour of intra-abdominal organ. Its exact nature of origin is not known. **But it is often associated with** mucinous cyst adenoma of the ovary, mucocele of the appendix and gallbladder and intestinal malignancy.

Spontaneous perforation of mucinous cyst may lead to implantation of the cells of low grade malignancy on the peritoneum. Or else, the mesothelium of the peritoneum is converted to high columnar epithelium with secretory activity. The cell type is similar to mucinous cyst adenoma.

Even after removal of the ovarian tumour, these cells continue to secrete mucin. There is a tendency of recurrence. *The prognosis is poor due to inanition,*

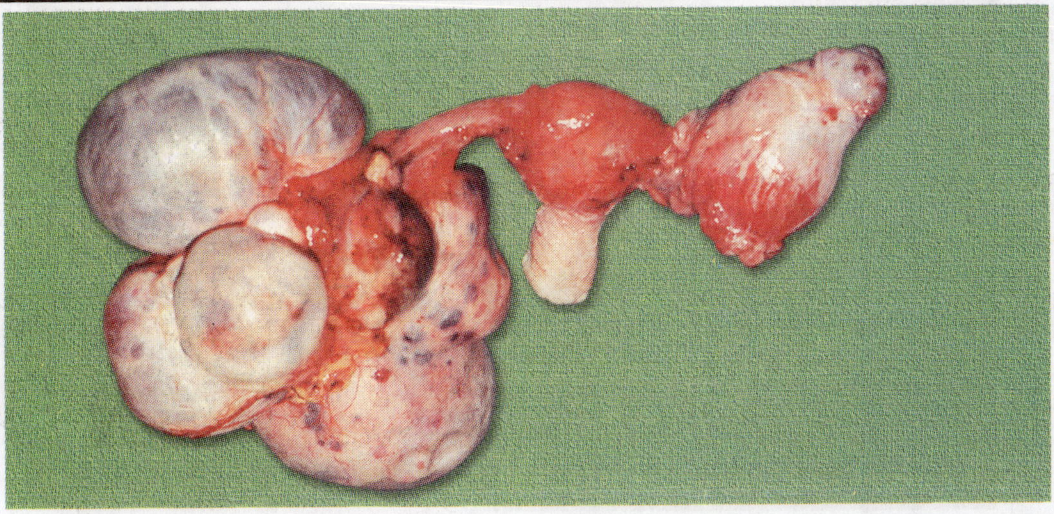

Fig. 20.14. Bilateral ovarian tumour in a perimenopausal woman treated by total hysterectomy with bilateral salpingo-oophorectomy

infection and intestinal obstruction. Treatment remains unsatisfactory.

Hysterectomy, bilateral salpingo-oophorectomy with removal of mucin, peritoneal implants along with appendix is recommended. Recurrence is high unless implants are removed entirely.

Malignancy : The malignancy rate varies. **The malignant potentiality is maximum in serous cyst adenoma specially of papillary variety and least in dermoid.** The former gives rise to adenocarcinoma and the latter to squamous cell carcinoma.

MANAGEMENT OF A BENIGN OVARIAN TUMOUR

Once an ovarian tumour is diagnosed, the patient should be admitted for operation — sooner the better. This is because, **the complication can occur at any time and the nature of the tumour cannot be assessed clinically.** A clinically benign tumour may turn into a malignant one at operation. In others, even a benign tumour removed may be proved malignant on histological examination.

Differentiation between benign and malignant ovarian tumours could be made by clinical examination, ultrasonography, laparotomy and finally by biopsy (see p. 283).

Guidelines for surgery in an apparently benign tum

- **Incision** should be vertical paramedian sufficiently big enough to deliver the cyst intact. An attempt to tap a cyst to minimise its size and to deliver it with a small incision is to be condemned. The content may be mucinous, sebaceous material, infective or malignant fluid which contaminates the peritoneal cavity. The longitudinal incision also allows adequate exposure in the upper abdomen.
- **To inspect** the nature of the peritoneal fluid — clear, straw colour, haemorrhagic or infective. A sample of the fluid or peritoneal washings should be sent for cytological examination.
- **To deliver the tumour** intact and to note it carefully about its nature (see Table 20.2 on p. 283).
- **To inspect and to palpate** the other ovary, pelvic organs, omentum, liver, under surface of diaphragm and para-aortic group of lymph glands.
- **To proceed** for the definitive surgery (see below).
- To **cut the tumour** and inspect the inner side for any evidence of malignancy. In suspected cases, the facility of frozen section is invaluable (Table 20.2 on p. 283).

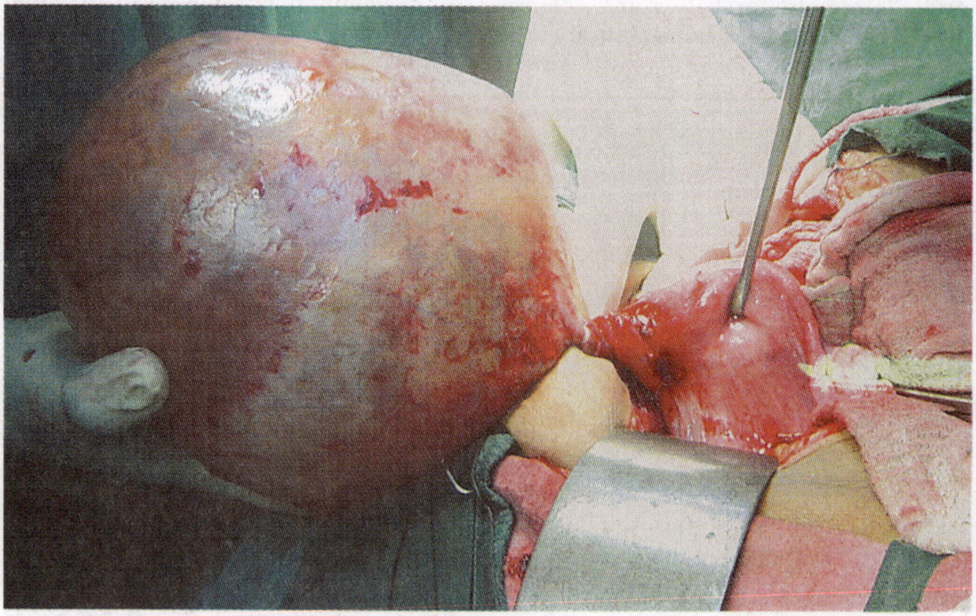

Fig. 20.15. Torsion of the pedicle of an ovarian tumour. Note the turns in the pedicle and stretched Fallopian tube

- It is not prudent to bisect the contralateral ovary, if it looks absolutely normal.

Definitive surgery

In young patients

- Ovarian cystectomy leaving behind the healthy ovarian tissue is the operation of choice.
- Ovariotomy (salpingo-oophorectomy) is reserved for a big tumour that has destroyed almost all the ovarian tissues or for a gangrenous cyst.
- If both the ovaries are involved, ovarian cystectomy should be done at least in one ovary.
- Retention of the uterus for possible ART may be considered when bilateral ovariotomy has to be done.

In parous women around 40 years

- Total hysterectomy with bilateral salpingo-oophorectomy is to be done (Fig. 20.14).

In between these two extremes of age

Individualisation is to be done as regards the nature of surgery. Due consideration is to be given about the reproductive and menstrual function.

In all cases, the entire tumour is to be sent for histological examination. If a part is to be sent, **a small piece from the comparatively solid or thick capsule is to be selected.**

BORDERLINE EPITHELIAL TUMOURS OF THE OVARY

Borderline malignant epithelial tumours have got some but not all the features of malignancy. They are of low malignant potential. The characteristic features are :

- They constitute 10-20 per cent of all epithelial tumours of the ovary.
- There is stratification of epithelial cells of the papillae.
- There is epithelial cell pleomorphism.
- Presence of papillary projection on the external surface.
- Detachment of cellular clusters from the sites of origin.
- Increased cellular mitotic activity.
- Presence of nuclear atypia of varying degrees.
- No invasion of ovarian stroma.
- Generally they are found in the younger age group and carry good prognosis.

Treatment : Unilateral oophorectomy is optimum specially for the young women. When there is bilateral ovarian involvement or peritoneal spread, total hysterectomy with bilateral salpingo-oophorectomy and excision of the involved peritoneum are done. Risk of recurrence is low.

PAROVARIAN CYST (Fig. 20.16)

Parovarian cyst may **arise either from the vestigeal remnants of Wolffian in the mesosalpinx or from the peritoneal inclusions or from tubal epithelium (Fig. 20.16).**

The ovary is separated and the uterine tube is stretched over the cyst. The cyst is unilocular; the wall is thin and contains clear fluid. The wall consists of connective tissue lined by a single layer of cuboidal or flat epithelium. There may be a thin muscle tissue along with secretory epithelium suggesting tubal origin.

The cysts are always benign. The **presenting features are like those of benign ovarian tumour. It can undergo torsion like that of ovarian tumour (Fig. 36.64).**

Removal of the tumour, when burrows in the broad ligament, needs a cautious approach as the ureter is either placed at the bottom or on the top of the cyst. An incision is made anterior and parallel to the round ligament (see Fig. 34.8). Enucleation of the tumour is done leaving behind the ovary. Haemostasis at the base is achieved by ligature taking care not to injure the ureter.

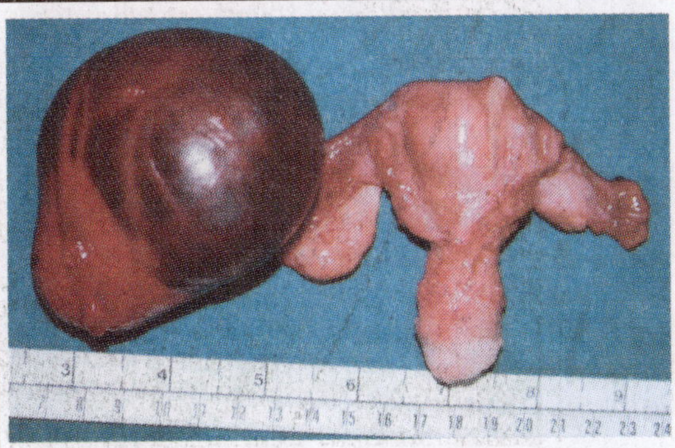

Fig. 20.16. Parovarian cyst (right). The ovary is seen separated and the uterine tube is stretched over the cyst

KEY POINTS

- The functional cysts of the ovary are predominantly follicular cyst and corpus luteum cyst. Follicular cysts are the most common and the initial management is conservative. Treatment of unruptured corpus luteum cyst is conservative.
- Ovarian cystic mass 8 cm or more after menopause or before puberty or a solid tumour at any age indicates laparotomy.
- Theca lutein cysts are due to excessive gonadotrophin (endogenous or exogenous) stimulation of the ovaries. Fifty per cent of molar pregnancies and 10 per cent of choriocarcinomas have associated bilateral theca lutein cysts (p. 349). They usually regress spontaneously with normalisation of serum hCG level.
- The following criteria must be fulfilled for conservative management of an ovarian cyst : (i) Asymptomatic. (ii) Unilateral. (iii) Size < 8 cm. (iv) Unilocular cyst without any solid area. (v) Normal CA 125. (vi) No ascites. Followed by — (vii) Ultrasound re-examination at 3-6 months time.
- Mucinous cyst adenoma accounts for 20-25 per cent of all ovarian tumours. They are bilateral in 10 per cent and chance of malignancy is 5-10 per cent.

  The content is mucin — a glycoprotein with high content of neutral polysaccharides.

  It is lined by tall columnar epithelium with deep stained basal nucleus without cilia, the structure like that of endocervix.
- Serous cyst adenoma accounts for 40 per cent of ovarian tumours. It is bilateral in 40 per cent and chance of malignancy is about 40 per cent.

  It is lined by cubical epithelium. In papillary type, the lining epithelium is like that of Fallopian tube.
- Dermoid cyst accounts for 15-20 per cent amongst ovarian tumours. It is bilateral in 15-20 per cent. Chance of malignancy is least — 1-2 per cent. If an ovarian cyst is lying anterior to uterus, it is likely to be dermoid.
- Meigs' syndrome is ascites and hydrothorax in association with fibroma of the ovary.
- Ovarian tumour is commonly confused with full bladder, pregnancy, fibroid or ascites.
- Torsion of the pedicle is the commonest complication of benign cystic ovarian tumour and the rarest one is malignancy.

  Pseudomyxoma peritonei is usually associated with mucinous cyst adenoma of the ovary, mucocele of the appendix and gallbladder and intestinal malignancy.
- The malignancy is highest in papillary variety of serous cyst adenoma being adenocarcinoma and lowest one in dermoid being squamous cell carcinoma.
- In young women, conservative surgery, either ovarian cystectomy or ovariotomy (oophorectomy) is to be done. In patient around 40 and above, total hysterectomy with bilateral salpingo-oophorectomy is justified.
- Borderline epithelial tumours of the ovary are of low malignant potential. Though there is cellular mitotic activity and nuclear atypia (see p. 291), stromal invasion is absent. Unilateral oophorectomy is the optimum treatment specially for a young woman. In elderly women total hysterectomy, bilateral salpingo-oophorectomy and omentectomy are done. Chemotherapy is not usually considered following surgery.
- 5 years survival rate for patients with borderline epithelial ovarian cancer (grade O) is close to 100 per cent.
- In all cases, the tumour is subjected to histopathological study to note the nature of the tumour and to exclude malignancy.

Endometriosis and Adenomyosis

21

ENDOMETRIOSIS

Definition

The presence of functioning endometrium (glands and stroma) in sites other than uterine mucosa is called endometriosis. It is not a neoplastic condition, although malignant transformation is possible.

These ectopic endometrial tissues may be found in the myometrium when it is called endometriosis interna or **adenomyosis**. More commonly however, these tissues are found at sites other than uterus and are called endometriosis externa or generally referred to as endometriosis.

As adenomyosis have different pathogenesis and appears to behave quite differently, the entity is dealt with separately.

Prevalence

During the last couple of decades, the prevalence of endometriosis has been increasing both in terms of real and apparent. **The real one** is due to delayed marriage, postponement of first conception and adoption of small family norm. **The apparent one** is

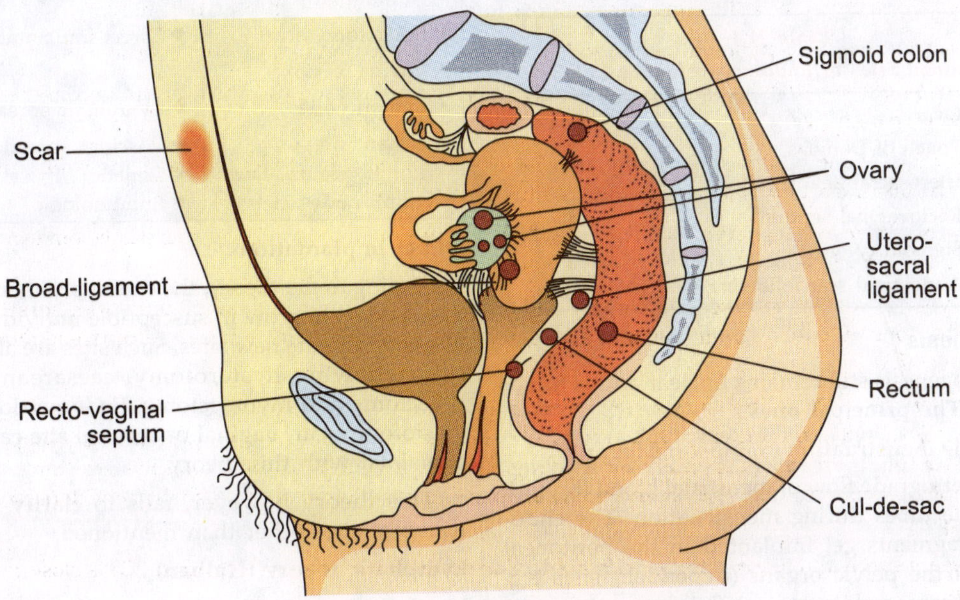

Fig. 21.1. Common sites of endometriosis

due to increased use of diagnostic laparoscopy as well as hightened awareness of this disease complex amongst the gynaecologists.

The prevalence is about 10 per cent. However, prevalence is high amongst the infertile women (30-40%) as based on diagnostic laparoscopy and laparotomy.

Sites (Table 21.1)

- **Abdominal** • **Extra-abdominal** • **Remote**

Abdominal

It can occur at any site but is usually confined to the abdominal structures below the level of umbilicus. **Common structures involved in order of frequency are ovary, pouch of Douglas, uterosacral ligament, broad ligament, rectovaginal septum, rectum and pelvic lymph nodes.** Rare sites are gut, appendix, ureter and urinary bladder. The levels of gonadal steroids are much higher in the ovary than in other peritoneal surface.

Extra-abdominal

The common sites are abdominal scar of hysterotomy, caesarean section, tubectomy and myomectomy, umbilicus, episiotomy scar, vagina and cervix.

Remote sites are pleura, lungs, deep tissues of arms and thighs.

Table 21.1
Common Sites of Endometriosis (Fig. 21.1)

- Ovary
- Pouch of Douglas
- Uterosacral ligament
- Rectovaginal septum
- Sigmoid colon
- Abdominal scar following hysterotomy.

Pathogenesis

The pathogenesis still remains unclear and is full of theories. **The principal ones :**

Retrograde menstruation (Sampson's theory)

There is retrograde flow of menstrual blood through the uterine tubes during menstruation. The endometrial fragments get implanted in the peritoneal surface of the pelvic organs (dependent sites e.g. ovaries, uterosacral ligaments). Subsequently, cyclic growth and shedding of the endometrium at the ectopic sites occur under the influence of the endogenous ovarian hormones. Retrograde menstruation *per se* is unlikely to produce endometriosis. Probably, a genetic factor or favourable hormonal milieu is necessary for successful implantation and growth of the fragments of endometrium. While this theory can explain pelvic endometriosis, it fails to explain the endometriosis at distant sites.

Coelomic metaplasia (Meyer and Ivanoff)

Chronic irritation of the pelvic peritoneum by the menstrual blood may cause coelomic metaplasia which results in endometriosis. Alternatively, the müllerian tissue remnants may be trapped within the peritoneum. They could undergo metaplasia and be transformed into endometrium.

This theory can explain endometriosis of the abdominal viscera, the rectovaginal septum and the umbilicus.

Table 21.2
Theories to explain endometriosis at different sites

Sites	Theory
• Pelvic endometriosis • Pelvic peritoneum	◆ Retrograde menstruation ◆ Coelomic metaplasia
• Abdominal viscera • Rectovaginal septum • Umbilicus	◆ Coelomic metaplasia
• Abdominal scar • Episiotomy scar • Vagina, cervix	◆ Direct implantation
• Lymph nodes	◆ Lymphatic spread
• Distant sites (Lungs, pleura, skin, lymph nodes, nerves)	◆ Vascular spread ✱ Genetic ✱ Immunologic

Direct implantation

According to the theory, the endometrial or decidual tissues start to grow in susceptible individual when implanted in the new sites. Such sites are abdominal scar following hysterotomy, caesarean section, tubectomy and myomectomy. Endometriosis at the episiotomy scar, vaginal or cervical site can also be explained with this theory.

This theory however, fails to clarify endometriosis at sites other than mentioned.

Lymphatic theory (Halban)

It may be possible for the normal endometrium to metastasise the pelvic lymph nodes through the draining lymphatic channels of the uterus. This could explain the lymph node involvement.

Vascular theory

This is sound at least to explain endometriosis at distant sites such as lungs, arms or thighs.

Genetic and immunological factors

Genetic basis of endometriosis probably accounts for less than 10 per cent of the patients. There is 6-7 times increased incidence in first degree relatives. Multifactorial inheritance is thought. However, a defect of local cellular immunity may be responsible for the ectopic tissue to grow in abnormal sites only in susceptible women.

Peritoneal macrophages normally remove the menstrual debris by phagocytosis. Pelvic endometriosis is associated with a **subclinical peritoneal inflammation** resulting in increase in peritoneal fluid. In patients with endometriosis, the activated macrophages secrete several factors like cytokines, interleukin–1, α TNF, integrins and angiogenic factors. These factors promote the growth of endometrial cells over the ectopic sites. Ectopic endometrium is more resistant to apoptosis. Furthermore activated macrophages reduce sperm motility, increase sperm phagocytosis and interfere with fertilisation.

Thus, it is certain that, not all cases of endometriosis at different sites can be explained by a single theory.

Pathology

General considerations

- The endometrium (glands and stroma) in the ectopic sites has got the potentiality to undergo changes under the action of ovarian hormones.
- While proliferative changes are constantly evidenced, the secretory changes are conspicuously absent in many; may be due to deficiency of steroid receptors in the ectopic endometrium.
- Cyclic growth and shedding continue till menopause. The periodically shed blood may remain encysted or else, the cyst becomes tense and ruptures.
- As the blood is irritant, there is dense tissue reaction surrounding the lesion with fibrosis. If it happens to occur on the pelvic peritoneum, it produces adhesions and puckering of the peritoneum.
- If encysted, the cyst enlarges with cyclic bleeding. The serum gets absorbed in between the periods and the content inside becomes chocolate coloured. Hence, the cyst is called chocolate cyst which is commonly located in the ovary. **Chocolate cyst may also** be due to haemorrhagic follicular or corpus luteum cyst or bleeding into a cyst adenoma. For this reason, the term endometrial cyst or endometrioma is preferred to chocolate cyst.

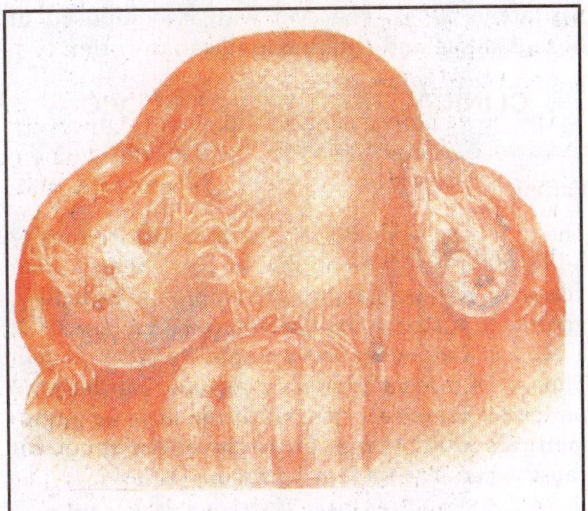

Fig. 21.2. The appearance of pelvic endometriosis. Note the black dots and puckered peritoneum

- In spite of dense adhesions amongst the pelvic structures, the **fallopian tubes remain patent**.

Naked eye appearance

The appearance of the lesion depends to a great extent on the organ(s) involved, extent of the lesion and reaction of the surrounding tissues.

Pelvic endometriosis

Typically, **there are small black dots, the so called *'powder burns'* seen on the uterosacral ligaments and pouch of Douglas (Fig. 21.2)**. Fibrosis and scarring in the peritoneum surrounding the implants is also a typical finding. **Other subtle appearances are** : *red flame shaped areas, red polypoid areas, yellow brown patches, white peritoneal areas, circular peritoneal defects*. These lesions are thought to be more active than the "powders burn" areas.

The ovaries are frequently involved usually bilaterally. The endometriomas (chocolate cysts) are of varying sizes and are visible as bluish colourations. The ovaries get adherent to the pelvic structures including rectum and sigmoid colon (see p. 301).

Microscopic appearance

There is presence of endometrial tissue — **both glands and stroma**. Due to pressure effect, the lining epithelium of the cyst may be absent or flattened (cuboidal) or replaced by granulation tissue. Adjacent to the lining epithelium, there may be presence of large polyhedral **phagocytic cells, laden with blood pigment** — **haemosiderin** (pseudoxanthoma cells). The cyst wall is composed of fibrous tissue and compressed ovarian cortex.

CLINICAL FEATURES OF PELVIC ENDOMETRIOSIS

Patient profile

The age is between 30-45. The patients are mostly nulliparous or have had one or two children long years prior to appearance of symptoms. Infertility, voluntary postponement of first conception until at a late age and higher social status are often related. Thus, it is more common in private than hospital patients. There is often family history of endometriosis. Outflow tract obstruction is an important cause when it is seen in teenagers (10%).

Symptoms

- About 25 per cent of patients with endometriosis have no symptom, being accidentally discovered either during laparoscopy or laparotomy.
- Symptoms are not related with extent of lesion. Even when the endometriosis is widespread, there may not be any symptom; conversely, there may be intense symptoms with minimal endometriosis.
- Depth of penetration is more related to symptoms rather than the spread. Lesions penetrating more than 5 mm are responsible for pain, dysmenorrhoea and dyspareunia.
- Non-pigmented endometriotic lesions compared to the classic pigmented "powder burns" lesions produce more prostaglandin F (PGF) and hence are more painful.
- The symptoms are mostly related to the site of lesion and its ability to respond to hormones. Midline lesions are more symptom producing. Degree of pain is not related to the severity of endometriosis.

Dysmenorrhoea (50%)

There is progressively increasing secondary dysmenorrhoea. The pain starts a few days prior to menstruation; gets worsened during menstruation and takes time, even after cessation of period, to get relief of pain, (co-menstrual dysmenorrhoea). Pain usually begins after few years pain-free menses. The site of pain is usually deep seated and on the back or rectum.

Increased secretion of PGF 2α, thromboxane β_2 from endometriotic tissue is the cause of pain.

Abnormal menstruation (60%)

Menorrhagia is the predominant abnormality. If the ovaries are also involved, polymenorrhoea or epimenorrhagia may be pronounced. There may be premenstrual spotting.

Infertility (40-60%)

Whether endometriosis causes infertility or infertility produces endometriosis is not clear. Endometriosis is found in 20-40 per cent of infertile women, whereas in about 40-50 per cent patients with endometriosis suffer from infertility. The multiple factors involved in producing infertility have been depicted in p. 224 (Table 16.2).

Dyspareunia

The dyspareunia is usually deep. It may be due to stretching of the structures of the pouch of Douglas or direct contact tenderness. As such, it is mostly found in endometriosis of the rectovaginal septum or pouch of Douglas and with fixed retroverted uterus.

Chronic Pelvic pain

The pain varies from pelvic discomfort, lower abdominal pain or backache. The cause may be multifactorial. These include — (i) Inflammation in the peritoneal implants due to cyclic bleeding. (ii) Action of inflammatory cytokines released by the macrophages. (iii) Irritation or invasion of nerves. The pain aggravates during period.

Abdominal pain

There may be variable degrees of abdominal pain around the periods. Sometimes, the pain may be acute due to rupture of chocolate cyst.

Other symptoms

The symptoms are related to the organ involved. The symptoms are cycle associated.

- Bladder — frequency, dysuria or even haematuria
- Sigmoid colon and rectum — painful defecation (dyschezia), diarrhoea, rectal bleeding or even melena.
- Chronic fatigue, perimenstrual symptoms (bowel, bladder).

Abdominal examination

Abdominal palpation may not reveal any abnormality. A mass may be felt in the lower abdomen arising from the pelvis — enlarged chocolate cyst or tubo-ovarian mass due to endometriotic adhesions. The mass is tender with restricted mobility.

Pelvic examination

Bimanual examination may not reveal any pathology. **The expected positive findings are** — pelvic tenderness, nodules in the pouch of Douglas, nodular feel of the uterosacral ligaments, fixed retroverted uterus or unilateral or bilateral adnexal mass of varying sizes (Fig. 21.3).

Speculum examination may reveal bluish spots in the posterior fornix.

Rectal or rectovaginal examination is often helpful to confirm the findings.

DIAGNOSIS

Clinical diagnosis is by the classic symptoms of progressively increasing secondary dysmenorrhoea, dyspareunia and infertility. This is corroborated by the pelvic findings of nodules in the pouch of Douglas, nodular feel of the uterosacral ligaments, fixed retroverted uterus and unilateral or bilateral adnexal mass. However, physical examination has poor sensitivity and specificity. Many patients have no abnormal findings on examination.

Serum marker CA 125 — A moderate elevation of serum CA 125 is noticed in patients with severe endometriosis. It is not specific for endometriosis, as it is significantly raised in epithelial ovarian carcinoma (see p. 363). However, it is helpful to assess the therapeutic response and in follow up of cases and to detect any recurrence after therapy. Its low sensitivity and specificity restricts its use for routine screening (see p. 369, 497, 615).

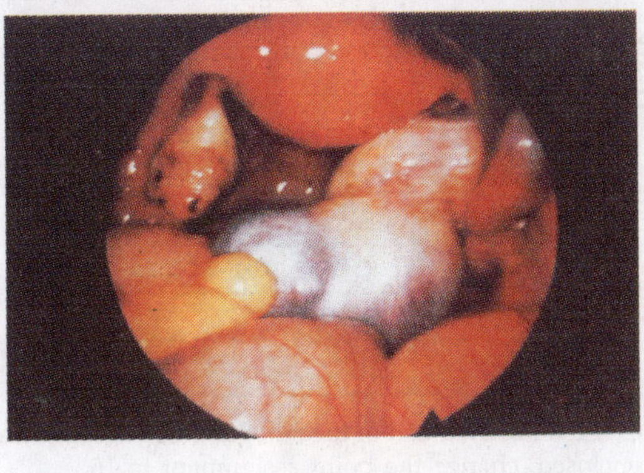

Fig. 21.3. Laparoscopic view of pelvic endometriosis : left ovary-endometriotic implants, right ovary-chocolate cyst

Imaging

Ultrasonography is not much helpful to the diagnosis. TVS can detect ovarian endometriomas. Transvaginal (TVS) and Endorectal ultrasound are found better for rectosigmoid endometriosis.

Computed tomography (CT) and magnetic resonance imaging (MRI) are expensive and are not much helpful to the diagnosis (p. 114).

Confirmation is by double puncture **laparoscopy (Gold standard)** or by laparotomy. The classic lesion of pelvic endometriosis is described as *'powder burns'* or *'match stick'* spots on the peritoneum of the pouch of Douglas (see p. 295). Findings may be recorded on video or DVD (RCOG-2006) Microscopically some of these lesions contain endometrial glands, stroma and haemosiderin-laden macrophages.

Biopsy confirmation of excised lesion is ideal but negative histology does not exclude it. None of the imaging techniques including ultrasound, can diagnose specifically the peritoneal endometriosis. Emperic medical treatment is usually not recommended except for pain relief and to reduce menstrual flow.

DIFFERENTIAL DIAGNOSIS

- **Chronic pelvic infection** is most often confused with symptomatic endometriosis. The clinical presentation is almost similar. Laparoscopy is helpful in actual diagnosis.

- **Ovarian endometrioma (chocolate cyst)** : Ovary is the most common site for endometriosis. It starts with a superficial endometriotic implant over the ovarian surface. The endometriotic tissue gradually invades the ovarian stroma. Cyst formation is due to periodic shedding and bleeding from the implant.

Leakage of this altered blood along with inflammation, leads to adhesion formation with the adjacent structures. Fallopian tubes may be affected. Epithelial lining of the cyst contain endometrial glands and stroma. Due to pressure effect the lining epithelium may be flattened. When the cyst ruptures the characteristic thick, tarry fluid (chocolate material) escapes.

If asymptomatic, may be confused with **benign ovarian tumour** and in symptomatic one, with **malignant ovarian**. Presence of nodules in the pouch of Douglas further confuses the diagnosis. **Ultrasonography** showing homogeneous internal echoes may be helpful (see Fig. 21.4). **Laparoscopy** differentiates one from the other. Too often, the diagnosis is made only during laparotomy.

• **Rupture of the chocolate cyst** : During operation, while separating the adhesions, the cyst invariably ruptures with escape of chocolate coloured blood. The rupture of the cyst can occur spontaneously causing acute abdomen with clinical features suggestive of acute ectopic. Acute abdomen **is confused with** torsion or rupture of the ovarian tumour, disturbed ectopic pregnancy, appendicitis or diverticulitis.

COMPLICATIONS OF ENDOMETRIOSIS

The following complications may occur :

- Endocrinopathy — This may be mostly responsible for infertility (Table 21.3).
- Rupture of chocolate cyst
- Infection of chocolate cyst
- Obstructive features :
  - Intestinal obstruction
  - Ureteral obstruction → hydroureter → hydronephrosis → renal infection
- Malignancy is rare, the commonest one being adenoacanthoma.

Table 21.3
Endocrinopathy in endometriosis

- Corpus luteum insufficiency (p. 230).
- Luteolysis due to ↑ PGF2α.
- Luteinised unruptured follicle (LUF) (p. 230).
- Anovulation.
- Elevated prolactin level.
- Double LH peak.

Staging

The diagnosed endometriosis should be appropriately staged based on laparoscopic findings.

- To predict prognosis. • To choose therapy.
- To evaluate the treatment protocol.

The scoring is (revised) by the American Fertility Society and is presented in Table 21.4. **The stage is determined by adding specific points given to each.**

Limitations of AFS staging

- Laparoscopy or Laparotomy has to be done.
- Interobserver and intraobserver variation.
- No correlation between the extent of disease and the degree of symptoms.
- Staging has not been correlated with fertility outcome.
- Staging has not been correlated with optimum mode of therapy.

TREATMENT OF ENDOMETRIOSIS

Endometriosis needs to be treated as it is a progressive disease (30-60%).

• **Preventive** • **Curative**

Preventive

The following guidelines may be prescribed to prevent or minimise endometriosis :

- To avoid tubal patency test immediately after curettage or around the time of menstruation.
- Forcible pelvic examination should not be done during or shortly after menstruation.

Table 21.4
American Fertility Society scoring system of endometriosis (revised)

	Endometriosis	< 1 cm	1-3 cm	> 3 cm
Peritoneum	Superficial	1	2	4
Peritoneum	Deep	2	4	6
Ovary	R Superficial	1	2	4
Ovary	Deep	4	16	20
Ovary	L Superficial	1	2	4
Ovary	Deep	4	16	20
	Posterior cul-de-sac obliteration	Partial	Complete	
		4	40	
	Adhesions	< 1/3 Enclosure	1/3-2/3 Enclosure	> 2/3 Enclosure
Ovary	R Filmy	1	2	4
Ovary	Dense	4	8	16
Ovary	L Filmy	1	2	4
Ovary	Dense	4	8	16
Tube	R Filmy	1	2	4
Tube	Dense	4*	8*	16
Tube	L Filmy	1	2	4
Tube	Dense	4*	8*	16

* If the fimbriated end of the fallopian tube is completely enclosed, change the point assignment to 16.

• ***Stage I*** (minimal) = 1-5 • ***Stage II*** (mild) = 6-15
• ***Stage III*** (moderate) = 16-40 • ***Stage IV*** (severe) = > 40.

The findings are depicted in a pictorial chart.

- Married women with family history of endometriosis are encouraged not to delay the first conception but to complete the family.

Curative : The objectives are :

- To abolish or minimise the symptoms — pelvic pain and dyspareunia.
- To improve the fertility.
- To prevent recurrence.

But, it is difficult to achieve the objectives because of obscure aetiology and unpredictable life history. The results of treatment are difficult to evaluate because of lack of uniform staging or grading. **The following facts are to be borne in mind.**

- Asymptomatic in good number of cases.
- Subjective symptoms are not proportionate to objective signs.
- Frequent association with infertility.
- Remission during pregnancy and menopause.

Prerequisites prior to therapy are accurate diagnosis with the help of laparoscopy along with staging and pictorial documentation.

Treatment options for Pelvic Endometriosis :

- **Expectant Management** (observation only)
- **Medical Therapy** : • Hormones • Others
- **Surgery** : • Conservative • Definitive
- **Combined Therapy** : • Medical and Surgical

Determinants of treatment options

- Age of the patient.
- Size and extent of lesions.
- Severity of symptoms.
- Location of disease.
- Desire for fertility.
- Results of previous therapy.

Expectant treatment

Endometriosis is a progressive disease in about 30-60 per cent of women. It is not possible to predict in which woman it will progress. Some form of treatment is often needed regardless of the clinical profile and to arrest the progress of the disease. However in women with minimal to mild endometriosis role of any treatment is controversial. Cumulative pregnancy rate is similar when expectant treatment is compared with conservative surgery. Case selection is important (see Table 21.5).

Table 21.5
Case selection for expectant treatment

- Minimal endometriosis with no other abnormal pelvic finding.
- Unmarried.
- Young married who are ready to start family.
- Approaching menopause.

Protocols for Expectant Management

Observation with administration of non-steroidal anti-inflammatory drugs or prostaglandin synthetase inhibiting drugs are used to relieve pain. Ibuprofen 800-1200 mg or mefenamic acid 150-600 mg a day is quite effective.

The married women are encouraged to have conception. Pregnancy usually cures the condition. This is due to absence of shedding and decidual changes in the ectopic endometrium causing its necrosis and absorption.

Hormonal treatment

The aim of the hormonal treatment is **to induce atrophy of the endometriotic implants**. It should be considered suppressive rather than curative because of high recurrence rate.

The mechanism of endometrial atrophy is either by producing *'pseudopregnancy'* (combined oral pills) or by *'pseudomenopause'* (Danazol) or by *'medical oophorectomy'* (GnRH agonists). The hormonal use is gratifying in superficial peritoneal implants and endometriomas of less than 1 cm.

The drugs used are combined oestrogen and progestogen (oral pill), progestogens, danazol and GnRH analogues. All the drugs are used continuously to produce amenorrhoea and as such individualisation of the dose is required.

Combined oestrogen and progestogen

The low dose contraceptive pills may be prescribed either in a cyclic or continuous fashion with advantages in young patients with mild disease who want to defer pregnancy. It causes endometrial decidualisation and atrophy (see p. 187). It may induce amenorrhoea. It relieves dysmenorrhoea. **Anastrozole** an aromatase inhibitor is found to reduce the growth and pain of endometriosis (p. 508).

Progestogens : It causes decidualisation of endometrium and atrophy (see p. 187). High doses may suppress ovulation and induce amenorrhoea.

Oral route is commonly used. Injectable preparations as depot form should be withheld in patients wishing to conceive. Ovulation may remain suspended for several months following withdrawal of the therapy. The side effects (see p. 510) are well-tolerated. The drug is comparatively cheaper than danazol. **Progesterone Antagonists** (Mifepristone 50-100 mg/day) has also been found effective.

Levonorgestrel-releasing-IUCD when used, is found to reduce dysmenorrhoea, pelvic pain, dyspareunia and menorrhagia significantly. It is specially useful for rectovaginal endometriosis.

Danazol (p. 504)

Danazol therapy is to be started from the day 5 of the menstrual cycle. The dose (600-800 mg daily) is variable and depends upon the extent of the lesions but should be adequate enough to produce amenorrhoea. **The patient should use barrier methods of contraception** to avoid virilisation of a female fetus in accidental pregnancy. *Resolution of endometriotic lesions has been seen in about 80% of cases but the recurrence rate is high (40%).* The side effects are at times intense and intolerable to the extent of discontinuation of the therapy. A few often persist even after the therapy. The drug is costlier than progestogen. **Gestrinone** (p. 505) has got the same mechanism of action like that of danazol. The side effects are less than danazol. Administration is simple, twice a week (see Table 21.6).

GnRH analogues (p. 500)—When used continuously act as medical oophorectomy, a state of hypo-oestrinism and amenorrhoea. The goal is to maintain a reduced level of serum oestrogen (30-45 pg/ml) so that growth of endometriosis is suppressed. The side effects are more tolerable than danazol. The drugs have got limited availability and costliest of all the drugs used. Long-term therapy (more than 6 months) should be avoided (see add-back therapy p. 502).

Results : The efficacy of the hormone therapy is judged by relief of symptoms, reduction of the

Table 21.6
Hormones used in endometriosis

Drugs	*Dose*	*Mechanism*	*Side effects*
Combined oestrogen progestogen (oral pill)	1-2 tab 6-9 months	Pseudopregnancy	Tolerated (see ch. 29)
Progestogens (p. 508) *Oral* • Medroxyprogesterone acetate • Dydrogesterone • Norethisterone *IM* • Medroxyprogesterone *IUCD* • Levonorgestrel-releasing-IUCD (p. 459)	 10 mg thrice daily × 6-9 months 10-20 mg daily × 6-9 months 10-30 mg daily × 6-9 months 150 mg 3 months interval × 2	Pseudopregnancy	Tolerated (see p. 510)
Danazol (p. 504)	400-800 mg orally in 4 divided doses × 6-9 months	Pseudomenopause	Less tolerated (see p. 505)
Gestrinone (p. 504)	1.25 or 2.5 mg twice a week × 6-9 months	Pseudomenopause	Well tolerated (see p. 505)
GnRH analogues (p. 500)	• Leuprolide 3.75 mg IM monthly × 6 months • Naferelin 200 µg intranasally daily × 6 months • Goserelin 3.6 mg depot IM monthly × 6 months	Medical oophorectomy	Well tolerated (see p. 501)

volume of the lesions as revealed by second look laparoscopy, improvement of fertility and prevention of recurrence. For quick relief of symptoms and reduction of the volume of the lesion, GnRH analogues are the best. Progestogens take some time to achieve these objectives. Danazol is placed midway between the two.

Taking every aspect together (pain relief, pregnancy rates, recurrence rates, costs and side effects), no single medical treatment is superior to others.

Following medical suppression or other conservative surgery, residual endometriotic lesions may regenerate once the ovarian function is reestablished. **Overall recurrence rate is about 40 per cent after 5 years.**

SURGICAL MANAGEMENT OF ENDOMETRIOSIS

Indications

- Endometriosis with severe symptoms unresponsive to hormone therapy.
- Severe and deeply infiltrating endometriosis to correct the distortion of pelvic anatomy.
- Endometriomas of more than 1 cm.

Surgery may be conservative or definitive.

CONSERVATIVE SURGERY

Conservative surgery is planned to destroy the endometriotic lesions in an attempt to improve the symptoms (pain, subfertility) and at the same time to preserve the reproductive function.

Laparoscopy is commonly done to destroy endometriotic lesions by excision or ablation by electrodiatherapy or by laser vaporisation. **Conservative surgical treatment in minimal to mild endometriosis (ablation plus adhesiolysis) improves the fertility outcome.** Laparoscopic uterosacral nerve ablation (LUNA) is done when pain is very severe. The advantage of laser is to cut the tissues precisely with least chance of damage to the underlying vital structures. Great deal of technical expertise is essential to avoid injury to the ureters.

Surgical treatment improves fertility and symptoms in women with moderate and severe endometriosis.

OVARIAN ENDOMETRIOMAS (see Fig. 21.4)

- **Small endometrioma (< 3 cm)** is aspirated laparoscopically. The cyst cavity is irrigated with normal saline. Cyst wall epithelium is destroyed by laser vaporisation.
- **Large endometrioma (≥ 4 cm)** is often associated with extensive adhesion to other pelvic structures. Laparoscopy is necessary for ovarian cystectomy and adhesiolysis.

Results : Laparoscopic cystectomy is effective in relieving pain in about 74% cases of mild to moderate disease. Pregnancy rate is observed in about 60% cases with moderate and 35% cases with severe disease. Restoration of normal pelvic anatomy improves fertility in cases with severe endometriosis. High pregnancy rate is observed within first 6 months of conservative surgery.

Infertility associated with endometriosis : When there is no improvement of infertility due to endometriosis with the usual treatment, couple should be counselled for ART (p. 243). Controlled ovarian hyperstimulation with IUI, IVF, GIFT and ICSI are the different methods (see p. 244).

Definitive surgery

Definitive surgery is indicated in women with **advanced stage endometriosis** where there is : (i) No prospect for fertility improvement. (ii) Other forms of treatment have failed. (iii) Women with completed family.

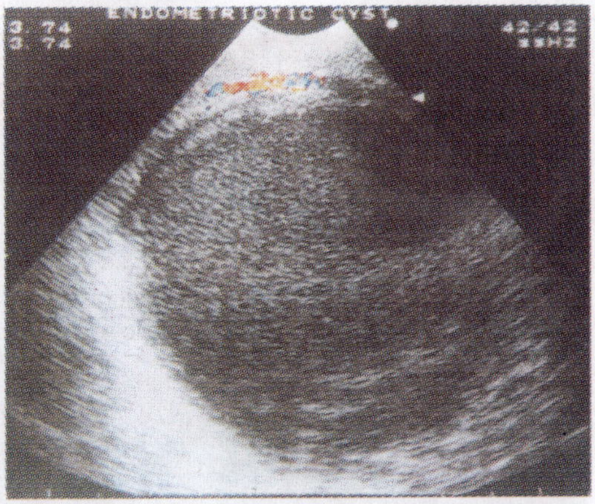

Fig. 21.4. Colour Doppler Scan (TV) of an ovarian endometrioma (chocolate cyst). Internal echoes are homogeneous. Increased vascularity is seen at the ovarian hilus

Definitive surgery means hysterectomy with bilateral salpingo-oophorectomy along with resection of the endometrial tissues as complete as possible.

Combined medical and surgical

Preoperative hormonal therapy aims at reduction of the size and vascularity of the lesion which facilitate surgery. The idea of **postoperative hormonal therapy** is to destroy the residual lesions left behind after surgery and to control the pain. But it does not improve fertility. It is generally avoided.

Duration of therapy is usually 3-6 months preoperatively and 3-6 months postoperatively. Improvement of fertility following one year of surgical treatment for pelvic endometriosis is approximately 39% for stage I, 31% for stage II, 30% for stage III and 25% for stage IV disease respectively. Overall risk of recurrence is 40% by 5 years time.

Emperical treatment of pelvic pain with the presumptive diagnosis of pelvic endometriosis may be given with combined oral contraceptives.

ENDOMETRIOSIS AT SPECIAL SITES

- **Abdominal scar**
- **Umbilicus**
- **Bladder and ureter**
- **Gut**
- **Cervix and vagina**
- **Lung**

Scar (Fig. 21.5) : It usually manifests following abdominal hysterotomy, caesarean section, myomectomy or even tubectomy. Implantation theory can explain its entity.

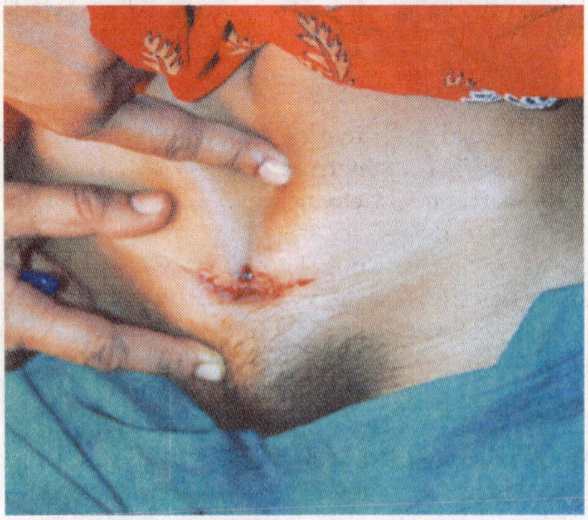

Fig. 21.5. Bleeding from a scar endometriosis. The patient was examined during her menstruation

The patient complains of painful nodular swelling over or adjacent to the scar which increases in size and often bleeds during periods. The size is variable, nodular feel, tender with restricted mobility. Associated pelvic endometriosis is usually absent. The same type of nodular swelling can be found over episiotomy scar. **Treatment** is by excision. Hormone therapy is ineffective.

Umbilicus : There is nodular painful swelling which increases in size and becomes tender during period. At times, bleeding may also occur. Coelomic metaplasia theory can explain its origin.

Treatment is by excision.

Bladder : The patient complains of dysuria, frequency, haematuria and lower abdominal pain specially during periods. Cystoscopic examination reveals blue area of the mucosa. IVP may reveal ureteric stricture and hydroureteric or even hydronephrotic changes on the affected side.

Treatment is not much effective with hormones. Local excision of the bladder wall and repair should be done. In ureteric involvements, the segment of the ureter is to be excised followed by implantation of the ureter to the bladder.

Gut : The rectum, sigmoid colon or even the small intestine are the common sites. Coelomic metaplasia theory can explain the endometriosis at these sites. **The mucosa is not involved, a differentiating feature from malignancy.**

The patient complains of periodic colicky pain on defecation or at times bleeding per rectum specially during periods. Associated pelvic endometriosis is a constant feature. There may be even features of subacute intestinal obstruction.

Rectal examination and investigations like sigmoidoscopy and barium enema confirm the diagnosis.

Lung, pleura, and **brain** are the rare sites. This may cause catamenial pneumothorax or seizures during mens.

Treatment : Hormone treatment may be effective. If it fails, surgery may have to be done. In young patients, resection anastomosis and in patients above 40, removal of the ovaries may help regression of the lesions.

Cervix and vagina : The lesions are usually due to implantation of the endometrium over the trauma inflicted at operation or following delivery. The only complaint may be dyspareunia. The lesion is revealed by speculum examination. Confusion may arise with carcinoma cervix. There is, bleeding on touch in carcinoma. Confirmation is done by biopsy. **Treatment** by hormone is ineffective. Surgical excision may be required.

ADENOMYOSIS

Definition

Adenomyosis is a condition where there is ingrowth of the endometrium, both the glandular and stromal components, directly into the myometrium.

Causes

The cause of such ingrowth is not known. It may be related to repeated childbirths, vigorous curettage or excess of oestrogen which produces cystic glandular hyperplasia of the endometrium. In some, only the basal endometrium, while in others the functional zone as well invades the myometrium. Pelvic endometriosis co-exists in about 40 per cent.

Pathology

The growth and tissue reaction in the endometrium depend on the response of the ectopic endometrial tissues to the ovarian steroids. If the basal layer is only present, the tissue reaction is much less, as it is unresponsive to hormones. But, if the functional zone is present which is responsive to hormones, the tissue reaction surrounding the endometrium is marked. There is hyperplasia of the myometrium producing diffuse enlargement of the uterus, sometimes symmetrically but at times, more on the posterior wall. The growth may be localised or may invade a polyp (adenomyomatous).

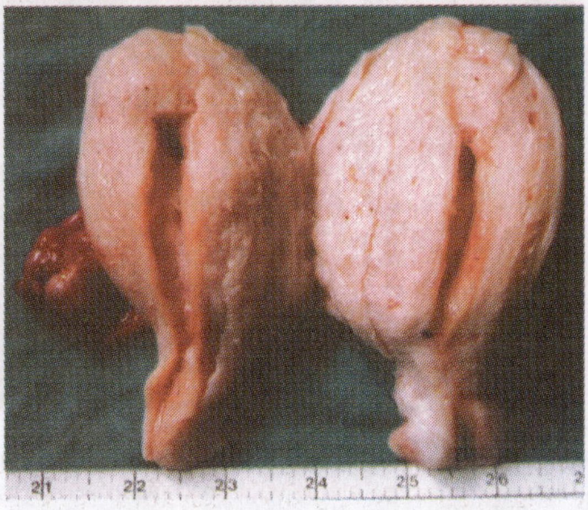

Fig. 21.6. Specimen of adenomyosis

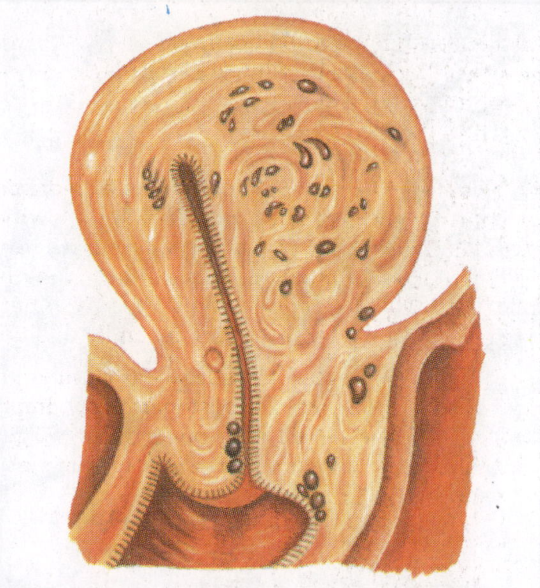

Fig. 21.7. Adenomyosis. Note the absence of capsule and presence of dark spots

Naked eye appearance

There is diffuse symmetrical enlargement of the uterus; the posterior wall is often more thickened than the anterior one. The size usually does not increase more than a large orange (12-14 weeks pregnant uterus). On cut section, there is thickening of the uterine wall. The cut surface presents characteristic trabeculated appearances. **Unlike fibroid, there is no capsule surrounding the growth**. There may be visible blood spots at places (Figs 21.6 and 21.7).

Histological examination

Histological examination reveals glandular tissue like that of endometrium surrounded by stromal cells in the myometrium. The ectopic endometrial tissue should be separated from the underlying basal endometrium. The response of the ectopic endometrial tissue to ovarian hormones is minimal as the invasion is predominantly in the basal layer (Fig. 21.8).

Clinical features

In about one-third, it remains asymptomatic being discovered on histological examination.

Patient profile : The patients are usually parous with age usually above 40.

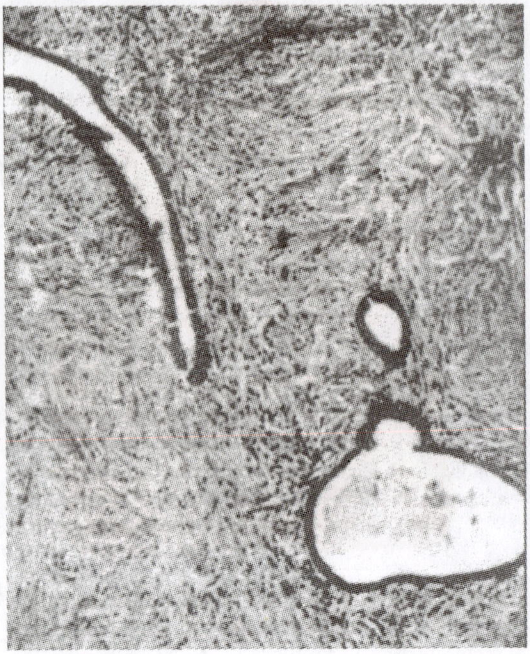

Fig. 21.8. Histologic picture of adenomyosis

Symptoms

Menorrhagia (70%) — The excessive bleeding is due to increased uterine cavity, associated endometrial hyperplasia and inadequate uterine contraction.

Dysmenorrhoea (30%) — Progressively increased colicky pain during period is probably due to disturbed myometrial contraction rather than bleeding from the ectopic endometrial tissues.

Dyspareunia or frequency of urination — may be present.

Signs : Abdominal examination may reveal a hypogastric mass arising out of the pelvis and occupying the midline. The size usually does not exceed 14 weeks pregnant uterus.

Pelvic examination — reveals uniform enlargement of the uterus.

The findings, however, may be altered due to associated fibroid or pelvic endometriosis.

Ultrasound and Colour Doppler (TVS) characteristics are : (i) Heterogenous echogenecity. (ii) Hypoechoic myometrium with multiple small cysts in the myometrium (bleeding). (iii) Increased vascularity within the myometrium (see Fig. 21.9).

Magnetic Resonance Imaging : It is more specific to the diagnosis. A thickened junctional zone is present on MRI.

Treatment

The treatment is surgical. There is little place of hormone therapy. Treatment with progestins or cyclic oestrogen and progestin have got little benefit. **Levonorgestrel–releasing-IUS** (p. 459) is found to improve the menorrhagia and dysmenorrhoea.

Conservative surgery includes partial resection of the adenomyomata.

As the patients are usually parous and aged, total hysterectomy with or without salpingo-oophorectomy is the treatment of choice.

STROMAL ENDOMETRIOSIS

This is a rare condition where the endometrial stromal cells, without glandular components, are present in places other than uterine mucosa.

Pathogenesis

The stromal cells extend into the myometrium along the course of the lymphatics and muscle bundles. There may be extension of stromal cells along the lymphatics and veins to the broad ligaments. As there is a chance of recurrence, it is considered as locally malignant. The uterus is uniformly enlarged

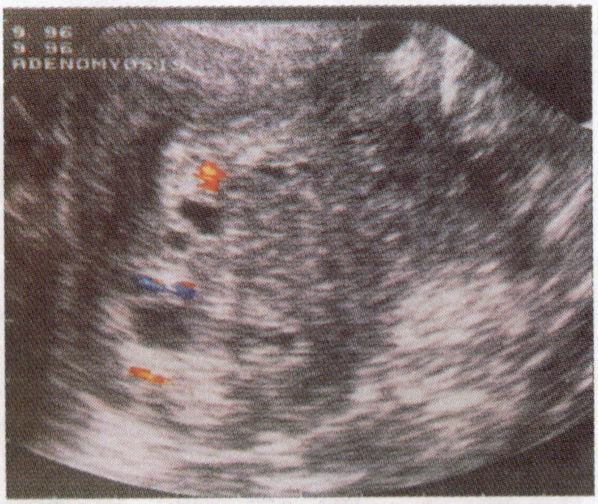

Fig. 21.9. Transvaginal Colour Doppler Scan showing diffusely enlarged uterus with anechoic cysts. 'Swiss cheese' pattern with increased vascularity is suggestive of adenomyosis

as in adenomyosis. Microscopic examination reveals round and oval cells of endometrial stroma.

Clinical features

- Menorrhagia, irregular bleeding and often postmenopausal bleeding may occur.
- Variable degrees of pelvic pain
- Suprapubic swelling.

Pelvic examination — reveals the enlarged uterus.

Treatment

Hysterectomy with bilateral salpingo-oophorectomy is the effective surgery. In younger patients, the ovaries may be preserved.

Radiotherapy may be needed in proved cases following its recurrence or incomplete surgery.

KEY POINTS

➤ The presence of functioning endometrium (stroma and glands) in sites other than uterine mucosa is called endometriosis. Endometriosis is a disease seen in the reproductive years of a woman as its growth depends on oestrogen.

The incidence is about 10 per cent but incidence is high (30-40%) amongst infertile women as based on diagnostic laparoscopy and laparotomy. The commonest abdominal site is ovary followed by pouch of Douglas and uterosacral ligaments (organs on the dependent part of the pelvis).

Abdominal scar is the commonest site of endometriosis following hysterotomy, caesarean section, tubectomy or myomectomy (Fig. 21.5).

➤ The disease is full of theories and no one single theory can explain endometriosis at all sites. Genetic basis and defect of local cellular immunity may be implicated (Table 21.2). In spite of dense adhesions amongst the pelvic structures, the fallopian tubes are usually patent. In pelvic endometriosis, typically there are small black dots — 'powder burns' or "gunshot" seen on uterosacral ligaments and pouch of Douglas. Other lesions are flame-shaped polypoidal, haemorrhagic and white patches.

About 25 per cent have got no symptom. Symptoms are not related to the extent of lesion. Severity of endometriosis and the degree of pelvic pain are not always proportional. Unlike primary dysmenorrhoea, the pain lasts for many days before and after the menstruation.

Dysmenorrhoea is associated in 50 per cent, menorrhagia in 60 per cent and infertility in 40-60 per cent. Endometriosis is found in 30-40 per cent of infertile women.

Clinical diagnosis is by the classic symptoms of progressively increasing dysmenorrhoea, dyspareunia, infertility and feel of nodules in the pouch of Douglas. Confirmation is by laparoscopy or laparotomy.

➤ Histologic diagnosis of endometriosis is ideal. Microscopic diagnostic features are : presence of endometrial glands, stroma and haemosiderin-laden macrophages.

Double puncture laparoscopy is considered the 'gold standard' for the diagnosis.

The cardinal features of endometriosis — pain, infertility and adhesion are due to activation of peritoneal macrophages by several factors like cytokines, interleukin-1, prostanoids and others (see p. 295).

The natural course of the disease is ill understood. It is progressive in about 30-60 per cent patients and for the remainder it is either static or resolve spontaneously. Unfortunately it is impossible to predict in which patient it will progress.

Serum marker CA 125 is helpful in follow up cases of proved endometriosis.

The pelvic endometriosis should be appropriately staged based on laparoscopic findings and depicted in a pictorial chart.

Endometriosis is often associated with tubal and ovarian damage (see Table 21.4). There is also pelvic adhesions so that there is no tubal motility and no ovum pick-up. However, endometriosis does not cause recurrent pregnancy loss. These combined factors along with endocrinopathy (Table 21.3) may be responsible for infertility. However, the association of minimal to mild endometriosis and infertility is controversial.

KEY POINTS

The complications include endocrinopathy (LPD, anovulation, LUF or elevated prolactin level) rupture chocolate cyst, infection of the cyst or obstructive features (intestinal or ureteric).

Other complications of endometriosis are : Acute abdomen due to rupture of chocolate cyst, infection of the cyst, colorectal obstruction and ureteral obstruction.

The short-term goals of treatment for endometriosis are : (i) relief of pain and (ii) improvement of fertility. The long-term goal is to prevent progression or recurrence of the disease.

The effect of danazol is by its 'pseudomenopause' response. The side effects are due to its androgenic and anabolic properties (see p. 504).

GnRH agonists produce 'Medical oophorectomy' and the side effects are due to the oestrogen deprivation (see p.500). 'Add back' therapy is suggested with chronic use of GnRH agonists.

Expectant treatment is extended to unmarried or young married with no abnormal pelvic findings. Endometriosis causes pelvic inflammation. So the drugs used are non-steroidal, anti-inflammatory drugs ($NSAID_S$) or prostaglandin synthetase inhibitors.

- The hormonal treatment should be considered suppressive rather than curative. The mechanism of atrophy can be explained by pseudopregnancy or by pseudomenopause or by medical hypophysectomy (see p. 300). The commonly used hormones are given in the Table 21.6.

The objective of medical therapy is to create amenorrhoea (hypo-oestrogenic state). Aromatase inhibitors (letrozol 2.5 mg daily) are used to inhibit aromatase which converts androgens to oestrogens. Oestrogen promotes its growth (p. 299, 508).

The overall fertility rate and the recurrence rate is about 40 per cent.

Conservative surgery in endometriosis includes removal of all macroscopic endometriosis, lysis of adhesions and restoration of normal pelvic anatomy. The surgery is preferably done by laparoscopy (diathermy, laser vaporisation). Endoscopic laser surgery is the best in selected cases for the treatment of pain and to prevent the disease progress.

- Ovarian endometriosis (< 3 cm) is treated by laparoscopic cyst aspiration. The cyst wall is vaporised to destroy the mucosal lining. Large ovarian endometrioma (> 3 cm) is treated by laparoscopic ovarian cystectomy. Laparoscopic adhesiolysis should be done at the same time. Laparoscopic ovarian cystectomy improves fertility.

Preoperative normal treatment with GnRh analogue may reduce the vascularity and the extent of the disease.

- Postoperative medical treatment should not prevent pregnancy as the chance of pregnancy is highest during the first 6-12 months after the conservative surgery.

Definitive surgery includes total hysterectomy with bilateral salpingo-oophorectomy. Laparotomy is done for advanced stage disease or in women who has completed her family.

- Postoperative oestrogen replacement therapy after total hysterectomy and bilateral oophorectomy may be given 3 months after surgery. The risk of recurrence is very low.

- Adenomyosis primarily occurs in parous women over the age of 35.

Adenomyosis is associated with pelvic endometriosis in 40 per cent. Menorrhagia (70%) and dysmenorrhoea are the chief complaints. Uterus is diffusely enlarged (2-3 times). Uterine size > 14 weeks gestation is rare.

Hormone treatment is often ineffective. Levonorgestrel-releasing IUS (p. 459) is found to improve menorrhagia and dysmenorrhoea. Hysterectomy is the effective treatment.

Premalignant Lesions 22

PREMALIGNANT VULVAL LESIONS

Premalignant vulval lesions include :

- Vulval intraepithelial neoplasia (VIN).
- Paget's disease.
- Lichen sclerosus.
- Squamous cell hyperplasia.
- Condyloma accuminata (see p. 152).

VULVAL INTRAEPITHELIAL NEOPLASIA (VIN)

The different degrees of VIN are :

VIN–I : Corresponds to mild cellular atypia. The lesion is limited to the deeper one-third of the epithelium.

VIN–II : Corresponds to moderate cellular atypia. The lesion is limited upto middle-third of the epithelium.

VIN–III : Corresponds to severe cellular atypia and carcinoma-*in-situ*. The abnormal cells involve whole thickness of the epithelium. There is no stromal invasion.

The following facts are to be borne in mind :

- It is more frequent in patients in the age group 20-40, i.e., at a younger age group compared to vulval carcinoma. **The average age is as low as 33 years.**
- There is some racial predisposition.
- It is often related with STD such as condyloma accuminata, herpes simplex virus II, gonorrhoea, syphilis or Gardnerella vaginalis.
- Viral aetiology is not confirmed. HPV 6 and 11 are associated with vulval condylomas. HPV 16, 18, 31, 35 are associated with VIN lesions.
- There is increased prevalence of associated CIN (10-80%).
- Regression frequently occurs in young woman, during pregnancy or when it is caused by viral infection.
- Rarely progresses to invasive carcinoma.

DIAGNOSIS

The chief complaints may be pruritus vulvae, lump or bleeding from a vulval ulcer. It may be even symptomless.

Local examination reveals a lesion in the vulva with white, grey, pink or dull red colour. Lesions look rough, raised from the surface and often multifocal. Application of 5 per cent acetic acid turns VIN lesions white with punctuation and mosaic patterns. These changes are best seen with a colposcope.

Confirmation of diagnosis is done by biopsy. Usually 3-5 mm diameter dermal punch is taken under local anaesthetic. The small amount of bleeding is controlled using Monsel's solution (ferrous sulphate). Larger biopsy when required may be taken using a scalpel. Multiple site biopsies are useful.

A complete pelvic examination is to be done. **To exclude vaginal or cervical neoplasia, cytologic evaluation has to be performed.**

Histology

The cells exhibit features of malignancy. There is complete loss of polarity and stratification. Cellular immaturity, nuclear abnormalities and mitotic activity vary depending upon the grade of VIN.

There is hyperkeratosis, acanthosis (hyperplasia of epidermis) and chronic inflammatory cell infiltration. Koilocytes (see p. 108) may be present. The rete ridges are large and elongated. Basement membrane remains intact. There is no evidence of involvement of the dermis.

Treatment of VIN

The fact remains that VIN has got low malignant potential. The risk of progression to invasive disease is less than 10 per cent. Hence conservative management is generally accepted.

Medical

Medical treatment is done for young woman to control the symptoms. Topical fluorinated steroid ointment can be applied twice daily for a period of about 6 months. Commonly used preparations are 0.1 per cent triamcinolone acetonide, or 0.1 per cent betamethasone valerate. Local application of chemotherapy in the form of 5 per cent 5-fluorouracil (5-FU) cream may be used in recurrent lesions. The result is however unsatisfactory.

Whatever therapy is employed, it is mandatory for regular follow up. Biopsies to be taken freely whenever an abnormal area is detected.

Surgery

The following types of surgery may be employed :

- Local excision — **Wide local excision** with 1 cm margin is reserved in young patient with localised lesion.
- Laser therapy — CO_2 laser vaporisation is gaining increasing popularity in the treatment of vulval epithelial atypia. It gives better cosmetic results with lower recurrence rate.

In multifocal lesion, **skinning vulvectomy** using laser can destroy tissues to a depth of 3-4 mm. The wide raw surface is covered with skin graft to improve the cosmetic results.

- Simple vulvectomy — It is employed in diffuse type specially in postmenopausal women (see p. 577).

PAGET'S DISEASE

This is a special type of VIN. The lesion grows horizontally within the epidermis. The rete ridges tend to push into the dermis without actually penetrating it.

The characteristic histologic picture is presence of Paget cells in the epidermis. The cells are large — round or oval in shape with abundant pale cytoplasm. There may be presence of mucopolysaccharides in most of the cells. Nuclear mitotic figures are rare.

Associated adenocarcinoma of apocrine gland is present in about 10 per cent of the cases. **There is high incidence (30%) of associated carcinomas of other organs (breast, cervix, ovary, GI tract and bladder).**

Symptoms are mainly pruritus, vulvar soreness, pain or bleeding.

Local examination reveals—labia majora appear red, scaling, with elevated lesion. There may be associated white lesions. The skin is usually indurated.

Treatment

Simple vulvectomy is done. Multiple biopsies are to be taken to exclude associated adenocarcinoma of the apocrine glands. If it is found positive, bilateral lymph node dissection should be done at a second stage.

VAGINAL INTRAEPITHELIAL NEOPLASIA (VAIN)

Pathology

VAIN–I : There is minimal loss of stratification and polarity of the cells.

VAIN–II : Epithelial abnormality extends onto the middle-third of the epithelium.

VAIN–III : Carcinoma-*in-situ*—There is loss of polarity and stratification through all layers. Basement membrane remains intact.

Diagnosis

- **Vaginal scrape cytology**
- **Colposcopy**
- **Biopsy**

Management

(a) Local excision for biopsy is diagnostic and therapeutic also. This is suitable for a small lesion.

(b) 5 Fluorouracil (5-FU) cream is to be applied at night for a period of 5-10 days and to be repeated every 2 weeks for 2-3 courses.

(c) Ablation therapy is by :

- **Electrocautery**
- **Laser (see p. 115)**

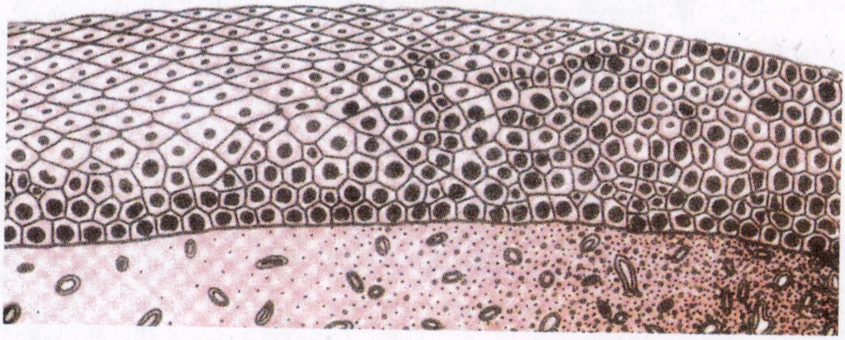

Fig. 22.1. Normal stratified squamous epithelium of the ectocervix on the left is progressed to CIN on the right through various degress of dysplastic changes

CERVICAL INTRAEPITHELIAL NEOPLASIA (CIN)

Nomenclature

Rubin (1910) introduced the term **'carcinoma-*in-situ*'** as a forerunner of invasive carcinoma.

Walters and **Regan** (1956) put forward the concept of **dysplasia** (mild, moderate and severe) — a stage of preinvasive process prior to carcinoma-*in-situ*.

Richart in 1967 brought-forth the concept of **cervical intraepithelial neoplasia (CIN)**. CIN is a histopathological condition where part or whole thickness of cervical squamous epithelium is replaced by cells showing varying degrees of atypia.

World Health Organisation (WHO) in 1975 classified the CIN into three categories correlating with former gradings of dysplasia and CIS. The grading is done according to the thickness occupied by the undifferentiated cells.

Bethesda system (1988) classified cytologic abnormalities of premalignant lesions into three categories : (a) atypical squamous cells (ASC), (b) low grade squamous intraepithelial lesions (LSIL) and (c) high grade squamous intraepithelial lesion (HSIL) (see p. 109, ch. 9). LSILs include CIN I and the changes of HPV (Koilocytic atypia).

The cytologic and histologic correlation of mild, moderate and severe dysplasia, carcinoma-*in-situ*, CIN and the Bethesda's system have been mentioned in Table 22.1. However, there is considerable degree of overlapping regarding the precise definition of each category of intraepithelial neoplasia. There is no sharp morphologic boundary between them. This creates disagreements in the diagnosis of severity of the lesion.

Table 22.1
Correlation of dysplasia, CIN (WHO) and Bethesda System

Dysplasia	*CIN*	*Limit of histologic changes*	*Bethesda*
Mild	CIN I	Basal one-third	LSIL
Moderate	CIN II	Basal half to two-third	HSIL
• Severe	CIN III	• Whole thickness except one or two superficial layers	HSIL
• CIS	CIN III	• Whole thickness	HSIL

Thus, the newer terminology CIN, is intended to emphasise that the **disease is a continuum and reflects the prognostic significance, if left untreated** (Fig. 22.1).

Squamocolumnar junction (SCJ) is the meeting point of columnar epithelium, that lines the endocervical canal, with squamous epithelium that lines the ectocervix (Fig. 22.3). This SCJ is a dynamic point. It moves up and down in relation to different phases of life, e.g. puberty, pregnancy and menopause.

In presence of oestrogen the vaginal epithelium accumulates glycogen. The lactobacilli act on glycogen to produce the acid pH (lactic acid) of vagina.

Scheme 1
Pathogenesis of CIN and invasive carcinoma

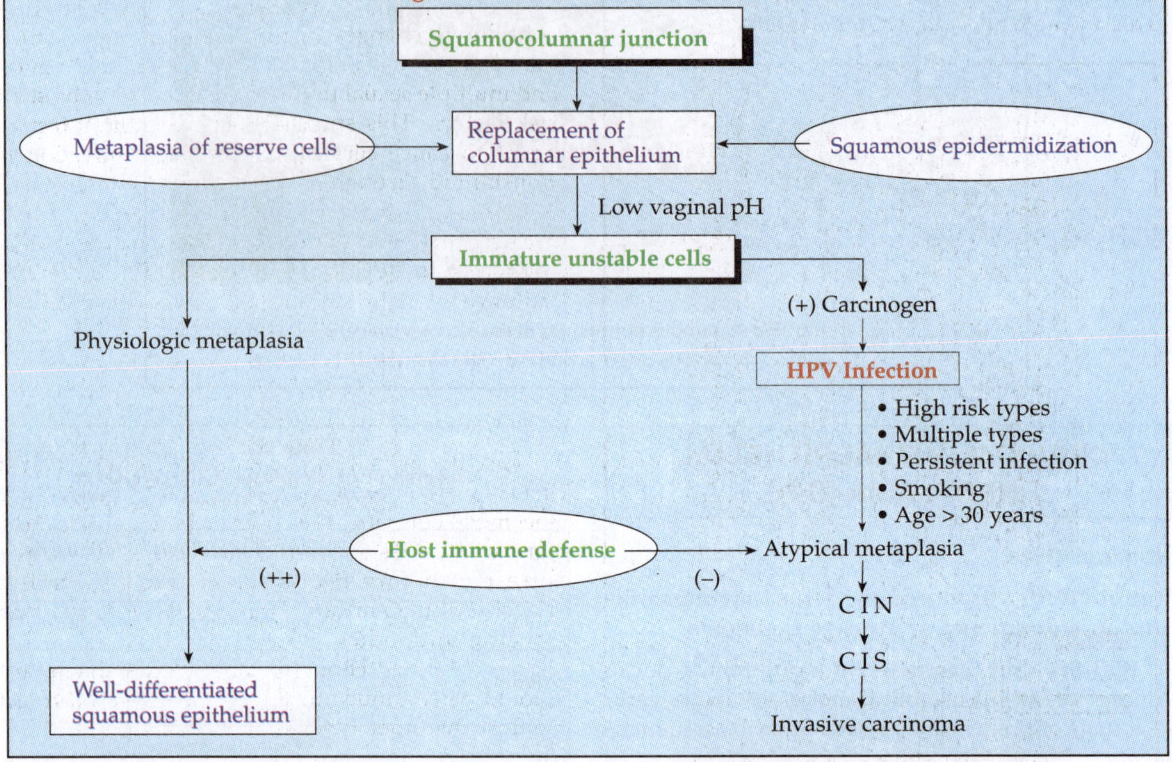

The **metaplasia** extends from the original SCJ (now squamosquamous) outside to the newly developed (physiologically active) SCJ (now squamocolumnar) inside (Fig. 21.3). This area is defined as **transformation zone (TZ)**.

Pathogenesis

The process of carcinogenesis starts at the **'transformation zone' (TZ)**. The zone is not static but in a dynamic state. Two mechanisms are involved in the process of replacement of endocervical columnar epithelium by squamous epithelium.

- By squamous metaplasia of the subcolumnar reserve cells (Fig. 22.2).
- Squamous epidermidisation by ingrowth of the squamous epithelium of the ectocervix under the columnar epithelium.

Initially, the squamous cells are immature but ultimately become mature and indistinguishable to the adjacent squamous epithelium.

This metaplastic process is very active at the time of menarche and during and after first pre-

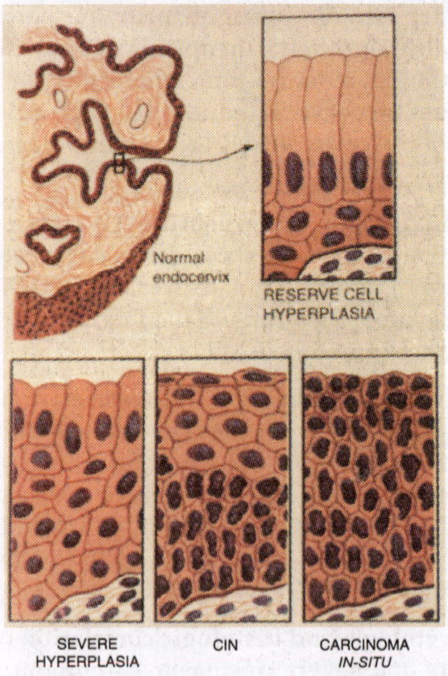

Fig. 22.2. Continuum of changes from reserve cell hyperplasia to carcinoma-*in-situ* through severe hyperplasia, CIN and CIS

gnancy. These periods are of high oestrogenic phase which lowers the vaginal pH. The acid pH probably is an important trigger for the metaplastic process. This metaplastic cells have got the potentiality to undergo atypical transformation by trauma or infection.

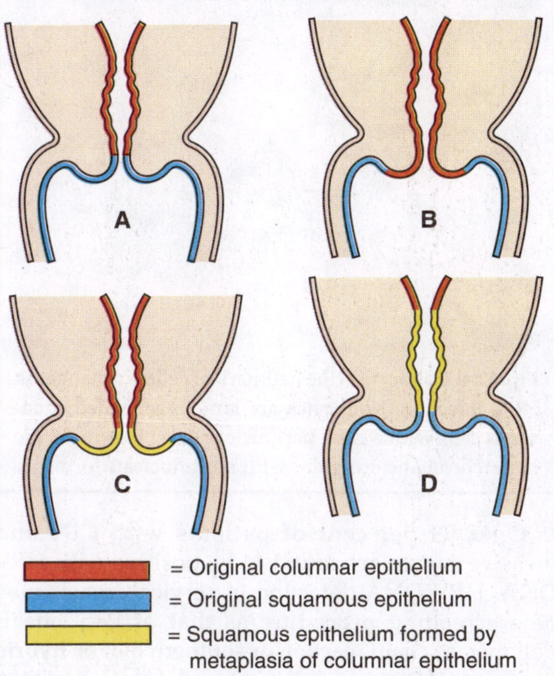

Fig. 22.3. (A) Before puberty, the ectocervix is covered with squamous epithelium. (B) Hightened oestrogenic activity exposes the columnar epithelium onto the ectocervix. (C) Replacement of columnar epithelium by squamous epithelium to form TZ. New squamo-columnar junction is situated at or slightly outside the external os during reproductive period. (D) Indrawing of the squamo-columnar junction and the TZ well into the cervical canal following menopause

The prolonged effect of carcinogens can produce continuous changes in the immature cells which may lead to malignancy. Early age sexual activity and multiple sexual partners are the most consistent risk factors. This suggested HPV as the infective agent to cause cervical cancer. HPV infection is transmitted through sexual activity. **Women may be immuno compromised due to genetic, iatrogenic or infective (HIV) factors.** These women are at high risk to develop persistent HPV infection. **Ultimately the important factors in the genesis of cervical cancer are : (i) Infection with high risk HPV (ii) Multiple types of HPV (iii) Persistence of infection (iv) Age > 30 years (v) Smoking and (vi) Compromised host immuno defense.**

Vaccines against HPV is found effective against the acquisition of **HPV types 16, 18**. These two are the most common HPV types related to cancer cervix. Vaccines should be given before the exposure e.g. before the onset of sexual activity. Vaccination resulted high titres of HPV type specific antibodies. **Vaccines are effective for atleast 3.5 years**. However, screening with Pap test should be continued as the vaccine do not protect against the other types of HPV.

Life cycle of unstable epithelium (Scheme—2)

The cases of CIN I or II may revert back to normal and these are most often related to infection or removed during biopsy. Some however, either remain static or progress to CIN III.

CIN III however, is more susceptible to progress into invasive carcinoma. This is more so in cases of carcinoma-*in-situ*.

Scheme - 2 : Life cycle of unstable cervical epithelium

Cervical epithelium	CIN I	CIN II	CIN III/CIS
Regression to normal (%)	60	40	30
Persistence (%)	30	35	50
Progression to CIN III/CIS (%)	10	20	—
Progression to invasion (%)	< 1	5	20

Duration of disease progression (years)	Normal	CIN I, II	CIN III/CIS	Invasion
	0	5	10	20
Age of the patient (year)		25-30	30-35	40-45

Thus, it is apparent that some of these epithelial atypia either remain stationary, regress or even progress to invasive carcinoma.

The real problem, at least to a clinician, to ascertain which one and how long the mild or moderate dysplasia takes to proceed to invasive carcinoma without passing through CIS. As such, even a CIN I or II should not be ignored, but to be followed up carefully.

Epidemiology

Prevalence : CIN is predominantly a disease of younger women. The mean age for carcinoma-*in-situ* is about 30 years, about 15 years less than that of invasive carcinoma. CIN like invasive carcinoma is most often related to some risk factors.

Table 22.2 : Risk factors for CIN and cervical cancer

- Early sexual intercourse (≤ 16 years).
- Early age of first pregnancy.
- Too many births/too frequent.
- Low socioeconomic status.
- Multiple sexual partners.
- Sexually transmitted diseases.
- Infection : HPV (16, 18, 31, 33), HIV, chlamydia.
- Immunosuppressed (HIV positive) individuals.
- Husband whose previous wife died of cervical malignancy.
- Oral pill users.
- Smoking habits.

Infectious agents: The causative agents appear to be transmitted to the susceptible women during intercourse. Two viruses are implicated as casual agents.

HUMAN PAPILLOMA VIRUS (HPV)

HPV is epitheliotropic and plays an important role in the development of CIN. HPV infected cells **(koilocytes)** are characterised by enlarged cells with perinuclear halos. The nucleus is large, irregular and hyperchromatic (Fig. 22.4). Depending on their oncogenic potential, HPV types are broadly grouped into two. More than 130 HPV types have been identified.

- High oncogenic risk—Types 16, 18, 31, 33, 35, 45, 56.
- Low oncogenic risk—Types 6, 11, 42, 43.

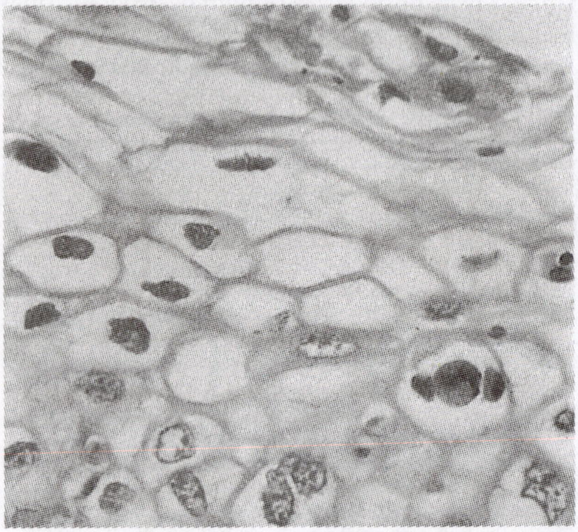

Fig. 22.4. Koilocyte is the hallmark of cellular changes in HPV infection. Koilocytes are large, vacuolated squamous cells with a clear perinuclear halo. The nuclei are hyperchromatic, irregular with multinucleate forms

Over 99 per cent of patients with CIN and invasive cancer are found to be positive with HPV DNA. HPV DNA detection in cervical tissues may be a screening procedure as that of Pap smear. Polymerase chain reaction or southern blot or **hybrid capture (HC)** technique is used for HPV DNA detection.

Pathogenesis of HPV Infection: HPV is epitheliotropic. Cervical epithelium → Infection (Latent/Active with virus replication) → Oncogenic HPV DNA integration to human genome → up-regulation of viral oncogenes → expression of E_6 and E_7 oncoproteins → Interference of tumour suppressor genes (p53 and Rb) → host cell immortalisation and HPV induced neoplastic transformation. HPV DNA is found in 99% of all squamous cell carcinomas.

HPV Triage Strategy includes : (i) Pap Smear test (LBC p. 109) → An atypical smear (after exclusion of infection) (ii) HPV testing → high risk HPV positive (iii) Colposcopy. This triage strategy can detect CIN II and III lesions effectively and reduces the load of colposcopy clinic.

Herpes simplex virus type II (HSV-2) infection is not proved convincingly as an aetiological factor for CIN.

DIAGNOSIS OF CIN

Cytologic screening

Exfoliative cytology (Papanicolaou and Traut–1943)

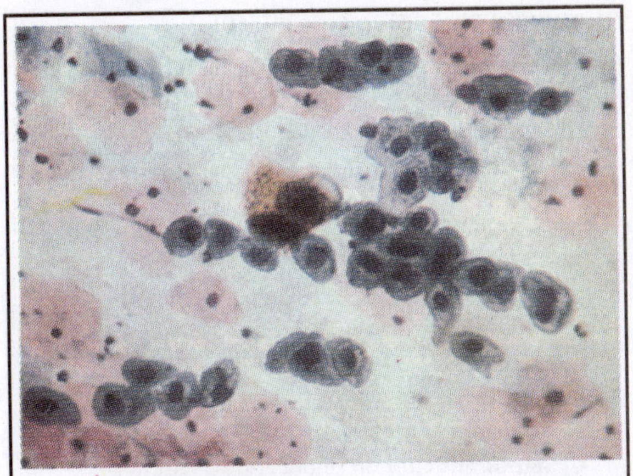

Fig. 22.5. Smear showing dyskaryotic cells

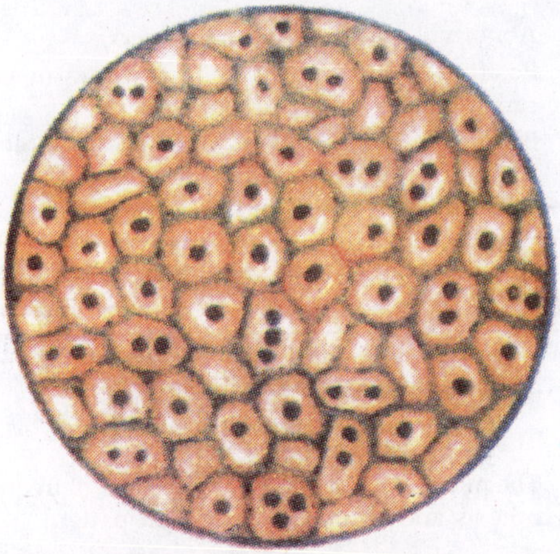

Fig. 22.6. Typical mosaic pattern in carcinoma-*in-situ*

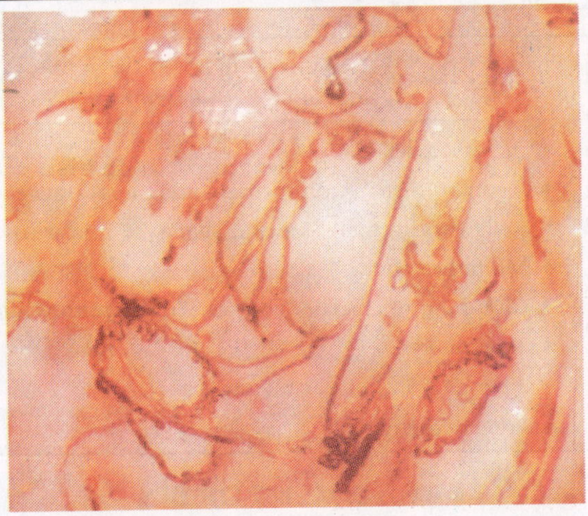

Fig. 22.7. Atypical blood vessels in invasive carcinoma

has become the gold standard for screening. The smear should contain cells from SCJ, TZ and the endocervix. Ayre's spatula and an endocervical brush is used for the purpose. Cells are spread on a single slide and fixed immediately (see p. 107).

(i) Dyskaryotic cells (p. 108) are atypical cells with hyperchromatic large nuclei having abundant cytoplasm (Fig. 22.5).

(ii) Carcinoma-*in-situ* cells contain hyperchromatic nuclei, coarse chromatin and lesser cytoplasm. There may be multiple nuclei and abnormal mitotic figures (Table 22.4).

Mild dyskaryotic smear is correlated with CIN II/III lesion in about 50 per cent of cases. Severe dyskaryosis is correlated with about 90 per cent of CIN II/III (Table 22.5).

HPV testing using hybrid capture method can reliably detect the high risk HPV types within hours. However, only about 2-5 per cent of women diagnosed with HPV DNA will ever develop CIN.

Visual inspection with acetic acid (VIA)

A speculum is introduced and acetic acid is applied to the cervix. Those women with aceto white lesions are considered for colposcopic examination and/or biopsy.

Colposcopy

Colposcopy is *in situ* examination of the cervix with a low magnification (6-16 times) microscope (Fig. 22.7). It is complementary and not a substitute for cytology. Cytology is the laboratory method while colposcopy is the clinical method of detection. Cytology evaluates the morphological changes of the exfoliated cells. Colposcopy evaluates mainly the changes in the terminal vascular network of the cervix which reflect the biochemical and metabolic changes of the tissue. In fact, cytology identifies the patient having cervical neoplasm, colposcopy identifies the site where from biopsies are to be taken.

Satisfactory colposcopic examination includes visualisation of the original SCJ, columnar epithelium, and the transformation zone in entirety. For procedure of colposcopy see p. 112.

Indications

- Those having abnormal cytology.
- Those with grossly abnormal cervical lesions even if cytology is negative.
- Those with postcoital bleeding even if the smear is negative.

Abnormal colposcopic findings are :

- **White epithelium** — leukoplakia.
- **Aceto white epithelium** — epithelium turning white following application of 3-5 per cent acetic acid.
- **Punctuation** — dilated capillaries which appear on the surface as dots.
- **Mosaic** — capillaries encircling polygonal shaped blocks of epithelial cells (Fig. 22.6)
- **Atypical blood vessels** with irregular diameter and branching are suggestive of invasive carcinoma (see Fig. 22.7)
- **Irregular surface contour** with ulceration and friability.

Cervicography

Photographs are taken from the cervix with a specially designed camera called cervicoscope. Film is developed, projected and is viewed by an expert colposcopist. Similar to colposcopy, cervix is treated with 5 per cent acetic acid before photography. It is complementary to cytology and colposcopy. It is also helpful where cytology service is not available.

Biopsy

Colposcopy available

- If colposcopy detects a suspicious area, biopsy is to be taken under its guidance.
- Endocervical curettage is mandatory whether or not the entire transformation zone can be seen.

Colposcopy not available

- Employing iodine solution (Schiller's 0.3% or Lugol's 5%), multiple punch biopsies are taken from the unstained areas.
- Alternatively, ring biopsy is taken from the squamocolumnar junction and subjected to serial sections.

Along with the above procedures, endocervical curettage has to be done to make the diagnosis more accurate.

Triage screening : (i) Liquid based thin layer cytology (p.109) evaluation → Atypical squamous cells.
(ii) Hybrid capture 2 for HPV DNA (see p. 313).
(iii) HPV DNA Test → Positive (High risk viruses) → Colposcopy → Biopsy; Negative → Repeat smear after one year

Diagnostic conisation (see p. 560)

In fact, the need for diagnostic cone biopsy has been reduced at least 80 per cent by the use of colposcopically directed biopsies (Table 22.3).

Table 22.3
Indications of diagnostic conisation

Colposcopy available

- Entire limits of the lesion not seen.
- Transformation zone not seen.
- Evidences of microinvasion on biopsy, colposcopy or cytology.
- Significant CIN on endocervical curettage.
- Normal colposcopic findings with abnormal cytology/biopsy.

Colposcopy not available

- Abnormal smear with healthy cervix.
- Positive diagnosis of CIS to exclude invasive carcinoma.
- Biopsy report is inconsistent with cytologic findings.

Table 22.4
The classic histologic picture of CIS (Fig. 22.8)

- The entire epithelial layer is affected.
- There is loss of stratification and polarity.
- The cells vary in size and shape.
- The nuclei stain deeply with presence of frequent mitosis and abnormal chromatin pattern.
- The nuclei are larger and hyperchromatic with scanty cytoplasm.
- The basement membrane remains intact.

Table 22.5
Common features of a dyskaryotic cell

- Increased cell size.
- Pleomorphism — different staining appearance.
- Cells vary in their size and shape.
- Multinucleation.
- Clumping of chromatin — varying degree.
- Aneuploidy.
- Alteration in nuclear membrane.
- Perinuclear halo.

TREATMENT OF CIN

- **Preventive**
- **Definitive**

Preventive

- To delay sexual exposure until the cervical epithelium, specially in the transformation zone, has attained physiological maturity.
- To maintain adequate local hygiene and to treat adequately any vaginal infection.
- To use condom specially during early sexual life.
- To maintain penile hygiene as it may be the reservoir for high risk HPV.
- Reducing or quitting smoking reduces CIN.
- **HPV vaccine (Gardasil)** is approved to all school girls (9-15 years) and women (16-26 years). It is a quadrivalent (HPV types 16, 18, 6 and 11) vaccine. This gives protection against HPV type 16 and 18 which are responsible for 70 per cent of all cervical cancer and type 6 and 11 which cause nearly 90 per cent of all genital warts. 3 doses (0, 2, 6 months) are given. Immunity persists for 3.5 years.

Definitive treatment

The treatment modalities depend on :

- Age of the patient. • Desire for reproduction.
- Risk factors present. • Degree of dysplasia.
- Facilities available for follow up such as colposcopy and/or cytology.

Treatment options are :

(a) *Observation with repeat smear and colposcopy every 4-6 months.*

(b) *Local ablative methods*
- Cryotherapy
- Cold coagulation
- Electrodiathermy
- Laser vaporisation

(c) *Excisional methods*
- Large loop (electrosurgical) excision of transformation zone (LLETZ).
- Cone excision—using a knife or laser.

(d) *Hysterectomy*—abdominal or vaginal.

CIN I

Women with CIN I, confirmed on biopsy, may be kept under observation with Pap smear follow up at 6 months or HPV DNA test at 12 months. If both the tests are negative annual screening is done. Women with persistent CIN I after 24 months should be treated with a local ablative method.

CIN II

The fact that over a prolonged follow up, about 10-15 per cent of CIN I and II progress to CIS. Then again, it is quite impossible to predict which one will remain stationary and which one will progress to severe dysplasia or CIS. **As such, CIN II is commonly treated with LLETZ.**

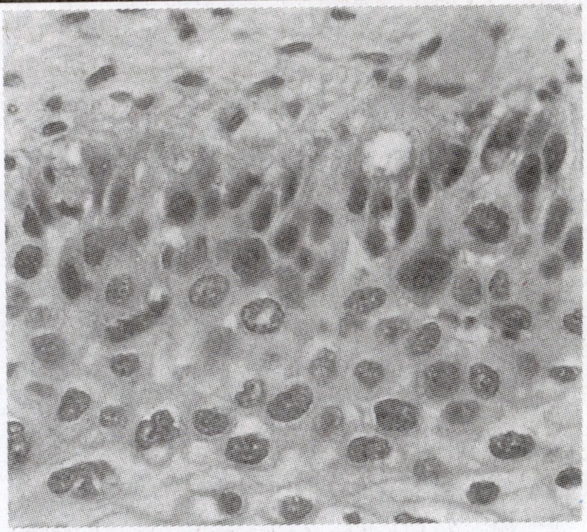

Fig. 22.8. Histology of carcinoma-*in-situ* of cervix. Marked nuclear abnormalities are seen throughout most of the thickness. Abnormal mitotic figures are present

CIN III and CIS

Patient desirous for reproduction

The basic concept is that CIN is a superficial lesion. As such, complete destruction of the lesion is considered to be a satisfactory treatment.

Pretreatment accurate evaluation about the extent of lesion and exclusion of invasive carcinoma with the available gadgets (cytology, colposcopy and directed biopsy) is a sine-qua-non to get a good result. Recurrence rate is high in cases of large lesions or those involving the endocervical glands.

Destruction of the local lesion

The following criteria should be fulfilled :

- The entire lesion is visualised within the transformation zone.
- There is no suggestive feature of microinvasion or invasion.
- There is no endocervical glandular involvement.
- The cytology and histology should correspond.

This is possible by one of the following methods. After the method employed, the patients are to be followed up regularly.

- **Cryotherapy** acts on the principle of crystallising the intracellular water at temperature of –90°C (see p. 562). It uses either nitrous oxide or carbon dioxide. Depth of tissue destruction is 5 mm. This method is ideal for minor degree and localised CIN lesions. Double freeze technique increases the effectiveness of cryotherapy.

Scheme 3

Evaluation of cervical cytology screening

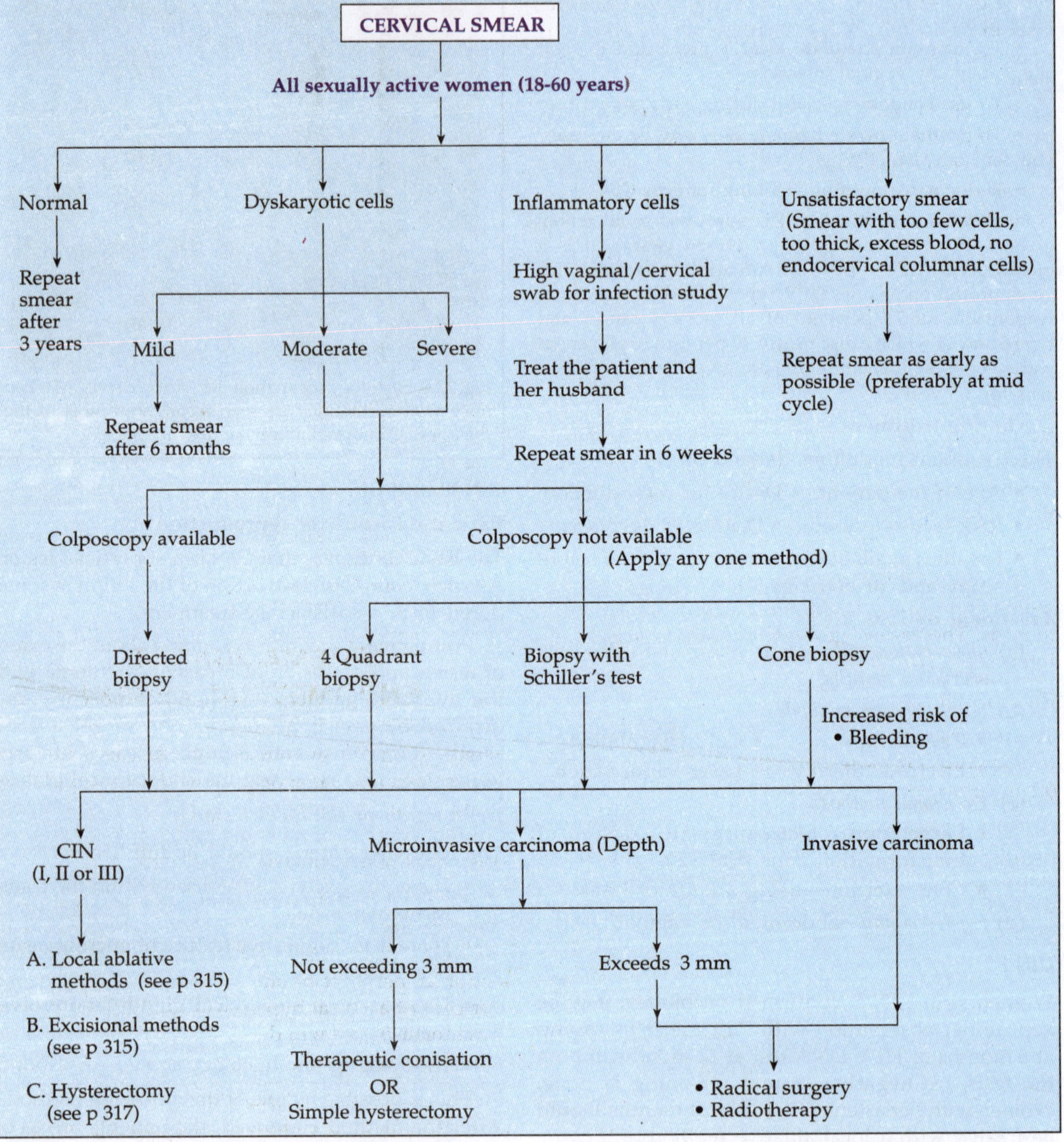

• **Cold coagulation** destroys cervical tissue at a temperature of 100-120°C. It does not need any anaesthesia. Depth of tissue destruction is about 4 mm.

• **Electrodiathermy** destroys cervical tissue up to a depth of 8-10 mm using a unipolar needle electrode. It is done under general anaesthesia.

• **Carbon dioxide laser** through colposcopic guidance — can destroy the epithelium by vaporisation up to a depth of 7 mm. The method is of choice when CIN extends onto the vaginal fornices.

The major advantages of laser vaporization are — (a) preservation of transformation zone for subsequent follow up, (b) precision control technique in depth and breadth and (c) rapid healing.

Excision

Conisation (see p. 560 ch. 34)

While cold knife conisation is commonly done but laser excision cone biopsy is preferable, as it can be done as outpatient under local anaesthesia with colposcopic guidance. Blood loss is also less. Conisation for CIN is as effective as hysterectomy provided the cone margins are free of disease. Complications like haemorrhage, infection, cervical stenosis or incompetence depend on the length of cone excised.

Large loop excision of the transformation zone (LLETZ) or Loop electrosurgical excision procedure (LEEP)

A loop (2-3 cm) of very thin stainless-steel wire is used for excision of the TZ. Blended current (cutting and coagulation), low voltage output is used. It is a simple and quicker procedure. It is done under local anaesthesia. Tissue up to a depth of 10 mm or more can be removed and sent for histological examination. Complications are minimal as compared to cone excision.

Follow up protocol includes an initial posttreatment cytology at 6 months and then repeated at 12 months. Thereafter cytology is repeated at 3 yearly intervals.

Recurrence

The recurrence rate is about 3–5 per cent and development of invasive carcinoma ranges between 0.1-0.4 per cent.

Any recurrence of vaginal intraepithelial neoplasia diagnosed with colposcopic follow up, requires treatment by excision biopsy, carbon dioxide laser vaporisation or topical 5-Fluorouracil (5-FU).

Hysterectomy

- CIN lesion associated with other gynaecologic problems like prolapse, fibroid, pelvic inflammatory disease or endometriosis.
- CIN extends into the vagina.
- Persistent dyskaryotic smear even with treatment.
- Patients with CIN 3.
- Patients with poor compliance for follow up.
- Cancer phobia.

Removal of vaginal cuff is done, if the lesion extends to the vaginal fornices.

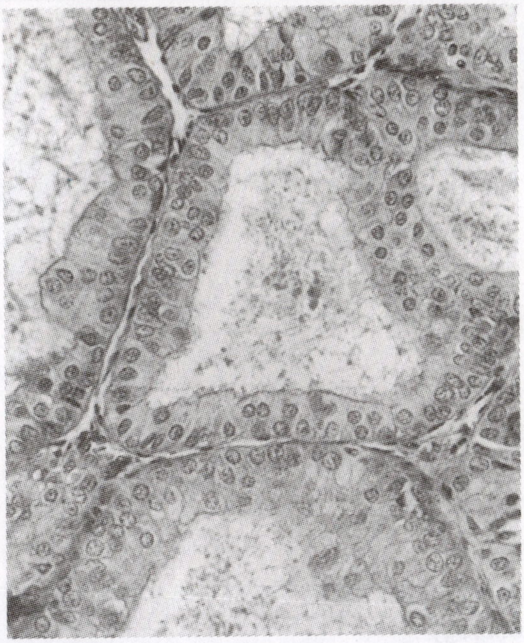

Fig. 22.9. Complex endometrial hyperplasia with nuclear stratification and cytological atypia. The glands are dilated. Mitosis is present in stroma also

PREMALIGNANT ENDOMETRIAL LESION

There is ample evidence that both endometrial hyperplasia and carcinoma are oestrogen dependent. Long-term unopposed oestrogen, particularly around the time of menopause, often leads to various types of endometrial hyperplasia (Fig. 22.9).

Risks : A significant number of such cases will develop invasive carcinoma during the period of 2-8 years (Table 22.6). It has been estimated that about 25 per cent of adenomatous hyperplasia, 50 per cent of atypical hyperplasia and 100 per cent of carcinoma-*in-situ* will develop endometrial carcinoma, if left untreated.

Table 22.6
Classification of Endometrial Hyperplasia (ISGP) (precursors to endometrial carcinoma)

Type of hyperplasia	Progression to cancer (%)
Simple (cystic without atypia)	1
Complex (adenomatous without atypia)	3
Simple (cystic with atypia)	8
Complex (adenomatous with atypia)	29

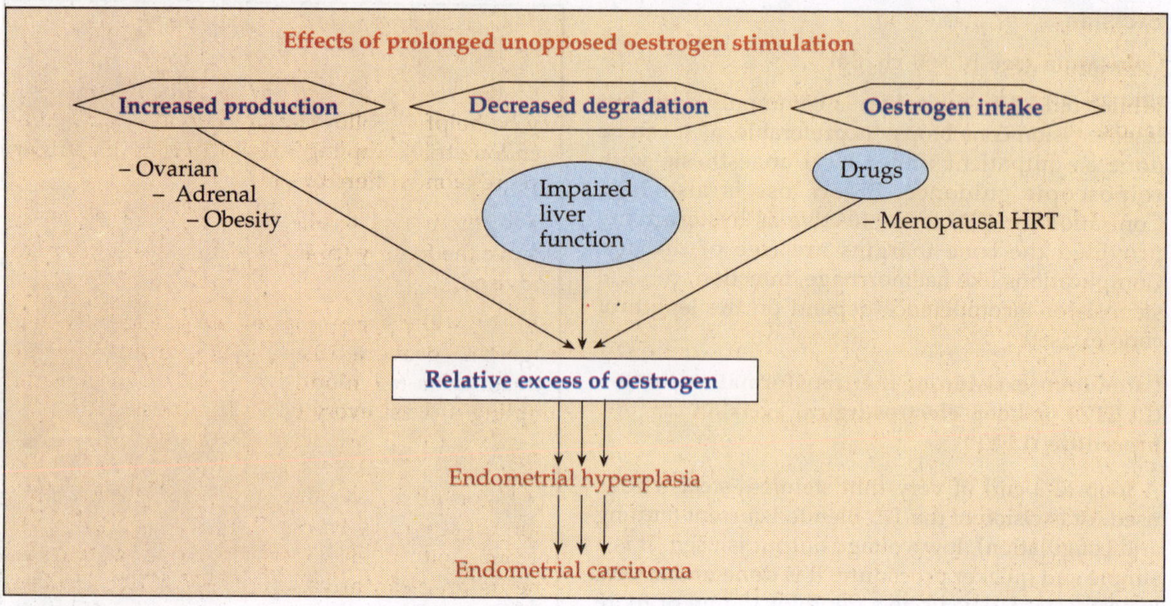

Aetiology

Endometrial hyperplasia develops in women of 40-50 years. Amongst numerous factors, unopposed oestrogen appears to be the primary factor. Premenopausal persistent anovulation is almost a constant factor. In the postmenopausal women with obesity, peripheral conversion of androgens into oestrogen is a risk factor. Long-term oestrogen stimulation in condition of polycystic ovarian syndrome or feminising ovarian tumour may predispose to endometrial cancer (Table 22.7).

Table 22.7 : Risk factors

- Unopposed oestrogen stimulation
- Delayed menopause
- Diabetes
- PCOS
- Obesity
- Nulliparity
- Hypertension
- Previous radiation therapy
- Family history of endometrial carcinoma, carcinoma of breast, ovary or colon
- Tamoxifen therapy

Table 22.8 : Protective factors

- Multiparity
- Normal weight
- Combined oral contraceptive use
- Progestogen therapy
- Menopause ≤ 49 years

Diagnosis

- There is no classic symptom of premalignant lesions. But the constant feature is abnormal perimenopausal uterine bleeding and ultimate diagnosis is by uterine curettage and histology.
- Accidental diagnosis is made during investigation of infertility, DUB, PCOS or excised specimen of removed uterus.
- Diagnosis by screening procedures extended to 'at risk' women is not as effective like that of CIN. Vaginal pool smear, endometrial aspiration (pipelle endometrial sampling), endometrial biopsy (curettage) and vaginal ultrasound (see p. 113) are the different methods available for screening.

Histology

Simple hyperplasia : Endometrium is thick. The glands are dilated and have out pouching and invaginations. They are crowded and have irregular outlines. The stroma is more dense and cellular.

Complex hyperplasia (Fig. 22.9) : Endometrium is thicker. The gland are crowded and arranged back to back with reduced stroma. Most glands have irregular outlines. There are papillary processes and intraluminal bridges within the glands. Epithelial pseudostratification is present.

Atypical hyperplasia : The endometrial glands have cytologic atypia. The gland outlines are of complex hyperplasia in type. The nuclei of the glands show enlargement, irregular size and shape, hyperchromasia and coarse chromatin.

Carcinoma-*in-situ*

Commonly describes a lesion with severe cytologic as well as architectural abnormalities of the glands.

Management

- **Preventive** • **Definitive treatment**

Preventive

- To maintain ideal body weight.
- Oestrogen use in non-hysterectomised women should be restricted. The combined oestrogen-progestogen preparations reduce the risks than oestrogen alone.
- Screening of 'at risk' women mentioned earlier should be done by periodic endometrial sampling.

Definitive treatment

Treatment depends on :

- **Age of the patient**
- **Histologic type of hyperplasia**

Young patient with cystic or adenomatous hyperplasia:

- **Cyclic progestogen therapy** for 6-9 months may be helpful. Follow up at interval of 6 months by endometrial sampling is essential to note whether its regression is there or not.
- **Induction of ovulation** in cases of PCOS to improve the fertility (p. 442, 450) in a young woman, is advised.
- **Atypical hyperplasia** requires therapy with a progestin (provera 10 mg bid) continuously or cyclically for 6-9 months. Periodic endometrial sampling at least every 6 months is essential.

Perimenopausal and postmenopausal women:

- **Hyperplasia without atypia**: Continuous progestin therapy may be considered. However, hysterectomy with bilateral salpingo-oophorectomy is done as an alternative as the risk of carcinoma increases with age.
- **Moderate to severe atypical hyperplasia** and also those women who fail to respond with progestin therapy should be considered for hysterectomy.

KEY POINTS

➤ The premalignant lesions of the vulva include vulval intraepithelial neoplasia (VIN), Paget's disease, lichen sclerosus, squamous hyperplasia and condyloma accuminata.

The average age of VIN is 33 years and it rarely progresses to invasive carcinoma.

For confirmation of carcinoma-*in-situ*, 3-5 mm diameter dermal punch biopsy is taken under local anaesthetic. Alternatively colposcopic examination and biopsy may be done after application of 5 per cent acetic acid.

Surgery for carcinoma-*in-situ* includes — wide local excision, skinning vulvectomy, simple vulvectomy and laser therapy. Regular follow up is mandatory.

Paget's disease is often associated with carcinoma breast. Simple vulvectomy is the surgery.

Predisposing factors for VAIN include infection with HPV, herpes virus II, immunosuppression or radiation.

➤ Vaginal intraepithelial neoplasia (VAIN) is diagnosed by exfoliative cytology, colposcopy and biopsy. The treatment is by 5-Fluorouracil cream or by ablation therapy by cryosurgery or laser.

➤ Richart in 1967 brought-forth the concept of cervical intraepithelial neoplasia (CIN) and replaced the terminology of cervical dysplasia. CIN is a spectrum of premalignant changes in the cervical epithelium showing varying degree of cellular atypia. It is a continuum of changes that begin with mild atypia and may progress too CIS. There is no sharp boundary between them.

Pap smear (cytology) is the gold standard for screening and has reduced the incidence of invasive carcinoma of cervix by about 80 per cent and the mortality by 70 per cent.

The false-negative rate of Pap smear is about 5-15 per cent. Liquid based cytology is found to be superior (p. 109).

KEY POINTS

Squamous intraepithelial lesion (SIL) is a cytologic term, used in Bethesda classification (1988). LSIL corresponds to HPV infection and CIN I whereas HSIL corresponds to CIN II, CIN III and CIS.

The squamocolumnar junction (SCJ) is a dynamic level that lies near the external os during the reproductive life. It moves further down during pregnancy and recedes up into the endocervical canal after menopause.

The process of pathogenesis starts at the 'transformation zone'. The replacement of columnar epithelium of the zone is by squamous epithelium by two mechanisms — by squamous metaplasia of the subcolumnar reserve cells or by squamous epidermidisation. The acid pH is probably an important trigger for the metaplastic process. This metaplastic cells can undergo atypical transformation by trauma or infection, if the host response is poor.

The risk of progression of CIN to invasive carcinoma is variable. The risk of malignant progression is lowest with CIN I – 1 per cent, moderate with CIN II – 5 per cent and highest with CIN III – 20 per cent. It is indeed difficult to ascertain which type of CIN and with what time CIN lesions will proceed to invasive carcinoma.

The mean age of CIN is about 30 years. Some of the documented risk factors are early sexual intercourse, early age of first pregnancy, too many and too frequent births, low socioeconomic status, multiple sexual partners, immunosuppressed (HIV positive) individuals, STD, husband whose previous wife died of cervical malignancy, oral pill users, smoking habits, etc.

- The exact cause of CIN is unknown. HPV infection is an increased risk factor. Human papilloma virus (HPV) types having high oncogenic risk are : 16, 18, 31, 33, 58 and 68. Not all women with HPV infection progress to CIN and HPV infection may regress spontaneously.
- Cytologic and colposcopic findings are aids to the diagnosis but biopsy is only confirmatory.
- The triage strategy (p. 314) includes Pap smear test (p. 109) → atypical smear → HPV DNA assay using hybroid capture 2 → High risk HPV → Colposcopy (p. 312). This strategy eliminates the need for unnecessary colposcopic exams and also frequently repeated Pap smears, when it is negative.
- Colposcopy is the examination of the cervix with magnification (6-16 times). Colposcopy is done when the Pap smear is abnormal. Biopsy is indicated when the colposcopic findings (see p. 314) are abnormal. Conisation of the cervix (p. 560) is performed when there is any discrepancy of cytology, colposcopy and biopsy reports.

The aim of therapy is to destroy all the abnormal (CIN) areas. Cryotherapy, cold coagulation, Electro-diathermy, Laser and LLETZ all can destroy the lesion. In cases with completed family, hysterectomy is the preferred treatment. In conservative surgery, long-term follow-up should be done.

Microinvasive carcinoma requires a conisation specimen. Conisation is as effective as hysterectomy for CIN, provided the cone margins are free of disease.

- Follow up of patients treated for CIN is cytology at 6 months and then repeated at 12 months. There after cytology is repeated at 3 yearly intervals. The risk of recurrence of CIN following initial therapy is about 3-5 per cent.
- CIN lesions detected during pregnancy needs to be evaluated in puerperium as such a lesion may regress spontaneously.
- The premalignant endometrial lesions include simple hyperplasia, complex hyperplasia, atypical simple hyperplasia and atypical complex hyperplasia (WHO). In young patients with cystic or glandular hyperplasia, cyclic progestogen therapy for 6-9 months may be helpful. If regression fails to occur or in perimenopausal women, hysterectomy with bilateral salpingo-oophorectomy should be done.

Atypical hyperplasia in peri or postmenopausal women is considered for hysterectomy.

Genital Malignancy

23

General consideration

There is wide range of geographical variation in the incidence of major genital malignancies, the reason is far from clear. In USA (1985), cancer of the breast, ovary and uterus accounts for 51 per cent of all cancers among females. These sites accounted for 28 per cent of all deaths caused by cancer. In most of the developed countries, cancer of the breast tops the list in female malignancies; **whereas in the developing countries, including India, genital malignancies top the list**. There is also not only wide variation in the incidence but also in the distribution and life time risk of the major genital malignancies (Tables 23.1 to 23.3).

Table 23.1
Incidence of major genital malignancies per 100,000 women

	Developed countries	*Developing countries*
Carcinoma cervix	4–15	30–40
Carcinoma body	10–20	5
Carcinoma ovary	12–15	4–6

Table 23.2
Distribution of genital malignancy (%)

	Developed countries	*Developing countries*
Carcinoma cervix	60	80
Carcinoma body	25–30	5
Carcinoma ovary	10	10–15

Table 23.3
Life time risk of pelvic malignancy

	Carcinoma cervix	*Carcinoma body*	*Carcinoma ovary*
USA			
• Black	1.9	1.2	1.0
• White	0.9	2.7	1.4
UK			
• Scotland	1.2	0.8	1.3
Japan	1.8	0.3	0.5
India (Bombay)	2.2	0.2	0.8

VULVAL CARCINOMA

Incidence

The lesion is rare, about 1.7 per 100,000 females. The distribution varies from 3-5 per cent amongst genital malignancy.

Aetiology

The aetiology remains unclear. But the following factors are often related.

- Usually occurring in postmenopausal women with a median age of 60.
- More common amongst whites.
- Increased association with obesity, hypertension, diabetes and nulliparity.
- Associated local lesions such as chronic vulval dystrophy specially of atypical type are implicated.
- Human papilloma virus (HPV) DNA (type 16, 18) has been detected in patients with invasive vulval cancer.

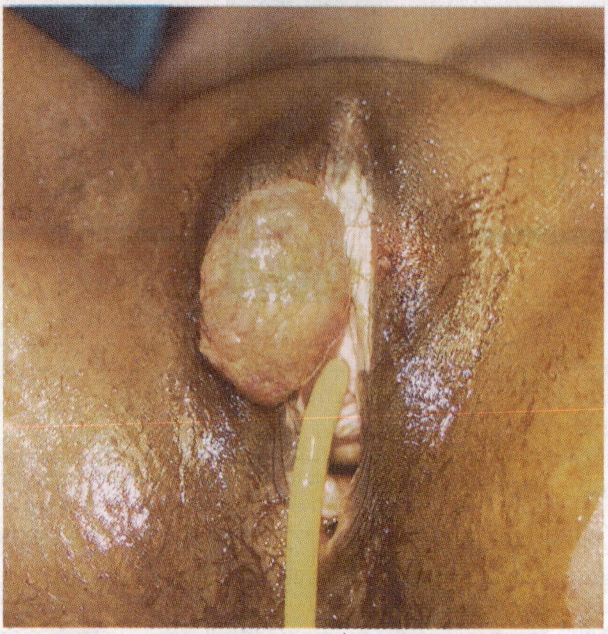

Fig. 23.1. Vulval carcinoma on labium majus (commonest site)

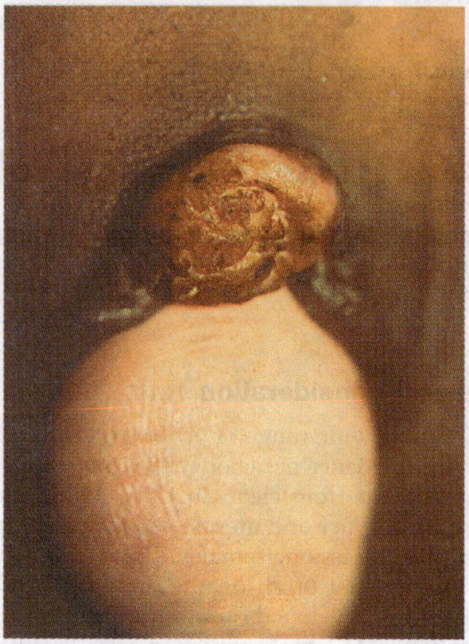

Fig. 23.2. Procidentia associated with carcinoma clitoris (second common site of vulval malignancy)

• Vulval cancer may have a casual relation with condyloma accuminata (HPV 6, 11), Herpes simplex virus type 2 (HSV-2), syphilis and lymphogranuloma venereum.

• Chronic pruritus usually preceeds invasive vulval cancer.

• Chronic irritation of the vulva by chemical or physical trauma associated with poor hygiene may be a predisposing factor.

• Other primary malignancies have been observed in about 20 per cent of cases with vulval cancer. Cervix is most commonly affected, other sites are breast, skin or colon.

Pathology

Sites

• The commonest site is labium majus followed by clitoris and labium minus. Anterior two-thirds are commonly affected. Malignant ulcer on the contralateral side may be multifactorial (Figs. 23.1 and 23.2).

Naked eye

• Ulcerative—The features are raised everted edges, sloughing base with surrounding induration. This is common.

• Hypertrophic—The overlying skin may be intact or it ulcerates sooner or later. This is rare.

Histology

• In majority, about 90 per cent, it is well-differentiated squamous cell carcinoma (Fig. 23.3). Melanoma is observed in about 5 per cent of cases. Rarely, there may be adenocarcinoma if the Bartholin's gland is involved. Other rare types are basal cell carcinoma and sarcomas.

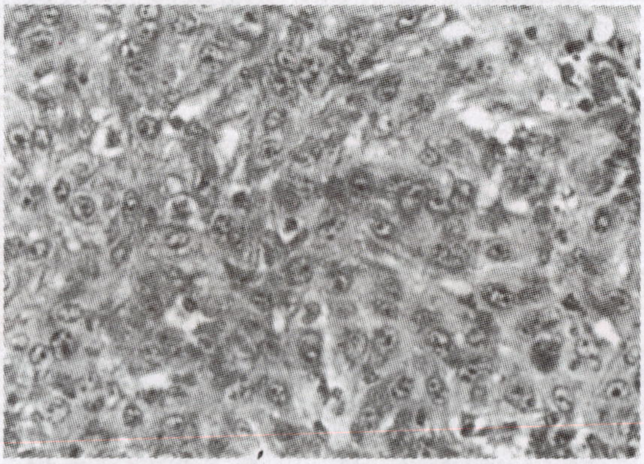

Fig. 23.3. Histologic picture of vulval squamous cell carcinoma

Spread

Direct :The direct spread occurs to the urethra, vagina, rectum and even to pelvic bones. As the disease progresses, other sites in the vulva may develop neoplasia, so that multifocal sites do occur.

Lymphatics : It is the commonest method of spread of lesion. It is estimated that in about 50 per cent, the lymph glands are involved by the time the patient consults the physician. **The following facts are to be borne in mind**:

- The lymphatic spread is primarily by embolisation and only at a late stage, the spread is by permeation to fill the lymphatic channels.
- Contralateral metastases are not infrequent (25%) as the lymphatics of the vulva cross the midline.
- When the ipsilateral nodes are not involved from a lesion located on one side, spread to the contralateral groin node is very unlikely.
- The lymph node involvement follows a sequential pattern. The lymphatics of labia → superficial inguinal lymph nodes → deep inguinal lymph nodes → pelvic nodes.
- Pelvic nodes are secondarily involved in about 20 per cent with affected inguinal nodes. The **nodes involved are** obturator, external iliac, hypogastric and common iliac.
- Lymphatics of the clitoris, anus and recto-vaginal septum may drain directly into the pelvic lymph nodes.
- Involvement of pelvic nodes, bypassing the inguinal lymph nodes, is less than 3 per cent.
- Incidence of lymph gland involvement is directly related to the site, size of the lesion and the depth of stromal invasion (see Table 23.4). Chance of bilateral lymph node involvement also increases when the midline structures (clitoris, perineum) are involved.
- Histologically proved groin node involvement is present in 25 per cent when missed on clinical assessment. In almost 25 per cent, the nodes are histologically negative when clinically thought to be involved. Approximate incidence of lymph node involvement is given in Table 23.4.
- Regional lymph nodes are assessed clinically and also by using MRI (p. 115), **sentinel node lymphoscintigraphy** (p. 328), ultrasound and PET (p. 115).

Blood borne : This is rare but may occur in advanced cases.

Table 23.4
Depth of stromal invasion and groin lymph node involvement in squamous cell carcinoma of vulva

Depth of invasion (mm)	*Per cent with positive nodes*
<1	0
1–2	7.5
2.1–3	10.0
3.1–5	30

Clinical features

Patient profile

The patients are usually postmenopausal, aged about 60 years often with obesity, hypertension and diabetes.

Symptoms :

- Pruritus vulvae
- Swelling with or without offensive discharge
- Difficulty in urination
- Vulval ulceration
- Bleeding
- Pain

Signs

- Vulval inspection reveals an ulcer or a fungating mass on the vulva. The ulcer have a sloughing base with raised, everted and irregular edges and it bleeds to touch. Surrounding tissue may be oedematous and indurated.
- Associated vulval lesions mentioned earlier may be present.
- Inguinal lymph glands of one or both the sides may be enlarged and palpable. The enlargement may also be due to infection.
- Clinical examination of the pelvic organs, including the cervix vagina urethra and rectum must be done. This is due to the co-existent other primary cancers in the genital tract.

Diagnosis

The diagnosis is confirmed by biopsy.

- When a definite growth is present, the biopsy is to be taken from the margin.
- In cases of vulval dystrophy, the sites are from multiple areas usually from the fissures or persistent red areas or from stained areas following toluidine blue test.

Differential diagnosis

The lesion is confused with :

- Condyloma accuminata
- Syphilitic ulcer
- Tubercular ulcer
- Lymphogranuloma venereum
- Soft sore.

Staging

The staging is based on clinical examination **and includes only the primary carcinoma, excluding melanoma**. The FIGO classification is widely used.

Clinical staging based on FIGO (1995)	
Stage-0	Carcinoma-*in-situ*, intraepithelial carcinoma (VIN 3)
Stage-I	Tumour confined to the vulva and/or perineum – 2 cm or less in greatest dimension. Nodes are not palpable.
	IA. Stromal invasion no greater than 1 mm
	IB. Stromal invasion greater than 1 mm
Stage-II	Tumour confined to the vulva and/or perineum – more than 2 cm in greatest dimension. Nodes are not palpable.
Stage-III	Tumour of any size with —
	(i) Adjacent spread to the lower urethra and/or the vagina or the anus and/or
	(ii) Unilateral regional node metastasis
Stage-IV	(A) Tumour invades any of the following :
	Upper urethra, bladder mucosa, rectal mucosa, pelvic bone and/or bilateral regional node metastasis.
	(B) Any distant metastasis including pelvic lymph nodes.

Causes of death

- Uraemia — from ureteric obstruction due to enlarged common iliac and para-aortic nodes
- Rupture of the femoral vessels by the overlying involved inguinal lymph glands
- Sepsis.

Management

Prophylactic

- Adequate therapy for non-neoplastic epithelial disorders of the vulva (see chapter 17).
- Adequate therapy for persistent pruritus vulvae in postmenopausal women (see p. 528).
- Frequent use of multiple biopsies in conservative treatment of VIN.
- Liberal use of simple vulvectomy in postmenopausal women with VIN where follow up facilities are not available.

Definitive treatment

- ***Microinvasive lesion***

There is increased incidence of lymph node involvement in lesion of more than 1 mm invasion. It is thus prudent to perform **radical vulvectomy with bilateral groin node dissection in all cases of stromal invasion more than 1 mm.**

However, if the invasion is less than 1 mm, wide local excision with or without ipsilateral groin lymphadenectomy may be done with follow up. Generally, there is no lymph gland involvement (see Table 23.4). Tumour free surgical margin should be at least 1 cm to prevent local recurrence.

- ***Frank invasion***

Radical vulvectomy with bilateral inguinofemoral lymphadenectomy is the ideal surgery (see p. 578). Three separate incision (one for radical vulvectomy and one each for groin node dissection) approach is currently preferred instead of en-block approach (Fig. 33.14).

Pelvic node metastases are rare unless inguinofemoral nodes are involved. Pelvic lymphadenectomy in cases of positive deep node involvement is omitted in preference to external radiation on the groin and pelvis — in the form of 4500 to 5000 cGy, usually 4-6 weeks after surgery.

Negative **sentinel lymph node (p. 328)** biopsy for micromatastasis may avoid extensive lymphadenectomy. Radical vulvectomy is often associated with major long-term morbidity, sexual dysfunction and loss of body image (see p. 579). Radical local excision of the vulva is considered to be an alternative to radical vulvectomy with equal result.

- ***If the general condition is poor and/or in presence of medical diseases***

The following principles may be adopted :

- Two stage operation is preferred. Total vulvectomy followed by at a later date, bilateral inguinofemoral lymphadenectomy.
- Total vulvectomy followed by full pelvic and groin irradiation (megavoltage therapy).

• Neoadjuvant chemotherapy — chemotherapy followed by surgery, radiotherapy or both.

• *Technically inoperable or recurrent lesion*
  - **Chemotherapy** (cisplatin, bleomycin, 5-FU) can be used as radiation sensitiser.
  - **Chemoradiation therapy** may be combined as primary therapy or following surgical excision of the tumour.
  - **Radiotherapy** can be used as a primary therapy for advanced disease.

Results

With negative groin nodes, the 5 year survival rate for invasive carcinoma ranges from 90-100 per cent.

With positive groin nodes, the survival rate falls to 20-55 per cent. **With positive pelvic nodes**, the survival rate falls even below 20 per cent.

Prognostic factors for vulval squamous cell carcinoma

• Clinical stage of the disease.
• Site of the tumour (p. 322).
• Depth of stromal invasion.
• Lymph node involvement (inguinofemoral and pelvic).
• Tumour diameter and differentiation.
• DNA ploidy status (as discussed in p. 366).

Prognosis

Approximate 5-year survival rate in squamous cell carcinoma is tabulated in Tables 23.5A.

Table 23.5A		Table 23.5B	
Stage	*Survival (%)*	*Survival by node status (5 years)*	
I	90–100	Negative nodes	80–100%
II	75–85	Positive inguinal	30–50%
III	35–45	Femoral nodes	30–50%
IV	20–30	Positive pelvic nodes	10–20%

Melanoma is the second common vulval cancer. The common sites are the clitoris and labia minora. It may arise from a junctional nevus. Radical vulvectomy and bilateral regional lymphadenectomy (en-block) is the preferred treatment. Pelvic lymphadenectomy does not alter the prognosis. Radiation therapy, adjuvant chemotherapy, or immunotherapy are ineffective. Overall prognosis is poor.

BARTHOLIN'S GLAND CARCINOMA

The surgery is like that of squamous cell carcinoma of the vulva. In addition, part of the lower vagina, levatores ani and the ischiorectal fat are to be removed. Prognosis in a case of Bartholin gland carcinoma is similar to squamous cell carcinoma when compared stage for stage of the disease.

VAGINAL CARCINOMA

• **Primary** • **Secondary**

PRIMARY

Incidence

The incidence of primary vaginal carcinoma is very rare (about 0.6 per 100,000 women). It constitutes about 1 per cent of genital malignancies. **The primary vaginal carcinoma should fulfil the following criteria.**

• The primary site of growth is in the vagina.
• The cervix and the vulva must not be involved.
• There must not be clinical evidence of metastatic disease.

Aetiology

Exact aetiology is unknown. Following factors are often related.

• HPV may have a causal relationship.
• Progression from vaginal intraepithelial neoplasia (VAIN).
• Women with history of cervical cancer (multicentric neoplasia).
• Diethyl stilboesterol (DES) is related with clear cell adenocarcinoma of the vagina. This is found in those who had history of intrauterine exposure to diethyl stilboesterol.
• Previous irradiation therapy to the vagina or immunosuppression.
• Prolonged use of pessary.
• More common amongst whites than blacks.

Pathology

Site

The commonest site is in the upper-third of the posterior wall.

Naked eye

The growth may be ulcerative or fungative.

Histopathology

Squamous cell carcinoma accounts for more than

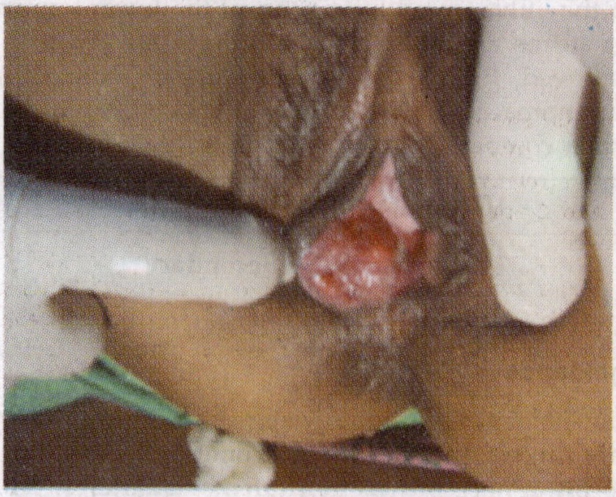

Fig. 23.4. Vaginal carcinoma

90 per cent of the cases. The rest are adenocarcinoma, melanoma and sarcoma.

Spread is by direct continuity, by lymphatics (see p. 29 anatomy) and rarely, blood borne. Inguinofemoral lymph nodes and pelvic lymph nodes are commonly involved. Haematogenous spread involves the lungs, liver or the bones.

Clinical features

The mean age of the patient is about 55 years.

Symptoms

- May be asymptomatic, being accidentally discovered during routine screening procedures.
- Abnormal vaginal bleeding including postcoital bleeding is conspicuously present as an early symptom.
- Foul smelling discharge per vaginam.

Signs

- Speculum examination reveals an ulcerative, nodular or exophytic growth.
- The cervix looks apparently normal.

Diagnosis

- During screening procedure to find an abnormal cytology.
- Colposcopic examination and targeted biopsy are helpful for patients with abnormal cytology or unexplained vaginal bleeding.
- Biopsy from clinically suspected lesion.

Staging

The clinical staging as outlined by FIGO is tabulated below :

Staging of vaginal carcinoma FIGO (1995)

Stage-0	Carcinoma-*in-situ*.
Stage-I	Carcinoma is limited to the vaginal wall.
Stage-II	Carcinoma has involved subvaginal tissue but has not extended to the pelvic wall.
Stage-III	Carcinoma has extended to the pelvic wall.
Stage-IV	Carcinoma has extended beyond the true pelvis or has involved the mucosa of the bladder or rectum.
	(a) Adjacent organs are involved (bladder, rectum).
	(b) Distant organs are involved.

Treatment

Radiotherapy or surgery or the combination is the accepted modality of therapy for invasive primary carcinoma of the vagina. Choice depends on the clinical stage, anatomical location and size of the lesion.

- **Growth limited to the upper-third**

Radical hysterectomy, partial vaginectomy and bilateral pelvic lymphadenectomy is the treatment of choice (as that of stage IB carcinoma cervix).

- **Growth limited to the lower-third**

Radical vulvectomy with removal of bilateral inguinofemoral lymph nodes along with partial vaginectomy.

- **Growth limited to middle-third**

Radiation by external beam therapy with intracavity or interstitial radiation. Care is to be taken to prevent bladder or rectal injury.

Pelvic exenteration operation (see p. 336) is done when there is failure with radiation therapy.

Radiotherapy

Radiation therapy is widely used as a primary treatment for invasive vaginal cancer. External radiation with 4500 to 5000 cGy is administered on the pelvis encompassing the vagina. Additional 3000 to 4000 cGy is delivered locally in the form of interstitial therapy (brachytherapy) with iridium.

Teletherapy (external radiation) reduces the tumour volume and sterilises the regional (pelvic and inguinofemoral) lymph nodes. Complication of radiotherapy (see p. 486) include vaginal stenosis, bladder and rectal fistula.

Cure rate

Overall 5-year survival rate ranges from 80 per cent for stage I disease to 10 per cent for stage IV disease.

CLEAR CELL ADENOCARCINOMA

Primary vaginal adenocarcinoma is rare. This is found in adolescent girls who have had history of intrauterine exposure to diethyl stilboestrol in the first trimester of pregnancy.

The approximate risk of an offspring to develop the clear cell adenocarcinoma of the vagina following DES exposure is I in 1000 or less.

These patients are more likely to develop vaginal adenosis (see p. 521) but, rarely clear cell adenocarcinoma.

The lesion usually involves the upper-third of the anterior vaginal wall. The cervix may also be involved.

Treatment

Radical hysterectomy, vaginectomy with pelvic lymphadenectomy is the treatment of choice.

Radiotherapy is reserved for advanced cases.

SECONDARY

Secondary vaginal malignancy follows carcinoma vulva, cervix or urethra by direct spread. Metastases in the lower-third of the anterior vaginal wall or vault occur in cases of choriocarcinoma (Fig. 22.12) or endometrial carcinoma.

CARCINOMA CERVIX

Magnitude of the problem

- Incidence of cervical cancer is steadily declining in the developed world.
- Pap smear has reduced the incidence of cervical cancer by nearly 80 per cent and death by 70 per cent.
- Cervical cancer is a preventable disease as the different screening, diagnostic and therapeutic procedures are effective.
- At present throughout the globe, there are nearly 1 million women each year having cervical cancer.
- Cancer cervix is the most common cancer in women of the developing countries where screening facilities are inadequate.

Incidence

In most of the developing countries carcinoma of the breast and cervix are the leading sites of malignancies in female and are major public health problems.

In India, twelve population based cancer registries (PBCRs) showed cancer breast was the most common followed by cancer of the cervix (ICMR-2004). In female cancers, relative proportion of cancer breast varied between 21 and 24 per cent whereas that of cancer cervix was between 14 and 24 per cent.

Major factors affecting the prevalence of carcinoma cervix in a population are economic factor, sexual behaviour and degree of effective mass screening.

Epidemiology

This has been discussed in CIN (p. 309). In India, the prevalence is more amongst the comparatively younger age group. Carcinoma cervix is rare in women who are sexually not active (nuns, virginal women). Male circumcision is only partially protective against cervical carcinogenesis.

Gross pathology

The site of the lesion is predominantly in the ectocervix (80%) and the rest (20%) are in the endocervix.

Naked eye

- Exophytic — These arise from the ectocervix and form friable masses almost filling up the upper vagina in late cases (Fig. 23.8).
- Ulcerative — The lesion excavates the cervix and often involves the vaginal fornices (Fig. 23.5).
- Infiltrative — These are found in endocervical growth. They cause expansion of the cervix, so that it becomes barrel-shaped.

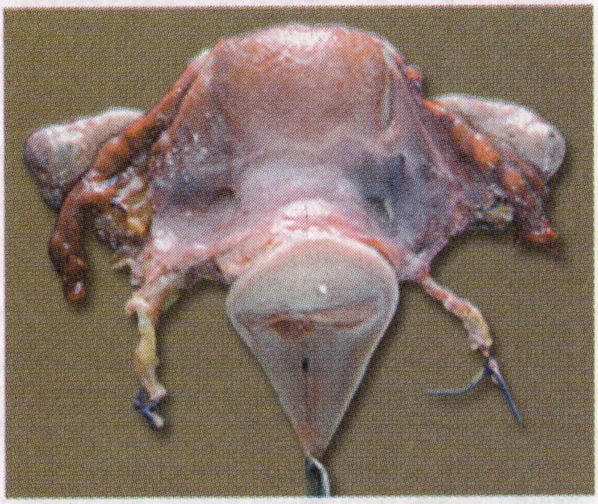

Fig. 23.5. Ulcerative type of cervical malignancy with a friable growth on the posterior lip. Radical hysterectomy done

Histopathology (Fig. 23.6)

The commonest variety is squamous cell carcinoma (85-90 per cent) either well-differentiated or moderately or poorly differentiated. These arise from the ectocervix. **The sources of the squamous epithelium which turn into malignancy are**—squamocolumnar junction, healing erosion, squamous metaplasia of the columnar epithelium and squamous cell rests in the ectocervix.

- Squamous cell carcinoma is further subdivided histologically into three groups : (i) large cell keratinising, (ii) large cell non-keratinising and (iii) small cell type. Patients with small cell type have got poor prognosis compared to the large cell types.

- Adenocarcinoma (10-15%) develops from the endocervical canal, either from the lining epithelium or from the glands.

- Currently increased number of cervical adenocarcinomas are observed specially in the younger age group. The majority (80%) of them are purely endocervical type. The remainders are endometrioid, clear cell, adenosquamous or a mixed type. *Adenomamalignum* is an extremely well-differentiated adenocarcinoma with favourable prognosis.

Mode of spread

By direct extension : The growth spreads directly to the adjacent structures, to the vagina and to the body of the uterus. It extends laterally to the parametrium, paracervical and paravaginal tissues. Here the tumour cells surround and compress the ureter. It may spread backwards along the uterosacral ligament, to involve the rectum or forwards to involve the base of the bladder, specially in endocervical growth.

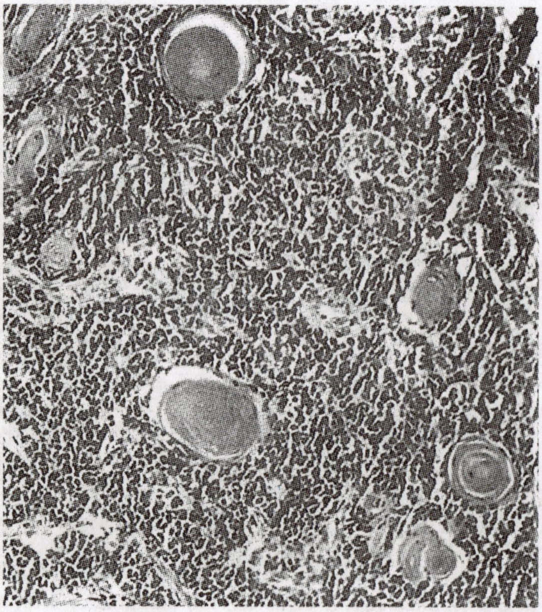

Fig. 23.6. Histology of squamous cell carcinoma of the cervix (small cell type). Keratin pearls are seen.

By lymphatics : **The primary group involved are** — parametrial nodes, internal iliac nodes, obturator, external iliac nodes and sacral nodes. **The secondary nodes involved are** — common iliac group, the inguinal nodes and paraaortic nodes (Table 23.6).

Sentinel lymph node is the first node that drains a primary tumour. In most cases (85%) there is a single sentinel lymph node (see p. 577). This node can be detected by intraoperative lymphatic mapping injecting methylene blue dye into the tumour or lymphoscintigraphy using technetium 99.

By blood stream : Blood borne metastasis is late and usually by veins rather than the arteries. Lungs, liver or bone are usually involved.

By direct implantation : Direct implantation of the cancer cells at operation on the vault of the vagina or abdominal or perineal wound is very rare.

The risk of ovarian metastases in stage I squamous cell carcinoma of the cervix is 0.5 per cent and it is 1.7 per cent for adenocarcinoma.

Table 23.6
Involvement of lymph nodes in different stages (Approximate)

Stage	*Pelvic nodes (%)*	*Paraaortic nodes (%)*
0	0	0
Ia_1 (< 3 mm)	0–0.5	0
Ia_2 (3-5 mm)	5	< 1
Ib	16	2
II	30	15
III	44	30
IV	55	40

Staging : **The purposes of staging are** to determine the prognosis, to formulate the line of treatment and to compare the results of one to the other.

The fallacies are — difficult to assess the lymph node involvement on clinical examination which adversely affects the prognosis. There is also difficulty in differentiation of inflammatory and malignant induration of the parametrium.

Table 23.7
Staging procedures allowed by FIGO

- Inspection of cervix and vagina
- Pelvic examination (vaginal, rectovaginal) under anaesthesia
- Lymph node palpation
- Colposcopy
- Biopsy
- Endocervical curettage
- Conisation
- Hysteroscopy
- Chest X-ray
- Skeletal X-ray
- Intravenous pyelogram
- Barium enema
- Cystoscopy
- Proctoscopy

Ultrasonography, lymphangiography, CT and MRI, PET, Radionucleotide scanning studies, Laparoscopy/ Laparotomy are optional and not to be used for FIGO staging.

Staging of cervical cancer is based principally on clinical examination. Pelvic examination (speculum, bimanual and rectal examination) should be done under anaesthesia. The routine supplementary investigations include X-ray chest, intravenous pyelography, cystoscopy and proctoscopy. In cases of suspected pelvic inflammation, a course of antibiotic should be given prior to clinical staging.

Final staging cannot be changed once therapy has begun. If any doubt exists as to which stage should be assigned, the lower stage should be chosen.

CT scan, MRI, Positron Emission Tomography (PET), Lymphangiography (p. 115) can detect involvement of the pelvic or periaortic lymph nodes and parametrium. MRI is helpful to detect parametrial extension and to define the tumour volume. But these findings do not change FIGO stage of disease.

The clinical staging as recommended by FIGO is tabulated below :

FIGO (1995) staging of carcinoma of the cervix

	PREINVASIVE CARCINOMA
Stage-0	Carcinoma-*in-situ* or intraepithelial carcinoma (cases of stage 0 should not be included in any therapeutic statistics).
	INVASIVE CARCINOMA
Stage-I	Carcinoma strictly confined to the cervix (extension to the corpus should be disregarded).
Stage-Ia	Preclinical carcinoma of the cervix, that is, those diagnosed only by microscopy.
Stage-Ia$_1$	Minimal microscopically evident stromal invasion, not exceeding 3 mm.
Stage-Ia$_2$	Microscopically measured invasion greater than 3 mm and no greater than 5 mm and no wider than 7 mm (Depth of invasion should not be more than 5 mm taken from the base of the epithelium, either surface or glandular, from which it originates and a second dimension, the horizontal spread must not exceed 7 mm). Larger lesions should be staged as Ib.
Stage-Ib	Lesions of greater dimensions than stage Ia$_2$ whether seen clinically or not. Vascular space involvement should not alter the staging but should be specifically recorded so as to determine whether it should affect treatment decisions in the future.
Stage-Ib$_1$	Lesion not exceeding 4 cm in size.
Stage-Ib$_2$	Lesion exceeds 4 cm in size.
Stage-II	The carcinoma extends beyond the cervix but has not extended to the pelvic wall. The carcinoma involves the vagina, but not the lower-third.
Stage-IIa	No obvious parametrial involvement
Stage-IIb	Obvious parametrial involvement
Stage-III	The carcinoma has extended to the pelvic wall. On rectal examination, there is no cancer-free space between the tumour and the pelvic wall. The tumour involves the lower-third of the vagina. All cases with hydronephrosis or nonfunctioning kidney are included.
Stage-IIIa	No extension to the pelvic wall but to the lower-third of vagina.
Stage-IIIb	Extension onto the pelvic wall and/or hydronephrosis or nonfunctioning kidney.
Stage-IV	The carcinoma has extended beyond the true pelvis or has clinically involved the mucosa of the bladder or rectum.
	A bullous oedema as such does not permit a case to be alloted to stage IV.
Stage-IVa	Spread of growth to adjacent organs.
Stage-IVb	Spread to distant organs.

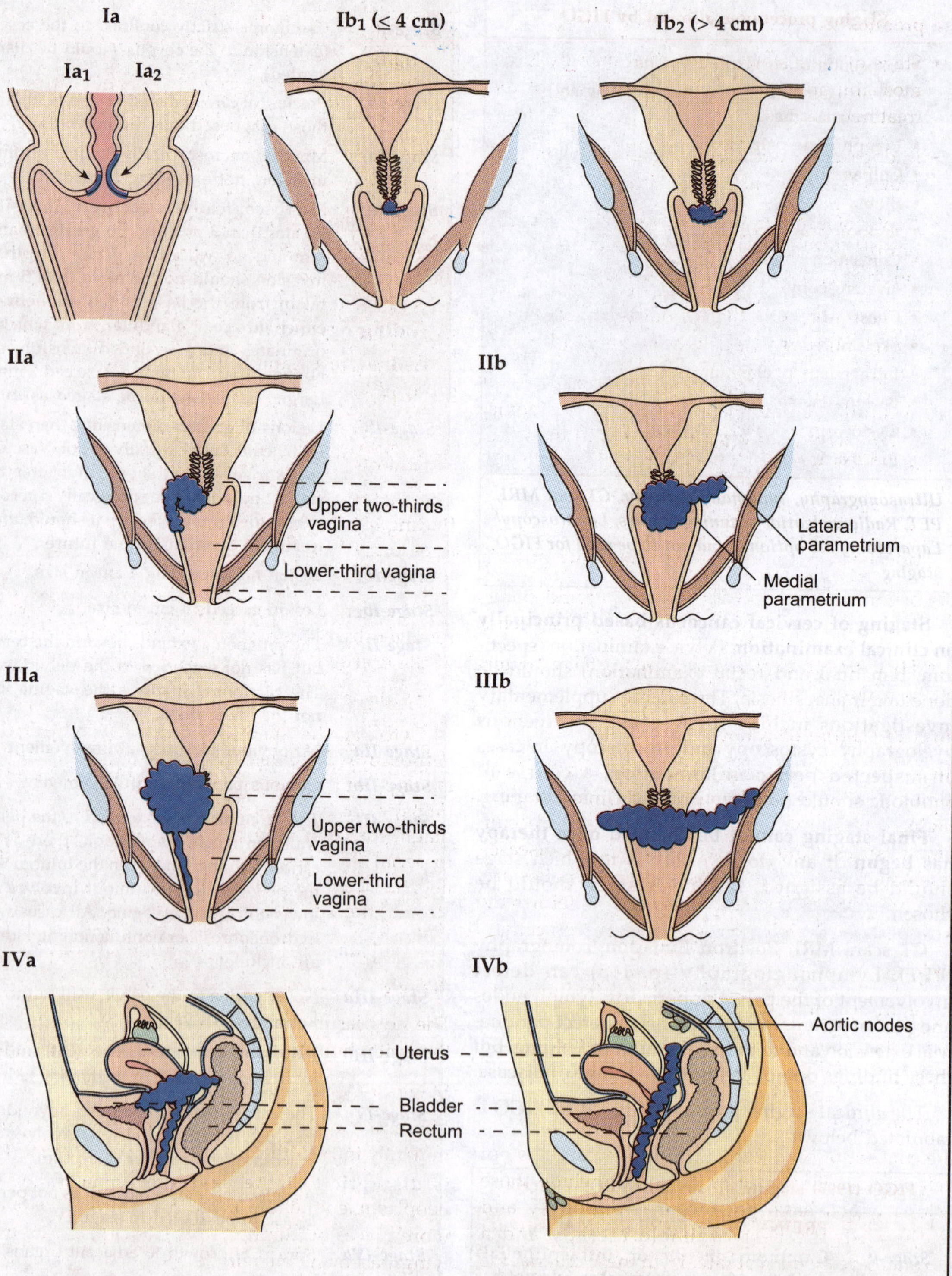

Fig. 23.7. Diagrammatic representation of staging of carcinoma cervix according to FIGO (see p. 329)

Prognosis

The prognosis depends on the following :

- Stage of the lesion at the initial therapy is the most important factor in the outcome of the treatment.
- Endocervical tumour is diagnosed late and grows faster.
- Depth of tumour invasion when <1 cm, less lymph nodes are involved and improved survival is observed.
- Tumour size more than 4 cm is associated with more lymph node metastasis and poor survival.
- Well-differentiated squamous cell carcinoma grows slowly and metastasises late than the anaplastic type.
- Young age is usually associated with poorly differentiated squamous cell carcinoma or adenocarcinoma and is prognostically poor.
- Lymph node involvement (pelvic and para-aortic) reduces the survival rate by 50 per cent.
- HPV positive younger patients have better prognosis.

Surgical staging of cancer cervix :

There are often discrepancies between clinical staging and surgicopathological findings. Surgical staging can minimise this by identifying the occult tumour spread and also the extra pelvic disease. Assessment of the pelvic and paraaortic nodes are done by surgical approach. This is done either by extra peritoneal approach or by laparoscopically.

Diagnosis

- Early carcinoma
- Advanced carcinoma/Late carcinoma.

Early carcinoma (Table 23.8)

Nomenclature

The concept of early carcinoma of the cervix is not well-defined. Presumably, it should include those lesions which have got minimal morbidity and deaths with the best available therapy and a maximal 5-year survival rate. With these criteria, the following stages as per FIGO classification are included in the category of early carcinoma.

Table 23.8 : Early carcinoma

Stage	*5-year survival rate (%)*
Ia_1	98.7
Ia_2	95.9
Ib_1	90.4
Ib_2	79.8

Thus all these have got a 5-year survival rate ranging between 80-100 per cent. Stage II reduces the 5-year survival rate to as low as 55-70 per cent. As such, **it is inappropriate to include any lesion extending beyond the cervix as early carcinoma**.

As the presentation of the case differs, these are grouped as :

- **Preclinical**
- **Clinical**

Preclinical

There may not be any symptom nor any pelvic finding to raise any suspicion. The cervix may look apparently healthy. The diagnosis is made by the following :

- Incidental on histological examination of tissues removed by biopsy, portio amputation or removal of the uterus.
- During screening procedures.

Cytologically suspicious smear is subjected to colposcopy followed by directed biopsy. In the absence of colposcopy, **Schiller's test** directed biopsy is to be taken. If a positive lesion is found, diagnostic conisation has to be done and subjected to serial sections. Depending upon the degree of neoplastic changes and or its invasion to the adjacent stroma, the lesions are diagnosed as follows :

- **Stage 0**
- **Stage Ia**
- **Stage Ib**

Stage 0

The neoplastic changes involve whole thickness of the epithelium **but the basement remains intact.**

Stage Ia (Microinvasive carcinoma)

Microinvasive carcinoma is one which is predominantly intraepithelial carcinoma, except that **there is disruption of the basement membrane**. The neoplastic epithelium invades the stroma in one or more places but limited upto 5 mm from the overlying basement membrane. As such, the depth of invasion is measured by using a microscope with an ocular micrometer.

The malignant cells maintain their connection with the overlying intraepithelial neoplasm. The cords of malignant cells may become confluent or invade the lymphovascular channels, irrespective of depth of penetration.

The mean age is 38-42 years.

In majority, the entity is asymptomatic. There may be blood stained discharge, intermenstrual, postcoital or postmenopausal bleeding. The cervix may look abnormal like erosion, eversion or cervicitis.

The diagnosis is made only on cone biopsy of the cervix. Initial screening may be done with cytology, colposcopy and directed biopsy along with endocervical curettage.

The patient with microinvasive carcinoma may be treated even with conservative surgery when there is no risk of lymph node metastasis.

Stage Ib : The invasion of the malignant cells to the underlying stroma exceeds 5 mm. There is no clinical manifestation and the cervix may look apparently normal.

- **Clinical : Stage Ib (overt)**

Symptoms : The duration of symptoms is not proportionate to the stage of the disease.

- Menstrual abnormalities in the form of contact bleeding or bleeding on straining (during defecation), intermenstrual bleeding are very much suspicious, specially over the age of 35.
- Excessive white discharge which may be at times offensive.

Signs

Speculum examination reveals :

- Either a red granular area which looks like an ectopy (erosion) extending from the external os or a **nodular growth** or **an ulcer**. The lesion bleeds on friction. **It should be done prior to bimanual examination.** The cervical lesion may not be visible due to bleeding from the friable lesion caused by digital examination.

Bimanual examination reveals the lesion is indurated, friable and bleeds to touch. Cervix is freely mobile.

Rectal examination reveals the parametrium absolutely free.

Confirmation of diagnosis is by biopsy

Ancillary aids for confirmation of staging :

- Cystoscopy
- X-ray chest
- Intravenous pyelography
- Proctoscopy.

All these give a negative finding and as such, the clinical staging of Ib is thereby confirmed.

Advanced carcinoma/Late carcinoma

All cases of carcinoma with stage II and onwards are arbitrarily called advanced carcinoma considering the reduced 5-year survival rate compared to earlier stages. In fact, in India, this group comprises about 80 per cent of the total cervical carcinoma patients attending the hospitals for treatment.

PATIENT PROFILE

The patients are usually multiparous, in premenopausal age group. They have previous history of postcoital or intermenstrual bleeding which they ignored.

Symptoms : As previously mentioned, the duration of symptoms is not proportionate to the stage of the disease. However, the following symptoms may be evident depending upon the extent of the lesion.

- **Irregular or continued vaginal bleeding** which may at times be brisk
- **Offensive vaginal discharge.**
- **Pelvic pain** of varying degree — This may be either due to involvement of uterosacral ligament leading to backache or deep seated pain due to involvement of sacral plexus.
- **Leg oedema** is due to progressive obstruction of lymphatics and/or iliofemoral veins by the tumour.
- **Bladder symptoms** include frequency of micturition, dysuria, haematuria or even true incontinence due to fistula formation.
- **Rectal involvement** is evidenced by diarrhoea, rectal pain, bleeding per rectum or even rectovaginal fistula (see Fig. 23.7).
- **Ureteral obstruction** is due to progressive growth of tumour laterally. There may be frequent attacks of pyelonephritis due to ureteric obstruction.

Ultimately, the patient may be **cachectic, anaemic with oedema legs and uraemia develops.**

Speculum examination reveals the nature of the

growth, ulcerative or fungating which bleeds to touch.

Bimanual examination reveals the induration and extent of the growth to the vagina and to the sides. The induration of the bladder base may be felt through the anterior fornix in advanced cases.

Rectal examination is invaluable to note the involvement of the parametrium and its extent in relation to the lateral pelvic wall. Nature of induration is to be noted carefully. **If it is smooth**, the possibility of inflammation has to be excluded and antibiotics has to be given prior to final assessment for staging. **In malignancy, the induration is nodular**. Incidental involvement of the rectum has to be noted.

For confirmation of diagnosis, *biopsy* is mandatory (see p. 560). If the lesion is small, wedge biopsy is taken which should include a portion of the healthy tissue as well. If it is big, a bit may be taken from a comparative noninfective area. There may be brisk haemorrhage which can be effectively controlled by plugging.

DIFFERENTIAL DIAGNOSIS

At times, the growth may be confused with :

- Cervical tuberculosis (p. 140).
- Syphilitic ulcer (p. 144).
- Cervical ectopy (p. 257).
- Products of conception in incomplete abortion.
- Fibroid polyp (p. 275).

COMPLICATIONS

The following complications may occur sooner or later, as the lesion progresses.

- Haemorrhage.
- Frequent attacks of ureteric pain, due to pyelitis and pyelonephritis and hydronephrosis.
- Pyometra — specially with endocervical variety.
- Vesicovaginal fistula.
- Rectovaginal fistula — This is comparatively rare because of the interposition of the pouch of Douglas. The rectum may be involved either through the uterosacral ligament or through rectovaginal septum.

Causes of death

The patient may die of :

Uraemia — This is due to ureteric obstruction following parametrial involvement. There is hydroureter and hydronephrosis. Infection supervenes, thereby further compromising kidney functions.

Haemorrhage — The vaginal bleeding from the growth may be brisk or continuous. This leads to anaemia and ill health.

Sepsis — Localised pelvic or generalised peritonitis may occur which may be fatal.

Cachexia — The cumulative effect of the factors mentioned leads to cachectic condition. The cancerous tissues have got depressant action on general metabolism.

Metastases to the distant organs commonly observed are : lung (36%), lymph nodes (30%), bone (16%) and abdominal cavity (7%). These may be fatal.

MANAGEMENT OF CARCINOMA CERVIX

- **Preventive** • **Curative**

Preventive

Primary prevention

It involves identifying the causal factors and eliminating or preventing those from exerting their effects. These are easy to enumerate, but difficult to implement in practice.

- **Identifying 'high risk' female**
  - Early sexual intercourse.
  - Early age of first pregnancy.
  - Too many births/too frequent birth.
  - Low socioeconomic status.
  - Poor maintenance of local hygiene.
  - Sexually transmitted oncogens (HPV and HSV type II).
- **Identifying 'high risk' males**
  - Multiple sexual partners.
  - Previous wife died of cervical carcinoma.

It is indeed an uphill task to prevent these epidemiological factors often associated with invasive carcinoma cervix. However, cancer consciousness, propagandas, proper health education of the population, specially amongst the poor socioeconomic group could be important steps in prevention.

• **Use of condom** during early intercourse, raising the age of marriage and of first birth, limitation of family, maintenance of local hygiene and effective therapy of STD may be positive steps in prevention.

• **Removal of cervix during hysterectomy** as a routine for benign lesion is a definite step in prevention of stump carcinoma. The incidence may be as high as 1 per cent.

• **Prophylactic recombinant HPV vaccine** is approved to all school girls (9-15 years) and women (16-25 years). See p. 315.

Secondary prevention : It involves identifying and treating the disease earlier in the more treatable stage. **This is done by screening procedures**. The details have been described in chapter 8 and 21. The abnormal cervical pathology likely to progress to invasive carcinoma can be detected. Its effective therapy reduces dramatically the incidence of invasive carcinoma in areas where it has been implemented. Even when the invasive carcinoma is detected, it is so early that a 85-100 per cent 5-year survival rate could be achieved.

Down staging screening (WHO 1986)

Down staging for cervical cancer is **defined as** "the detection of the disease at an earlier stage when it is still curable. Detection is done by nurses and other paramedical health workers using a simple speculum for visual inspection of the cervix".

The "downstaging screening" is an experimental approach suggested by WHO as an alternative to regular cytologic screening. In the developing countries, where effective mass screening cannot be extended and the majority of cases of carcinoma cervix are diagnosed at an advanced stage, 'down staging screening' offers at least an **early detection of disease**. **Compared to cytological screening it is suboptimal.** But in places where prevalence of cancer is high and cytological screening is not available, "down staging screening" is useful. **The strategy is however, not expected to lower the incidence of cancer cervix, but it can certainly minimise the cancer death through early detection**.

Downstaging procedure : A female primary health care worker is trained for 2-3 weeks to perform speculum examination. They are trained to distinguish a normal cervix from an abnormal one.

Characters of a normal cervix : Pink in colour, round in shape, smooth surface and does not bleed on touch. Whereas an **abnormal cervix has the following characters** : Reddish, red or white area of patch, growth or ulcer on the surface and bleeds on touch.

Once the abnormality is suspected, the case is referred to a centre where diagnosis and treatment of premalignant and malignant lesions are done.

Curative : Ideally, the management of the patient with cervical cancer is a team approach. Both the gynaecologist and radiooncologist should review the patient along with the biopsy report and the plan outlay be individualised. Due consideration should be given to :

- General condition of the patient.
- Stage of the disease.
- Facilities available – surgical and radiotherapy.
- Wish of the patient to be judiciously complied with.

Table 23.9 : Pretreatment Evaluations

History
Physical examination
• General condition • Tumour staging
Blood values
• Complete haemogram, Biochemical studies, Electrolytes, Tumour marker (SCC)
Liver function tests
• Serum proteins and liver enzymes
Radiologic studies
• X-ray chest • IVP • Barium enema (in advanced stage)
Cystoscopy (as indicated)
Treatment decision should be made jointly by the Gynaecologist and the Radiotherapist

Pretreatment evaluation

Irrespective of the treatment modalities (surgery or radiotherapy) the following evaluations are to be made apart from those already done (Table 23.7) for staging purposes (Table 23.9).

Serum marker (see p. 497)

SCC (Squamous Cell Carcinoma) antigen is the

Table 23.10
BRACHYTHERAPY TECHNIQUES

	Amount of radium placement	*No. of application*	*Duration*
Paris technique	Intrauterine tandem 33.3 mg — one Vaginal ovoid 13.3 mg — two or three	One	120 hours
Manchester technique	Intrauterine tandem 30-50 mg Vaginal colpostat 30-50 mg	Two	72 hours each at interval of 7 days
Stockholm technique	Intrauterine tandem 50 mg — one Vaginal plaque — 65-80 mg	Three	24 hours each at weekly interval

serum marker. Although, the antigen is not specific, it has been useful as a means to monitor treatment response and to predict tumour recurrence.

Pretreatment preparations

Irrespective of the methods of treatment, general health of the patient must be improved. Due attention is to be paid to correct anaemia and malnutrition. This not only makes the patient sufficiently fit to withstand surgery but rise in haemoglobin percentage improves the tissue oxygenation needed for effective ionising effect of irradiation.

TREATMENT MODALITIES OF CARCINOMA CERVIX

The types of treatment employed for the invasive carcinoma are as follows :

- Primary surgery
- Primary radiotherapy
- Chemotherapy
- Combination therapy.

Surgery

The types of surgery employed in invasive carcinoma are :

Radical hysterectomy (Fig. 23.8)

John Clark (1898) first did the operation while working as a resident in Johns Hospkins Hospital. This operation is commonly done abdominally and is known by different names (**Wertheim** of Viena–1898, **Okabayashi** of Japan–1921, **Meigs** of USA–1944). **Extensive vaginal operation** was subsequently developed to minimise the mortality and morbidity from abdominal approach. Pelvic lymph nodes are removed by bilateral extra-peritoneal approach. This operation is also popularly known by different names (**Schauta** of Viena–1902, **Mitra** of India–1957). There have been several modifications of the techniques of radical hysterectomy and bilateral pelvic lymphadenectomy at present.

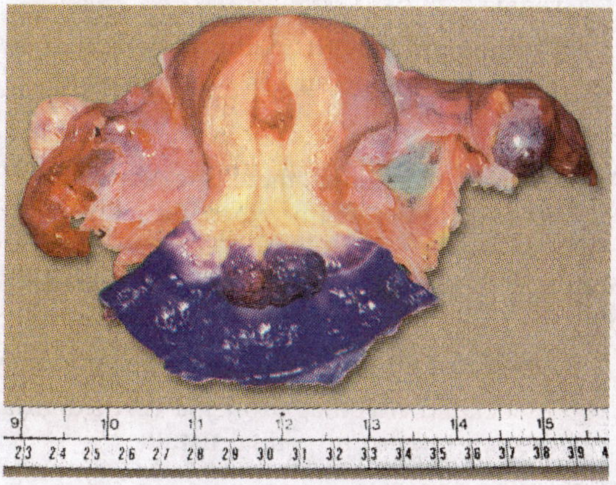

Fig. 23.8. Exophytic type of cervical squamous cell carcinoma — radical hysterectomy done

The surgery includes (Fig. 34.13) removal of the uterus, tubes and ovaries of both the sides (ovaries may be spared in young women), upper half of vagina, parametrium (most of cardinal and uterosacral ligaments) and the draining primary cervical lymph nodes (parametrial, obturator, internal and external iliac groups and sometimes common iliac. **Sacral group is not removed**). Paraaortic lymph node evaluation is done. Any enlarged paraaortic lymph node is sampled and sent for frozen section biopsy. Radiation therapy is to be considered if lymph nodes are found involved. Generally **negative sentinel lymph nodes may allow omission of lymphadenectomy of the nodal basin.**

Limitation : It is ideally limited to early stage disease (Table 23.11).

Advantages of surgery over radiotherapy

- Spread of the disease can be determined more thoroughly by surgicopathological staging.
- Surgical staging (Laparotomy or Laparoscopy) and assessment of paraaortic and pelvic nodes, can predict the survival rate accurately.
- Preservation of ovarian function, if desired specially in a young woman.
- Ovaries may be transposed out of the radiation field if radiation is considered in the postoperative period.
- Retention of more functional and pliable vagina.
- Psychologic benefit to the patient that her cancer bearing organ has been removed.

Special indications

As previously mentioned, there is no superiority of surgery over radiotherapy when the patients are placed in ideal circumstances. But there are conditions where **radiotherapy is contraindicated** and only the surgical treatment has to be extended.

- Associated PID acute or chronic, pelvic kidney.
- Associated myoma, prolapse (procidentia), ovarian tumour or genital fistula.
- Young patient.
- Vaginal stenosis — placement of radiation source is inadequate.
- Recurrence after irradiation.
- Surgery is preferred for those with adenocarcinoma or adenosquamous carcinoma.

Postoperative complications

Major postoperative complications as observed following total abdominal hysterectomy have been discussed (see p. 568). **Other complications include :** ureteric fistula (about 1%), vesicovaginal fistula (0.5%), bladder dysfunction, cystitis pyelonephritis and rectal dysfunction. There may be lymphocyst in the pelvis, lymphoedema of one or both the legs, dyspareunia and recurrence. The mortality rate of the procedure is less than 1 per cent.

Bladder dysfunction (atony) is a known complication. This is due to damage of the sympathetic and parasympathetic fibers to and from the bladder and urethra. Continuous catheterisation for bladder drainage is maintained for a period of 6–10 days.

Neuropathies due to nerve injuries (Femoral, Obturator, Sciatic, Genito femoral, Ilioinguinal, Lateral femoral cutaneous and Pudendal nerves.

Lymphocyst formation is a frequent complication. Tissue fluid, lymph and blood are collected to form the cyst following radical hysterectomy. Lymphocyst is best diagnosed by ultrasound. Rarely it may be of large size to cause pain and ureteral or venous obstruction. Adequate suction drainage of the retroperitoneal space postoperatively is an important preventive measure. Majority resolve spontaneously. Sometimes it may drain through vagina. Rarely needle aspiration is needed when the size is large or it produces symptoms.

• Pelvic exenteration

This type of ultraradical surgery is named after **Brunschwig**. This procedure is done in a very selective case only :

- Stage IVA disease.
- Central pelvic recurrent carcinoma (biopsy proven) without any metastasis.
- Completely resectable tumour mass.
- Absence of ureteral obstruction, sciatic pain or unilateral leg oedema.
- Woman should be psychologically and physically adjusted to cope with urinary and faecal stomas.

Contraindications of pelvic exenteration are extra-pelvic spread of disease with distant metastasis to liver, lungs or bones.

Types

- **Anterior exenteration** — It consists of radical hysterectomy, removal of urinary bladder and implantation of ureters either in the sigmoid colon or into an artificial bladder made from an ileal loop (ileal bladder).
- **Posterior exenteration** — It consists of radical hysterectomy, removal of rectum and a permanent colostomy.
- **Complete or total** — It consists of combination of anterior and posterior exenteration with a permanent colostomy and an ileal bladder. The operative mortality of such type of operation is about 10-20 per cent and with a 5-year survival rate of about 10 per cent only.
- **Laparoscopic radical hysterectomy** — It is a new procedure. Laparoscopic Assisted Radial Vaginal Hysterectomy (LARVH) combined with laparoscopic pelvic lymphadenectomy is done for early invasive disease. Ovarian vessels, round ligaments and uterine vessels are divided abdominally. The procedure is then completed vaginally as a modified version of Schauta's Radical vaginal hysterectomy.

Primary radiotherapy

Cancer of the cervix was the first cancer of an internal organ to be treated with ionising radiation using radium by Margaret Cleves in 1903. **Primary therapy (chemoradiation)** is given in locally advanced (stage IIB to IVA) disease (see below).

External photon beam radiation and brachytherapy are the two main methods (see p. 484).

The advantages of radiotherapy as a primary modality of treatment are :

- Wider applicability in all stages of carcinoma cervix.
- Survival rate 85%, comparable with that of surgery in early stages.
- Less primary mortality and morbidity.
- Individualisation of dose distributions/requirement possible.

- **Early stages**

Brachytherapy technique is employed (ch. 30). Small radioactive sources, mainly radium sulphate is mixed with some inert powder and packed in small needles or tubes. These are used for interstitial, intracavitary or surface applications. Radiation sources for intracavitary radiation are Radium (226Ra), Cesium (137Cs) or Cobalt (60Co). The container is made up of platinum, gold or alloy steel to absorb alpha and beta particles and allowing the gamma rays to sterilise the cancer cells. In carcinoma cervix, the tandems are inserted in the uterine cavity and the ovoids and colpostats are placed in the vaginal vault under anaesthesia. Different methods of brachytherapy are in vogue (see Fig. 23.9).

In Paris and Manchester techniques, the source strength is smaller but exposure time is increased. The vaginal source is away from the cervix. They are used with either preloaded or after loaded special applicators. One treatment period in Paris technique is 96-200 hours as compared to Stockholm technique where each application is 24-28 hours in duration (see Table 23.10). Manchester system, which is a modification of the Paris technique, delivers constant isodose at different depths, regardless of the size of the uterus and vagina.

In Stockholm technique (Fig. 23.9), large high intensity source with less exposure time is given, but the vaginal source is closer to the cervix.

These three basic techniques are followed all through the world in the brachytherapy for carcinoma cervix. After loading remote control technique (see p. 484) is used for calculated dose distribution and to prevent radiation hazard. Fletcher-Suit after loading modification system is widely used these days.

Drawbacks of radiotherapy are : Intestinal and urinary strictures, fistula formation (2-6%), vaginal fibrosis and stenosis causing dyspareunia, radiation menopause (p. 57), fibrosis of bowel and bladder. **Ovarian transposition (ovariopexy)** well out of the range of pelvic irradiation may be done to avoid radiation menopause. For other complications of radiation (see p. 486).

Calculation of the dose (see p. 488) : The radium dose is conventionally calculated with respect to the amount of radiation received at two arbitrary points A and B. **Point A** is 2 cm cephalic and 2 cm lateral to the external os and is the point of crossing of the uterine artery and ureter. **Point B** is 2 cm cephalic and 5 cm lateral at the same plane and is approximately the site of obturator gland (Fig. 30.2).

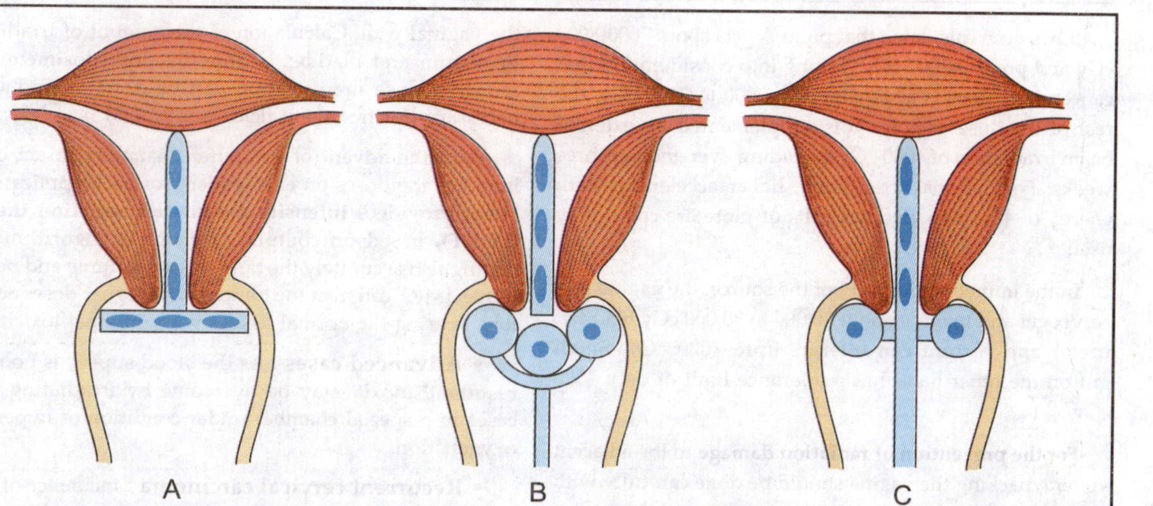

Fig. 23.9. Different methods of brachytherapy — A. Stockholm technique, B. Paris technique, C. Manchester technique

Table 23.11
Treatment modality of microinvasive (Stage Ia) and early invasive (Stage Ib, IIa) carcinoma of the cervix

Depth of invasion	*Stage*	*Pelvic lymph node involvement*	*Surgery*
• Minimal stromal invasion. • Depth of invasion < 1 mm.	Ia1	0 – 0.2%	• Simple hysterectomy. • Therapeutic conisation, if the patient so desires, provided strongly motivated for long-term follow up. Surgical margin must be free of disease.
• Invasion ≤ 3 mm. • No lymph-vascular space involvement.	Ia1	0.6%	• Extrafascial hysterectomy (Type I). • Therapeutic conisation in exceptional cases (see above).
• Stromal invasion 3-5 mm and horizontal spread 7 mm. • Lymphovascular involvement irrespective of depth of penetration.	Ia2 Ia1/Ia2	6.5%	• Radical trachelectomy (p. 339). • Modified Radical (Type II) hysterectomy with pelvic lymphadenectomy.
• Stromal invasion exceeds 5 mm.	Ib, IIa	16%	• Radical hysterectomy, pelvic lymphadenectomy (Type III) with paraaortic lymph node evaluation. External radiation if the nodes are positive OR Primary Radiation with concomitant platinum based chemotherapy.

Type I — Extrafascial hysterectomy; pubocervical ligament is incised allowing lateral deflection of the ureter. **Type II** (Modified radical). Medial half of the Mackenrodt and Uterosacral ligaments along with selective (clinically enlarged palpable) lymph nodes and upper-third (2 cm.) of vagina are removed; **Type III** (Radical hysterectomy) — The uterine artery is ligated at its origin (internal iliac artery). Uterosacral and Cardinal ligaments are resected at their attachments to the sacrum and pelvic side wall. Bilateral pelvic lymphadenectomy is done. The upper half of the vagina is resected. **Type IV** (Extended radical hysterectomy) — see p. 576. **Type V** (Partial exenteration) see p. 336.

It has been calculated that point A gets about 7000-8000 cGy and point B 2000 cGy. Taking into consideration that cancerolytic dose is approximately 7000 to 7500 cGy, the rest of the dose at point B is supplemented by external beam irradiation of 4000 cGy spreading over another three weeks. For external irradiation, linear accelerator with energy of 4 million electron volts or more are commonly used.

In the immediate vicinity of the source, the vagina and cervix get and tolerate about 20,000 to 30,000 cGy bladder, ureter and rectum can tolerate upto 7000 cGy. Small gut on the other hand has a tolerance limit of only 4500 cGy.

For the prevention of radiation damage to the adjacent viscera, packing the vagina should be done carefully with gauze around the vaginal ovoids or needles. Recent development of tungsten inserts with plastic applicator (colpostats) has minimised excess gamma irradiation of the vaginal wall. Calculation of the amount of irradiation in rectum and bladder is done by dose dosimeter and required dose modification can be done as and when necessary (for treatment field—see p. 488).

With the advent of computer dosimetry, exact calculation of the doses on each patient for each application is being provided. **Intensity modulated radiation therapy (IMRT),** based on computer generated algorithms can distinguish accurately the target tissue volume and normal tissue. IMRT can treat the tumour with higher doses accurately, sparing the normal tissues with minimal toxicity.

- **Advanced cases** : As the blood supply is poor, the resultant anoxia may be overcome by irradiating these cases in a special chamber under condition of hyperbaric oxygenation.

- **Recurrent cervical carcinoma** : Incidence of recurrence or persistent disease after therapy is about 35%. Whole pelvic irradiation with external beam radiotherapy has been advocated.

- **Carcinoma detected after simple hysterectomy**

Diagnosis of invasive carcinoma after simple hysterectomy should be treated with pelvic irradiation to a dose of 4500 rads in 5 weeks. Vault irradiation is given thereafter.

- **Stump carcinoma** : Transvaginal tandem with external beam radiotherapy is recommended.
- **Complications of radiotherapy**

Perforation of the uterus may result during introduction of uterine tandem. Radiation reactions have been discussed in detail in ch. 30 (see p. 486).

Combination therapy

In the combination therapy, either the surgery or the radiotherapy precedes or follows the other.

- *Surgery followed by radiotherapy*
  - This is indicated in cases with **positive lymph nodes** detected following surgery.
  - **Accidental discovery of invasive carcinoma cervix** of a uterus removed by simple hysterectomy.
  - When **positive tissue resection margin** is present.

The objective of this form of therapy is to sterilise the cancer cells in the pelvic lymph nodes. The fact remains that even by pelvic lymph node dissection it is not possible to remove all the positive nodes Radiation dose is reduced to 4500 cGy in 24 fractions over 5 weeks.

In such cases **adjuvant chemoradiation** — is found superior to adjuvant radiation alone (see below).

- *Radiotherapy followed by surgery*
  - **Endocervical carcinoma** with barrel-shaped cervix.
  - **Bulky tumour** : Radiotherapy controls sepsis, the growth shrinks and the tumour resectability is improved.

The surgery should be done either *within 10 days* or *6 weeks* following radiotherapy. Due to fibrosis, operation may be difficult and delay in vault healing. Chance of ureteric fistula is more. **The either of the combined therapy produces comparable 5-year survival rate.**

Neoadjuvant chemotherapy

Three cycles of platinum-based combination therapy followed by radical hysterectomy and lymphadenectomy has improved the resectability of the bulky 4 cm (stage Ib_2 and bulky IIa) disease. **The drugs used are in combination of Cisplatin, Ifosfamide, Paclitaxel or Vinorelbine.**

Laparoscopic Assisted Vaginal Radical Trachelectomy with Pelvic and Aortic Lymphadenectomy (LARVT) was designed (Daniel Dargent 1987) to treat early invasive cervical cancer (Stage Ia_2, Ib_1). This is done in a young woman where fertility and childbearing function is to be preserved. Initially pelvic and aortic lymph node dissection is done. **Vaginal radical trachelectomy is done only when these nodes are negative**. Laparoscopic approach is similar to LARVH (p. 336). Vaginal part includes resection of cervical, vaginal, paracervical and paravaginal tissues. Vaginal cuff is resected circumferentially about 2 cm below the cervicovaginal junction. Ideally the resected cervical tissue margins should be free of disease as evaluated by frozen section.

PLANNING OF TREATMENT MODALITIES

A. **Early Invasive Carcinoma (early stage disease).**

B. **Relatively Advanced Stage Disease.**

C. **Advanced Stage Disease.**

(A) **Early Stage Disease** : See Table 23.11 (p. 338)

(i) Stage Ia — See Table 23.11 (p. 338).

(ii) Stage Ib — See Table 23.11 (p. 338).

For **early stage disease**, the survival rate following treatment with either by radical hysterectomy and pelvic lymphadenectomy or with primary radiation (see p. 336) with concurrent chemotherapy (chemoradiation) are almost equal.

Radical trachelectomy (resection of the cervix) and lymphadenectomy **in early stage (Ia_1, Ia_2, Ib_1) with small tumour volume ($\leq$ 2 cm) has been done** in a selected case to preserve fertility.

(B) **Relatively Advanced Stage**

(i) Stage IIa — See Table 23.11 (p. 338).

(ii) Stage IIb — See below.

(C) **Advanced Stage Disease**

(i) **Locally advanced** :

Stage IIa to IVa : Primary chemoradiation (external beam plus brachytherapy) with concomitant cisplatin-based combined chemotherapy.

(ii) **Disseminated :**

Stage IVb : (i) Chemotherapy—Single or multiple agent. (ii) Palliative Radiation.

Concurrent chemoradiation includes radiation and weekly cisplatin-based combination chemotherapy.

Cisplatin-based concurrent chemoradiation is used as a treatment of choice in : (a) Early stage (Ia_2, Ib, IIa) disease after radical hysterectomy. (b) As a primary treatment for patients with bulky (≥ 4 cm.) tumour, (stage Ib and IIa) and (c) Locally advanced (stage IIb to IVa) disease as a primary therapy. Chemotherapy sensitises the cancer cells to radiation and improves the survival rate.

PALLIATIVE TREATMENT

Palliative treatment is primarily aimed to provide comprehensive care for relief of symptoms along with treatment of cancer in the advanced stage.

A purulent or foul vaginal discharge is treated with antimicrobial vaginal creams or suppositories.

Bleeding — Palliative radiation therapy (180-200 cGy/day) or chemotherapy may be used to relieve symptoms of pain or bleeding. Tight vaginal pack soaked in Monsel's solution (Ferric Subsulphate) against the cervix may control bleeding temporarily.

Pain — Palliation of pain is done either by reducing the pain stimulus or by raising the pain threshold. Pain from bone metastasis is mainly due to prostaglandin production. It is best controlled by using nonsteroidal anti-inflammatory drugs (NSAIDs). Palliative radiation with 3000 cGy over five treatment course may be an alternative. Anxiolytiç (benzodiazepines) or antidepressant drugs (amitriptyline) may be helpful to raise the pain threshold. Opioid (oral morphine 3-10 mg) combined with paracetamol or aspirin, given at a regular interval (4-5 hrs) is widely used to reduce pain perception.

Neuropathic pain is difficult to manage. Regional blockade with local anaesthetic techniques has been considered in some cases. Pudendal block is helpful for lower pelvic and perineal pain. Intrathecal (spinal, epidural) opioids are appropriate for pain from any region. Unilateral cordotomy (C 1-2) is considered for widespread pain which is refractory.

CARCINOMA OF CERVIX AND PREGNANCY

Incidence of invasive carcinoma of the cervix is about one in 2500 pregnancies.

Diagnosis is often late. Cone biopsy may be necessary for confirmation. **Complications of cone biopsy include** : haemorrhage, abortion, preterm labour and infection (see p. 561).

Management : The following points are taken into consideration before actual management : (A) period of gestation, (B) survival of the fetus and (C) wishes of the patient.

(A) **Patient with microinvasive carcinoma** may be followed up to term. Patient is revaluated following delivery and treated as in the nonpregnant state.

(B) **Advanced stage** : In the first trimester, treatment modality is the same as in the nonpregnant state. In late pregnancy, following maturity, fetus is delivered by classical caesarean section. Subsequent treatment with either radical surgery or radiotherapy is the same as in the nonpregnant state.

Prognosis : Clinical stage of the disease is the single most important prognostic factor. Stage for stage survival outcome appears to be no different between pregnancy and nonpregnant state (for details see author's Textbook of Obstetrics, ch. 21).

RESULTS OF THERAPY FOR CARCINOMA CERVIX

The result of therapy is expressed in terms of 5-year survival rate. The over all 5-year survival rate is tabulated in Table 23.12.

Table 23.12

Stage	5-year survival rate (%)
IIa	76.0
IIb	73.3
IIIa	50.5
IIIb	46.4
IVa	29.6
IVb	22.0

There is about 30 per cent recurrence after 5 years. The recurrence **sites are** in the side wall of the pelvis and central pelvis. **A patient is declared cured if remains well even after 10 years following initial therapy**. The chance of survival rate of the patient after the symptoms appear, if left untreated, is about 2 years.

Recurrent cervical cancer

Risk factors for recurrent disease are : Large tumour

size, lymph-vascular space invasion, positive lymph nodes, advanced stage disease.

Most common site of recurrence is pelvic side wall. Features of disease recurrence are : pain in the pelvis, back, unilateral leg oedema ureteral obstruction, vaginal bleeding, palpable tumour in the pelvis and lymphadenopathy. Single agent or multiagent chemotherapy with cisplatin, paclitaxel or Ifosfamide is used. Palliative radiation therapy may be used who have been treated initially with surgery.

Follow up : The majority of the recurrences occur in the first two years. As such, the follow up protocols should be at 3-4 months interval for the first two years then at 6 months interval for next 2 years and there after annually. Thorough physical examination is done including examination of supraclavicular and inguinal lymph nodes. Cervical or vaginal cytology is performed. X-ray chest is done annually.

STUMP CARCINOMA

When the carcinoma develops in the cervical stump left behind after subtotal hysterectomy, it is called stump carcinoma. **In true stump carcinoma**, malignancy develops 2 years after primary surgery. If it occurs earlier to that, it is presumed that the carcinoma was present at the time of primary surgery and as such it is called coincidental, residual or false stump carcinoma.

The incidence may be as high as 1 per cent. It is difficult to stage the disease.

There is also difficulty in the **treatment**. Dense adhesions of bladder, rectum and also ureters with the stump make the operation difficult and risky. The radiation therapy is also technically difficult, because of absence of uterus and close proximity of bladder and rectum to the radiation source. Radical parametrectomy, removal of cervix, upper vagina and pelvic lymphadenectomy is done in early stage disease.

External beam radiation therapy is given when the cervix is short. Vaginal radium application (vaginal ovoids) is also used. The prognosis is unfavourable. The 5-year survival rate varies from 30-60 per cent.

ENDOMETRIAL CARCINOMA

Incidence

The incidence is higher amongst the white population of United States and lowest in India and Japan. In North America, amongst the whites, carcinoma body is the leading site of genital malignancy followed by ovary and cervix. In USA, a woman has about 1 per cent chance of developing endometrial carcinoma during her lifetime. In India, it ranks third amongst genital malignancy next to cervix and ovary.

While in the Western countries, there has been increased incidence of carcinoma body relative to cervical one and the ratio becomes almost 1:1; in India, the incidence still remains low and the ratio ranges *between 1 : 8 and 1 : 15.* **The high prevalence of cancer cervix may be due to** early marriage, multiparity, poor local hygienic care and childbirth trauma to the cervix.

The higher incidence in the Western countries may be real or apparent. The real one is due to high expectation of life and injudicious use of oestrogen in postmenopausal women and the apparent one is due to its detection, out of increased awareness amongst the gynaecologists.

Aetiology

The following are found to be related to carcinoma body of the uterus :

- **Oestrogen** — Persistent stimulation of endometrium with unopposed oestrogen is the single most important factor for the development of endometrial cancer.
- **Age** — About 75 per cent are postmenopausal with a median age of 60 (c.f. Carcinoma cervix is more common in perimenopausal period). About 10 per cent of women with postmenopausal bleeding have endometrial cancer.
- **Parity** — It is quite common in unmarried and in married, nulliparity is associated in about 30 per cent. (c.f. – Carcinoma cervix is associated more with multiparae).
- **Late menopause** — The chance of carcinoma increases, if menopause fails to occur beyond 52 years.
- **Corpus cancer syndrome** — encompasses – obesity, hypertension and diabetes.
- **Obesity** leads to high level of free oestradiol as the sex hormone binding globulin level is low.
- **Unopposed oestrogen stimulation** in conditions such as functioning ovarian tumours (granulosa cell) or polycystic ovarian syndrome (PCOS) is associated with increased risk of endometrial cancer. Unopposed oestrogen replacement therapy (see p. 318) in postmenopausal women is associated with increased risk of endometrial cancer. Use of cyclic progestin reduces the risk. Prior use of combined oral contraceptives reduces the risk significantly (50%).

• **Tamoxifen** is antioestrogenic as well as weakly oestrogenic. It is used for the treatment of breast cancer. Increased risk of endometrial cancer is noted when it is used for a long time due to its weak oestrogenic effect.

• **Family history or personal history** of colon, ovarian or breast cancer increases the risk of endometrial cancer. Genetic inheritance (Lynch 11 syndrome family) is currently thought (see p. 496).

• **Fibroid** is associated in about 30 per cent cases.

• **Endometrial hyperplasia** precedes carcinoma in about 25 per cent cases.

Pathology

Naked eye — The uterus may be smaller, normal or even enlarged (due to myohyperplasia, myometrial involvement, pyometra or associated fibroid). Two varieties are found :

• **Localised** • **Diffuse**

Localised :The usual site is on the fundus. It is either sessile or pedunculated. Myometrial involvement is late.

Diffuse : The spread is through the endometrium. The myometrium is commonly invaded; may invade to reach the serosal coat (Fig. 23.10).

Microscopic appearances

The following varieties are noted :

- Adenocarcinoma (endometrioid 80%) (Fig. 23.11).

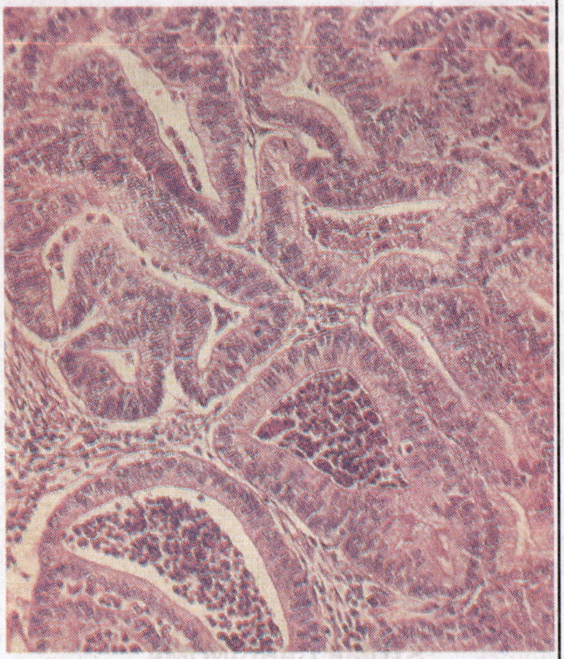

Fig. 23.11. Adenocarcinoma of the endometrium, the commonest histologic type. There is significant cellular mitotic activity. The glands are arranged back-to-back.

- Adenocarcinoma with squamous elements.
- Uterine papillary serous carcinoma (5-10%).
- Mucinous adenocarcinoma (5%).
- Clear cell adenocarcinoma (5%).
- Secretory carcinoma (1%).
- Squamous cell carcinoma.
- Mixed carcinoma.

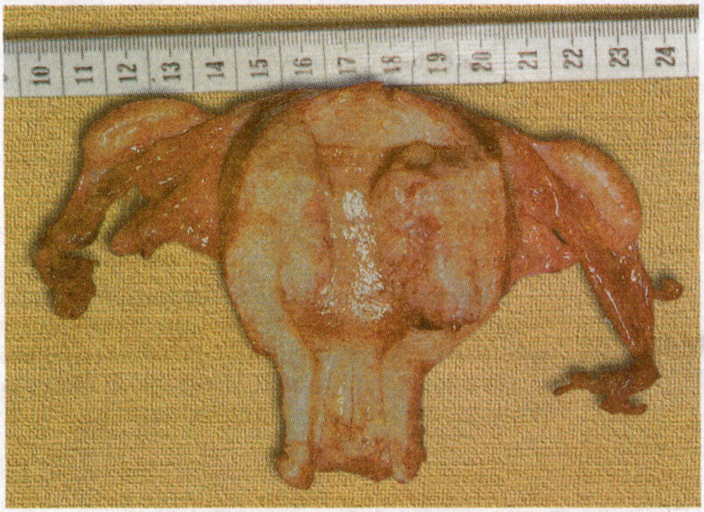

Fig. 23.10. Diffuse type of endometrial carcinoma
[By courtesy Dr. (Mrs.) Pampa Sarkar]

Spread

Direct

As it is slow growing, it is confined to the stroma for a long time but eventually, it spreads in all directions. Thus, it may infiltrate the myometrium and spread to the parametrium or into the peritoneal cavity. It may spread downwards to involve the cervix in about 15 per cent.

Lymphatic

The lymphatic spread is usually late. Lymphatic spread involves **pelvic, paraaortic (through infundibulopelvic ligament) and rarely inguinal**

and femoral (through lymphatics of round ligament) nodes.

Lymph node metastasis depends on the degree of tumour differentiation, myometrial invasion, tumour size and the surgical pathological stage of the disease. Pelvic lymph node involvement in stage I disease varies from about 4 per cent in grade 1 and 2 disease with superficial myometrial involvement to about 40 per cent with grade 3 tumour with deep myometrial invasion. Approximately 50 per cent of the patients with pelvic lymph nodes will have paraaortic lymph node metastasis. In stage II disease incidence of pelvic lymph node metastasis increases to 30-45 per cent. Lymph node metastasis is the most important prognostic factor.

The **tubes and ovaries** are involved (3-5%) either by direct spread or by lymphatics.

The vagina is involved in about 10-15 per cent cases. The metastasis to the lower-third of the anterior vaginal wall is probably through lymphatic or by retrograde venous flow. The vault metastasis following hysterectomy may be due to direct implantation or may be explained by previous lymphatic or venous embolism.

Blood borne

Blood borne spread occurs late. The common sites of metastases are lungs, liver, bones and brain.

Staging

The staging is based on clinical examination supplemented by fractional curettage and is that adopted by FIGO (1989). Approximately 75 per cent patients present with stage I disease.

Clinical staging for invasive endometrial carcinoma (FIGO–1971)

Stage I	The carcinoma is confined to the corpus.
Stage Ia	The length of the uterine cavity is 8 cm or less.
Stage Ib	The length of the uterine cavity is more than 8 cm.
	Histological subgroup of Stage I
G_1	Highly differentiated adenocarcinoma.
G_2	Moderately differentiated adenocarcinoma with partly solid areas.
G_3	Predominantly solid or entirely undifferentiated carcinoma.
Stage II	The carcinoma has involved the corpus and the cervix but has not extended outside the uterus.
Stage III	The carcinoma has extended outside the uterus but not outside the true pelvis.
Stage IV	The carcinoma has extended outside the true pelvis or has obviously involved the mucosa of the bladder or rectum. A bullous oedema as such does not permit a case to be alloted to stage IV.
Stage IVa	Spread of the growth to the adjacent organs.
Stage IVb	Spread to distant organs.

CLINICAL FEATURES

Patient profile

The patient is usually a nullipara, likely to be postmenopausal. There may be history of delayed menopause. She may be obese; likely to have hypertension or diabetes (Table 23.13).

Symptoms

- Postmenopausal bleeding (75%) which may be slight, irregular or continuous. The bleeding at times may be excessive.
- In premenopausal women, there may be irregular and excessive bleeding.
- At time, there is watery and offensive discharge due to pyometra.
- Pain is not uncommon. It may be colicky due to uterine contractions in an attempt to expel the polypoidal growth.
- Few patients (< 5%) remain asymptomatic.

Signs : The patient presents with the features as mentioned in patient profile. There may be varying degrees of pallor.

Pelvic examination

Speculum examination reveals the cervix looking healthy and the blood or purulent offensive discharge escapes out of the external os.

Bimanual examination reveals — The uterus is either atrophic, normal or may be enlarged due to spread of the tumour, associated fibroid or pyometra. The uterus is usually mobile unless in late stage, when it becomes fixed.

Rectal examination corroborates the bimanual findings.

Regional lymph nodes and breasts are examined carefully.

DIAGNOSIS OF ENDOMETRIAL CARCINOMA

The following guidelines are prescribed:

- A case of postmenopausal bleeding is considered to be due to endometrial carcinoma unless proved otherwise.
- Finding a benign condition to account for postmenopausal bleeding does not negate a thorough investigation to rule out carcinoma. The two lesions may co-exist.
- History and clinical examination are to be recorded, as mentioned earlier.
- **Endometrial biopsy** – using a Sharman curette or a soft, flexible, plastic suction cannula (pipelle) has been done with reliability (90%). This is done as an outpatient procedure (Fig. 9.22).
- **Papanicolaou smear** is not a reliable diagnostic test for endometrial carcinoma. It is positive only in 30 per cent cases of endometrial cancer.
- **Ultrasound and colour doppler (TVS)**: Findings suggestive of endometrial carcinoma are — (i) Endometrial thickness > 5 mm. (ii) Hyperechoic endometrium with irregular outline. (iii) Increased vascularity with low vascular resistance. (iv) Intrauterine fluid. However, it cannot replace definitive biopsy.
- **Hysteroscopy** — helps in direct visualisation of endometrium and to take target biopsy. Its role in diagnosis is yet to be established.
- **Fractional curettage** — is not only **the definite method of diagnosis** but can detect the extent of growth. This is done under anaesthesia with utmost gentleness to prevent perforation of the uterus. If pyometra is detected, the procedure is withheld for about one week to avoid perforation and systemic infection.

The Orderly steps for fractional curettage:

- Endocervical curettage (ECC).
- To pass an uterine sound to note the length of the uterocervical canal.
- Dilatation of the internal os.
- Uterine curettage at the fundus and lower part of the body. The endometrial tissue is usually profuse and often dark colour.
- Finally, a polyp forceps is introduced in case any endometrial polyp has escaped the curette.

The specimens, so obtained, should be placed in **separate containers**, labelled properly and submitted for histological examination.

- **Computed Tomography (CT) scan** of pelvis and abdomen may be used to detect lymph node metastases (p. 114).
- **Magnetic Resonance Imaging (MRI)** can detect myometrial invasion (see p. 625).
- **Positron Emission Tomography (see p. 115).**

Surgical staging

Increased inaccuracy of clinical staging and the importance of prognostic factors some of which can only be identified surgically, result in introduction of surgicopathological staging by FIGO in 1989.

Surgical staging of endometrial carcinoma (FIGO 1989)

	Description
Stage Ia (G123)	Tumour limited to endometrium
Stage Ib (G123)	Invasion < 1/2 myometrium
Stage Ic (G123)	Invasion > 1/2 myometrium
Stage IIa (G123)	Endocervical glandular involvement only
Stage IIb (G123)	Cervical stromal invasion
Stage IIIa (G123)	Tumour invades serosa and/or adnexae and/or positive peritoneal cytology
Stage IIIb (G123)	Vaginal metastases
Stage IIIc (G123)	Metastases to pelvic and/or para-aortic lymph nodes
Stage IVa (G123)	Tumour involves bladder and/or bowel mucosa
Stage IVb (G123)	Distant metastases including intra-abdominal and/or inguinal lymph node

Depending upon the percentage of solid component, G1 has ≤ 5% (solid, nonsquamous component), G2 has 6–50% and G3 has > 50% of these features.

MANAGEMENT OF ENDOMETRIAL CARCINOMA

- **Preventive** • **Curative**

PREVENTIVE

Primary prevention includes:

- Strict weight control beginning early in life
- To restrict the use of oestrogen after meno-

pause in nonhysterectomised women. If at all it is needed, cyclic administration of progestogen preparations are added and continued under supervision.

• Education as regard the significance of irregular bleeding per vaginam in perimenopausal and postmenopausal period.

Secondary prevention includes :

• Screening of 'high risk' women at least in menopausal period to detect the premalignant or early carcinoma is a positive step.

Methods

• The cytologic specimens are obtained by either endometrial aspiration or endometrial lavage. If suspicious cells are detected, histological specimen is obtained by uterine curettage.

• The presence of abnormal endometrial cells in vaginal pool cytology requires a diagnostic curettage.

• Judicial hysterectomy in premalignant lesions of the corpus (see p. 319).

Table 23.13
'High risk' factors for Endometrial Cancer

- Late menopause.
- Nulliparity.
- Unopposed oestrogen therapy.
- History of persistent anovulation (PCOS).
- History of irregular and excessive premenopausal bleeding.
- Obesity, diabetes, hypertension.
- Personal or family history of breast, ovary, colon or endometrial cancer.
- Atypical endometrial hyperplasia (p. 317).
- Tamoxifen therapy.
- Radiation menopause.

CURATIVE

Pretreatment work up

As the patients are usually aged, obese and often complicated with medical disorders, careful systemic examination and necessary investigations are mandatory before formulating the line of treatment. Along with a gynaecologic oncologist, a physician's help may be needed.

Pretreatment preparations (Table 23.14).

The same protocol as mentioned in cases of carcinoma cervix is to be followed.

TREATMENT MODALITIES OF CARCINOMA ENDOMETRIUM

- **Surgery**
- **Radiotherapy**
- **Chemotherapy**
- **Combined therapy**

Table 23.14 : Preoperative evaluation

- Blood examination — Haemoglobin percentage, total and differential count, postprandial sugar, urea, creatinine and electrolytes.
- Urine — Routine examination for – protein, sugar and pus cells.
- ECG and X-ray chest for cardiopulmonary assessment.
- Pelvic ultrasonography.
- Magnetic resonance imaging (optional) to assess the extrauterine spread of the disease and the degree of myometrial invasion.
- Liver and renal function tests.
- Steroid receptor status.
- Serum marker – CA 125.

SURGERY

Extrafascial hysterectomy is the preferred treatment for endometrial carcinoma confined to the body. The surgery includes removal of the uterus, tubes and ovaries of both the sides and cuff of vagina. Removal of vaginal cuff is not essential as it neither improves the survival nor reduces the recurrence rate.

IN STAGE I, SURGERY IS THE MAINSTAY OF TREATMENT

Surgical procedures (surgical staging p. 344)

• **Incision** longitudinal midline or paramedian is of choice for better exposure.

• **Peritoneal washings** are taken for cytology.

• **Thorough exploration** of liver, diaphragm, omentum, pelvic organs, pelvic and paraaortic lymph nodes, is done.

• **Suturing** the cervix and fimbrial end of the fallopian tubes to prevent tumour cells spillage during operation are not essential.

• **Not to hold** the uterus by a vulsellum. Instead, traction is given by placing long straight artery forceps on either side of uterine cornu (Fig. 34.4).

• **Total abdominal hysterectomy (extrafascial)** with bilateral salpingo-oophorectomy is performed.

• **Uterus** is cut opened in the operating room – for evaluation of tumour size, cervical extension and myometrial invasion.

• **Presence of big tumour (>2 cm)**, cervical extension, poor tumour differentiation and myometrial invasion (>1/2 thickness) as determined by frozen section biopsy, indicates pelvic and paraaortic lymph node sampling.

• **Lymph node sampling** of the following areas are done : (i) Common iliac (ii) External iliac (iii) Internal iliac (iv) Obturator and (v) Paraaortic.

• **Vaginal hysterectomy** may be done selectively (stage I, with well-differentiated tumour) in patients with uterovaginal prolapse or with extreme obesity.

• **Laparoscopic assisted** vaginal hysterectomy (LAVH) with bilateral salpingo-oophorectomy and lymph node sampling are done for staging and treatment of endometrial carcinoma (stage I).

In Stage II, Carcinoma

• **Radical hysterectomy** (see p. 335) or **Radiation** (external pelvic and intracavitary cesium) therapy followed by extrafascial hysterectomy (see above) in 6 weeks time is recommended.

RADIOTHERAPY

The primary treatment by radiotherapy is indicated in :

- Women found medically unfit for surgery.
- Surgically inoperable disease.
- Those with high-risk of recurrence.
- **Patients with Stage III and IV :**

  Whole abdomen is irradiated (3000 cGy) shielding the kidneys, with a pelvic boost (2000 cGy) and additional dose (1500 cGy) to the paraaortic lymph nodes.

Contraindications radiotherapy : Presence of a pelvic mass, pelvic kidney, pyometra, pelvic abscess, previous laparotomies and/or adhesions with bowel and prior pelvic radiation.

COMBINED THERAPY (SURGERY AND RADIATION)

Combined therapy has shown high degree of success in this disease.

Extrafascial hysterectomy followed by irradiation therapy 4-6 weeks after surgery, in a selected case, is done **to prevent tumour recurrence**.

• **No myometrial invasion stage Ia** (G1, 2) : Observation only.

• **Myometrial invasion < 1/2 thickness (stage Ib or stage Ia G3 disease)** : Vaginal vault radiation (6000-7000 cGy) using colpostats after loading techniques.

• **Myometrial invasion > 1/2 thickness (stage Ic)** : Whole pelvis external beam radiation (4500-5000 cGy) over 5-6 weeks plus vaginal cuff boost.

• **Lymph node metastasis (stage IIIb, IIIc)** : Extended field (pelvic, common iliac and paraaortic nodes) radiation. Paraaortic radiation dose is 4500 to 5000 cGy. It improves the survival rate.

Stage III and IV Endometrial Cancer

Whole abdomen irradiation (3000 cGy with kidney shielding) plus 1500 cGy to the paraaortic nodes and 2000 cGy to the pelvis.

• **External pelvic and intracavitary radiation followed by extended hysterectomy** 6 weeks later in cases of :

– Highly anaplastic tumour

– Growth extending to the cervix

CHEMOTHERAPY

Chemotherapy is used in advanced and recurrent cases or in metastatic lesions.

• **Progestogens** — are widely used. The response is good in well-differentiated carcinoma with adequate oestrogen and progesterone receptors (see p. 508).

Any one of the drugs – 17 hydroxyprogesterone caproate (1 gm/wk. I M), medroxy progesterone acetate (1 gm/wk. I M or 150 mg/day oral) or megesterol acetate (160 mg/day orally) is of use. The drug is to be continued for at least 3 months. If responsive, may be continued for longer period with reduced doses.

• **Tamoxifen is** a nonsteroidal agent with anti-oestrogenic as well as weakly oestrogenic properties. It is used 10 mg twice daily along with progestogen therapy. It blocks the tissue oestrogen receptor. It is effective in patients with hormone receptor positive tumours (see p. 508).

• **Cytotoxic drugs** — are being tried either singly or in combination but without any superiority over the hormonal therapy. The drugs commonly used are adriamycin, cisplatin, carboplatin, paclitaxel and cyclophosphamide (see ch. 30, Table 30.7).

Recurrent disease

Common sites for recurrence are the vagina and the pelvis. The extrapelvic metastases are seen in the lung, lymph nodes (aortic), liver, brain and bones. Majority (60%) of recurrences are seen within 2 years of initial therapy.

- Radiation therapy is the choice for isolated recurrence following surgical treatment.
- Exenterative surgery for recurrent endometrial cancer is of limited value.
- Hormonal therapy and chemotherapy (see p. 489) have been used depending on the individual case.

Follow up of patients

Following initial therapy, patient is examined every 4 months for the first 2 years, every 6 months for next 2 years and thereafter annually. Evaluation of symptoms, thorough clinical examination and X-ray chest (annual) are essential. Other investigations are : mammography (annual) and CT, MRI when clinically indicated. Regular estimation of serum CA 125 may be helpful in some cases.

Table 23.15
Prognostic factors in endometrial adenocarcinoma

- Age at diagnosis (older the patient poorer the prognosis).
- Stage of the disease.
- Histologic type (typical adenocarcinomas — better prognosis, papillary serous carcinoma — poor prognosis).
- Histologic differentiation.
- Histologic grade (p. 344) : grade 3 tumours have 5 times more risk of recurrence and low 5 year survival rate.
- Myometrial penetration.
- Lymphovascular space invasion.
- Lymph node metastasis.
- Extension to cervix.
- Peritoneal cytology.
- Tumour size (>2 cm → more lymph node metastasis).
- Hormone receptor status (receptor positive tumours have got better prognosis).
- Ploidy status — aneuploid tumours have got poor prognosis compared to diploid tumours.
- Oncogene expression — HER – 2/neu, poor prognosis (see ch. 30, p. 496).

Place of hormone replacement therapy

Oestrogen replacement therapy to combat the oestrogen deficiency symptoms following treatment of endometrial cancer is a debatable issue. In a patient with severe postmenopausal symptoms progestin (medroxy progesterone acetate, 5-10 mg daily) may be a choice. Non-hormonal therapy (clonidine) can also be used (p. 58). Urogenital symptoms can be improved using topical oestrogen (p. 60).

Prognosis

The poorly differentiated tumour, the greater degree of myometrial penetration, lymphovascular space invasion and the advanced stages are prognostically poor. Aneuploid tumours are prognostically worst. Histologically non-endometrioid tumours are aggressive and carry increased risk of recurrence. The prognostic factors to be considered are tabulated in Table 23.15.

Table 23.16 : 5-year survival rate

Stage	*Overall survival rate (%)*
I	81 – 91
II	67 – 77
III	30 – 60
IV	5 – 20

GESTATIONAL TROPHOBLASTIC NEOPLASIA (GTN)

Gestational Trophoblastic Neoplasia (GTN) is a spectrum of abnormal growth and development of the trophoblasts that continue even beyond the end of pregnancy. GTN encompasses persistent hydatidiform mole, invasive mole, choriocarcinoma and a rare entity of placental site trophoblastic tumour (Table 23.17).

Diagnosis of postmolar GTN is made when the hCG level plateaus for 3 or more consecutive weeks or reelevates. **This may occur in 15-20 per cent following hydatidiform mole.** Some, however, follow abortion, ectopic and even normal pregnancy.

Persistent Gestational Trophoblastic Neoplasia (GTN) : Persistent GTN is evidenced by persistence of trophoblastic activity following evacuation of molar pregnancy. **This is clinically diagnosed** when the patient presents with (a) Irregular vaginal bleeding. (b) Subinvolution of the uterus. (c) Persistence of theca lutein cysts and (d) Level of hCG either plateaus or reelevates after an initial fall. After molar evacuation serum β hCG becomes normal in about 7-9 weeks.

Postmolar GTN of serious nature may be either invasive mole or choriocarcinoma but **GTN after non-molar pregnancy is always a choriocarcinoma**.

Incidence

The incidence of GTN is about 1 in 5000 pregnancies in oriental countries and 1 in 50,000 in Europe and North America. More than fifty per cent occur after molar pregnancy, about 25 per cent after abortion and/or ectopic pregnancy and a few after normal pregnancy. **Non-metastatic (locally invasive) lesions develop in 15 per cent and metastatic lesions develop in about 4 per cent of patients after molar evacuation.**

Placental site Trophoblastic tumour

The tumour arises from the trophoblast of the placental bed. Incidence is about 1 per cent of all patients with GTN. 15-20 per cent of these patients develop metastases. Syncytiotrophoblast cells are generally absent, instead intermediate trophoblast cells predominant. β hCG secretion is low but human placental lactogen (hPL) is secreted and this is monitored during the follow up. **The entity is not responsive to chemotherapy. Hysterectomy is the preferred treatment. Serial serum hPL** may be a reliable marker and hPL is useful for immunohistochemical staining to confirm the diagnosis.

INVASIVE MOLE
(Chorioadenoma destruens)

Invasive mole comprises about 15 per cent of all GTN.

The prominent features of this type of mole are invasive and destructive potentialities. Invasive mole shows abnormal penetration through the muscle layers of the uterus. The uterine wall may be perforated at multiple areas showing purple, fungating growth with massive intraperitoneal haemorrhage. The neoplasm may invade the pelvic blood vessels and metastasises to vagina or distant sites as like those in choriocarcinoma.

Diagnosis

- **On laparotomy** — (a) Perforation of the uterus through which purple fungating growth is visible. (b) Haemoperitoneum.

- **Histology** — There is penetration of the uterine wall by the hyperplastic trophoblastic cells which **still retain villus structures. There is no evidence of muscle necrosis** (Fig. 23.12). The materials for uterine curettage are often deceptive as the lesion may be deep inside the myometrium.

- **Persistent high level** of urinary or serum hCG.

Table 23.17
Gestational trophoblastic neoplasia (GTN)

- Persistent hydatidiform mole
- Invasive mole
- Choriocarcinoma
- Placental site trophoblastic tumour

- **Non-metastatic disease (confined to the uterus)**
- **Metastatic disease:**

A. Low risk (good prognosis)
- Disease is present < 4 months duration
- Initial serum hCG level < 40,000 mIU/ml
- Metastasis limited to lung and vagina
- No prior chemotherapy

B. High risk (poor prognosis)
- Long duration of disease (> 4 months)
- Initial serum hCG > 40,000 mIU/ml
- Brain or liver metastasis
- Failure of prior chemotherapy
- Following term pregnancy
- WHO score ≥ 7 (see p. 351)

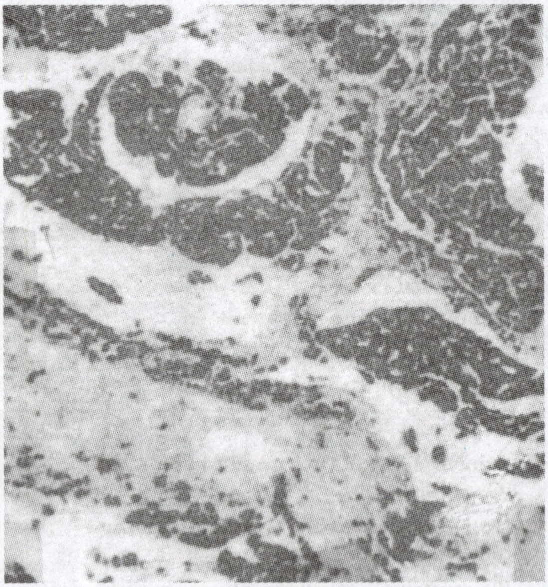

Fig. 23.12. Histological section of invasive mole showing structures of villi with marked trophoblastic proliferation deep in myometrium

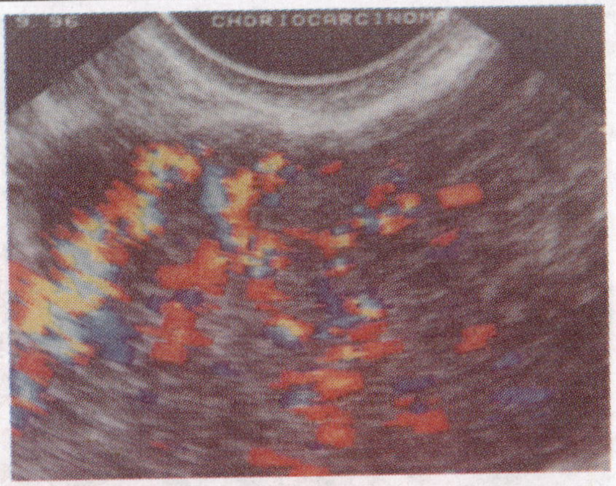

Fig. 23.13. Transvaginal colour Doppler scan of choriocarcinoma showing randomly dispersed vessels

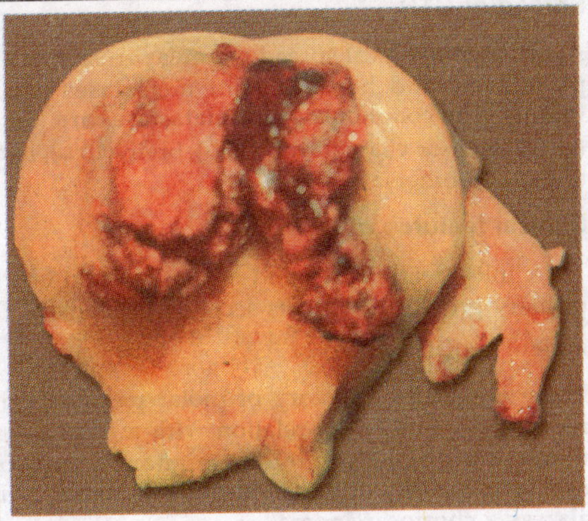

Fig. 23.14. Choriocarcinoma of diffuse type

CHORIOCARCINOMA

Choriocarcinoma is a highly malignant tumour arising from the chorionic epithelium. It should be remembered that it is not a tumour of the uterus which is secondarily involved.

About 3-5 per cent of all patients with molar pregnancies develop choriocarcinoma. Amongst all patients with choriocarcinoma, around 50 per cent develop following a hydatidiform mole, 30 per cent occur after a miscarriage or an ectopic pregnancy and 20 per cent after an apparently normal pregnancy. **Trophoblastic disease following a normal pregnancy is either choriocarcinoma or PSTT and not a benign or invasive mole.**

Pathology : The primary site is usually any where in the uterus. Rarely, it starts in the tube or ovary. Ovarian choriocarcinoma (non-gestational) may also be associated with malignant teratoma or dysgerminoma.

Naked eye appearances (Fig. 23.14)

The lesion is usually localised nodular type. It looks red, haemorrhagic and necrotic. At times, the lesion is diffuse involving the entire endometrium. The nodular type may be located deep in the myometrium with overlying endometrium intact. This often gives the false-negative diagnosis on uterine curettage.

Microscopic appearance (Fig. 23.15)

There are anaplastic sheets or columns of trophoblastic cells invading the uterine musculature. There are **evidences of necrosis and haemorrhage. Villus pattern is completely absent.**

Ovarian enlargement : Bilateral lutein cysts are present in about 30 per cent. These are due to excessive production of chorionic gonadotrophin.

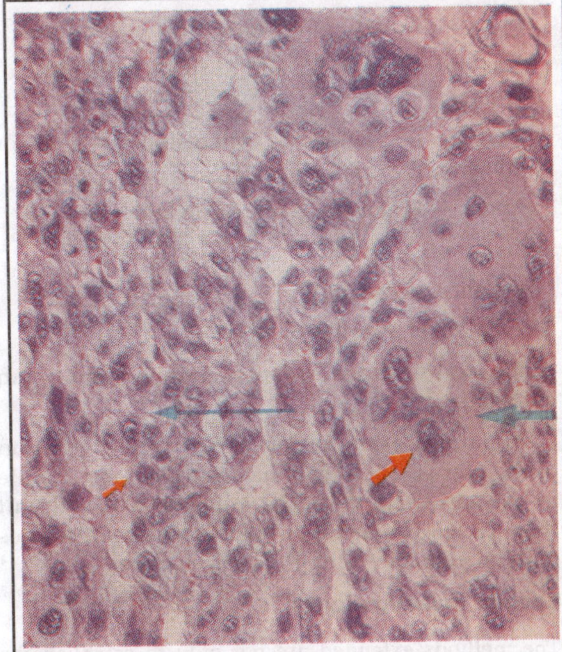

Fig. 23.15. Histologic picture of choriocarcinoma. The cytotrophoblast cells are well-defined with clear cytoplasm (thin arrow). The syncitiotrophoblast cells are arranged in sheets of multi-nucleated cytoplasm (thick arrow)

Spread of GTN

Apart from the local spread, vascular erosion takes place early and hence distant metastases occur rapidly. **The common sites of metastases are** lungs (80%), anterior vaginal wall (30%), brain (10%), liver (10%) and others.

Clinical features of GTN

The clinical features depend on the location of the primary growth and on its secondary deposits.

Patient profile

There is usually a history of molar pregnancy in recent past. Rarely, its relation with a term pregnancy, abortion or ectopic pregnancy may be established. **GTN after a non-molar pregnancy is always a choriocarcinoma**.

Symptoms

The following are the usual symptoms :

- Persistent ill health.
- Irregular vaginal bleeding, at times brisk.
- Continued amenorrhoea.

Other symptoms due to metastatic lesions are :

Lung — Cough, breathlessness, haemoptysis.

Vaginal — Irregular and at times brisk haemorrhage.

Cerebral — Headache, convulsion, paralysis or coma.

Liver — Epigastric pain, jaundice.

Signs

- Patient looks ill.
- Pallor of varying degrees.

Physical signs are evident according to the organ involved.

Bimanual examination reveals subinvolution of the uterus. There may be a purplish red nodule in the lower-third of the anterior vaginal wall (Fig. 23.16). Unilateral or bilateral enlarged ovaries may be palpable through lateral fornices.

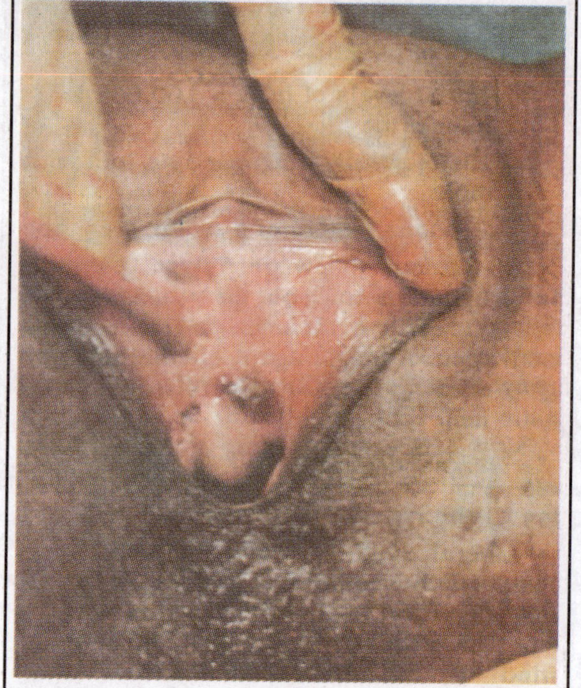

Fig. 23.16. Note the purplish red metastatic nodule in the lower third of anterior vaginal wall (sub-urethral). Metastases may occur in vaginal fornices also.

Special investigations

The methods extended are not only to establish the diagnosis but also to note the metastatic sites which help in staging.

hCG titres : Irrespective of the site of lesion — non-metastatic or metastatic, β hCG levels are raised both in the 24 hour urine and serum. Excess of 2 mIU/ml in serum is of value, if pregnancy is excluded. If following primary treatment of molar pregnancy, the hCG titres remain elevated or become positive after a negative report, it is very much suggestive of developing choriocarcinoma provided pregnancy is excluded. Metastatic brain lesion is suspected when the ratio of hCG in spinal fluid/in serum is more than 1 : 60.

Chest X-ray : X-ray shows 'cannon ball' shadow or 'snow storm' appearance due to numerous tumour emboli (Fig. 23.17). Pleural effusion may be present.

Pelvic sonography : Sonography helps not only to localise the lesion but to differentiate GTN from a normal pregnancy.

Diagnostic uterine curettage : Pretherapy D and C reduces the intrauterine tumour bulk. However, routine D and C for histologic diagnosis is not required. It reveals the characteristic histological pattern (p. 359). It is emphasised that, the curetted material may not reveal the diagnosis in all the cases, as the lesion may be deep in the myometrium or the uterus may not be the primary site. One should be very careful and alert while doing uterine curettage as brisk haemorrhage may occur for which a life saving hysterectomy may have to be done.

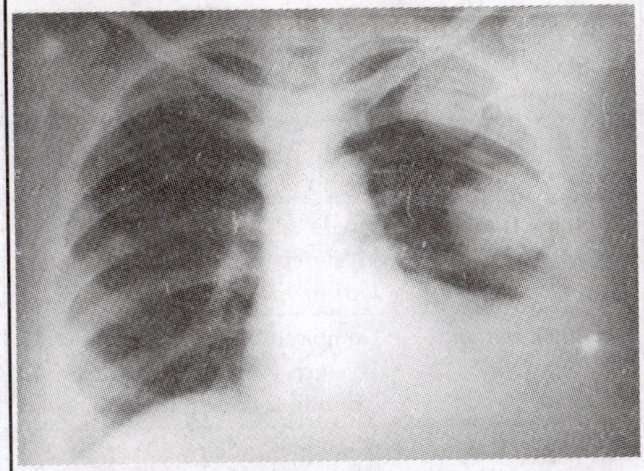

Fig. 23.17. Cannon ball shadow in the left apical and mid region of the lung with pleural effusion in choriocarcinoma [*By courtesy — Eden Hospital, M.C.H., Calcutta*]

WHO Prognostic Scoring System of Gestational Trophoplastic Disease as modified by FIGO (2000)

Parameter	Score			
	0	1	2	4
Age (years)	< 39	> 39	—	—
Antecedent pregnancy	Mole	Abortion	Term	—
Interval (month)‡	< 4	4 – 6	7 – 12	≥ 13
Pretreatment hCG (IU/L)	< 10^3	10^3–10^4	10^4–10^5	> 10^5
Largest tumour (cm)	< 3	3 – 5	> 5	—
Site of metastases	Lung Pelvis	Spleen Kidney	GI tract Liver	Brain
No. of metastases detected	—	1–4	5–8	> 8
Previous chemotherapy	—	—	Single drug	Multiple drugs

Total score = < 6 is low risk and a total score ≥ 7 is high risk.
‡ Interval : Time between antecedent pregnancy and start of chemotherapy.

For diagnosis of metastases :

Vaginal nodules

• Excision biopsy or biopsy should not be done. Massive haemorrhage following resection, may need packing or selective embolisation.

Cerebral : • The ratio of hCG levels in spinal fluid and serum is higher than 60.
• CT scan or MRI.

Liver : • CT scan.

Metastases to other sites are uncommon when pelvic examination and chest X-ray are normal. However, chest CT may show micrometastases which are not visible on a chest radiograph.

Staging : The anatomic staging for gestational trophoblastic tumours (GTT) as described by FIGO is tabulated below :

FIGO Anatomic staging for GTT	
Stage I	The lesion is confined to the uterus.
Stage II	The lesion spreads outside the uterus but is confined to the genital organs.
Stage III	The lesion metastasises to the lungs.
Stage IV	The lesion metastasises to sites such as brain, liver or gastrointestinal tract.

The drawbacks of the anatomic staging are :

- As the site of lesion cannot be located precisely, even though hCG is elevated, it is not logical to categorise the lesion to be as stage I.
- It does not help in treatment.
- The prognosis is poorly correlated.

MANAGEMENT OF GTN

• **Preventive** • **Curative**

Preventive

• **Prophylactic chemotherapy** in 'at risk' women following evacuation of molar pregnancy may be considered. It prevents uterine invasion or metastasis. 'At risk' women are :

– Age of patient > 35 years.
– Initial levels of serum hCG ≥ 100,000 IU/ml.
– hCG level fails to become normal by 7-9 weeks time or there is re-elevation.
– Histologically diagnosed as infiltrative mole.
– Evidence of metastases irrespective of the level of hCG.
– Previous history of a molar pregnancy.
– Woman who is unreliable for follow up.

Disadvantage of routine chemotherapy is unnecessary exposure of the toxic drugs to all women who may not need it. Majority (80-90%) of women do not develop persistent GTN.

• **Meticulous follow up** following evacuation of hydatidiform mole is essential for at least 6 months to detect early evidences of trophoblastic reactivation.

A single agent chemotherapy is highly effective in non-metastatic and low-risk metastatic GTN

• **Selective hysterectomy** in hydatidiform mole over 35 years. There is 4 fold reduction in the risks of choriocarcinoma.

• **Diagnostic uterine curettage** in unexplained abnormal bleeding, 8 weeks following term delivery or abortion.

• In suspected cases, serum hCG is to be determined.

Curative

• **Chemotherapy** • **Surgery** • **Radiation**

Chemotherapy

The advent of chemotherapy has revolutionised the treatment of both the non-metastatic and metastatic lesion of choriocarcinoma. Chemotherapy is now the mainstay in the treatment.

Whether a single agent (Table 23.19) or multidrug regimen (Tables 23.20 and 23.21) to be used, depends on the risk factor present. **In general, patients with non-metastatic (low risk) and good prognosis disease are treated effectively with single agent therapy (Methotrexate or Actinomycin). The patients with poor prognosis metastatic disease should be treated with combination drug regimen (EMA-CO regimen).**

Whatever drugs are used, the basic formalities are to be followed as tabulated in Table 23.18.

Table 23.18
Formalities to be followed during therapy

Blood counts Liver function Kidney function	Daily
X-ray chest	To repeat only if hCG titre plateaus or rises
Serum/urine hCG	Weekly
• Treatment course should not be repeated if : – WBC < 3000 cu mm – Polymorphonuclear leucocytes < 1500 cu mm – Platelet counts < 100000 cu mm – Significant elevation BUN, SGPT	
• Continue treatment at 1-3 weekly interval until three consecutive negative weekly hCG titres.	

Management of GTN needs thorough assessment of the extent of the disease. **Chemotherapy regimen is decided** on the consideration of anatomic staging (p. 351), risk factor assessment (p. 348) and WHO prognostic scoring (p. 351).

Management of GTN

A. Stage I Low risk GTN	• Single agent chemotherapy.
High risk or Resistant	• Combination therapy. • Family completed→hysterectomy.
B. Stage II and III Low risk GTN	• Single agent chemotherapy. • Hysterectomy (Family completed) to reduce tumour mass.
High risk or Resistant	• Combination therapy • Hysterectomy — to reduce (trophoblastic) tumour mass
C. Stage IV	• Combination chemotherapy. • Surgery (hepatic resection, craniotomy). • Radiation (cerebral metastasis)

Table 23.19
Single drug regimen in low-risk cases

Methotrexate	1-1.5 mg/kg	IM/IV	Days 1, 3, 5 and 7
Folinic acid	0.1-0.15 mg/kg	IM	Days 2, 4, 6 and 8
The courses are to be repeated at interval of 7 days			

Table 23.20 : MAC protocol in low-risk cases

Methotrexate	1-1.5 mg/kg	IM/IV	Days 1,3,5 and 7
Folinic acid	0.1-0.15 mg/kg	IM	Days 2,4,6 and 8
Actinomycin D	12 μg/kg	IV	Days 1-5
Cyclophosphamide	3 mg/kg	IV	Days 1-5
The courses are to be repeated at interval of 2 weeks			

In poor prognosis metastatic disease best results are obtained with EMA-CO protocol (Table 23.21).

Table 23.21
EMA-CO protocol in poor prognosis metastatic disease

	Drug	*Dose*
Day 1	Etoposide	100 mg/m^2 in 200 ml saline infused over 30 minutes.
	Actinomycin D	0.5 mg IV bolus
	Methotrexate	100 mg/m^2 bolus followed by 200 mg/m^2 IV infusion over 12 hours.

Table 23.21 contd. from previous page
EMA-CO protocol in poor prognosis metastatic disease

	Drug	*Dose*
Day 2	Etoposide	100 mg/m² in 200 ml saline infused over 30 minutes.
	Actinomycin D	0.5 mg IV bolus.
	Folinic acid	15 mg IM every 12 hrs. for 4 doses beginning 24 hours after starting methotrexate.
Day 8	Cyclophosphamide	600 mg/m² IV in saline over 30 minutes.
	Vincristine (oncovin)	1 mg/m² IV bolus.

The course will restart after 7-14 days, if possible. Generally 2 additional courses are given after the hCG levels become normal.

During chemotherapy serum hCG levels should be done at one week interval. Chemotherapy should be changed if there is no fall in hCG titre by at least 25 per cent after a treatment cycle.

Place of Hysterectomy : Primary hysterectomy has got a limited place. Chemotherapy alone is successful in curing 85 per cent of patients with non-metastic and good prognosis metastatic GTN.

Patients with non-metastatic or good prognosis metastatic disease, **hysterectomy decreases the number of courses of chemotherapy**.

The overall indications are :

- Lesions confined to the uterus in women aged above 35 years to improve the efficacies of chemotherapy.
- Localised uterine lesion resistant to chemotherapy.
- Intractable bleeding or accidental uterine perforation during uterine curettage.

It is preferable to start chemotherapy → surgery on day 3 → followed by chemotherapy as per schedule.

Type of surgery :

- Total hysterectomy is enough. The ovaries are usually not involved and if involved, can be effectively cured with postoperative chemotherapy.
- Lung resection in pulmonary metastasis in drug resistant cases.
- Craniotomy for control of bleeding.

Radiation : Patients with brain metastases require whole-brain radiation therapy (3000 cGy over 10 days). Intrathecal high dose methotrexate may be administered to prevent haemorrhage and for tumour shrinkage.

Liver metastasis — Interventional radiology (hepatic artery ligation or embolisation) or whole liver radiation (2000 cGy over 10 days) along with chemotherapy may be effective. Hepatic metastasis has a poor prognosis.

Transplacental metastases to the fetus is rare and the prognosis is poor.

Prognosis : The cure rate is almost 100 per cent in low risk and about 70 per cent in high risk metastatic groups.

Recurrences : For non-metastatic GTN : 2-3 per cent; 'Good prognosis' metastatic disease : 3-5 per cent and 'Poor prognosis' disease : 21 per cent. Recurrence following 12 months of normal hCG level is < 1 per cent.

Prevention of recurrent disease

Additional cycle of chemotherapy following normalisation of hCG level, should be given as follows : For non-metastatic disease — one cycle; for good prognosis metastatic disease — two cycles; for poor prognosis metastatic disease — three cycles.

Future childbirth : There is no adverse effect on the subsequent pregnancy provided the conception occurs after 1 year of completion of chemotherapy. **Pregnancy** should be confirmed by USG early and hCG to be measured 6 weeks after delivery to exclude persistent GTN. Incidence of placenta accreta is increased.

Follow up is mandatory for all patients at least for 2 years. Serum hCG is measured weekly until it is negative for three consecutive weeks. Thereafter it is measured monthly for 6 months and 6 monthly thereafter for life. Increased risk for the development of secondary malignancies after treatment with multiple agent chemotherapy have been observed.

SARCOMA UTERUS

Incidence : Sarcoma of the uterus is rare and constitutes about 3 per cent of uterine malignancy.

Classification of uterine sarcomas
(Gynaecologic Oncology Group)

- Leiomyosarcomas.
- Endometrial stromal sarcomas.
- Malignant mixed müllerian tumour (Homologous and Heterologous).
- Other uterine sarcomas.

The commonest one arises from the intramural part. The consistency is soft and friable. The cut surface shows haemorrhage and irregular margins. There is no whorl appearance nor any capsule.

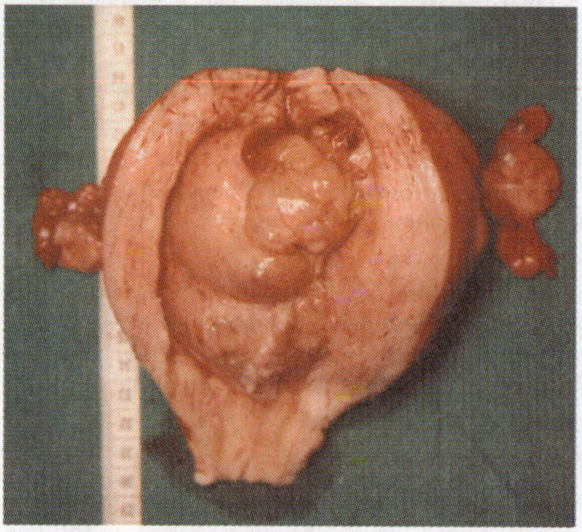

Fig. 23.18. Endometrial stromal sarcoma of uterus

Tumours with more than 10 mitotic figures/10 high-power field have poor prognosis.

Endometrial stromal tumours arises from endometrial stromal cells. **Depending on mitotic activity endometrial stromal tumours are of three types** : (i) endometrial stromal nodule (mostly benign), (ii) endolymphatic stromal myosis (low grade malignancy) and (iii) endometrial stromal sarcoma (high grade malignancy).

Leiomyosarcomas are of different clinicopathologic types. **Intravenous leiomyomatosis** — where benign smooth muscle grows into venous channels within the broad ligaments, uterine and iliac veins. Prognosis following surgery is excellent.

Leiomyomatosis peritonealis disseminata – where benign smooth muscle nodules grow over the peritoneal surfaces. It is thought to arise from the metaplasia of subperitoneal mesenchymal stem cells to smooth muscle, fibroblasts, myofibroblasts under the influence of oestrogen and progesterone.

Sarcomatous change of fibroid occurs in about 0.1 per cent cases. When it does, the fibroid becomes soft. The cut section shows yellowish appearance with haemorrhage and cystic degeneration. **The whorl appearance is lost (Fig. 23.18).**

Malignant mixed müllerian tumours (MMMT) of the uterus usually forms a large fleshy mass protruding into the uterine cavity with a broad base. Majority (90%) presents with postmenopausal bleeding.

Microscopic appearance : Uterine sarcomas may be pure (single cell type) or mixed (more than one cell type). The tumour is termed *homologous when* the tissue elements are native (smooth muscle) or *heterologous when* tissue elements are not native (cartilage, striated muscle, bones). This is due to the totipotent nature of endometrial stromal cells.

Histologically, three types of cells are seen — spindle, round or combination of the two along with giant cells. **The commonest is spindle cell type (Fig. 23.19).**

Malignant mixed müllerian tumour is evidenced by presence of **both the structures of sarcoma and carcinoma (carcinosarcoma).**

Spread

- Blood borne — This is the commonest mode of spread. The organs involved are liver, lungs, kidneys, brain, bones, etc.
- Directly to the adjacent structures.
- Lymphatic spread to the regional lymph glands.

Clinical features

Patient profile : The age is usually between 40-60 years. There may be history of pelvic irradiation either for induction of menopause or malignancy.

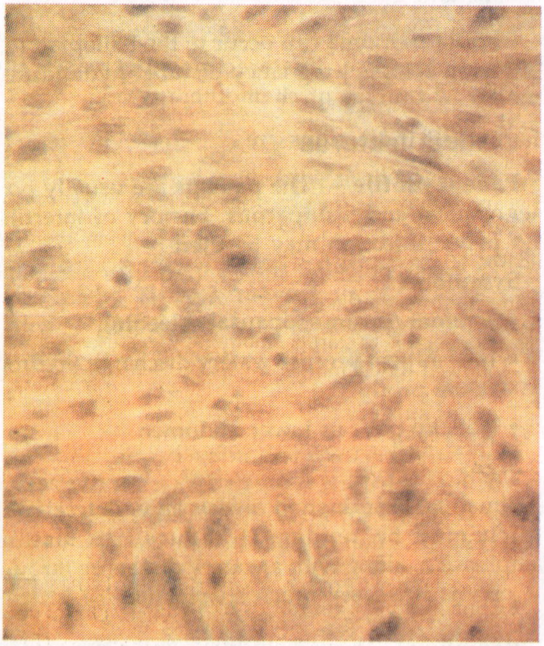

Fig. 23.19. Microscopic picture of leiomyosarcoma showing large spindle-shaped cells with pleomorphic nuclei. There is moderate cellular atypia

Symptoms : There is no specific symptom.

- Irregular premenopausal or postmenopausal vaginal bleeding.
- Abnormal vaginal discharge — offensive, watery associated at times with expulsion of fleshy necrotic mass.
- Abdominal pain — due to involvement of surrounding structures.
- Pyrexia, weakness and anorexia.

Suspected sarcomatous change in a fibroid is evidenced by :

- Postmenopausal bleeding.
- Rapid enlargement of fibroid.
- Recurrence following myomectomy or polypectomy.

Pelvic examination : There is no specific finding. The uterus may be enlarged and irregular. Parametrium may be thickened and indurated.

Speculum examination may reveal a polypoidal mass protruding out through the external os.

Diagnosis

- Diagnosis is made usually following histological examination of the removed uterus.
- Diagnostic uterine curettage may reveal the mucosal form of sarcoma.
- Histologic examination of the removed polyp.

Treatment

- Total hysterectomy with bilateral salpingo-oophorectomy is to be done. This should be followed by external pelvic radiation.

Leiomyomatosis peritonealis disseminata

Total abdominal hysterectomy, bilateral salpingo-oophorectomy, omentectomy and excision of gross disease should be done. Overall prognosis is satisfactory.

- If the cervix is also involved, radical hysterectomy should be done.
- **Radiation therapy** (adjuvant) preoperative or postoperative is helpful to decrease the pelvic recurrence in endometrial stromal sarcoma and MMMT.
- **Several chemotherapeutic agents** have been tried in cases with metastatic disease. Doxorubicin, dimethyl-triazeno-imidazole carboxamide (DTIC), cisplatin gemcitabine, docetaxel and ifosfamide are the drugs used either singly or in combination with varying response.
- Watchful expectancy may be extended in cases of sarcoma detected accidentally from the well-capsulated fibroid following myomectomy.

Prognosis

The prognosis is unsatisfactory. The 5-year survival rate ranges from 10-30 per cent. Sarcoma in fibroid has got a better prognosis.

SARCOMA BOTRYOIDES
(Embryonal rhabdomyosarcoma)

This is special type of mixed mesodermal tumour (rhabdomyosarcoma) commonly arising from the cervix and sometimes from the vagina or the uterus. It may affect both the adult and the child (usually before the age of 5).

Clinical features

The presenting features are :

- Blood stained watery vaginal discharge
- Anaemia and cachexia
- Vaginal examination reveals pinkish, grape-like polypoidal soft growth arising from the cervix. It may often fill up the whole vagina.

Diagnosis is confirmed by histologic appearances of loose myxomatous stroma, pleomorphic malignant cells with occasional striated rhabdomyoblasts.

Treatment

Intravenous administration of VAC therapy (vincristine, actinomycin-D, cyclophosphamide) and radiation has been found very much effective. The drugs should be administered every 2 weeks over a period of 6 months. Chemotherapy with local resection of the disease give better result. The results of radical surgery are relatively poor.

Prognosis : Local recurrence and distant metastases are common. Prognosis is poor.

CARCINOMA FALLOPIAN TUBE

- **Primary** • **Secondary**

PRIMARY

Primary carcinoma of the fallopian tube is very rare. The incidence of tubal carcinoma is less than 0.5 per cent of gynaecological malignancies.

Pathology

The site is usually in the ampullary part and the

mucosa is commonly affected. The fimbrial end usually gets blocked resulting in hydrosalpinx or haematosalpinx (Fig. 36.57). It is mostly unilateral (80%).

Microscopic appearance — It is mostly adenocarcinoma.

Spread

Apart from direct spread, the lymphatic spread to the regional lymph glands (paraaortic) usually occurs. Blood borne spread to distant organs can occur in late stages.

Choriocarcinoma can occur in the fallopian tube following ectopic pregnancy or tubal hydatidiform mole.

Clinical features

Patient profile — The patients are usually postmenopausal and nulliparous. History of infertility and pelvic infection may be there.

Symptoms

- Vaginal (postmenopausal) bleeding.
- Intermittent profuse watery discharge (hydrops tubae profluens).
- Colicky pain in lower abdomen.

Signs

Bimanual examination reveals an unilateral mass which may be tender. If reduced in size on compression, along with a watery discharge through the cervix, it is very much suspicious.

Diagnosis

- Most often accidentally discovered on laparotomy and histologic examination of the excised tube.
- Clinical features — as mentioned earlier.
- Suspected features are :
  - Persistent postmenopausal bleeding with uterine pathology being excluded by curettage.
  - Persistent positive Papanicolaou smear with a negative cervical and endometrial pathology.
- Laparoscopy — In cases of persistent postmenopausal bleeding with a negative uterine pathology.
- Ultrasound can help in the preoperative diagnosis.

Treatment

Total hysterectomy with bilateral salpingo-oophorectomy along with omentectomy. This should be followed by external pelvic radiation. In advanced cases, radiotherapy and/or chemotherapy is considered (see ch. 30).

Prognosis

The prognosis is unfavourable mostly due to late diagnosis. The 5-year survival rate ranges between 25-40 per cent.

SECONDARY

This is more common (90%) than the primary. **The common primary sites are** ovary, uterus, breast and gastrointestinal tract.

The mode of spread from the ovary or uterus is probably by lymphatics rather than a direct one.

MALIGNANT OVARIAN TUMOURS

Incidence

Ovarian malignancy constitutes about 15-20 per cent of genital malignancy. It is more prevalent in USA and Scandinavian countries but much less in Oriental or Latin American and Asian countries including Japan and India. Approximately, 1 in every 70 newborn females in the United States will live to develop ovarian cancer. Twenty per cent of ovarian neoplasms are malignant. **It is more common amongst nulliparous.** It is the fourth most common cause of cancer deaths in women exceeded only by breast, colon and lung malignancies.

Epidemiology

Highest incidence is recorded in the industrialised countries (Sweden, USA and UK). There is significant reduction in the risk with increasing parity. Nulligravidas carry a higher risk for ovarian malignancy. Incessant ovulation theory (Fathalla, 1971) suggests repeated

Incidence and Death Rate of Ovarian Cancer for different countries

Countries	*Incidence per 100,000*	*Death rate per 100,000*
Sweden	14.9	12.9
Norway	14.2	9.5
US (White)	13.3	7.3
UK	11.1.	9.1
India	4.6	
Japan	2.7	2.1

ovulatory trauma to the ovarian epithelial lining is a promoting factor for carcinogenesis. Combined oral contraceptive pills reduce the risk significantly as also repeated pregnancies. The role of ovulation inducing drugs is yet uncertain. Use of coffee, tobacco, alcohol and dietary fat has been implicated. Association of ovarian cancer with talc and asbestos has also been mentioned. Breastfeeding, tubal ligation and hysterectomy have been associated with reduction in the risk.

GENETICS AND OVARIAN MALIGNANCY

Hereditary ovarian cancer occurs in two forms :

(i) **Hereditary breast ovarian cancer syndrome** (BOC) is observed in 80-95 per cent cases of all familial ovarian cancers. BRCAI (chromosome 17q) and BRCA2 (chromosome 13q) gene mutations are observed in majority of such cases (serous not mucinous carcinoma). These patients present at an earlier age.

(ii) **Hereditary nonpolyposis colorectal cancer (HNPCC)** — is an autosomal dominant transmission. Women with HNPCC (Lynch II syndrome) have life time risk of about 50% for endometrial cancer and 12% for ovarian cancer. The risks of other cancers like genitourinary in addition to HNPCC are high. It is due to mutations in three DNA mismatch repair genes (MLH1, MSH2 and MSH6).

However, majority of epithelial ovarian cancers are not familial or hereditary. **Familial cancer account for less than 10 per cent of all ovarian cancers (p. 496).**

Pathology of Ovarian Malignancy

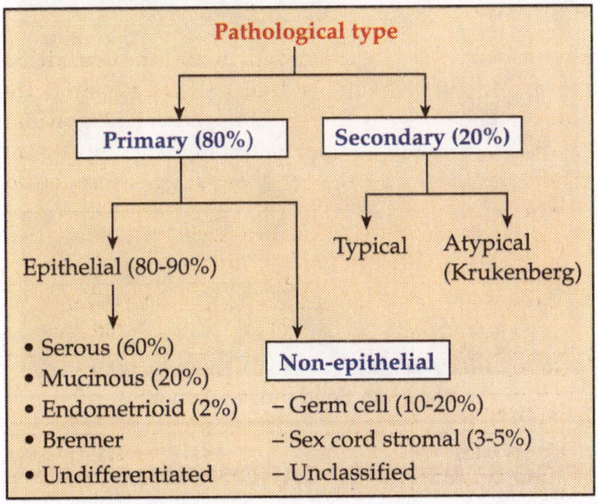

General considerations

Malignant epithelial tumours constitute about 90 per cent of all primary ovarian carcinomas. The nonepithelial malignant tumours such as gonadal stromal or germ cell tumours are indeed rare, present special problems in extremes of age and are of pathologist's curiosity. These will be dealt separately. **Thus, in the discussion to follow, only the malignant epithelial tumours will be described.**

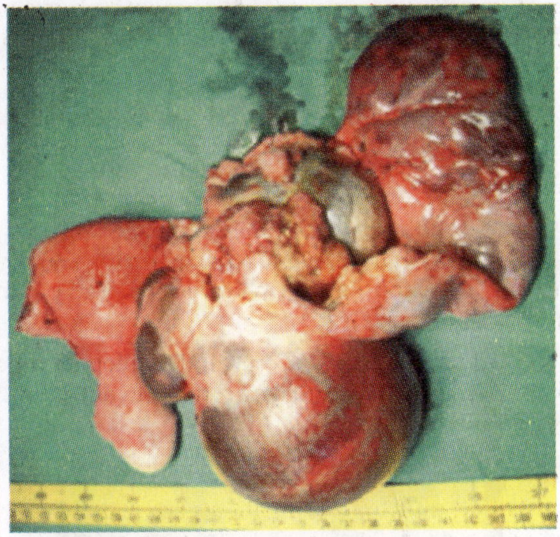

Fig. 23.20. Cut section of a mucinous cyst adenocarcinoma. The tumour was multi locular with polypoid growths

Primary epithelial

Malignant epithelial tumours include both cystic and solid types. **These are bilateral in about 50 per cent** (Fig. 23.24). Cystic is more common than solid. These may arise *de novo* as malignant or more commonly, they result from malignant changes of benign cystic tumours.

Endometrioid carcinoma is associated with endometrial carcinoma in 20 per cent and ovarian endometriosis in 10 per cent cases. In less than 5 per cent, it may arise from the endometrial cyst.

Cystic

Naked eye appearances — The wall of the cystic tumour becomes shaggy. There may be papillary projection at places. Cut section shows solid areas with haemorrhage at places. The papillae become friable, the base becomes broad and indurated. In mucinous type, it is filled up with gelatinous material (Fig. 23.20).

Microscopic picture — The histologic appearance in each type is tabulated in Table 23.22.

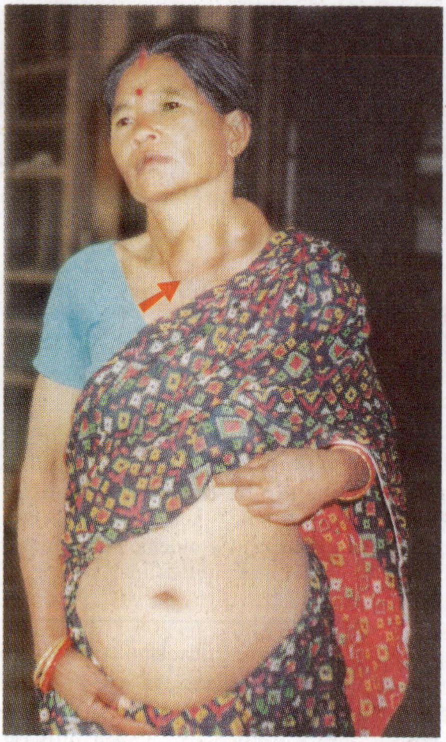

Fig. 23.21. Case of advanced ovarian malignancy with enlarged left supraclavicular glands (Virchow's gland) [*By courtesy* — Dr. A Halder, Asst. Professor, Dept. G&O., N.B.M.C&H., Sushrutnagar, Darjeeling].

Table 23.22

Type of tumour	*Histologic picture*
Serous cyst carcinoma	Adenocarcinoma
Mucinous cyst carcinoma	Adenocarcinoma (Fig. 23.22)
Malignant dermoid	Squamous cell carcinoma
Endometrioid or Adenoacanthoma	Adenocarcinoma

Solid (Fig. 23.23)

It attains a moderate size. The external surface is smooth and often lobulated. Subserous blood vessels may be prominent. Cut section shows greyish granular appearance, at times brain-like. There may be irregular cystic spaces due to necrosis.

Microscopic appearance reveals adenocarcinoma or carcinoma without adenomatous pattern.

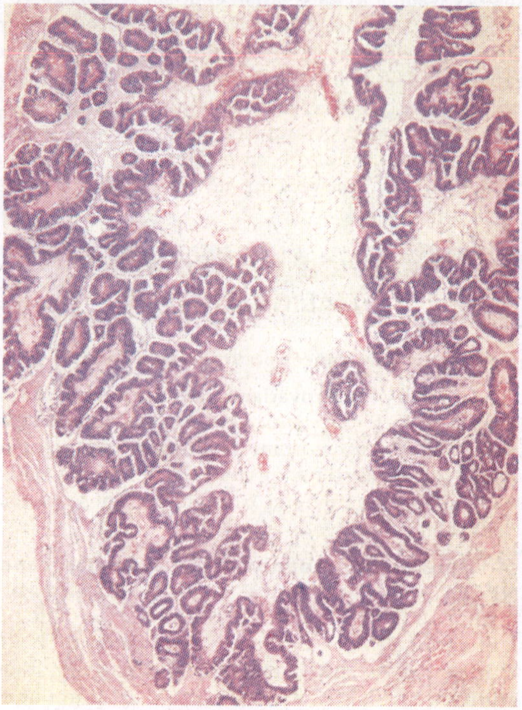

Fig. 23.22. Histologic picture of serous cyst adenocarcinoma. Long papillary outgrowths are seen. There is considerable cellular mitotic activity. This lace-like pattern characterised by slit-like spaces between the papillae is due to extensive coalescence of papillae

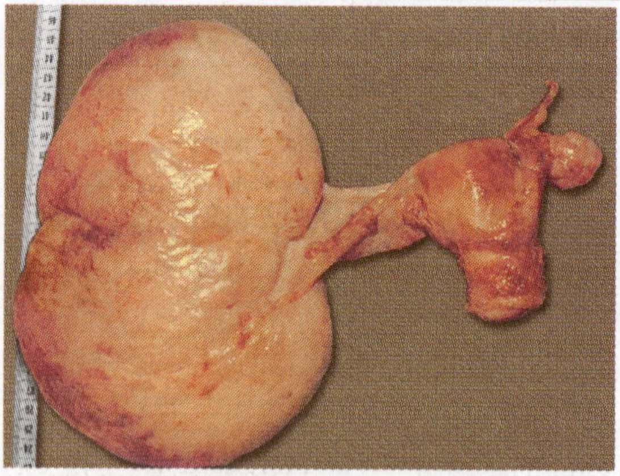

Fig. 23.23. Solid ovarian tumour

FIGO STAGING OF CARCINOMA OVARY

The staging aims at :

- Better choice of adjuvant therapy
- Better assessment of prognosis

The staging is done following laparotomy (staging laparotomy) and is followed as per FIGO (1988).

Spread

Natural path of spread : The tumours spread along the peritoneal surface to involve ovarian, parietal and intestinal peritoneal surfaces as well as the under surface of the diaphragm, particularly on the right side. The modes of spread are :

- **Transcoelomic**
- **Lymphatics**
- **Direct**
- **Blood borne**

Transcoelomic

Implantation of malignant cells occurs by :

- Direct exfoliation of cells as in papillary cyst adenocarcinoma.
- Penetration of tumour capsule.
- Rupture of the capsule.

The exfoliated cells in the peritoneal fluid flow along the paracolic gutters.

Multiple secondary deposits are formed on the peritoneal surfaces specially in the pouch of Douglas, in the omentum, diaphragm, retroperitoneal nodes and serous surfaces of the abdominopelvic organs.

Lymphatics

The lymphatic spread is to the draining lymph nodes namely paraaortic and superior gastric nodes. The pelvic nodes may be involved through peritoneal permeation into the subperitoneal lymphatics (Table 23.23). **The left supracalvicular nodes are enlarged due to** obstruction of the efferent lymphatic channel of the nodes by the tumour emboli, as it enters the thoracic duct just prior to its drainage into the left subclavian vein (Fig. 23.21).

STAGING OF CARCINOMA OF THE OVARY (FIGO – 1988)	
Stage I	Growth limited to the ovaries (a) Growth limited to one ovary; no ascites No tumour on the external surface; capsule intact (b) Growth limited to both ovaries; no ascites. No tumour on the external surfaces; capsule intact. (c) Tumour either stage Ia or Ib, but tumour on surface of one or both ovaries; or with capsule ruptured; or with ascites present containing malignant cells or with positive peritoneal washings.
Stage II	Growth involving one or both ovaries with pelvic extension (a) Extension and/or metastases to the uterus and/or tubes (b) Extension to other pelvic tissues (c) Tumour either Stage IIa or IIb, but tumour on surface on one or both ovaries; or with capsule(s) ruptured or with ascites present containing malignant cells or with positive peritoneal washings.
Stage III	Tumour involving one or both ovaries with peritoneal implants outside the pelvis and/or positive retroperitoneal or inguinal lymph nodes. Superficial liver metastasis equals stage III. Tumour is limited to the true pelvis but with histologically proven malignant extension to small bowel or omentum. (a) Tumour grossly limited to the true pelvis with negative nodes but histologically confirmed microscopic seeding of abdominal peritoneal surfaces. (b) Tumour involving one or both ovaries with histologically confirmed implants of abdominal peritoneal surfaces with none exceeding 2 cm in diameter. Nodes are negative. (c) Abdominal implants greater than 2 cm in diameter and/or positive retroperitoneal or inguinal nodes.
Stage IV	Growth involving one or both ovaries with distant metastases. If pleural effusion is present, there must be positive cytology to allot a case to stage IV. Parenchymal liver metastasis equals stage IV.

Table 23.23 : Lymph node involvement in ovarian malignancy (%)

Stage	Paraaortic (%)	Pelvic (%)
I and II	20	30
III and IV	65	67

Direct

After the capsule is broken, the spread occurs directly to the adjacent organs such as tubes, broad ligament, intestines, omentum and uterus.

Blood borne

The blood stream metastasis is late and the involved organs are lungs, liver, bones, etc.

Clinicopathologic explanation

Ascites : Ascites is due to obstruction of peritoneal fluid outflow principally through the diaphragm. There is also increased transudation of serum across the peritoneal surfaces. The secretion is not from the tumour bearing peritoneum but from the tumour-free areas.

Liver : The involvement of liver is usually blood borne when the guts are involved.

Contralateral ovary (Fig. 23.24)

The contralateral ovary is involved in majority of metastatic ovarian malignancy. Even in primary malignancy, the contralateral involvement may be due to retrograde lymphatic spread through para-aortic glands. Direct implantation or multicentric origin may also be a possibility.

Uterus : The body is mostly affected either due to lymphatics or through transtubal spread. The cervical involvement is rare.

Right sided pleural effusion : More ascitic fluid reaches the right subdiaphragmatic space along the wider right paracolic gutter. This is facilitated by the increased negative suction created by liver during respiration. The fluid so collected can pass freely across the diaphragm. This is because of free communication of submesothelial network of lymphatic capillaries with the corresponding plexuses on the thoracic surface of the diaphragm underlying the pleura on the right side → right pleural effusion. Alternatively, there is more presence of wide pleuroperitoneal sinuses on the right side and hence producing right pleural effusion.

CLINICAL FEATURES

Patient profile : Although, no age is immune to ovarian malignancy, but about 60 per cent of ovarian neoplasms in postmenopausal and about 20 per cent in premenopausal women are malignant. There is increased association of nulliparity and with a family history.

Symptoms

In its early stage, ovarian carcinoma is a notoriously silent disease. The presenting complaints are usually of short duration and insidious in onset. Symptoms are not specific.

- Feeling of abdominal distension and vague discomfort.
- Features of dyspepsia such as flatulence and eructations.

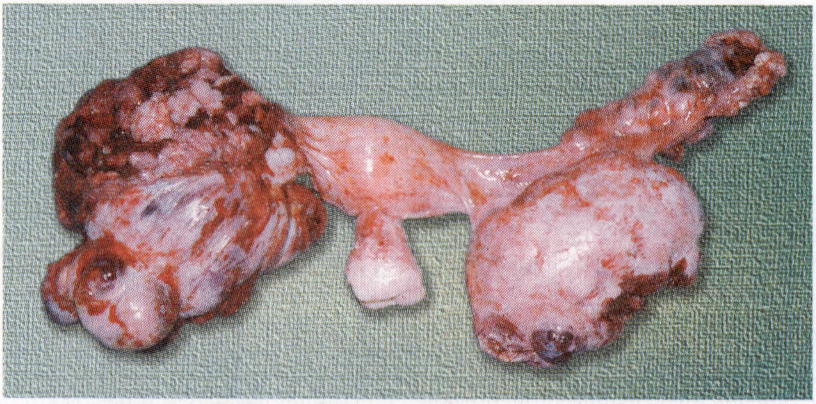

Fig. 23.24. Bilateral malignant epithelial tumours of the ovary
(By courtesy Dr. Biswajit Ghosh, Burnpur)

- Loss of appetite with a sense of bloating after meals.
- In pre-existing tumour.
  - Appearance of dull aching pain and tenderness over one area.
  - Rapid enlargement of the tumour.

Gradually, more pronounced symptoms appear. These are :

- Abdominal swelling which may be rapid.
- Dull abdominal pain.
- Sudden loss of weight.
- Respiratory distress — may be mechanical due to ascites or due to pleural effusion.
- Menstrual abnormality is conspicuously absent except in functioning ovarian tumours (mentioned later in the chapter).

Signs : The following are the findings in an established case of ovarian malignancy.

General examination reveals :

- Cachexia and pallor of varying degree.
- Jaundice may be evident in late cases.
- Left supraclavicular lymph gland (Virchow's) may be enlarged.
- Oedema leg or vulva is characteristic of malignant and not of benign neoplasm.

Per abdomen

- Liver may be enlarged, firm and nodular.
- A mass is felt in the hypogastrium; too often it may be bilateral. It has got the following features :
  - Feel — solid or heterogenous.
  - Mobility — mobile or restricted.
  - Tenderness — usually present.
  - Surfaces — irregular.
  - Margins — well-defined but the lower pole is usually not reached.
  - Percussion — usually dull over the tumour; may be resonant due to overlying intestinal adhesions.

Per vaginam

- The uterus is separated from the mass felt per abdomen.
- Nodules may be felt through the posterior fornix. If it is more than 1 cm, the diagnosis of malignancy is almost certain.

Special investigations

Investigation aims at :

- To confirm malignancy preoperatively.
- To identify the extent of lesion.
- To detect the primary site.

To confirm malignancy

- Cytologic examination for detection of malignant cells is carried out from the fluid collected by abdominal paracentesis or "cul-de-sac" aspiration.
- Tumour marker : In epithelial carcinoma, there is no specific tumour marker. But, elevated CA-125 level > 65 U/ml with a pelvic mass may be suggestive. Other biomarkers are : CA-19-9, CA-15-3, OVXI may be suggestive.

To identify the extent of lesion

- **Straight X-ray** chest to exclude pleural effusion and chest metastasis.
- **Barium enema** to detect any lower bowel malignancy.
- **Cytologic examination** of thoracocentesis fluid.
- **Sonography** is of limited help but can be employed to detect involvement of the omentum or contralateral ovary.
- **Computed Tomography (CT)** is helpful for retroperitoneal lymph node assessment and detection of metastasis (liver, omentum). It helps in staging of ovarian carcinoma (see p. 624).
- **Magnetic Resonance Imaging (MRI)** is helpful to determine the nature of ovarian neoplasm and also for the retroperitoneal lymph nodes and detection of metastasis. It can also detect relapse of the tumour following initial treatment.
- **Positron Emission Tomography (PET)** can differentiate normal tissues from cancerous tissues. It is more sensitive than CT or MRI (p. 115).
- Intravenous pyelography.
- Examination under anaesthesia.
- Diagnostic uterine curettage.

To detect the primary site

- Barium meal X-ray.
- Gastroscopy/colonoscopy.
- Mammography.

Diagnosis

- Clinical.
- Ancillary aids.
- Operative findings.
- Histologic confirmation.

Clinical—**Clinical diagnosis in early stage is very much deceptive because of :**

- **No age specificity** — Although more prevalent beyond the age of 45 (40% of ovarian neoplasms are malignant), no age is immune to ovarian cancer. All physicians must be aware of the possible significance of persistent gastrointestinal symptoms in women over the age of 40 with a history of ovarian dysfunction.

- **No specific symptom** — It may remain asymptomatic in about 15 per cent when first diagnosed.

- **Unrelated to duration of symptoms — Even with symptoms** of short duration may have extensive spread, conversely a long-standing tumour may remain benign.

- **Unrelated to the size of the tumour** — A big tumour may remain benign for a long time whereas, a small enlarged ovary may be found malignant.

The cumulative effects of such vagaries explain the fact that at the time of diagnosis, about 70 per cent of patients with epithelial carcinomas have metastases outside the pelvis. **The most common sites of metastases are — peritoneum (85%), omentum (70%), contralateral ovary (70%), liver (35%), lung (25%) and uterus (20%).**

In established and or advanced cases of malignancy, the clinical features as mentioned earlier are enough to arrive at a diagnosis.

Ancillary aids

- Detection of malignant cells from the ascitic fluid collected by abdominal paracentesis or cul-de-sac aspiration is a positive proof of abdominal malignancies. When combined with presence of a pelvic mass almost confirms ovarian malignancy.

- Noninvasive methods such as MRI or CT scan has not yet proved to be much useful in diagnosis. Transvaginal sonography improves the detection rate (see p. 113).

- Examination under anaesthesia may be useful in doubtful cases specially in an obese patient.

- Laparoscopy too, has got limited scope in confirmation of malignancy. It can just detect a neoplasm.

- Elevation of serum CA 125 beyond 35U/ml. may be suggestive.

Operative findings

- Nature of peritoneal fluid.

While haemorrhagic fluid is very much suggestive but a clear or straw colour fluid cannot rule out malignancy.

- Nature of the tumour—differentiation between a benign and malignant tumour may be possible clinically, with a laparotomy findings and with ultrasonographic criteria (see p. 283).

- Metastatic nodules on the peritoneal surfaces and omentum.

Histological diagnosis

All ovarian tumours irrespective of its nature must be subjected to histologic examination. This not only confirms the diagnosis but also identifies the type and grade of malignancy.

MANAGEMENT OF EPITHELIAL OVARIAN CANCER

- **Preventive** • **Curative**

Preventive

Primary prevention : Because of dearth about the knowledge of epidemiology of ovarian cancer, the primary prevention cannot be clearly formulated. However the preventive measures are :

(i) **Genetic screening for BRCA 1 and BRCA 2** for women with high risk for ovarian and breast cancer.

(ii) **Annual mammographic screening** for women with strong family history of breast cancer.

(iii) **Periodic screening** for other malignancies (colonoscopy, endometrial biopsy) for women with Lynch II syndrome.

(iv) **Combined oral contraceptive pills** as a preventive measure is recommended to a woman specially belonging to Lynch type II families.

(v) **Prophylactic oophorectomy along with hysterectomy** specially in **'high risk' women** (Table 23.24) is a preventive measure against ovarian malignancy. **The cases include :**

- Nulliparous women aged > 45 years.
- A woman of any age who has a history of ovarian, endometrial or colonic carcinoma in first degree relative (mother and sister).

- Grossly abnormal ovary in premenopausal group (ovarian volume > 20 cm^3).
- Woman who had one ovary removed for benign neoplasm.
- Previous history of breast carcinoma.
- Any woman with radiation induced menopause.

Guidelines for management of an enlarged ovary

- An ovarian enlargement of ≥ 8 cm during childbearing period deserves careful follow up.
- In postmenopausal women any ovarian enlargement should be assessed by serum CA-125 and transvaginal sonography.
- Cysts that are simple, unilocular, ≤ 8 cm in diameter with normal serum CA-125 — can be managed conservatively. Women should be under follow up with ultrasound scan and serum CA-125 at an interval of 4 months.
- Early laparotomy is indicated in cases :
  - The ovary enlarges progressively beyond 8 cm while under observation.
  - Any symptomatic ovarian tumour regardless of size.

Secondary prevention (screening for ovarian cancer)

Natural history of the disease is not well-understood. There is no preinvasive stage like that of cervical intraepithelial neoplasia. As such, screening aims at detecting early ovarian malignancy in asymptomatic women. Till date no specific method of screening for early detection of epithelial ovarian cancer is available.

Screening procedures : *Clinical* — Regular and periodic clinical examination of the 'high risk' group is done. Bimanual pelvic examination in an asymptomatic woman may detect an adnexal mass. However clinical examination is not very specific.

Tumour markers : CA 125 is a glycoprotein has been used for screening of epithelial cancers of the ovary. Value more than 35 U/ml is suggestive of epithelial ovarian cancer. It is also used for monitoring a patient during chemotherapy and for follow up. But it is not a tumour specific antigen. There are several other conditions, where level of CA-125 is raised :

- Normal woman (1%).
- Carcinomas of the breast, lung, colon and endometrium.
- Endometriosis.
- Pelvic inflammatory disease.
- Peritonitis.

The serum level of CA–125 falls after surgical resection of the tumour or following chemotherapy. Elevated level indicates bulky residual disease or tumour recurrence or resistant clones to chemotherapy. Serum half life of CA–125 is 20 days.

Other tumour markers of value are macrophage colony-stimulating factors (M-CSF), OVXI, HER-2/ neu and inhibin (see p. 497).

Ultrasound imaging : Transvaginal colour Doppler imaging has been able to differentiate benign from malignant tumours by assessment of its vascular supply and intratumoural blood flow. Increased neoangiogenesis in ovarian malignancy causes central neovascularity. Study of **vascular parameters** e.g. Pulsatility Index (PI) < 1.0 or Resistive Index (RI) < 0.4 increases the risk of malignancy.

Recently **three dimensional**, contrast enhanced, power Doppler sonography is found to be more diagnostic.

- **Risk of Malignancy Index (RMI)** : **RMI = U × M × CA 125**; U = USG score (one point each for : multilocular cyst; solid areas; metastasis; ascites; bilateral lesions), M = 3 (postmenopausal women) and CA 125 level in U/ml. The risk of cancer is 75% when the RMI value is > 250 (see p. 543).

Table 23.24 : 'High risk' women
• Age group 40–60 years.
• Familial cancers : Breast, endometrial, ovarian, colorectal.
• History of removal of benign ovarian tumour or breast carcinoma.
• Postmenopausal palpable ovary (volume > 8 cm^3).
• Relative or absolute infertility.
• Dysgenetic gonad.
• Fertility drugs use (incessant ovulation).
• Women workers in asbestos related industries.

Protective factors for ovarian malignancy

- Combined oral contraceptives.
- Pregnancy.
- Tubal ligation, hysterectomy.
- Breastfeeding.

TREATMENT OF MALIGNANT OVARIAN TUMOUR

- **Surgery**
- **Chemotherapy**
- **Radiotherapy**
- **Combined therapy**

SURGICAL TREATMENT OF OVARIAN CANCER

Surgery is the keystone in the primary treatment of ovarian malignancy.

The aims are :

• To stage the disease (staging laparotomy) accurately thereby allowing better choice of adjuvant therapy and a better assessment of prognosis.

• To perform effective surgical removal.

Practical guidelines

• **Liberal vertical incision** to minimise chance of rupture of the tumour and to facilitate better exploration.

• **To note the character of the ascitic fluid** if any, and to collect sample for cytology. If appreciable fluid is not available, then a sample of peritoneal wash with 100 ml saline in the subdiaphragmatic area is to be collected.

• **A systematic (visual and manual) exploration** — palpation of liver, gastrointestinal tract, subdiaphragmatic area, omentum and paraaortic lymph nodes. This is done in a clockwise fashion starting from the caecum.

• **Pelvic exploration** — nature of the tumour, extent of adhesions, condition of the contralateral ovary, uterus and tubes and palpation of pelvic lymph nodes.

• **Any metastatic deposit** over the peritoneal surfaces, under surface of the diaphragm should be biopsied. Pelvic and paraaortic lymph node sampling should be done.

• **In the absence of any metastatic disease**, multiple peritoneal biopsy, scraping from the diaphragm for cytology should be taken. Occult metastasis has been found in about 10-40 per cent of early stage (stage I and II) epithelial ovarian cancer.

PRIMARY SURGERY

A. Early stage disease (Stage Ia, G_1, G_2) :

(a) **Young woman** → unilateral oophorectomy (fertility sparing surgery) → Routine follow up and monitoring → Completion of family → Removal of the uterus and the other ovary.

(b) **Elderly woman** → Hysterectomy and bilateral Salpingo-oophorectomy.

(c) **In Stage Ia, G_3 disease and others stage I** : Staging Laparotomy → Hysterectomy and bilateral Salpingo-oophorectomy. Chemotherapy is considered for most patients.

B. Advanced stage disease : Exploratory Laparotomy → **cytoreductive or debulking surgery**. This includes : Total abdominal hysterectomy bilateral salpingo-oophorectomy, complete omentectomy and resection of any metastatic tumour (Fig. 36.60). Cytoreductive surgery is aimed to reduce the tumour load. Lesser the residual tumour volume (< 1 cm), better is the survival.

Maximum cytoreductive surgery may need resection of a segment of bowel, bladder or the lymph nodes. Removal of omental cake by cytoreductive surgery improves the result of subsequent chemotherapy or radiotherapy. Large tumour masses have huge number of poorly oxygenated cells in the "resting" phase (Go) (see p. 488), those are resistant to any type of therapy. Lesser the residual tumour mass (< 5 mm) higher the survival rate. Appendectomy is done in cases with mucinous ovarian cancer.

ADJUVANT CHEMOTHERAPY

A. **In stage Ia (Grade I)** epithelial carcinoma → no adjuvant chemotherapy.

B. **In all other stage I disease** → adjuvant chemotherapy with carboplatin and paclitaxel for six cycles.

C. **Advanced stage disease**

Combination chemotherapy : Paclitaxel (175 mg/m^2) and carboplatin (400 mg/m^2).

Patients who are hypersensitive to paclitaxel, topotecan 1 mg/m^2 for 5 days, every 3 weeks or Gemcitabine 800 mg/m^2, every 3 weeks is given.

Chemotherapy : Chemotherapy is used widely following surgery to improve the result in terms of survival. Drugs are given for five or six cycles at 3-4 weekly interval (see p. 495).

Single agent — Alkylating agents (melphelan, cyclophosphamide, ifosfamide) are commonly used (see Table 23.25).

Platinum compounds (cisplatin, carboplatin) are the **most effective drugs** in terms of tumour response and survival rate (see p. 495). Like alkylating agents they cause cross linkage of DNA strands. **They can be used either singly or in combination with paclitaxel (see below).**

Taxane derivatives (paclitaxel, docetaxel) are found to be very effective in ovarian cancer (see p. 492). Paclitaxel is derived from the bark of the pacific yew tree. Docetaxel is semisynthetic and its side effects are (less peripheral neuropathy). Taxane derivatives prevent cell division by polymerisation of microtubules and making them excessively stable. They are found to be effective even in cisplatin resistant ovarian cancer. **Paclitaxel is recommended as the primary treatment of all epithelial ovarian cancer following optimal cytoreductive surgery.**

Table 23.25 : Recommended drugs and doses used as a single agent

Drug	*Dose*	*Route*	*Cycle*	*Interval*
Melphelan	200 µg/kg per day for 5 days.	oral	6	4 weeks
Cisplatin	75 mg/M²	IV	6	4 weeks
Carboplatin	400 mg/M²	IV	6	4 weeks
Paclitaxel	175 mg/M²	IV	6	4 weeks

The recommended drugs and doses for chemotherapy of ovarian carcinoma (CAP and CP) is tabulated below :

Table 23.26
Recommended drugs and doses of chemotherapy (CAP and CP)

Drugs	*DOSE*	
	CAP	CP
Cyclophosphamide (C)	500 mg/m²	750-1000 mg/m²
Adriamycin (A)	50 mg/m²	
Cisplatin (P)	50 mg/m²	50-100 mg/m²

Drugs are given IV on day 1 every 4 weeks interval as toxicity permits (see ch. 25, p. 497)

In **combination chemotherapy**, drugs acting in different ways on the cell cycle (see p. 489), with different toxicities, are combined. Therefore efficacy is expected to be more and chance of drug resistance is low. **Currently paclitaxel and carboplatin combination chemotherapy is found to have better survival rate in advanced ovarian cancer (Tables 23.26 and 23.27).**

Efficacy of **docetaxel** has been found similar to paclitaxel. **Topotecan** has got similar efficacy.

Intraperitoneal chemotherapy is used only for minimal (< 2 cm) or microscopic residual disease. The drugs can penetrate only few millimetres. Moreover, serum levels are similar to those seen after IV chemotherapy. Currently cisplatin and paclitaxel are used. There is no distinct benefit of intraperitoneal cisplatin and paclitaxel over their intravenous use.

Table 23.27
Recommended Drugs and doses of chemotherapy (CP)

Drugs	*Dose*	*Cycle*	*Interval*
Carboplatin (CP)	400 mg/M² or AUC 5	6	4 weeks
Paclitaxel (T)	135 mg/M²	6	4 weeks

Primary chemotherapy for advanced ovarian cancer may be considered before cytoreductive surgery. It is considered for a selected patient who presents with huge ascites and/or pleural effusions. Chemotherapy (Paclitaxel and Carboplatin) often dry up ascites and effusions. Postoperative morbidity is then reduced.

High-dose chemotherapy along with bone marrow transplant or peripheral stem cell support has been used to improve the survival rate. It can be used in refractory cases or in cases with persistent disease following primary surgery or as a first line treatment.

Radiotherapy: There is very little scope of radiotherapy as an adjunct to surgery because of the advent of chemotherapy. Total abdominopelvic irradiation is rarely employed now.

Radioactive isotopes (see p. 484) : In early cases of ovarian cancer, radioactive phosphorous (^{32}P) is instilled into the peritoneal cavity. The isotopes are taken up by macrophages and the radiation effects are limited to superficial 4-6 mm of peritoneal lining. ^{32}P acts by emitting β-rays. Bowel complications are increased.

Hormone therapy: Tamoxifen, leuprolide acetate (GnRH agonist), Aromatase inhibitors are being studied in relapsed cases of ovarian tumour.

Immunotherapy: With the use of cytokines, interferon or interleukin-2 is under trial. Herceptin, an antibody, when used along with chemotherapy improves the response rate. This is specially helpful in a patient whose ovarian cancer over expresses HER-2/neu oncogene or mutated p. 53 tumour suppressor gene.

Human tumour stem cell assay has been developed *in vitro*. Growth of cultured cells *in vitro* and their response against a variety of chemotherapeutic agents are then tested. Such clonogenic assays may be useful in selection of appropriate chemotherapy.

Gene and Molecular therapy — see page 496.

SECONDARY SURGERY

Second look surgery either by laparoscopy or laparotomy may be employed to patients who have received treatment for ovarian cancer. The aims are :

- To confirm "cure" and to stop chemotherapy.
- To assess the response of chemotherapy.
- To change the drugs when found resistant.

When to be done? It is employed either after 12 courses of chemotherapy or after 1 year of primary therapy.

A laparoscopy prior to laparotomy is advised. Currently, CT, MRI and serum CA-125 are being evaluated as an alternative to second look laparotomy. A positive findings eliminate unnecessary laparotomy. But, if gross tumour is not visualised, biopsy specimens and cytology sampling are taken. When laparotomy is done, sampling of the peritoneal fluid/washing, multiple biopsy at different areas, residual omentectomy, sampling of palpable pelvic and paraaortic lymph nodes are to be done. Second line therapy includes secondary cytoreduction (debulking) and second line chemotherapy. Better survival rate following second look surgery is however questionable. As such the value of second-look procedures is debated.

Secondary Cytoreductive Surgery may be done in some selected cases where (i) There is no response or partial response to primary chemotherapy. (ii) Recurrence following primary cytoreductive surgery and chemotherapy. (iii) Following initial suboptimal debulking followed by chemotherapy. This is also called "Interval debulking" and (iv) Clinically persistent tumour at second-look laparotomy. Optimal cytoreduction during secondary surgery, improves survival rate significantly.

Reasons for difficulties in the management of ovarian cancers

- Late diagnosis.
- Large tumour mass.
- Extent of tumour spread is often unknown.
- Limitations of cytoreductive surgery.
- Variable chemosensitivity.
- Radiation dose restriction by neighbouring organs.
- Tumour cells are freely mobile within the peritoneal cavity.

Prognostic factors in ovarian malignancy

- Surgical stage of the disease — worse beyond stage II (Table 23.28).
- Histological type — endometrioid tumour has got a higher survival rate than serous type because the former tumour is highly well-differentiated.
- Histological grade of the tumour — higher the grade, poorer the prognosis.
- Peritoneal cytology — positive malignant cells, higher the risk.
- Presence of ascites — higher the risk.
- Presence of metastatic disease before cytoreductive surgery — poor the prognosis and shorter the survival.
- Volume of residual tumour after primary surgery — when < 5 mm better the prognosis.
- Ploidy status – diploid tumours are prognostically better compared to aneuploid tumours.
- Degree of oncogene expression (see p. 496 chap. 30).

Table 23.28

Stage	*Approximate 5-year survival (%)*
I	75 – 90
II	60 – 70
III	20 – 40
IV	5 – 10

PRIMARY PERITONEAL CARCINOMA

Papillary serous Carcinoma of the Peritoneum is a rare type of primary peritoneal adenocarcinoma (PPA). It constitutes 7-20% of all epithelial ovarian carcinoma.

Criteria for diagnosis of PPA (GOG 1993)

- The ovaries are either absent or normal in size (< 4 cm diameter).
- Extra-ovarian sites are more involved than that of the ovarian surfaces.
- Microscopically the ovaries are either not involved or exhibit cortical implants < 5 mm in depth.
- The histologic and cytologic tumour character is serous type. FIGO staging for ovarian carcinoma is followed. Management is according to ovarian carcinoma grade and staging. Prognosis is generally poor.

GERM CELL TUMOURS OF THE OVARY

Germ cell tumours constitute about 15-20 per cent of all ovarian neoplasm and they are the second common ovarian tumours. For classification see p. 281. They have got varying degrees of malignant potentiality. About 3 per cent of these tumours are malignant. Germ cell tumours occur predominantly in children and young adults. They arise from embryonic germ cells.

Dysgerminoma

Dysgerminoma is the commonest (30-40%) malignant germ cell tumour. It arises from undifferentiated form of germ cells. It is often (5%) associated with dysgenetic gonad (see Ch. 27). The counter part of dysgerminoma in male is seminoma. Majority (75%) of the tumours occur before the age of 30 years.

hCG assays are often positive, confusing the diagnosis with pregnancy. It may coexist with pregnancy (20-30%). Dysgerminoma may be associated with choriocarcinoma or endodermal sinus tumour. Tumour markers α-fetoprotein (AFP) and hCG may be positive in that situation. Karyotyping is needed specially when a premenarcheal girl presents with a pelvic mass.

Pathology: The shape is usually round or oval and is usually 5-15 cm in diameter; feel is boggy, at times it is firm rubbery. It may be bilateral (10%). Cut section shows pink or yellow colour. Microscopic appearance reveals uniform large round cells (monotonous pattern), arranged in cords or clumps with abundant clear cytoplasm. Nuclei are large, irregular and hyperchromatic with varying degree of mitosis. There is intense infiltration of lymphocytes and plasma cells in the fibrous septum (Fig. 23.25). In more than 50 per cent, they are potentially malignant.

Clinical features are not specific for the tumour.

Treatment: Majority (75%) of dysgerminomas are confined to one ovary and are stage I at the time of diagnosis.

In a young patient where preservation of fertility is desired, laparotomy for surgical staging and unilateral salpingo-oophorectomy is done. If there is any suspicion of involvement to the other ovary, bisection of the contralateral ovary and excisional biopsy should be done. The tumour is sensitive to both chemotherapy and radiotherapy. Systemic chemotherapy is the treatment of choice, where fertility is to be preserved, even in the presence of metastatic disease.

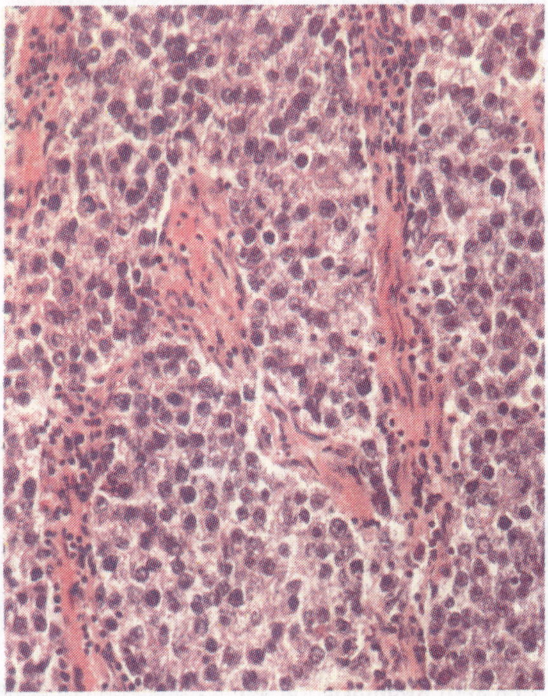

Fig. 23.25. Histologic picture of dysgerminoma cells are mostly uniform (monotonous pattern) in size. The stroma is dense with lymphocytic infiltrate

Types of malignant germ cell tumour

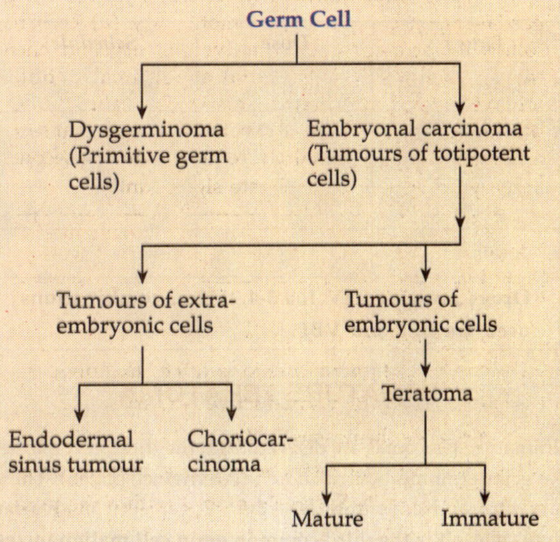

Different chemotherapeutic agents are used either singly or in combination (see ch. 30). Carboplatin 400 mg/M², IV, every 4 weeks, for 6 courses have been used as a single agent therapy where the tumour have been removed completely. BEP (Bleomycin, Etoposide and Cisplatin), VBP (Vinblastin, Bleomycin and Cisplatin), VAC (Vincristine, Actinomycin and Cyclophosphamide) are the commonly used drugs for the germ cell tumours. The most effective chemotherapeutic regimens used are BEP, VBP and VAC (see Table 23.29 and p. 494). Combination chemotherapy has significantly improved the survival rate.

Patient with Y chromosome as detected on karyotyping should have both the ovaries (gonads) removed.

Radiotherapy : Loss of fertility is a problem with radiation therapy. So radiation therapy is not used in young patients.

Recurrent disease is treated either with combination chemotherapy or radiation therapy. Combination chemotherapy with POMB-ACE (Vincristine, bleomycin, methotrexate, cisplatin, etoposide, actinomycin D and cyclophosphamide) is preferred (see p. 495). Radiation therapy is considered for patients who had been treated with combination chemotherapy earlier.

Overall prognosis following unilateral oophorectomy in early stage disease (stage Ia) and following cisplatin-based combination chemotherapy in advanced disease, is good.

Table 23.29 : Recommended drugs and doses of chemotherapy (BEP, VBP)

Drugs	*Dose*	*Schedule*
Bleomycin (B)	15 units/M²	every week
Etoposide (E)	100 mg/M²	on days 1-3, every 4 weeks
Cisplatin (P)	100 mg/M²	every 3 weeks
Vinblastin (V)	12 mg/M²	every 3 weeks

Drugs are given IV for 3-4 cycles, combinations used are BEP and VBP.

IMMATURE TERATOMA

Immature teratomas are derived from the three germ layers — ectoderm, mesoderm and endoderm (see p. 286). These are rare and constitute less than 1 per cent of ovarian teratomas. **It is the third common germ cell malignancies.** It is commonly (50%) seen in women between the ages of 10 and 20 years and rarely seen after menopause. Immature teratomas are almost never bilateral.

Pathology : Varying grades of undifferentiated tissue elements are present. Prognosis depends on the quantity of immature neural tissue elements. The prognosis of immature teratoma depends mainly on the tumour grade and the stage of the disease. Grade 3 tumour has poor prognosis. Serum AFP levels may be raised. Mature teratoma carries excellent prognosis.

Treatment : Unilateral oophorectomy with surgical staging is the optimum treatment when the tumour is confined to one ovary. For elderly women hysterectomy and bilateral salpingo-oophorectomy is ideal. **Adjuvant chemotherapy** for patients beyond stage IaGI is indicated. BEP (see above) is preferred, though VAC regimen is also effective.

ENDODERMAL SINUS TUMOUR (YOLK SAC TUMOUR)

These tumours arise from the primitive yolk sac.

It is observed mostly between 15-20 years of age. **It is the second most common (20%) malignant germ cell tumour of the ovary.** Endodermal sinus tumours are unilateral and are usually solid, more than 10 cm in diameter.

Characteristic histological feature is the presence of cystic spaces lined by flattened epithelium. Within this space a tuft of vascular tissue is often seen. This is called **Schiller-Duval body**. Eosinophilic, hyaline bodies containing alphafetoprotein and other proteins are also constant microscopic feature.

It is highly malignant and spreads to the adjacent structures rapidly. It is usually solid and cut section shows gelatinous or haemorrhagic areas. It is composed of yolk sac endoderm and extra-embryonic mesoblasts. Association with dysgerminoma should be kept in mind.

Treatment : Surgical staging and unilateral salpingo-oophorectomy is generally the treatment of choice. All patients need subsequent chemotherapy. Total hysterectomy and contralateral salpingo-oophorectomy does not improve the prognosis in any way.

Chemotherapy : Routine use of combination chemotherapy has improved the survival significantly. Different combination regimens (VAC, VPB and POMB–ACE) are used (see p. 495). Combinations containing platinum-based compounds are associated with better response and survival.

The tumour produces alphafetoprotein which is an useful marker (serum level above 20 µg/ml) to monitor regression and detect recurrence.

NON-GESTATIONAL OVARIAN CHORIOCARCINOMA

Ovarian choriocarcinoma may be gestational, arising from ovarian pregnancy or metastases from the uterine choriocarcinoma. It may be non-gestational arising from one element of a solid teratoma. Pure non-gestational choriocarcinoma of the ovary is extremely rare. Most patients present before 20 years of age. Isosexual precocious puberty (p. 49) is common (50%). It consists of both cytotrophoblasts and syncitiotrophoblasts and **secretes gonadotrophins (hCG) which is utilised as a marker** in diagnosis and follow up.

Unlike gestational choriocarcinoma, it is not so sensitive to methotrexate. As such, surgery is the primary treatment to be followed by chemotherapy. Combination chemotherapy (MAC, BEP) have been used. Prognosis is poor.

GONADOBLASTOMA

It is a rare ovarian tumour. It consists of germ cells and gonadal stromal cells. Dysgerminoma is present in 50 per cent of cases. Patients often present with primary amenorrhoea, virilism or genital abnormalities. Karyotype is usually 45, X or 46,XX/46,XY. It is bilateral in 30% of cases.

Treatment is surgical removal of the tumour and also the contralateral ovary. Prognosis is excellent.

MIXED GERM CELL TUMOURS

Presence of more than one germ cell element (at least two) is considered in this group. Dysgerminoma is the most common (70-80%) tissue element. Complete surgery followed by chemotherapy (VBP, MAC or VAC) is advised.

Chemotherapy in germ cell tumour

Combination chemotherapy has improved the survival following conservative surgery in malignant germ cell tumours of the ovary. Patients with stage-Ia disease need close follow-up only. Following combination regimens have been used most commonly. BEP (bleomycin, etoposide and cisplatin), VBP (vinblastin, bleomycin and cisplatin) MAC (methotrexate, actinomycin-D and cyclophosphamide), VAC (vincristine, actinomycin-D and cyclophosphamide) and POMB-ACE (cisplatin, vincristine, methotrexate, bleomycin, actinomycin-D, cyclophosphamide and etoposide). For details see p. 495.

Menstrual function, fertility and other endocrine function have been found normal following use of these drugs.

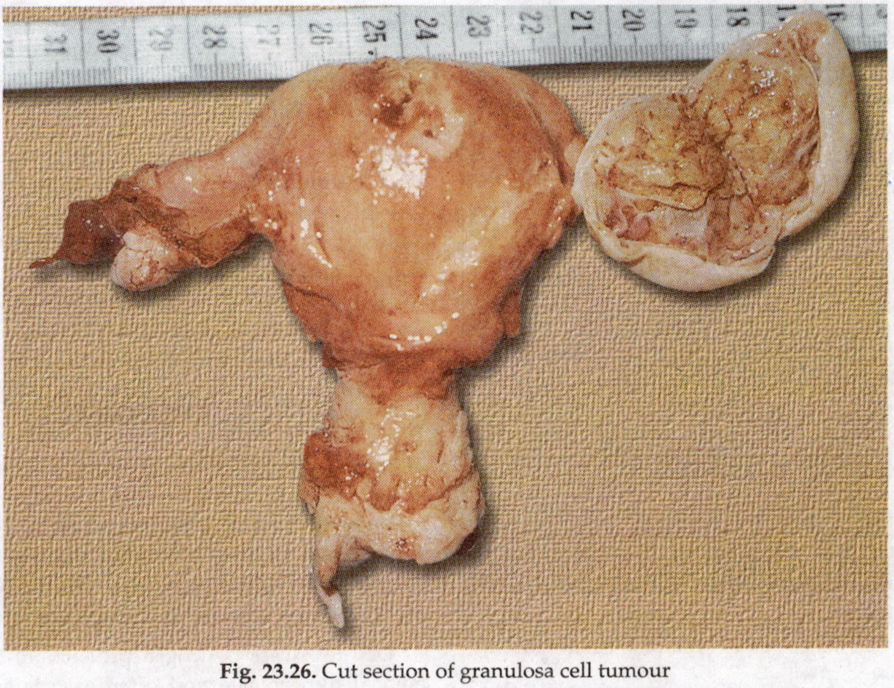

Fig. 23.26. Cut section of granulosa cell tumour

SEX CORD STROMAL TUMOUR

- Granulosa cell tumours.
- Thecomas, fibromas.
- Sertoli-Leydig cell tumours (androblastoma).
- Gynandroblastoma (mixed).

Sex cord stromal tumours constitute 5 per cent or less of all ovarian neoplasms. Peak incidence is over the age of 50. As 15-30 per cent of these tumours produce hormones, they are also known as *'functioning tumours'*.

GRANULOSA CELL TUMOURS

Granulosa cell tumours constitute 2 per cent of all ovarian neoplasms. The tumour originates from the 'rests' of primitive granulosa cells unused in folliculogenesis. **It is the commonest ovarian stromal tumour.**

It is bilateral only in 2 per cent of cases and is a slow growing tumour. The size varies, so also the consistency — may be solid or cystic. **Cut section** is characteristically yellow or orange (Fig. 23.26) due to its lipid content.

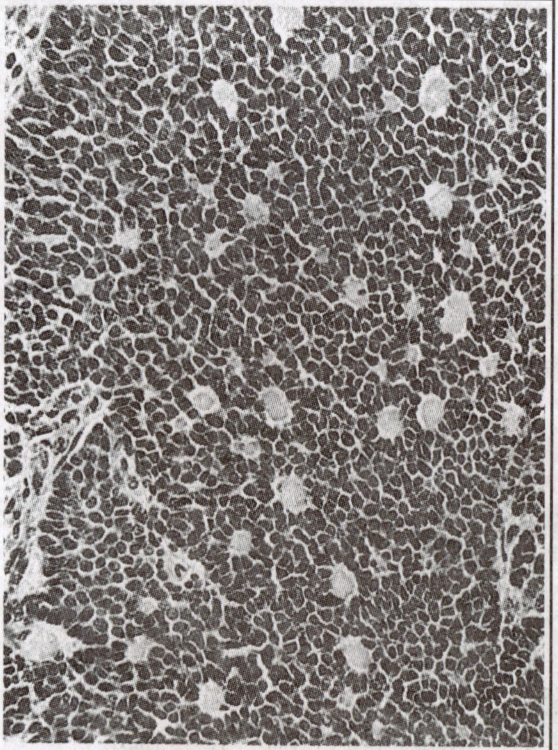

Fig. 23.27. Histologic picture of granulosa cell tumour. Presence of Call-Exner bodies (microfollicular pattern) are diagnostic

Microscopic appearance (Fig. 23.27)

The cells are round or polygonal with granular eosinophilic cytoplasm with ill-defined borders. The tumour cell nuclei are variable in size but they are pale, usually grooved or folded and are called **"Coffee bean" nuclei**. Some cells are luteinised containing large polyhedral lipid cells. The cells are arranged in a number of architectural pattern but commonly in folliculoid type. The granulosa cells are arranged in small clusters around a central cavity. These structures are called **Call-Exner bodies and are pathognomonic of granulosa cell tumour.** The juvenile tumour has less number of Call-Exner bodies and less number of "Coffee bean" nuclei compared to the adult variety. The tumour cells secrete inhibin and it is an useful marker for the disease (see p. 497).

As the tumour produces oestrogen, there may be associated endometrial hyperplasia (50%). Unopposed oestrogenic stimulation leads to development of endometrial carcinoma in about 5-10 per cent of cases.

Clinical features : It occurs in all ages, 10 per cent prior to puberty, 40 per cent during childbearing period and 50 per cent in postmenopausal women.

Apart from the non-specific features due to tumour mass, it produces **effects caused by hyperoestrinism which differs with ages.**

- Prior to puberty — Precocious puberty (p. 49).
- Childbearing period — Abnormal uterine bleeding.
- Postmenopausal — Bleeding (p. 532).

The features of precocious puberty revert back to normal after removal of the tumour. Patient may present with **acute abdomen** as these tumours have the propensity to rupture.

Treatment : Laparotomy and surgical staging is done (see p. 364). Unilateral salpingo-oophorectomy is the optimum treatment for children or women in the reproductive age. Metastatic disease and recurrences have been treated with BEP (p. 495) chemotherapeutic regimens. Overall prognosis is good. Life time follow-up is essential as recurrence can occur as late as 30 years.

THECOMA

Thecoma is predominantly a lesion of postmenopausal age. It may occur as a distinct entity or mixed with granulosa cell tumour. External appearance looks like a fibroma. Cut surface shows islands of yellow tissue separated by grey fibrous septa. Microscopic picture reveals cells like that of cortical stroma with areas of granulosa cells.

Due to excess oestrogen production, there is endometrial hyperplasia and often associated with endometrial carcinoma. It is responsible for postmenopausal bleeding. Rarely it may cause ascites or Meig's syndrome.

Treatment is surgical removal — total hysterectomy with bilateral salpingo-oophorectomy. In younger age group, conservative surgery may be employed considering the fact that it is mostly benign.

Fibroma in the ovary is usually observed in the postmenopausal women. It is derived from the stromal cells and are similar to thecomas. Less than 10% are bilateral. Meig's syndrome (Ascites, pleural effusion and ovarian fibroma) is seen in about 1% of cases (see p. 285, 616).

SERTOLI-LEYDIG CELL TUMOUR (ANDROBLASTOMA, ARRHENOBLASTOMA)

Sertoli-Leydig cell tumour is very rare and accounts for less than 0.5 per cent of all ovarian tumours.

They probably arise from the male directed cell rests in the hilum of the ovary, from granulosa cells or from teratomas. The tumour produces predominantly androgens (80%) and in some cases oestrogen.

The tumours are small, usually unilateral (90%) and solid in consistency. Cut surface shows yellowish tinge with areas of haemorrhage and necrosis. Microscopic picture often resembles to various testicular cells such as Sertoli and Leydig cells.

Clinical features : The androgens produced by the tumour first lead to **defeminisation** — atrophy of the breasts and uterus and amenorrhoea followed by **masculinisation (50%)**. This is evidenced by male type of distribution of hair, hoarseness of voice, breast atrophy, hirsutism, baldness and clitoral enlargement. Serum testosterone level is elevated.

Treatment is surgical removal of the tumour. The menstruation and fertility may return but the virilising features fail to regress. Unilateral oophorectomy for younger age group is optimum. For older patients total hysterectomy with bilateral salpingo-oophorectomy is ideal. **Adjuvant therapy** is needed for poorly differentiated tumour. Combination chemotherapy (VAC or VBP) is needed for recurrent disease. Tumour removal results in rapid resolution of most hormonal effects except deepening of voice and clitoromegaly.

GYNANDROBLASTOMA

This is a very rare type of tumour. It contains both granulosa cell (oestrogenic) or Sertoli-Leydig cell (androgenic) types. Usually it has got a benign course. Surgical removal is the optimum treatment.

METASTATIC TUMOURS OF THE OVARY

Metastatic tumours of the ovary constitute about 5 per cent of all ovarian tumours.

The common primary sites from where metastases to the ovaries occur are gastrointestinal tract (pylorus, colon and rarely small intestine), gallbladder, pancreas, breast and endometrial carcinoma. Two types of secondary ovarian growth

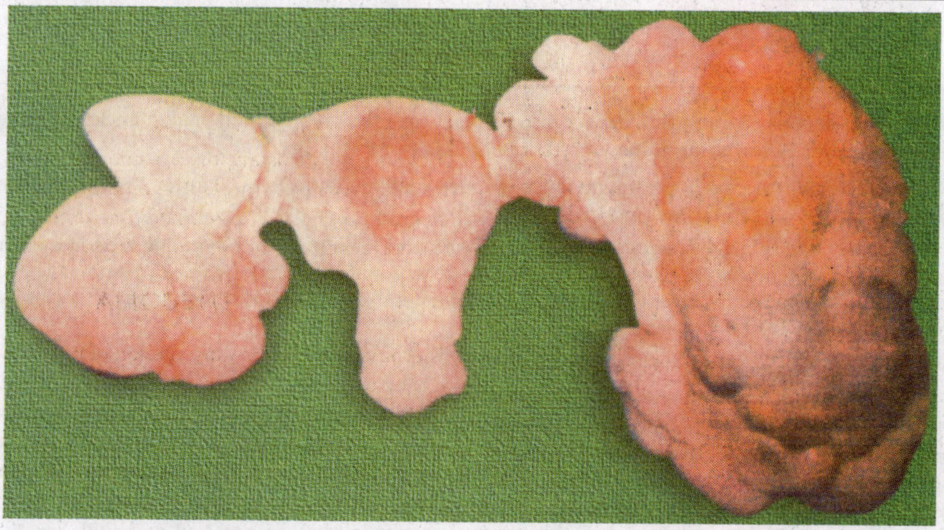

Fig. 23.28. Naked eye appearance of Krukenberg tumour *(Presented by Dr. Sagar/Dulal Sinha)*

occur. Krukenberg tumour constitutes about one-third of all metastatic ovarian cancers.

The mode of spread from the primary growth is through retrograde lymphatics or by implantation from metastases within the peritoneal cavity. The malignant cells from the stomach reach the superior gastric group of lymph glands which also receive the lymphatics of the ovaries.

These are usually bilateral, solid with irregular surfaces (Fig. 23.28). Peritoneal metastases are present, so also ascites. The omentum is involved and becomes solid.

Typical : Histologic picture same as that of primary one.

Atypical : The **atypical one is Krukenberg tumour** in which the histological picture differs from that of the primary one.

Naked-eye appearance : The tumour is usually bilateral, solid with smooth surfaces and usually maintaining the shape of the ovary. They typically form rounded or reniform, firm white masses. Sometimes they are bosselated and may attain a big size. There is no tendency of adhesion (i.e. capsule remains intact) (Fig. 23.28).

The cut surfaces usually look yellow or white in colour with cystic space at places due to degeneration. Cut surface has waxy consistency.

Histologically, the stroma is highly cellular. The mucin within epithelial cells compresses the nuclei to one pole, producing 'signet ring' appearance. The scattered 'signet ring' looking cells are characteristics of Krukenberg tumour (Fig. 23.29).

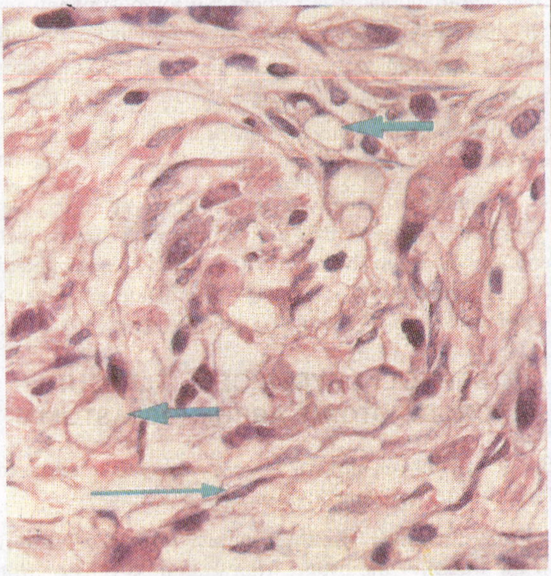

Fig. 23.29. Histologic picture of Krukenberg tumour showing characteristic 'signet-ring' appearance. The signet-ring cells contain the eccentric nuclei and abundant pale cytoplasm.

In most patients with Krukenberg's tumours, the prognosis is poor. Median survival being less than a year. Rarely, no primary site can be identified and the Krukenberg's tumour may be a **primary tumour**.

KEY POINTS

- In most of the developed countries, cancer of the breast tops the list in female malignancies, whereas in the developing countries including India, genital malignancies top the list.
- Vulval cancer usually occurs in postmenopausal women with median age of 60 years. Vulval cancer accounts for 3-5 per cent of all genital malignancies.

  The commonest site is labia majora followed by clitoris and labia minora. Ulcerative type is the commoner than the hypertrophic type. In 85 per cent, it is well-differentiated squamous cell carcinoma. The spread is predominantly by lymphatic both ipsilateral and contralateral (25%). Involvement of pelvic nodes bypassing the inguinal is less than 3 per cent.

  Causes of death are due to uraemia, rupture of the femoral vessels and sepsis.

  Microinvasive lesion of less than 1 mm requires wide local excision and follow up as metastasis to regional nodes are rare. Invasion of more than 1 mm requires radical vulvectomy with bilateral groin node dissection.

  Frank invasive carcinoma should be dealt with by radical vulvectomy with bilateral inguinofemoral lymphadenectomy. Pelvic lymphadenectomy is omitted in preference to radiation on the groin and pelvis - 4500 to 5000 cGy 4-6 weeks after operation. With negative groin nodes, the 5-year survival ranges from 90-100 per cent; with positive groin nodes, the survival rate falls to 20-55 per cent and with positive pelvic nodes, the survival rate is only 20 per cent.

KEY POINTS

- Prognosis of vulval carcinoma depends on many factors (p. 325). HPV positive younger patients tend to have a better prognosis.
- Melanoma comprise 5 per cent of vulval cancer and overall 5-year survival is about 50 per cent. Basal cell vulvar carcinoma is treated by wide local excision.
- Primary carcinoma of vagina is rare and most vaginal cancers are metastatic. The commonest site is in the upper-third of the posterior wall. The mean age is 55 years. Squamous cell carcinoma accounts for 90 per cent of the cases. 5-year survival rate is about 40-45 per cent.

  Clear cell adenocarcinoma is seen in adolescent girls, who have had history of intrauterine exposure to diethyl stilboestrol. Radical hysterectomy, vaginectomy with pelvic lymphadenectomy is the surgery.
- Surgery (see p. 326) is the treatment of choice for upper vaginal, low stage tumour in younger patients. However, radiation is used widely as a primary therapy. Ideally, 7000-75000 cGy is administered in less than 9 weeks.
- In most of the developing countries, including India, carcinoma of the cervix is the most common malignancy in the female. It ranks first, the second being breast carcinoma. The site of lesion is predominantly ectocervix (80%). The commonest histologic type is squamous cell carcinoma (85-90%) and about 10-15 per cent are adenocarcinomas.

  Squamous cell carcinomas have a viral (HPV) and veneral association unlike that of adenocarcinomas.

  The primary groups of lymph gland involvement are parametrial, internal iliac, obturator, external iliac and sacral nodes.

  Preclinical invasive carcinoma is diagnosed by cytology, colposcopy and directed biopsy. If positive lesion is found, diagnostic conisation and serial section has to be performed to establish the diagnosis. Definitive diagnosis of microinvasive carcinoma is made by cervical conisation. The cone margins must be free of disease when conservative therapy is undertaken. Clinical presentation of early carcinoma includes menstrual abnormalities – intermenstrual bleeding or contact bleeding or excessive white discharge. Speculum examination reveals the lesion on the ectocervix which bleeds on friction.

  Causes of death are uraemia, haemorrhage, sepsis, cachexia and metastases to the lung.

  Primary prevention includes identifying 'high risk' women, and 'high risk' males, use of condom during early intercourse and removal of cervix during hysterectomy. Secondary prevention involves in screening programme and identifying the precancerous lesions or invasive lesion at its treatable stage.
- The prognosis of carcinoma cervix depends on many factors (p. 29) of which stage of the disease is important. Cancer cervix is a locally invasive tumours. It spreads primarily to pelvic tissues, then to pelvic and para-aortic lymph nodes. Rarely haematogenous spread to liver, lungs and bones may occur. Currently, advanced stage tumours are treated by chemoradiation. Cisplatin 40 mg/m^2 weekly is used along with radiation (teletherapy and brachytherapy). Complications of radiotherapy (p. 486) may occur more than 1 year after therapy.

  Radical hysterectomy can be performed upto stage IIA. This is specially used for a younger patient to preserve her ovarian function and to avoid vaginal fibrosis.

  Survival outcome of treatment following surgery or radiation for stage IB/IIA is the same (85%).

  Results of therapy in term of 5-year survival, is gratifying in early stages – 95 per cent in stage Ia, reduced to 70 per cent in stage II and 45 per cent in stage III and 24 per cent in stage IV (see Table 23.12).

  Radical trachelectomy can be done in young women to preserve fertility as an alternative to radical hysterectomy. The disease must be in early stage (IA_2 or small $IB_1 \leq 2$ cm). A therapeutic lymphadenectomy is also performed.
- Leg pain along the distribution of sciatic nerve and unilateral leg swelling are suggestive of pelvic recurrence of carcinoma cervix.
- The incidence of stump carcinoma is about 1 per cent. The 5-year survival rate is 30-60 per cent.
- For women with carcinoma cervix during pregnancy, survival rate is not different stage for stage when compared with the non-pregnant state.

KEY POINTS

- Carcinoma body ranks third amongst genital malignancies next to cervix and ovary. In USA, it is the leading site of genital malignancies followed by ovary and cervix.

  75 per cent are postmenopausal with the median age of 60. Nulliparity is associated in 30 per cent.

- Use of combined oral contraceptive is a known protective factor whereas chronic unopposed oestrogen stimulation is a known predisposing factor for endometrial carcinoma (see Tables 23.13, 22.8).

  Corpus cancer syndrome encompasses obesity, hypertension and diabetes. Fibroid is associated in 30 per cent. Endometrial hyperplasia precedes carcinoma in 25 per cent. The commonest histological type is adenocarcinoma. The pelvic and/or paraaortic glands are involved in about 10 per cent in Stage I.

  Postmenopausal bleeding is the predominant feature (75%). In premenopausal women, irregular bleeding is too often related. Once suspected, fractional curettage is to be done, not only to diagnose but to determine the extent of the lesion. The important primary prevention includes restriction of injudicious use of oestrogen after menopause in nonhysterectomised women.

  Secondary prevention includes screening of 'high risk' women at least in menopausal period and liberal hysterectomy in pre-malignant lesions of the corpus.

  Mainstay in the treatment of carcinoma body is total abdominal hysterectomy and bilateral salpingo-oophorectomy. In stage II, radical hysterectomy has to be done. Adjuvant radiation is considered depending on the surgical stage of the disease, myometrial invasion and histologic grade (p. 346).

  Primary radiotherapy is the treatment in surgically risk patients and in advanced stages.

  Chemotherapy is used in advanced and recurrent cases or in metastatic lesions.

  Progestogens are widely used in well-differentiated carcinoma with adequate oestrogen and progesterone receptors. Antioestrogen, tamoxifen is often used along with progestogens to improve the result.

  Prognosis of endometrial cancer depends on many factors (Table 23.15) of which depth of myometrial invasion and tumour grade are the most important ones. Younger women with endometrial cancer have a better prognosis when compared with the older women.

- Gestational trophoblastic neoplasia (GTN) encompasses persistent hydatidiform mole, invasive mole, choriocarcinoma and placental site trophoblastic tumour.

  The incidence of GTN is about 1 in 5,000 pregnancies in Oriental countries and 1 in 50,000 in Europe and North America. Fifty per cent occur after molar pregnancy, 25 per cent after abortion and ectopic and 25 per cent after normal pregnancy. Nonmetastatic lesions develop in 15 per cent and metastatic lesions develop in about 4 per cent of patients after molar evacuation.

  Trophoblastic cells normally regresses within 3 weeks following delivery. Women treated for GTT should not become pregnant for 6-12 months after the treatment. This helps to assess the level of β-hCG and treatment response. Diagnosis of postmolar GTN is made when the hCG level plateaus for 3 or more consecutive weeks or re-elevates.

  The invasive mole is diagnosed on laparotomy and on histology showing hyperplastic trophoblastic cells maintaining villous structures without evidences of muscle necrosis. In choriocarcinoma, the hyperplastic trophoblastic column of cells invade the muscles. There are evidences of haemorrhage and muscle necrosis. The villous pattern is lost.

  The commonest site of metastases is lung, followed by anterior vaginal wall, brain and liver.

- Recurrence rate of GTN following treatment (hCG level reached normal) is 5 per cent for metastatic good prognosis cases and is 1-2 per cent for nonmetastatic cases (see Table 23.17).

  Primary surgery has got limited place. Hysterectomy is indicated in women aged more than 35 years to improve the efficacy of chemotherapy or to control intractable bleeding. Total hysterectomy is to be done on day 3 of a course of chemotherapy.

KEY POINTS

There is no adverse effect on subsequent pregnancy, if it occurs after 1 year of chemotherapy. The damaged cells are likely to be washed by this time. Pregnancy should be confirmed by USG early and serum hCG should be measured 6 weeks after delivery to exclude persistent GTN.

- Prophylactic chemotherapy can prevent uterine invasion and metastasis. But it is given selectively.
- Low risk GTN cases (see Table 23.17) are usually treated by single-agent chemotherapy. Whereas high-risk metastatic cases are treated with multiple-agent chemotherapy (see p. 352). Non-metastatic and low-risk metastatic GTN cases are completely curable by chemotherapy.
- The commonest site of uterine sarcoma is the intramural part.

  The commonest mode of spread is blood borne. Total hysterectomy with bilateral salpingo-oophorectomy is the surgery. This is followed by external pelvic radiation. Mitotic figure is an important prognostic factor for leiomyosarcoma of the uterus. Patients with mitotic rate of less than 5/10 HPF behave as a benign lesion but mitotic rate of more than 10 per 10 HPF are frankly malignant and have got worst prognosis.
- Sarcoma botryoides is a special type of mixed mesodermal tumour arising from the cervix. The child, before the age of 5, may be affected. Chemotherapy gives better result than radical surgery.
- Primary carcinoma of the fallopian tube is rarest. It is mostly unilateral (80%). Associated haematosalpinx is often present. Classic traid of adnexal mass, intermittent profuse watery discharge (hydrops tubae profluens) and vaginal bleeding is considered pathognomonic for tubal carcinoma. USG/Laparoscopy is suggestive and biopsy is confirmatory. Persistent postmenopausal bleeding and/or positive vaginal cytology for adenocarcinoma, in the absence of endometrial carcinoma, the diagnosis of tubal carcinoma should be considered.

  Total hysterectomy with bilateral salpingo-oophorectomy along with omentectomy followed by whole pelvic radiation is the treatment. The prognosis is not good.

  Secondary carcinoma (metastatic) is common (90%), the primary sites are from ovary, uterus, breast or gastro-intestinal tract.
- There is wide geographical variation in the incidence of ovarian malignancy. Incidence is high in Scandinavian countries and USA, low in Asian countries (India, Japan).

  Serous cyst adenomas are the most common epithelial tumours. Serous adenocarcinomas have the worst prognosis of epithelial adenocarcinomas.

  Twenty per cent of ovarian neoplasms are malignant. Malignant epithelial tumours constitute about 90 per cent of all primary ovarian carcinomas. The primary mode of spread of epithelial ovarian carcinoma is transcoelomic and it spreads to the visceral and parietal peritoneum, diaphragm and to the retroperitoneal nodes.

  Endometrioid carcinoma is associated with endometrial carcinoma in 20 per cent and ovarian-endometriosis in 10 per cent cases.

  The common primary sites of metastatic ovarian malignancies are gastrointestinal tract, gallbladder, breast and endometrial carcinoma. The tumour may be typical or atypical (Krukenberg). The primary sites of Krukenberg are stomach, large bowel and breast. The spread to the ovaries is by retrograde lymphatics. Histologically, it is confirmed by presence of 'signet ring' looking cells.

  Patients with familial cancer syndrome (Lynch type I and II) have a higher risk of developing epithelial ovarian cancer. Mutations of BRCA 1 gene (17 q) and BRCA II gene (13 q) have been observed. Inherited ovarian malignancies account for about 5 per cent of epithelial ovarian cancers (see p. 357).

  The efficacy of screening procedure is not well-documented. However, periodic internal examination supplemented by transvaginal colour Doppler sonography to note the ovarian volume, blood flow and estimation of CA 125 in 'high risk' population, can reveal the lesion at the early stage. Gene mutation study for detection of genetic inheritance is not currently recommended.

KEY POINTS

High-risk women are : family history of ovarian, endometrial or breast carcinoma, history of removal of ovarian or breast neoplasm, presence of pelvic tumour in adolescent and perimenopausal women and postmenopausal palpable ovary (volume $\geq$ 8 cm^3).

Protective factors for ovarian epithelial adenocarcinomas are : combined oral contraceptives, pregnancy, tubal ligation, hysterectomy and breastfeeding.

Ovarian enlargement less than 8 cm in diameter in a menstruating women is most commonly functional.

Surgery is the keystone in the primary treatment of ovarian malignancy. The aims are staging of the disease and to perform maximum surgical removal.

The ideal definitive surgery is total hysterectomy with bilateral salpingo-oophorectomy with infracolic omentectomy. In exceptional cases, conservative surgery of unilateral salpingo-oophorectomy is justified.

Debulking surgery with residual tumour nodules < 1 cm. confers better survival advantage even in advanced stage disease. CT, MRI and PET are effective for detecting residual tumour and the retroperitoneal nodes.

Second look surgery either by laparoscopy or laparotomy is employed either after 12 courses of chemotherapy or after 1 year of primary therapy.

The 5-year survival rate for patients with borderline epithelial ovarian cancer (grade 0) is close to 100 per cent (p. 291). For other stages see Table 23.26.

Chemotherapy is being widely used following surgery to improve the result in terms of survival.

Platinum compounds (cisplatin, carboplatin), either alone or in combination, prolong the survival rate. Taxane derivatives (paclitaxel, docetaxel) are effective in cisplatin resistant ovarian cancer. Treatment with carboplatin and paclitaxel for 3-6 cycles is desirable for most patients.

The ovarian antigen CA-125 is useful to monitor the patient during chemotherapy and for follow up.

The prognosis of epithelial ovarian carcinoma depends on many factors (see p. 366). Over expression of oncogene (HER-2/neu) has been associated with poor prognosis.

- Germ cell tumours occur in young women. They are the second most common type of ovarian neoplasm. Most common germ cell tumour is the benign cystic teratoma (dermoid). It is bilateral in 10-15 per cent cases.
- Dysgerminoma is the most common malignant germ cell tumour. It is bilateral in 10 per cent cases. The tumour is highly sensitive to radiation.
- Fibroma is the most common benign solid ovarian tumour.
- Endodermal sinus tumour is highly malignant occurring at a median age of 19. Alpha fetoprotein is the tumour marker. Treatment is surgery followed by chemotherapy.
- Non-gestational ovarian choriocarcinoma is highly malignant. hCG is the tumour marker. It is not responsive to chemotherapy. The treatment is surgery followed by chemotherapy.
- Multi-agent chemotherapy (VAC, VBP, CAP) has improved the survival rate as well as childbearing function in patients with malignant germ cell tumours.
- Granulosa cell tumour produces oestrogen and may be associated with endometrial hyperplasia or endometrial carcinoma. It occurs 10 per cent prior to puberty and 40 per cent in postmenopause. It produces precocious puberty and postmenopausal bleeding. Thecoma is predominantly postmenopausal. There is excess oestrogen production.
- Sertoli-Leydig cell tumour (previously called arrhenoblastoma) is very rare, it arises from the male directed cell rests in the hilum of the ovary, from granulosa cells or from teratomas. The tumour produces androgens (80%) and in some cases oestrogen.

Urinary Problems in Gynaecology

24

ANATOMY OF VESICOURETHRAL UNIT

The bladder and urethra should be considered as a single unit with two major functions — storage of urine and voiding of urine.

Though the two organs are anatomically separate entities but integrated with complex functional interplay.

The descriptive anatomy of the urinary bladder and urethra has been described in Chapter 1. **The anatomic and physiologic peculiarities involved in storage and voiding of urine are to be discussed here.**

BLADDER

The bladder muscles — called detrusor consist of three layers of muscles (Fig. 24.1).

- **Outer longitudinal** — The muscles course downwards from the fundus to bladder neck. At the level of bladder neck, it forms a sling. With this arrangement, it forms an active and dominant role in both storage and voiding.
- **Middle circular** — It is more prominent in the lower part of the bladder.
- **Inner longitudinal** — It courses downwards from the fundus of the bladder and continues in the form of spirals upto the midurethra.

Recent studies, however, suggest that there is

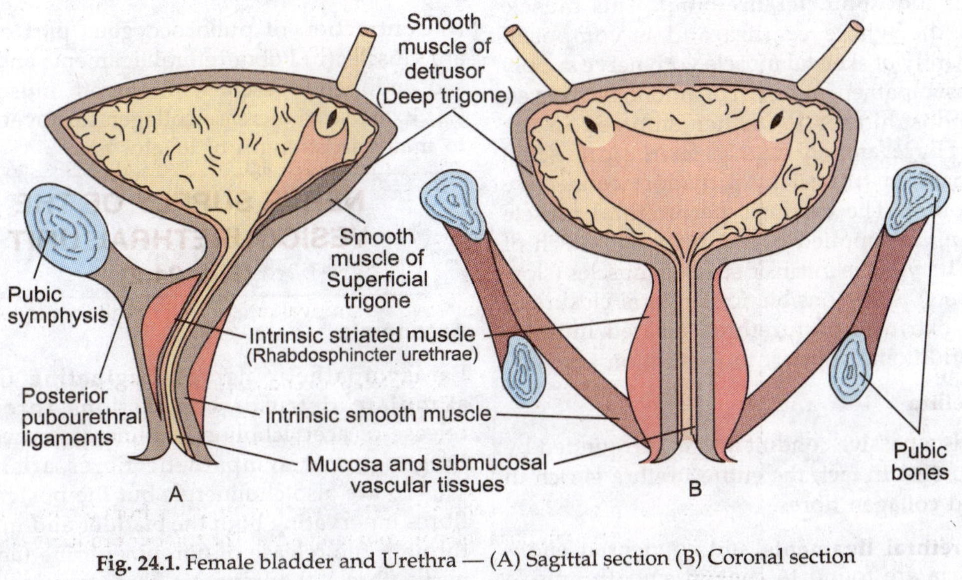

Fig. 24.1. Female bladder and Urethra — (A) Sagittal section (B) Coronal section

frequent interchange of fibres between the bundles and the separate layers are not distinctly defined.

From a functional point of view, the detrusor appears to contract as a single syncytial mass. The detrusor muscles are shown to contain significant amount of acetylcholinesterase.

Trigone

The smooth muscle has got two distinct layers. The deeper one is similar to detrusor. The superficial layer is relatively thin. Traced distally, it fades out in the proximal urethra. It is devoid of acetylcholinesterase but have more cholinergic nerve supply.

Bladder neck

The muscle bundles are largely oblique or longitudinal. They appear to have little or no sphincteric action.

URETHRA

From the functional point of view, the anatomic length of the urethra is divided into three parts.

Proximal urethra

It is weakest part of the urethra. Inner longitudinal muscle of the detrusor fades out in this part of the urethra. It fails to withstand the rise of intravesical or intra-abdominal pressure.

Midurethra (Fig. 24.1)

This is the strongest part of the urethra. This part has got an additional support by the intrinsic striated muscle (rhabdosphincter urethrae). This muscle encircles the whole urethra and is composed predominantly of skeletal muscle with nerve supply from parasympathetic division of autonomic nerves. This rhabdosphincter is further enforced in the upper part by levator ani muscles (extrinsic muscles) being separated from it by a distinct connective tissue septum. The extrinsic periurethral muscle (levator ani) is supplied by the perineal branch of pudendal nerve. The intrinsic striated muscles (slow twitch fibers) is responsible for urethral closure at rest. The extrinsic periurethral striated muscles provide additional support to urethra on stress.

Distal urethra

This part is a passive conduit and is surrounded by collagen tissue. In fact, the entire urethra is rich in elastic and collagen fibres.

Pubourethral ligaments and condensed endopelvic fascia are found to contain smooth muscle fibres. They work together to maintain the normal anatomic support and prevent hypermobility of bladder neck and urethra.

Submucous layer of the urethra

Submucous layer is the vascular layer which by its plasticity helps in urethral compression.

Two venous plexi are identified in the submucous coat. A distal one which varies little with age and a proximal one beneath the bladder neck which undergoes marked changes with age. In the reproductive period, these vessels give a cavernous appearance to the submucosa which disappears in the postmenopausal period. **This urethral vascular system plays a significant role in the maintenance of resting urethral pressure.**

Mucous layer of the urethra

Mucosa is arranged in longitudinal folds that allow apposition and distension.

Support to bladder neck and urethra

Support is maintained by intrinsic and extrinsic factors.

Intrinsic factors

(i) Intrinsic rhabdosphincter urethrae (Fig. 24.1). (ii) Urethral submucosal venous plexus (cavernous plexus). (iii) Urethral smooth muscles. (iv) Sympathetic activity to maintain urethral tone by α-adrenergic receptors. (v) Estrogen to increase collagen connective tissue.

Extrinsic factors

(i) Contraction of pubococcygeus part of levator ani muscle; (ii) Pubourethral ligaments and condensed endopelvic fascia with smooth muscle fibres; (iii) Exercise to increase collagen turnover and also to maintain strength of levator ani.

NERVE SUPPLY OF THE VESICOURETHRAL UNIT (Fig. 24.2)

Autonomic

Parasympathetic nerves originating from S_{2-4} stimulate detrusor contractions through the release of acetylcholine (cholinergic nerve fibres). Preganglionic sympathetic fibres arising from T_{10} - L_2 are also cholinergic but the postganglionic fibres innervating both the bladder and urethra act through the release of norepinephrine (adrenergic nerve fibres). β-adrenergic fibres terminate mainly

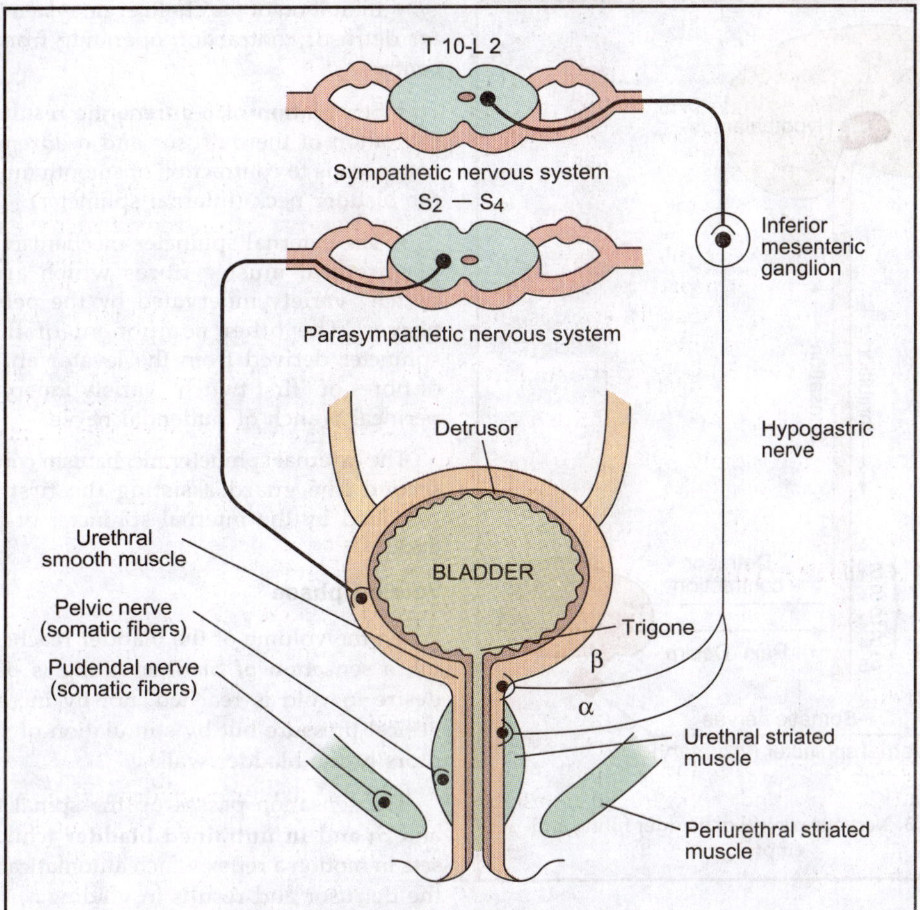

Fig. 24.2. Nerve supply of the vesicourethral unit

in the bladder and α-adrenergic mostly in the urethra. The former component relaxes both the bladder and urethra and latter one contracts only the urethra. α receptors are located mainly in the bladder base and are responsible for detrusor contraction. β receptors are located mainly on the fundus of the bladder and cause detrusor relaxation.

The sympathetic is concerned mainly with the filling and storage phase of micturition. Parasympathetic supply (acetylcholine) is responsible for detrusor contraction and normal voiding.

Somatic

The somatic supply to the striated muscle of urethra is through the pudendal nerve. The rhabdosphincter is supplied by pelvic splanchnic nerves travelling with the parasympathetic fibres. Extrinsic periurethral striated muscle is supplied by the motor fibres of the pudendal nerves.

PHYSIOLOGY OF MICTURITION

The bladder and urethra should be considered as a single unit with two main functions :

- **Storage of urine**
- **Voiding of urine**

Storage phase

The urine comes into the bladder drop by drop through the ureteric openings. As the bladder fills, the walls stretch to maintain a constant muscle tone. The bladder usually fills at the rate of 0.5-5 ml/min. from the ureters. The intravesical pressure is raised to remain at almost steady level of about 10 cm of water even with a volume of about 500 ml.

The intravesical pressure is kept lower than that of the urethra by delicately coordinated relaxation of detrusor muscle. **This is possible through number of mechanisms.**

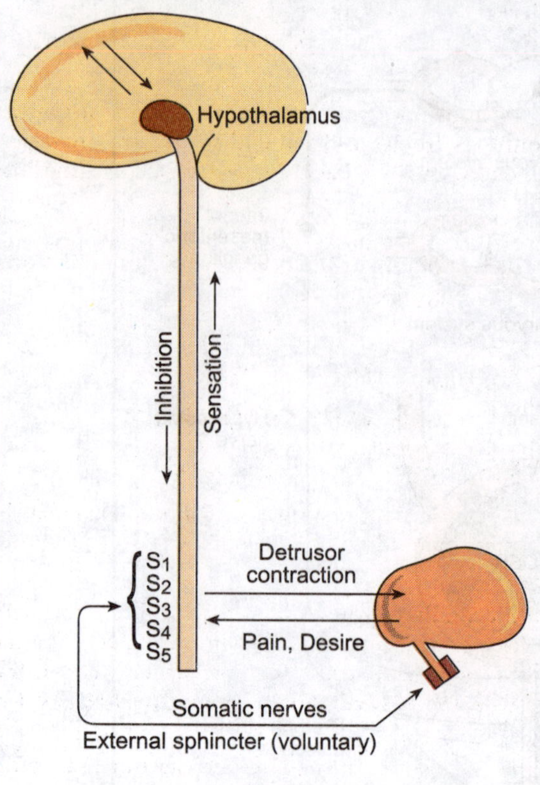

Fig. 24.3. Nervous control of bladder filling and emptying

- Proximal urethral musculature acts like a sphincter by maintaining tonic contraction.
- Stretching of the detrusor reflexly contracts the sphincteric muscles of the bladder neck.
- Inhibition of the cholinergic system responsible for detrusor contraction operating from the spinal centres.
- Stimulation of β-adrenergic results in further relaxation of the detrusor and α-adrenergic dominance leads to contraction of smooth muscles round the bladder neck (internal sphincter).
- The external sphincter mechanism consists of periurethral muscle fibres which are of "slow twitch" variety innervated by the pelvic efferent nerves. The other component of the external sphincter derived from the levator ani, composed of fibres of "first twitch" variety innervated by the perineal branch of pudendal nerve.

The external sphincter mechanism contributes the second line guard assisting the first line guard provided by the internal sphincter of the bladder neck.

Voiding phase

When the volume of the bladder reaches about 250 ml, a sensation of bladder filling is perceived. A desire to void is reached, not by increased intravesical pressure but by stimulation of stretch receptors in the bladder wall.

The sensation passes up the spinal roots S2, S3 and S4 **and in untrained bladder** (children), there sets in motion a reflex which automatically contracts the detrusor and results in voiding.

But in the trained adults, this urge can be suppressed especially if the time or place is not convenient. Because in adults, the reflex spinal arc is under control of the hypothalamus and higher areas

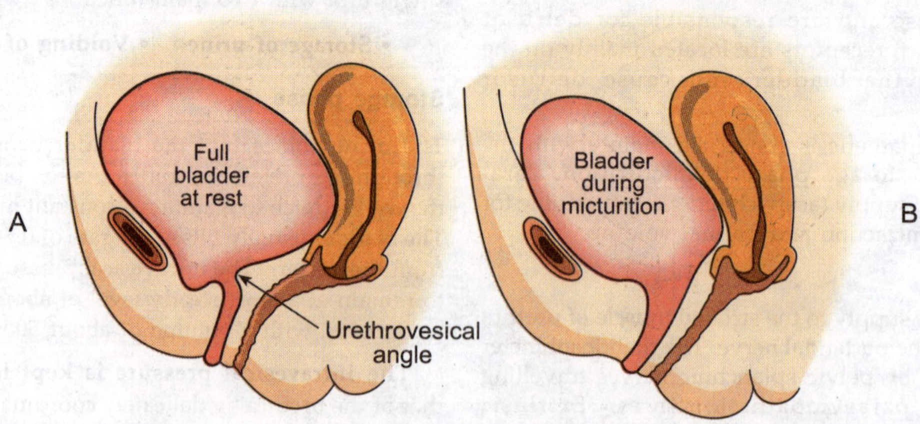

Fig. 24.4. Radiographic tracing of the bladder and urethra — (A) At rest (B) During micturition

of the brain (anterior part of the frontal lobes). Cerebral control of micturition is complex but is predominantly controlled by pontine centre. Action of detrusor can therefore, be voluntarily inhibited (Fig. 24.3).

When the time or the place is convenient, the higher centres via the hypothalamus no longer inhibit the detrusor and the bladder changes from its passive to active role. The detrusor contracts to raise the intravesical pressure to 30-50 cm of water. The pressure is further raised to about 100 cm of water by voluntary contraction of the abdominal muscles.

The series of chronologic events to follow in the process of micturition are :

The diaphragm is fixed; the abdominal muscles are contracted and the pelvic floor is relaxed.

↓

Immediately following this or possibly as a consequence of them, there is drop of intraurethral pressure. This drop is due to skeletal muscle relaxation and sympathetic blockade. Bladder base descends with obliteration of posterior urethrovesical angle (normal 100°) (Fig. 24.4).

↓

Detrusor contraction starts.

↓

Funnelling of the bladder neck and upper urethra, i.e. dilatation of the urethra from above down.

↓

Urine leaks into the upper urethra.

↓

External urethral sphincter opens voluntarily or is overwhelmed by the raised intravesical pressure.

↓

Voiding

↓

At the end of micturition, the proximal urethra contracts from the distal end to the urethrovesical junction, milking back the last drop of urine into the bladder.

↓

The anatomy of the base and posterior urethrovesical angle is restored.

↓

Finally, the external sphincter closes.

URINARY CONTINENCE

Mechanism of urinary continence

The mechanism responsible for maintenance of urinary continence in the females is still ill-understood.

Normally, intraurethral pressure at rest and with stress is much higher (20-50 cm of water) than the intravesical pressure (10 cm of water). **The intraurethral pressure at rest is maintained by the following** :

- Apposition of the longitudinal mucosal folds.
- Submucosal vascular plexus (hermetic seal).
- Abundant deposition of collagen and elastic tissues throughout the circumference of the urethra.
- Tonic contraction of the smooth muscles in the proximal urethra and bladder neck.
- Rhabdosphincter in the midurethra and levator ani muscles.

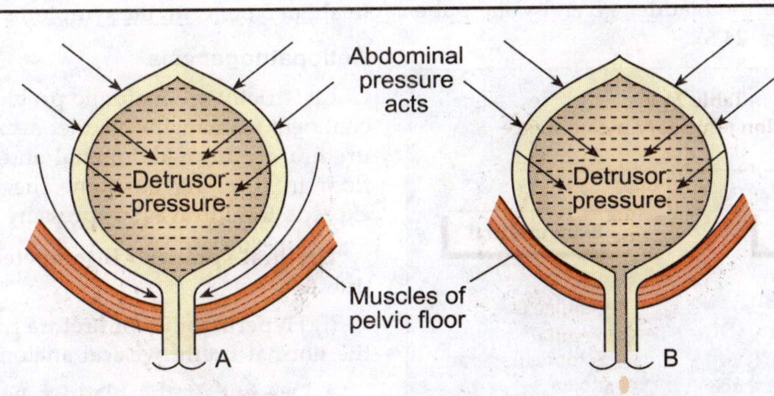

Fig. 24.5. (a) Normally any increase in intra-abdominal pressure compresses the upper urethra. **(b)** If the bladder neck descends, this does not occur

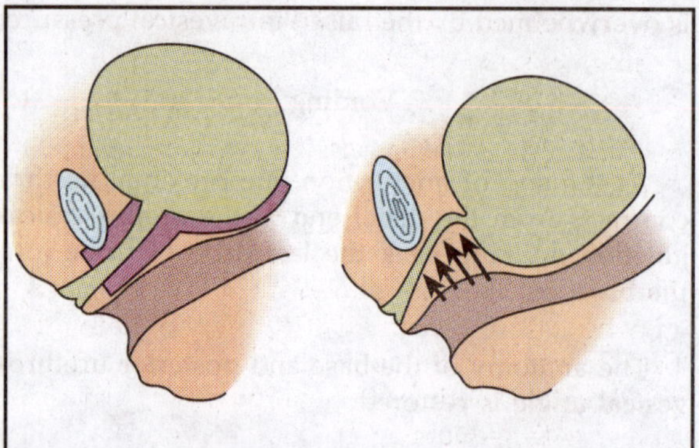

Fig. 24.6. Kinking of the urethra during stress pulling the bladder neck upwards and forwards

Approximately, one-third of the resting urethral pressure is due to rhabdosphincter effects, one-third to smooth muscle effects and one-third to its vascular plexus.

During stress, with rise of intra-abdominal pressure, the escape of urine is prevented by the additional factors :

(i) Centripetal force of intra-abdominal pressure transmitted to the proximal urethra which occurs as long as the bladder neck remains above the pelvic diaphragm (Fig. 24.5).

(ii) Reflex contraction of the urethral striated sphincter and periurethral striated musculature during stress.

(iii) Kinking of the urethra due to :

- Bladder base rocks downwards and backwards
- Bladder neck is pulled upwards and forwards behind the symphysis pubis due to preferential better support to the posterior wall of the urethra than to the base of the bladder given by the pubocervical fascia (Fig. 24.6).

Table 24.1
Classification of urinary incontinence

Urethral	Extra urethral
• Urethral sphincter incompetence (GSI)	Acquired
• Detrusor instability (DI)	• Fistulae (see p. 401)
• Mixed (GSI and DI)	Congenital
• Over-flow incontinence (acute and chronic)	• Ectopic ureter and others
• Functional and others (UTI)	
• Congenital (epispadius)	

URINARY INCONTINENCE

Urinary incontinence is defined as objectively demonstrable involuntary loss of urine so as to cause hygienic and/or social inconvenience for day to day activity.

Pathophysiology of Urinary Incontinence — Basic pathology of incontinence is the rise of intravesical pressure over that of maximum urethral pressure. It may be due to mechanical injury to the supports of the bladder neck following childbirth, trauma (surgery), or due to ageing. Instability of the detrusor muscles, may also be associated.

Stress urinary incontinence (SUI) is defined as involuntary escape of urine from the external urinary meatus due to sudden rise in intra-abdominal pressure. The term, 'urethral sphincter incompetence' seems to be appropriate as it signifies the basic pathology (Table 24.1).

GENUINE STRESS INCONTINENCE (GSI)

Definition

Genuine stress incontinence (GSI) is defined, according to the international continence society (ICS) as involuntary urethral loss of urine when the intravesical pressure exceeds the maximum urethral pressure **in the absence of detrusor activity**. The diagnosis of GSI should be made following urodynamic assessment only.

Incidence

The reported incidence in the Western countries is as high as 40 per cent in association with prolapse. In about 5 per cent, the symptoms may be annoying.

Aetiopathogenesis

GSI is strictly an anatomic problem. In the normal continent woman, the bladder neck and the proximal urethra are intra-abdominal and above the pelvic floor in standing position. The urethral pressure exceeds the intravesical pressure.

Urethral sphincter incompetence is principally due to :

(i) Hypermobility of urethra due to distortion of the normal urethrovesical anatomy.

- Descent of the bladder neck and proximal urethra which normally lies above the urogenital diaphragm, hinders rise of intraurethral pressure during straining (Fig. 24.5).

(ii) Lowered urethral pressure — Lowered intraurethral pressure at rest below the intravesical pressure.

Risk factors for stress urinary incontinence

- **Developmental weakness** of the supporting structures maintaining the bladder neck and proximal urethra in position. There may be genetic variations in collagen and other connective tissues which normally maintain anatomic and physiologic aspect of the vesicourethral unit.
- **Childbirth trauma** causing damage of the pelvic floor and pubocervical fascia. Denervation of the smooth and striated components of the sphincter mechanism also operates. **The injury is more common in gynaecoid and least in android pelvis.**
- **Pregnancy** — It is probably functional in nature and related to high level of progesterone.
- **Postmenopausal** — Oestrogen deficiency leads to atrophy of the supporting structures along with diminished periurethral vascular resistance.
- **Trauma** — Injury to symphysis pubis due to fracture or following symphysiotomy.
- **Following surgery** like anterior colporrhaphy, local repair of VVF or bladder neck surgery, there may be fibrosis of the urethra and urethral musculature.
- **Obesity.**

Morbid anatomic changes

In GSI, the main defects are:

- Intrinsic sphincter dysfunction.
- Bladder base becomes flat and lies in line with the posterior wall of the proximal urethra.
- Descent of the proximal urethra.

The net effect of these changes is to lower the intraurethral pressure as in early stage of micturition. Thus, even a small rise of intravesical pressure during stress, allows the urine to escape out.

GSI is the ultimate symptom of varying severity due to anatomic urethral hypermobility (80%) and/or intrinsic sphincter deficiency (20%).

Clinical features

Patient profile: The patients are usually parous, may be postmenopausal. Often the complaints date back to the last childbirth or some vaginal plastic operation. Sometimes the symptoms may be combined with frequency or urge incontinence. The patient may be obese.

Symptoms: The only symptom is escape of urine with coughing, sneezing or laughing. **The loss of urine has got the following features**:

- Brief and coincides precisely to the period of raised intra-abdominal pressure.
- Unassociated with a desire to pass urine.
- Rarely, occurs in supine position or during sleep.
- Patients are fully aware of it.
- The amount of loss is small.

Details of medical history (e.g. diabetes, chronic pulmonary disease, neurological disease), surgical history (spine or genitourinary tract), current medications (sedatives, antipsychotics) must be noted. Because these have direct bearing on urinary incontinence.

Local examination: Pelvic examination should be done with the bladder full.

- Some degree of pelvic relaxation with cystocele or cystourethrocele is usually evident.
- Stress test — When the patient is asked to cough, a few drops of urine are seen escaping from the external urethral meatus. If the escape is not

Table 24.2
Difference in clinical presentation

Stress Incontinence	Urge Incontinence (sensory)	Detrusor Instability
• Leakage of urine coincides with stress • No prior urge to void • Amount — small • Patient — fully aware of it • Micturition — normal	• Unable to control the escape of urine, once there is urge to void • Amount — large • Patient — aware of the urge • Urgency and frequency	• The incontinence may occur abruptly even without a full bladder • Amount — large • Patient — not aware of it • Frequency and nocturia

detected in supine position, the examination is to be conducted in standing position.

• Q-tip test — The Q-tip test has been tried to predict SUI. A sterile (lubricated with 2% xylocaine jelly) cotton tipped swab is introduced to the level of bladder neck through the urethra. Then the patient is asked to sit and cough (valsalva). If there is marked upward elevation (>30°) of the cotton tipped swab, urethra is considered hypermobile. Unfortunately the test is imprecise to the diagnosis of SUI.

Differential diagnosis

Sometimes, there may be clinical confusion with other forms of incontinence such as urge or detrusor instability. The differentiating features are tabulated in Table 24.2.

Special investigations (Table 24.4)

The investigations aim at :

- To confirm the diagnosis
- To rule out associated pathology.

Midstream urine examination — This should be a routine prior to urodynamic studies to avoid risk of flaring up the infection during invasive procedures. The infection, if present, must be treated effectively. Haematuria, if present, must be thoroughly evaluated with malignant cell cytology, cystourethroscopy and intravenous urography (IVU).

Pad test — An one hour extended pad test is recommended in cases when the clinical stress test is negative.

The patient wears a preweighed sanitary pad, drinks about 500 ml of water and rests for 15 minutes. She then performs exercises like walking or climbing stairs for 30 minutes. This is to be followed by provocative exercises such as bending, jumping, coughing, etc. for another 15 minutes. After a period of hour, the sanitary pad is removed and weighed. **An increase in weight by 1 gm is considered as significant loss.**

Frequency volume chart (urinary diary) — Patient is asked to record her fluid intake, output, episodes of leakage in relation to time and activity. It should be recorded at least for 7 days. This diary gives an idea about daily urine output, number of voids per day and functional bladder capacity.

Urodynamic study

If the stress incontinence is the only symptom, there may not be any need for detailed urodynamic studies. **However, the evaluation is needed in** (i) presence of mixed symptomatology (GSI and detrusor instability), (ii) associated frequency/nocturia/voiding difficulties, (iii) associated neuropathy or (iv) previous failed surgery.

Uroflowmetry

The procedure is simple. The time period of total voiding is recorded by a stop watch and the amount of urine is estimated. **The normal flow rate is 15-25 ml/sec.** If the flow rate drops to less than 10 ml/sec, it indicates atonic bladder or urethral obstruction which can be confirmed by cystometry. The residual urine is to be estimated. Flowmeters can be used to produce a graphic record.

Low peak flow rate (< 15 ml/sec) associated with increased detrusor pressure (> 50 cm H_2O) with prolonged voiding time indicates outflow obstruction.

In stress incontinence, urinary flow rate is normal with nil or insignificant residual urine.

If the uroflowmetry is normal, the next step is to submit the patient to cystometry to exclude detrusor instability or urge incontinence.

Cystometry (Filling and Voiding cystometry)

Cystometry evaluates the behaviour of the bladder during filling and voiding (Table 24.3).

Principle — Pressure catheters with electronic microtip transducer are used. One pressure catheter is introduced into the bladder. An additional catheter is placed in the bladder to fill it up. Another rectal or vaginal pressure catheter is introduced to measure the intra-abdominal pressure. Measurements of total intravesical pressure (P_{ves}), intra-abdominal pressure (P_{abd}) and true detrusor pressure (P_{det}) are done. Rectal pressure (P_{abd}) is subtracted from total intravesical pressure (P_{ves}) to obtain true detrusor pressure (P_{det}).

Technique — Patient sits on the study coach. Normal saline is infused inside the bladder through the filling catheter at the rate of 50-100 ml/min. Continuous recording of fluid volume infused and pressure change is done. Patient may be asked for standing, coughing or heel bouncing, for provocation. During voiding cystometry, filling catheter is removed. Total volume voided, urine flow rate and pressure (P_{abd}, P_{ves} and P_{det}) are recorded. Urge incontinence during filling cystometry indicates detrusor instability. Ambulatory urodynamic studies are thought to be more reliable.

In GSI, the cystometric evaluation is normal. The values are abnormal in detrusor instability and sensory urge incontinence.

Table 24.3
Normal findings in cystometry

• Residual volume	... 0-50 ml
• First sensation of urination	... 150-200 ml
• Capacity	... 400-600 ml
• Intravesical pressure on filling and standing	... 0-15 cm H_2O
• Absence of systolic detrusor contraction	
• No leakage on coughing	
• Able to interrupt the urine flow on command	
• Maximum detrusor pressure during voiding	... < 70 cm H_2O
• Peak urinary flow rate	... > 15 ml/sec.

Abnormal cystometry : (i) Urine leaks on caughing. No rise in detrusor pressure → GSI. (ii) Detrusor contractions during filling phase → Detrusor instability.

Ambulatory monitoring using microtip pressure transducers is found to increase the detection of overactive bladder. This test is more physiological.

Urethral pressure profiles

For a continent woman urethral pressure must be higher than the bladder pressure. Urethral pressure profile test is performed with a special catheter having microtip pressure transducers, which is slowly pulled down from the bladder (filled with 250 ml of normal saline) along the urethra to outside. The transducer measures the intravesical and urethral pressure while it is pulled down. This pressure profile is represented as a curve called urethral pressure profile (Fig. 24.7). Maximum urethral closure pressure is obtained by subtracting intravesical pressure from maximum urethral pressure. Unfortunately correlation between urethral pressure and severity of incontinence is poor.

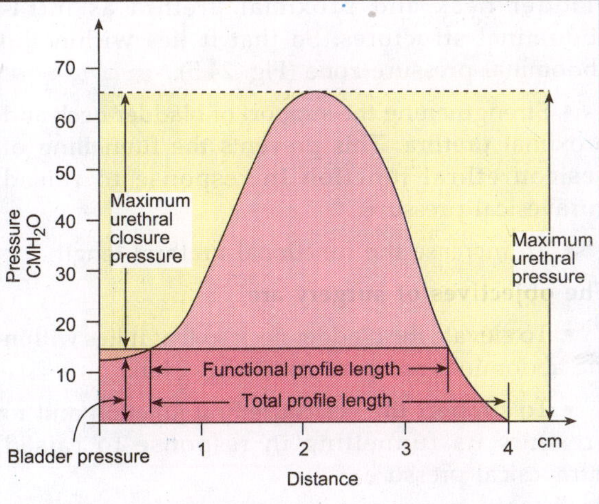

Fig. 24.7. Urethral pressure and urethral closure pressure profiles

Abnormalities are :

- Functional length of the urethra is decreased usually well below 3 cm.
- Peak urethral pressure decreases in both supine and erect position.
- Intravesical pressure rises to a greater extent than intraurethral pressure during strain.
- During strain, there is **significant lowering of the urethral closure pressure. This is pathognomonic of GSI.**

Leak-point pressure test : It gives an idea about sphincteric strength.

Method : Patient is asked to strain when the bladder is filled up to a reasonable volume (200 ml) to increase intravesical pressure. The minimum pressure (cm H_2O) at which leakage is observed is recorded as 'Valsalva leak-point pressure'. If no leakage is observed even at the highest pressure exerted (cm H_2O), it is recorded as "no leakage".

Cystoscopy and urethroscopy — are not done as a routine but can be performed in selected cases. The common indications are (i) any history of haematuria; (ii) suspected neoplasm; (iii) suspected fistula; (iv) history of urgency and frequency to rule out interstitial cystitis and reduced bladder capacity.

Table 24.4
Diagnosis of GSI

- Clinical stress test — positive.
- Pad test — positive.
- Midstream urine analysis — normal.
- Urinary diary (volume frequency chart).
- Uroflowmetry — normal.
- Cystometry — normal.
- Significant lowering of urethral closure pressure during strain.
- Leak-point pressure (Valsalva) test — positive.
- Cystourethroscopy — negative finding.
- Videocystourethrography — bladder neck funnelling.
- Transvaginal endosonography — altered anatomical relationship (descent) of urethrovesical junction and bladder base.

Videocystourethrography (VCU) — It is not a routine procedure. Special indications are (i) history of failure of previous surgery and (ii) to exclude diverticula and sacculation. Contrast media (35% urograffin) is used. Anatomical relationship of bladder neck, urethra and bladder base are assessed. Similar information can be obtained from transvaginal endosonography.

Intravenous urography (IVU) — is not a routine procedure. Indications of IVU are (i) patient with neuropathic bladder; (ii) to rule out congenital anomalies, calculi or fistulae.

Transvaginal endosonography is widely used to assess the anatomy of bladder neck, urethra, bladder wall thickness. Rectal, perineal and recently intraurethral probes with three dimensional image are becoming more promising.

Grade of GSI (clinical)

Grade I : Incontinence on cough or sneeze;
Grade II : With mild exercise;
Grade III : Even with change of posture.

Treatment : • Preventive • Definitive

Preventive : Prevention includes avoidance of repeated childbirth trauma and delay in second stage of labour. Management of obesity, diabetes, chronic pulmonary and neurological diseases are the essential steps in prevention.

Definitive : The treatment aims at :

- Restoration of the function of the muscles of the urethrovesical junction.
- Strengthening the support of the urethra.

• **Conservative** • **Surgical**

Conservative

To improve the tone of the pelvic floor muscles :

- Pelvic floor exercise — Basic principle is to strengthen the muscular part of rhabdosphincter and pelvic floor muscle. This will bring back the urethral pressure. Physiotherapy will not, however, strengthen the involuntary muscles of the bladder base and proximal urethra for which surgery is required.

The pelvic floor exercises are in the form of drawing up the anus and tightening the vagina for stopping micturition. This should be done about 100 times a day for several months.

The suitable cases are — GSI of minor degree in cases of recent delivery having poor pelvic muscular tone.

— Use of vaginal devices : Pessaries, bladder neck support prosthesis.

— Use of vaginal cone with weight ranging from 20-100 gm.

— Electrical stimulation — activation of the pelvic floor muscles by stimulation of pudendal nerves.

— Diet control in obese patient.

Drugs

Oestrogen — It is useful in postmenopausal patient. It improves the urethral closure pressure by increasing the collagen support and vascular pulsations of the submucosal plexuses. Oestradiol 2 mg per day orally is effective. Oestrogen replacement improves the effectiveness of sympathomimetic drugs when used.

Sympathomimetic drugs (α-adrenergic drugs) — α-adrenergic drug improves the tone of urethra and bladder neck and thereby symptoms are improved. Imipramine 10-25 mg, orally twice daily or Ephedrine 15-30 mg, orally twice daily is effective. The periurethral levator ani muscles having both the type-I (slow-twitch) and type-II (fast-twitch) fibres are responsible for maintaining continence against sudden increased abdominal pressure.

Paraurethral implants — Implants using Teflon increase the functional length of the urethra. Periurethral injection of GAX collagen (glutaraldehyde cross-linked bovine collagen) is effective in GSI of minor degree. It prevents premature bladder neck opening.

Surgery

The principles of surgery are :

- Restoration of normal anatomy to maintain bladder neck and proximal urethra as intraabdominal structures. So that it lies within the abdominal pressure zone (Fig. 24.5).
- Strengthening the support of bladder neck and proximal urethra. This prevents the funnelling of vesicourethral junction in response to raised intravesical pressure.
- To increase the functional urethral length.

The objectives of surgery are :

- To elevate the bladder neck so that it lies within the abdominal pressure zone (Fig. 24.5).
- To support the vesicourethral junction and to prevents its funnelling in response to raised intravesical pressure.

Surgery for GSI varies widely. Procedures could be vaginal (anterior colporrhaphy) or abdominal (elevation of the bladder neck) or combined (endoscopic bladder neck suspension or sling procedures). No one single procedure can be ideal for all women. Individualisation should be done depending on her age, severity of symptoms and ultimately the experience of the surgeon. Ideally all patients must be reviewed on the basis of her clinical presentation and urodynamic features.

Kelly's cystourethroplasty (Howard Kelly-1914) (Fig. 24.8)

This is the common surgical procedure employed in GSI with success.

The technique consists of meticulous exposure of the urethra and the bladder neck vaginally. This is followed by plicating the pubocervical fascia with vertical mattress sutures using 'O' catgut or Vicryl along the proximal urethra and bladder neck. These sutures will strengthen the urethral pressure and assist elevation of the bladder neck.

Advantages are — (i) simple procedure; (ii) less time is required; (iii) correction of co-existent cystocele; (iv) specially suited for women who are elderly and medically unfit for prolonged surgery.

Disadvantage — Long-term success rate is low (50-60%).

Retropubic cystourethropexy (colposuspension)

Principle of all these operations is to restore the normal anatomy (elevation) of the urethrovesical junction and to prevent the hypermobility of bladder neck. Long-term (5 years) success rate for retropubic cystourethropexy is 80–90 per cent.

Surgical treatment of GSI

- Kelly's urethroplasty (p. 387)
- Retropubic urethropexy
  - MMK (p. 388)
  - Burch (p. 388)
- Needle urethropexy (p. 388)
  - Pereyra, Raz, Stamey
- Suburethral sling
  - Aldridge (p. 389)
- Midurethral sling
  - TVT (p. 388)
  - TOT (p. 389)

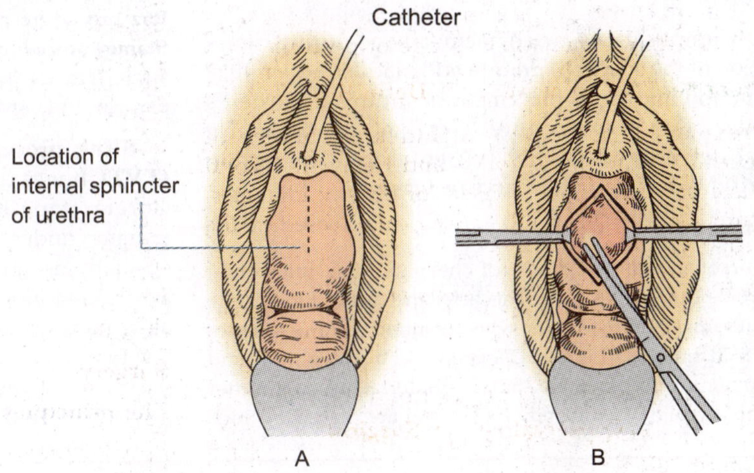

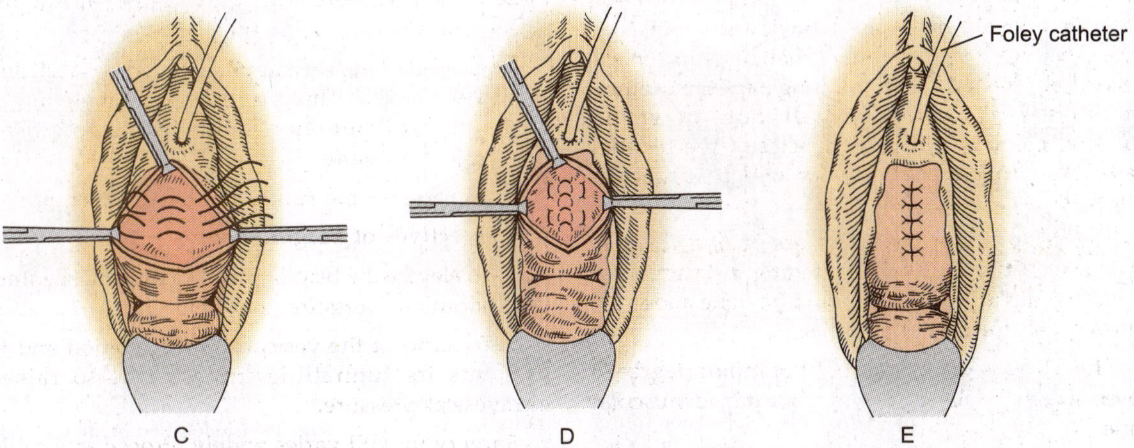

Fig. 24.8. Surgical procedure — Cystourethroplasty *(Kelly's type)*

There are several modifications of this operation. This procedure is performed suprapubically (through low abdominal incision) to reach the space of Retzius.

(a) *Marshall-Marchetti-Krantz (MMK 1949)* — The principle is to achieve elevation of the urethrovesical junction. Paraurethral and paravesical endopelvic fascia are stitched to the periosteum at the back of the symphysis pubis [Fig. 24.9A(b)].

(b) In *Burch (1961) colposuspension* the same endopelvic fascia and/or the lateral vaginal fornix is sutured to the ipsilateral iliopectineal ligament [Cooper's ligament, Fig. 24.9A(a)]. Vaginal vault mobility is essential. Mild cystocele is corrected with this procedure.

Laparoscopic bladder neck suspension has been done exactly by the same way as that of an open Burch.

Complications are (i) haemorrhage during dissection of the space (ii) urethra and bladder neck injury due to injudicious placement of sutures (iii) osteitis pubis (MMK procedure) (iv) voiding difficulty (v) detrusor instability (vi) enterocele formation (vii) VVF (viii) failure and recurrence.

Procedure

Dorsolithotomy position of the patient is made and urological drape is used. This helps the surgeon to operate with fingers in the vagina when required. Foley's catheter (18-20 size) is inserted. Dissection of bladder neck and upper urethra is done. Suture material used is either polyglycolic or ethibond. 3-4 sutures are placed on each side at 0.5 cm apart. Haemostasis is checked and sutures are tied. Drainage at the retropubic space is left and suprapubic catheter is inserted.

(c) *Endoscopic bladder neck suspension (colposuspension)* — This procedure is simple and takes little time (Fig. 24.9B). There are various modifications of this operation following original description by Pereyra later on by Raz and Stamey. This procedure suspends the paraurethral and paravesical tissue on either side of bladder neck to the rectus sheath. It primarily corrects the anatomic hypermobility of the bladder neck and urethra.

Procedure : Dissection at the bladder neck region is done vaginally to expose the endopelvic fascia. A small suprapubic incision is made. Sutures are passed between vagina and anterior abdominal wall on either side of the bladder neck with a specially designed long needle (under cystoscopic guidance). Suture material used is proline. In **Raz** procedure part of vaginal wall is incorporated. In **Stamey** procedure a buffer is used below the pubocervical fascia (Fig. 24.9B). Long-term success rate is around 50 per cent. It is specially suited for elderly women.

Sling procedures: **Tension-free Vaginal Tape (TVT).** It was devised by Nilson 1998. A marlex or Goretex tape is passed vaginally in a 'U' shape manner, under the midurethra to the either side with specially designed needles (Fig. 24.10). The needles are passed along the back of the pubic bone to the skin incision one on either side of the mid-line. Cystoscopy is done at the end of the procedure. Dissection is minimal and the tape is not sutured to any structure (tension-free). This acts by improving

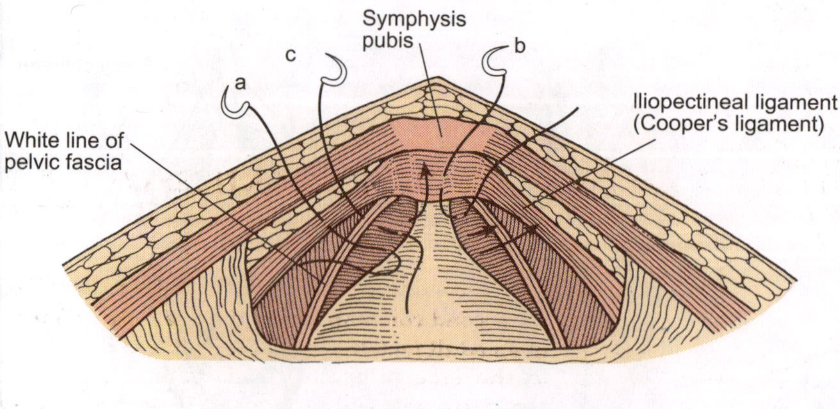

Fig. 24.9A. Colposuspension (Burch operation).
a = Burch colposuspension, b = MMK procedure,
c = Colposuspension using the white line of pelvic fascia

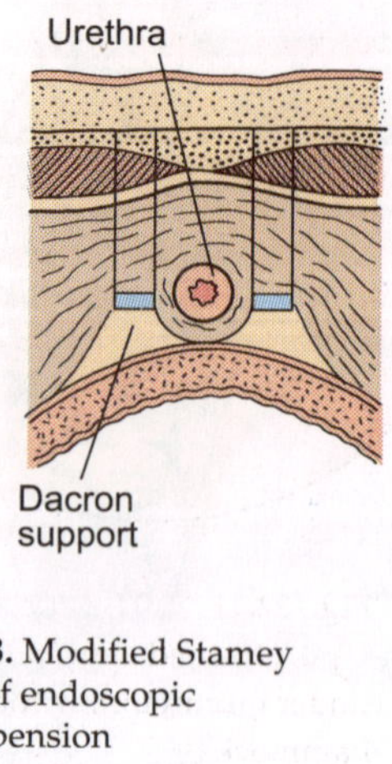

Fig. 24.9B. Modified Stamey method of endoscopic colposuspension

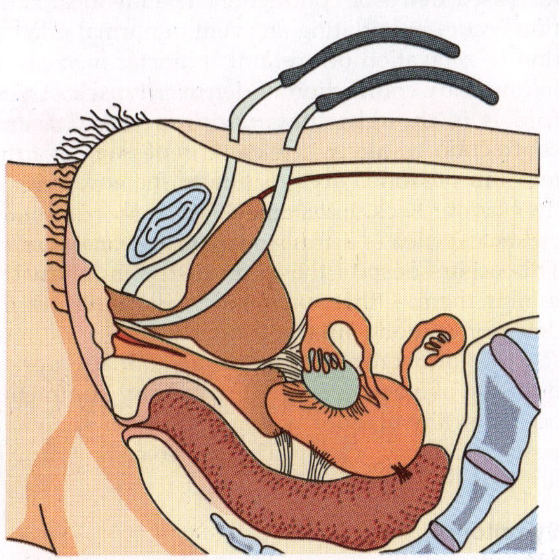

Fig. 24.10. TVT procedure with needles in position. The tape is left tension-free under the urethra

the midurethral support. TVT increases urethral-coaptation by kinking the urethra during increased intra-abdominal pressure. This is less invasive and operative time is short. Common complications are : injury to bladder, retropubic haematoma, sling erosion and overactive bladder. Success rate is about 80-90 per cent at 3 years.

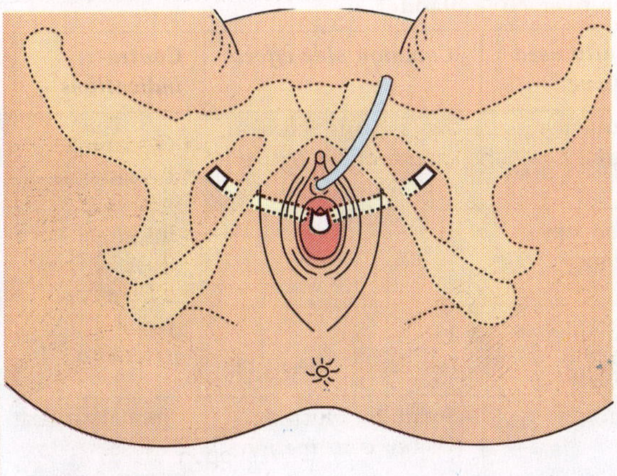

Fig. 24.11. TOT procedure showing the tunnel, the tape attached and pulled through. The tape is left under midurethra without any tension to support it as a hammock

Tension-free Obturator Tape (TOT)

It is a minimally invasive procedure designed by Delorme (2001) to support the urethra as a hammock. A 2 cm. incision is made in the vagina over mid the urethra. A tunnel is created out to the obturator foramen on either side. A multifilament microporous polypropylene tape is fed through the trocar which passes from the thighfold through the obturator foramen from outside to inside along the tunnel. It is finally brought round the vaginal incision. The procedure is repeated on the other side and the tape is left tension-free under the midurethra. It acts similar to a natural hammock supporting the urethra. As it avoids the retropubic space, complications are less. It can be performed under the local anaesthetic. There is no need to perform cystoscopy in TOT procedure. Success rate is similar to that of TVT. The same procedure can be performed from inside to outside (*de Laval-2003*).

Other sling procedures are not used as a primary procedure but may be employed for complicated cases of sphincter incompetence (failed surgery, reduced vaginal capacity and mobility). **Sling operations work by compressing the urethra at the urethrovesical junction**. The materials used for sling are — (i) organic, (autogenous) — rectus sheath (Aldridge procedure), fascia lata or (ii) inorganic — silastic, marlex, goretex. Combined approach,vaginal and abdominal (retropubic space) is made. Sling is passed around the bladder neck and is fixed to rectus sheath under **minimal tension to act as a hammock**. Overall success rate is 70 per cent. Disadvantages are voiding difficulties, detrusor instability and sling erosion.

Salvage procedures are suggested where all other procedures have failed hopelessly. Only a small percentage of woman will need this.

The procedures are :

- Implantation of artificial sphincter
- Urinary diversion.

URGE INCONTINENCE

Incidence

Urge incontinence due to detrusor instability (DI) is the **second common cause of urinary incontinence in an adult female**, the first being the GSI. However in the elderly group, DI is commonest. DI is associated with GSI in about 10-15 per cent of cases when urodynamic studies are done. Overall incidence of DI is 10 per cent. It may be :

- Motor urge incontinence (overactive bladder)
- Sensory urge incontinence.

OVERACTIVE BLADDER
(Detrusor instability)

Definition

An overactive bladder is defined by the International Continence Society as "one that is shown objectively to contract spontaneously or on provocation during the filling phase while the patient is attempting to inhibit micturition". Among the elderly women, overactive bladder is the commonest cause of urinary incontinence.

Aetiology

The condition is largely functional and psychosomatic in origin. The patient may be of emotionally labile type or passing through a phase of anxiety, stress, etc. Sometimes, a hypertonic detrusor is even stimulated by bodily movements like getting up from sitting or lying position. **The causative factors are**:

- Idiopathic — majority.
- Psychosomatic.
- Following surgery for incontinence.
- Detrusor hyper-reflexia (neuropathic) — Multiple sclerosis, spinal injuries, early parkinsonism, diabetic neuropathy, cerebrovascular accident, etc.

Pathophysiology

The pathophysiology is obscure. There may be increased alpha-adrenergic activities causing increased detrusor contraction. The identical situation occurs in initiating an event of normal micturition — relaxation of urethral sphincter mechanism followed by contraction of detrusor muscle. Therefore it is thought that inappropriate detrusor contraction results when there is passage of urine into the proximal urethra due to incompetence of the bladder neck. Incompetent bladder neck → urine in proximal urethra → detrusor overactivity → incontinence. This occurs despite the effort of the individual to inhibit them. Other explanation is change in the detrusor smooth muscle property (due to atherosclerosis or neuropathy) that leads to inappropriate detrusor overactivity. The involuntary contraction occurs at any bladder volumes — either spontaneously or on provocation. There is preceding drop in urethral pressure.

Symptoms

There is involuntary loss of urine without any prior urge to urinate. **Most common symptoms are urgency, frequency (> 7 times/day), nocturia (> once/night) and bed wetting**. It should be remembered that the entity is too often associated with genuine stress incontinence (Table 24.7).

Special investigations

(a) **Maintenance of urinary diary** (frequency volume chart see p. 384) for 1 week.

(b) **A careful neurological examination** is made to exclude neurological disorders. One has to look for perineal sensation, pelvic muscle tone and

Table 24.5 : Drugs used in overactive bladder

Nature	*Drugs with dosage*	*Specially used to relieve*	*Common side effects*	*Contra-indications*
Anti-cholinergic Musculotropic relaxants	Oxybutynin chloride 5 mg thrice daily (Anti-muscarinic)	• Frequency • Urgency	Dry mouth and skin, constipation, blurred vision	• Glaucoma • Myasthenia gravis • Intestinal obstruction • Ulcerative colitis • Urinary retention
Anti-muscarinic (Detrusor selective)	Tolterodine 1-2 mg, P.O., BID	• Frequency • Urgency	— Do —	
Anti-muscarinic (Detrusor selective)	Solifenacin 5-10 mg, P.O. daily	• Frequency • Urgency	— Do — flatulence, chest pain	
Tricyclic (Antidepressants)	Imipramine hydrochloride 50 mg at night.	Nocturia	Sedation, blurred vision, constipation	Coronary artery disease, hypertension.
Synthetic antidiuretic hormone analogue	DDAVP (Desamino deoxy arginine vasopressin) Intranasally 20-40 μg at night.	Nocturnal enuresis	Fluid retention, hyponatraemia. Rhinitis, Nausea.	Cardiac insufficiency.

Table 24.6
Common causes of urgency, urge incontinence, frequency of micturition

Gynaecological	• Genitourinary prolapse • GSI • Menopause (tissue atrophy due to oestrogen deficiency) • Pelvic mass • Pregnancy
Urological	• Urinary tract infection • DI • Urethral syndrome • Interstitial cystitis
Medical	• Diabetes • Neurological lesions (multiple sclerosis, Alzheimer's disease) • Diuretic therapy
Psychological and idiopathic	

bulbocavernous reflex to know the integrity of the sacral reflex S2-4 (gentle clitoral stroke should produce anal sphincter contraction). Cranial nerves are examined.

(c) **Midstream examination** of urine for culture and sensitivity test.

(d) **Uroflowmetry**.

In idiopathic group, the flow rate is high and the voiding time is short.

(e) **Cystometry**.

- Urge to pass urine is provoked at a much lower bladder filling of 100-175 ml of water.
- True detrusor pressure increases by more than 15 cm of water during bladder filling with 200 ml of fluid.

(f) **Cystourethroscopy** : This is to exclude the associated local pathology. The findings are normal except for a diminished bladder capacity.

Treatment

General measure

- Psychosomatic problems should be treated by psychotherapy.
- Other medical problems (neurological, diabetes) should be properly attended.

Behavioural therapy

- To limit the intake of fluid to 1 litre/day.
- To reduce tea and coffee.
- Bladder retraining.

When combined with stress incontinence, unstable bladder is to be treated first before proceeding to surgical correction for stress incontinence.

Failed surgical treatment of stress incontinence is to be evaluated for the presence of unstable bladder.

Bladder retraining : This is useful in idiopathic group. This can be achieved by bladder drill, biofeedback or hypnotherapy.

In bladder drill, the patient is instructed to void by the clock at progressively increasing intervals over a 6-week time period. The initial response is quite good but the failure rate is high. Simultaneous anticholinergic drug therapy improves the result. The drill is, however, not useful where neurologic disease is responsible for unstable bladder.

Drug therapy : Aims are to — (i) Inhibit bladder contractility, (ii) Increase bladder neck and urethral resistance.

The drugs (Table 24.5) have mostly got anticholinergic properties, thereby minimises detrusor irritability. When administered along with bladder retraining, there is improvement of results.

The other drugs used are : Trospium chloride (atropine derivative with antimuscarinic effects) and Propiverine (anti-cholinergic and calcium channel blocker). Both are effective with less side effects.

In addition, the peri or postmenopausal women are often helped by oestrogen therapy. It has shown to raise the sensory threshold.

Transvesical phenol : In idiopathic detrusor instability aqueous phenol (6%) is injected in the bladder base beneath the epithelium through a cystoscope.

Surgery : In intractable cases not relieved by drugs or bladder irritability due to neurologic disease, surgery may be of help. This is in the form of denervation (to interrupt the nervous pathways), augmentation cystoplasty (to increase bladder capacity) or urinary diversion (ideal conduit).

Sensory urge incontinence (Table 24.7)

It is the involuntary leakage of urine per urethra accompanied by or immediately preceded by

Table 24.7
Clinical presentation and diagnosis of GSI and urge incontinence (sensory and motor)

	Stress	Urge incontinence (sensory)	Overactive bladder (OAB)
Definition	Involuntary escape of urine when intravesical pressure exceeds maximum urethral pressure in the absence of detrusor activity.	Unable to control the escape of urine once there is urge to void.	Leakage of urine due to detrusor over activity during the filling phase while the patient tries to inhibit it.
Clinical presentation			
• Stress prior to leakage	Always present	Nil	Nil
• Urge prior to leakage	Nil	Present	Present except in neurologic disease
• Awareness	Present	Present	Not present
• Control of loss	Can control	Can control with adequate encouragement	Cannot control despite strong encouragement
• Amount	Small	Large	Large
Midstream urine examination	Not informative	Evidences of infection	Usually non-informative
Uroflowmetry	Normal	Normal	High in idiopathic group
Cystometry	During strain, there is significant lowering of the urethral pressure. (Urethral pressure profile)	Normal	• Urge to pass urine is provoked at much lower bladder filling. • Detrusor pressure is increased during filling.
Cystourethroscopy	Normal	Offending factor present	Diminished bladder capacity
Lateral cystourethrography	Funnelling of the proximal urethra.	Normal	Normal

urgency. Sensory urge incontinence is unassociated with detrusor contraction until urination is initiated. This occurs in a stable bladder and without any anatomic descent of urethra and bladder neck (Fig. 24.5).

Mixed incontinence of stress and urge may be present. Urodynamic studies are indicated in such a case (p. 384). In such a situation, symptoms are prioritised and then treatment is initiated. Conservative management should be tried first. However, in many women (50-60%), urge symptoms are improved after mid-urethral sling procedure (p. 388).

PAINFUL BLADDER SYNDROME (PBS)

It is a chronic inflammatory condition resulting in painful voiding. According to the International Continence Society (2002), **PBS is defined** as the presence of suprapubic pain related to bladder filling associated with other symptoms like frequencey, in the absence of urinary tract infection or other pathology. Therefore urgency and pain are the two important diagnostic criteria of painful bladder syndrome. PBS is more prevalent in women than in men.

Interstitial cystitis, is considered within the spectrum of PBS.

Symptoms : The clinical presentation varies widely. Symptoms include urgency, frequency, pelvic and lower urinary tract pain, dyspareunia and urinary incontinence.

Diagnosis : PBS is a diagnosis of exclusion. The differential diagnosis includes cystitis, trigonitis, tuberculosis, overactive bladder (OAB), bladder stones, or cancer, diverticula, and urogenital atrophy due to oestrogen deficiency.

Treatment : As the diagnosis of PBS is difficult, treatment is directed to control the symptoms mainly.

- **Diet** : Alcohol, spices, citrus and caffeinated drinks are avoided as they are found to increase bladder inflammation and pain.
- **Drugs** : Urinary tract analgesics like hyoscyamine, phenyl salicylate may reduce urethral irritation.
- **Surgery** : Bladder instillation therapy — with agents like steroids, sodium bicarbonate, heparinoids and dimethyl sulfoxide has been found to be helpful. They need to be repeated weekly for a minimum of 6 weeks.

– *Hydrodistension* : Cystoscopy and hydrodistension of bladder is used in refractory cases of PBS. Glomerulations (petechial haemorrhages) may be seen in the bladder mucosa after hydrodistension.

- **Other treatments** : Tricyclic antidepressants, transcutaneous electrical nerve stimulation (TENS) and acupuncture have been tried as neuromodulation.

OVERFLOW INCONTINENCE

This occurs as a result of prolonged and neglected retention. Its mechanism is probably the overdistension of the bladder pulls open the internal sphincter. There may be compensatory detrusor hypertrophy.

The causes of overflow incontinence are the same as retention of urine which will be mentioned later in the chapter.

Urodynamic findings

Uroflowmetry reveals low flow rate and significant residual urine.

Cystometry reveals large capacity of the bladder and no rise of detrusor pressure during voiding.

Treatment

Surgical treatment of obstruction, if any, has to be done.

In cases of non-obstructive group, continuous catheter drainage is required. Intermittent clamping of the catheter is to be done prior to its removal. Following removal of the catheter, the residual urine has to be measured. It should not be more than 100 ml, preferably 50 ml. If more than 100 ml, the continuous drainage is reinstituted.

REFLEX INCONTINENCE

This is found in paraplegics where the cerebral control of micturition is lost over local reflex.

Urodynamic studies reveal — low flow rate of urine and significant residual urine. There is high urethral pressure.

Treatment is by continuous catheter drainage.

VOIDING DISORDER

Definition

Difficulty in emptying the bladder is due to dysfunction of effective detrusor contraction and/or urethral sphincter mechanism. Anuria must be excluded. Normally for complete emptying of bladder, pelvic floor muscle (levator ani) and urethral sphincter (intrinsic rhabdosphincter) must relax and at the same time the detrusor must contract. Voiding difficulties may lead to **retention of urine** either **acute** *(inability to void more than 12 hours without catheterisation)* or **chronic** *(inability to empty the bladder more than 50 per cent of its volume).*

Retention of urine

Causes

1. **Postoperative**—the commonest cause of retention in gynaecology.

Following any operation on the vagina or perineum.

The factors operating are :

- Obstructive due to postoperative oedema in the neighbourhood of the stitch line.
- Reflex spasm of bladder sphincters specially following anterior colporrhaphy.
- Reflex spasm of the levators following perineorrhaphy.
- Postoperative vaginal packing so often given following vaginal plastic operations.

Following radical operation :

- Denervation of the nerve supply of the bladder which travels from S2,3,4 in the parametrium. This especially happens in Wertheim's operation, where extensive dissection of the parametrium is carried out.

2. **Obstructive conditions intrinsic to the urethra**

- Cicatrical stenosis following operations for repair of a urethrovaginal fistula or caruncle.
- Urethral angulation in cases with big cystocele.
- Bladder neck obstruction in postmenopausal women.
- After sling operation for stress incontinence.
- Cancer of the urethra, bladder neck, vulva, paraurethral cyst and tumour.

3. **Bladder detrusor may fail to contract**

- *Diseases* — multiple sclerosis (detrusor-sphincter dyssynergia), Parkinson's disease, neuropathy.
- *Drugs* — epidural anaesthesia antidepressant, ganglion blockers.
- *Psychogenic* — hysteria, fear, modesty or shyness.

4. **Spasm of external sphincter**

- Nervousness and embarrassment or unaccustomed position.
- Perineal injuries due to operation.
- Urethritis.

5. **Gynaecological causes (Table 24.8)**

A pelvic tumour or a mass in the pelvis may produce retention of urine. The diagnosis is usually made by giving attention to associated symptoms.

Lateral urethrocystography has demonstrated that the bladder neck remains in its original pelvic position and the retention is caused by the tumour interfering with the opening of internal sphincter of the urethra.

Investigations should be designed on the basis of aetiology. Neurological examination should done as a routine.

Management

The treatment aims at :

- To relieve the symptom
- To treat the primary cause, when present.

Acute retention

Catheterisation is to be done by using an autoclaved soft rubber catheter. Due aseptic precautions are to be taken as described in chapter 9 (p. 105).

If the patient fails to pass urine normally again after 8 hours, a self-retaining catheter is to be introduced for continuous drainage for at least 24-48 hours.

Chronic retention

In cases of chronic retention with marked over-distension of the bladder, it is better to put a self-retaining catheter, sooner the better. The number of days, it is to be kept, depends on the regaining of the bladder tone. This is determined by the amount of residual urine. Under no circumstances, the residual urine should exceed 100 ml, preferably below 50 ml.

URINARY TRACT INFECTIONS

About 20 per cent of all women have urinary tract infections (UTI) during their lifetime. As such, it requires special attention by the obstetricians/gynaecologists to prevent serious consequences arising out of it. The cases are often overlooked or ignored when the manifestations are minor. Moreover, in cases of asymptomatic bacteriuria, the infection remains in the urinary tract for a long period of time only to flare up to produce pyelo-

Table 24.8
Provisional diagnosis of gynaecological pathology with retention of urine

Period of life	Associated disorders	Provisional diagnosis
Postmenarchal	Primary amenorrhoea	Cryptomenorrhoea (see p. 431)
Childbearing period	Short period of secondary amenorrhoea	Retroverted gravid uterus (p. 195)
	Menorrhagia	Uterine fibroid impacted in POD (p. 273)
	No menstrual abnormality	Impacted ovarian tumour, cervical or broad ligament fibroid
	Irregular bleeding with pain	Pelvic haematocele
	Irregular bleeding with fever	Pelvic abscess (p. 171)

nephritis in significant cases. As such, due attention should be paid even in asymptomatic patients having significant bacteriuria.

Prevalence

The prevalence of UTI upto 11 years is about 1 per cent for boys and 3 per cent for girls. In older girls, there is 10-fold increase in incidence as compared to boys. However, around 55 years the incidence in men and women is almost equal. The incidence of asymptomatic bacteriuria in female is about 4 per cent. In pregnancy, it rises to 10 per cent.

Table 24.9
Protective mechanisms in female

- Vulval apposition
- Apposition of the urethral mucosal folds
- Role of rhabdosphincter and pelvic floor muscles in maintaining urethral tone
- Inflow of urine from kidneys
- Protective bladder mucosa — immunologically resistant to infection
- Periodic voiding.

Increased chance of UTI in females compared to males is due to:

- Short urethra (4 cm).
- Close proximity of the external urethral meatus to the areas (vulva and lower-third of vagina) contaminated heavily with bacteria.
- Sexual intercourse.
- Catheterisation.
- **Aggravating factors during pregnancy are**:

Stasis of urine in bladder → multiplication of bacteria → influx of the infected urine into the ureters and renal pelves due to laxity of the vesicoureteral sphincters due to oedema.

Organisms

The commonest organism is *Escherichia coli* which is present in about 80-90 per cent cases. Others are *Pseudomonas, Klebsiella, Proteus, Enterococci, Staphylococcus*, etc.

Predisposing factors

- **The lower urethra is colonised** with bacteria early in life but the bacteria are non-pathogenic. The protective effect of oestrogen is also lacking.
- **Sexual intercourse** increases the ascent of the organisms from the lower urethra into the bladder.
- **Full bladder** — Provided bladder is kept empty completely and regularly, there is least chance of UTI. But certain circumstances favour atonicity of the bladder and urinary stasis as in pregnancy, puerperium and following major pelvic surgery or pelvic tumours producing outflow tract obstruction.
- **Catheterisation** — This is probably the commonest cause of introducing the organisms from the lower urethra into the bladder whatever meticulous aseptic technique being taken. It has been observed that an indwelling catheter kept for 24 hours will produce bacteriuria in 50 per cent and if left for 4 days will lead to bacteriuria in 100 per cent of cases.
- **Hypo-oestrogenic state** as in postmenopausal women — when defence of the bladder and urethral mucosa is diminished.
- **Immunocompromising disorders** like diabetes mellitus.

Routes of infection

- **Ascending** • **Haematogenous** • **Lymphatic**

Ascending — is the commonest route of infection. The organisms from the anorectal region, lower vagina and vulva gain access to the urethra and thence to the bladder and kidneys.

Haematogenous — spread involving the kidneys is from the intestine or septic tonsils or other septic foci.

Lymphatic — spread is either from the adjacent ascending colon or genital organs (cervicitis). The kidneys may be affected from the bladder through periureteral lymphatics.

Thus, while the urethra and bladder are mostly affected by direct ascending infection, the kidneys are usually secondarily affected following cystitis. The infection is either by influx of the infected urine through the ureters or through periureteral lymphatics.

Clinical presentations

Asymptomatic bacteriuria

The term asymptomatic bacteriuria is used when a bacterial count of the same species over 10^5/ml in midstream specimen of urine on two occasions is detected without symptom of urinary infection. Counts less than 10^5/ml indicate contamination of urine from the urethra or external genitalia. Nearly 30 per cent of women with asymptomatic bacteriuria develop symptoms of UTI at a later date, if left untreated.

The entity is found related with high incidence of urinary tract abnormality — congenital or acquired. The woman runs a greater risk of developing chronic renal lesion later in life.

Lower urinary tract infection

Urethritis : The symptoms include dysuria, frequency and urgency of micturition. Pain is typically scalding during the act of micturition. Urethra is tender on palpation. Often, pus may be squeezed out from the urethra.

Apart from clean catch midstream urine for culture, the expressed pus should be submitted for Gram stain for intracellular diplococci suggestive of gonorrhoea and culture for *Chlamydia* and *Neisseria gonorrhoeae*.

Urethral syndrome : It is a chronic form of urethritis probably due to urethral hypersensitivity or UTI. The symptoms include dysuria, frequency and urgency of micturition. Urethroscopy reveals reddened, chronically inflamed urethral mucosa and spasm of the bladder neck. Benzodiazepines, Amitriptyline. Antibiotics (doxycycline) and oestrogen replacement therapy give short-term relief. Progressive urethral dilatation has been the treatment of choice. Spontaneous remission has also been noted.

Cystitis : Cystitis is the most common of the urinary tract infections.

Symptoms include dysuria, frequency and urgency of micturition and pain. It produces painful micturition specially at the end of the act. There may be suprapubic tenderness and may have constitutional upset.

Investigations : Midstream clean catch urine for microscopic examination, culture and drug sensitivity is to be done in every case.

Microscopic examination usually reveals plenty of pus cells and occasional red blood cells. The culture will detect the organism within 24 hours and it usually exceeds 10^5/ml of urine.

Sterile pyuria (negative culture in presence of plenty of pus cells) alerts the possibility of tubercular infection. In suspected tuberculosis, at least three early morning urine specimens have to be collected and cultured.

The presence of red blood cells in the absence of pus cells or negative culture suggests pathology other than infection.

Apart from midstream urine, other methods of collection of urine are — suprapubic needle aspiration and urethral catheterisation.

Pyelitis : Symptoms include acute aching pain over the loins and fever with chills and rigor. There is frequency of micturition and dysuria. There may be anorexia, nausea or vomiting.

The patient looks ill with dry tongue. The pulse rate is proportionate with temperature. There is varying degrees of loin tenderness.

Investigations : Midstream urine examination reveals plenty of pus cells and red blood corpuscles. Culture will detect the organism.

- Blood examination shows leucocytosis; urea and creatinine level may be raised.

In chronic or recurrent urinary tract infections, more extended investigative protocols such as intravenous pyelography and cystoscopy is indicated.

Prevention

The following guidelines are prescribed in an attempt **to prevent infection to lower urinary tract**.

- **To maintain proper perineal hygiene**. This consists of cleansing the vulvar region at least daily, wiping the rectum away from the urethra.
- **Prophylaxis of the coital infection** — To void urine immediately following coitus. A single dose of nitrofurantoin 50 mg following coital act is an effective means of prophylaxis. This is helpful in women who have history of postcoital exacerbation of infection.
- **Catheter infection** — Whatever aseptic measures are taken, use of catheter favours introduction of infection. This is equally applicable to indwelling catheter. As such, the following formalities should be made while an indwelling catheter is placed.
  - The use is to be judiciously decided.
  - Bacteriological monitoring — periodic and after removal of the catheter.
  - Plenty of fluid intake.
  - Postmenopausal sexually active women should receive HRT.

Management

The principles in the management are :

- To isolate the organism and drug sensitivity, if time permits prior to antimicrobial therapy.
- To administer effective drug for an adequate length of time.
- To prevent reinfection.

General measures : Bed rest is imposed. Light easily digestable diet is prescribed. The patient should be properly hydrated and the fluid intake should be 3-5 litres a day.

Antimicrobial agents : The appropriate drug sensitive to the organism should be administered in adequate doses. The duration of therapy should be for a period of about 7-10 days. The possibility of impaired renal function and the nephrotoxicity of the drug should be kept in mind. **One negative culture two weeks after the course of therapy is considered cure.**

In persistent infection, more effective agents like quinolones (ciprofloxacin) acid or aminoglycosides (amikacin) may have to be used. Outflow tract obstruction, if present, may have to be dilated.

In reinfection, the appropriate drug is to be continued for at least 2 weeks. This is to be followed by nitrofurantoin 50 mg or norfloxacin 400 mg daily for 4-6 months.

DYSURIA

Definition

Dysuria or difficulty in passing urine is a common symptom in gynaecology. The difficulty may be painful — or merely mechanical.

Causes

The causes of mechanical difficulty are :

- All the factors leading to retention of urine are usually preceded by difficulty.
- Uterine prolapse with big cystocele.

Painful micturition is associated with :

- Causes in the bladder.

The bladder lesions include — cystitis due to infection with *Esch. coli* or tuberculosis, stone, radiation cystitis, papilloma or carcinoma.

Cystitis or other lesions in the bladder cause painful micturition especially at the end of the act.

- Causes in the urethra.

Here, the pain is scalding during the act. Urethral lesions responsible are — urethritis due to specific or non-specific organisms, tender caruncle, prolapse of urethral mucosa, kraurosis, urethral carcinoma, etc.

- Postoperative causes of dysuria may be due to :
  - Cystitis or urethritis
  - Precipitated by catheterisation
  - Trauma around the bladder neck and urethra.

FREQUENCY OF URINATION

The frequency of micturition is a common complaint in women. **The bladder irritability may be caused by :**

- Local diseases
- Mechanical factors
- Nervous factor

Local diseases

They operate by direct irritation of the bladder detrusor or heighten the stretch receptors in the wall.

- Diseases inside the bladder :

Cystitis either bacterial or allergic, tubercular; calculus and foreign bodies, trigonitis, papilloma or carcinoma.

- Diseases of the anterior vaginal wall and cervix — by causing congestion and irritation of the trigone :

These include chronic cervicitis, endometriosis of anterior vaginal wall or anterior lip of cervix, carcinoma cervix involving the bladder, etc.

- Urethral conditions can reflexly cause bladder irritability.
- Trauma during catheterisation, operation or due to trauma of the external urethral meatus during coitus "honeymoon cystitis".

Mechanical factors

- Displacement of bladder can stimulate the stretch receptors in the wall. **In cystocele, the frequency is typically only diurnal** because the displacement and irritation disappear on rest.
- Pelvic and lower abdominal tumours such as myoma, ovarian cyst produce diurnal frequency if they are mobile and nocturnal frequency, if impacted.
- Incomplete emptying of the bladder results in immediate desire to void again, e.g. in cystocele and postoperative retention.
- Bands and adhesions in the uterovesical pouch.

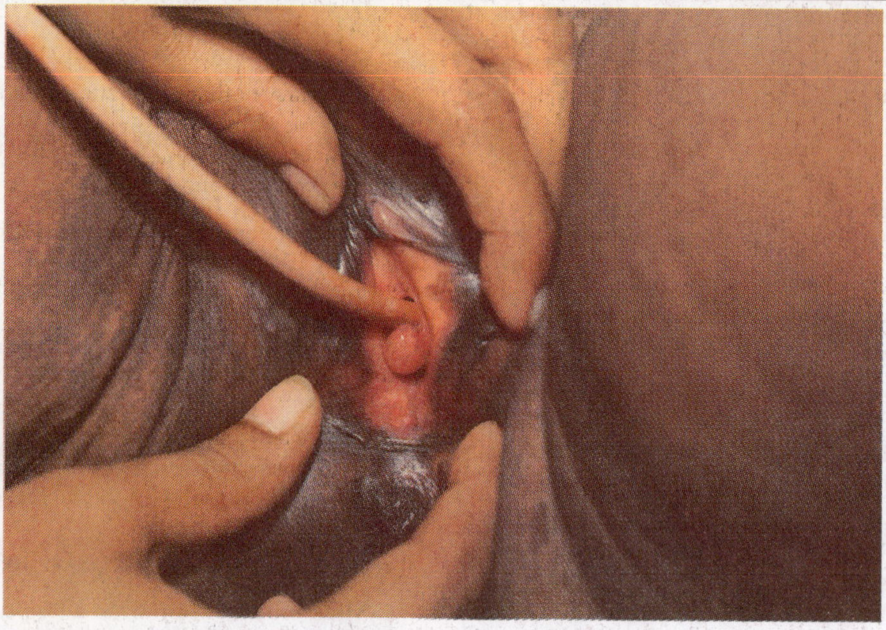

Fig. 24.12. Urethral caruncle

URETHRAL CARUNCLE (Figs 24.12 and 24.13)

Definition

It is a benign lesion of the urethra, clinically characterised by a pedunculated, reddish-looking mass protruding out of the external urethral meatus.

Pathogenesis

It is presumably infective in origin and usually confined to postmenopausal women. It is usually single and arises from the posterior wall of the urethra.

Naked eye : The size is small, usually not exceeding 0.5 cm. It looks reddish (Fig. 24.12).

Microscopic appearance : It consists of vascularised granulation tissue covered by transitional or stratified squamous epithelium. **Three types are described** — granulomatous, angiomatous and papillomatous depending upon the histologic appearance.

Clinical features

The patients are usually postmenopausal.

Symptoms include :

- Irregular bleeding per vaginam.
- Urinary complaints such as painful micturition, frequency or even retention.
- Dyspareunia.

Signs

A small angry red-looking, pea-shaped mass protruding out of the external urethral meatus. It may be tender or bleeds to touch.

Differential diagnosis

The lesion is often confused with prolapse of the urethral mucosa and urethral malignancy (Fig. 24.14).

Treatment

Excision biopsy is the definitive surgery. The raw area may be sutured or cauterised. Continuous bladder drainage is required for a few days.

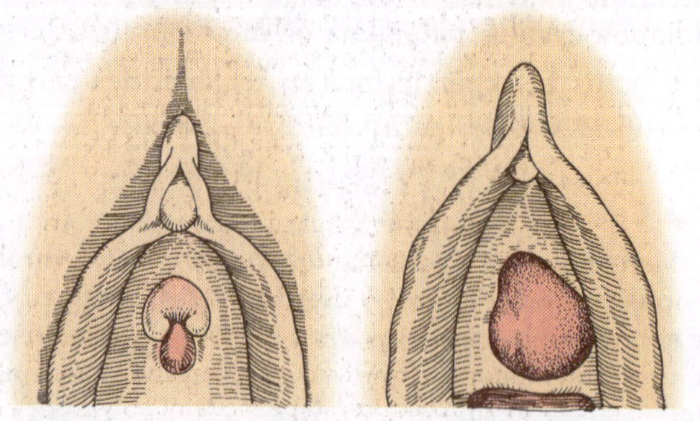

Fig. 24.13. Urethral caruncle

Fig. 24.14. Prolapse urethral mucosa

KEY POINTS

- The sympathetic supply to the bladder is concerned mainly with the filling and storage of urine. The parasympathetic is important for normal voiding.
- Parasympathetic nervous system (acetylcholine receptor) activate detrusor contraction. Sympathetic system in bladder (β receptor) causes relaxation and in the urethra (α receptor) causes contraction.
- Urethral sphincters for continence are (i) intrinsic rhabdosphincter urethrae (containing slow twitch fibres) and extrinsic sphincter of levator ani (containing both slow and fast twitch fibres).
- Intrinsic urethral sphincter maintains urethral closure at rest, where as extrinsic sphincter maintain urethral closure during stress (cough, sneeze).
- Normally urethral closure pressure is maintained effectively. Any rise in intra-abdominal pressure transmitted equally to the bladder and the proximal urethra. This mechanism maintains the pressure gradient [see Figs. 24.5(a) and (b)].
- Approximately one-third of the resting urethral pressure is due to rhabdosphincter effects, one-third to smooth muscle effects and one-third to submucous vascular plexus of the urethra.
- The intravesical pressure is about 10 cm of water and is much lower than the urethral pressure (20–50 cm of water).
- Normally first sensation of urination is felt at 150-200 ml of bladder volume and functional bladder capacity is 400–600 ml.
- Urinary incontinence is either urethral or extraurethral in origin (see Table 24.1).
- Nearly 30 per cent of women suffer from some degree of urinary incontinence during their life time.
- GSI is defined as involuntary urethral loss of urine when intravesical pressure exceeds the maximum urethral pressure in the absence of the detrusor activity.
- Genuine stress incontinence (GSI) is due to anatomic hypermobility of bladder neck and urethra (80%) and also due to urethral intrinsic sphincteric incompetence (20%).
- GSI is often confused with urge incontinence (sensory) and detrusor instability (motor) (Tables 24.2 and 24.7). During strain, there is significant lowering of the urethral closure pressure. This is pathognomonic of GSI.
- Thorough urodynamic investigations are essential in certain conditions (see p. 384) to get maximum benefit of treatment.
- Patient with urodynamic features of both GSI and DI, DI is to be treated first.
- UTI must be treated before any urodynamic investigation.
- IVU, cystourethroscopy or videocystourethrography should not be performed as a routine investigation.
- USG (transvaginal, perineal or intraurethral) is becoming more informative (see p. 386) in assessing a patient with urinary symptoms.
- Cystometry confirms the diagnosis of DI but GSI is a diagnosis of exclusion.
- Vaginal delivery causes damage to anatomical supports of the bladder neck, urethra and the pelvic floor nerves. It is an important cause for genitourinary prolapse and GSI.
- Individualisation of a patient for a particular type of incontinence surgery is essential. Important deciding factors are (i) severity of symptoms, (ii) patient's age, (iii) associated complications, (iv) experience of the surgeon.
- The objectives of the surgical treatment are to elevate the bladder neck along with proximal urethra and to support the vesicourethral junction to prevent funnelling during stress. Surgical treatment of GSI vary depending on an individual patient (Figure p. 387).
- Approximate success rate (5 years) for individual procedure is : cystourethroplasty 50-60 per cent cystourethropexy MMK 80-90 per cent , Burch 85-90 per cent, endoscopic bladder neck suspension 50 per cent. In TVT procedure a tape made of polypropelene is placed U-shaped under the midurethra, lying tension-free (see p. 389). Overall cure rate of this procedure is 84-90 per cent. Injury to the bladder (during trocar insertion), haemorrhage in the retropubic space, tape rejection or erosion are the complications.

KEY POINTS

- TOT is a simple procedure where a polypropylene tape is placed under the mid-urethra. The tape passes through the obturator foramen either from outside in (TOT) or from inside-out (TVT-O). It maintains the natural suspension of the urethra. As it avoids the retropubic space, the complications are less. It can be done under local anaesthetic. Success rate is similar to that of TVT (p. 389).
- Detrusor overactivity is defined as an unstable bladder, objectively to contract spontaneously or on provocation during the filling phase while the patient is attempting to inhibit it. It is the second common cause of urinary incontinence in adult female, the first being GSI. It is the most common cause in elderly women. The diagnosis is based on urodynamic assessment.
- The aetiology of overactive bladder (OAB) is largely functional and psychosomatic in origin. True detrusor pressure increases by more than 15 cm of water during bladder filling even with 100-175 ml of fluid.
- OAB has got spontaneous remissions and exacerbations.
- Bladder retraining, behavioural therapy and anticholinergic drugs (p. 391) are effective to control symptoms of OAB on majority of patients. Dosage of anticholinergic drugs need to be increased gradually to a level as to produce side effects (Table 24.5). Anticholinergic agents decrease detrusor activity.
- PBS (p. 392) is a chronic inflammatory condition associated with urgency and painful voiding. It is a diagnosis of exclusion. Urinary tract infection must be ruled out. Treatment is directed to control the symptoms. Diet and drugs (to control inflammation), surgery and neuro-modulation therapy are the options.
- Sensory urge incontinence is usually associated with infection or foreign body. The treatment is by appropriate antibiotic therapy and HRT in postmenopausal women.
- Important causes of urgency, urge incontinence and frequency of micturition are gynaecological, urological or medical disorders (Table 24.6).
- There is increased risk of UTI in females than in males (see p. 394). The commonest organism is *Escherichia coli*.
- Recurrent UTI need to be investigated with cystoscopy and intravenous urography. In a chronic case, following an appropriate drug therapy for 2 weeks, nitrofurantoin 50 mg or norfloxacin 400 mg daily bed time for 3-4 months is to be continued.
- Urethral syndrome is a chronic form of painful micturition due to urethral hypersensitivity or UTI.
- Negative culture in presence of plenty of pus cells alerts to the possibility of tubercular infection.
- The presence of red blood cells in the absence of pus cells or negative culture suggests pathology other than infection.
- Apart from midstream urine, other methods of collection of urine are suprapubic needle aspiration and urethral catheterisation.
- Voiding disorders are defined as difficulty in emptying bladder due to dysfunction of effective detrusor contraction and/or sphincter mechanism.
- Low peak flow rate (< 15 ml/sec.) associated with increased detrusor pressure (> 50 cm of H_2O), with prolonged voiding time indicates outflow obstruction.
- Retention of urine may be acute (inability to void over 12 hours without catheterisation) or chronic (inability to empty bladder more than 50% of its volume). Desire to void is felt at a bladder volume of 150-200 ml and functional bladder capacity is 400-500 ml.
- Common causes of retention of urine in gynaecology are : postoperative, retroverted gravid uterus, impacted uterine fibroid or ovarian tumour in the POD, cervical fibroid or cryptomenorrhoea.

  Investigations and management (p. 394) for retention of urine should be designed according to the aetiology (Table 24.8).
- Urethral caruncle is a benign lesion arising from posterior wall of the urethra. It is commonly seen in postmenopausal women. Histologically it may be granulomatous, angiomatous or papillomatous in type. Excision biopsy is the definitive surgery.

Genital Fistulae

25

GENITOURINARY FISTULA

Definition

A fistula is an abnormal communication between two or more epithelial surfaces. Genitourinary fistula is an abnormal communication between the urinary and genital tract either acquired or congenital with involuntary escape of urine into the vagina.

The incidence is estimated to be as high as 0.5-3 per cent amongst gynaecological admissions in referral hospitals of the developing countries. The incidence is however, much less in the affluent countries.

Types : The communication may occur between the bladder, urethra or ureter and genital tract. Accordingly, the following types are described (Fig. 25.1).

Bladder

- Vesicovaginal (commonest)
- Vesicourethrovaginal
- Vesicouterine
- Vesicocervical.

Urethra

- Urethrovaginal.

Ureter

- Ureterovaginal
- Ureterouterine
- Ureterocervical.

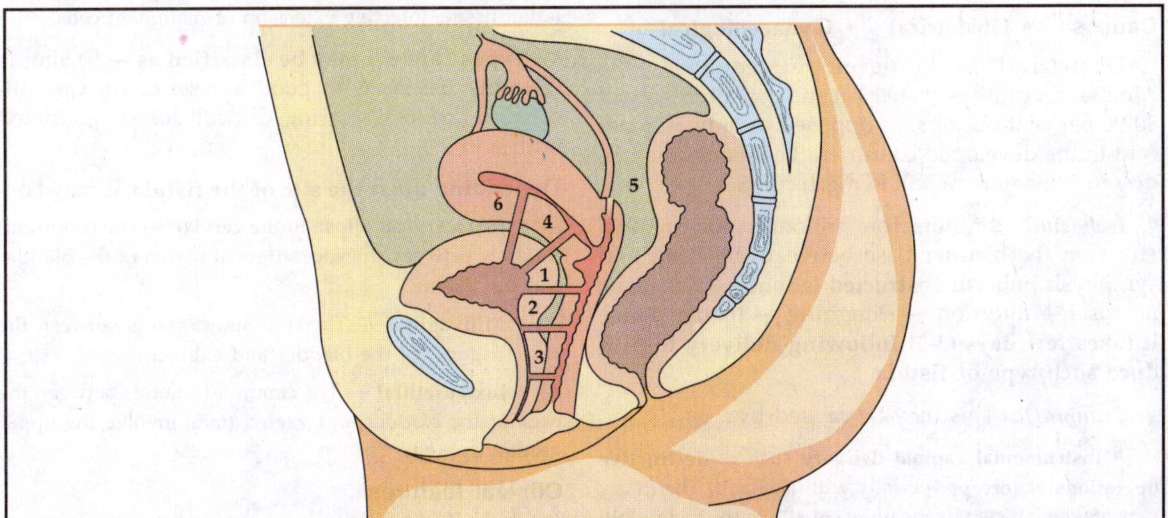

Fig. 25.1. Types of genitourinary fistula — (1) Vesicovaginal (2) Vesicourethrovaginal (3) Urethrovaginal (4) Vesicocervical (5) Ureterovaginal (6) Vesicouterine

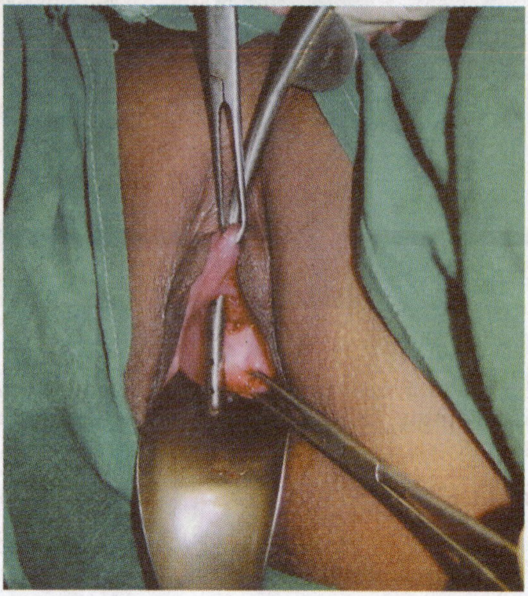

Fig. 25.2. Midvaginal obstetric fistula (VVF). It was of moderate size to allow a metal catheter which is clearly visible [*By courtesy Dr. P. Mukherjee, Professor, Dept of G&O, IPGME&R, Kolkata*]

Vesicovaginal fistula (VVF)

Definition : There is communication between the bladder and the vagina and the urine escapes into the vagina causing true incontinence (Fig. 25.2). **This is the commonest type of genitourinary fistula.**

Causes : • **Obstetrical** • **Gynaecological**

Obstetrical : In the developing countries, the commonest cause is obstetrical and constitutes about 80-90 per cent of cases, as opposed to only 5-15 per cent in the developed countries. The fistula may be due to ischaemia or following trauma.

Ischaemic : It results from prolonged compression effect on the bladder base between the head and symphysis pubis in **obstructed labour** → ischaemic necrosis → infection → sloughing → fistula. **Thus, it takes few days (3-5) following delivery to produce such type of fistula.**

Traumatic : This may be caused by :

- **Instrumental vaginal delivery** such as **destructive operations** or **forceps** specially with Kielland. The injury may also be inflicted by the **bony spicule** of the foetal skull in **craniotomy operation.**
- **Abdominal operations** such as hysterectomy for rupture uterus or Caesarean section specially a repeat one or for caesarean hysterectomy. The injury may be direct or ischaemic following a part of the bladder wall being caught in the suture.

This type of direct traumatic fistula usually follows soon after delivery.

Gynaecological :

Although a rarity in the developing countries, it is the commonest type met in the developed ones and accounts for more than 80 per cent of fistulae.

- **Operative injury** likely to produce fistula includes operations like anterior colporrhaphy, abdominal hysterectomy for benign or malignant lesions or removal of Gartner's cyst.
- **Traumatic** — The anterior vaginal wall and the bladder may be injured following fall on a pointed object, by a stick used for criminal abortion, following fracture of pelvic bones or due to retained and forgotten pessary.
- **Malignancy** — Advanced carcinoma of the cervix, vagina or bladder may produce fistula by direct spread.
- **Radiation** — There may be ischaemic necrosis by endarteritis obliterans due to radiation effect, when the carcinoma cervix is treated by radiation. Apart from overdose or malapplication, it may occur even with accurate therapy. It takes usually long time (1-2 years) to produce such fistula.
- **Infective** — Chronic granulomatous lesions such as vaginal tuberculosis, lymphogranuloma venereum, schistosomiasis or actinomycosis may produce fistula.

Thus, the fistula tract may be lined by fibrous, granulation tissue, infective extension or malignant cells.

Types : **Fistula may be classified as** — (i) Simple (Healthy tissues with good access) or (ii) Complicated (tissue loss, scarring, difficult access, associated with RVF).

Depending upon the site of the fistula, it may be :

- **Juxtacervical (close to the cervix)** — The communication is between the supratrigonal region of the bladder and the vagina.
- **Midvaginal** — The communication is between the base (trigone) of the bladder and vagina.
- **Juxtaurethral** — The communication is between the neck of the bladder and vagina (may involve the upper urethra as well).

Clinical features

Patient profile : In the developing countries, obstetrical fistula being common, the patients are usually young primiparous with history of difficult labour or instrumental delivery in recent past. In others, it is related with the relevant events.

Symptoms

• Continuous escape of urine per vaginam (true incontinence) is the classic symptom. The patient has got no urge to pass urine. However, if the fistula is small, the escape of urine occurs in certain position and the patient can also pass urine normally. Such history has got a positive correlation with the related events mentioned in the aetiology.

• There is associated pruritus vulvae.

Signs :

Vulval inspection

- Escape of watery discharge per vaginam of ammoniacal smell is characteristic.
- Evidences of sodden and excoriation of the vulval skin.
- Varying degrees of perineal tear may be present.

Internal examination : If the fistula is big enough, its position, size and tissues at the margins are to be noted.

At times, there may be varying degrees of vaginal atresia so as to make the fistula inaccessible.

Speculum examination : A Sims' speculum in Sims' position gives a good view of the anterior vaginal wall when the vagina becomes ballooned up by air because of negative suction.

- The size, site and number of fistula.
- Often, the bladder mucosa may be visibly prolapsed through a big fistula (Fig. 25.2).
- A tiny fistula is evidenced by a puckered area of vaginal mucosa.

Associated clinical features that may be present in cases of such fistula are :

- Secondary amenorrhoea of hypothalamic origin (Menstruation resumes following successful repair).
- Foot-drop due to prolonged compression of the sacral nerve roots by the fetal head during labour.
- Complete perineal tear or rectovaginal fistula.

Confirmation of diagnosis

The diagnosis is most often made from the typical history and local examination. But, sometimes confusion arises in a case of tiny fistula for which additional methods are to be employed (Table 25.2). **The confused clinical conditions are** stress incontinence, ureterovaginal and urethrovaginal fistula.

To confirm the diagnosis, following are helpful :

- EUA is needed for better evaluation.
- The patient is placed in Sims' or knee chest position and while examining the anterior vaginal wall, bubbles of air are seen through the small tiny fistula when the woman coughs.

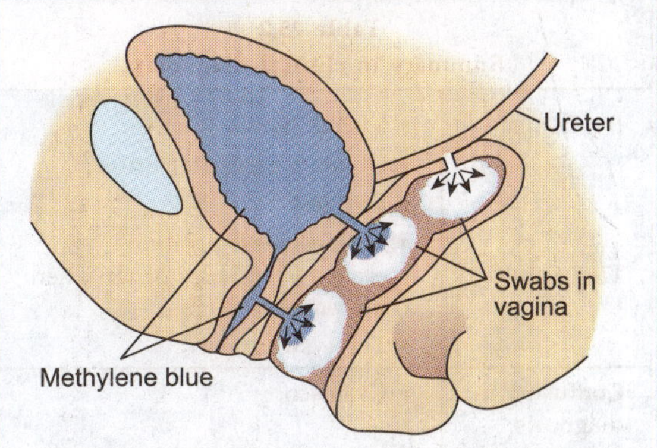

Fig. 25.3. Three swab test using methylene blue

- **Dye test** — A speculum is introduced and the anterior vaginal wall is swabbed dry. When the methylene blue solution is introduced into the bladder by a catheter, the dye will be seen coming out through the opening.
- A metal catheter passed through the external urethral meatus into the bladder when comes out through the fistula not only confirms the VVF but ensures patency of the urethra.
- **Three swab test** — The three swab test not only confirms the VVF but also differentiates it from ureterovaginal and urethrovaginal fistula.

Procedure of three swab test (Fig. 25.3)

Three cotton swabs are placed in the vagina — one at the vault, one at the middle and one just above the introitus. The methylene blue is instilled into the bladder through a rubber catheter and the patient is asked to walk about for about 5 minutes. She is then asked to lie down and the swabs are removed for inspection (Table 25.1).

Table 25.1 : Three swab test

Observation	*Inference*
Upper most swab soaked with urine but unstained with dye. The lower two fistula swabs remain dry.	Ureterovaginal fistula
Upper and lower swabs remain dry but the middle swab stained with dye.	Vesicovaginal fistula
The upper two swabs remain dry but the lower swab stained with dye.	Urethrovaginal fistula

Table 25.2
Summary in clinical diagnosis

Big fistula	• Visible fistula tract • Obvious escape of urine • Dye test
Tiny fistula	• In knee-chest position escape of bubbles of air when the patient coughs • Three swab test
Confusion in diagnosis	• Cystoscopy

Investigations

Imaging studies

❑ **(A)**

(1) **Intravenous urography** : for the diagnosis of ureterovaginal fistula.

(2) **Retrograde pyelography** : for the diagnosis of exact site of ureterovaginal fistula.

❑ **(B)**

(1) **Cystography** — not done in cases with VVF. It may be done in a complex fistula or vesicouterine fistula where uterine cavity (lateral view) may be seen.

(2) **Endoscopy studies** : Cystourethroscopy is not routinely done. The added information are : Exact level and location of the fistula and its relationship to ureteric orifices and bladder neck.

Treatment of old VVF

• Preventive • Operative

Preventive

Obstetric fistula in the developing world can be prevented with safe motherhood initiative **(WHO-1987)**. Gynaecological fistula — can be prevented with better anticipation and improved surgical skill.

The following guidelines are prescribed :

• Adequate antenatal care is to be extended to screen out 'at risk' mothers likely to develop obstructed labour.

• Anticipation, early detection (partograph) and ideal approach in the method of delivery in relieving the obstruction.

• Continuous bladder drainage for a variable period of about 5-7 days following delivery either vaginally or abdominally in a case of long-standing obstructed labour.

• Care to be taken to avoid injury to the bladder during pelvic surgery — obstetrical or gynaecological.

Immediate management : Once the diagnosis is made, continuous catheterisation for 6-8 weeks is maintained. This may help spontaneous closure of the fistula tract. Unobstructed outflow tract helps epithelialisation, provided the tissue damage is minimum. The management of genitourinary fistula may need a team approach both by the gynaecologists and the urologists.

Operative

Local repair of the fistula is the surgery of choice.

• Preoperative assessment

• Preoperative preparations

• Definitive surgery.

Preoperative assessment

• Fistula status — Assessment is done as regards the site, size, number, mobility and status of the margins of the fistula. If necessary, the examination may be conducted under general anaesthesia.

• Urethral involvement is assessed by introducing a metal catheter through external urethral meatus into the bladder.

• To ascertain the position of the ureteric openings in relation to a big fistula, cystoscopy is indicated. The patient is placed in knee-chest position when the bladder becomes distended with air (Kelly's air cystoscopy).

• **To exclude associated rectovaginal fistula or complete perineal tear.**

• Complete haemogram and urea, creatinine (renal function) estimation are done.

Preoperative preparations

• As the patients are usually from poor socioeconomic status, and socially outcasted the improvement of the general condition is essential prior to surgery.

• Local infection in the vulval skin should be treated by application of bland ointment or glycerine.

• Urinary infection, if any, should be corrected before hand. It is difficult to collect urine for culture and sensitivity. It is preferable to collect urine for the same from the indwelling catheter kept following the surgical repair. Preoperative collection is best to be done through ureteric catheterisation.

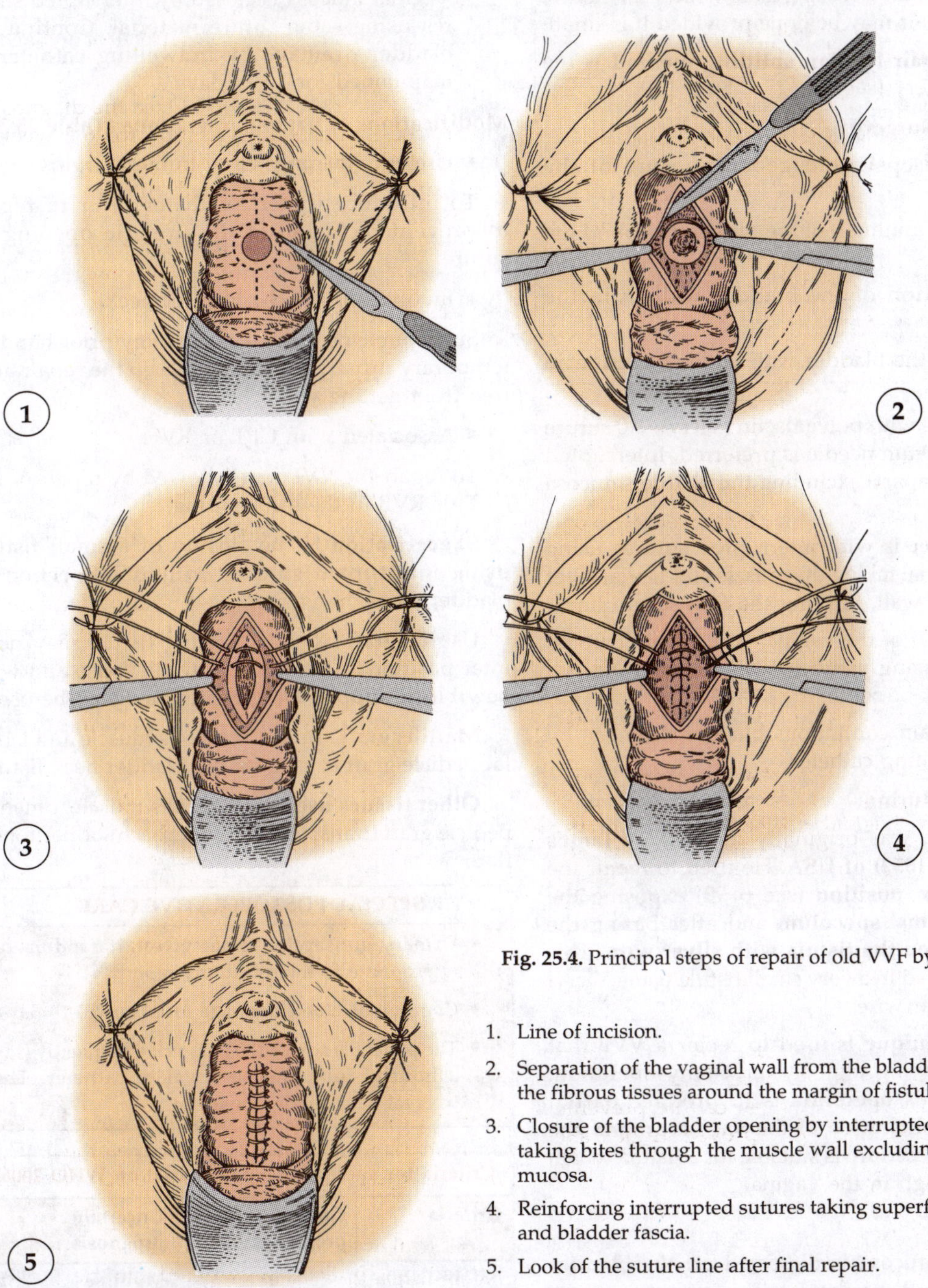

Fig. 25.4. Principal steps of repair of old VVF by flap method

1. Line of incision.
2. Separation of the vaginal wall from the bladder. To excise the fibrous tissues around the margin of fistula.
3. Closure of the bladder opening by interrupted sutures taking bites through the muscle wall excluding the bladder mucosa.
4. Reinforcing interrupted sutures taking superficial muscle and bladder fascia.
5. Look of the suture line after final repair.

Urine collected through vaginal speculum will not serve the purpose because of contamination. It is advised to start urinary antiseptics at least 3-5 days prior to surgery.

Definitive surgery **— (Old obstetric VVF).**

Time : The ideal time of surgery is after 3 months following delivery. By this time, the general condition improves and local tissues are likely to be free from infection. Further delay is likely to produce more fibrosis and unnecessary prolongs the misery of the patient.

Surgical fistula if recognised within 24 hours, immediate repair may be done provided it is small.

- **Local repair by flap splitting method** is the preferred surgery (see Fig. 25.4, Step 1-5).

Principles of surgery:

- Perfect asepsis and good exposure of the fistula.
- Excision (minimal) of the scar tissue round the margins.
- Mobilisation of the bladder wall from the vagina.
- Suturing the bladder wall without tension in two layers.

First layer is with polygalactin (Vicryl) 2-0 suture (p. 607) on a 30mm needle is preferred. Interrupted stitches (3mm apart) excluding the bladder mucosa are done.

Second layer is with interrupted sutures using the same material taking the muscle and fascial layer of the bladder wall, burying the first suture line.

- Apposition of the vaginal wall by interrupted sutures using same suture material No. 'O' (Fig. 25.4).
- To maintain continuous bladder drainage by an indwelling catheter.

Paring and suturing

This operation was originally devised by **James Marion Sims (1852) of USA**. He used to repair the fistula in **Sims' position** (see p. 99) exposing the fistula with **Sims' speculum** and after paring the margins, **sutured the fistula with silver wire**. This may be employed in a very small fistula using Vicryl instead of silver wire.

Latzko technique is used to repair a VVF that develops following total hysterectomy operation. Principle of this operation is to produce partial colpocleisis (obliteration of the vagina around the fistula). This procedure is suitable for a fistula which is small and high in the vagina.

Principal steps:

- Vaginal mucosa is dissected off the bladder wall around the fistula site.
- The fistula tract is excised.
- Bladder mucosal edges are approximated with interrupted sutures (2-0 Vicryl).
- Two additional suture layers are used to appose the muscle and fascia.
- Vaginal mucosa is closed by interrupted sutures using same suture material. Continuous bladder drainage by indwelling catheter is maintained for 10-14 days.

Modifications of vaginal operations (Table 25.3)

- Ureteric openings close to the margins.

To introduce ureteric catheter prior to repair to prevent inclusion of the ureteric opening in suture.

- Involvement of the bladder neck.

Suprapubic or vaginal cystostomy prior hand as temporary urinary diversion to keep the repair area free from getting wet.

- Associated with CPT or RVF.

To repair the VVF first followed by repair of the CPT or RVF in the same sitting.

Saucerisation is the closure of a small fistula using interrupted stitches without dissection of bladder from the vagina.

Use of graft: Repair of a big fistula may need inter position of tissue grafts to fill space and with new blood supply. Different tissues may be used.

Martius graft: Bulbocavernous muscle and labial fat pedicle graft is used for big bladder neck fistula.

Other tissues used are Gracillis muscle, omental pedicle graft (transperitoneal approach) or peritoneal flap.

SPECIAL POSTOPERATIVE CARE

- Urinary antiseptics either given at random or appropriate to the sensitivity report.
- Continuous blood drainage for about 10-14 days.
- The patient is advised to pass urine frequently (say 2 hourly) following removal of catheter. The interval is gradually increased.

Criteria for successful repair (based on WHO 2006)

Criteria	Good prognosis prognosis	Uncertain prognosis
No. of fistula	Single	Multiple
Site	Vesicovaginal fistula (VVF)	Rectovaginal fistula (RVF), Mixed (VVF and RVF)
Size	< 4 cm	> 4 cm
Urethral involvement	Absent	Present

Table contd. next page

Criteria for successful repair (based on WHO 2006) *(contd. from previous page)*

Criteria	Good prognosis	Uncertain prognosis
Vaginal scarring	Absent	Present
Tissue loss	Minimal	Extensive
Ureter involvement	Ureters are draining inside the bladder, not into the vagina	Ureters are draining into the vagina
Circumferential defect (urethra completely separated from the bladder)	Absent	Present

Advice during discharge

- To pass urine more frequently.
- To avoid intercourse for at least 3 months.
- To defer pregnancy for at least 1 year.
- If conception occurs, to report to the hospital and must have mandatory antenatal check up and hospital delivery. **A successful repair should have an abdominal delivery.**

If repair fails, local repair should again be attempted after 3 months. The fistula may become smaller when the second attempt may be successful. In cases of repeated failures, before declaring the case as irrepairable, it is preferable to have a second opinion or to consult an urologic surgeon. This might avert the last resort to go for urinary diversion — implantation of ureters into the pelvic colon or ileal bladder (preferred).

Table 25.3
Other routes of repair of bladder fistula

- Transperitoneal — Vesicouterine fistula.
- Transvesical — fistula unapproachable per vaginam, specially employed by urologic surgeon.
- Transperitoneal or transvesical approach is preferred when the fistula margins are close to the ureteral orifices. This is done for proper dissection and to avoid injury to the ureter. This approach is also used when ureteroneocystostomy is done or omental graft is used.

Principles in the management of gynaecological VVF

- Detected during operation : To repair immediately in two layers.
- Detected in the postoperative period : To put an indwelling catheter for about 10–14 days. If fails, repair is to be done after 3 months.
- Malignant or postradiation fistula : Any of the following may relief the symptoms — (1) Ileal bladder, (2) Anterior exenteration, (3) Colpocleisis.
- Infective fistula : Eradication of the specific infection be done first followed by local repair.

URETHROVAGINAL FISTULA

Causes

- Part or whole of the urethra is involved along with bladder. The causes are the same as those of VVF.
- Small isolated urethrovaginal fistula is caused by :
  - Injury inflicted during anterior colporrhaphy, urethroplasty, suspension or sling operation for stress incontinence.
  - Residual fistula left behind following repair of vesicourethrovaginal fistula.

Diagnosis : The patient has got urge to pass urine but the urine dribbles out into the vagina during the act of micturition. A sound or a metal catheter passed through the external urethral meatus when comes out through the communicating urethrovaginal opening confirms the diagnosis. In cases of confusion in diagnosis with VVF or ureterovaginal fistula, three swab test (mentioned earlier) may be employed.

Treatment : Surgical repair in two layers followed by continuous bladder drainage as outlined in repair of VVF is satisfactory. Prior suprapubic or vaginal cystostomy ensures better success. In cases of complete destruction of the urethra, reconstruction of urethra is to be performed. Stress urinary incontinence has been observed in 10-15 per cent cases following successful repair of VVF.

URETERIC INJURY IN GYNAECOLOGIC SURGERY

Ureteric injury through rare has got considerable morbidity. It is an important cause for litigation.

Causes : • Acquired • Congenital

Acquired : This is common and usually follows trauma during pelvic surgery. Although commonly associated with difficult surgery like abdominal hysterectomy in cervical fibroid, broad ligament fibroid, endometriosis, ovarian malignancy or radical hysterectomy, it may be injured even in apparently simple hysterectomy abdominal or vaginal (rare).

Congenital : The aberrant ureter may open into the vault of vagina, uterus or into urethra.

INJURY TO THE URETER DURING GYNAECOLOGICAL SURGERY

Because of close anatomical association between ureter and genital organs, ureteric injury is not uncommon during gynaecological surgery. Overall incidence is 0.5-1 per cent of all pelvic operations. About 75 per cent of ureteral injury result from gynaecological operations and 75 per cent of them occur following abdominal gynaecological procedures.

Important anatomical locations where ureteric injury is more common.

- At the level of infundibulopelvic ligament — where ureter runs parallel to ovarian vessels at the same place. Ureter forms the posterior boundary of ovarian fossa. Any inflammatory or malignant processes will involve the ureter.
- Deep in the pelvis, below the level of ischial spine, where ureter lies lateral to the peritoneum of uterosacral ligament.
- At the level of internal cervical-os, 1.5 cm lateral to the cervix where uterine artery crosses the ureter from above.
- Over the anterior vaginal fornix, within the ureteric tunnel of cardinal ligament (tunnel of Wertheim) where it turns anteriorly and medially to enter the bladder.
- Where it traverses through the musculature of bladder (intravesical part).
- Any congenital malformation (duplex ureter) makes it more vulnerable to injury at any of these sites.

Nature of ureteral Injury

Severity of ureteric injury may be any of the following types :

- Simple kinking or angulation – causing obstruction.
- Ischaemic injury resulting from trauma to ureteric sheath endangering its blood supply.
- Ligature incorporation.
- Crushing injury by clamps followed by necrosis.
- Transection — either partial or complete.
- Segmental resection either accidental or planned.
- Thermal injury during minimally invasive surgical procedure when diathermy (monopolar or bipolar) or laser energy is used (see p. 585).
- Injury by staplers during Laparoscopic surgery.

Gynaecological operations and Ureteric injury

Risk of injury is more where pelvic anatomy is distorted due to presence of any pelvic pathology. Common pathological conditions are :

- Cervical fibroid or low corporeal fibroid (p.575)
- Broad ligament tumour (p. 573).
- Pelvic endometriosis (p. 570).
- Gynaecological malignancy (p. 576).
- Pelvic haematoma.
- Tubo-ovarian mass, pelvic adhesions.
- Reapplication of a clamp to the pedicle of uterine artery following its initial slip.
- Presacral neuronectomy (endoscopic).
- Ovarian remnant (see p. 532) — when needs removal.
- Radical hysterectomy (p. 576).
- Vaginal hysterectomy (rare) (p. 211).
- Colposuspension (p. 387).
- LAVH (p. 570, 585).

Diagnosis : Signs and symptoms are subtle and often overlooked. Fever, flank pain, haematuria, abdominal distension, urine leakage (vaginally), peritonitis, ileus and retroperitoneal urinoma should raise the suspicion.

(a) *Escape of urine through vagina* following the operative procedure is suspicious.

(b) The patient has got *urge to pass urine and can pass urine normally.*

(c) *Three swab test* differentiates it from VVF (Table 25.1)

(d) *Intravenous indigo carmine test* — if the urine in the vagina is unstained following three swab test, indigo carmine is injected intravenously. If urine becomes blue (generally within 4-5 minutes) the diagnosis of ureterovaginal fistula is established.

(e) *Cystoscopy* — Should be performed to determine the side of ureterovaginal fistula. There is no spurt of urine from the ureteric orifice of the affected side.

(f) When a *ureteric catheter* is passed under cystoscopic guidance, obstruction is met when the catheter tip reaches the site of injury.

(g) *Excretory urography (IVU)* confirms the side and site of fistula. The tract of ureterovaginal fistula is also outlined.

(h) *Renal ultrasound* is a noninvasive method. Hydronephrosis and retroperitoneal urinomas when seen, are helpful to the diagnosis.

(i) *Computed Tomography (CT)* showing contrast extravasation is the most consistent to the diagnosis.

Per operative detection of ureteral laceration can be made by seeing the leakage of dye at the site, following intravenous injection of indigo carmine. When the ureter is ligated or kinked, gradually increasing ureteric dilatation will be noticed, instead of dye leakage.

MANAGEMENT OF URETERIC INJURY

• Preventive • Operative

Preventive measures

A thorough knowledge of pelvic anatomy is essential. Where there is any doubt, the following measures may be of help if taken either during preoperative or intraoperative period.

• Intravenous urography (preoperative) — is helpful in certain situation (e.g. pelvic tumours), to ascertain the course of the ureters. Any congenital abnormality is also revealed.

• Placement of ureteral catheters (preoperative or intraoperative) to facilitate detection and dissection of ureters. Unfortunately in a fibrotic pelvic condition (endometriosis) palpation may be difficult.

• Direct visualisation and/or palpation of ureters throughout its pelvic course wherever possible.

• Uriglow — ureteric catheters within built incorporated light source for better localisation has been tried.

• Adequate exposure of pelvic organs is a must. Inadequate incision leads to inadequate exposure and dissection. This may lead to blind clamping or suturing.

• Meticulous care during dissection — not to damage the sheath of ureter so that longitudinal vessels are not destroyed.

• To follow the important axiom of surgery — any important structure at risk of inadvertent injury must be carefully dissected and adequately exposed.

• To avoid blind clamping of blood vessels.

Operative

Management of ureteric injury depends on the following factors — (a) Time of detection : intraoperative or postoperative (b) Type and severity of injury (c) Anatomical level (d) Mobility of the ureter and bladder (e) Pathology leading to ureter injury (f) Patient's general condition and prognosis.

Principles of Ureteric Repair

- Not to damage the ureteric sheath and its blood supply during dissection.
- Ureteric mobilisation and tension-free anastomosis.
- Watertight closure with fine absorbable suture.
- Sent with a ureteric catheter.
- Passive drain at the anastomotic site to prevent urine accumulation.

Management when injury is recognised during operation

Ureteral sheath denudation : No intervention, rarely ureteral stenting (double J or Pig tail), if a long segment is involved.

Ureteral kinking (due to closely placed sutures) : Immediate removal of suture.

Ureteral ligation : Deligation immediately → assessment of viability by blood flow and ureteral peristalsis. Ureteral stenting may be needed if any doubt.

Ureteral crushing (clamp injury) : Remove the clamp → check the viability → ureteral stenting → extraperitoneal drainage at the site is placed.

Ureteric transection

Partial : Primary repair over ureteral stent placement.

Complete : (i) In the middle-third → end-to-end anastomosis over an ureteral stent (uretero-ureterostomy) following adequate mobilisation of both the segments. Otherwise ureteroileal interposition is done. (ii) In the lower-third → ureteroneocystostomy with psoas hitch over an ureteral stent.

Ureteric implantation into the bladder must be done without any tension. High mobilisation of bladder is needed and bladder dome is sutured to the psoas muscle on that side (**psoas hitch**). To prevent vesicoureteric reflux, ureter is implanted through submucosal tunnel in the posterior wall of the bladder.

Bladder flap procedure (modified Boari-Ockerblad) is an alternative when the ureter is short or the injury is at the level of pelvic brim. An obliquely placed bladder flap is outlined. The flap is rolled into a tube and the ureter is reimplanted in the submucosal tunnel without tension.

Alternatively **ureteroileoneocystostomy** would be done.

Thermal injury : Depending upon the severity it may need resection and management according to transection.

Complications following repair of ureteric injury

(i) Stricture. (ii) Infection. (iii) Ureteric obstruction. (iv) Reflux of urine. (v) Stent or Boari flap complications.

RECTOVAGINAL FISTULA

Definition : Abnormal communication between the rectum and vagina with involuntary escape of flatus and/or faeces into the vagina is called rectovaginal fistula (RVF). See Fig. 25.5.

Causes : **• Acquired • Congenital**

Acquired :

Obstetrical — (a) Incomplete healing or unrepaired recent CPT is the commonest cause of RVF.

(b) Obstructed labour — The rectum is protected by peritoneum of pouch of Douglas in its upper-third, by the perineal body in the lower-third and by the curved sacrum in the middle-third. However, if the sacrum is flat, during obstructed labour the compression effect produces pressure necrosis → infection → sloughing → fistula.

(c) Instrumental injury inflicted during destructive operation.

Gynaecological : (a) Following incomplete healing of repair of old CPT (commonest).

(b) Trauma inflicted inadvertently and remains unrecognised in operations like — perineorrhaphy, repair of enterocele, vaginal tubectomy, posterior colpotomy to drain the pelvic abscess, reconstruction of vagina, etc.

(c) Fall on a sharp pointed object.

(d) Malignancy of the vagina (common), cervix or bowel.

(e) Radiation.

(f) Lymphogranuloma venereum or tuberculosis of the vagina.

(g) Diverticulitis of the sigmoid colon → abscess → bursts into the vagina.

(h) Crohn's disease involving the anal canal or lower rectum.

Congenital : The anal canal may open into the vestibule or in the vagina.

Diagnosis

- Involuntary escape of flatus and or faeces into the vagina. If the fistula is small, there is incontinence of flatus and loose stool only but not of hard stool.
- Rectovaginal examination reveals the site and size of the fistula.
- Confirmation may be done by a probe passing through the vagina into the rectum. If necessary, methylene blue dye is introduced into the rectum

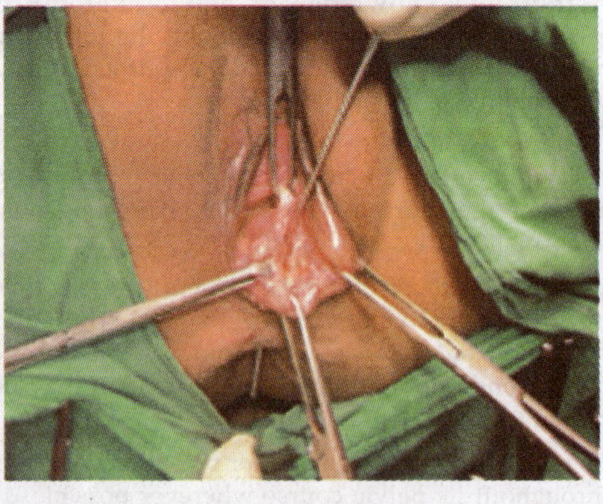

Fig. 25.5. Rectovaginal fistula (RVF) following traumatic forceps delivery. It was of moderate size so as to pass a metal probe through the vagina and it is clearly seen to come out through the anus

which is seen escaping out through the fistula into the vagina. Examination under anaesthesia may be conducted to facilitate clinical diagnosis (see Fig. 25.5).

Investigations :

- Barium enema.
- Barium meal and follow through may be needed to confirm the site of intestinal fistula.

Sigmoidoscopy and proctoscopy are helpful for the diagnosis of inflammatory bowel disease or for taking biopsy of fistula edge.

Treatment : • **Preventive** • **Definitive**

Preventive : Preventive aspects include good intranatal care, identification of CPT and its effective repair. Consciousness about the possible injury of the rectum in gynaecologic surgery mentioned and its effective and appropriate surgery minimise the incidence of fistula.

Definitive surgery includes :

- Situated low down — to make it a complete perineal tear and repair it as that of CPT.
- Situated in the middle-third — repair by flap method.

Repair by flap method — Repair is commonly done transvaginally. The scar-margin is excised. Vaginal wall separated from the underlying rectal wall. This wide tissue mobilisation helps repair without any tension. Repair is done in layers. Pre- and postoperative bowel management are similar to that in repair of CPT.

- Situated high up — Preliminary colostomy → local repair after 3 weeks → closure of colostomy after 3 weeks.
- The preoperative preparations of one stage vaginal repair are like those mentioned in repair of CPT.

KEY POINTS

- The incidence of genitourinary fistula ranges between 0.5-3 per cent amongst gynaecological admission of the developing countries. Vesicovaginal fistula is the commonest one.
- The majority (80-90%) is obstetrical following ischaemia due to obstructed labour (p. 402). In the developed countries, the fistula is mostly gynaecological (80%).
- The fistula is best revealed in Sims' position using Sims' speculum (Sims' triad p. 406). In tiny fistula, diagnosis is made by three swab test. The test also differentiates it from ureterovaginal fistula.

  Local repair by flap splitting method between 3–6 months following delivery is the preferred surgery. Continuous bladder drainage for 10–14 days following surgery should be a must p. 406). Special postoperative care is essential for success.

  If repair fails, local repair should be attempted after 3 months. In traumatic fistula specially gynaecological, the repair should be done immediately during primary surgery. However, if detected in the postoperative period, the continuous bladder drainage is to be kept for about 10–14 days failing which repair is to be done after 3 months. There are some favourable factors for successful repair (Table on p. 406)
- Ureterovaginal fistula is common following difficult abdominal hysterectomy for cervical or broad ligament fibroid, endometriosis, ovarian malignancy or radical hysterectomy (see p. 408). It may also occur following vaginal hysterectomy or otherwise, in a case of simple hysterectomy. There are some anatomical locations as well as pelvic pathologies where ureteric injury is more likely (see p. 408). Nature of ureteric injury may vary from kinking to complete transection. Three swab test differentiates it from a tiny VVF (p. 403). Further investigations are needed to confirm the diagnosis and also to know the side and site of injury (see p. 408). End-to-end anastomosis during surgery or ureteroneocystostomy is the preferred surgery in late cases.
- Rectovaginal fistula is common following incomplete healing or unrepaired recent complete perineal tear. Other cause of RVF are obstetric, gynaecological or congenital (p. 410).
- Diagnosis (p. 410) is important as regard the site and size of fistula.
- Definitive surgery for RVF may be as that of a repair of a CPT or by flap method or repair with prior colostomy (p. 411).

Genital Tract Injuries

26

Introduction

The genital tract and the adjacent pelvic organs are subjected to strain of vaginal delivery either spontaneous or assisted. The injury is more in areas of inadequate antenatal and intranatal care. The patients may have full recovery from the injuries but a substantial number may produce permanent legacies which lead to major gynaecologic problems. The following are some of such major obstetric legacies (Table 26.1).

All are dealt in appropriate chapters; only the severe form of perineal injuries — i.e. old complete perineal tear will be dealt within this chapter. It has to be borne in mind that with improved antenatal and intranatal care, majority of the complications could be prevented. It is thus appropriately considered that obstetrics is a branch of preventive medicine.

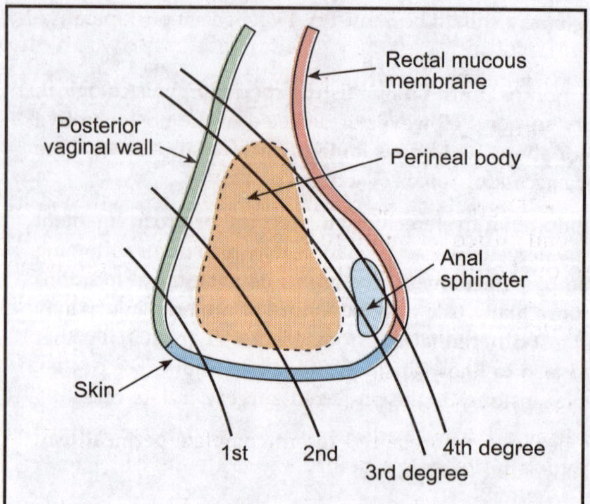

Fig. 26.1. Diagrammatic representation showing different degrees of perineal tear (from author's Textbook of Obstetrics)

Table 26.1
Obstetric legacies leading to gross gynaecologic problems

- Genital prolapse
- Perineal injuries including complete perineal tear
- Genitourinary and rectovaginal fistula
- Tender perineal and vaginal scar
- Backache
- Eversion cervix with cervicitis
- Ill health and chronic debilitating state

OLD COMPLETE PERINEAL TEAR (CPT)

Definition

Tear of the perineal body involving the sphincter ani externus with or without involvement of the anorectal mucosa is called **complete perineal tear**. It is called old when passed beyond an arbitrary period of 3 months following the injury (Fig. 26.1).

Classification of Perineal Tears (RCOG–2007)	
Grade	**Features**
First degree	Laceration of vaginal epithelium or perineal skin.
Second degree	Involvement of the perineal body but not the anal sphincter.
Third degree	Disruption of the anal sphincter complex (both external and internal).
Fourth degree	Injury to the anal sphincter complex with tear of the anal epithelium.

Aetiology

- Obstetrical
- Gynaecological

Obstetrical : Perineal injury (3° and 4°) results from **over stretching** or **sudden stretching** of the perineum during child birth. It is more common when the perineum is **inelastic**.

RISK FACTORS FOR THIRD DEGREE TEARS (RCOG–2007)

- Primigravida
- Big baby (> 3 kg)
- Face to pubis delivery
- Midline episiotomy
- Forceps delivery
- Outlet contraction with narrow pubic arch
- Shoulder dystocia
- Precipitate labour
- Scar in the perineum
- Prolonged second stage

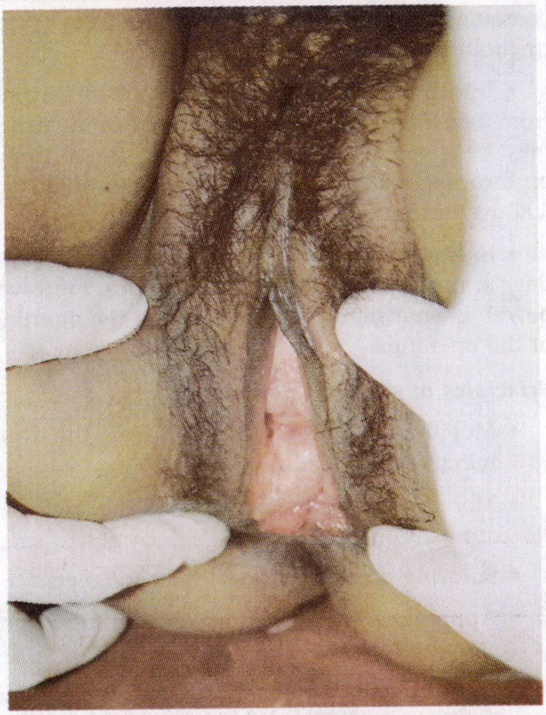

Fig. 26.2. Old complete perineal tear. Note the absence of perineum and the pinkish vaginal mucosa is continuous with reddish rectal mucosa

Gynaecological

Direct injury on the perineum by fall may lead to trauma on the perineum to the extent of CPT.

Table 26.2

Structures torn through are :

- Posterior vaginal wall or perineal skin.
- Perineal muscles.
- Perineal body.
- Anal sphincter complex.
- Varying degrees of anorectal mucous membrane.

Clinical features

Patient profile

Patients are usually primiparous with a history suggestive of inadequate care during childbirth.

Symptoms

The chief complaints are :

• Inability of hold the flatus and faeces. While incontinence of flatus is invariable but that of faeces depends on the extent of damage of the external anal sphincter. If the damage is slight, there is incontinence of only loose stool but if the damage is severe, there is incontinence of hard stool as well.

• Soreness over the perianal region is due to constant irritation by the stool. It is often surprising that, the condition may remain asymptomatic for many years and only discovered accidentally during pelvic examination. Over activity of the levator ani makes the patient continent with the stool; the incontinence of flatus being ignored.

Signs

Inspection of the perineum reveals

• There is absence of perineum. Vaginal and rectal mucous membranes are found to be continuous, only separated by a bridge of fibrous tissue **(rectal mucosa is reddish and the vaginal one is pinkish in colour) (Fig. 26.2)**.

• Visible dimple on the skin on either side of the fused mucosa may be present. These represent the retracted torn ends of the sphincter ani externus which have got subcutaneous attachment.

Radial wrinkling of the skin is present only on the posterior aspect of the anal opening.

Palpation : There is absence of the sphincteric grip evidenced when a finger is introduced into the rectum. The anal canal is separated from the vagina only by a septum.

It is surprising that in spite of deficit of the perineum, there is no prolapse. This is because of overactivity of the levator ani muscle. If prolapse is found along with CPT, it is more likely pre-existing.

Differential diagnosis

A rectovaginal fistula situated low down may at times be confused with complete perineal tear. This is specially in cases where overlying skin remains intact. **Rectovaginal fistula causes more inconvenience to the patient than CPT**.

Treatment

• **Preventive** • **Operative**

Preventive : Proper conduct in the second stage of labour taking due care of the perineum when it is likely to be damaged is the effective step to prevent undue lacerations (Table 26.3).

The prevention of the perineal injuries in normal delivery includes :

- More attention should be paid not to the perineum but to the controlled delivery of the head.
- Delivery by early extension is to be avoided. Flexion of the head is to be maintained till the suboccipt comes under the symphysis pubis so that lesser suboccipitofrontal (10 cm) diameter emerges out of the introitus.
- Spontaneous forcible delivery of the head is to be avoided by assuring the patient not to bear down during contractions, pressing on the head and the perineum by the palms and giving inhalation analgesics, if available.
- To deliver the head in between contractions.
- To perform timely episiotomy.
- To take care during delivery of the shoulders as the wider bisacromial diameter (12 cm) emerges out of the introitus.

Table 26.3
Prophylaxis to perineal injuries during delivery

- Delivery of the head by early extension is to be avoided.
- Controlled delivery of the flexed head in between uterine contractions.
- Timely and judicious mediolateral episiotomy specially in primigravidae, occipito-posterior, face, breech or forceps delivery.

Operative : The definitive surgery is repair of the perineal tear with restoration of the perineal body (perineorrhaphy).

This should preferably be done between 3-6 months following the injury. The best time of repair is however, within 24 hours of the injury.

By 3 months time, the local infection subsides, general condition of the patient improves and the baby can be kept at home. If kept more than 6 months, there is more fibrosis on the margins and unnecessary prolonged inconvenience to the patient.

Preoperative investigations

There is no special preoperative investigation except the stool should be examined for evidence of intestinal infestations like hookworm, Ascaris or *E. histolytica* which are rampant in the tropical countries. Their presence needs eradication prior to surgery.

Preoperative preparations

- The patient is admitted at least 3 days prior to surgery.
- The patient should have low residual diet consisting of milk, bread, lime-whey for 2 days prior to surgery.
- Intestinal antiseptics are prescribed starting from 2 days prior to surgery. Any one of the drugs may be given — neomycin 250 mg thrice daily, erythromycin 500 mg thrice daily, metronidazole 400 mg thrice daily.
- Enema and bowel wash are given daily, for two days prior to operation. The idea is to clear the lower bowel. Enema should not be given in the morning of the operation.

Principles of surgery (Flap method)

- Mobilisation of the rectal wall from the overlying vaginal wall.
- Mobilisation of the torn ends of the sphincter ani externus.
- Suturing of the rectal wall in two layers.
- Approximation of the torn ends of the sphincters by interrupted sutures.
- Apposition of the musculofascial structures of the perineal body by 2-3 interrupted sutures.
- Apposition of the vaginal wall and skin of the perineum by interrupted sutures.

Steps of operation (Fig. 26.3)

Preliminaries

As in anterior colporrhaphy.

Actual steps

Mobilisation of the rectum and anal sphincter

- Two Allis tissue forceps are placed on either side of the fused rectovaginal mucosa and are retracted laterally by the assistant.
- An incision is made over the fused mucosa extending from one end to the other. [Fig. 26.3(1)].
- Two Allis forceps are placed on either side on the lower end of the labium minus.
- Incision over the fused mucosa is extended upwards from each end upto the lower end the labium minus.
- The posterior vaginal wall is dissected off from the rectum and the rectum is well-mobilised. [Fig. 26.3(2)].
- Two more Allis forceps are placed beyond the skin dimple on either side. Incision is made from each end of the fused mucosa downwards over the skin dimple (site of torn end of the sphincter ani externus).

The incision lines now look almost to the letter 'H'.

- Torn end of the anal sphincter of each side is held by Allis forceps and is well-mobilised. [Fig. 26.3(4)].

Repair : Prior to repair, the scar tissue on the rectal margins is to be excised.

- The rectal wall is sutured by interrupted sutures using polygalactin (Vicryl) No. '2-0' with round body a-traumatic needle starting from the apex. The knots are placed inside the lumen. [Fig. 26.3(2)].
- The pararectal fascia is approximated over the first layer by interrupted sutures using the same suture materials. [Fig. 26.3(3)].
- The torn ends of the sphincter ani externus are approximated infront of the repaired rectum by a figure of eight suture using polydioxanone (PDS) No. '2-0'. This is enforced by one or two interrupted sutures. [Figs 26.3(4) and 26.3(5)]. Results of repair of EAS either by an overlapping or an end to end approximation method, are the same.

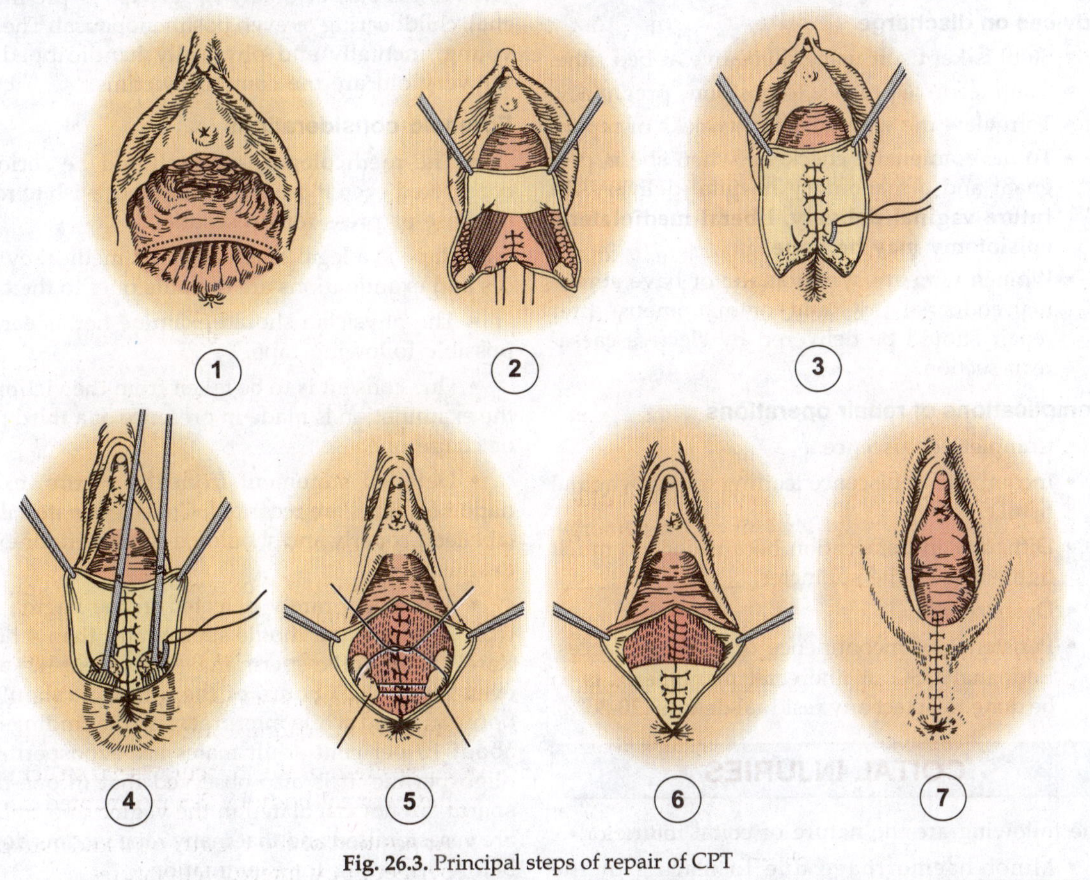

Fig. 26.3. Principal steps of repair of CPT

- Redundant portion of the vaginal mucosa is excised.
- Two or three interrupted sutures are placed through the fibromuscular tissues of the perineal body using Vicryl No. 'O' [Fig. 26.3(6)].
- The rest of the steps are like that of perineorrhaphy.

Special postoperative care

- Non-residual diet is given from 3rd day onwards; the full diet is given on 6th day.
- Bowel should not be moved for about 4-5 days.
- Lactulose 10 ml twice daily beginning on the second day and increasing the dose upto 30 ml on the 3rd day is a satisfactory regimen to soften the stool.
- If the patient fails to pass stool and is having discomfort, compound enema (olive oil or liquid paraffin, glycerine and normal saline, each 4 oz) may be given by a rubber catheter.
- Antibiotics (cefuroxime 1.5 gm and metronidazole 500 mg – IV) are used to cover the perioperative period.
- Intestinal antiseptics should be continued for about 5 days (see above).

Advices on discharge

- Stool is kept soft using a laxative at bed time.
- Contraceptive practice to postpone pregnancy.
- To review the woman after 6 weeks of repair.
- To have antenatal check up when she is pregnant and a mandatory hospital delivery. **In future vaginal delivery, liberal mediolateral episiotomy may be done.**
- Women who are symptomatic or have abnormal endoanal USG and/or manometry after repair should be delivered by elective caesarean section.

Complications of repair operations

- Complete dehiscence.
- Incomplete dehiscence leading to rectovaginal fistula.
- Difficulty in defaecation because of too much tightening of the sphincter.
- Dyspareunia.
- Peristence of incontinence of flatus or faeces. Endoanal USG or anorectal manometry is to be done to detect any residual defects (20-30%).

COITAL INJURIES

The following are the nature of coital injuries :

- Minor haemorrhage due to tearing of the hymen or bruising of the vagina or urethra may occur at defloration. No treatment is usually required.
- Severe haemorrhage may occur, if the tear spreads to involve the vestibule or the region of the clitoris. Lacerations of the anterior vaginal wall may occur usually following rape.
- Very rarely, rupture of the vault of the vagina may occur to expose the peritoneal cavity. This usually occurs in — (a) rape, (b) very young girls, (c) postmenopausal atrophy and (d) following vaginal/abdominal hysterectomy. Bowels and omentum may prolapse through the ruptured vault and cause shock and peritonitis.

Management : Small tears need no treatment; only pressure application is enough. Larger lacerations have to be repaired. If the vault has ruptured, it is preferable to perform laparotomy and repair the vault and to tackle any associated pathology.

RAPE VICTIMS

The victims may be of any age groups — pre-menarchal, childbearing or even postmenopausal. The very young, mentally and physically handicapped and the very old are the common victims.

Forensic considerations

- The medicolegal issues should be seriously considered even if the victim does not wish to report the case or press for prosecution.
- Rape is a legal diagnosis. The medical evidences and examinations are of value only to the court.
- The physician should examine her as early as possible following rape.
- Due consent is to be taken from the victim and the examination is made in presence of a third party or chaperone.
- Detailed statement from the victim, examination findings are recorded. Collected materials are labelled properly and should be submitted for expert examination.
- Sperm are rarely detected in the vagina later than 72 hours and motile sperm later than 4 hours. Rarely non-motile sperm may be present in vagina even after 12-20 hours of the attack. It should be borne in mind while interpretating the findings that about 10 per cent adult males are azoospermic or oligospermic. It is also observed that in one-third, sperm are not ejaculated in the vagina and millions are vasectomised and that many rape victims douche before reporting for examination.

Management

Management aims at :

- To treat any local injury
- To perform appropriate tests
- To prevent infection and STD
- To prevent pregnancy
- Medicolegal procedure
- To provide emotional support to the victim.

MEDICOLEGAL PROCEDURES
• To document history in detail. • To examine her thoroughly and to note the injuries. • To collect the clothings, hair samples by combing pubic hair and finger nail scrapings. • To collect samples for sperm, acid phosphatase from the affected site (vagina, rectum, pharynx). • To send specimens to forensic authorities with record.

Local injuries : The injuries may be in the form of bruises, lacerations around the neck, buttocks or vulva. Extensive lacerations in the area of hymen, vagina, urethra even the vaginal vault may be there. There may be major injuries specially in young virgins or premenarchal girls. The injuries should be repaired under general anaesthesia. In premenarchal girls, to increase the vaginal defence, small dose of oestrogen is given orally daily for two weeks (0.01 mg ethinyl oestradiol).

To prevent infection and STD

Infection may be genital as well as extragenital (pharynx). **Rape victim runs the risk of infection with gonorrhoea, syphilis, chlamydia, trichomonas, HIV, Hepatitis B and others (see ch. 11).** Blood for serological test for syphilis and cervical and urethral smear for *gonococcus* are to be collected for bacteriological study. Cultures of cervical mucous should also be done for microbiological study.

Since about 6 weeks must elapse after exposure before the serology becomes positive, a positive test at the first visit indicates that the victim has already been exposed. If negative, the test is to be repeated after 6 weeks. Drugs commonly used for the prevention of STD are given in the Table 26.4.

Table 26.4 Drugs used for prevention of infection and STD
• Ceftriaxone 250 mg IM is given — single dose. Plus • Doxycycline 100 mg orally two times a day for 7 days.

To prevent pregnancy

Due care is to be taken to prevent pregnancy. **This is however not applicable** in premenarchal girls, in women protected by 'pills' or IUD or permanent sterilisation. If the patient is at risk of pregnancy emergency contraception is advised (see p. 471).

Medicolegal procedures : Details of history and examination specially the injuries are documented. All clothings and undergarments are collected and labelled properly. Smears of vaginal secretions are made to document the presence of sperm, acid phosphatase and for DNA typing. Collected swabs are refrigerated until they are processed. Pubic hair combings is done to obtain pubic hair of the assaulter. Finger nail scrapings are obtained for DNA typing of the perpetrator.

To provide emotional support

To treat the psychic trauma (rape trauma syndrome), which usually lasts for a variable period — sympathetic handling, assurance, tranquilizers, and antidepressant drugs are of help.

The acute phase lasts for hours to days. The victim may present with features of fear, depression, guilt, sleeplessness and eating disorders.

The late phase or the reorganisation phase consists of nightmares, flash backs or phobias. It may last for months to years. The victim is allowed to express her feelings, anxieties and fears. She should be reassured as far as possible. Other health care personnel may be involved to counsel her if needed. Follow up visit should be planned within 4–6 weeks before she is discharged.

Follow up

The follow up should be arranged in 1–4 weeks. The protocols to be maintained are :

- Serological test for syphilis.
- Test of cure by culture for gonorrhoea.
- Urine test for pregnancy, if suspected.
- Reassurance and support.

DIRECT TRAUMA

Accident, as falling astride on any sharp or pointed object, is not uncommon specially in young girls. It may produce bruising of the vulva or at times give rise to vulval haematoma (Fig. 26.4).

Major accident may involve fracture pelvic bones causing injuries to pelvic viscera like bladder or rectum apart from vagina. There may be supralevator haematoma.

Even, fall on a sharp object may produce the above picture or perforate the vaginal wall with injury of the surrounding viscera.

Management : Assessment of the general condition and the nature and extent of the injuries inflicted should be done first. Small vulval haematoma, if not spreading may be left alone but if it is a big one or spreading, along with resuscitative measures, the haematoma is to be tackled under general anaesthesia.

This includes scooping of the blood clots after giving an incision, secure haemostasis and obliteration of the dead space by interrupted mattress sutures.

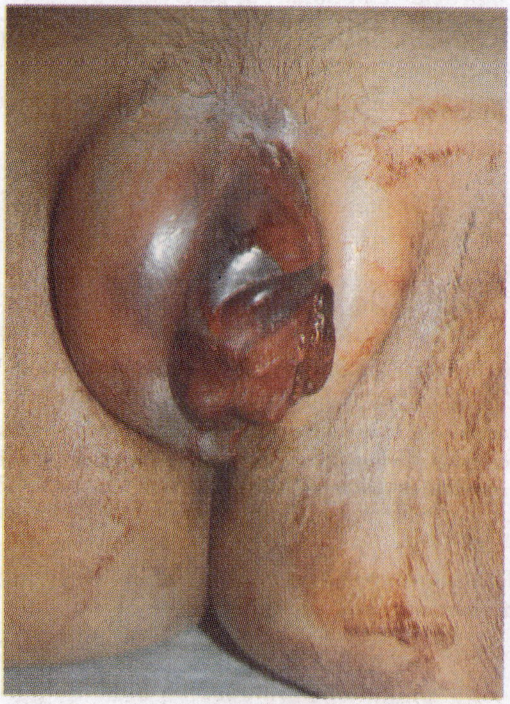

Fig. 26.4. A 17 year-old-girl suffered extensive vulval haematoma following a fall on a chair

In supralevator haematoma or in cases of suspected gut injuries, laparotomy is indicated and appropriate measures taken.

FOREIGN BODIES

Various types of foreign bodies may be placed either in the vagina or uterus and retained for a prolonged period often unnoticed by the patient. The articles so placed are either introduced by the patient or at times by a physician. Such articles are of varying nature, to mention only a few of them.

In the vagina

- Coins, toys, small stones either introduced out of curiosity by children or perversion in adults.
- Forgotten menstrual tampoon or diaphragm, cervical cap or condom used as contraceptives.
- Articles introduced to procure abortion.
- Packs, swabs or dressings.
- Forgotten pessary.

In the uterus

- Retained IUCD for a long time.
- Old gauze packs.
- Articles inserted for procuring abortion.

Effects : The effects depend upon the nature of the foreign body, duration of its existence and amount of tissue damage.

Any material left inside invites infection. This specially happens in rubber goods, foreign bodies, swabs or gauze packs. There is foul smelling discharge.

Retained and forgotten pessary may cause vaginitis, sloughing and ulceration. It may produce vesicovaginal fistula and may be a precursor of vaginal carcinoma. **Prolonged retention of IUD may cause** menorrhagia, irregular bleeding and if left even in postmenopausal period, may produce pyometra or postmenopausal bleeding.

Management : Once diagnosed, the foreign body is to be removed. In children, it may not be easy and it is better to expose the vagina under general anaesthesia using aural or nasal speculum.

INSTRUMENTAL INJURIES

Uterine injury in gynaecologic conditions is rather uncommon compared to pregnant uterus. However, injuries do happen with all types of instruments used in cervical dilatation and uterine curettage operation.

Cervical injuries may be inflicted by the vulsellum or by a dilator specially in nulliparous cervix. There may be at times brisk haemorrhage. **Late sequela includes cervical incompetency.**

Body of the uterus is commonly injured by sound, dilator or curette or during insertion of IUD. Apart from inadvertent injuries, the likely susceptible conditions are :

- Small and soft uterus during lactation
- Postmenopausal uterus
- Infected uterus • Pyometra • Malignancy

Dangers : There may not be any appreciable alteration of the general condition and the condition is left unnoticed. But it may be associated with :

- Brisk haemorrhage either intraperitoneal or revealed.
- Spreading infection (peritonitis).
- Injury to the gut.

Management

Once diagnosis is made, the operative procedure is to be stopped. Further management depends on :

- Type of instrument causing injury
- Pathology in the uterus
- Effect on the patient.

Non-infective/non-malignant

Observation

Pulse and blood pressure are to be observed periodically and to administer antibiotics. Evidences of peritonitis are to be looked for. Laparoscopy can give a good guide for observation or interference.

Interference

- Deteriorating general condition
- Suspected gut injury
- Features of developing peritonitis.

Infective/malignant

- In infective uterus, there is chance of spreading peritonitis. Observation may be done under cover of antibiotics but if unresponsive, laparotomy is preferred.
- In malignancy or pyometra, laparotomy and definitive surgery have to be seriously considered.

KEY POINTS

- Obstetric legacies leading to gross gynaecologic problems include — genital prolapse, perineal injuries, fistula, backache, chronic cervicitis and ill health.
- Gross injury to the perineum is mostly due to mismanaged second stage of labour.
- Incomplete perineal tear, there is absence of perineum and the vaginal and rectal mucous membranes are found to be continuous.
- The definitive surgery is perineorrhaphy. The best time is within 24 hours of injury and in late cases between 3-6 months. Bowel preparations are to be done prior to surgery.
- Minor haemorrhage due to tearing of the hymen is the commonest coital injury. Severe injury results from rape in very young girls or postmenopausal atrophy.
- Rape is a legal diagnosis. Due consent is to be taken from the victim and the examination is made in presence of a third party or chaperone. **Management of rape victims aims at** — treatment of the local injuries, prevention of infection and STD, prevention of pregnancy, medicolegal procedures and emotional support to the victim (see p. 417). To prevent infection ceftriaxone (250 mg IM-single dose) and doxycycline (100 mg P.O.B.D. for 7 days) are given. Emergency contraception is advised if the victim is at risk of pregnancy (chapter 29, p.471).
- Direct injury to the vulva may at times produces haematoma which requires resuscitation and exploration under general anaesthesia. **Foreign bodies** — placed in the vagina for a prolonged period are pessary and diaphragm or cervical cap used as contraceptives. IUD may be forgotten and retained for a prolonged period in the uterus. Once diagnosed, the foreign bodies are to be removed.
- Uterine injury in gynaecologic surgery is relatively uncommon compared to pregnant uterus. Interference is indicated in deteriorating general condition, suspected gut injury and with the features of developing peritonitis. In infective or malignant condition, laparotomy is seriously to be thought of.

Intersex

27

Definition

Intersexuality may be defined as the presence of both male and female external and or internal genital organs in the same individual causing confusion in the diagnosis of true sex. The incidence is about 2 per 1,000.

Embryological consideration

The development of the gonads and the genitalia has been described in chapter 3. Only its schematic representation is depicted below.

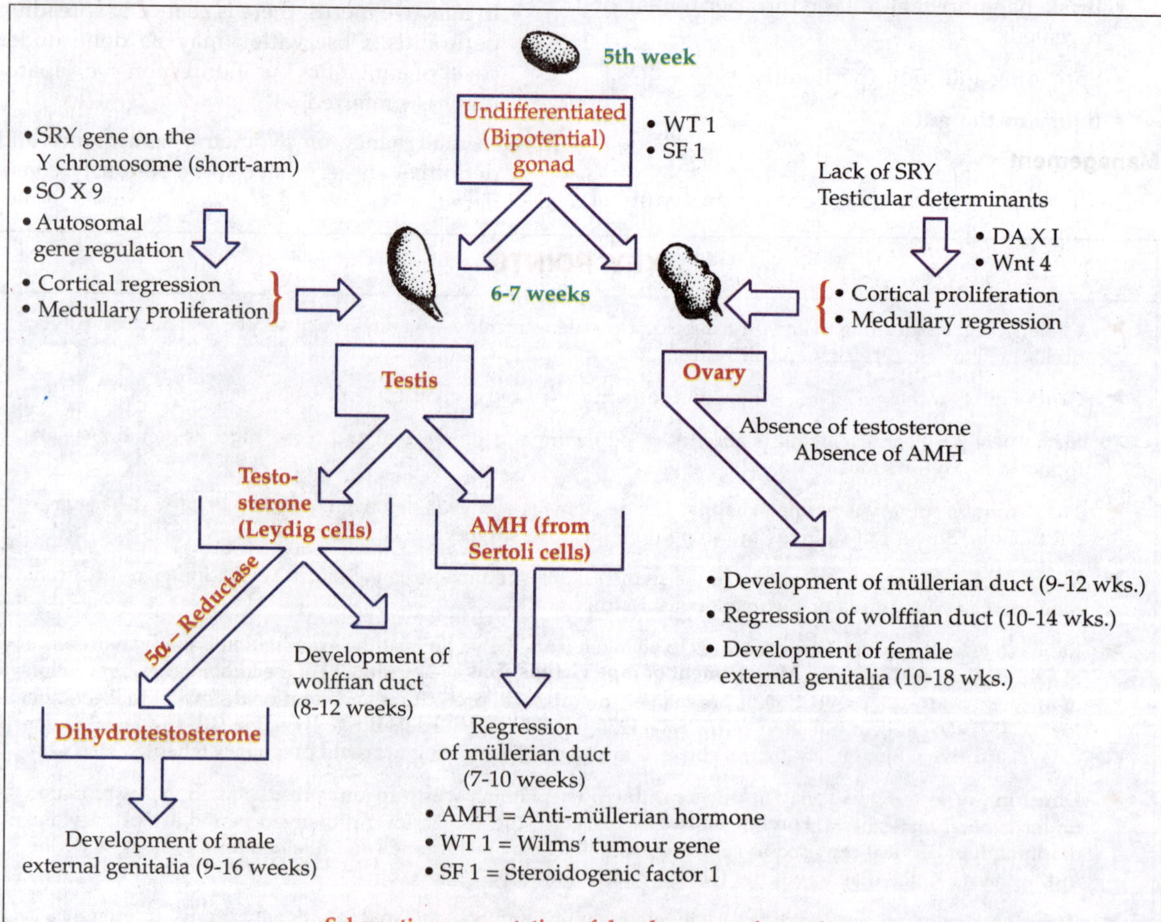

Schematic representation of development of gonads

Determination of sex

In determining the sex, the following factors are to be considered — (1) Genetic sex (2) Chromosomal sex (3) External and internal anatomic sex (4) Gonadal sex (5) Hormonal sex (6) Psychologic sex (7) Sex of rearing.

In the newborn, the diagnosis of the apparent sex is determined by the appearance of the external genital organs. In the adolescence however, in addition to the appearance of external genitalia, sex of rearing, psychogenic sex and the appearance of secondary sex characters should be taken into consideration.

Nomenclature

- Female intersex or female pseudohermaphrodite — An association of female gonads with male external genitalia.
- Male intersex or male pseudohermaphrodite. – An association of male gonads with female external genitalia.
- True hermaphrodite — An individual possessing both ovaries and testes with ambiguity of genital organs.

AETIOLOGY, CLINICAL PRESENTATION AND DIAGNOSIS

- Female intersex.
- Disorders of gonadal development.
- Male intersex.
- True hermaphroditism.

FEMALE INTERSEX

(a) Adrenogenital syndrome (congenital adrenal hyperplasia) (Fig. 27.1)

Aetiology

It is an autosomal recessive disorder. It is due to inborn error of adrenal steroid metabolism, commonly due to 21-hydroxylase (95%) and rarely due to 11-hydroxylase or 3β hydroxy steroid dehydrogenase deficiency. There is lack of cortisol production resulting in excess of ACTH production from the pituitary. ACTH in turn, stimulates the adrenal to produce excess androgens with virilisation of female offspring. Associated aldosterone deficiency may lead to excess salt depletion. There is often history of affection of sibling. The girls are potentially fertile.

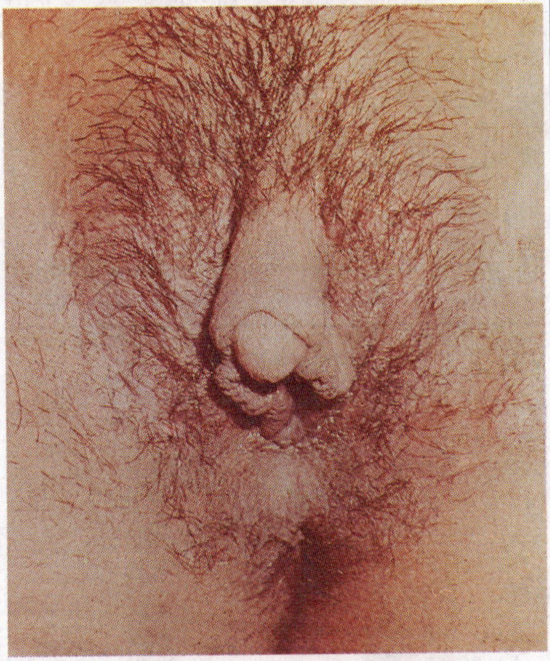

Fig. 27.1. Enlarged clitoris, fused labia minora in adrenogenital syndrome [*By courtesy* : Prof. B. N. Chakravorty, IRM, Kolkata]

Clinical presentation

Ambiguity of sex at birth — Cases of ambiguity of sex detected at birth are due to adrenogenital syndrome unless proved otherwise.

- Hirsutism and amenorrhoea may be the presenting features around puberty in milder form.

Diagnosis at birth

The suspected anatomic abnormalities include :

- An enlarged clitoris (Fig. 27.1).
- Presence of penile urethra or hypospadius.
- Associated metabolic abnormality — salt wasting (hyponatraemia, hyperkalaemia) and hypotension may be present.
- Fusion of the labia minora.
- The presence of any one or more of the above features necessitates further investigations for confirmation of an early diagnosis.

Investigations

- Sonographic evaluation of internal genitalia shows presence of uterus, fallopian tubes, and vagina. The gonads are ovaries.

- Sex chromatin study reveals positive Barr body.
- Karyotype is 46, XX.
- Serum estimation
  - 17 hydroxy-progesterone (17 OHP) is elevated to beyond 800 ng/ml.
  - Electrolyte values are estimated to check the possibility of their depletion and producing "salt loosing syndrome" (sodium and chloride – low, potassium – raised).

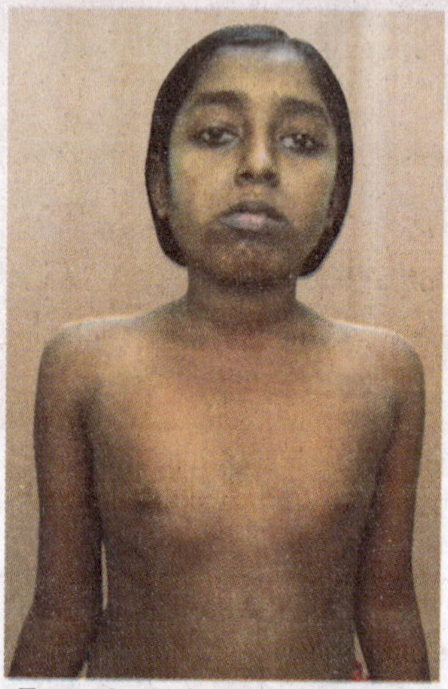

Fig. 27.2A. Turner's syndrome in a 16 year old girl with poor secondary sexual characters

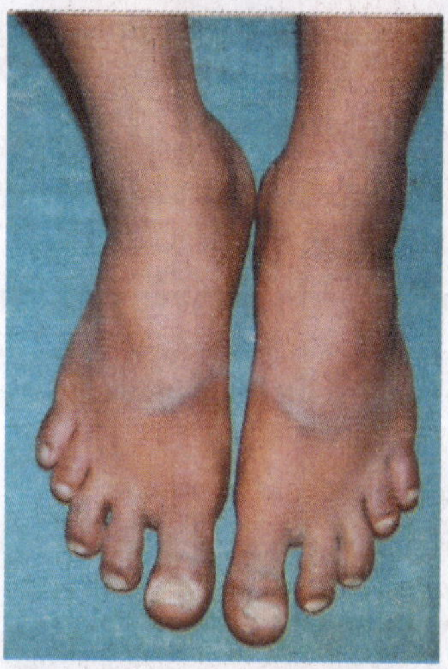

Fig. 27.2B. Deformity of the metatarsal bones in Turner's syndrome [*By courtesy* : Dr. S. Chaudhury, Asst. Professor, Dept. of Obst. and Gynae., N.R.S. Medical College, Kolkata]

- Urinary excretion of pregnanetriol and 17 Ketosteroids are markedly elevated.

(b) Masculinisation due to increased androgen in maternal circulation

Drug induced androgenicity is very rare nowadays. Progestogens used in early pregnancy complication has too often been implicated. But, the newer progestogens have got least adverse effect. Danazol used in endometriosis may produce virilisation in female offsprings, if continued during accidental pregnancy. Rarely, the androgen source may be adrenal tumour, androgen secreting tumour or Cushing's syndrome of the mother.

There may be confusion in diagnosis of sex at birth. The history of intake of androgenic drug is often present. The source of excess androgen can be detected by appropriate investigations. To rule out adrenogenital syndrome, serum 17 hydroxy-progesterone is to be measured. **This is not elevated in any of the conditions mentioned.**

DISORDERS OF GONADAL DEVELOPMENT

Gonadal dysgenesis

The term is employed for patients with female habits in whom the gonads are imperfectly developed.

It is due to cytogenetic abnormality. The germ cells either fail to develop or fail to reach the gonads. The gonads are represented by white streaks without any germ cell.

TURNER'S SYNDROME (Henry Turner — 1938)

The cases usually present as primary amenorrhoea with delayed secondary sex characters.

The syndrome is characterised by short stature (height < 150 cm), webbing of the neck, cubitus valgus, broad shield chest, low hair line on the neck, short fourth metatarsals and poor development of secondary sex characters. They are mentally retarded and often associated with coarctation of aorta (Figs 27.2A and B).

Renal anomalies (horse shoe kidneys) and multi-glandular autoimmune disorders are common. 45X is the commonest chromosomal abnormality and 99 per cent of fetuses are aborted.

Vagina, uterus and fallopian tubes are present. The uterus is small but is responsive to exogenous oestrogen. Gonads are 'streaks' (fibrous tissue) without any follicle nor any potentiality to produce hormone (chromosomally incompetent ovarian failure). Associated autoimmune disorders like Hashimoto's thyroiditis, Addison's disease, hypothyroidism are common.

Investigations : Confirmation of the clinical diagnosis is by the following.

- Sex chromatin study is negative.
- Karyotype is 45, XO.
- Serum E_2 is very low.
- Serum FSH and LH are elevated.
- Autoantibodies may be present (see p. 444, ch. 28).

Thus, there is hypergonadotrophic hypogonadism state.

Mosaic variety — In mosaic variety, the classic features of Turner are absent. The individual is of normal height. Ovaries are 'streaks' with few follicles. Occasionally, menstruation can occur for few cycles until the follicles are exhausted. Pregnancy has also been recorded.

- Sex chromatin is doubtful.
- Karyotype is 46, XX/45, XO.

Structural abnormality of X chromosome

Deletion of genetic material from short arm of 'X' chromosome leads to somatic features of Turner's syndrome (short stature). Loss of the long arm near the centromere leads to primary amenorrhoea.

Pure gonadal dysgenesis or gonadal agenesis

The patients usually present as primary amenorrhoea with delayed development of secondary sex characters. **The stature is average**.

The vagina, uterus, and tubes are present although infantile. Gonads are bilateral 'streaks' without any potentiality to produce hormones. The uterus is however sensitive to exogenous oestrogen.

As these patients have got no gonads, a female phenotype is expected regardless of the chromosomal complement.

- Sex chromatin is doubtful.
- Karyotype is either 46, XX or 46, XY.

Mixed gonadal dysgenesis

Some present with the problem of ambiguous external genitalia at birth. Usually, the patients come around puberty for features of masculinisation or primary amenorrhoea.

There are features of partial masculinisation of the external genitalia. The gonad of one side is testis and on the other side a 'streak'.

The karyotype is usually 45, X0/46, XY.

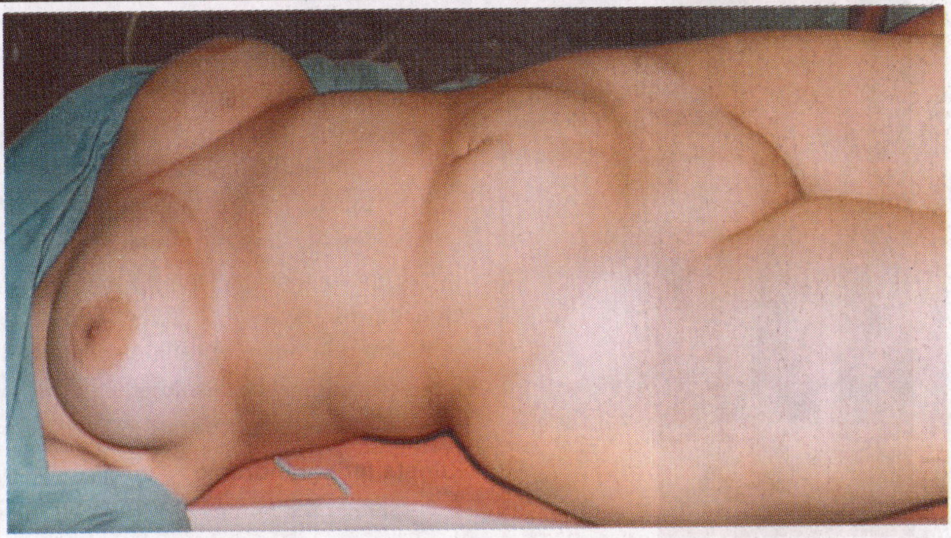

Fig. 27.3. A case of androgen insensitivity syndrome. Breasts are well-developed, absent pubic hair [*By courtesy* : Prof. B. N. Chakravorty, IRM, Kolkata]

MALE INTERSEX

Androgen insensitivity syndrome (Testicular feminisation)

The condition is inherited as a X-linked recessive gene. The underlying pathology is the inability of the endorgans to respond to androgens. Either, there is lack of androgen cytosol receptor or the receptor is defective (mutated).

- The cases are rarely diagnosed prior to puberty.
- Usually presents with primary amenorrhoea and or infertility.
- They are phenotypically and psychologically female.
- Breast development is adequate (Fig. 27.3).
- The nipples are small with pale areola.
- There is eunuchoidal tendency (long arms, big hands and feet).
- Absent or sparce of axillary and pubic hair (Fig. 27.3).

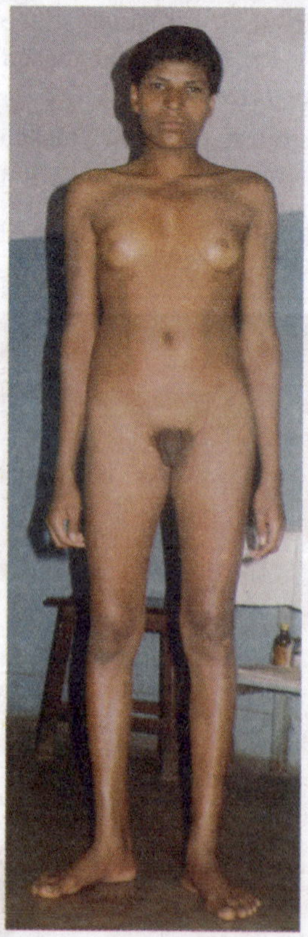

Fig. 27.4. A case of Klinefelter's syndrome having gynaecomastias [*By courtesy : Dr. B. Ghosh, Burnpur*]

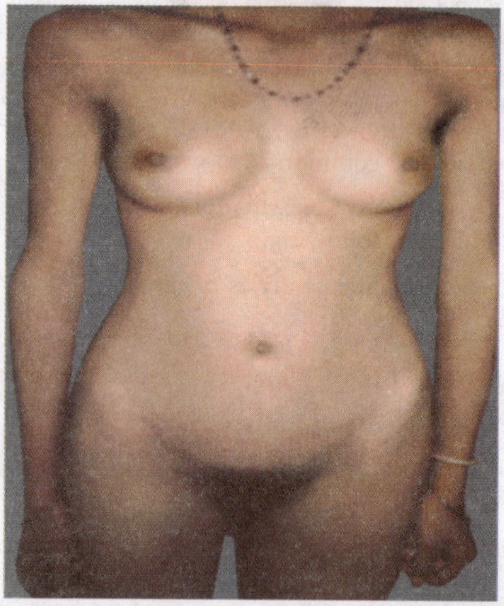

Fig. 27.5. A case of sex reversal 47,XXY female Klinefelter [*By courtesy* : Prof. B. N. Chakravorty, IRM, Kolkata]

- External genitalia looks female.
- Vagina is short and blind (Fig. 27.7). The upper two-thirds of vagina, uterus and tubes are absent due to the effect of AMH. The gonads (Sertoli cells) secrete AMH (Anti-müllerian hormone).
- Gonads (testes) are either placed in the labia, or inguinal canal or intra-abdominal (Figs. 27.6 and 27.7).

Investigations

- Sex chromatin is negative.
- **Karyotype is 46, XY.**
- Serum testosterone is within average for normal males.
- Serum E2 level is high normal for males.
- Serum LH level is normal or slightly elevated.
- Confirmation of diagnosis is by gonadal biopsy.

Gonadal biopsy

- Seminiferous tubules are small, hyalinised.
- Spermatogenesis is absent.
- Leydig cells and Sertoli cells are normal.

Klinefelter's syndrome

The patients are eunuchoid in build, infertile with small penis, testis and varying degrees of gynaecomastias (Fig. 27.4). The features at times become confusing when first seen in adolescence (Fig. 27.5).

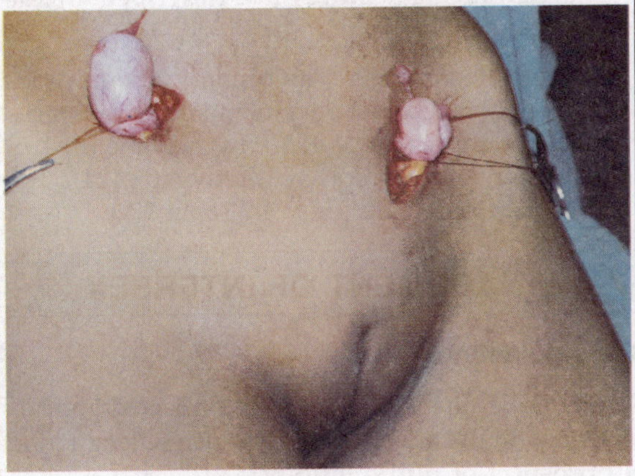

Fig. 27.6. Testicular feminisation — bilateral inguinal gonads [*By courtesy*: Prof. B. N. Chakravorty, IRM, Kolkata]

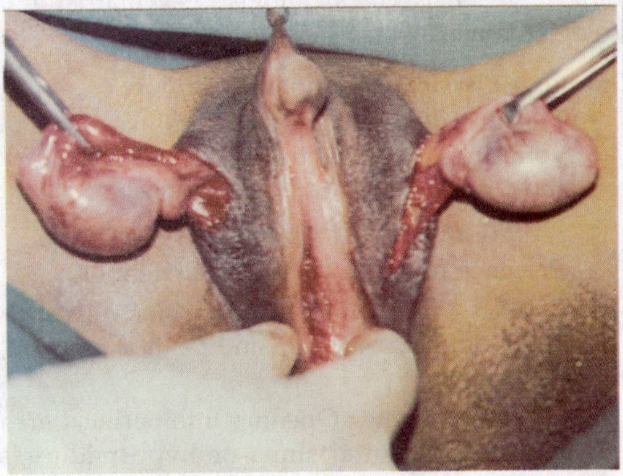

Fig. 27.7. Bilateral labial gonads (testes) and short blind vagina in testicular feminisation [*By courtesy* : Prof. B. N. Chakravorty, IRM, Kolkata]

- Sex chromatin is positive.
- Karyotype is XXY or XXXY.
- Genitalia—small and infantile. Genital ducts are wolffian.
- Serum gonadotrophins are elevated.

Cases of sex reversal 47, XXY female Klinefelter have been recorded (Fig. 27.5). Breasts are well-developed and secondary sexual characters are female (Fig. 27.5).

TRUE HERMAPHRODITISM

The condition is common among Bantu tribes in southern part of Africa.

The entity is due to chromosomal defect and genetic cause.

Types

Both the testicular and ovarian tissues are present in an individual in different combinations.

- Ovotestis on each side(commonest).
- Testis on one side, ovary on the other.
- Testis or ovary on one side and ovotestis on the other.

It is probable that fertilisation by a sperm carrying one 'X' chromosome which contains some male determining material from 'Y' gives rise to this condition.

- The common presentation is ambiguity of external genitalia.
- The internal structures depend on the degree of differentiation of the associated gonad on that side.
- 75 per cent develop gynaecomastia and nearly 50 per cent menstruate.

Investigations

- Sex chromatin is usually positive.
- Karyotype is usually 46, XX (70%), rest are 46, XY and rarely mosaic XX/XY.
- Confirmation of diagnosis is by gonadal biopsy.

DIAGNOSIS OF INTERSEX

At birth : Most cases of ambiguous genitalia detected at birth are due to either congenital adrenal hyperplasia (21-hydroxylase deficiency) or to androgenic drugs administered to the mother in early pregnancy.

At puberty : **Most cases presented at puberty are** late manifestations of congenital adrenal hyperplasia, those of gonadal dysgenesis and rarely male intersex (testicular feminisation). In these conditions, the child is reared up as girl and she is brought to the clinician either for poor development of secondary sex characters or for primary amenorrhoea with or without hirsutism.

Diagnosis of Ambiguous Genitalia : It is a major diagnostic problem. Combined approach by endocrinologist, geneticist, neonatologist, psychiatrist and urologist is needed.

Thorough Physical Examination to note :

- Life threatening conditions with features of vomiting, dehydration, diarrhoea, or shock must be excluded (adrenal failure).
- Height and secondary sexual characters.
- Presence of vagina or urogenital sinus.
- Length of phallus : In a normal newborn clitoris measures < 1 cm and penis is < 2.5 cm, in length.
- Urethral meatus : Opening into perineal area or into urogenital sinus or hypospadias is noted.
- Labioscrotal folds – degree of fusion is noted.
- Location of gonads — Gonads may be felt in the inguinal or in the labial region.

Table 27.1 : Differentiation of a normal looking girl presenting with primary amenorrhoea having normal breast development but absent uterus

Characters	Androgen Insensitivity Syndrome	Müllerian Agenesis (M-R-K-H Syndrome)
1. Sexual hair (pubic and axillary)	Absent or sparce	Normal female
2. Primary amenorrhoea	Present	Present
3. Vagina	Short and blind	Absent
4. Clitoris	Enlarged	Normal female
5. Gonads :		
• Structure	Testes	Ovary
• Location	Inguinal, Labial or Abdominal	Abdominal
6. Breasts	Developed	Developed
7. Serum Testosterone level	Slightly elevated	Normal female
8. Müllerian system	Absent	Absent or rudimentary
9. Wolffian system	Absent	Absent
10. Karyotype	46, XY	46, XX
11. Associated anomalies	Rare	Skeletal 12% and Urological (renal) 47%

The diagnostic features are described in the Table 27.2.

A normal looking girl with primary amenorrhoea who have normal breast development but no uterus may be either a case of M-R-K-H syndrome (p. 435) or testicular feminisation syndrome (p. 424). The diagnostic features are given in Table 27.1.

MANAGEMENT OF INTERSEX

Basic guidelines

Gender assignment rests on — (i) projected appearance of genitalia after puberty, (ii) penile length and (iii) prospect of future fertility.

• It is always better to diagnose the correct nature of intersex at birth or as early as possible. This is essential not only to correct the underlying disorders promptly but also to avoid the adverse psychological effect on the child and the family.

• If the diagnosis remains uncertain or the corrective surgery is deferred for the future, the baby should be reared up as female.

(1) **Management of adrenogenital syndrome** Hydrocortisone 10-20 mg/m^2 body surface area per day is given to suppress the excess ACTH secretion. Mineralocorticoid (fluorocortisone) is also given in cases with 21-hydroxylase deficiency. Cases with salt loss must be replaced carefully. Thereafter, a long-term therapy with corticosteroid is essential to suppress the adrenocortical hyperfunction.

Once the neonate is stable, surgery to reduce the enlarged clitoris (reduction clitoroplasty) may be done. Reconstructive surgery includes clitoroplasty and vaginoplasty. Timing of surgery is debated. However, it is recommended to perform vaginoplasty with the onset of puberty. However, the reproductive potentiality remains unaffected, if treated early. **Prenatal diagnosis** is possible with chorion villus sampling at early weeks (9-12) of pregnancy using DNA probes. 17-OHP level in the amniotic fluid (amniocentesis) is elevated. Prenatal therapy with dexamethasone or termination of pregnancy is the option.

(2) **In cases of gonadal dysgenesis**, karyotyping should be done. The presence of 'Y' chromatin necessitates removal of the gonads as there is chance of dysgerminoma, seminoma or gonadoblastoma in such gonads. Substitution therapy using cyclic oestrogen and progestogen will help to develop secondary sex characters.

Turner's syndrome

- Exogenous growth hormone (GH) can increase the height.
- Low dose oestrogen (conjugated oestrogen 0.625 mg) orally daily for 25 days with progestin (medroxy progesterone acetate 5 mg daily) for last 10 days is started after 13 years of age.

(3) In cases of androgen insensitive syndrome, the individual should be reared up as a girl. The ectopic gonads (testes) are to be removed (Figs. 27.6 and 27.7) as the risks of gonadal malignancy (gonadoblastoma or dysgerminoma are high (5-10%). Vaginoplasty is done after the growth is completed (16-18 years) with development of secondary sex characters. After gonadectomy, long-term oestrogen replacement therapy should be prescribed for its effect on vaginal epithelium, osteoporosis and cardiovascular system (see p. 437).

Appropriate counselling is done. It may be psychologically traumatic to disclose the diagnosis either to the patient or to the parents. They should be told that as the gonads are abnormal and they should be removed.

(4) In rare variety of true hermaphrodite, the change of sex depends on sex of rearing, psychologic and the anatomic sex. The genitalia inconsistent with sex assignment should be surgically removed or modified. In general, it is possible to change the external genitalia from male to female but not from female to male. Management depends upon the phenotype. The gonads are to be removed to be followed by substitution therapy.

UTERINE HERNIA SYNDROME

In this condition uterus and tubes are found in an inguinal hernia sac. Gonads are testes and are undescended. The affected individual is a male with 46, XY karyotype. This is due to failure of AMH function or secretion.

TESTICULAR REGRESSION SYNDROME (SWYER SYNDROME)

- The individual presents with primary amenorrhoea.
- External genitalia are female.
- Internal genital organs are female.
- Secondary sexual characters are absent.
- Karyotype 46, XY.
- Gonads are fibrous due to failure of development or regression.

It is thought to be due to mutation in SRY gene at the Y chromosome. Gonadectomy is recommended. Oestrogen and progestin therapy is given for development of secondary sex characters.

Table 27.2 : Entity, clinical presentation and diagnosis of intersex

Entity	Clinical presentation	Diagnostic criteria
Adrenogenital syndrome	– Ambiguity of sex at birth	– Sonographic evaluation of internal genital organs – Karyotype 46, XX – Serum 17 hydroxy-progesterone ↑ – Urinary pregnanetriol ↑ > 5 μg/100 ml
—do— (mild form)	– Virilism and amenorrhoea at puberty	– Karyotype 46, XX – Serum 17 hydroxy-progesterone ↑
Masculinisation due to androgen excess in maternal circulation	– Ambiguity of sex at birth	– History of drug intake – Karyotype 46, XX – Serum 17 hydroxy-progesterone — normal.

Table 27.2 contd. next page

Table 27.2 : Entity, clinical presentation and diagnosis of Intersex *(contd. from previous page)*

Entity	Clinical presentation	Diagnostic criteria
Gonadal dysgenesis • Turner's syndrome	– Primary amenorrhoea – Poor secondary sex characters – Short stature – Webbing of neck – Cubitus valgus – Genitalia underdeveloped	– Sex chromatin 45, XO – Bilateral 'streak' gonads – Serum : E2 ↓ and FSH ↑
Mosaic Turner	– Primary/secondary amenorrhoea – Average height – Poor sec. sex characters – Genitalia under developed	– Sex chromatin 45, XO/46, XX – Bilateral 'streak' gonads
• Pure gonadal dysgenesis	– Primary amenorrhoea – Delayed sec. sex characters – Average height – Genitalia-underdeveloped	– Sex chromatin — 46, XX or 46, XY – Bilateral 'streak' gonads
• Mixed gonadal dysgenesis	• At birth : – Ambiguity of sex • At puberty : – Virilism with amenorrhoea – Ext. genitalia – partial masculinisation Int. genitalia may be unilateral müllerian development	– Karyotype — – 45 XO/46 XY – Gonads — testis on one side and on the other side a 'streak'
Testicular feminisation	– Primary amenorrhoea – Infertility – Phenotypically female – Breast development – good – Ext. genitalia-female	– Axillary and pubic hair scanty or absent – Short, blind vagina – Gonads — Labial, inguinal or abdominal – Karyotype – 46, XY – Gonads are testes
Klinefelter's syndrome	– Eunuchoid – Infertility (azoospermia) – Gynaecomastia	– Ext. genitalia — male – Genital ducts — wolffian – Gonads — testes (small) – Sex chromatin — positive – Karyotype — 47 XXY
True hermaphroditism	– Ambiguity of sex at different phase of early life – Amenorrhoea	– Karyotype is usually 46, XX; may be 46, XY or 46, XX or 46, XX/46, XY – Gonadal biopsy is confirmatory – Common — ovotestes

KEY POINTS

- The incidence of intersex is about 2 per 1,000.
- Female intersex is association of female gonads with male external genitalia.
- Male intersex is association of male gonads with female external genitalia.
- True hermaphrodite is an individual possessing both ovaries and testes with ambiguity of genital organs.
- Female intersex is due to congenital adrenal hyperplasia (commonest) or due to increased androgen in maternal circulation.

  Ambiguity of sex at birth is due to adrenogenital syndrome unless proved otherwise. The entity is confirmed by elevated serum 17 hydroxy-progesterone and urinary pregnanetriol with karyotype 46, XX. Prenatal diagnosis can be made by CVS or amniocentesis using DNA probe.
- Disorders of gonadal development include — gonadal dysgenesis, gonadal agenesis and mixed gonadal dysgenesis.
  - Turner's syndrome is the commonest variety of gonadal dysgenesis. The individual is short (< 60"), absence of secondary sex characters with webbing of the neck and having 'streak' gonads. Karyotype is 45, XO with low serum E2 and elevated serum FSH. There may be mosaic Turner with karyotype-46, XX/45 XO. In pure gonadal dysgenesis, the karyotype is either 46, XX or 46, XY. In mixed gonadal dysgenesis, the karyotype is usually 45, XO or 46, XY.
- About one-third of women with gonadal dysgenesis have major cardiovascular or renal abnormalities. Individuals with gonadal dysgenesis should have karyotyped done to determine the presence of Y chromosome.
- Male intersex (Testicular feminisation) is rarely diagnosed prior to puberty. The patient is phenotypically female with short blind vagina and gonads (testes) are in the labia or inguinal canal or intra-abdominal. Sex chromatin is negative. Karyotype is 46, XY. Confirmation is by gonadal biopsy (structures of testis). Gonadal oestrogen secretion induces normal pubertal feminisation and breast development.

  In Klinefelter's syndrome, the sex chromatin is positive and the karyotype is XXY or XXXY. Serum gonadotrophin is elevated.
- In true hermaphrodite, ovotestis is the commonest presentation. Sex chromatin is positive. Karyotype is usually 46, XX or 46, XY. Confirmation is by gonadal biopsy.
- A normal looking girl with primary amenorrhoea, who have normal breast development but absent uterus, may be either a case of Mayer-Rokitansky-Küster-Hauser syndrome or androgen insensitivity syndrome (p. 426, Table 27.1).
- Gonadal dysgenesis and uterovaginal anomalies are the common causes of primary amenorrhoea.
- **Management of intersex**
  - Congenital adrenogenital syndrome should be treated energetically by hydrocortisone or dexamethasone. Apart from reduction clitoroplasty, the corrective surgery should be deferred till puberty (p. 426).
  - Cases of gonadal dysgenesis should be treated by substitution therapy with oestrogen and progestogen. In presence of 'Y' chromosome, gonadectomy should be done to prevent malignancy.
  - In testicular feminisation, gonadectomy is to be done after the development of secondary sex characters (puberty) to be followed by oestrogen supplementation therapy (p. 427).
  - In true hermaphrodite, the genitalia inconsistent with sex assignment should be surgically removed or modified (p. 427).

28

Amenorrhoea

Definition

Amenorrhoea literally means absence of menstruation. It is a symptom and not a disease.

There are at least five basic factors involved in the onset and continuation of normal menstruation. These are :

- Normal female chromosomal pattern (46XX).
- Co-ordinated hypothalamo-pituitary ovarian axis.
- Anatomical presence and patency of the outflow tract.
- Responsive endometrium.
- Active support of thyroid and adrenal glands.

Clinical types

For descriptive purposes, the following types are conveniently described (vide scheme below). This will help the clinicians to sort out the clinicopathological entity.

PHYSIOLOGICAL

Before puberty

The pituitary gonadotrophins are not adequate enough to stimulate the ovarian follicles for effective steroidogenesis → oestrogen levels are not sufficient enough to cause bleeding from the endometrium.

During pregnancy

Large amount of oestrogens and chorionic gonadotrophins secreted from the trophoblasts suppress the pituitary gonadotrophins → no maturation of the ovarian follicles.

During lactation

High level of prolactin → inhibits ovarian response to FSH → no follicular growth → hypo-oestrogenic

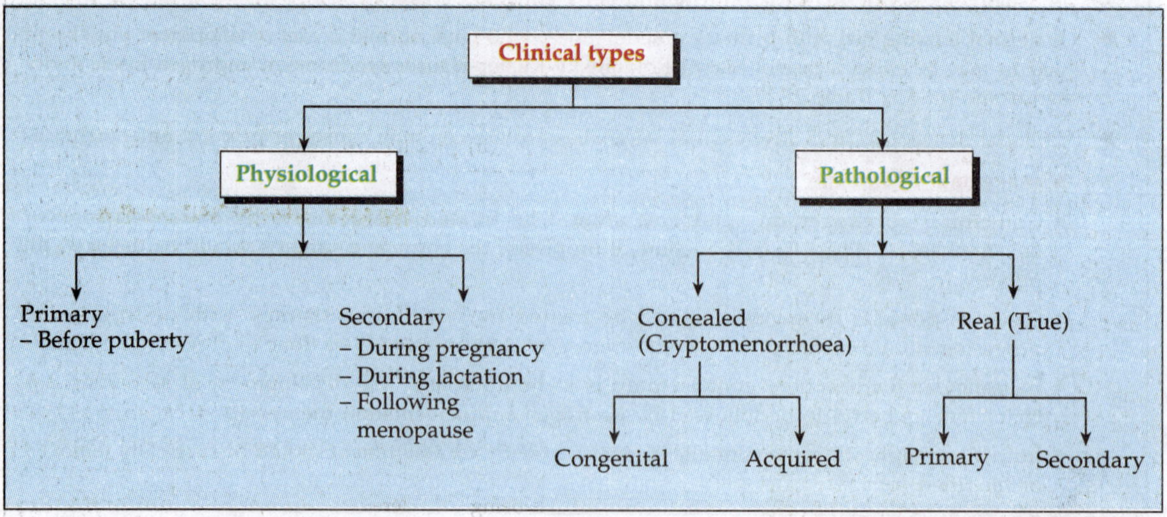

state → no menstruation. If the patient does not breastfeed her baby, the menstruation returns by 6th week following delivery in about 40 per cent and by 12th week in 80 per cent of cases. If the patient breastfeeds her baby, the menstruation may be suspended in about 70 per cent until the baby stops breastfeeding.

Following menopause

No more responsive follicles are available in the ovaries for the gonadotrophins to act. As a result, there is cessation of oestrogen production from the ovaries with elevation of pituitary gonadotrophins.

PATHOLOGICAL

CRYPTOMENORRHOEA

In cryptomenorrhoea, there is periodic shedding of the endometrium and bleeding but the menstrual blood fails to come out from the genital tract due to obstruction in the passage.

Causes

• Congenital • Acquired

Congenital

- Imperforate hymen
- Transverse vaginal septum
- Atresia of upper-third of vagina and cervix.

Morbid pathological changes, clinical features and treatment of the congenital aetiology have been described in the ch. 4.

Acquired

- Stenosis of the cervix following amputation, deep cauterisation and conisation.
- Secondary vaginal atresia following neglected and difficult vaginal delivery.

Pathology : There is only accumulation of blood in the uterine cavity resulting in haematometra. In neglected cases, the blood may enter the tubes whose fimbrial ends get blocked resulting in distension of the tubes by blood → haematosalpinx.

Clinical features : The patients with history of any of the aetiological factors mentioned earlier, complain of :

- Amenorrhoea dated back from the events.
- Periodic pain lower abdomen.

Pelvic examination reveals the offending lesion either in the vagina or cervix. The uterus is symmetrically enlarged.

Treatment

Simple dilatation of the cervix so as to drain the collected blood is enough. In cases of secondary atresia of the vagina, reconstructive surgery is to be performed, to maintain the patency.

SUMMARY OF CRYPTOMENORRHOEA

Cryptomenorrhoea is a condition where the menstrual blood fails to come out from the genital tract due to obstruction in the passage.

Causes

The commonest cause is congenital due to imperforate hymen. The acquired cause is rare due to cervical stenosis following amputation, conisation or deep cauterisation.

Pathophysiology

If the site of obstruction is low down in the vagina, the accumulated blood results in haematocolpos → haematometra → haematosalpinx. If the obstruction is at the cervix, it will produce haematometra → haematosalpinx. **Haematocolpos produces marked elongation of the urethra** → retention of urine.

Clinical features

The patient aged about 13-15 (congenital type) complains of periodic pain lower abdomen. Haematocolpos is usually associated with urinary problems to the extent of retention of urine. Abdominal examination reveals an uniform globular mass in the hypogastrium. Vulval inspection reveals the bulging hymen. Rectal examination confirms the fullness of the vagina and uterine mass.

Management

(i) Cruciate incision of the hymen and drainage of blood (see Fig. 4.4).

(ii) Dilatation of the cervix in stenosis.

PRIMARY AMENORRHOEA

Definition : A young girl who has not yet menstruated by her 16 years of age is having primary amenorrhoea rather than delayed menarche. The normal upper age limit for menarche is 15 years.

In view of lower mean age of menarche, currently a cut off value at 13 years (in the absence of secondary sexual characters) and 15 years (with secondary sexual characters) is being considered.

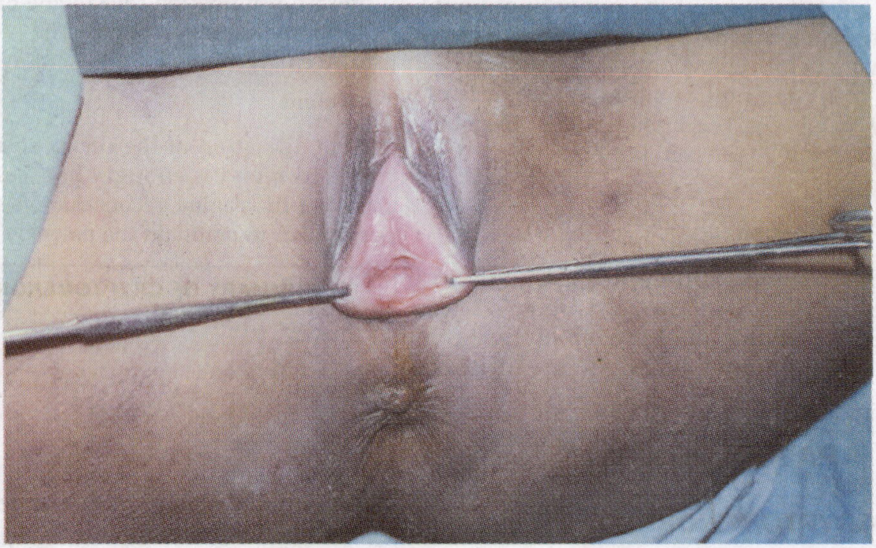

Fig. 28.1. Complete absence of vagina [*By courtesy* : Prof. K.M. Gun]

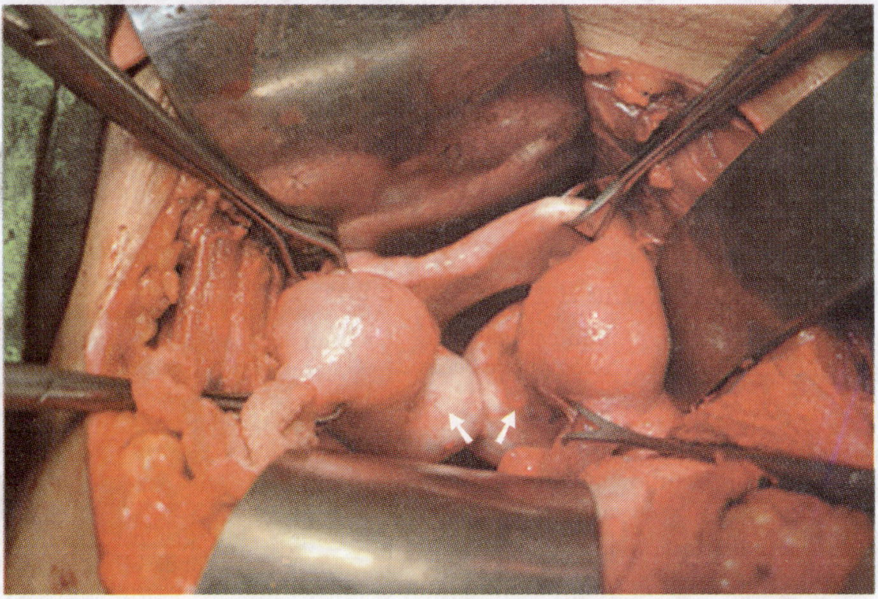

Fig. 28.2. Müllerian agenesis with small uterine knobs one on either side. Normal ovaries are seen (arrow). Cervix and vagina were absent in this case [*By courtesy* : Dr. P.K. Biswas, Associate Professor, Department of Obstetrics & Gynaecology, N.R.S. Medical College, Kolkata]

Causes : The **causes of primary amenorrhoea are** grouped as follows :

A. Hypogonadotrophic hypogonadism

(i) *Delayed puberty* — delayed GnRH pulse reactivation.

(ii) *Hypothalamic and pituitary dysfunction* — Gonadotrophin deficiency due to stress, weight loss, excessive exercise, anorexia nervosa, chronic disease (tuberculosis).

(iii) *Kallmann's syndrome* — inadequate GnRH pulse secretion — reduced FSH and LH (see p. 445).

(iv) *Central nervous system tumours* — craniopharyngioma → reduced GnRH secretion → reduced FSH and LH.

B. Hypergonadotrophic hypogonadism

(i) *Primary ovarian failure* (see p. 444).

(ii) *Resistant ovarian syndrome* (see p. 444).

(iii) *Galactosemia* : Due to premature ovarian failure (see p. 444).

(iv) *Enzyme deficiency (17 α hydroxylase deficiency)* — characterised by ↓ cortisol and ↑ ACTH, ↑ mineralocorticoids production. There is hypertension with hypernatraemia and hypokalaemia. The individual may be 46 XX or 46 XY with primary amenorrhoea and no secondary sexual characters.

(v) *Others* — Gonadotrophin receptor mutations – rarely FSH and/or LH levels are high as the respective receptor may be absent or mutated.

C. Abnormal chromosomal pattern

- Turner's syndrome (45 X) (Figs. 27.2A and B).
- Various mosaic states 45 X/46 XX.
- Pure gonadal dysgenesis (46 XX or 46 XY) — Phenotypically female with streak gonads. Stature is average with some secondary sexual characters.
- Androgen insensitivity syndrome (Testicular feminisation syndrome), 46 XY (see Fig. 27.3).
- Partial deletions of the X chromosome (46 XX).

When part of one X chromosome is missing — deletion of long arm of X chromosome (Xq^-) leads to streak gonads and amenorrhoea but no somatic abnormalities. Deletion of short arm of X chromosome (Xp^-) usually leads to somatic features similar to Turner's syndrome.

D. Developmental defect of genital tract

- Imperforate hymen (Fig. 4.2).
- Transverse vaginal septum.
- Atresia upper-third of vagina and cervix (Fig. 4.4).
- Complete absence of vagina (Fig. 28.1).
- Absence of uterus MRKH syndrome (Fig. 28.2 and Table 27.1).

E. Dysfunction of thyroid and adrenal cortex

- Adrenogenital syndrome (Figs. 27.1 and 32.1).
- Cretinism.

F. Metabolic disorders

- Juvenile diabetes.

G. Systemic illness

- Malnutrition, anaemia
- Weight loss • Tuberculosis.

H. Unresponsive endometrium

- Congenital
  - Uterine synechiae (tubercular).

INVESTIGATIONS

The basic disorders responsible for primary amenorrhoea almost always have some specific clinical manifestations. The diagnosis and management of cryptomenorrhoea of congenital variety has already been described in chapter 4. **Only the true primary amenorrhoea is dealt with here.**

When to start investigation?

The following guidelines may be of help :

(i) No period by 16 years of age in the presence of normal secondary sex characters.

(ii) No period by the age of 14 in the absence of growth or development of secondary sex characters.

However, the formula may not be applicable in all cases. A patient may come with typical features suggestive of Turner and there is no point to defer the investigation or a patient of 14 with absence of vagina should not be told to come after 2 years for investigation. Even in primary amenorrhoea, the possibility of pregnancy should be kept in mind, as pregnancy can occur even prior to menarche. **The investigation protocols can be grouped as :**

History, Clinical examination, Special investigations

• History

Certain types of primary amenorrhoea are of heredofamilial in nature. Delayed menarche or androgen insensitivity syndrome often runs in family, the later one is often found in multiple sibs of the same family and their maternal aunts.

Medical diseases : Genital tuberculosis or diabetes though rare, may be responsible for primary amenorrhoea. Such type of amenorrhoea is usually associated with hypogonadism.

Other features : Abnormal loss or gain in weight within short span of time is suggestive of some metabolic disorders.

• Clinical examinations

With few exceptions, the physical signs are so apparent that the clinical diagnosis of aetiological factors of primary amenorrhoea does not seem to be difficult. The diagnosis of some common causes based on clinical examinations are tabulated in Table 28.1.

Table 28.1
Diagnosis of primary amenorrhoea based on clinical examinations

Physical appearance	Ext. genitalia	Internal genitalia	Probable diagnosis
• Sec. sex characters • Stature			
– Normal breast development – Normal sexual hair – Average stature	– Normal	– Absence of vagina – Absent uterus	• Müllerian agenesis (Mayer-Rokitansky–Küster-Hauser syndrome)
—do—	—do—	– Normal	• Unresponsive endometrium — receptor defect (Rare) • Uterine synechiae (Rare)
– Poor breast development – Scanty pubic hair – Average stature	– Underdeveloped	– Underdeveloped (vaginal rugosity absent)	• Hypogonadotrophic – hypogonadism
– Tall and lanky	—do—	—do—	• Primary ovarian failure
– Poor sec. sex characters – Stature — short – Webbing of the neck and cubitus valgus present – Congenital malformations of cardiac, renal or great vessels (coarctation of aorta)	—do—	—do— 'Streak' gonads	• Turner's syndrome
– Phenotypically female Average height Delayed sec. sex. characters	Normal	Bilateral 'streak' gonads	• Pure gonadal dysgenesis
– Normal breast development without areolar pigmentation – Scanty pubic and axillary hair – Average stature	– Labial or inguinal gonads (Figs. 27.6 and 27.7)	– Short blind vagina – Absence of uterus	• Androgen insensitivity syndrome
– Normal phenotypically female – Average stature	– Labial fusion – Enlargement of clitoris	– Normal	• Adrenogenital syndrome (Late onset)
– Features of hypogonadism • Short stature • Mental retardation • Obesity	– Underdeveloped	– Underdeveloped	• Cretinism due to hypothyroidism • Hypothalamo-pituitary dysfunction (rare) (Hypogonadotropic hypogonadism) – Kallmann syndrome – Prader – Labhardt– Willi syndrome – Laurence – Moon – Bardet – Biedl syndrome (rare)

Table 28.2

Special investigations in a case of primary amenorrhoea to corroborate clinical diagnosis

Probable diagnosis	Investigations	Findings
Müllerian agenesis (Mayer-Rokitansky–Küster–Hauser syndrome)	– Ultrasonography – Laparoscopy – Karyotype – IVP	Uterus — absent Tubes — present Ovaries — normal 46, XX Urinary tract abnormalities (30%)
Unresponsive endometrium	* – Progesterone challenge test – H S G / Hysteroscopy – Hormonal studies	Negative Normal uterine cavity Normal
Uterine synechiae	– Progesterone challenge test – H S G – Hysteroscopy	Negative Honeycomb appearance Direct visualisation
Tubercular (see p. 137)	– Blood — ESR – X-ray — Chest – Mantoux test – Endometrial biopsy	Raised May have positive finding Positive (usually) Positive lesion may be detected.
Hypogonadotrophic – hypogonadism	– Progesterone challenge test – Serum gonadotrophins	Positve Low < 5 mlU/ml
Primary ovarian failure (see p. 444)	– Karyotype – Serum oestradiol – Serum gonadotrophins – Ovarian biopsy (ovaries — small/streak) ovarian biopsy is not essential for diagnosis.	46, XX Low (< 20 pg/ml) Elevated > 40 mlU/ml (i) Afollicular (common), (ii) follicular or (iii) autoimmune (lymphocytic infiltration) type. Follicles are present in resistant ovarian syndrome.
Turner (p. 422)	– Laparoscopy – Serum gonadotrophins – Karyotype	'Streak' gonads high 45, X O or 45, XO/46, XX
Androgen insensitivity syndrome (p. 424)	– Laparoscopy – Serum testosterone – Karyotype – Gonadal biopsy	Uterus — absent Tubes — absent Equal to normal males 46, XY Testicular structure
Adrenogenital syndrome (p. 421)	– Karyotype – Serum 17 hydroxy-progesterone – Urinary pregnanetriol	46, XX Elevated (> 8 ng/ml). Elevated
Thyroid dysfunction (Hypo)	– Serum TSH – T_3, T_4	Elevated Lowered
Diabetes	– Blood sugar	Elevated

* The test is performed by administrating Inj. Progesterone in oil 75 mg IM or Tab. medroxyprogesterone 10 mg daily for 10 days. Withdrawal bleeding usually occurs within 10 days, if the test is positive.

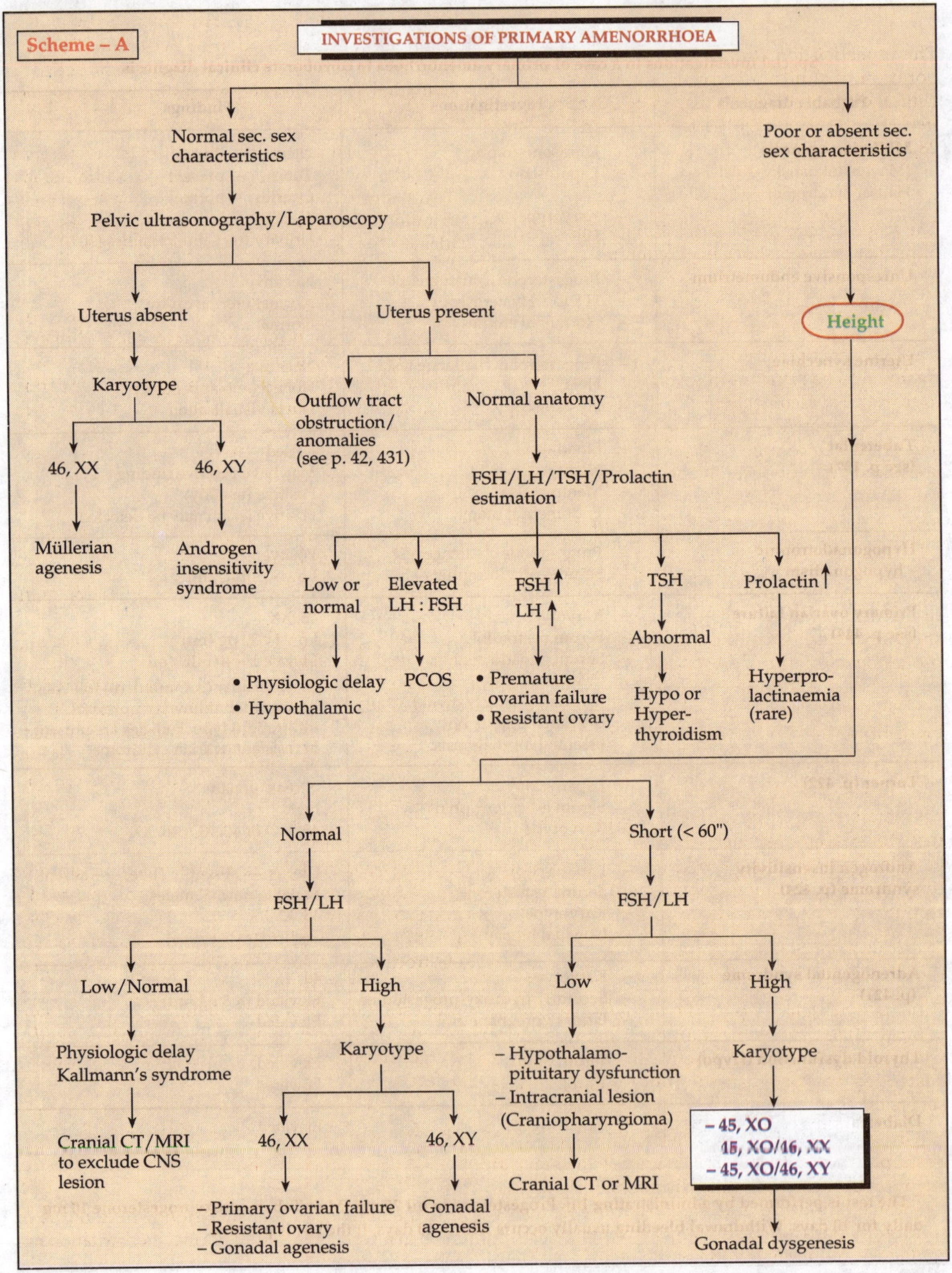
Scheme – A
INVESTIGATIONS OF PRIMARY AMENORRHOEA
Normal sec. sex characteristics
Poor or absent sec. sex characteristics
Pelvic ultrasonography/Laparoscopy
Uterus absent
Uterus present
Height
Karyotype
Outflow tract obstruction/anomalies (see p. 42, 431)
Normal anatomy
46, XX
46, XY
FSH/LH/TSH/Prolactin estimation
Müllerian agenesis
Androgen insensitivity syndrome
Low or normal
Elevated LH : FSH
FSH ↑ LH ↑
TSH
Prolactin ↑
Abnormal
• Physiologic delay
• Hypothalamic
PCOS
• Premature ovarian failure
• Resistant ovary
Hypo or Hyper-thyroidism
Hyperpro-lactinaemia (rare)
Normal
Short (< 60")
FSH/LH
FSH/LH
Low/Normal
High
Low
High
Physiologic delay Kallmann's syndrome
Karyotype
– Hypothalamo-pituitary dysfunction
– Intracranial lesion (Craniopharyngioma)
Karyotype
Cranial CT/MRI to exclude CNS lesion
46, XX
46, XY
– 45, XO
45, XO/46, XX
– 45, XO/46, XY
Cranial CT or MRI
– Primary ovarian failure
– Resistant ovary
– Gonadal agenesis
Gonadal agenesis
Gonadal dysgenesis

- **Special investigations**

The investigation should be restricted for corroboration of clinical diagnosis and in cases where clinical diagnosis remains disputed. The appropriate investigation protocol is tabulated in the Table 28.2.

MANAGEMENT

The scope of therapeutic success in the management of primary amenorrhoea is very limited.

Development anomalies

Complete agenesis of vagina

Vaginal reconstruction is the accepted form of treatment. The principle of vaginal reconstruction is to create an avascular space between the bladder and rectum. The patency is to be maintained by a mould and graft. **The commonly used materials for graft** are skin or amniotic membranes. The result is quite satisfactory so far as the coital act is concerned. **The ideal time of operation** is prior to or soon after marriage.

Chromosomal abnormalities

In Turner or other types of gonadal dysgenesis, short-term use of combination of oestrogen and progestogen is indicated at least for development of breasts (see p. 427). **The gonads of XY gonadal dysgenesis should be removed** for its increased development of seminoma or dysgerminoma (see p. 427).

In androgen insensitivity syndrome, the ectopic gonads are to be removed after the secondary sex characters are well-developed, because they may turn to malignancy. Substitution therapy after gonadectomy is indicated to maintain the secondary sex characters. Hormone replacement therapy with conjugated equine oestrogen (premarin 0.625 mg daily) is adequate (see p. 427).

Hypothalamopituitary ovarian axis defect

Patients with delayed puberty, following exclusion of other causes, should be counselled and reassured. Otherwise puberty may be induced using oral oestrogen and progestin therapy when there is severe delay.

Gross defects in the form of adiposogenital dystrophy or pituitary dwarfism are not amenable to any form of therapy. In mild disorders, it is possible to induce ovulation and menstruation either by treatment with gonadotrophins or with GnRH analogues. Individuals with isolated gonadotrophin deficiency (Kallmann's syndrome) can be treated for induction of menstruation or ovulation. Pulsatile administration of GnRH is used for induction of ovulation. Oestrogen and progestin therapy is given for menstruation.

Hypothalamic-pituitary tumours (craniopharyngioma) may need surgical excision or radiotherapy. Team approach involving a gynaecologist, an endocrinologist, a neurosurgeon and a radiotherapist is ideal.

Thyroid and adrenal dysfunction

Gross thyroid hypoplasia (cretinism) does not respond to thyroid replacement therapy. However, mild hypothyroidism may have good result with replacement therapy. Adrenogenital syndrome with enlarged clitoris should be treated by surgical removal of clitoris (clitoroplasty) as early as possible to avoid psychological problems. Corticosteroid therapy should be continued for a prolonged period.

Corticosteroid replacement therapy is given for 17 α hydroxylase deficiency state.

Prolactinomas need to be treated with dopamine agonists (see p. 450).

Metabolic and nutritional

Diabetes and tuberculosis are to be treated by antidiabetic and antitubercular drug respectively. Correction of anaemia and improvement of nutrition status may resume menstruation. Correction of malabsorption, weight loss stress and chronic diseases are to be done when indicated.

Unresponsive endometrium

Uterine synechiae of tubercular origin should be treated by antitubercular drugs supplemented by adhesiolysis and IUCD insertion. Hysteroscopic (see p. 587) release of adhesions using scissors or electrocautery can be done. To prevent recurrence of adhesion formation, high dose oestrogen and progestin therapy is given monthly for withdrawal bleed. There is no known treatment as yet for congenital unresponsive endometrium (receptor defect).

SECONDARY AMENORRHOEA

Definition

It is the absence of menstruation for 6 months or more in a woman in whom normal menstruation has been established.

The physiological and cryptomenorrhoea has been described earlier in the chapter. Only the true secondary amenorrhoea will be discussed here.

Aetiology : The causes of true secondary amenorrhoea with the possible mechanism are outlined in Table 28.3.

Clinical features and diagnosis

Uterine factors

Tubercular endometritis : The family history or past history of tuberculosis in the patient herself may or may not be present. Physical and pelvic examination may not be informative. The diagnosis is often accidentally made following diagnostic curettage or at laparotomy or laparoscopy.

Uterine synechiae (Syn: Asherman's syndrome)

There is formation of adhesions following postabortal and puerperal curettage and also following diagnostic curettage in dysfunctional uterine bleeding. Rarely, it follows tubercular endometritis. Menstrual abnormalities include hypomenorrhoea, oligomenorrhoea or amenorrhoea. Progesterone challenge test is negative. Hysterosalpingography shows honeycomb appearance (Fig. 36.72). Hysteroscopy reveals the extent of adhesions directly.

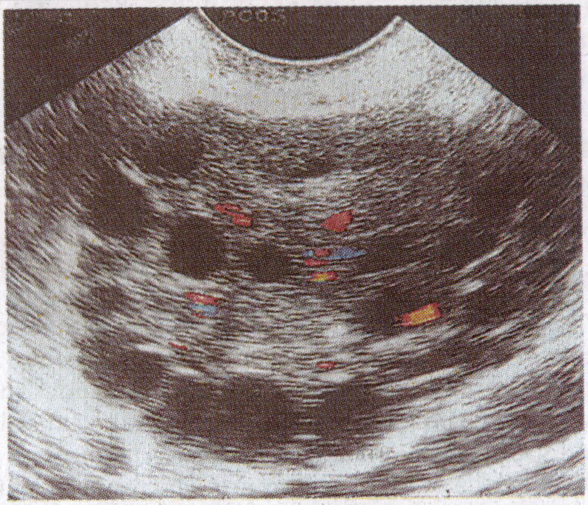

Fig. 28.3. Colour Doppler (TV) Scan showing numerous small cysts with increased ovarian stroma and vascularity — typical of PCOS

Table 28.3 : Aetiopathogenesis of secondary amenorrhoea

Aetiology		Mechanism
Uterine factors		
• Tubercular endometritis	—	Destruction of the endometrium or inhibition of ovarian function by tubercular toxin.
• Postradiation	—	Destruction of the endometrium
• Synechiae	—	Intrauterine adhesions → viscerocortical reflex → amenorrhoea
• Surgical removal	—	Ablation of endometrium by laser, resectoscope (see p. 589)
Ovarian factors		
• Polycystic ovarian syndrome (PCOS)	—	Tonically elevated LH → Increased androgen production from the theca cells and stroma of the ovaries → Decrease SHBG → increased unbound oestrogens and androgens → Pituitary sensitivity to GnRH is increased → Preferential increased production of LH, decreased production of FSH due to inhibin. Disturbed adrenal function is also implicated in androgen excess. A state of hyperandrogenism produces amenorrhoea by its antioestrogenic action.
• Premature ovarian failure	—	Absence of follicle or accelerated rate of depletion of follicles in the ovaries.
• Resistant ovarian syndrome (Savage's syndrome)	—	Follicles are present but are resistant to gonadotrophins (defect in FSH receptor).
• Hyperoestrogenic state	—	The oestrogen level remains high and there is no fluctuation.
– Persistent follicles in metropathia – Feminising tumour of the ovary (Granulosa cell tumour)		As such, so long as endometrial support is not lost, amenorrhoea continues.

Table 28.3 contd. next page

Cause	Mechanism
• Masculinising tumour of the ovary (Sertoli-Leydig cell tumour)	— Androgen excess opposes the effect of oestrogen on the endometrium. (p. 371)
• Hypo-oestrogenic state	
– Ablation of the ovaries	— Removal of the site of production of oestrogens.
– Pelvic radiation	— Makes the ovaries unresponsive to gonadotrophins.
Pituitary factors	
• Adenoma (Prolactinoma) • Cushing's disease • Acromegaly	— Microadenoma usually associated with hyperprolactinaemia. It either inhibits ovarian steroidogenesis directly or inhibits pituitary gonadotrophin release (see p. 445).
• Sheehan's syndrome • Simmond's disease (unrelated to pregnancy)	— There is partial or complete destruction of the pituitary by ischaemia caused by venous thrombosis following severe postpartum haemorrhage and shock. The principal hormones affected are growth hormone, gonadotrophins, TSH, adrenocorticotrophins and prolactin.
Hypothalamic factors	
• Psychogenic shock, stress, anorexia nervosa, strenuous exercise, pseudocyesis, etc.	— Inhibit the release of GnRH or affect dopamine metabolism. There is low level of oestrogen and LH but FSH level remains normal (see below).
• Congenital malformation. • Trauma : Accidents, surgery or radiotherapy. • Infection : Tubercular or sarcoid granulomas. • Tumours : Craniopharyngioma, meningioma.	Lead to hypogonadotrophic hypogonadism. There may be hyperprolactinaemia due to altered dopamine inhibition. Tumours of the hypothalamus or pituitary need surgical excision or radiotherapy. Management needs a team approach including a neurosurgeon, a radiotherapist and an endocrinologist.
Adrenal factors	
• Adrenal tumour or hyperplasia	— Androgen excess opposes the effect of oestrogen on the endometrium.
• Cushing syndrome	— —do— —do—
Thyroid factors	
• Hypothyroid state	— Raised TSH and hyperprolactinaemia by direct action of TRH on the galactophore cells in the pituitary.
General disease	
Malnutrition, tuberculosis, chronic nephritis, diabetes, etc.	— Probably affecting the hypothalamopituitaryovarian axis.
Iatrogenic	
• Contraceptive pills (post pill amenorrhoea)	— Suppression of GnRH release.
• Psychotrophic phenothiazine derivative drugs	— Dopamine receptor blocking agents raise the prolactin level.
• Antihypertensive drugs like reserpine or dopamine antagonists.	— Dopamine depleting agents raise the prolactin level.

Table 28.4 : Common causes of secondary amenorrhoea

Hypothalamus	Pituitary	Ovary	Uterine	Systemic
• **Stress** • Post pill • Sudden change in weight — either too much loss or too much gain • Psychotrophic and anti-hypertensive drugs	• Adenoma • Sheehan's	• **PCOS** • **Premature ovarian failure**	• Synechiae	• Malnutrition • **Hypothyroid state** • Diabetes

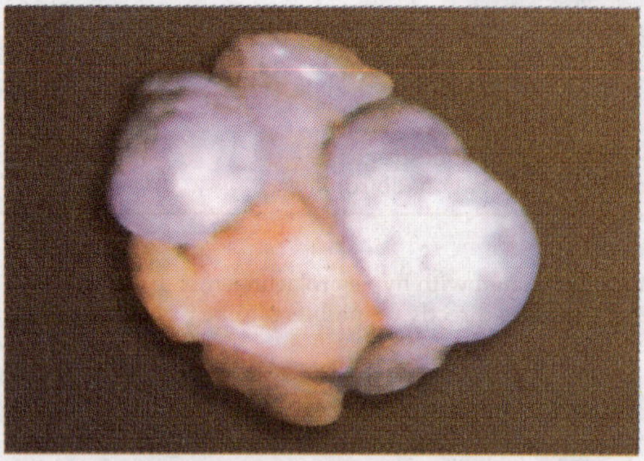

Fig. 28.4. Bilateral polycystic ovarian enlargement in PCOS [*By courtesy* : Dr. N. Chowdhury]

Ovarian factors

POLYCYSTIC OVARIAN SYNDROME (PCOS)

Polycystic ovarian syndrome (PCOS) was originally described in 1935 by Stein and Leventhal as a syndrome manifested by amenorrhoea, hirsutism and obesity associated with enlarged polycystic ovaries.

This heterogenous disorder is characterised by excessive androgen production by the ovaries mainly, which interferes with the reproductive, endocrine and metabolic functions. **PCOS is a multifactorial and polygenic condition**. *Diagnosis is based upon the presence of any two of the following three criteria* (ASRM/ESHRE, 2003).

- Oligo and/or anovulation.
- Hyperandrogenism (clinical and/or biochemical).
- Polycystic ovaries.

Other aetiologies (adrenal) are to be excluded. The incidence varies between 0.5-4 per cent, more common amongst infertile women. It is prevalent in young reproductive age group (20-30%).

Pathology : Typically, the ovaries are enlarged. Ovarian volume is increased $\geq$ 10 cm^3. Stroma is increased. The capsule is thickened and pearly white in colour. Presence of multiple ($\geq$ 12) follicular cysts measuring about 2-9 mm in diameter are crowded around the cortex (Fig. 28.4).

Histologically, there is thickening of tunica albuginea. The cysts are follicles at varying stages of maturation and atresia. There is theca cell hypertrophy (stromal hyperthecosis). Patient may present with features of diabetes mellitus (insulin resistance).

Clinical features

The patient complains of increasing obesity (abdominal), menstrual abnormalities in the form of oligomenorrhoea, amenorrhoea or DUB and infertility. There may be hirsutism and acne (Fig. 28.5). Virilism is rare. The patient may not always be obese.

Acanthosis nigricans is characterised by specific skin changes due to insulin resistance. The skin is thickened and pigmented. Commonly affected sites are nape of the neck, inner thighs, and axilla (see Fig. 28.6).

HAIR-AN syndrome in patients with PCOS is characterised by hyperandrogenism, insulin resistance and acanthosis nigricans.

Internal examination reveals bilateral enlarged cystic ovaries which may not be revealed due to obesity.

Investigations

- Sonography — Transvaginal sonography is specially useful in obese patient. Ovaries are enlarged in volume ($\geq$ 10 cm^3). Increased number (> 12) of peripherally arranged cysts (2-9 mm) are seen (Fig. 28.3).
- Serum values :
  - LH level is elevated and/or the ratio LH : FSH is > 3 : 1.
  - Raised level of oestradiol and oestrone — The oestrone level is markedly elevated.

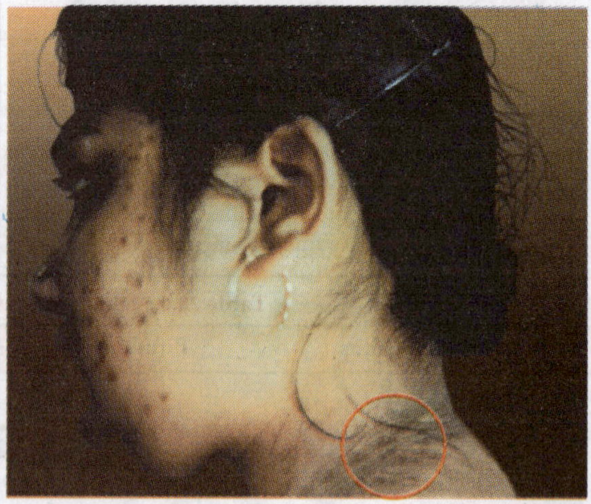

Fig. 28.5. Hirsutism, acne, acanthosis nigricans in PCOS [*By courtesy* : Prof. B. N. Chakravorty, IRM, Kolkata]

   - SHBG level is reduced.
   - Androstenedione is elevated.
   - Raised serum testosterone (> 150 ng/dl) and DHEA–S may be marginally elevated.
   - **Insulin Resistance (IR)** : Raised fasting insulin levels > 25 μ IU/ml and levels of serum insulin response > 300 μ IU/ml at 2 hours postglucose (75 gm) load, suggests IR (p. 547).

- Laparoscopy — Bilateral polycystic ovaries are characteristic of PCOS (Fig. 28.4).

Pathophysiology

Exact pathophysiology of PCOS is not clearly understood. It may be discussed under the following heads (Scheme 6) :

(a) Hypothalamic — pituitary compartment abnormality.

(b) Androgen excess (p. 544).

(c) Anovulation.

(d) Obesity and insulin resistance.

(e) Long-term consequences.

Hypothalamic-Pituitary Compartment in PCOS

- Increased pulse frequency of GnRH leads to increased pulse frequency of LH. **Leptin**, a peptide, secreted by fat cells and by the ovarian follicle, in presence of hyperinsulinaemia may be responsible for this.
- GnRH is preferential to LH rather than FSH.
- Increased pulse frequency and amplitude of LH results in tonically elevated level of LH.
- FSH level is not increased. This is mainly due to the negative feedback effect of chronically elevated oestrogen and the follicular inhibin.

Scheme –1

Hypothalamus → Increased pulse frequency of GnRH → Pituitary sensitivity to GnRH↑ → Increased pulse frequency of LH (preferential) compared to FSH → LH(↑) : FSH (↓)

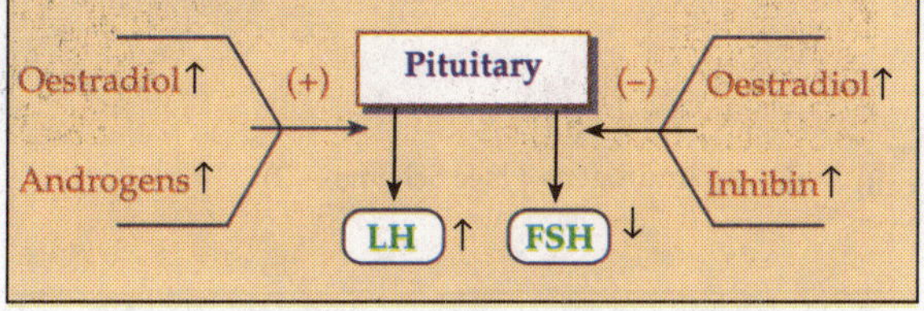

Scheme — 2

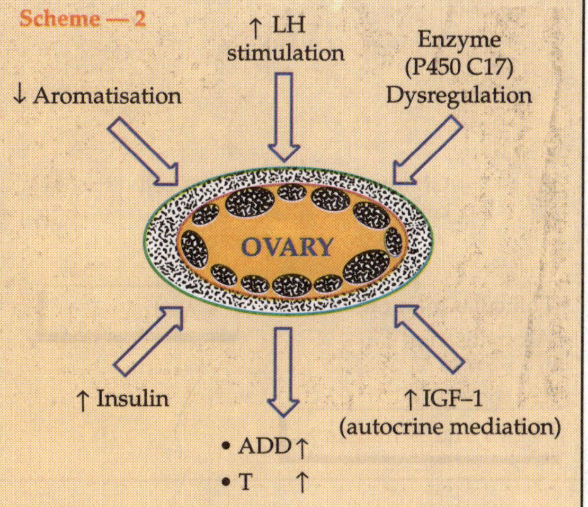

ADD = Androstenedione, T = Testosterone
IGF = Insulin growth factor

Scheme — 3

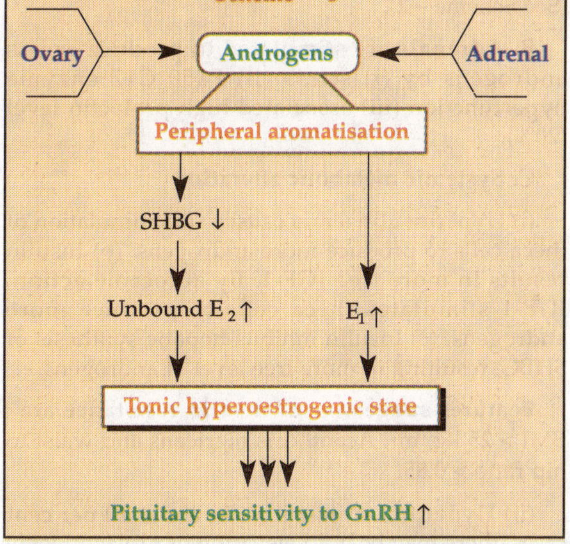

- Increased free oestradiol due to reduced sex hormone binding globulin (SHBG) bears positive feedback relationship to LH.
- The LH : FSH ratio is increased.

Androgen excess

Abnormal regulation of the androgen forming enzyme (P450 C 17) is thought to be the main cause for **excess production of androgens from the ovaries** and adrenals. The principal sources of androgens are (A) Ovary (B) Adrenal (C) Systemic metabolic alteration.

A. **Ovary** produces excess androgens due to — (i) stimulation of theca cells by high LH (ii) P450

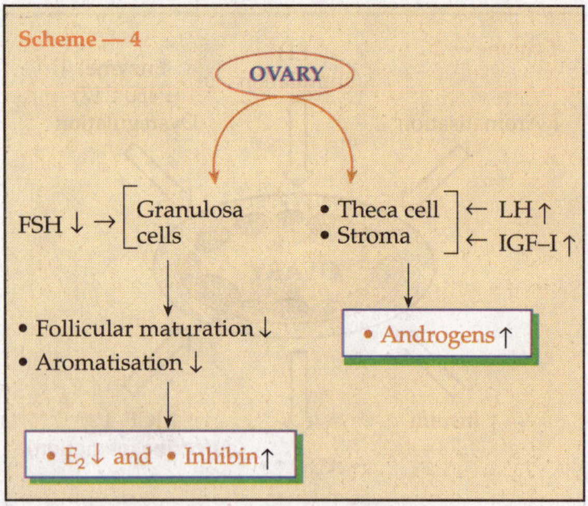

C17 enzyme hyperfunction (iii) defective aromatisation of androgens to oestrogen (iv) stimulation of theca cells by IGF-1 (insulin growth factor-1) (See Scheme – 2).

B. **Adrenals** are stimulated to produce excess androgens by (i) stress (ii) P450 C17 enzyme hyperfunction (iii) associated high prolactin level (20%).

C. **Systemic metabolic alteration**

(i) **Hyperinsulinaemia causes** : (a) Stimulation of theca cells to produce more androgens. (b) Insulin results in more free IGF-1. By autocrine action, IGF-1 stimulates theca cells to produce more androgens. (c) Insulin inhibits hepatic synthesis of SHBG, resulting in more free level of androgens.

Features suggestive of insulin resistance are : BMI > 25 kg/m^2, Acanthosis nigricans and waist to hip ratio > 0.85.

(ii) **Hyperprolactinaemia** : In about 20 per cent cases, there may be mild elevation of prolactin level due to increased pulsitivity of GnRH or due to dopamine deficiency or to both. The prolactin further stimulates adrenal androgen production.

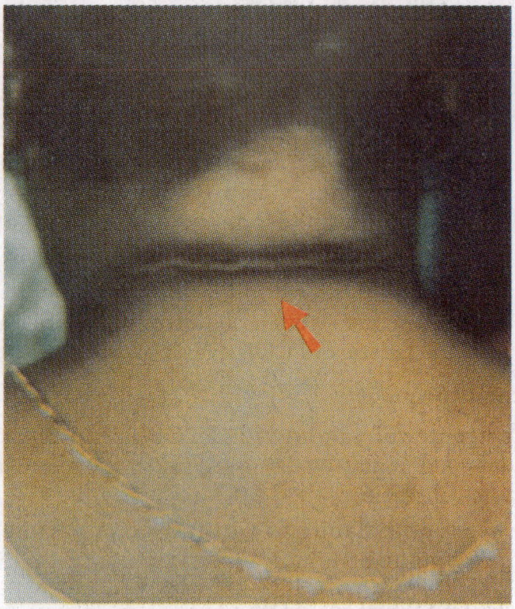

Fig. 28.6. Acanthosis nigricans in PCOS
[*By courtesy* : Prof. B. N. Chakravorty, IRM, Kolkata]

Whatever may be the aetiology, the endocrinologic effects of PCOS produce a vicious cycle of events as shown in the Scheme – 6.

Anovulation : Because of low FSH level, follicular growth is arrested at different phases of maturation (2-10 mm diameter). The net effect is diminished oestradiol and increased inhibin production. **Due to elevated LH**, there is hypertrophy of theca cells and more androgens are produced either from theca cells or stroma.

There is defective FSH induced aromatisation of androgens to oestrogens.

Follicular microenvironment is therefore more androgenic rather than oestrogenic.

Unless there is oestrogenic follicular microenvironment, follicular growth, maturation and ovulation cannot occur. There is huge number of

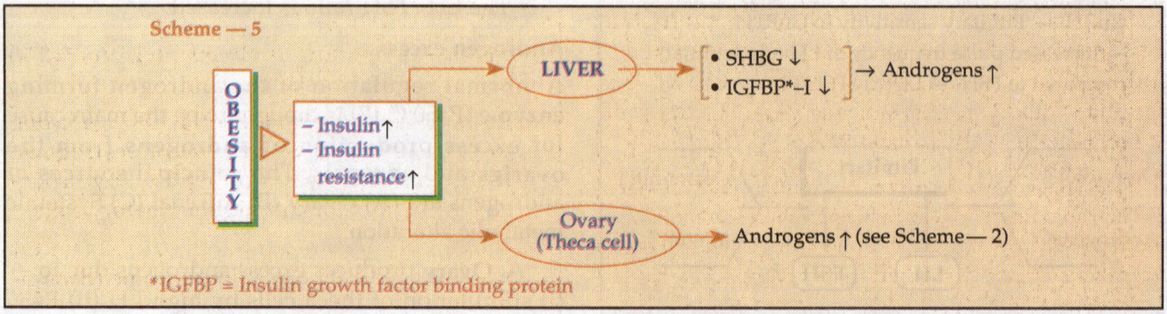

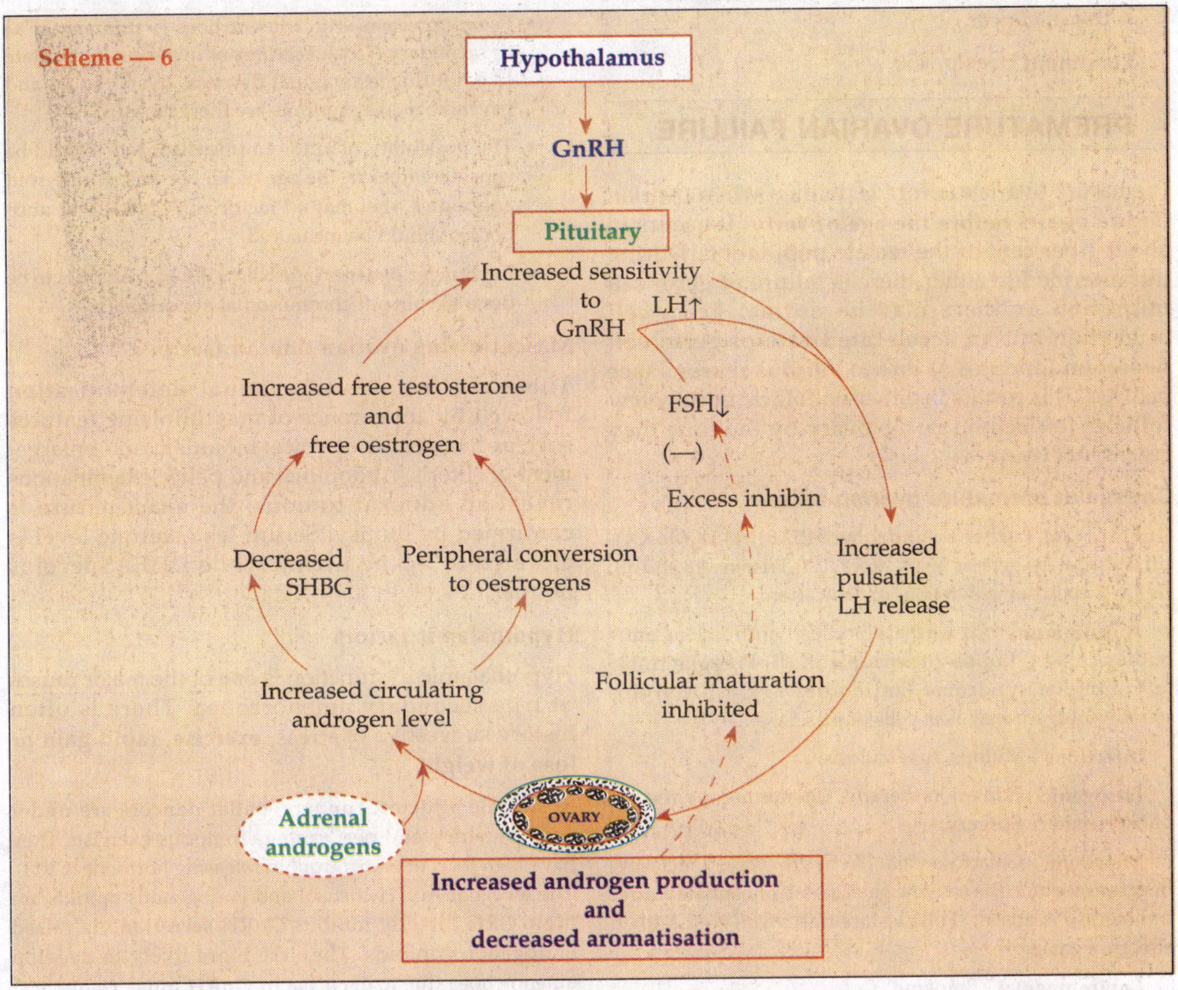

atretic follicles that contribute to increased ovarian stroma (hyperthecosis). LH level is tonically elevated without any surge. LH surge is essential for ovulation to occur.

Obesity and Insulin resistance

Obesity (central) is recognised as an important contributory factor. Apart from excess production of androgens, obesity is also associated with reduced SHBG. It also induces insulin resistance and hyperinsulinaemia which in turn increases the gonadal androgen production. PCOS is thought to have a dominant mode of inheritance as about 50 per cent of first degree relatives have PCOS.

Aetiology of insulin resistance is unknown. Mutations of the insulin receptor gene in the peripheral target tissues and reduced tyrosine autophosphorylation of the insulin receptor, is currently thought to be an important cause. Increased central body fat leads to android obesity.

Long-term consequences in a patient suffering from PCOS includes:

The **excess androgens** (mainly androstenedione) either from the ovaries or adrenals are peripherally aromatised to oestrone (E_1). There is concomitant **diminished SHBG. Cumulative excess unbound E_2 and oestrone results in a tonic hyperoestrogenic state**. There is endometrial hyperplasia.

Possible late sequelae are:

- Risk of developing **diabetes mellitus (15%)** due to insulin resistance.
- Risk of developing **endometrial carcinoma** due to persistently elevated level of oestrogens. Oestrogen effects are not opposed by progesterone because of chronic anovulatory state.
- Risk of **hypertension and cardiovascular disease** due to abnormal lipid profile (dyslipidaemia).

- Breast cancer.

Treatment : See p. 450.

PREMATURE OVARIAN FAILURE

Premature ovarian failure is defined when ovarian failure occurs **before the age of forty**. It occurs in about 1 per cent of the female population. During intrauterine life either there is failure of germ cell migration or there may be normal germ cell migration but an accelerated rate of germ cell depletion (apoptosis) due to various reasons (see below). This results in either no follicle or only few follicles left behind in the ovary by the time they reach puberty.

Causes of premature ovarian failure

Genetic : (i) Turner's syndrome (45X0), (45X/46XX), (ii) Gonadal dysgenesis 46XX, 46XY, (iii) Trisomy 18 and 13, (iv) X-chromosome deletion, translocation.

Autoimmune : (i) Autoantibodies : antinuclear antibodies (ANA), Lupus anticoagulant, (ii) Polyglandular autoimmune syndrome (antibodies against thyroid, parathyroid, adrenal, islet cells of pancreas).

Infections : Mumps, tuberculosis.

Iatrogenic : Radiation therapy, Chemotherapy (cyclophosphamide), Surgery.

Metabolic : Galactosaemia, 17α hydroxylase deficiency. In galactosaemia, the enzyme galactose-1-phosphate uridyl transferase is absent. Follicles are destroyed to the toxic effects of galactose.

Environmental : Smoking.

FSH receptor absent or postreceptor defect (Savage's syndrome).

Idiopathic :

Diagnosis/Investigations

- History of amenorrhoea in less than 35 years of age.
- Serum gonadotrophin level (FSH > 40 m IU/ml) is high.
- Serum E_2 level is low (< 20 pg/ml).
- Karyotype abnormality (see above).
- Organ specific humoral antibody (antithyroid commonest).
- Ovarian biopsy (afollicular, follicular and autoimmune variety) is not essential to the diagnosis. In autoimmune variety, there is perifollicular lymphocyte infiltration. In **resistant ovarian syndrome**, follicles are present. FSH receptor is either absent or defective.
- Patient presents with amenorrhoea — primary (25%) or secondary (75%). Features of hypoestrogenic state like hot flushes, vaginal dryness, dyspareunia and psychological symptoms are there (see p. 57).
- The possibility of autoimmune disorders should be considered below the age of 35. For this, antithyroid antibodies, rheumatoid factor and antinuclear antibodies should be measured.
- In younger patients (age below 30) karyotype is to be done to rule out chromosomal abnormality.

Masculinising ovarian tumour (see p. 371)

There are features of gradual defeminisation followed by appearance of masculinising features such as hoarseness of voice, hirsutism and enlargement of clitoris. Abdominal and pelvic examinations reveal an adnexal tumour; the exact nature is confirmed by biopsy. Serum testosterone level is elevated to > 2 ng per ml while DHEAS level is normal.

Hypothalamic factors

Hypothalamic dysfunction is one of the major causes of true secondary amenorrhoea. There is often history suggestive of **stress, exercise, rapid gain or loss of weight**.

Female athletes, runners, ballet dancers are under constant stress and performing strenuous exercise. They have high level of corticotrophin releasing hormone (CRH). The levels of ACTH cortisol and endogenous opioids are high. CRH directly inhibits GnRH secretion via raised endogenous opioids. They are more likely to develop amenorrhoea due to **decrease in GnRH pulse frequency**. According to body weight hypothesis, body weight should be above critical level to achieve menarche and regular menstruation. To achieve menarche, body fat should reach 17 per cent of the body weight. And for regularity of menstruation body fat should be maintained at least at 22 per cent. Reduction of body fat by about one-third will result in menstrual abnormality. Menstruation becomes irregular when the BMI is < 19 kg/m^2.

These subjects are hypoestrogenic and have got elevated prolactin and cortisol level. Leptin level is found low.

Anorexia nervosa is a state of self imposed starvation. This is a psychosexual problem where the patient suffers from the illusion of excessive body fat and distorted body image. Patient denies food and is markedly under weight. Amenorrhoea is the rule. Constipation is common. Release of GnRH is affected. **FSH and LH levels are low, cortisol level is high**. This may be a life-threatening disorder.

Obesity — Obese women so often suffer from irregular

menstrual bleeding. Excess number of fat cells in obese women, convert peripheral androgens to oestrogen (aromatisation). There is also low level of sex-hormone binding globulin, which helps free androgens to be converted to oestrone. Obesity with polycystic ovarian disease can cause oligomenorrhoea or amenorrhoea (see p. 440).

Kallmann syndrome — Embryologically GnRH neurones develop in the ectodermal olfactory placode before they migrate finally to the hypothalamus. GnRH neurones are absent due to partial or complete agenesis of olfactory bulb (olfactogenital dysplasia). This disorder is characterised by hypogonadotrophic hypogonadism, anosmia and colour blindness. There may be associated cleft lip and palate. Patients present with primary amenorrhoea. Mode of inheritance is thought to be 'X' linked. Menstruation can be induced with combined oestrogen and progestin therapy. Induction of ovulation is successful with exogenous gonadotrophins.

Pituitary factors

Adenoma

In adenoma either micro or macro, there is usually associated inappropriate galactorrhoea (p. 548), secondary amenorrhoea and infertility. There may be headache with disturbed vision.

Serum prolactin level is raised beyond 100 ng/ml. X-ray sella turcica may reveal space occupying lesion. CT or MRI scan is more informative.

Hyperprolactinaemia and amenorrhoea

Prolactin inhibits GnRH pulse secretion. Gonadotrophin levels are suppressed. Hyperprolactinaemia inhibits ovarian steroidogenesis.

Pituitary adenoma (Prolactinoma)

Prolactin is a protein hormone having 199 amino-acids with a molecular weight of 23,000 daltons. Prolactin has got various forms, called as 'little' or (monomer), "big" (dimer) or "big big" (multimeric) prolactin respectively. Little prolactin has got more biological activity. Prolactin is synthesized and released primarily by the lactotrophs located in the anterior pituitary gland. **Extrapituitary sites of PRL production include** decidua, endometrium, lungs, etc. Prolactin secretion from the anterior pituitary is under the inhibitory control of dopamine. Dopamine produced in the arcuate nucleus of the hypothalamus and is released in the portal hypophyseal vessels. Hyperprolactinaemia is commonly due to pituitary adenomas (microadenoma or macroadenoma). There are other various causes of hyperprolactinaemia (see Table 33.17). Normal plasma level of prolactin is 1–20 ng/ml.

Causes of hyperprolactinaemia

A. Physiological

- Stress and exercise (raised endogenous opioids)
- Stimulation of the nipples
- Sleep
- Idiopathic

B. Hypothalamus and pituitary

- Craniopharyngioma
- Tuberculosis
- Hypothyroidism
- Multiple endocrine disorder (Cushing's syndrome, Acromegaly)
- Pituitary adenomas
- Resection of pituitary stalk

C. Drugs — (↓) Decreased hypothalamic PIF

- Phenothiazines
- Metoclopramide
- Methyldopa
- Reserpine
- Antidepressants
- Oestrogens

D. Others

- Renal failure — (↓) Decreased PRL clearance
- Cirrhosis of liver — (↑) Increased PRL production
- Idiopathic

Diagnosis of pituitary adenomas

Prolactin level is more than 100 ng/ml is often associated with prolactinoma. Most of the adenomas are microadenoma (diameter less than 1 cm). "Coned down" and lateral views of the sella turcica by radiography can detect gross abnormalities, calcification of tumour. Microadenomas rarely progress to macroadenomas. Computerised tomography (CT) is helpful for macroadenomas. Magnetic resonance imaging (MRI) with better resolution can diagnose even microadenomas.

Visual field examination is essential to detect any compression effect on the optic nerves.

Treatment : See p. 450.

Sheehan's syndrome : There is history of severe postpartum haemorrhage, shock or severe infection. Depending upon the degree of anterior pituitary necrosis, the features vary. **The common manifestations are** falling lactation, loss of pubic and axillary hair, lethargy, hypotension, secondary amenorrhoea and atrophy of the breasts and genitalia. Gonadotrophin level is low, so also T_3, T_4 and cortisol. The

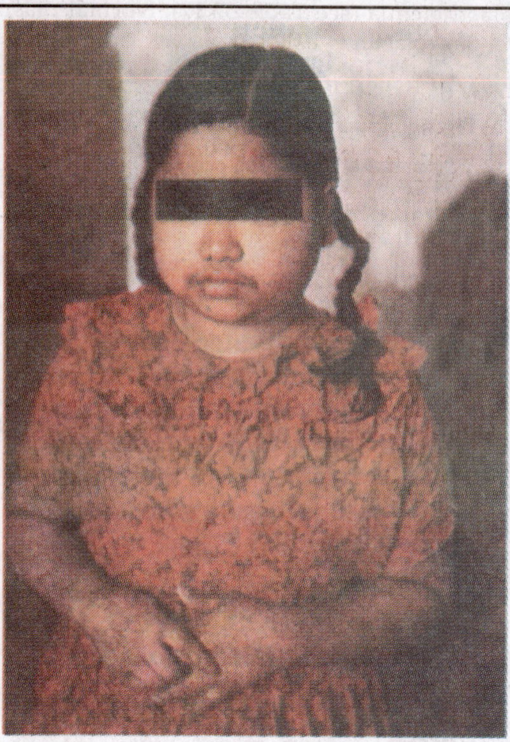

Fig. 28.7. A case of Cushing syndrome with mild hirsute [*By courtesy* : Prof. K.M. Gun]

hormones affected in order of frequency are, growth hormone (GH), gonadotrophins (FSH and LH), TSH and ACTH. The syndrome may develop slowly over 8—10 years time.

Management

Replacement therapy with appropriate hormones including corticosteroid and thyroid are needed. Fertility can be achieved in these women with hMG and hCG. Clomiphene is ineffective.

Adrenal tumour or hyperplasia

There is secondary amenorrhoea, infertility, acne and features of defeminisation followed by virilisation (hoarseness of voice, hirsutism and enlargement of clitoris). In both the conditions there is excess production of androgens. Serum level of DHEA–S correlate well with daily urinary 17 KS excretion. **Rise of serum DHAS and urinary 17 ketosteroid levels are suppressed with dexamethasone 2 mg daily for 2 days in adrenal hyperplasia but not in tumour**. For confirmation of the diagnosis of tumour, IVP, MRI, CT scan or sonography is helpful.

Level of serum testosterone > 200 ng/dl is suggestive of an ovarian androgen secreting tumour. Whereas level of DHAS > 800 μg/dl is suggestive of an adrenal tumour. Urinary 17 ketosteroid excretion is high in a case with adrenal tumour. Ovarian neoplasm could be diagnosed with ultrasonographic examination (Endo vaginal or abdominal).

Late onset congenital adrenal hyperplasia (CAH) is due to enzyme defect (21 hydroxylase, 11β hydrolase or 3β hydroxy steroid dehydrogenase) and leads to excess androgen production. But there is relative decrease in cortisol production. 21 hydroxylase deficiency is most common (90%). It is an autosomal recessive disorder.

Serum (morning sample) level of 17 hydroxy progesterone 17 OHP > 800 ng/dl is diagnostic of 21 hydroxylase deficiency. Level of serum 17 OHP < 200 ng/dl virtually rules out the diagnosis of CAH. There is significant rise in 17 OHP level following ACTH stimulation test.

Cushing syndrome

Cushing first described the syndrome in 1932. Androgens are formed as intermediate products in the synthesis of cortisol. The elevated cortisol level found in Cushing syndrome encompasses two distinct pathologic entities.

- Cushing disease (ACTH dependent).
- Adrenal tumour (ACTH independent).

In Cushing disease, there is excess production of ACTH from the anterior pituitary or from ectopic sites. Basophil adenoma (microadenoma) is present in about 75 per cent of cases. The increased ACTH causes hyperstimulation of adrenal cortex leading to its hyperplasia which in turn leads to excess production of cortisol and androgens.

ACTH independent causes (adrenal adenoma or cancer) may be iatrogenic (high dose corticosteroid therapy) or adrenal tumour.

The cause of adrenal mischief is cortisol secreting adenoma which produces excess cortisol. The androgen production is usually less but may be markedly elevated in presence of adrenal carcinoma.

Symptoms include weakness, oligomenorrhoea, amenorrhoea, acne and hirsutism. Virilism is rare. **Signs include** — moon facies, centripetal obesity and abdominal striae (Fig. 28.7).

The syndrome is often associated with hypertension, osteoporosis and insulin dependent diabetes.

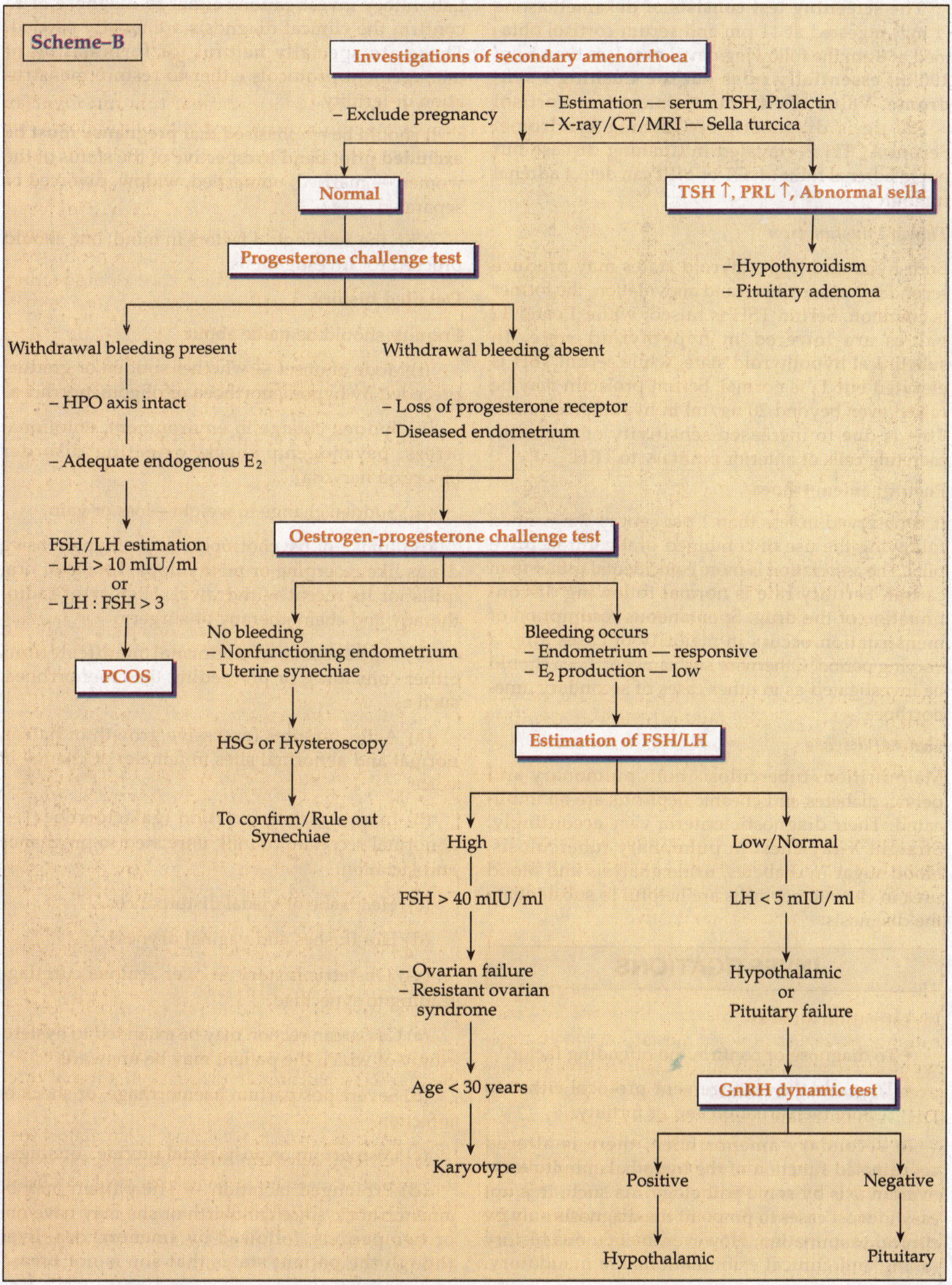
Scheme–B
Investigations of secondary amenorrhoea
– Exclude pregnancy
– Estimation — serum TSH, Prolactin
– X-ray/CT/MRI — Sella turcica
Normal
TSH ↑, PRL ↑, Abnormal sella
– Hypothyroidism
– Pituitary adenoma
Progesterone challenge test
Withdrawal bleeding present
Withdrawal bleeding absent
– HPO axis intact
– Adequate endogenous E2
– Loss of progesterone receptor
– Diseased endometrium
FSH/LH estimation
– LH > 10 mIU/ml
or
– LH : FSH > 3
PCOS
Oestrogen-progesterone challenge test
No bleeding
– Nonfunctioning endometrium
– Uterine synechiae
Bleeding occurs
– Endometrium — responsive
– E2 production — low
HSG or Hysteroscopy
To confirm/Rule out Synechiae
Estimation of FSH/LH
High
FSH > 40 mIU/ml
– Ovarian failure
– Resistant ovarian syndrome
Age < 30 years
Karyotype
Low/Normal
LH < 5 mIU/ml
Hypothalamic or Pituitary failure
GnRH dynamic test
Positive
Negative
Hypothalamic
Pituitary

The screening test consists of dexamethasone (1 mg) ingested at 11 pm and serum cortisol obtained at 8 am the following day. **Level less than 5 μg/100 ml essentially rules out the Cushing's syndrome.** Value of 24 hour urinary free cortisol > 250 μg is diagnostic of Cushing syndrome. Serum ACTH is elevated in Cushing disease but not in adrenal tumour. CT or MRI can detect adrenal tumour.

Thyroid dysfunction

Both hypo-and hyperthyroid states may produce secondary amenorrhoea and anovulation, the former is common. Serum TSH is raised, while T_3 and T_4 values are lowered in hypothyroid state. In subclinical hypothyroid state, while serum TSH is elevated but T_4 is normal. Serum prolactin may be raised even beyond 20 ng/ml in hypothyroid state. This is due to increased sensitivity of prolactin secreting cells of anterior pituitary to TRH.

Postpill amenorrhoea

It is observed in less than 1 per cent of the women following the use of combined oral contraceptive pills. The association is more coincidental rather than causal. Fertility rate is normal following discontinuation of the drug. Spontaneous resumption of menstruation occurs in majority of cases after a varying period. Otherwise such amenorrhoea should be investigated as in other cases of secondary amenorrhoea.

General disease

Malnutrition, tuberculosis both pulmonary and pelvic, diabetes and chronic nephritis are all implicated. Their diagnostic criteria vary accordingly. Straight X-ray chest in pulmonary tuberculosis, blood sugar in diabetes, urine analysis and blood urea in chronic nephritis are helpful to substantiate the diagnosis.

INVESTIGATIONS

Investigation aims at

- To diagnose or confirm the offending factor.
- To guide the management protocol either to restore menstruation and or fertility.

In secondary amenorrhoea, there is altered coordinated function of the hypothalamopituitary-ovarian axis by some pathology. As such, it is not easy in most cases to pinpoint the diagnosis only by clinical examination. However, meticulous history taking and clinical examinations are mandatory. Laboratory investigations either to diagnose or to confirm the clinical diagnosis are mostly needed. These are specially helpful for formulation of management protocols either to restore menstruation or fertility.

It should be emphasised that **pregnancy must be excluded** prior hand irrespective of the status of the women — married, unmarried, widow, divorced or separated.

With the aetiological factors in mind, one should proceed for investigations.

Detailed history

Enquiry should be made about :

(i) Mode of onset — whether sudden or gradual preceded by hypomenorrhoea or oligomenorrhoea.

(ii) Sudden change in environment, emotional stress, psychogenic shock, or eating disorder (anorexia nervosa).

(iii) Sudden change in weight—loss or gain.

(iv) Intake of psychotrophic or antihypertensive drugs like reserpine or methyldopa. Intake of oral 'pills' or its recent withdrawal. History of radiotherapy and chemotherapy or surgery.

(v) Appearance of abnormal manifestations either coinciding or preceeding the amenorrhoea, such as :

(a) Acne, hirsutes (excessive growth of hair in normal and abnormal sites in female) or change in voice.

(b) Inappropriate lactation (galactorrhoea) — abnormal secretion of milk unrelated to pregnancy and lactation.

(c) Headache or visual disturbances.

(d) Hot flushes and vaginal dryness.

(vi) Obstetric history — over zealous curettage leading to synechiae.

(a) Caesarean section may be extended to hysterectomy of which the patient may be unaware.

(b) Severe postpartum haemorrhage, or shock or infection.

(c) Postpartum or postabortal uterine curettage.

(d) Prolonged lactation — The patient may be amenorrhoeic since childbirth or she may have one or two periods, followed by amenorrhoea. Even though the patient states that she is not breastfeeding her baby, a patient enquiry may reveal that she is putting the baby to the breast at night. This is sufficient to make the patient remain amenorrhoeic.

(vii) Medical history of tuberculosis (pulmonary or extra pulmonary), diabetes, chronic nephritis or overt hypothyroid state should be enquired.

(viii) Family history — Premature menopause often runs in the family (mother or sisters).

General examination

The following features are to be noted :

(i) Nutritional status.

(ii) Extreme emaciation or marked obesity.

(iii) Presence of acne or hirsutes.

(iv) Discharge of milk from the breasts.

Abdominal examination

(i) Presence of striae associated with obesity may be related to Cushing disease.

(ii) A mass in the lower abdomen.

Pelvic examination

(i) Enlargement of clitoris.

(ii) Adnexal mass suggestive of tubercular tubo-ovarian mass or ovarian tumour.

With the above methods, either a probable diagnosis is made or no abnormality is detected to account for amenorrhoea. **The latter group is much more common and these are investigated as outlined below**.

Even though there is no inappropriate galactorrhoea, serum prolactin, TSH estimations and X-ray sella turcica are mandatory. **If these are normal, the following protocols are followed**.

Step – I

Progesterone challenge test is employed. **If withdrawal bleeding occurs, it proves**— (i) the intact hypothalamopituitaryovarian axis and (ii) there is adequate endogenous oestrogens (serum E_2 level more than 40 pg/ml) to promote progesterone receptors in the endometrium. (iii) Anatomically patent outflow tract and (iv) Endometrium is responsive.

Estimation of serum LH and FSH is to be done to diagnose PCOS. In PCOS, LH is > 10 mIU/ml and/or LH : FSH ratio is > 3.

If withdrawal bleeding fails to occur, it signifies — (i) lack of progesterone receptors in the endometrium or (ii) diseased endometrium. To differentiate between the two, one is to proceed to step II.

Step – II

Oestrogen–progesterone challenge test — Ethinyl oestradiol 0.02 mg. or conjugated equine oestrogen 1.25 mg is to be taken daily for 25 days. Medroxyprogesterone acetate 10 mg daily is added from day 15-25. Alternately, one course of oral contraceptive pill is given and to observe whether withdrawal bleeding occurs or not.

If there is no bleeding, it signifies local endometrial lesion such as uterine synechiae. This is to be confirmed by **HSG or hysteroscopy**.

If withdrawal bleeding occurs, it indicates the presence of responsive endometrium but the endogenous oestrogen production is inadequate. As such, to determine whether the underlying defect lies in the ovary or in the pituitary, one is to proceed to step III.

Step – III

Estimation of serum gonadotrophins is to be done. If the level of serum FSH is more than 40 mIU/ml, the case is one of premature ovarian failure or resistant ovarian syndrome. Ovarian biopsy is not recommended to confirm the diagnosis or to differentiate the two entities.

If, however, the level of FSH is either normal or low, it signifies pituitary dysfunction. Whether the disturbed pituitary function is primary or secondary to hypothalamus, one should proceed to step IV.

Step – IV

GnRH dynamic test — If with GnRH administration, there is rise of pituitary gonadotrophins, it is probably a case of hypothalamic dysfunction (see p. 500). In cases of primary pituitary disorder, there will be no rise of gonadotrophins. The result is however inconclusive.

If possible, pituitary tumour have to be excluded by X-ray sella turcica, CT or MRI, scan even though the prolactin level is normal.

MANAGEMENT

I. No abnormality detected

• The patient is not anxious about amenorrhoea and or fertility. No treatment is required. Only assurance is given and too often, menstruation resumes within a year or so.

• The patient is anxious for amenorrhoea but not for fertility.

(i) With normal endogenous oestrogen : Oral combined steroidal contraceptives are prescribed and to be continued for at least three cycles.

(ii) With low endogenous oestrogen : Ethinyl oestradiol 0.02 mg or conjugated equine oestrogen 1.25 mg daily is to be taken for 25 days. Medroxyprogesterone acetate 10 mg daily is added from day 16-25.

• The patient is anxious for fertility.

Husband's semen analysis in primary infertility and the tubal factor of the women are to be evaluated prior to induction of ovulation either using clomiphene or gonadotrophins (details in ch. 15).

II. Cases with detectable cause

(i) **Anxiety and stress** — may be corrected by assurance and psychotherapy.

(ii) **Systemic illness and malnutrition** : To improve the health status and appropriate therapy for systemic illness.

(iii) **Exercise induced** amenorrhoea is cured with limitation of activity and appropriate diet.

III. POLYCYSTIC OVARIAN SYNDROME (PCOS)

Management of PCOS needs individualisation of the patient. It depends on her presenting symptoms, like menstrual disorder, infertility, obesity, hirsutism or combined symptoms. Patient counselling is important. **Treatment is primarily targeted to correct the biochemical abnormalities** (Table 28.5).

Table 28.5
Biochemical abnormalities associated with PCOS

– Hyperandrogenism	– Hyperinsulinaemia
– Hypersecretion of LH	– Hyperprolactinaemia
– High serum oestrogens (Oestradiol, oestrone)	– Low FSH – Low serum SHBG
– Androgenic follicular microenvironment	– Low serum progesterone – Hyperlipidaemia

Weight reduction in obese patients is the first line of treatment. Body mass index (BMI) < 25 improves menstrual abnormalities, hirsutism and infertility. It reduces insulin and androgen levels.

Fertility not concerned

• **Androgen excess (see p. 544)** — Combined oral contraceptive pills are effective. Progestin suppresses LH and oestrogen improves SHBG, reducing free testosterone level. Norgestrel containing pill is avoided because of its high androgenicity. Newer progestins (desogestrel) are best suited (Table 29.8).

– GnRH agonists – Leuprolide acetate 3.75 mg IM or Goserelin 3.6 mg SC every four weeks can be used to suppress ovarian steroid production (see p. 500).

– Cyproterone acetate, spironolactone, ketoconazole, flutamide, finasteride are the other antiandrogens that can be used for the management of **hirsutism** (see p. 512 and 544).

– **Hyperinsulinaemia** is treated to reduce the risks of cardiovascular disease and diabetes mellitus (see below). **Endometrium** should be protected against the unapposed effects of oestrogen (see p. 510).

Patient wanting pregnancy

• **Ovulation induction** is usually achieved by clomiphene citrate with or without dexamethasone or bromocriptine. In unresponsive cases, pure FSH or HMG along with hCG may be administered backed up with monitoring facilities (see ch. 16).

Insulin sensitisers : Women with PCOS and hyperinsulinaemia with BMI > 25, ovulate satisfactorily when clomiphene is combined with metformin. Metformin 500 mg thrice daily is found to correct the biochemical abnormalities (hyperinsulinaemia and hyperandrogenism) — see Table 28.5. Pioglitazone and rosiglitazone are also being used in cases resistant to metformin.

Surgery (Fig. 28.8)

Surgery is the alternative procedure for PCOS who are resistant to medical therapy. Endoscopic cauterisation or CO_2 laser vapourisation (see p. 583) of multiple cysts has replaced the conventional wedge resection of the ovaries (see p. 570). Pregnancy rates following ovarian diathermy are higher.

IV. Hyperprolactinaemia, Inappropriate galactorrhoea

Treatment—*Medical* : Bromocriptine (lysergic acid derivative) a dopamine agoinst is the drug first choice. Dose of 1.25 mg orally, bed time, is started for the first week and then increased gradually. Common side effects of the drug are giddiness, nausea, vomiting, headache, constipation and orthostatic hypotension. Other drugs used with

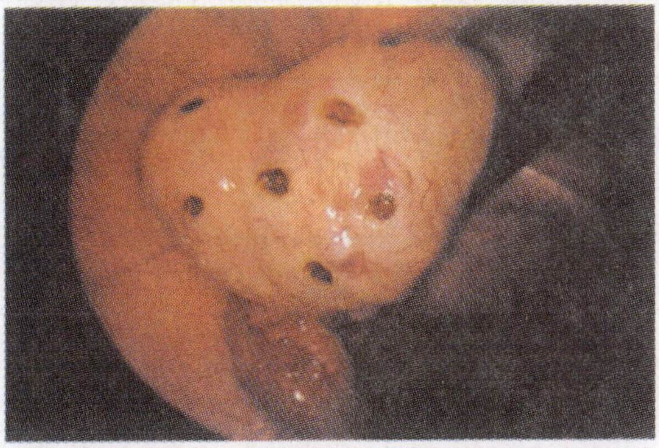

Fig. 28.8. Laparoscopic ovarian drilling using laser

minimum side-effects are pergolide (50–150 mg daily) and carbergoline (0.25 mg once or twice weekly). There is shrinkage of the tumour with therapy. Bromocriptine can be continued safely in pregnancy when required. **Surgery** is considered when there is failure of medical therapy. Transnasal — transphenoidal excision is done. Complications of surgery are : meningitis, diabetes insipidus, leakage of CSF and recurrence. Radiation therapy is not commonly preferred (see also p. 549).

V. Premature ovarian failure

- To prevent or to minimise postmenopausal health hazards, HRT should be judiciously employed (see p. 61).
- In proved cases of autoimmune disorders, corticosteroids may be of help.
- Fertility potentiality is far and remote. However, induction of ovulation may be hopefully tried in presence of follicle. This may be achieved by administration of sequential oestrogen and progesterone or by use of GnRH agonist, followed by administration of gonadotrophins for ovulation induction.
- Spontaneous recovery and pregnancy have been reported in an occasional case of premature ovarian failure.
- IVF with donor's oocyte with total replacement of hormones may be hopefully tried with occasional success.
- In the presence of 'Y' chromosome, gonadectomy is to be done to avoid malignancy.

VI. Adrenal disorders

Treatment of Cushing's Disease : Pituitary tumour is treated by transsphenoidal resection or by external beam radiation. Excess cortisol due to adrenal tumour is cured by simple adrenalectomy. Many patients need medical therapy either before or after surgery to maintain normal cortisol level. Mitotane (adrenocorticolytic drug) may be used to produce medical adrenalectomy. Enzyme inhibitors like amnioglutethimide or metyrapone has been used to block excess cortisol production. Ketoconazole inhibits adrenal steroid biosynthesis. It is also used for long-term benefit.

Adult onset adrenal hyperplasia — Dexamethasone replacement therapy is given. A dose of 0.25–0.5 mg may be adequate. Periodic serum cortisol level is to be checked and is maintained at > 2 μg/dL.

VII. Hypothyroid state should be treated by thyroxine.

VIII. Hyperandrogenic state — Suppression of hyperandrogenism can be achieved using — oral contraceptives, glucocorticoids or antiandrogen preparations (details in Tables 33.14 and 33.16).

IX. Uterine synechiae — Adhesiolysis followed by insertion of IUD is effective. Addition of oral contraceptive pills for three months may help in regeneration of the endometrium.

X. Ovarian tumour — Appropriate surgery is done (see p. 371).

XI. Anorexia nervosa needs multidisciplinary approach. Behavioural therapy, psychiatric consultation are helpful. Hospitalisation may be needed in severe cases.

RESULTS

The following conclusions are made about the fate of the patients having amenorrhoea.

In primary amenorrhoea, more investigations are often done to find out the cause with minimal effect. In fact, in most of the cases where menstruation occurs are the young girls whose menarche is delayed in onset.

In secondary amenorrhoea, with comparative fewer investigations, the result is satisfactory. But the percentage of cures falls steeply as the duration of amenorrhoea lengthens. However, with or without treatment, spontaneous resumption of menstruation occurs in about 60 per cent cases of secondary amenorrhoea of more than one year's duration.

KEY POINTS

- Amenorrhoea is physiological before puberty, during pregnancy and lactation and following menopause.
- The most common cause of amenorrhoea is hypothalamic dysfunction.
- Commonest cause of cryptomenorrhoea is imperforate hymen. The symptoms include periodic lower abdominal pain and occasional retention of urine. The treatment is cruciate incision of the hymen and drainage of blood (see p. 42).
- Common causes of primary amenorrhoea are abnormal chromosomal pattern, development defect of genital tract and disturbed function of the hypothalamopituitaryovarian axis.

  As such detailed history, clinical examination and specific investigations most often clinch the diagnosis of primary amenorrhoea (see Tables 28.1 and 28.2 and scheme–A).
- Women with primary amenorrhoea due to hypogonadotrophic hypogonadism should have CT scan to rule out CNS lesion. Karyotyping is not needed.

  The scope of therapeutic success in the management of primary amenorrhoea is very limited.

  XY gonads should be removed for its increased risk of malignancy. Substitution oestrogen therapy should be prescribed for the development and maintenance of secondary sex characters.
- Common causes of secondary amenorrhoea are hypothalamic dysfunction, PCOS, stress, premature ovarian failure and hypothyroid state (see Table 28.3).
- Individuals with gonadal dysgenesis and X chromosomal abnormality are less than 150 cm in height.
- Majority of women with PCOS have android obesity (BMI > 25), elevated levels of biologically active LH. About 40 per cent of women with PCOS have hyperinsulinaemia and impaired glucose tolerance and androgen excess (p. 440).
- Presence of two out of the three following criteria is essential to define PCOS (ESHRE/ASRM): (1) Oligo-and/or anovulation. (2) Hyperandrogenism (clinical or biochemical). (3) Polycystic ovaries.
- In polycystic ovarian syndrome (PCOS), there is excess androgen production by the ovaries. Typically, the ovaries are enlarged, capsule is thickened with multiple cysts along with hypertrophy of theca cells (stromal hyperthecosis) (p. 440).
- Management of PCOS needs patient individualisation (see p. 450). Weight reduction is an important step. Correction of hyperandrogenaemia (p. 547), hyperprolactinaemia (ch. 450), hyperinsulinaemia and elevated LH levels (see p. 450) are the others. Metformin ameliorates the biochemical abnormalities. Ovulation induction has higher success when clomiphene is combined with metformin (insulin sensitising agent). In refractory cases, laparoscopic ovarian diathermy or laser vapourisation of multiple cysts of the ovaries is better than wedge resection (p. 450).
- Long-term risk of PCOS patients, if left untreated includes, diabetes mellitus, dyslipidaemia, hypertension and endometrial carcinoma, breast carcinoma (p. 443).
- Common causes of uterine synechiae are tubercular endometritis, overzealous postabortal or puerperal curettage (p. 438).
- Level of serum FSH can differentiate hypogonadotrophic hypogonadism from oestrogen deficiency due to ovarian failure (p. 444).
- Serum FSH level > 40 mIU/ml, establishes the diagnosis of ovarian failure or hypergonadotrophic hypogonadism (p. 444).
- Women with müllerian abnormalities have associated renal abnormalities in about one-third of cases.
- When uterine bleeding fails to occur after progestin therapy, level of endogenous oestradiol is below 40 pg/ml (p. 449).

KEY POINTS

- When withdrawal bleeding occurs following progestin challenge test, it suggests : (i) intact hypothalamopituitaryovarian axis, (ii) serum E_2 level is more than 40 pg/ml, (iii) outflow tract is present and is patent anatomically and (iv) endometrium is responsive.
- The triad for diagnosis of premature ovarian failure include amenorrhoea, raised gonadotrophins and low serum oestradiol. Karyotype should be done for younger (< 30 years) age group. Serum antibodies are positive in autoimmune variety. Ovarian biopsy is not essential to the diagnosis (p. 444, 451).
- Serum level (morning sample) of 17–OHP when > 8 ng/ml establishes the diagnosis of late onset congenital adrenal hyperplasia.
- Abnormal secretion of GnRH results in amenorrhoea is about 30 per cent of women. Stress induced amenorrhoea is due to increased level of opioids (β endorphin) in CNS, causing interference of GnRH release. Increased leptin level is associated with hypothalamic amenorrhoea.
- Weight loss when 15 per cent below the ideal, can cause amenorrhoea due to hypothalamic dysfunction.
- Exercise induced amenorrhoea is also due to reduced GnRH pulse secretion, resulting in decreased LH pulses.
- Hyperprolactinaemia is associated with anovulation, amenorrhoea or galactorrhoea. Causes of hyperprolactinaemia are many (see p. 445). Most common cause of mildly raised prolactin level is stress. Majority of women with hyperprolactinaemia, amenorrhoea and galactorrhoea will have prolactinoma. Most microadenomas (< 1 cm in diameter) do not enlarge with time. Bromocriptine shrinks 80-90 per cent of macroadenomas. Most common side effects of bromocriptine therapy are nausea, vomiting and orthostatic hypotension. Cabergoline is more effective and is better tolerated.
- Hyperprolactinaemia is present in 15 per cent of all anovulatory women. Nearly 60 per cent of all women with galactorrhoea have hyperprolactinaemia. Nearly 90 per cent of women with galactorrhoea amenorrhoea have hyperprolactinaemia. About 5 per cent of women with hyperprolactinaemia have hypothyroidism (p. 445).

  Bromocriptine treatment returns prolactin level to normal in 90 per cent, induces ovulation in 80 per cent and cures galactorrhoea in 60 per cent of cases (p. 450).

  Combined oral contraceptives do not stimulate the growth of prolactin secreting microadenomas.
- Pregnancy induced by bromocriptine is not associated with an increased risk of congenital malformation or multiple pregnancy (p. 450).
- Surgical treatment of prolactinomas is done when there is failure of medical treatment but long-term recurrence rate is about 20 per cent (p. 451).
- In masculinising ovarian tumour, serum testosterone is elevated to > 2 ng/ml while DHEA–S is normal. Elevated DHEA–S reflects adrenal androgen excess (p. 544). Serum levels of DHEA–S correlate well with daily urinary 17 KS excretion.
- In Sheehan's syndrome, there is failing lactation, loss of pubic and axillary hair, secondary amenorrhoea and atrophy of the breasts. Hormones affected in order of frequency are GH, FSH, LH, TSH and ACTH.

  In Cushing disease, there is excess production of ACTH leading to excess secretion of cortisol and androgen production. The symptoms of Cushing syndrome include weakness, amenorrhoea, acne and hirsutism; signs include moon facies, centripetal obesity and abdominal striae.

  The diagnosis of a case of secondary amenorrhoea is difficult to make out from the clinical examination scheme – B). Pregnancy must be excluded prior hand. Even though, there is no galactorrhoea, serum prolactin, TSH estimation and X-ray sella turcica are mandatory as the first step of investigation. When no abnormality is detected and the patient is not anxious about amenorrhoea and or fertility, no treatment is required (p. 447).

  In primary amenorrhoea, more investigations are often done to find out the cause with minimal effect. In secondary amenorrhoea, with comparative fewer investigations, the result is satisfactory (p. 436, 447).

Contraception

29

Introduction

Rapid population growth is a critical issue in most developing countries. Family planning matters save women's lives preventing unintended pregnancies. **Slower population growth conserves resources, improves health and living standards.**

Benefits of fertility control are interrelated. Benefits are : Improved quality of life, better health, less physical and emotional stress of life, better education, job and economic opportunities. Benefits are enjoyed by the couple, the children, other family members, the community and the country.

Contraception and fertility control are not synonymous. Fertility control includes both fertility inhibition (contraception) and fertility stimulation. While the fertility stimulation is related to the problem of the infertile couples, **the term contraception includes all measures, temporary or permanent, designed to prevent pregnancy due to the coital act.**

Ideal contraceptive methods should fulfil the following criteria — widely acceptable, inexpensive, simple to use, safe, highly effective and requiring minimal motivation, maintenance and supervision. No one single universally acceptable method has yet been discovered.

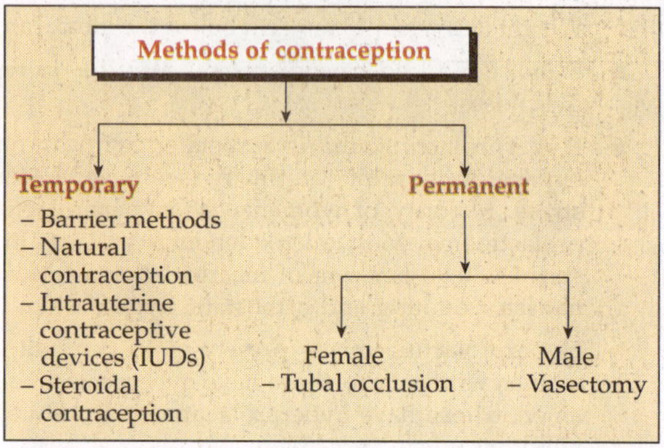

METHODS OF CONTRACEPTION

The various methods of contraception are schematically depicted above.

Table 29.1
Methods of contraception used by women of reproductive age in different countries

	METHODS USED (PER CENT)							
	Sterilisation							
Country (year)	*F*	*M*	*OC*	*IUD*	*Condom*	*Injectable*	*Others*	*Any method*
India (98-99)	34	2	2	2	3	–	5	48
Bangladesh (99-2000)	7	1	23	1	4	7	10	53
Sri Lanka (1987)	25	5	5	2	2	3	20	62
UK (2003-2004)	11	12	25	5	23	3	8	98

TEMPORARY

Temporary methods are commonly used to postpone or to space births. However, the methods are also frequently being used by the couples even though they have got strong desire for no more children (Table 29.2).

Table 29.2 : Failure rate of contraceptive methods in first 12 months of use

Methods	Pregnancy rate per 100 women years (approx.)
No method	80
Rhythm	24
Coitus interruptus	19
Lactational amenorrhoea	2
Condom (male)	14
Diaphragm	20
IUCD	0.1-3
Combined oral pill	0.1
Progestin only pill	1
DMPA and NET injectables	0.3
Norplant	0.1
Vasectomy	0.15
Tubectomy	0.5

Failure rate is further less when methods are used correctly and consistently

BARRIER METHODS

These methods prevent sperm deposition in the vagina or prevent sperm penetration through the cervical canal. The objective is achieved by mechanical devices or by chemical means which produce sperm immobilisation, or by combined means. The following are used :

- **Mechanical**
  - Male — Condom
  - Female — Condom, diaphragm, cervical cap
- **Chemical**
  - (Vaginal contraceptives)
  - Creams — Delfen (nonoxynol-9, 12.5%)
  - Jelly — Koromex, Volpar paste
  - Foam tablets — Aerosol foams, Chlorimin T or Contab, Sponge (Today)
- **Combination**
  - Combined use of mechanical and chemical

Condom (male)

Condoms are made of polyurethane or latex. Polyurethane condoms are thinner and suitable to those who are sensitive to latex rubber. It is the most widely practised method used by the male. In India, one particular brand (latex) is widely marketed as 'Nirodh'. The efficacy of condoms can be augmented by improving the quality of the products and by adding spermicidal agents during its use. **Protection against sexually transmitted disease is an additional advantage**. Occasionally, the partner may be allergic to latex.

Table 29.3 : Condom

Advantages
1. Cheaper with no contraindications.
2. No side effects.
3. Easy to carry, simple to use and disposable.
4. Protection against sexually transmitted diseases, e.g. gonorrhoea, chlamydia, HPV and HIV.
5. Protection against pelvic inflammatory diseases.
6. Reduces the incidence of tubal infertility and ectopic pregnancy.
7. Protection against cervical cell abnormalities.
8. Useful where the coital act is infrequent and irregular.

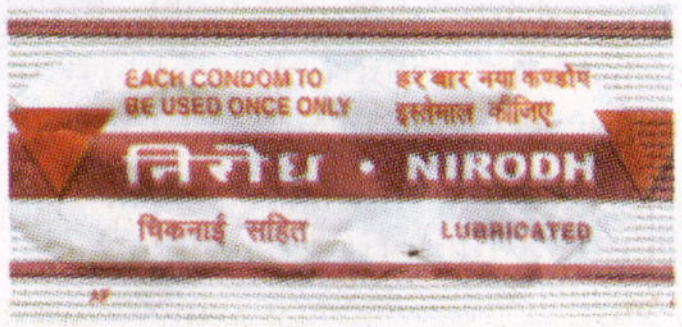

Disadvantages
1. May accidentally break or slip off during coitus.
2. Inadequate sexual pleasure.
3. To discard after one coital act.
4. Failure rate — 14 (HWY); 3 (HWY) when used correctly and consistently.

Precautions : (i) To use a fresh condom for every act of coitus. (ii) To cover the penis with condom prior to genital contact. (iii) Create a reservoir at the tip. (iv) To withdraw while the penis is still erect. (v) To grasp the base of the condom during withdrawal.

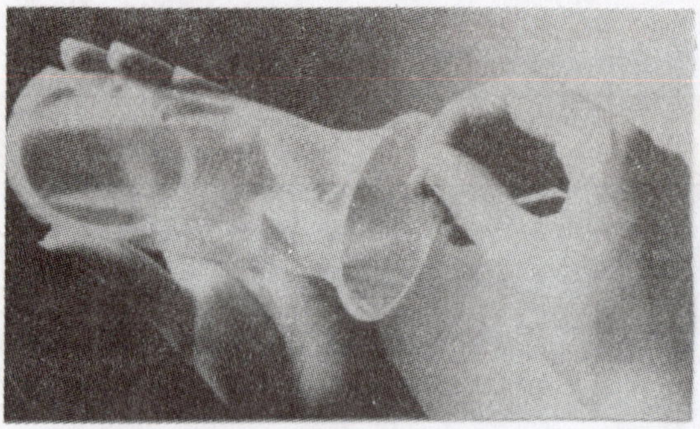

Fig. 29.1A. Female condom

The method is suitable for couples who want to space their families and who have contraindications to the use of oral contraceptive or IUD. These are also suitable to those who have infrequent sexual intercourse.

Female condom (Femidom) (Fig. 29.1A)

It is a pouch made of polyurethane which lines the vagina and also the external genitalia. It is 15 cm in length with one flexible polyurethane ring at each end. Inner ring at the closed end is smaller compared to the outer ring. It gives protection against sexually transmitted disease and pelvic inflammatory disease. It is expensive. Failure rate is about 3–5/HWY.

Use of condom : (1) As an elective contraceptive method. (2) As an interim form of contraception during pill use, following vasectomy operation (see later) and if an IUD is thought lost until a new IUD can be fitted. (3) During the treatment of trichomonal vaginitis of the wife, the husband should use it during the course of treatment irrespective of contraceptive practice. (4) Immunological infertility — male partner to use for three months. For other **non-contraceptive benefits** (Table 29.3).

Diaphragm (Table 29.4 and Fig. 29.1B)

It is an intravaginal device made of rubber with flexible metal or spring ring at the margin. Its diameter varies from 5-10 cm. It is not a popular method. It requires a medical or paramedical personnel to measure the size of the device. The distance between the tip of the middle finger placed in the posterior fornix and the point over the finger below the symphysis pubis gives the approximate diameter of the diaphragm. As it cannot effectively prevent ascent of the sperms alongside the margin of the device, additional chemical spermicidal agent should be placed on the superior surface of the device during insertion so that it remains in contact with the cervix. **The device is introduced upto 3 hours before intercourse and is to be kept for at least 6 hours after the last coital act.** Ill fitting and accidental displacement during intercourse increase the failure rate.

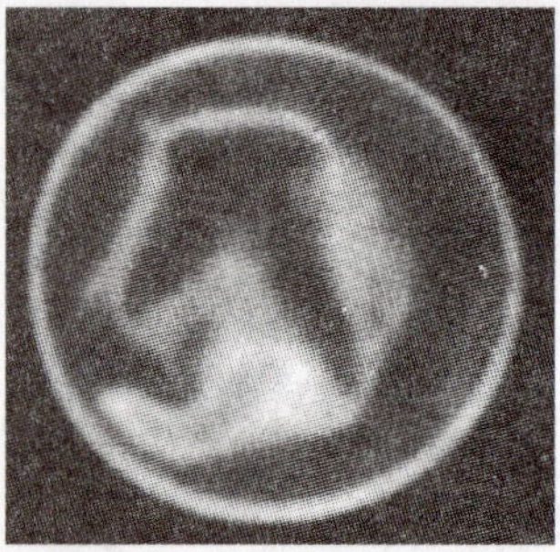

Fig. 29.1B. Commonly used conventional contraceptives (Diaphragm)

Vaginal Contraceptives (Fig. 29.1C)

Chemicals : Various spermicidal agents are available in the market either in the form of cream, jelly or foam tablet. These agents mostly produce sperm immobilisation when they come in contact and to some extent mechanically prevent sperm penetration through the cervical canal. **The cream or jelly** is introduced high in the vagina with the help of the applicator soon before coitus. **Foam tablets** (1-2) are to be introduced high in the vagina at least 5 minutes

Table 29.4 : Diaphragm

Advantages	Disadvantages
• Cheap.	• Requires help of a doctor or paramedical person to measure the size required.
• Can be used repeatedly for a long time.	• Risk of vaginal irritation and urinary tract infection are there.
• Used with spermicide reduces the incidence of PID/STD to some extent.	• Not suitable for women with uterine prolapse. *Failure rate—20 (HWY)*

Table 29.5 : Rhythm method

Advantages	Disadvantages
• No cost. • Lack of side effects. *Failure rate — 20-30 (HWY)*	• Difficult to calculate the safe period. • Compulsory abstinence from sexual act during certain periods. • Not applicable during lactational amenorrhoea or when the periods are irregular. • Higher rate of ectopic or congenital abnormality of the fetus because of chance of the union of the ageing sperm and ovum.

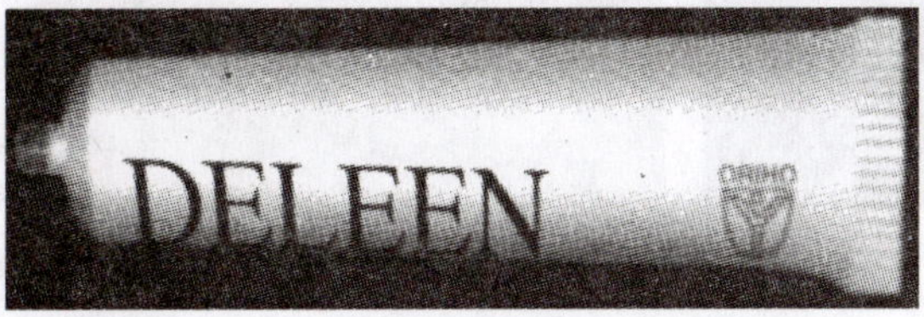

Fig. 29.1C. Vaginal contraceptive (Nonoxynol–9, 12.5%)

prior to intercourse. In isolation, it is not effective (26 HWY), but enhances the efficacy of condom or diaphragm when used along with it. There may be occasional local allergic manifestations either in the vagina or vulva.

Vaginal contraceptive sponge (Today)

It is made of polyurethane impregnated with 1 gm of nonoxynol-9 as a spermicide. Nonoxynol-9 acts as a surfactant which either immobilises or kills sperm. **It releases spermicide during coitus, absorbs ejaculate and blocks the entrance to the cervical canal. The sponge should not be removed for 6 hours after intercourse. Its failure rate is about 10/HWY.** Currently it is observed that nonoxynol-9 is partially effective in preventing cervical gonorrhoea, chlamydia or HIV infection. Moreover, it produces lesions in the genital tract when used frequently. Those lesions are associated with increased risk of HIV transmission.

Natural Contraception (Table 29.5)

Rhythm Method: This is the only method approved by the Roman Catholic Church. **The method is based on identification of the fertile period of a cycle and to abstain from sexual intercourse during that period.** The methods to determine the approximate time of ovulation and the fertile period include — (a) recording of previous menstrual cycles (calendar rhythm), (b) noting the basal body temperature chart (temperature rhythm) and (c) noting of excessive mucoid vaginal discharge (mucus rhythm). **The users of the calendar method** obtain the period of abstinence from calculations based on the previous twelve menstrual cycle records. **The first unsafe day is obtained** by subtracting 20 days from the length of the shortest cycle and **last unsafe day** by deducting 10 days from the longest cycle. **Users of temperature rhythm** require abstinence until the third day of the rise of temperature. **Users of mucus rhythm** require abstinence on all days of noticeable mucus and for three days thereafter.

Coitus Interruptus (Table 29.6)

It is the oldest and probably the most widely accepted contraceptive method used by man. **It necessitates withdrawal of penis shortly before ejaculation.** It requires sufficient self control by the man so that withdrawal of penis precedes ejaculation.

Table 29.6 : Coitus interruptus

Advantages	Disadvantages
• No appliance is required. • No cost. *Failure rate — 20 (HWY)*	• Requires sufficient self control by the man. • The woman may develop anxiety neurosis, vaginismus or pelvic congestion. • Chance of pregnancy is more : (a) Precoital secretion may contain sperm. (b) Accidental chance of sperm deposition into the vagina.

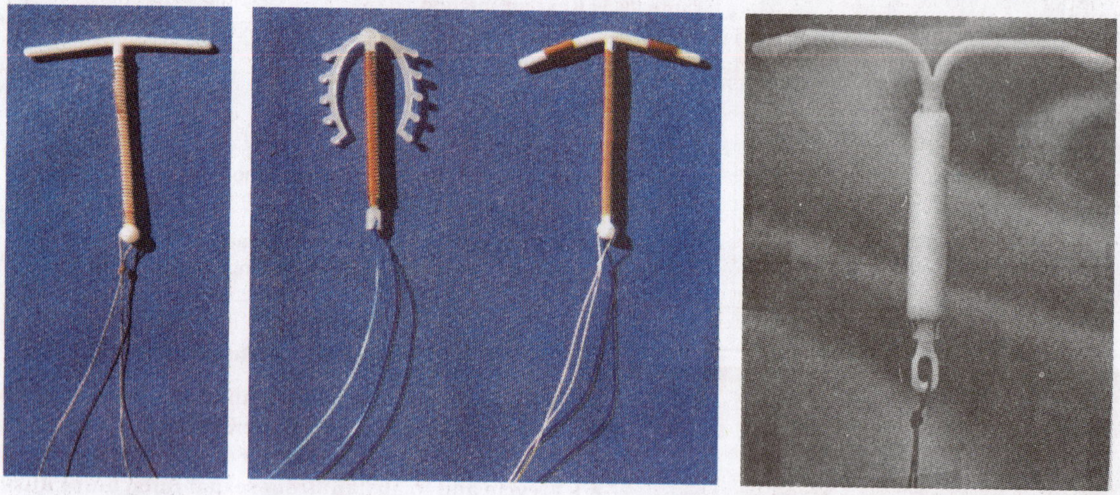

Cu T 200 A | Multiload 375 B | Cu T 380A C | Levonorgestrel containing IUD (LNG-IUS) D

Fig. 29.2. Commonly used IUD

Breastfeeding, Lactional amenorrhoea (LAM)

Prolonged and sustained breastfeeding offers a natural protection of pregnancy. This is more effective in women who are amenorrhoeic than those who are menstruating. The risk of pregnancy to a woman who is fully breastfeeding and amenorrhoeic is less than 2 per cent in the first 6 months. Otherwise, the failure rate is high (1–10%). Thus during breastfeeding, additional contraceptive support should be given by condom, IUCD or injectable steroids where available to provide complete contraception.

When the women is **full breastfeeding**, a contraceptive method should be used in the **3rd postpartum month and with partial or no breastfeeding, she should use it in the 3rd postpartum week**.

Fertility awareness based methods are :

(1) **Natural contraception** (Rhythm method, Coitus interruptus and Lactational amenorrhoea method).

(2) **Barrier method** (Condoms, diaphragm and spermicides).

INTRAUTERINE CONTRACEPTIVE DEVICES (IUD)

The intrauterine device have been used throughout the world. During the last couple of decades, however, there has been a significant improvement in its design and content. The idea is to obtain maximum efficacy without increasing the adverse effects. **The device is classified as open**, when it has got no circumscribed aperture of more than 5 mm so that a loop of intestine or omentum cannot enter and becomes strangulated if, accidentally, the device perforates through the uterus into the peritoneal cavity. Lippes loop, Cu T, Cu 7, Multiload and Progestasert are examples of open devices. **If closed devices**, like Grafenberg ring and Birnberg bow, accidentally enter the abdominal cavity, they have the potential of causing strangulation of the gut; and hence are obsolete. **The device may be non-medicated** as Lippes loop or **medicated (bioactive)** by incorporating a metal copper, in devices like Cu T-200, Cu T-380A, Multiload-250, Multiload-375 (Fig. 29.2).

Hormone containing IUD either releasing progesterone (progestasert) or levonorgestrel (LNG-IUS) has also been introduced. Nowadays the following medicated intrauterine contraceptive devices are in use :

• Cu T 200	• Multiload 250	• Multiload 375
• Cu T 380A	• LNG – IUS	• GyneFix

Description of the devices (Fig. 29.2)

Copper T 200 — The widely used medicated device is Copper T 200 B. It carries 215 sq mm surface area of fine copper wire wounded round the vertical stem of the device. Stem of the T-shaped device is made of a polyethylene frame. It has a polyethylene monofilament tied at the end of the vertical stem. These two threads are used for detection and removal. In spite of the copper being radio-opaque, additional barium sulphate is incorporated in the device. The device contains 124 mg of copper. The copper is lost at the rate of about 50 μg per 24 hours during a period of one year. It is supplied inside a sterilised sealed packet. **The device is to be removed after 4 years. Cu T 200** carries 200 sq mm surface area of wire containing 120 mg of copper and **is removed after 3 years. Apart from the use of Cu T as a contraceptive, it is used following synaecolysis.**

Cu T 380A — Cu T 380A carries 380 mm^2 surface area of copper wire wound around the stem (314 mm^2) and each copper sleeve on the horizontal arms (33 mm^2). The frame contains barium sulphate and is radio-opaque. Replacement is every 10 years.

Multiload Cu 250 — The device is available in a sterilised sealed packet with an applicator. There is no introducer and no plunger. The device emits 60–100 μg of copper per day during a period of one year. **The device is to be replaced every 3 years.**

Multiload–375 — It has 375 mm^2 surface area of Copper wire wound around its vertical stem. Replacement is every 5 years (Fig. 29.2).

Levonorgestrel intrauterine system (LNG-IUS) (Fig. 29.2D) — This is a T-shaped device, with polydimethylsiloxane membrane around the stem which acts as a steroid reservoir. Total amount of levonorgestrel is 52 mg and is released at the rate 20 μg/day. This device is to be replaced every 5 years. Its efficacy is comparable to sterilisation. It has many non-contraceptive benefits also (p. 463).

Progestasert — It is a progesterone (38 mg) containing IUD that releases progesterone 65 μg/day. It is to be replaced by after 1 year. Progestasert is no longer manufactured.

Lippes Loop — It is a non-medicated open intrauterine device. It is no longer used in India.

Mode of action

Mechanism of antifertility effect of all the IUDs is not yet clear. They act predominantly in the uterine cavity and do not inhibit ovulation. Probable factors are :

- **Biochemical and histological changes in the endometrium** — There is a non-specific inflammatory reaction along with biochemical changes in the endometrium which have got gametotoxic and spermolytic effect. Lysosomal disintegration from the macrophages attached to the device with liberation of prostaglandins also have antifertility effect.

- **There may be increased tubal motility** which results in quick migration of the fertilised ovum into the uterine cavity before the endometrium is receptive.

- **There may be impaired sperm ascent** probably due to local chemical effect affecting the sperm vitality and migration.

- **Copper devices** — Ionised copper has got an additional local antifertility effect by **preventing implantation through enzymatic interference.** Copper initiates the release of cytokines which are cytotoxic. Serum copper level is not increased. It seems that the progressive calcium deposition in the device prevents copper diffusion, if kept for longer period.

- **Levonorgestrel-IUS (Mirena)**— It induces strong and uniform suppression of endometrium. Cervical mucous becomes very scantly. Anovulation and insufficient luteal phase activity has also been mentioned. Serum progesterone level is not increased.

Contraindications for Insertion

The contraindications are—(1) Presence of pelvic infection. (2) Undiagnosed genital tract bleeding. (3) Suspected pregnancy. (4) Distortion of the shape of the uterine cavity as in fibroid or congenital uterine-malformation. (5) Severe dysmenorrhoea. (6) Past history of ectopic pregnancy. (7) Nullipara. (8) Within 6 weeks following caesarean section. (9) HIV (STD) positive women. (10) Significant immunosuppression. (11) Diabetes. Additionally for CuT : (12) Wilson disease and (13) Copper allergy. For LNG-IUS: (14) Hepatic tumour or hepatocellular disease (active). (15) Current breast cancer. (16) Severe arterial disease.

Time of insertion

(a) *Interval* (When the insertion is made in the interconceptional period beyond 6 weeks following childbirth or abortion)—**It is preferable to insert 2-3 days after the period is over.** But it can be inserted any time during the cycle even during menstrual phase which has certain advantages (open cervical canal, distended uterine cavity, less cramp). However, during lactational amenorrhoea, it can be inserted at any time.

(b) *Postabortal* — Following termination of pregnancy by suction evacuation or D and E, or following spontaneous abortion, the device may be inserted. The additional advantage of preventing uterine synaechia can help in motivation for insertion.

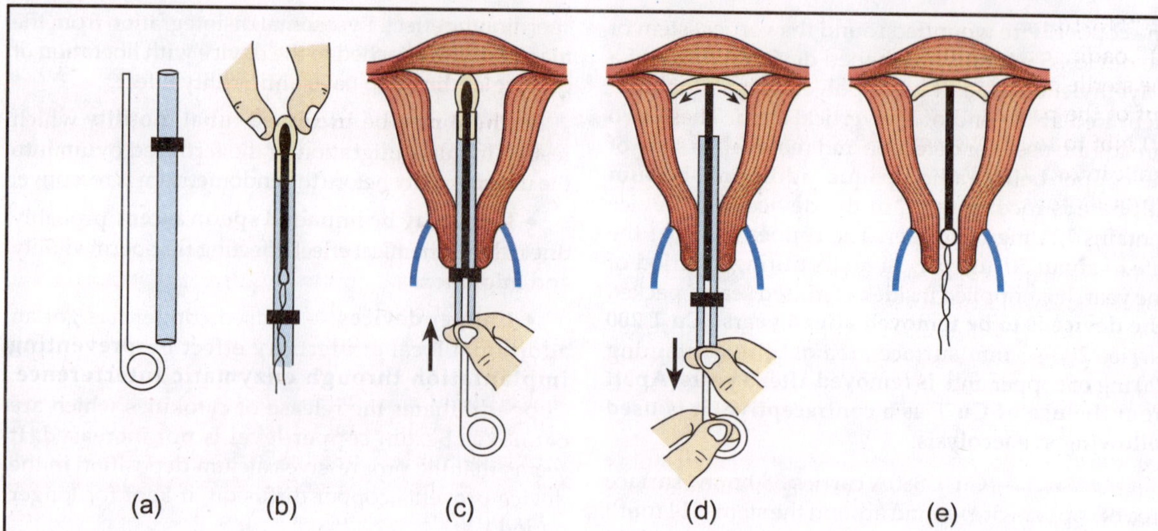

Fig. 29.3. Withdrawal technique of insertion of Cu-T

(c) ***Postpartum*** — Insertion of the device can be done before the patients are discharged from the hospital. Because of high rate of expulsion, it is preferable to withhold insertion for 6 weeks when the uterus will be involuted to near normal size.

(d) ***Postplacental delivery***—insertion immediately following delivery of the placenta could be done. But the expulsion rate is high.

Methods of Insertion (Figs. 29.3 and 29.4)

- **Cu T 200**
- **Cu T 380A**

(A) Preliminaries

(1) History taking and examinations (general and pelvic) to exclude any contraindication of insertion.

(2) Patient is informed about the various problems, the device is shown to her and consent is obtained.

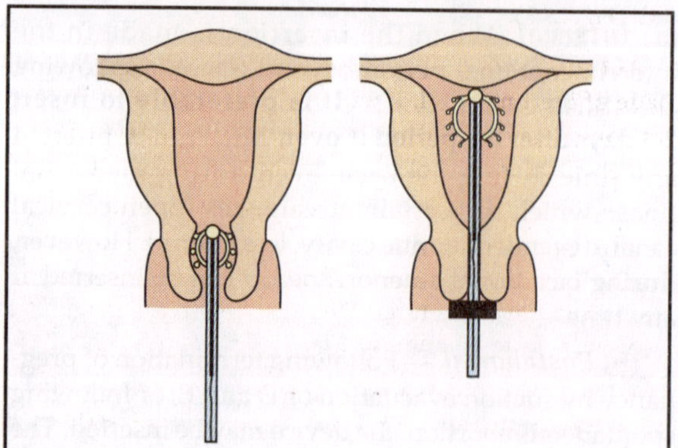

Fig. 29.4. Technique of insertion of Multiload IUCDs

(3) **The insertion is done in the outpatient department**, taking aseptic precautions without sedation or anaesthesia. To reduce cramping pain Ibuprofen (NSAID) may be given 30 min before insertion.

(4) **Placement of the device inside the inserter** — The device is taken out from the sealed packet. The thread, the vertical stem and then the horizontal stem folded to the vertical stem are introduced through the distal end of the inserter. The device is now ready for introduction. **"No touch" insertion method is preferred** (see below).

(B) Actual steps

(1) The patient empties her bladder and is placed in lithotomy position. Uterine size and position are ascertained by pelvic examination.

(2) Posterior vaginal speculum is introduced and the vagina and cervix are cleansed by antiseptic lotion.

(3) The anterior lip of the cervix is grasped by Allis forceps. A sound is passed through the cervical canal to note the position of the uterus and the length of the uterine cavity. The appropriate length of the inserter is adjusted depending on the length of the uterine cavity.

(4) The inserter with the device placed inside is then introduced through the cervical canal right upto the fundus and after positioning it by the guard, the inserter is withdrawn keeping the plunger in position. **Thus, the device is not pushed out of the tube but held in place by the plunger while the inserter is withdrawn (withdrawal technique Fig. 29.3).**

(5) The excess of the nylon thread beyond 2–3 cm from the external os is cut. Then the Allis forceps and the posterior vaginal speculum are taken off.

"No-touch" insertion technique includes : (i) Loading the IUD in the inserter without opening the sterile package. The loaded inserter is now taken out of the package without touching the distal end. (ii) Not to touch the vaginal wall and the speculum while introducing the loaded IUD inserter through the cervical canal.

Multiload Cu 250 : **Multiload 375** —The applicator with the device is just to be taken out of the sealed packet in a 'no-touch' method and **the same is pushed through the cervical canal upto the fundus of the uterus**. The applicator is then withdrawn (Fig. 29.4).

LNG-IUS : The arms of the device are released in the uterine cavity about 2 cm below the fundus. The details of insertion is to be followed as in the instruction package (Fig. 29.2D).

Instructions to the Patient

The possible symptoms of pain and slight vaginal bleeding should be explained. The patient should be advised to feel the thread periodically by the finger. The patient is checked after 1 month and then annually.

Complications

Immediate :

- **Cramp like pain** — It is transient but at times, severe and usually lasts for 1/2 to 1 hour. It is relieved by analgesic or antispasmodic drugs.
- **Syncopal attack** — Pain and syncopal attack are more often found in nulliparous or when the device is large enough to distend the uterine cavity.
- **Partial or complete perforation** — It is due to faulty technique of insertion but liable to be met with in lactational period when the uterus remains small and soft.

Remote :

- **Pain** — The pain is more or less proportionate to the degree of myometrial distension. A proper size of the device may minimise the pain.
- **Abnormal menstrual bleeding** — The excessive bleeding involves increased menstrual blood loss, prolongation of duration of period and intermenstrual bleeding. The patient may become anaemic and is of concern in one who is already anaemic. Iron supplement is advocated. **Menstrual loss is much less with the use of third generation IUDs (see p. 463)**.
- **Pelvic infection (PID)** — The risk of developing PID is 2-10 times greater amongst IUD users. The risk is more in the first 3 weeks. Infection with chlamydia and rarely with actinomyces are seen. Newer IUDs reduce the risk (see p. 463, 481).

Pain, abnormal uterine bleeding and PID are the principal factors related to its discontinuation (10-15%).

- **Spontaneous expulsion** — Spontaneous expulsion usually occurs within a few months following insertion, more commonly during the period, at times unnoticed by the patient. Failure to palpate the thread which could be felt before, is an urgent ground to report to the physician. **The expulsion rate is about 5 per cent.** The rate is, however, more following postabortal or puerperal insertions. The expulsion rate is markedly reduced in the successive years. Another device of appropriate size may be reintroduced and this is likely to be retained. **The newer IUDs have got less expulsion rate (see p. 463 and 481).**
- **Perforation of the uterus** — The incidence of uterine perforation is difficult to estimate but should not be more than 1 in 1000 insertions. Most perforations occur at the time of insertion but the migration may also occur following initial partial perforation with subsequent myometrial contraction. **It is however less common when the device is introduced by the withdrawal technique.**

Diagnosis : Non-visibility of the thread through the external os and the appearance of pelvic symptoms after a long asymptomatic period are suspicious. **Negative findings on exploration** of the uterine cavity by a probe is suggestive. **Ultrasonography** can detect the IUD in abdominal cavity and is better than radiography. **Straight X-ray,** anteroposterior and lateral view, following introduction of a radio-opaque probe (uterine sound) into the uterine cavity is conclusive. The device is found away from the opaque shadow placed in the uterine cavity, if it has perforated the uterine wall (Fig. 29.7).

Management : **Lippes loop** — As it is an open device made of inert material, it will cause no harm if left in the peritoneal cavity. Adhesions and intestinal injury are unlikely. But for psychologic reason or otherwise, **it is better to remove it by laparoscopy or by laparotomy**.

Copper device — A copper bearing device induces an intense local inflammatory reaction with adhesions with the surrounding structures. Thus, as soon as the diagnosis is made, it is to be removed by laparoscopy or laparotomy.

- **Pregnancy** — The pregnancy rate with the device *in situ* is about 2 per 100 women years of use. Lowest pregnancy rates are observed with Cu T 380A

(0.8–HWY) and LNG-IUS (0.2 – HWY). Should pregnancy occur with a device *in situ*, there is risk of ectopic pregnancy (1-2%). IUD can thus prevent an uterine but not an ectopic pregnancy. There is relative increased incidence of ovarian pregnancy specially with progestasert device. Third generation of IUDs like Cu T 380 A and LNG-IUS **give some amount of protection against an ectopic pregnancy**.

Management : **If the thread is visible** through the cervix it is best to remove the device. This will minimise such complications as abortion, sepsis and low birth weight baby. **However, if the thread is not visible** it is better to leave it alone after counselling with the patient about the risks involved in continuing pregnancy. The device is expected to be expelled spontaneously with the delivery of the after-births. There is no conclusive evidence of increased risk of fetal anomalies with copper devices.

Indications for removal

The indications for removal are — (1) Persistent excessive regular or irregular uterine bleeding. (2) Flaring up of salpingitis. (3) Perforation of the uterus. (4) IUD has come out of place (partial expulsion). (5) Pregnancy occurring with the device *in situ*. (6) Woman desirous of a baby. (7) Missing thread. (8) One year after menopause. (9) When effective lifespan of the device is over.

IUD removal is simple and can be done at any time. It is done by pulling the strings gently and slowly with a forceps.

Missing thread

The thread may not be visible through the cervical os due to — (a) Thread coiled inside (b) Thread torn through (c) Device expelled outside unnoticed by the patient (d) Device perforated the uterine wall and is lying in the peritoneal cavity. (e) Device pulled up by the growing uterus in pregnancy.

Methods of identification :

Pregnancy is to be excluded first —

1. **Ultrasonography** can detect the IUD either within the uterine cavity or in the peritoneal cavity (if perforated). It is preferred to radiography (Fig. 29.5).

2. **Hysteroscopy** can be used for direct visualisation of the uterine cavity and it could be removed simultaneously (Fig. 29.6).

3. **Sounding** the uterine cavity by a probe (Fig. 29.7).

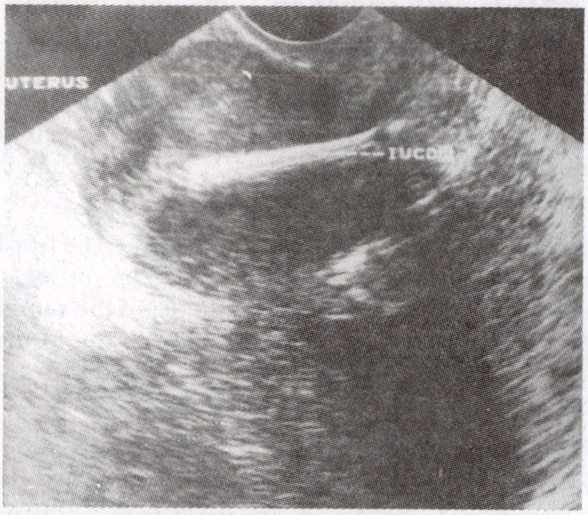

Fig. 29.5. Ultrasonogram showing the Cu T inside the uterine cavity. Thread was missing in this case

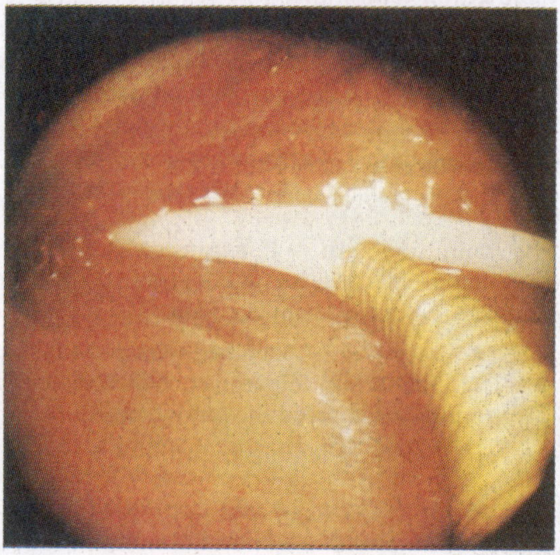

Fig. 29.6. Hysteroscopic view of IUCD in uterine cavity. The threads are coiled inside

4. If negative, **straight X-ray** after introducing radio-opaque probe (uterine sound) into the uterine cavity. This will not only reveal the presence or absence of the device but also its existence outside the uterine cavity (Fig. 29.7).

Removal

A. Device inside the uterine cavity : It can be removed by any of the following methods mentioned below :

(i) Specially designed blunt hook (Fig. 36.41).

(ii) Artery forceps (Fig. 36.28).

Table 29.7 : IUD (Cu devices and Hormone releasing IUDs)	
Advantages	**Disadvantages**
1. Inexpensive : Cu T-distributed free of cost through Government channel.	1. Require motivation.
2. Simplicity in techniques of insertion.	2. Limitation in its use.
3. Prolonged contraceptive protection after insertion (5-10 years) and suitable for the rural population of developing countries.	3. Adverse local reactions manifested by menstrual abnormalities, PID, pelvic pain and heavy periods. Beside effects are less with third generation of IUDs.
4. Systemic side effects are nil. Suitable for hypertensives, postpartum women and epileptics.	4. Risk of ectopic pregnancy.
5. Reversibility to fertility is prompt after removal.	*Failure rate — 0.1-2 (H W Y)*

(iii) Uterine curette (Fig. 36.13).

(iv) Hysteroscopically under direct vision (Fig. 29.6).

B. Outside the uterus but inside the abdominal cavity

(i) Laparoscopy (ii) Laparotomy (rarely).

Advantages of third generation of IUDs over the others (Cu T- 380A, Multiload 375 and Levonorgestrel IUS).

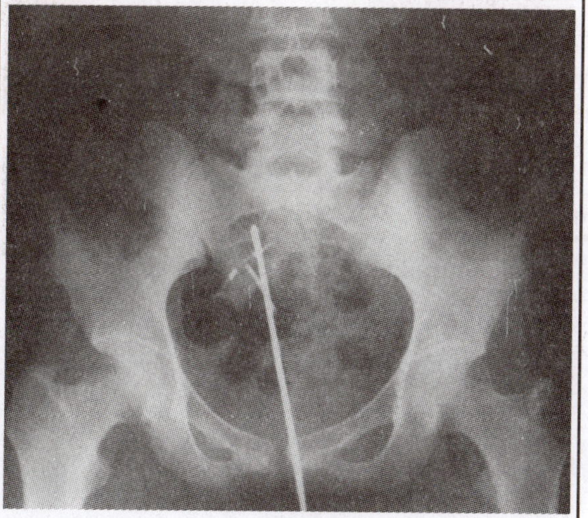

Fig. 29.7 : Straight X-ray of the pelvis with an uterine sound placed inside the uterine cavity — (a) the displaced IUCD seems inside the uterine cavity with AP view. Lateral view is needed for confirmation. [*By courtesy* : Dr. Swati Shirodkar, HOD, Dept. of Obst. Gyn., MGM Medical College, Aurangabad].

(1) Higher efficacy with lowest pregnancy rate (less than one per 100 women years).

(2) Longer duration of action (5–10 years).

(3) Low expulsion rate and fewer indications for medical removal.

(4) Risk of ectopic pregnancy is significantly reduced (Cu T –380A and LNG-IUS : 0.02 HWY).

(5) Risk of PID is reduced, anaemia is improved.

(6) **Non-contraceptive benefits specially with LNG-IUD** : (i) **Significant reduction** in menstrual blood loss, Menorrhagia, Dysmenorrhoea and Premenstrual Tension Syndrome (PMS). (ii) It can be used **in the treatment of** Endometrial hyperplasia, Adenomyosis, Uterine leiomyomas and Endometrial cancer. (iii) can be used **as an alternative to** hysterectomy for menorrhagia, DUB. (iv) it provides excellent benefits of **hormone replacement therapy** (HRT) when used over the transition years of reproduction to perimenopause. (Fibroplant p. 481).

Disadvantages of third generation of IUDs

- Expensive.
- LNG-IUS is not available through government channel in India currently.
- Malpositioning with long duration of use may cause pregnancy (failure) or expulsion.

SUMMARY OF IUD

Intrauterine contraceptive device is a widely acceptable reversible method of contraception for spacing of births. Amongst many, either a copper impregnated device like Cu T, multiload or a hormone releasing device like LNG-IUS is commonly used. **Its mode of action** is not clear. Probably, it produces nonspecific biochemical and histological changes in the endometrium and ionised copper has got spermolytic and gametotoxic effects. LNG-IUS induces uniform suppression of endometrium and produces very scanty cervial mucous. **It should not be used in newly married women or when any pelvic pathology is present**. The device can be introduced in the interval period or following abortion or following childbirth. The introduction is an outdoor procedure and can be done even by a trained paramedical personnel without anaesthesia. The technique employed is either "push-out" in Lippes loop or "withdrawal" in Cu T. **The immediate complications** include cramp-like pains or even syncopal attacks. **The delayed complications** include pelvic pain, menstrual irregularities, expulsion of the IUD or even perforation of the uterus. Complications are much less with third generation of IUDs. **The indications of its removal are**, missing threads, persistent pelvic pain, menorrhagia, pregnancy, displacement of the device and flaring up of pelvic infection. While Cu T 200 should be removed after 3-4 years, multiload 375 is replaced after 5 years, Cu T 380A after 10 years and LNG-IUS after 5 years. **The failure rate is** about 0.5-2 per HWY. Copper device can also be used as postcoital contraception and following synaecolysis.

STEROIDAL CONTRACEPTIONS

Enovid (norethynodrel 10 mg and menstranol 0.15 mg) was used in the first contraceptive field trial in Puerto Rico in 1956 by Pincus and his colleagues. Intensive pharmacological research and clinical trials were conducted during the following years to minimise the adverse effects of oestrogen without reducing the contraceptive efficacy, resulted in lowering the dose of oestrogen to a minimum of 20 μg or even 15 μg in the tablet.

COMBINED ORAL CONTRACEPTIVES (PILLS)

The combined oral steroidal contraceptives is the most effective reversible method of contraception. In the combination pill, **the commonly used progestins are either levonorgestrel or norethisterone or desogestrel and the oestrogens are principally confined to either ethinyl-oestradiol or menstranol** (3 methyl-ether of ethinyl-oestradiol). Currently 'lipid friendly', **third generation progestins,** namely desogestrel, gestodene and norgestimate are available. Some of the preparations available in the market are mentioned in the Table 29.8. Only Mala-N is distributed through government channel free of cost.

Mode of action

The probable mechanism of contraception are :

- **Inhibition of ovulation** — Both the hormones synergistically act on the hypothalamopituitary axis. The release of gonadotrophic releasing hormones from the hypothalamus is prevented through a negative feedback mechanism. There is thus no peak

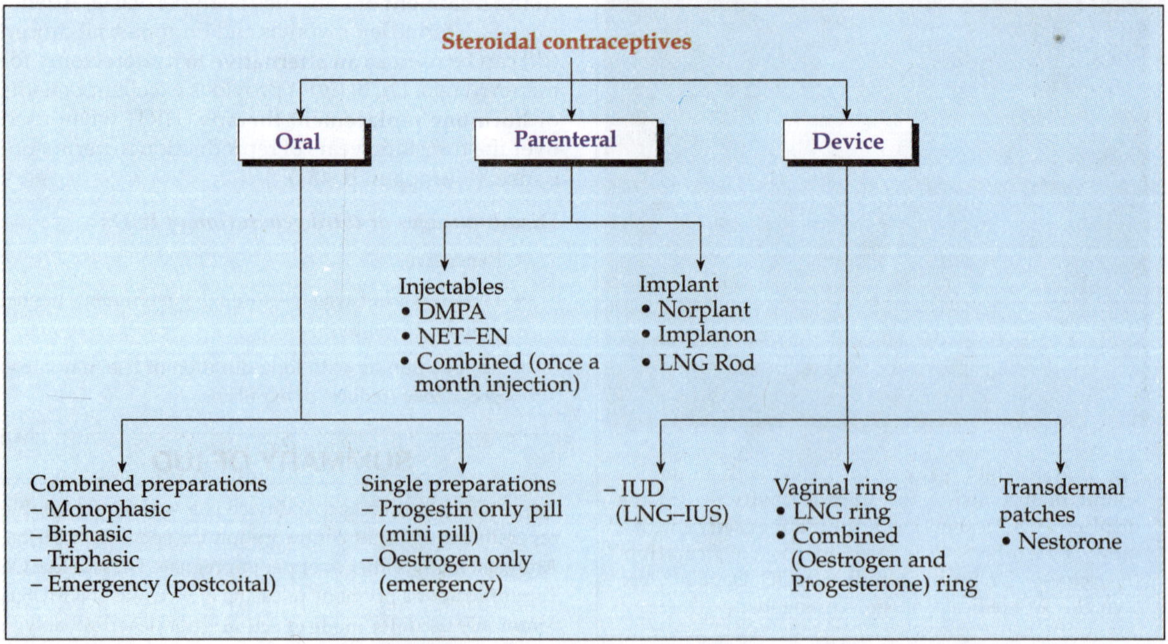

Table 29.8 : Some of the oral contraceptives and their composition

Commercial names	Composition		No. of tablets
	Progestins (mg)	Oestrogen (μg)	
1. Mala N (Govt. of India)	Levonorgestrel 0.15	Ethinyl oestradiol 30	21 + 7 iron tablets
2. Mala-D	Levonorgestrel 0.15	—do—	21 + 7 iron tablets
3. Femilon (Infar)	Desogestrel 0.15	Ethinyl oestradiol 20	21
4. Yasmin (Schering)	Drospirenone 3 mg (p. 509)	Ethinyl oestradiol 30	21

Depending on the amount of ethinyl oestradiol (E) and the types of progestin (P) used, pills are defined as : **1st generation** — with E 50 μg or more; **2nd generation** — with E 30-35 μg and P as levonorgestrel or norgestimate; **3rd generation** — with E 20-30 μg and P as desogestrel or gestodene. Low dose pills have E less than 50 μg.

release of FSH and LH from the anterior pituitary. So follicular growth is either not initiated or if initiated, recruitment does not occur.

- **Producing static endometrial hypoplasia** — There is stromal oedema, decidual reaction and regression of the glands.
- **Alteration of the character of the cervical mucus** (thick, viscid and scanty) so as to prevent sperm penetration.
- **Probably interferes** with motility and secretions of the fallopian tubes.

Thus, even though accidental breakthrough ovulation occurs, the other mechanisms prevent conception.

Oestrogen inhibits FSH rise and prevents follicular growth. It is also useful for better cycle control and to prevent breakthrough bleeding.

Progestin : Anovulatory effect is primarily by inhibiting LH surge. **It is also helpful to counteract the adverse effects of oestrogen on the endometrium** (endometrial hyperplasia and heavy withdrawal bleeding). It is also responsible for changes in the cervical mucus (vide supra).

Selection of the Patient

History and general examination should be thorough, taking special care to screen cases for contraindications (headache, migraine). Examination of the breasts for any nodules, weight and blood pressure are to be noted. **Pelvic examination** to exclude cervical pathology, is mandatory. Pregnancy must be excluded. **Cervical cytology** to exclude abnormal cells, is to be done. Thus, any woman of reproductive age group without any systemic disease and contraindications listed, is a suitable candidate for combined pill therapy. Growth and development of the pubertal and sexually active girls are not affected by the use of "pill".

How to prescribe a pill

Instruction : **New users** should normally start their pill packet **on day one of their cycle**. One tablet is to be taken daily preferably at bed time for consecutive 21 days. It is continued for 21 days and then have a seven days break, with this routine there is contraceptive protection from the first pill. Next pack should be started on the eighth day, irrespective of bleeding (same day of the week, the pill finished). **Thus, a simple regime of "3 weeks on and 1 week off" is to be followed**. Packing of 28 tablets, there should be no break between packs. Seven of the pills are dummies and contain either iron or vitamin preparations. However, a woman can start the pill up to day 5 of the bleeding. In that case she is advised to use a condom for the next 7 days. The pill should be started on the day after abortion. Following childbirth in non-lactating woman, it is started after 3 weeks and in lactating woman it is to be withheld for 6 months (see later in the chapter).

Follow up : The patient should be examined after 3 months, then after 6 months and then yearly. **The patient above the age 35 should be checked more frequently**. At each visit, any adverse symptoms are to be noted. Examination of the breasts, weight and blood pressure recording and pelvic examination including cervical cytology, are to be done and compared with the previous records.

Missed pills : Normally there is return of pituitary and ovarian follicular activity during the pill-free interval (PFI) of 7 days. Breakthrough ovulation may occur in about 20 per cent cases during the time. Lengthening of PFI due to omissions, malabsorption, or vomiting either at the start or at the end of a packet, increases the risk of breakthrough ovulation and therefore pregnancy.

Management : When a woman forgets to take **one pill** (late upto 24 hours), she should take the missed pill at once and continue the rest as schedule. There is nothing to worry.

When she **misses two pills** in the first week (days 1-7), she should take 2 pills on each of the next 2 days and then continue the rest as schedule. Extra precaution has to be taken for next 7 days either by using a condom or by avoiding sex.

If 2 pills are missed in the third week (days 15-21) or if more than two active pills are missed at any time, another form of contraception should be used as back up for next 7 days as mentioned above. She should start the next pack without a break.

If she misses any of the **7 inactive pills** (in a 28 day pack only) she should throw away the missed pills. She should take the remaining pills one a day and start the new pack as usual.

Drug interactions : Effectiveness of some drugs (Aspirin, oral anticoagulants, oral hypoglycaemics) are decreased and that for some other drugs (beta blockers, corticosteroids, diazepam, aminophylline) are increased by oral contraceptives.

Additional Contraception

To ensure cent per cent efficacy, additional mechanical contraceptives (usually condom) are to be used in the following circumstances :

(1) **When broad spectrum antibiotics like** ampi-

MEDICAL ELIGIBILITY CRITERIA FOR CONTRACEPTIVE USE (WHO/FRM/FPP—1996)

INDICATIONS OF COCs	CONTRAINDICATIONS OF COMBINED ORAL CONTRACEPTIVES (COCs)	
No restriction of use (WHO Category–1)	**Relative (WHO Category–2 and 3)**	**Absolute (WHO Category–4)**
• Age : Menarche to 40 years. • Postabortion. • Anaemia (iron deficiency, Malaria) • HIV or AIDS (additional to condom use). • GTN following normal hCG level. • History of ectopic pregnancy. • Endometriosis, Uterine fibroid, Ovarian or endometrial cancer. • Dysmenorrhoea, DUB. • PID. • Epilepsy. • Thyroid disease. • Varicose veins. • Tuberculosis. • Benign breast disease.	**A. WHO Category–2 : (Advantages outweigh the risks)** • Age ≥ 40 years. • Smoker < 35 years. • History of jaundice. • Mild hypertension. • Gallbladder disease. • Diabetes. • Sickle cell disease. • Headache. • Cancer cervix or CIN. **B. WHO Category–3 : (Risks outweigh the advantages)** • Unexplained vaginal bleeding. • Hyperlipidaemia. • Liver tumours (Benign). • Breastfeeding (postpartum 6 weeks to 6 months). • Heavy smoker (> 20 cigarettes/day). • Past breast cancer.	**(A) Circulatory diseases (Past or present)** • Arterial or venous thrombosis. • Severe hypertension. • History of stroke. • Valvular heart disease, Ischaemic heart disease. • Diabetes with vascular complications. • Migraine with focal neurologic symptoms. **(B) Diseases of the liver** • Active liver disease. • Liver adenoma, carcinoma. **(C) Others** • Pregnancy. • Breastfeeding (postpartum 6 weeks). • Major surgery or prolonged immobilisation. • Oestrogen dependent neoplasms, e.g. breast cancer.

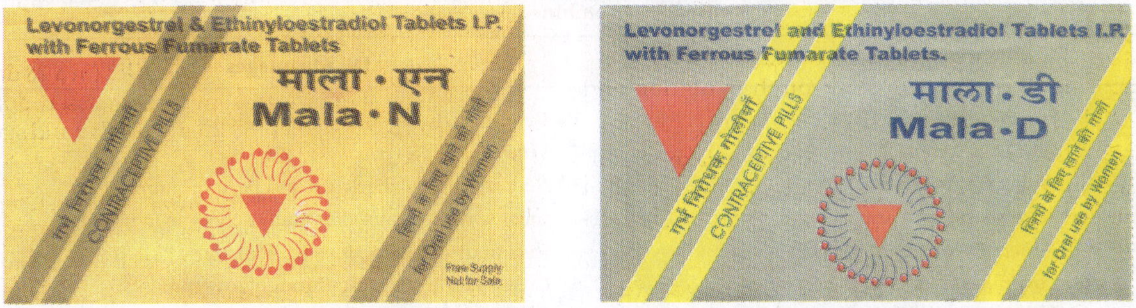

Fig. 29.8. Some commonly used oral contraceptives

cillin, amoxicillin, tetracycline, doxycycline are used — as they impair the absorption of ethinyl oestradiol.

(2) When enzyme inducing drugs are used, e.g. (a) barbiturates (b) all antiepileptic drugs except sodium valproate and clonazepam (c) rifampicin (d) ketoconazole (e) griseofulvin (f) ritonavir (g) nevirapine—under such circumstances high dose preparations (ethinyl oestradiol of 50 µg or more) are to be used to counter balance the increased liver metabolism.

Indications for withdrawal

While the majority tolerates the combined pill, in some susceptible individuals, gross adverse symptoms develop which necessitate its withdrawal. **The indications for withdrawal of the pill are** — (1) Severe migraine. (2) Visual or speech disturbances. (3) Sudden chest pain. (4) Unexplained fainting atack or acute vertigo. (5) Severe cramps and pains in legs. (6) Excessive weight gain. (7) Severe depression. (8) Prior to surgery (it should be withheld for at least 6 weeks to minimise postoperative vascular complications). (9) Patient wanting pregnancy.

How long can the pill be continued ?

Potential benefits of pills are greater when compared to risks, in a well-selected individual. A woman who does not smoke and has no other risk factor for cardiovascular disease, may continue the pill (with careful monitoring) until the age of fifty. This offers the dual advantages of effective contraception and hormone replacement therapy. However, for spacing of births, use of 3 to 5 years is considered enough and safe.

General and metabolic effects of combined oral contraceptives

The combined preparations containing oestrogen and progestin have got a wide range of metabolic activities which affect almost all the systems of the body. The changes are almost similar to those of pregnancy and almost completely revert back to normal after the drug is withdrawn. **The effects are related either to the oestrogen (OGN) or to the progestin (PGN) or to both (OGN + PGN) of the compounds**.

BENEFITS OF COMBINED ORAL CONTRACEPTIVES (COCs)

(a) **Contraceptive benefits** : (i) Protection against unwanted pregnancy (failure rate – 0.1 per 100 women year). (ii) Convenient to use. (iii) Not intercourse related. (iv) Reversibility. (v) Improving maternal and child health care.

(b) **Non-contraceptive benefits** : *Improvement of menstrual abnormalities* — (1) Regulation of menstrual cycle. (2) Reduction of dysmenorrhoea (40%). (3) Reduction of menorrhagia (50%). (4) Reduction of premenstrual tension syndrome (PMS). (5) Reduction of Mittelschmerz's syndrome. (6) Protection against iron-deficiency anaemia. **Protection against health disorders** — (7) Pelvic inflammatory disease (thick cervical mucous). (8) Ectopic pregnancy. (9) Endometriosis. (10) Fibroid uterus. (11) Hirsutism and acne. (12) Functional ovarian cysts. (13) Benign breast disease. (14) Osteopenia and postmenopausal osteoporotic fractures. (15) Autoimmune disorders of thyroid. (16) Rheumatoid arthritis. **Prevention of malignancies**—(17) Endometrial cancer (50%). (18) Ovarian cancer (40%). (19) Colorectal cancer (40%).

ADVERSE EFFECTS OF COMBINED ORAL CONTRACEPTIVES

The minor complications or ailments are —

Table 29.9 : Combined preparations

Advantages	Disadvantages
1. Highly effective.	1. Requires education and motivation.
2. Good cycle control.	2. Limitation in its use.
3. Well-tolerated in majority.	3. Requires initial check up and periodic supervision.
4. Additional non-contraceptive — benefits are many (p. 467).	4. Inconvenience caused by daily schedule in its use.
5. Low dose pill with 'lipid friendly' progestins further reduces the risk.	5. Risk of drug interactions (p. 466).
6. Reversibility rate is prompt.	6. Costly but free supply through government channel (Mala-N) *Failure rate—0.1 (HWY)*

• **Nausea, vomiting, headache (OGN) and leg cramps (PGN)** — These are transient and often subside following continuous use for 2-3 cycles.

• **Mastalgia (OGN + PGN)** — Heaviness or even tenderness in the breast is often transient.

• **Weight gain (PGN)** — Though progestins have got an anabolic effect due to its chemical relation to testosterone, use of low dose COCs does not cause any increase in weight.

• **Chloasma (OGN) and acne (PGN)** are annoying for cosmetic reasons. Low dose oral contraceptives improves acne as levonorgestrel preparations are less androgenic.

• **Menstrual abnormalities** — (a) ***Breakthrough bleeding (BTB)*** is commonly due to subthreshold blood level of hormones. Other causes of breakthrough bleeding in pill takers are (i) disturbance of drug absorption — diarrhoea, vomiting (ii) use of enzyme inducing drugs (mentioned earlier), missing pills, use of low dose pills (iii) pregnancy complications (miscarriage) (iv) diseases—cervical ectopy or carcinoma. Usually it settles after 3-4 cycles when there is no other specific cause for BTB. Exogenous oestrogen (conjugated oestrogen 1.25 mg or oestradiol 2 mg) given daily for 7 days can control the bleeding. Phasic pill preparation may be used. A pill containing higher dose of oestrogen, with different progestin could be helpful. (b) **Hypomenorrhoea (PGN)** — It is of little significance although disturbing to the patient. It is due to the local endometrial changes. (c) **Menorrhagia (OGN)** — It is usually pre-existing and use of compounds with progestin preponderance is helpful. (d) **Amenorrhoea (OGN or PGN)** — Post pill amenorrhoea of more than 6 months duration occurs in less than 1 per cent cases. The association is casual not causal. It is usually more in women with pre-existing functional menstrual disorders. Spontaneous resumption of menstruation occurs in majority of cases after a varying interval. A refractory case should be investigated as any other case of secondary amenorrhoea.

• **Libido** : Libido may be diminished **(PGN)** probably due to dryness of the vagina. More often, it may either remain static or at times, may even increase due to loss of fear of pregnancy.

• **Leucorrhoea** : It may be due to excessive cervical mucus secretion **(OGN)** or due to increased preponderancy of monilial infection **(OGN + PGN)**.

The major complications are :

• **Depression** : Low dose oestrogen preparations are not associated with depression.

• **Hypertension (OGN)** : Current low dose COC_S rarely cause significant hypertension. Pre-existing hypertension is likely to be aggravated. The effect on blood pressure is thought to involve the renin-angiotensin system. There is marked increase in plasma angiotensinogen. The changes however reverse back to normal 3-6 months after stoppage of pill.

• **Vascular complications (OGN)**:(a) *Venous thromboembolism (VTE)* — The overall risk is to the extent of 4-6 times more than the non-users. Pre-existing hypertension, diabetes, obesity and elderly patient (over 35 specially with smoking habits) are some of the important risk factors. Ethinyl oestradiol in preference to mestranol and the reduction of the dose of oestrogen compound to 20 μg in the pill markedly reduce the incidence.

Current studies estimate the annual number of nonfatal VTE per 100,000 users as : no COC use = 5, second generation COC = 15, COC containing desogestrel and gestodene = 30, pregnancy = 60. The absolute risk is very small compared to pregnancy. Carriers of factor V Leiden mutation have higher risk (8 fold) and use of COC increases the risk further (4 fold). (b) Arterial thrombosis — The high risk factors for myocardial infarction and stroke (ischaemic and haemorrhagic) are hypertension, smoking habit, age over 35 and high dose pills. COC containing less than 50 mg ethinyl oestradiol do not increase the risk of arterial thrombosis in the low risk women.

In the third world countries, cardiovascular risk factors such as smoking and high blood cholesterol are less prevalent specially in the vast rural populations. Genetic thrombophilia (factor V Leiden) is rare in non-caucasians. As such, the vascular complications are relatively unimportant.

- **Cholestatic jaundice** — Susceptibility is increased in women with previous history of idiopathic recurrent jaundice in pregnancy or hepatitis.

- **Neoplasia (OGN)** — Combined oral contraceptives (COCs) reduce the risk of ovarian (40% ↓) and endometrial (50% ↓) carcinoma. This protective effect persists for 10-15 years even after stopping the method following a use of 6 month to 1 year. No major association has been established between breast carcinoma and COC. Conclusions regarding association of COC and cervical carcinoma are not definite. However, pill users should have regular **cervical cytology screening. No increased risk of hepatocellular adenomas** have been found with low dose preparations. It gives protection against benign cystic breast disease and cystic ovaries.

General Metabolic Effects

- **Carbohydrate (PGN)** : Progestins impair glucose tolerance promoting insulin resistance and hyperglycaemia. This is particularly noticeable in preparations containing 150 μg or more levonorgestrel. Low dose COCs have no effect on insulin and glucose changes.

- **Protein (OGN)** : Oestrogen has got some stimulatory effect on the hepatic secretion of many proteins. The level of sex hormone binding globulin (SHBG) is increased.

- **Lipid (OGN)** : Plasma lipids and lipoproteins are increased. Total cholesterol and triglycerides are increased. Low dose oestrogen increases HDL cholesterol and decreases LDL cholesterol thereby exerts its protective effect against atherosclerosis. Progestins however decrease HDL cholesterol and increase LDL cholesterol thereby promote heart disease. Preparations with more selective, lipid friendly and third generation progestins namely desogestrel, gestodene or norgestimate, HDL level is some what elevated. Thus they have got very small atherogenic risk.

- **Vitamins and minerals** : Vitamin B_6, B_{12}, folic acid, calcium, manganese, zinc and ascorbic acid levels are decreased while Vit A and Vit K levels are increased.

Effects on Organs

- **Hypothalamopituitary axis** : Both FSH and LH levels remain low as found in early proliferative phase and remain throughout the cycle at such static low level.

- **Ovary** : Ovarian function remains quiescent with occasional evidence of breakthrough ovulation. There is evidence of fibrosis, progressive wastage of unripe ova with advancing age without evidence of corpus luteum. The endogenous hormones remain static at a low level.

- **Endometrium (PGN)** — Stromal oedema, decidual reaction and glandular exhaustion out of depletion of glycogen are more or less constant findings.

- **Cervix (PGN + OGN)** — Increased glandular hyperplasia and downgrowth of the endocervical epithelium beyond the squamocolumnar junction gives the appearance of an ectopy. There is evidence of cervical epithelial dysplasia or even carcinoma-*in-situ* in susceptible individuals (OGN). Cervical mucus becomes thick, viscid and scanty (PGN).

- **Uterus (OGN)**—Uterus may be slightly enlarged. The associated fibroid, if any, may undergo the same changes as those observed in pregnancy.

- **Vagina (PGN)**—Cytohormonal study reflects the picture of early luteal phase.

- **Other organs** : (i) *Liver* — The liver functions are depressed. (ii) *Gastrointestinal tract* — There is increased incidence of mesenteric vein thrombosis and ulcerative colitis. (iii) *Urinary* — There is increased incidence of urinary tract infection but is probably related to increase in sexual activity.

Effects on reproduction

- **Ovulation returns within 3 months of withdrawal of the drug in 90 per cent cases.**

- **Risk to fetus** : When COC is taken during early pregnancy inadvertently there is no greater risk of significant congenital anomaly. Risk of congenital abnormality in general is 2-3 per cent.

- **Lactation (OGN + PGN)** : Lactation is probably affected by a reduction in the milk production and also by alteration of the quality of the milk (reduction of protein and fat content). Moreover, significant amount of the steroids are ingested by the infant, the effects are as yet unknown. Mini-pill is a better alternative for the breastfeeders.

Triphasic Formulations of Combined Oral Pills

In these preparations, the hormonal doses of each compound vary over the course of the cycle. Minimum doses are provided for contraceptive effect in the early part of the cycle and slightly higher doses later in the cycle to prevent breakthrough bleeding. **It is an attempt to minimise undesirable side effects on lipid metabolism.** This is due to low total amount of steroids and the balanced oestrogen-progestogen relationship.

Triquilar tablets (Shering-AG) — First 6 tablets contain 0.05 mg levonorgestrel and 30 mg of ethinyl oestradiol; next 5 tablets contain 0.075 mg levonorgestrel and 40 mg ethinyl oestradiol; the last 10 tablets contain 0.125 mg levonorgestrel and 30 mg ethinyl oestradiol. It has to be taken like conventional 'pills'.

PROGESTIN ONLY CONTRACEPTION

PROGESTIN ONLY PILL (POP/MINI PILL)

POP is devoid of any oestrogen compound. It contains very low dose of a progestin in any one of the following form — Levonorgestrel 75 µg, norethisterone 350 µg, desogestrel 75 µg, lynestrenol 500 µg or norgestrel 30 µg. **It has to be taken daily from the first day of the cycle.**

Mechanism of action: It works mainly by making cervical mucous thick and viscous, thereby prevents sperm penetration. Endometrium becomes atrophic, so blastocyst implantation is also hindered. In about 2 per cent of cases ovulation is inhibited.

How to prescribe mini pill: The first pill has to be taken on the first day of the cycle and then continuously. It has to be taken **regularly and at the same time of the day**. There must be no break between the packs. **Delay in intake** for more than 3 hours, the woman should have missed pill immediately and the next one as schedule. Extra precaution has to be taken for next 2 days (see above).

Advantages: (1) Side effects attributed to oestrogen in the combined pill are totally eliminated. (2) No adverse effect on lactation and hence can be suitably prescribed in lactating women and as such it is often called "Lactation Pill". (3) Easy to take as there is no "On and Off" regime. (4) It may be prescribed in patient having hypertension, fibroid, diabetes, epilepsy, smoking and history of thromboembolism. (5) Reduces the risk of PID and endometrial cancer.

Disadvantages: (1) There may be acne, mastalgia, headache, breakthrough bleeding, or at times amenorrhoea in about 20-30 per cent cases. (2) All the side effects, attributed to progestins may be evident. (3) Simple cysts of the ovary may be seen, but they do not require any surgery. (4) Failure rate is about 0.5-2 per 100 women years of use. Failure is more in young compared to women over 40.

Contraindications: (i) Pregnancy, (ii) unexplained vaginal bleeding, (iii) recent breast cancer, (iv) arterial disease.

INJECTABLE PROGESTINS

The preparations commonly used are depomedroxy progesterone acetate (DMPA) and norethisterone enanthate (NET-EN). Both are administered intramuscularly within 5 days of the cycle. DMPA in a dose of 150 mg every three months or 300 mg every six months; NET-EN in a dose of 200 mg given at two-monthly intervals.

Mechanism of action: (1) Inhibition of ovulation — by suppressing the mid cycle LH peak (2) cervical mucous becomes thick and viscid thereby prevents sperm penetration (3) Endometrium is atrophic preventing blastocyst implantation.

Advantages: (1) It eliminates regular medication as imposed by oral pill. (2) It can be used safely during lactation. It probably increases the milk secretion without altering its composition. (3) No oestrogen related side effects. (4) Menstrual symptoms, e.g. menorrhagia, dysmenorrhoea are reduced. (5) Protective against endometrial cancer. (6) Can be used as an interim contraception before vasectomy becomes effective. (7) Reduction in PID, endometriosis, ectopic pregnancy and ovarian cancer.

Disadvantages: **Failure rate** for DMPA – (0-0.3) (HWY). There is chance of irregular bleeding and occasional phase of amenorrhoea. Return of fertility after their discontinuation is usually delayed for several months (4-8 months). However, with NET-EN the return of fertility is quicker. Loss of bone mineral density has been observed with long-term use of depot provera. However, it is reversible. **Other side effects are**: weight gain and headache.

Contraindications: Women with high-risk factors for osteoporosis and the others are same as in POP (see above).

IMPLANT

Norplant is a progestin only delivery system containing levonorgestrel. It is a long-term (up to 5 years) reversible contraception. It consists of six flexible closed capsules (made of polydimethyl siloxane 34 mm × 2.4 mm) and each contains 36 mg of levonorgestrel. It initially releases 85 µg and later on reduced to 30 µg levonorgestrel per day over 5 years (Fig. 29.9).

Mechanism of action: It inhibits ovulation in 90 per cent of the cycles for the first year. It has got its supplementary effect on endometrium (atrophy) and cervical mucous (thick) as well.

Insertion: The capsules are inserted subdermally, in the inner aspect of the nondominant arm, 6-8 cm above the

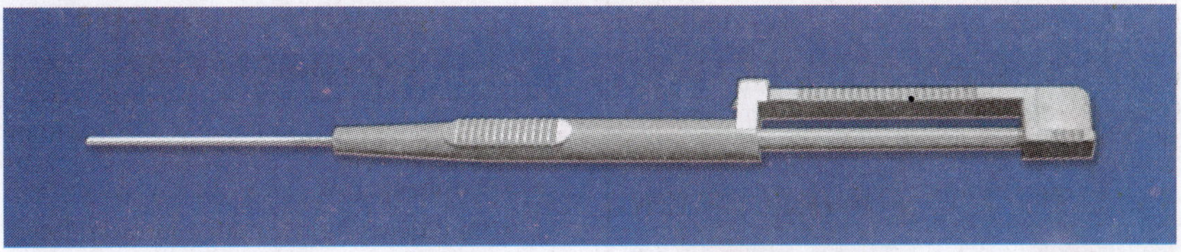

Fig. 29.9. Single implant rod — Implanon

elbow fold. It is done under local anaesthetic. It is ideally inserted on day one of a menstrual cycle, immediately after abortion and three weeks after postpartum.

Removal : Norplant should be removed within 5 years of insertion. Loss of contraceptive action is immediate (Fig. 29.9).

Advantages are the same as with DMPA. Others are (i) Highly effective for long-term use and rapidly reversible. (ii) suited for women who have completed their family but do not desire permanent sterilisation.

Efficacy is comparable to the combined pills. Failure rate is 0.1 per 100 woman years. This safe and effective method is considered as 'reversible sterilisation'.

Drawbacks : Frequent irregular menstrual bleeding, spotting and amenorrhoea are common. Difficulty in removal is felt occasionally. **Contraindications** are similar to POP (see above).

Implanon : Single implant rod (4 cm long), containing 68 mg of 3-keto-desogestrel (etonogestrel) is used. It releases the hormone about 67 μg, reduced to 30 μg per day over 3 years. Use of single rod makes implanon easier for insertion and removal (Fig. 29.9). It is inserted within D5 of the cycle. Efficacy of implanon is extremely high with Pearl indices of 0.01. This is an alternative to sterilisation and a rapidly reversible procedure. Side effects and contraindications are the same as that of norplant.

EMERGENCY CONTRACEPTION
(SYN : POSTCOITAL CONTRACEPTION)

- **Hormones**
- **IUD**
- **Anti-progesterone**
- **Others**

Indications of emergency contraception : Unprotected intercourse, condom rupture, missed pill, delay in taking POP for more than 3 hours, sexual assault or rape and first time intercourse, as known to be always unplanned. Risk of pregnancy following a single act of unprotected coitus around the time of ovulation is 8 per cent.

Hormones (Table 29.10)

Morning-after Pill : This is not true contraception, but has rightly been called interception, preventing conception in case of accidental unprotected exposure around the time of ovulation. **Any of the following drugs is used** — ethinyl-oestradiol 2.5 mg, premarin (conjugated oestrogen) 15 mg. The drug is taken orally twice daily for 5 days, beginning soon after the exposure but not later than 72 hours.

Combined hormonal regimen (Yuzpe method) is equally effective. Two tablets of Ovral (0.25 mg levo-norgestrel and 50 μg ethinyl oestradiol) should be taken as early as possible after coitus (< 72 hours) and two more tablets are to be taken 12 hours later.

Table 29.10
Postcoital contraceptives

Drug	Dose	Pregnancy rate (%)
Levonorgestrel	0.75 mg stat and after 12 hours	0–1
Ethinyl oestradiol 50 μg + Norgestrel 0.25 mg	2 tab stat and 2 after 12 hours	0–2
Conjugated oestrogen	15 mg BD × 5 days	0–0.6
Ethinyl oestradiol	2.5 mg BD × 5 days	0–0.6
Mifepristone	100 mg single dose	0–0.6
Copper IUDs	Insertion within 5 days	0–0.1

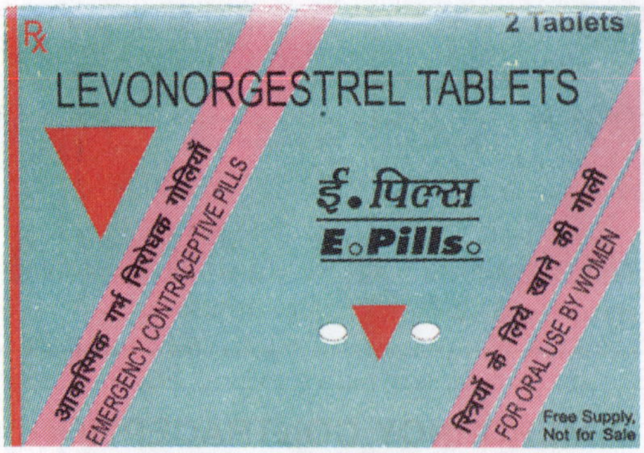

Fig. 29.10. Levonorgestrel pill

Levonorgestrel (E. Pills) 0.75 mg, two doses given at 12 hours interval, is very successful and without any side effects. The two tablets (1.50 mg) can be taken as a single dose also. The first dose should be taken within 72 hours (see Fig. 29.10).

No fetal adverse effects has been observed when there is failure of emergency contraception. However, induced abortion should be offered to the patient, if the method fails.

Mode of action : The exact mechanism of action of hormonal preparations remains unclear. The following are the possibilities :

- Ovulation is either prevented or delayed when the drug is taken in the beginning of the cycle.
- Fertilisation is interfered.
- Implantation is prevented (except E. Pills) as the endometrium is rendered unfavourable.
- Interferes with the function of corpus luteum or may cause luteolysis.

Drawbacks : Nausea and vomiting are much more intense with oestrogen use. Antiemetic (meclizine) should be prescribed.

Copper IUD : Introduction of a copper IUD within a maximum period of 5 days can prevent conception following accidental unprotectred exposure. This prevents implantation. Failure rate is about 0-1 per cent. Postcoital contraception is only employed as an emergency measure and is not effective if used as a regular method of contraception.

Anti-progesterone : Anti-progesterone (RU 486-Mifepristone) binds competitively to progesterone receptors and nullifies the effect of endogenous progesterone.

Dose : A single dose of 100 mg is to be taken within 17 days of intercourse. Implantation is prevented due to its anti-progesterone effect. Pregnancy rate is 0–0.6 per cent.

SUMMARY OF ORAL CONTRACEPTIVES

- **Combined pills**
- **Triphasic pill**
- **Emergency (postcoital) contraception**
- **Mini pill.**

• **Conventional combined preparations**—The widely used oral contraceptives consist of tablets containing oestrogen and progestin compounds. It is the most effective and reversible method of contraception. Each tablet usually contains 30 mg of ethinyl oestradiol and 1 mg of norethisterone or 0.3 mg norgestrel. **It has got trigger action**—(a) inhibition of ovulation, (b) production of static endometrial hypoplasia and (c) alteration of the character of the cervical mucus. **Its use is absolutely contraindicated in cases** with circulatory diseases, liver diseases, severe migraine and oestrogen dependent tumour. The pill should be started from the day one of a cycle and continued as "three weeks on and one week off" regime. Periodic check up is essential specially when prescribed in women above the age of 35. **The pill should be withdrawn** if complications arise such as severe migraine, chest pain, visual disturbances, etc.

The beneficial effects are relief of dysmenorrhoea, premenstrual tension, endometriosis, acne, hirsutism and lesser chance of ectopic and PID. It gives protection against ovarian and endometrial carcinomas.

The minor side effects are—nausea, vomiting, breakthrough bleeding, mastalgia, leg cramp, weight gain, hypomenorrhoea or amenorrhoea. The major complications are rare and include depression, hypertension and thromboembolic manifestations. The failure rate is about 0.1 per HWY.

• **Triphasic pill**—It has got lesser amount of steroids than the conventional monophasic tablets. There is lesser effect on lipid metabolism.

• **Emergency**—Following rape or accidental exposure, either levonorgestrel, 0.75 mg two doses at 12 hours interval or two tablets of the COC preparations are to be taken soon after coitus and two more tablets after 12 hours are quite effective in preventing conception. The first dose should be taken within 72 hours.

• **Mini pill**—The pill contains low doses of progestin—norgestrel 30 mg, levonorgestrel 75 µg or desogestrel 75 µg. It should be taken daily and can be safely prescribed during lactation. It is best suited where oestrogen is contraindicated.

STERILISATION

Permanent surgical contraception, also called voluntary sterilisation, is a surgical method whereby the reproductive function of an individual male or female is purposefully and permanently destroyed. **The operation done on male is vasectomy and that on the female is tubal occlusion, or tubectomy.**

Couple counselling

Couple must be counselled adequately before any permanent procedure is undertaken. Individual procedure must be discussed in terms of benefits, risks, side effects, failure rate and reversibility.

VASECTOMY (Fig. 29.11)

It is a permanent sterilisation operation done in the male where a segment of vas deferens of both the sides are resected and the cut ends are ligated.

Advantages: (1) The operative technique is simple and can be performed by one with minimal training. (2) The operation can be done as an outdoor procedure or in a mass camp even in remote villages. (3) Complications — immediate or late are few. (4) Failure rate is minimal — 0.15 per cent and there is a fair chance of success of reversal anastomosis operation (50%). (5) The overall expenditure is minimal in terms of equipment, hospital stay and doctor's training.

Drawbacks: (1) Additional contraceptive protection is needed for about 2-3 months following operations, i.e. till the semen becomes free of sperm. (2) Frigidity or impotency when occurs is mostly psychological.

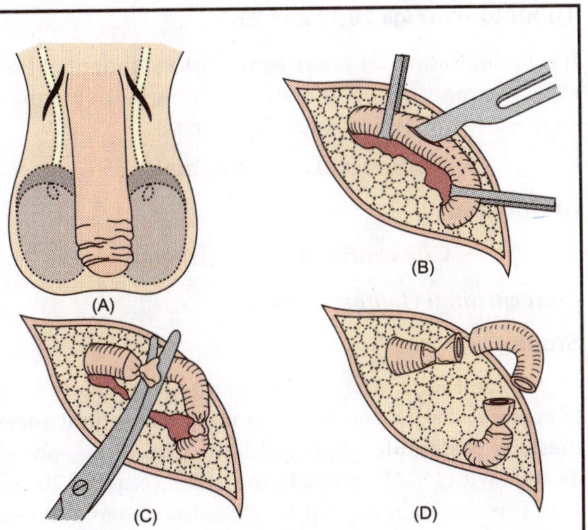

Fig. 29.11. Steps of vasectomy operation

Selection of candidates : **Sexually active and psychologically adjusted husband having the desired number of children is an ideal one.** Any misconception about the fear of castration, loss of hormones and impotency are to be removed by sympathetic conversation. Eczema or scabies on the scrotal area is a temporary contraindication. In the presence of hydrocele or inguinal hernia, vasectomy can be done only along with operative correction of these conditions.

Technique

Written consent of the person is a must and the surgeon should be convinced about the family structure of the couple. The operation is done as an outdoor procedure or in the camp. Premedication is usually not necessary. The local area is shaved and an antiseptic dressing is given with Savlon. **Full surgical asepsis has** to be maintained during operation.

The vas is palpated at the base of the scrotum and is lifted up by the thumb and index finger of the left hand. The area over the vas and the adjoining part are infiltrated with 1 per cent lignocaine (5-10 cc). Small vertical incision $1/2''$–$3/4''$ is given over the vas. After dissecting the dartos muscle and cutting the sheath, the vas is reached and is separated from the surrounding structure and lifted up by an Allis forceps. The vas is ligated at two places 1 cm apart by No. '00' chromic catgut and the segment of the vas in between the ligatures is cut. Haemostasis is secured and the skin is sutured by interrupted catgut. The same procedure is repeated on the other side. A scrotal suspensory bandage is worn. The patient is allowed to go home after $1/2$ an hour. If facilities are available, histological examination of the excised segment of the vas is done for confirmation (Fig. 29.11).

Advices : Antibiotic (Inj. Penidure LA 6 IM) is administered as a routine and an analgesic is prescribed. Weight lifting, heavy work or cycling is restricted for about two weeks, while usual activities can be resumed forthwith. For check up, the patient should report back after 1 week, or earlier, if complication arises. **Additional contraceptive should be used for 2-3 months.**

Precaution : **The man does not become sterile soon after the operation** as the semen is stored in the distal part of the vas channels for a varying period of about 2-3 months. **It requires about 20 ejaculations to empty the stored semen.** Semen should be examined once a month and then again at two months and **if the two consecutive semen analyses show an absence of**

spermatozoa, the man is declared as sterile. Till then, additional contraceptive (condom or DMPA) should be advised.

Complications

• *Immediate* — (1) Wound sepsis which may lead to scrotal cellulitis or abscess. (2) Scrotal haematoma.

• *Remote* — (1) Frigidity or impotency — It is mostly psychologic in origin. (2) Sperm granuloma is due to inflammatory reaction to sperm leakage. This can be prevented by cauterisation or fulguration of the cut ends. (3) Increase in sperm agglutinin in the circulation. (4) Spontaneous recanalisation.

No-scalpel vasectomy: It is performed under local anaesthetic. Stretched skin over the vas (as described above) is punctured with the sharp pointed end of a forceps instead of using a scalpel. Then the hole is increased and the vas is dissected out by using the tips of the forceps. The rest of the steps are as described above. No skin suturing is needed. It takes less time, helps faster recovery due to less tissue injury. However, it needs much skill on the part of the surgeon.

Percutaneous Vasocclusion (popular in China), is an effective and reversible method. Polyurethane elastomere is injected into the vas. It solidifies and forms a plug and blocks the sperm passage. The plugs can be removed under local anaesthetic.

Open ended vasectomy: The abdominal end of the resected vas is coagulated. The testicular end is left open. This will prevent congestive epididymitis.

FEMALE STERILISATION

Occlusion of the fallopian tubes in some form is the underlying principle to achieve female sterilisation. It is the most popular method of terminal contraception all over the world.

Indications

(1) **Family planning purposes**: This is the principal indication in most of the developing countries, India in particular. Intensive motivation is done and even cash incentives are provided to boost up the programme.

(2) **Socioeconomic**: An individual is adopted to accept the method after having the desired number of children.

(3) **Medicosurgical indications (therapeutic)**: Medical diseases such as heart disease, diabetes, chronic renal disease, hypertension are likely to worsen, if repeated pregnancies occur and hence sterilisation is advisable. During third time repeat Caesarean section or repair of prolapse operation, to avoid the risks involved in the future childbirth process, sterilisation operation should be seriously considered.

Time of operation

The operation can be performed:

(1) ***During puerperium (puerperal)***: If the patient is otherwise healthy, the operation can be done 24-48 hours following delivery. Its chief advantage is technical simplicity. Hospital stay and rest at home following delivery, are enough to help the patient to recover simultaneously from the two events, i.e. delivery and operation.

(2) ***Interval***: The operation is done beyond 3 months following delivery or abortion. **The ideal time of operation is following the menstrual period in the proliferative phase.**

(3) ***Concurrent with MTP***: Sterilisation is performed along with termination of pregnancy. This is mostly done specially in the urban centres.

Methods of female sterilisation:

Occlusion by resection of a segment of both the fallopian tubes (commonly called Tubectomy) is the widely accepted procedure. During recent years, occlusion of the tubes with rings or clips using a laparoscope is gaining popularity.

Hysterectomy during the childbearing period has got an incidental sterilisation effect but should not be done for sterilisation purpose.

Tubectomy (Figs 29.12 and 29.14)

It is an operation where resection of a segment of both the fallopian tubes is done to achieve permanent sterilisation. The approach may be:

• **Abdominal** • **Vaginal**

Abdominal

• **Conventional** • **Minilaparotomy**

Conventional (Laparotomy):

Steps

• **Anaesthesia**: The operation can be done under general or spinal or local anaesthesia. **In mass camp, local anaesthesia is preferable.** In case of local anaesthesia, premedication with Inj. Morphine 15 mg or Inj. Pethidine 100 mg with Phenergan 50 mg IM is to be administered at least 30-45 min prior to surgery. The incisional area is infiltrated with 1 per cent lignocaine.

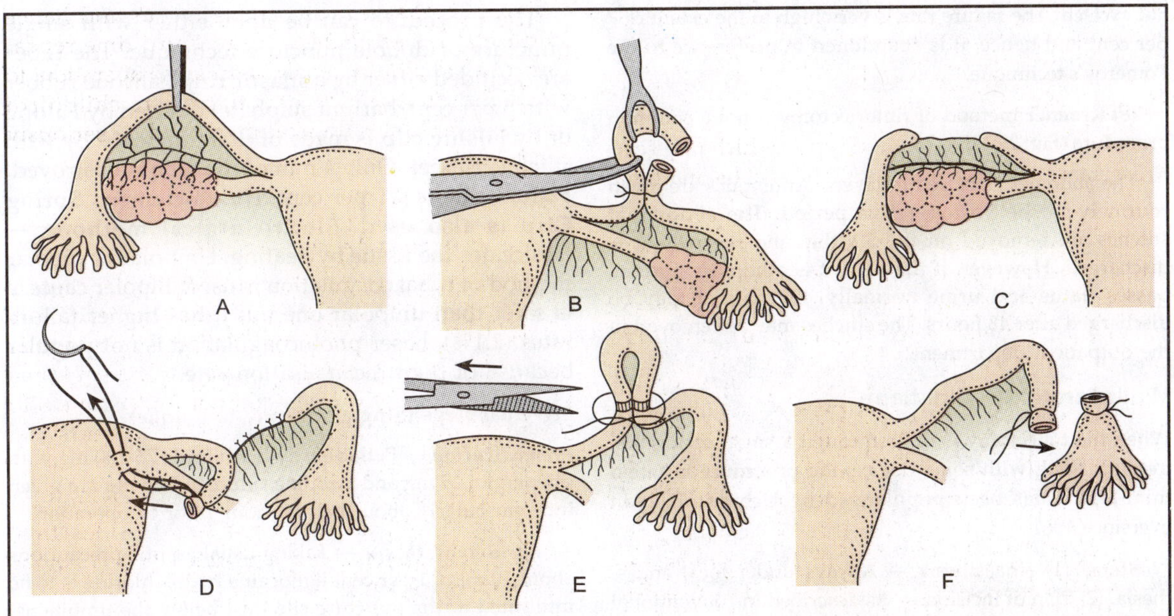

Fig. 29.12. Steps of tubectomy by **Pomeroy's method** : (A) A segment of the Fallopian tube is lifted up. (B) The loop is ligated with chromic catgut and is cut (about 1.5 cm). (C) End result of the operation — note wide separation. (D) **Irving procedure** : the medial cut end is buried in the myometrium posteriorly and the distal cut end is buried in the mesosalpinx. (E) **Madlener procedure.** (F) **Kroener procedure** : the ampullary end of the tube is ligated and resected

- **Incision** : **In puerperal cases**, where the uterus is felt per abdomen, the incision is made two fingers breadth (1") below the fundal height and in interval cases, the incision is made 2 fingers breadth above the symphysis pubis. The incision may be either midline or paramedian or transverse. The abdomen is opened by the usual procedure.

- **Delivery of the tube** : The index finger is introduced through the incision. The finger is passed across the posterior surface of the uterus and then to the posterior leaf of the broad ligament from where the tube is hooked out. **The tube is identified by** the fimbrial end and mesosalpinx containing utero-ovarian anastomotic vessels.

- **Techniques — (Fig. 29.12)** : (a) **Pomeroy's** : A loop is made by holding the tube by an Allis forceps in such a way that the major part of the loop consists mainly of isthmus and part of the ampullary part of the tube (at the junction of proximal and middle third). Through an avascular area in the mesosalpinx, a needle threaded with No. 'O' chromic catgut is passed and both the limbs of the loop are firmly tied together. About 1–1.5 cm of the segment of the loop distal to the ligature is excised. The tube is so excised as to leave behind about 1.5 cm of intact tube adjacent to uterus. **Segment of the loop removed is to be inspected to be sure that the wall has not been partially resected and to send it for histology.** The same procedure is repeated on the other side. Because of the absorption of the absorbable ligature, the cut ends become independently sealed off and are separated after a few weeks.

Advantages: It is easy, safe and very effective in spite of the simplicity of the technique. The failure rate is 0.1–0.5 per cent. The cut ends become independently sealed off and retract widely from each other (Fig. 29.12C).

(b) **Uchida technique** — A saline solution is injected subserosally in the mid portion of the tube to create a bleb. The serous coat is incised along the antimesenteric border to expose the muscular tube. The tube is ligated with No. O chromic catgut on either side and about 3-5 cm of the tube is resected off. The ligated proximal stump is allowed to retract beneath the serous coat. The serous coat is closed with a fine suture in such a way that the proximal stump is buried but the distal stump is open to the peritoneal cavity. No failure in this method has been observed so far.

(c) **Irving method** — The tube is ligated on either side and mid portion of the tube (between the ties) is excised. The free medial end of the tube is then turned back and buried into the posterior uterine wall creating a myometrial tunnel (Fig. 29.12D).

(d) **Madlener technique** (Fig. 29.12E) — It is the easiest method. The loop of the tube is crushed with an artery forceps. The crushed area is tied with black silk. **The loop is**

not excised. The failure rate is very high to the extent of 7 per cent and hence, it is abandoned in preference to the Pomeroy's technique.

(e) **Kroener** method of fimbriectomy is not a common procedure (Fig. 29.12F).

The abdomen is closed in layers. Antibiotics are given routinely in the postoperative period. The abdominal stitches are removed on the 5th day and the patient is discharged. However, if the patient is otherwise normal, passes flatus and urine normally, the patient may be discharged after 48 hours. The stitches may be removed in the outpatient department.

Minilaparotomy (Mini-Lap)

When the tubectomy is done through a small abdominal incision along with some device, the procedure is called mini-lap. It has been popularised by Uchida of Japan eversince 1961.

Steps : (1) Anaesthesia — Always under local anaesthesia. (2) Plan of incision — As described in conventional method but the incision should be $^1/_2$"–$^3/_4$". (3) Specially designed retractor may be introduced after the abdomen is opened. (4) Uterus is elevated or pushed to one side or the other by the elevator that has already been introduced transvaginally into the uterine cavity. This helps manipulation of the tube in bringing it close to the incisional area, when it is seized by artery forceps. (5) The appropriate technique of tubectomy is performed on one side and then repeated on the other side. (6) The peritoneum is closed by purse string suture.

Once conversant with the technique, it can be performed with satisfaction to the patient. It also benefits the organisation (turn over of the patient per bed is more than that in the conventional method). The patient is usually discharged within 24-48 hours.

Vaginal Ligation : Tubectomy through the vaginal route may be done along with vaginal plastic operation or in isolation. When done in isolation, **the approach to the tube is through posterior colpotomy.** Its limitation and relative merits and demerits in contrast to that of abdominal approach are given in the Table 29.11.

LAPAROSCOPIC STERILISATION

Laparoscopy is the commonly employed method of endoscopic sterilisation (Fig. 29.13). It is gradually becoming more popular — specially, in the camps. The procedure is mostly done under local anaesthesia. The operation is done in the interval period, concurrent with vaginal termination of pregnancy or 6 weeks following delivery. It should not be done within 6 weeks following delivery (Fig. 29.13).

The procedure can be done either with single puncture or double puncture technique. The tubes are occluded either by a **silastic ring** (silicone rubber with 5 per cent barium sulphate) devised by **Falope** or by **Filshie clip** is made of titanium lined by with silicone rubber. Only 4 mm of the tube is destroyed. Failure rate is 0.1 per cent. **Hulka-clemens Spring Clip** is also used. **Electrosurgical methods** — Desiccates the tissue by heating. Unipolar or bipolar method of tubal coagulation is used. Bipolar cautery is safer than unipolar one but it has higher failure rates (2.1%). Laser photocoagulation is not popular because of high recanalisation rate.

Principal steps (Single puncture technique)

Premedication — Pethidine hydrochloride 75-100 mg with phenergan 25 mg and atropine sulphate 0.65 mg are given intramuscularly about half an hour prior to operation.

Local anaesthesia — Taking usual aseptic precautions about 10 ml of 1 per cent lignocaine hydrochloride is to be infiltrated at the puncture site (just below the umbilicus) down upto the peritoneum. (If necessary, diazepam 10 mg is given intravenously slowly just prior to local anaesthesia).

Position of the patient — The patient is placed in lithotomy position. The operating table is tilted to approximately 15 degrees of Trendelenburg position. Usual aseptic precaution is taken as in abdominal and vaginal operations. The bladder should be fully emptied by a metal catheter. Pelvic examination is done methodically. An uterine manipulator is introduced through the cervical canal for manipulation for visualisation of tubes and uterus at a later step.

Producing pneumoperitoneum — A small skin incision (1.25 cm) is made just below the umbilicus. The Verres

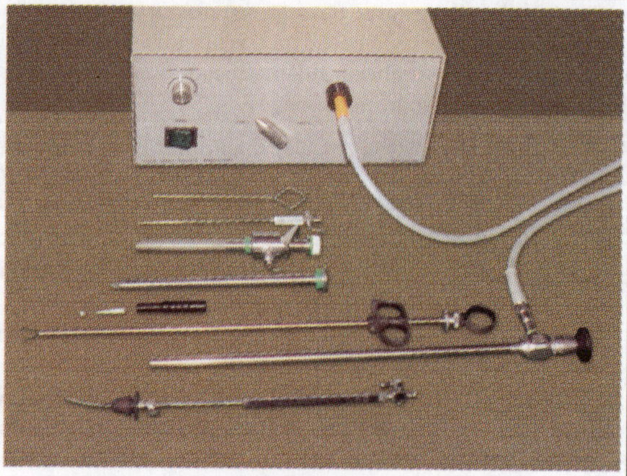

Fig. 29.13. Laparoscopic instruments for tubal sterilisation

Table : 29.11 : Female sterilisation

	Abdominal approach	Vaginal approach
Surgeon	Can be performed by any one conversant with surgery	Can be done only by a surgeon conversant with vaginal plastic operation
Time of operation	Can be done at any time, puerperal or interval	Interval period is most suited. May be done in other times, provided the uterus is smaller than 12 weeks.
Contraindication	Practically — nil	Associated TO mass, uterus—more than 12 weeks size.
Anaesthesia	Can be done under local anaesthesia	General or spinal anaesthesia is usually needed
Complication during operation	Easy to tackle	Difficult at times and laparotomy may be necessary
Duration of operation	Shorter time	Longer time
Complications :	Few	Few
Immediate	Wound infection, peritonitis—rare	Haemorrhage, revealed or broad ligament haematoma, injury to the rectum
Late	Incisional hernia, Failure rate—less	Dyspareunia, failure rate—more
Hospital stay	Longer—5–6 days Shorter with mini-lap (24–48 hours)	Shorter—24–48 hours

needle is introduced through the incision with 45° angulation into the peritoneal cavity. **The abdomen is inflated with about 2 litres of gas (carbon dioxide or nitrous oxide or room air or oxygen).**

Introduction of the trocar and laparoscope with ring loaded applicator—Two silastic rings are loaded one after the other on the applicator with the help of a loader and pusher. The trocar with cannula is introduced through the incision previously made with a twisting movement. The trocar is removed and the laparoscope together with ring applicator is inserted through the cannula.

The ring loaded applicator approaches one side of the tube and grasps **at the junction of the proximal and middle third of the tube.** A loop of the tube (2.5 cm) is lifted up, drawn into the cylinder of the applicator and the ring is slipped into the base of the loop under direct vision. The procedure is to be repeated on the other side (Fig. 29.14).

Removal of the laparoscope : After viewing that the rings are properly placed in position, the tubal loops looking white and there is no intraperitoneal bleeding, the laparoscope is removed. The gas or air is deflated from the abdominal cavity. The abdominal wound is sutured by a single chromic catgut suture.

Comments on Methods of Female Sterilisation

In the third world countries, mini-lap remains the mainstay in the National Family Planning Programme as a method of permanent sterilisation. It is safe, has

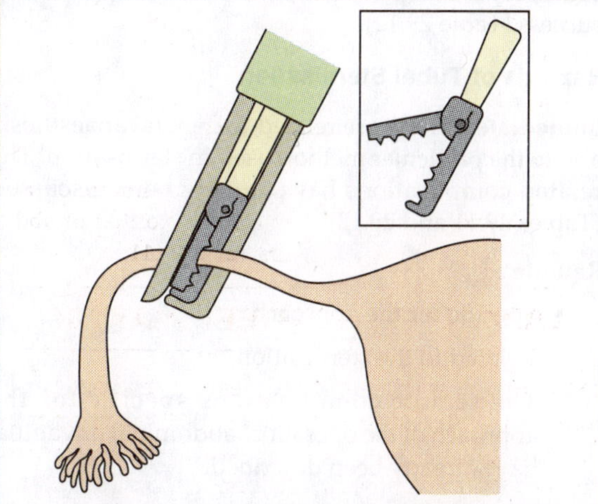

Fig. 29.14. Laparoscopic tubal sterilisation by Filshie clip. Filshie (GM Filshie) clip is made of titanium and the inner surfaces are lined with silicon. It is easier to apply and damage to the tube is less (see p. 479)

Table 29.12 : Mini-lap *vis-a-vis* laparoscopic sterilisation

	Mini-lap	Laparoscopic sterilisation
1. Cost	Minimal	Expensive instrument and requires adequate maintenance
2. Personnel	Any medical personnel with little surgical skill	Should only be performed by persons with special training
3. Assistance	Minimal or nil	Requires a teamwork consisting of medical and paramedical personnel
4. Selection of time	Any time — Puerperium, Interval, with MTP	Should not be done within 6 weeks following delivery or with enlarged uterus
5. Contraindication	Practically none. Can be done in conditions contraindicated for laparoscopy	Lung lesions, organic heart diseases, anticipated intra-abdominal adhesions, extreme obesity
6. Complication	Minimal but not life-threatening	Minimal but at times fatal : injury to bowels, blood vessels, surgical emphysema (see p. 580)
7. Hospital stay	3–5 days	3–4 hours
8. Failure rate	0.1–0.3%	0.2–0.6 %
9. Reversibility	Difficult due to adhesion formation. Success depends on the length the tube left behind, after excision (see p. 241)	Easier and effective. **Only 4 mm of the tube is destroyed with the Filshie clip (see p. 240, 477, and Fig. 29.14)**

wider applicability, is less expensive and has got a less failure rate compared to laparoscopic sterilisation. However, for a quick turn over in an organised mass camp, laparoscopic sterilisation offers a promising success (Table 29.12).

Hazards of Tubal Sterilisation

Immediate : These are related to general anaesthesia and to the particular method used in sterilisation. The related complications have already been discussed (Tables 29.11 and 29.12).

Remote :

- Specific for the approach.
- Related to the sterilisation.
- The remote complications specific for the approach of the operation, abdominal or vaginal have already been described.
- The complications related to sterilisation can be grouped into :
  - **General complications** : These include occasional obesity, psychological upset.
  - **Gynaecological** : (1) Chronic pelvic pain (2) Congestive dysmenorrhoea (3) Menstrual abnormalities in the form of menorrhagia, hypomenorrhoea or irregular periods. Pelvic pain, menorrhagia along with cystic ovaries **constitute a postligation syndrome**. It may be vascular in origin. However, the incidence, can be minimised, if the blood vessels adjacent to the mesosalpinx are not unduly disturbed. (4) Alteration in libido.

Failure rate :The overall failure rate in tubal sterilisation is about 0.7 per cent, **the Pomeroy's technique being the lowest 0.1-0.5 per cent**, in contrast to the Madlener's, being 1.5-7 per cent. The failure rate is increased when it is done during hysterotomy or during Caesarean section. The failure rate is also increased when it is done through vaginal route. Failure may be due to **fistula formation or due to spontaneous reanastomosis**.

Mortality following tubal sterilisation is estimated to be 72 per 100,000 for all methods. Laparoscopic procedures carried the mortality rate of 5-10 per

100,000 compared to 7 per 100,000 for puerperal ligations.

Reversibility : Informed consent must be obtained after **adequate counselling**. Couple must understand the permanency of the procedure, its occasional failure rate the risks and side effects and its alternatives. Unfortunately regret is not uncommon. Microsurgical techniques give excellent result for tubal reanastomosis. Pregnancy rates after reversal are high (80%) following use of clips and rings. Reversal of vasectomy with restoration of vas patency is possible up to 90 per cent of cases. But pregnancy rate is low (50%).

CONTRACEPTIVE PRESCRIPTION

Pregnancy carries an overall maternal mortality around 400 per 100,000 total births in the developing countries and the same in the developed countries is less than 10. Whereas annual number of deaths per 100,000 exposed to pill is 1.3 and with that of IUDs is 1. The risks of death from automobile driving is 1 in 6000 per year. **So the benefits of contraceptive use outweigh the risks.**

No one single universally acceptable method has yet been discovered. The individual should have the liberty to choose any of the currently available well-tested method, which may even vary at each phase in her reproductive life. If one compares the risks and benefits of any contraceptive, it is observed that more deaths occur as a result of unplanned pregnancies than from the hazards of any modern contraceptive method (excluding "Pill" users over 35 who smoke).

While selecting the method, one should take into consideration whether the couple intend to prevent further pregnancies or just to delay the next pregnancy. It does no good to select a method of high efficacy if it is not correctly and consistently used. **Acceptability is probably the most critical factor in the effectiveness of a contraceptive method. Couple (client) should be helped to make an informed choice.**

A clear account of the risks and the benefits for an individual method is given. Regular follow up and compliance with the instructions are to be ensured. It is also essential that an informed (verbal) consent is obtained and recorded.

Prescription

Conventional contraceptives can be safely prescribed during the entire reproductive period as elective choice or as an alternative to 'Pill' or IUD if they are contraindicated or unacceptable to the couple. As such only the advice regarding the use of 'Pill' or IUD during different phases of reproductive life is discussed.

Adolescent girls—low dose combined pills are most effective for the sexually active adolescents. It is the contraceptive of choice. However, DMPA or norplant may be an alternative where available.

Newly married couple : Provided there is not enough justification to prove early fertility, a highly effective and acceptable contraceptive should be prescribed. **IUD should not be prescribed** for its increased association with PID. As such 'Pill' is recommended provided there is no contraindication. Apart from effective contraception 'Pill' has got many noncontraceptive benefits as well.

Spacing of births

- **Postabortal**
- **Postpartum**
- **Interval**

Postabortal : The contraceptive practice should be started soon following the abortion process is completed. 'Pill' is the ideal; IUD is an alternative.

Postpartum : • **Nonlactating** • **Lactating**

Nonlactating—Contraceptive practice should be started after three weeks. 'Pill' is good; IUD is an equally effective alternative. Injectable depomedroxy progesterone acetate could be used as it is devoid of any oestrogen related side effects. Norplant (Levonorgestrel implant) could be prescribed if available.

Lactating — In fully lactating women (5-6 feeds and spending about 60 minutes in 24 hours), the contraceptive practice may be safely withheld for 10 weeks postpartum. For doubtful adverse effects of steroids on lactation and on the babies through the ingested milk, **'Pill' is better withheld. Minipill or injectable steroids** if available, is ideal. Alternatively, IUD can be inserted.

Interval : Below the age of 35, she can have her choice to either 'Pill' or IUD following adequate counselling. In women above the age of 35 specially who are smokers, IUD should be inserted in preference to 'Pill'. Injectables (DMPA) or implant (Norplant) where available is the other alternative.

To stop future pregnancies : The decision to advise permanent sterilisation should be judiciously given specially to the under-privileged women in the face of high perinatal and infant mortality rate. The cases are to be individualised. However, a two-child formula is usually recommended and as such, a couple having two children who have been fully immunised can have permanent sterilisation (husband or wife). If the couple is not motivated to undergo the sterilisation operation, any of the temporary methods is to be prescribed till the end of the reproductive period of the wife. Women who have completed their family but do not desire for permanent sterilisation, may use IUD (CU T 380A) or implant (norplant) if available.

Older women : Contraception should be prescribed to avoid unplanned pregnancy. Low dose pills can be continued till menopause (with monitoring) in the low-risk group. Progestin only pill, injectable progestin, LNG-IUS are the other alternatives. Barrier methods and vaginal spermicides can be used either as a primary or back up method. Usually fertility is reduced after 40 years of age.

Women at risk of STD should use condoms and spermicides even when they use another family planning method.

Women using enzyme inducers are advised to take COCs having more than usual dosage (see p. 467) or other method of contraception (injectables, IUDs).

Postcoital contraception when required as emergency, POP, IUD or other methods can be used (p. 471).

ONGOING TRIALS AND SELECTIVE AVAILABILITY

The following are used on trial basis or are available in selected countries :

Female

• **Centchroman (SAHELI)** — *Ormeloxifene* is a research product of Central Drug Research Institute of Lucknow, India. It is a non-steroidal compound with potent anti-oestrogenic and weak-oestrogenic properties. It is taken orally (30 mg) twice a week for first three months then once a week. It works primarily by preventing implantation of fertilised ovum. It does not inhibit ovulation.

Side effects are few. It is avoided in polycystic ovarian disease, with liver and kidney diseases and in tuberculosis. There may be a tendency of oligomenorrhoea. The failure rate is about 1-4 per 100 women years of use. Failure rate is less with increased doses. It is devoid of any significant adverse metabolic effect. This may also be used as an emergency contraceptive. It is sold in the market against prescription only and not over the counter.

Non-contraceptive use : Because of its potent anti-oestrogenic activity, centchroman is being currently tried in the management of dysfunctional uterine bleeding, endometrial hyperplasia, endometriosis and breast cancer. It is used as hormone replacement therapy (HRT), because of its weak oestrogenic property.

• **Combined injectable contraceptives (CICs)** — Both oestrogen and progestin are combined in these monthly injectables. Preparations available are : DMPA 25 mg with oestradiol cypionate 5 mg (Cyclofem) and NET-EN 50 mg with oestradiol valerate 5 mg (Mesigyna). Oestrogen has been incorporated to improve the menstrual cycle. Use of "natural" oestrogens in CICs has got favourable impact on lipid metabolism and cardiovascular effects compared to synthetic oestrogen used inj COCs. It is given within first 5 days of menstruation. Next injection should be on the same date of each month (4 week schedule).

Drawbacks—(i) Irregular or prolonged menstrual bleeding. (ii) Not suitable for nursing mothers.

• **Transdermal delivery systems** : *Nestorone (newer progestin)*—When used as a cream to the skin provides effective contraception. **Patch** delivers 150 μg of norelgestromin (progestin) and 20 μg ethinyl oestradiol daily. The patch is used weekly for 3 weeks and one week off for withdrawal bleeding. It is well-tolerated, safe and effective. **Drawbacks** : Patch detachment, skin reaction and high failure in overweight women (> 90 kg). It is applied over the buttocks, outer arm, or lower abdomen.

• **Vaginal ring**—Containing levonorgestrel covered by silastic tubing have been introduced. They are 5 and 6 cm in diameter. The vaginal ring delivers levonorgestrel (20 μg/day) to maintain a constant blood level like norplant. The rings are replaced by 90 days. Pregnancy rate is 3 per 100 woman years. This method is under woman's control.

• **Combined ring** — Soft, transparent ethylene vinyl ring (Nuva Ring) releases ethinyl oestradiol (15 μg) and etonogestrel (metabolite of desogestrel 0.12 mg) daily over a period of 21 days. It is then removed and after 1 week (after the withdrawal bleed) and a new ring is inserted. Pearl index is 0.65 and cycle control is good. The ring is 5 cm in diameter. Side effects are, headache, leucorrhoea, vaginitis and expulsion.

• **LNG Rod**—Recently developed implant with a total 150 mg of levonorgestrel (75 mg/rod) is found to be very effective for five years.

• **Uniplant** is a single rod implant, containing 55 mg of nomegestrol (newer progestin) with a release rate of 100 μg per day. It provides contraception for one year.

• **Biodegradable implants** are under study. **Capronor** (single capsule) releases levonorgestrel from the polymer E-caprolactone at a rate 10 times faster than from silastic. The longer capsule contains 26 mg of levonorgestrel and inhibits ovulation in about 50 per cent of cycles. Contraceptive efficacy is comparable to norplant. The capsule begins to disappear after 12 months.

• **Injectable contraceptive (biodegradable)** in the form of microspheres using Copolymer (Lactide-glycolide) have been studied. Hormone currently used in the microsphere (0.06 – 0.1 mm diameter) is either norethindrone or norethindrone combined with ethinyloestradiol. Injection is given over the gluteal muscle. Unlike implant, microspheres cannot be removed once injected.

• **LHRH** agonist (buserelin) and antagonist (cetrorelix) acts by preventing the pituitary response to the endogenous GnRH. They have the potential to arrest follicular growth and endometrial development. Unwanted side effects (loss of libido and hot flushes) are avoided using add-back therapy (see p. 502). Long-term effects are not known as yet.

- **Newer IUDs—A frameless IUD (Gynefix)** is made of six copper beads (330 mm^2 of Cu) on a monofilament polypropylene thread. The upper and lower beads are crimped onto the thread. The thread is knotted at one end which is embeded into the fundal myometrium to a depth of 1 cm. This anchors the device at the fundus. **The advantages** of the device (Fig. 29.15) over the framed ones are significant reduced risk of expulsion, dysmenorrhoea, bleeding and infection. Threadless (Butterfly) IUD is also found promising to reduce the risk of side effects (infection). It can be removed with a hook when required. This device is specially suited for nulligravid women.

- **Fibro plant (LNG) :** Similar to Mirena (see p. 459), a smaller version of Levonorgestrel System is currently being tested. Its small size is suitable for the perimenopausal women in whom the uterus shrinks. It releases LNG at the rate of 14 mcg/day. It is also used as a HRT for postmenopausal women.

TRANSCERVICAL STERILISATION

- **Quinacrine pellet**, 252 mg is inserted on two occasions one month apart into the uterine cavity transcervically through a hysteroscope during the proliferative phase. It is repeated in the next cycle. It acts as a sclerosing agent. Pregnancy rate is 2-3 per 100 woman years. Long-term results are awaited.

- **Essure** is a 4 cm long microcoil (spring like device) made of nickel-titanium alloy coil within which lie dacron fibres (Fig. 29.16).

It is inserted into each fallopian tube transcervically using a hysteroscope. The tube is blocked permanently when scar tissue grows into the device. Proper placement of essure is checked with ultrasound imaging three months after. Its success rate is similar to surgical sterilisation (99.74%). For the first three months the woman needs to use a temporary contraceptive method in addition, till the scar tissue is formed.

Anti hCG vaccine — The principle of hCG vaccine is to produce antibody which will block the action of hCG on ovaries and therefore, progesterone will not be produced. Immune approaches have been understudy for a long time without any promise.

Male

Testosterone or a combination of testosterone and progestin (monthly injection or implant) is found to suppress sperm production. Testosterone undecanoate is used and found successful.

- **GnRH analogues** produce a decline in sperm density, sperm mobility and a decrease in testosterone level. The marked loss of libido makes it unacceptable. Add-back therapy (testosterone) is used to overcome the side effects.

- **Gossypol** — It has been discovered in China; an extract from cottonseed. It acts directly on the seminiferous tubules inhibiting spermatogenesis. The side effects are fatigue, decreased libido and delayed recovery of sperm count. The serious side effects are hypokalaemic paralysis and cardiac arrhythmias.

Intra Vas Device (IVD) : Two plugs are implanted in each vas to block sperm transport through the vas deferens. Plugs could be removed to make it a reversible procedure. Its contraceptive effectiveness is being studied.

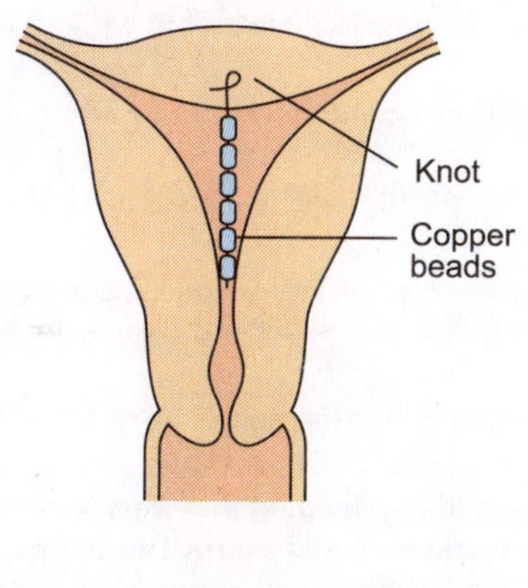

Fig. 29.15 : Frameless IUD (GyneFix) with the modified inserter

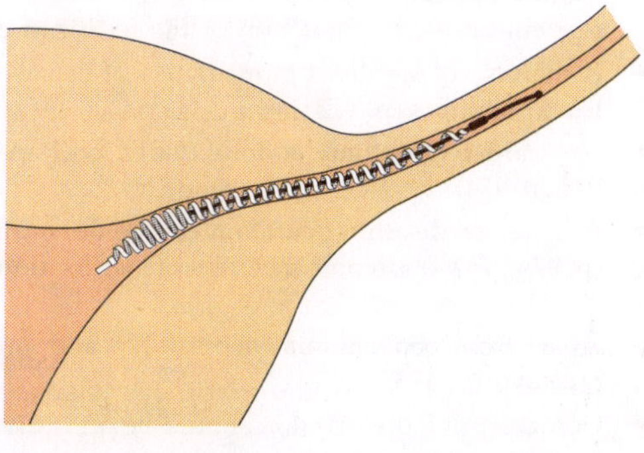

Fig. 29.16 : Essure device within the intramural portion of the Fallopian tube. It is inserted using a hysteroscope

KEY POINTS

- **Barrier methods** of contraception include condom, diaphragm and vaginal contraceptives (chemicals and sponge today).
- **Natural contraception includes**—rhythm method, coitus interruptus and breastfeeding (p. 457).
- **Conventional contraceptive methods** include use of condom, vaginal diaphragm, spermicidals and rhythm method.
- **The introduction of IUD** is an OPD procedure without anaesthesia taking full aseptic precautions. **'No touch' insertion** technique is preferred (p. 461).
- The **contraindications** of insertion of IUD are nulliparity, PID, suspected pregnancy, DUB or suspicious cervix. The pregnancy rate is about 0.5–2 HWY. There is risk of ectopic pregnancy 1–2 per cent. Third generation IUDs have minimal side effects and lowest pregnancy rate (p. 463).

  Immediate complications include pain, syncopal attack and uterine perforation. **Remote complications** include — pain, abnormal uterine bleeding, pelvic infection, spontaneous expulsion or even perforation of the uterus (p. 461).
- Indications **of removal of IUD are**—excessive uterine bleeding, flaring up of pelvic infection, uterine perforation, pregnancy, missing thread and patient desirous of a baby (p. 462).
- Apart from contraception, the IUD is used as interception and following synecolysis.
- The **replacement time** for CuT 200 B is 4 years, multiload 250 — 3 years, CuT 380A — 10 years, multiload 375 — 5 years and LNG–IUS is 5 years.
- LNG-IUS has got many **health benefits** (see p. 463). It is a very safe and effective method for prolonged use.
- **Combined oral contraceptives** are very reliable apart from their many other health benefits (see Page 467).
- **Absolute contraindications** of oral pills (p. 466), major side effects (p. 467) and indications of withdrawal of pills (p.467) have been discussed.
- The **newer low dose pills** with more specific and "lipid friendly" progestins reduce the health risk further.
- A woman who does not smoke and has no other risk factor for cardiovascular disease, may continue the pill (with careful monitoring) until the age of 50.
- **Low dose progestin pill (mini pill)** is advantageous in lactating women, as it has got no adverse effect on breast milk. It can be used as a suitable alternative where oestrogen is contraindicated (p. 470).
- **Overall safety of DMPA** is clearly greater than COC. Norplant and Implanon are safe and effective for long-term use. Both are considered as 'reversible sterilisation' (p. 470).
- **Emergency contraception** includes hormones, IUD and antiprogesterone (RU-486). Within 72 hours, hormonal preparations are effective; within 5 days, IUD is effective and Ru 486 should be taken within day 27 of cycle irrespective of the day and number of intercourse (p. 472).
- **Centchroman** in a nonsteroidal antioestrogenic compound used as once a week contraceptive pill. It acts by preventing the implantation of the fertilized ovum (p. 480).
- A man is not sterilised immediately after vasectomy. As such, additional condom should be advised for at least 3 months (p. 473).
- **No scalpel vasectomy** is done under local anaesthetic making a tiny picture over the stretched skin of the vas (p. 474).
- **Female sterilisation** operation can be done during puerperium, in interval period or concurrent with MTP (p. 474). Hysteroscopic methods of sterilisation include insertion of quinacrine pellet and Essure (microcoil), p. 481.
- Apart from conventional or mini-lap abdominal method, **laparoscopic sterilisation** is very popular and effective (p. 476).
- Contraceptive prescription should be on **individual basis**. In an individual, method may vary according to her phase of reproductive life. **Teenage girls, older women** and **sex workers** should also be protected (p. 479).
- It is hard to predict contraceptive trends in the immediate future as the results of contraceptive research are still unclear about the risks and benefits.

Radiotherapy, Chemotherapy, Immunotherapy and Genetherapy in Gynaecology

30

Introduction

Radiotherapy and chemotherapy are the important modalities of therapy for human cancers apart from surgery. Bias towards any particular one is unscientific. They may have a curative role (e.g. radiotherapy in carcinoma cervix and chemotherapy in gestational trophoblastic neoplasia) when used as a primary therapy. Combination of different therapeutic measures may be needed for the treatment of some malignancies to improve the outcome. Radiotherapy and or chemotherapy should be considered even for palliation of incapacitating symptoms when cure may not be achieved. The basic principles of radiotherapy and chemotherapy in relation to gynaecologic malignancies have been discussed in the chapter. Current understanding in immunotherapy and genetherapy have also been discussed.

RADIOTHERAPY

Radiotherapy means treatment of disease by ionising radiations producing biological damage to living tissues. Ionising radiations in sufficient dosage will affect the cells in two ways—(i) loss of clonogenic capacity (inability to proliferate) and (ii) cell death. **Marie Curie** and **Pierre Curie** from Pitchblende identified intense radioactivity of Radium in 1898.

Certain basic informations are necessary for proper understanding of the subject. Ionising radiation used for therapy may be (i) Electromagnetic radiation, (ii) Particulate radiation.

Electromagnetic radiation

This consists of quanta of energy and wavelength (photon radiation). They are of two types—X-rays and gamma rays. These electromagnetic waves travel in discrete bundles called 'Photons'.

- **Gamma rays** are produced spontaneously as a result of decay of the **atomic nucleus** of some radioactive isotopes. ^{60}Cobalt or ^{192}Iridium is a source of γ-rays.
- **X-rays** are produced **outside the atomic nucleus**. When fast moving electrons approach the fields around the nuclei of atoms of a target material (tungsten), they are deflected from their path. The energy thus emitted in the form of electromagnetic radiation (photons) is X-rays. Machines such as betatron (circular fashion) and linear accelerator (linear fashion) can accelerate electrons with high kinetic energy. Therefore X-rays generated by these machines are very high in energy.
- **X-rays and gamma rays** are collectively called photons. When photons interact with matter (tissue),

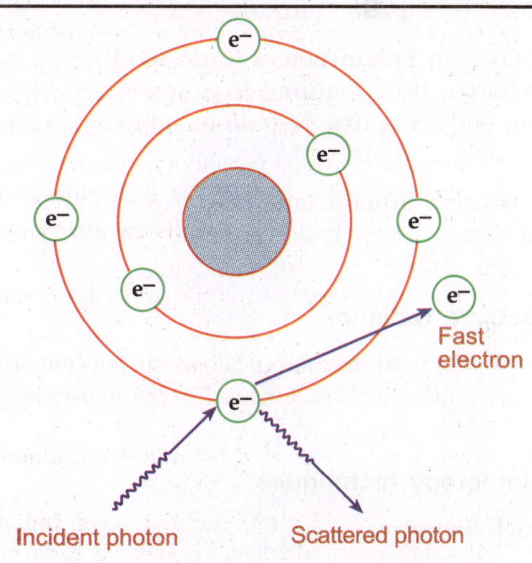

Fig. 30.1. Compton scattering

three effects are observed : (i) photoelectric effect, (ii) compton scattering and (iii) pair production. In human radiation therapy, **compton scattering** is the major interaction of photons with tissue (see Fig. 30.1). X-rays and gamma rays have shorter wavelength and high frequency. They have high kinetic energy. X-rays and gamma rays possess considerable power of tissue penetration depending on the photon energy and the density of the matter through which they pass. The photon energy produced from radioactive cobalt is 1.2 million electron volts (Mev). External photon beam radiation is usually derived from a linear accelerator (p. 487).

- **Isotopes** are atoms of an element with same number of protons but different number of neutrons at its nuclear core. Isotopes are stable or unstable. Unstable isotopes try to attain stability by ejection of particles. This process often produces ionising radiation with elaboration of alpha and beta particles and gamma rays.

- **Atoms** normally exist in neutral state. As such, the total number of positively charged particles at the nucleus (proton) and negatively charged particles at the orbit (electron) are equal.

- **Radioactive nuclei particles** give off alpha and beta particles and gamma rays.

- **Radium 226**, caesium 137, gold 198, iodine 125, cobalt 60, iridium 192 are used as radioactive sources for therapeutic purpose (Table 30.1).

- **Radioactive substances** are encapsulated to absorb alpha and beta particles leaving gamma rays to attain therapeutic purpose.

- **Oxygen Enhancement Ratio (OER)** : The ratio of radiation dose required for a given level of cell killing under hypoxic condition compared with the dose needed in air.

- **Inverse Square law** : Effect of radiation at a point varies inversely as the square of the distance from the source.

Particulate radiation

This consists of atomic subparticles such as electrons, protons and neutrons. Only electrons (β-rays) are used in radiotherapy.

Radiotherapy techniques

• Brachytherapy

Brachytherapy gives a very high dose of radiation from a source close to the tumour. The application may be (i) Intracavitary or (ii) Interstitial. Damage to normal tissues is less as there is rapid fall-off of radiation around the source (radiation dose falls with the source of the distance travelled).

Intracavitary : The devices for brachytherapy consist of hollow stem (intrauterine tandem) which is placed within the uterine cavity (Fig. 30.2). Specially designed devices used for vaginal placements are called vaginal ovoids or colpostats.

Table 30.1
Radioisotopes commonly used in gynaecological malignancies

Isotope	Energy (MeV)	Half-life
Cesium 137 (^{137}Cs)	0.662	30 yrs
Radium 226 (^{226}Ra)	0.8	1620 yrs
Cobalt 60 (^{60}Co)	1.173	5.3 yrs
Iridium 192 (^{192}Ir)	0.47	74 days
Gold 198 (^{198}Au)	0.411	2.69 days
Iodine 125 (^{125}I)	0.027	60 days
Phosphorus 32 (^{32}P)	0.698	14.3 days

The commonly used radioisotopes for brachytherapy are given in the Table 30.1.

Interstitial form of brachytherapy consists of placement of radioactive sources (needles, wires or seeds) within the tissues. Commonly used sources are Iridium-192 (^{192}Ir), Cesium-137 (^{137}Cs). Small volume of tumour, as in early cases of vaginal carcinoma, can be treated with the method. Normal tissues are spared from radiation injury.

• After loading technique

It is a modern development of brachytherapy to prevent radiation complications to the personnel. A mock insertion of applicators is performed and an X-ray is taken to note their exact position. After loading technique may be manual or by remote control. Later on, live radioactive sources are introduced by remote control in identical manner. Remote after loading system uses Selectron (^{137}Cs) or high dose Selectron (^{60}Co). Remote control systems allow complete protection of staff from radiation exposure.

• Teletherapy

Here a beam of electromagnetic wave or particulate radiation is directed to the tumour tissue from a distance (usually 100 cm). Cobalt 60 is the common teletherapy source for external beam radiation therapy, the other one is cesium 137. External radiation therapy is used to treat large volumes (tumour, lymph nodes, parametrium) of tumour (see p. 337). It is designed to deliver a uniform radiation dose to the tumour volume without 'hot' (excess dose) or 'cold' (under dose) spots. Accurate tumour localisation and volume measurement are essential. Greater the tumour volume, higher the radiation dose required.

- **Instillation of radioisotopes into the peritoneal or pleural cavity**

Radioactive isotopes of either gold or phosphorus, linked to carrier colloids, are commonly used in ovarian cancer. This can give radiation only to a depth of 4-8 mm. Radioactive chromic phosphate (^{32}P) emits pure β-rays and has got longer half life (14.3 days) and deeper penetration (8 mm) power compared to radio gold (^{198}Au). Small volume of tumour in the peritoneal or pleural cavity is treated with solution of radioisotopes.

Measurement of radiation

For radiotherapy, proper measurement and estimation of appropriate dose is essential.

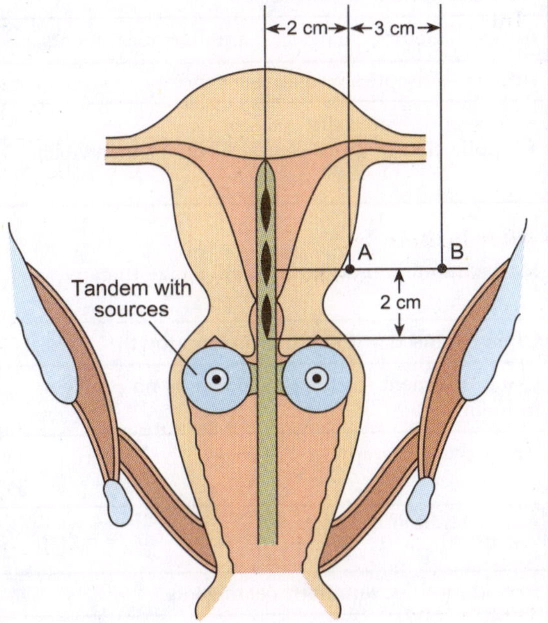

Fig. 30.2. Tandem and ovoid placement for carcinoma cervix (Manchester technique). Points A and B are the reference points (see p. 337)

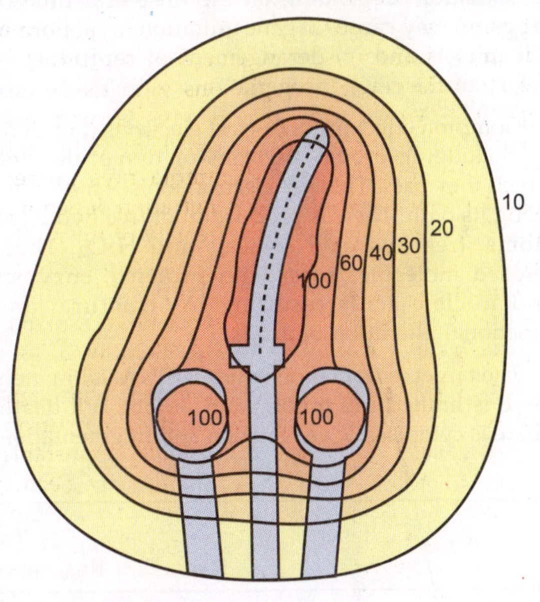

Fig. 30.3. Isodose distribution curve with intracavitary irradiation

Absorbed dose

Measurement of this dose is more important as it helps in ascertaining the actual amount of energy deposited at the point of therapy.

Radiation absorption dose (Gray) is the unit used to measure the amount of energy absorbed per unit mass of tissue. **One gray (Gy)** is equivalent to 1 Joule/kg which is equivable to 100 rads. Currently the term **centigray** (cGy) is used. One cGy is equivalent to one rad. Amount of radiation the patient receives is calculated by **dosimetry**. Homogeneous irradiation of tissues is desirable (Fig. 30.3). Primary tumour should receive high dose. Brachytherapy and teletherapy should be combined to provide adequate irradiation to the primary tumour as well as the pelvic lymph nodes and the parametrium (Fig. 30.2).

Biological effects of radiation (Radiobiology)

Radiation has got two actions :

(1) **Direct action** : Where the radiation is absorbed and it causes damage to DNA directly. This is the predominant mechanism of action of particulate radiation (neutrons).

(2) **Indirect action :** Where the radiation interact with other substance (H_2O) in the cell to produce radicals (OH^-) which in turn damage the cell.

Radiation, depending on the dose and time of exposure may cause (a) gene mutation (b) abnormal cell mitosis and (c) derangement of reproductive ability of the cell—"progeria".

Compton effect produces fast electrons (Fig. 30.1) by dislodging orbital electrons of tissue, through which they pass. This fast electron ionises molecules along its path. There is production of free hydrogen atoms, free hydroxyl radicals and H_2O_2. These ionised molecules react with proteins, enzymes and nucleic acids resulting in structural and functional alteration of a cell.

The target for radiation injury is DNA. Ultimately there is limited cell mitosis and mitotic cell death. There is cytoplasmic vacuolation and fragmentation. Ionising radiation also produces damage to nuclear and plasma membranes.

This effect of ionising radiation is common for both the normal and neoplastic tissues, encountered in the radiation path. Radiation complications are mainly due to interaction with the normal tissues (Table 30.2). When the radiation effect to a cell is sublethal, cellular DNA may undergo repair and the cell survives. Lethal effect kills the cell.

Radiation dose : According to the "inverse square law" there is reduction of radiation at a distance from the source in brachytherapy. This protects the normal tissues (see isodose distribution curve Fig. 30.3).

Table 30.2
Radiation Reactions and their Management

Early : Anorexia, nausea, vomiting, lassitude or even fever	• Antiemetics • Anti-histaminics
Diarrhoea (radiation enteritis)	Intravenous fluid therapy to correct electrolyte imbalance
Leucopenia and thrombocytopenia, anaemia	Haematinics, blood transfusion
Intestinal reaction such as enteritis, colitis, proctitis	Anti-spasmodics, analgesics, antidiarrhoeal agents
Urinary — cystitis, pyelitis, haematuria	Urinary antiseptics and analgesics
Skin reaction such as peeling often found in moist area of the vulva. This is almost absent in megavoltage radiotherapy.	• To keep the area dry • Application of 1 per cent aqueous gentian violet
Late (due to vasculitis and fibrosis) : Atrophic changes of vulval skin and vaginal stricture	Markedly minimised with megavoltage therapy
Radiation fibrosis	Often confused with recurrence of growth
Pathological fracture due to osteoporosis	Usual treatment for fracture. There is no problem in union
Intestine — stricture, bleeding per rectum, perforation, obstruction	Appropriate therapy
Malabsorption syndrome with megaloblastic anaemia	Administration of folic acid
Proctosigmoiditis	Steroid enemas, antidiarrhoeal agents
Fistula : Vesicovaginal *or* Rectovaginal Usually occurs 1-2 years following primary therapy	• Difficult to treat locally • Colpocleisis may be an alternative
Ovary	Radiation damage, menopausal symptoms

A planning computer calculates the field sizes, the dose from each field and the angles of the treatment machine. High energy machines spare the skin and deliver more radiation below the skin surface. Linear accelerators which delivery X-rays of 4-8 Mev are used currently. Treatment is carried out in a specially protected room. During the treatment time the patient should be alone and she is supervised using a television camera. Safety precautions of radiation are maintained.

Radiocurability is the elimination of tumour at the primary or metastatic site due to a direct effect of radiation.

Radiosensitivity means the response of the tumour to irradiation. Radiosensitivity is measured in terms of loss of cellular proliferative capacity due to the damage to DNA. Accumulation of sublethal injury following repeat radiation leads to ultimate DNA damage and cell death. **Radiosensitivity depends on several factors** :

- **Tissue hypoxia** — higher the hypoxic fraction of cells, the less is the radiation response. Hypoxic cells are more resistant to radiation compared to oxic cells.
- **Proportion of proliferating (clonogenic) cells** — Clonogenic cells are more radiosensitive.
- **Cell cycle** — mitotic cells and G2 cells are more radiosensitive compared to late S-phase cells.
- **Tumour specificity** certain tumours (dysgerminomas) are more radiosensitive than the others.
- **Tumour volume** — smaller the tumour volume → lesser the hypoxic cells → less the radiation dose better the radiation response.

Lesser the photon wavelength more is the penetrating power and energy of ionising radiation. Supervoltage and megavoltage radiation (^{60}Co, ^{137}Cs, ^{226}Ra, betatron, linear accelerator) have the following advantages over the orthovoltage one. They have higher energy of radiation, less skin injury, less lateral scattering and more tissue penetration at a greater depth. They are suitable for the deep seated tumours (e.g. carcinomas of the cervix and endometrium).

Fractionation : External beam radiotherapy is usually fractionated and is given once daily for five times a week. A dose of 180-220 cGy per fraction is used. This is based on the ability of the cells to accumulate and repair the sublethal injury. Tumour tissue takes longer time to recover from radiation damage compared to normal tissue. Fractionation allows **normal tissue** (intestinal mucosa, bone marrow) to repair sublethal injury (sparing effect). On the other hand irradiation results in accumulation of sublethal damage and ultimate loss of reproductive capacity in **tumour tissue**.

Radiation dose prescription should include the total dose, number of fractions with dose and time for each fraction (e.g. 40 Gy in 20 fractions given five times weekly can be given in 4 weeks at 2 Gy per fraction).

RECENT ADVANCES IN RADIATION THERAPY

High linear energy transfer : X-rays and γ-rays are less effective against hypoxic cells compared to oxygenated cells. **Fast neutrons** or negative π mesons (pions) or protons are very effective against the hypoxic cells. **Fast neutron** beam for radiotherapy are generated by the cyclotron and the D-T generator. The neutron is emitted with an energy of 14-16 Mev.

Negative π mesons (pions) with energies between 40 and 70 Mev have a depth range in tissue of about 6-13 cm. It has high biologic effectiveness and a low dependance on oxygen.

Electron Beam : High energy electron beams are produced by many linear accelerators. Electrons lose energy rapidly as they travel in tissues till their kinetic energy is reduced to zero at the maximum depth of penetration. Transcervical electron irradiation can be used for control of haemorrhage in cases with bleeding cervical carcinoma.

Radiopotentiators and hypoxic cell sensitisers

Compared to well-oxygenated cells, hypoxic cells require about three times the radiation dose, to obtain the same proportion of cell kill. Hypoxic cell can be sensitised to ionising radiation to improve the **Oxygen Enhancement Ratio (OER)** by different chemical compounds.

Number of chemotherapeutic agents have been found to potentiate the radiation effect and also to sensitise the hypoxic cells (Table 30.3). Exact mechanism is not well-

Table 30.3
Radiopotentiators, Hypoxic cell sensitises

Chemotherapeutic agents	Others
• Cisplatin	Misonidazole
• Bleomycin	Tumour Necrosis Factor (TNF)
• Chlorambucil	Interferon
• Doxorubicin	Acyclovir

understood. Use of hyperbaric oxygen to increase radiosensitivity is of doubtful benefit. More over this technique is cumbersome.

Radiation with computerised dosimetry can be increased to compensate for asymmetric parametrial disease. **Combining** pelvic radiation with concomitant chemotherapy (cisplatin) for locally advanced cervical cancer (stage IB to IVA) was found to improve survival rate compared to radiation alone.

Generally external beam radiation therapy is given when the primary tumour is bulky. This shrinks the tumour whereby intracavitary therapy is possible to achieve the total dose.

Intraoperative radiation of large fraction of 1500-2500 cGy are delivered directly to the area selected. Periaortic node irradiation (biopsy proven) at the time of staging laparotomy is being tried with encouraging initial results.

Hyperthermia is found helpful as an active antineoplastic agent and a significant radiosensitiser.

Three-Dimensional Treatment Planning (3-DTP) is a combination of traditional simulation and Computed Tomography (CT) imaging. Studies are underway.

Treatment field for carcinoma cervix

Superior border — between L_4 and L_5 to include the common iliac nodes. **Inferior border** — at the inferior margin of obturator foramen to include the obturator nodes. **Lateral borders** — 1 cm lateral to the margins of the bony pelvis.

Lead compensators are used in the path of external beam radiation to prevent over dose to the central portion of the pelvis which has received high dosage from brachytherapy.

Radiotherapy in Epithelial Ovarian Carcinoma

Role of postoperative radiotherapy in the management of epithelial ovarian carcinoma is no longer favoured. Chemotherapy has replaced radiotherapy both for the management of early and advanced disease. However it may be used in the following cases who fail to respond with chemotherapy.

(i) Metastatic deposits over the peritoneal surfaces

(ii) Lymph node metastasis

(iii) Palliation for painful recurrences in the pelvis or bone.

Moving strip technique is used to irradiate whole of abdomen. Presence of residual disease following debulking procedures in a case of ovarian carcinoma is treated with this technique. Whole abdomen is divided into contiguous strips of 2.5 cm wide area. Each strip is irradiated from front and back over 2 days and the field is gradually moved up. Cobalt 60 machine is generally used and a total tumour dose of 2600 to 2800 cGy is delivered. Pelvic boost of 2000 to 3000 cGy is given additionally. Kidneys and right lobe of liver are shielded with lead to reduce the dose to these organs. **Bulky residual disease (> 2 cm) is not suitable for radiotherapy.**

Use of radiotherapy for individual organ malignancy — see respective chapters.

Radiation reactions and their management — see Table 30.2. **Contraindications of radiotherapy** — see page 336.

CHEMOTHERAPY

General considerations

Mustard gas used in World War I, found to have tremendous effect on bone marrow suppression. This led to the concept of cytotoxic chemotherapy in the treatment of human cancer.

Use of cytotoxic chemotherapy has got the following objects :

- Complete remission of the tumour
- Partial remission (for a certain period) with improvement of median survival
- To prevent recurrence of the tumour
- To alleviate the symptoms, so as to improve the quality of life (palliation).

Effective chemotherapy is designed to kill selectively the malignant cells without producing serious irreversible harm to normal cells. The substances as yet available, damage both cancerous and normal tissues but in contradistinction to normal tissues, cancerous tissues cannot recover from the insult.

CELL KINETICS

Cell cycle time denotes the amount of time needed by a proliferating cell to progress through the cell cycle and produce a new daughter cell. Cell cycle times vary widely (12-217 hours) but are relatively constant for a specific tumour type.

Normal cells have the inherent capacity to multiply and this is controlled by various internal and external forces. There is also constant and balanced cell loss. Normal cells may be classified as :

- **Proliferating cells** (bone marrow, intestinal mucosa) — undergo constant cell division.

Gap 1 (G_1) (Synthesis of enzymes and regulatory proteins)	Postmitotic	4–24 hours (variable)
DNA Synthesis (S) and Replication		10–20 hours
Gap 2 (G_2) RNA synthesis Protein synthesis	Premitotic	2–10 hours
Mitosis (M)		0.5–1 hour
G_0 Resting phase		variable period

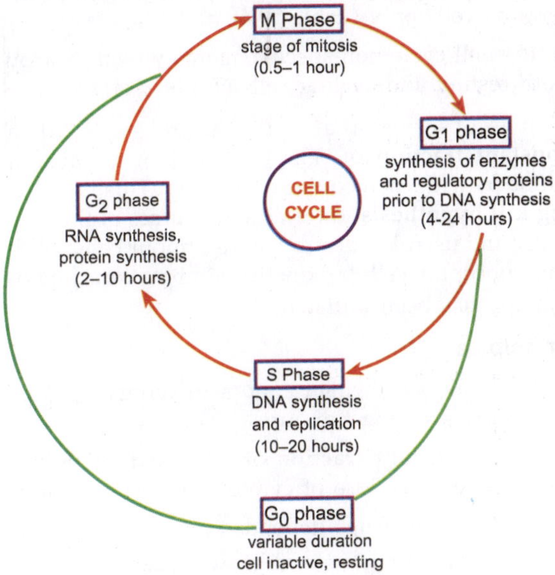

Fig. 30.4. The cell cycle and cell generation time

- **Quiescent cells** (liver)—can proliferate under special conditions (injury), otherwise they are in quiescent phase.
- **Static cells** (neurons)—rarely proliferate.

Cancer cells undergo uncontrolled and excessive proliferation compared to cell loss. Speed of cell division is the same compared to a normal cell.

Doubling time of human tumour is defined as the time taken by a tumour mass to double its size. Doubling time varies depending upon the specific type of the tumour. Tumour growth depends on growth fraction and cell death. **Growth fraction** is the number of cells in the tumour mass that are actively involved in the phase of cell division.

Gompertzian growth states that when a tumour volume increases in size, its mass doubling time becomes progressively longer.

Cell cycle—There are four phases of cell cycle. These are G_1, S, G_2 and M (Fig. 30.4). The duration of the cycle from M phase to M phase is called **generation time**. Tumour cells do not have faster generation time. Normal tissues have huge number of cells in the G_0 phase (out of cycle), in contrast to tumour cells, where more cells are in the active phase of cell division.

Cell cycle concept is very important for cancer chemotherapy. Dividing tumour cells are most sensitive to cytotoxic agents whereas cells in the G_0 are relatively insensitive (Fig. 30.4).

Varieties of malignancy

The credibility of the use of cancerolytic drugs depends upon the fact that in all malignancies, dissemination occurs at some stage of the disease and local treatment may not suffice. Proper understanding of cell cycle has evolved legitimate synergistic combinations of drugs with better cancer killing potentialities and less side effects (Fig. 30.3).

Table 30.4 : Drug activity in the cell cycle

Cell cycle	**Non-specific**	Cyclophosphamide, Cisplatin, Carboplatin
Cell cycle	**Specific :** On G_1	Actinomycin D
	On S phase	Methotrexate 5 FU Doxorubicin
	On G_2	Bleomycin, Etoposide
	On M phase	Vinblastine Vincristine Taxanes
	G_0	Nitrosoureas (BCNU, CCNU)

Broadly speaking chemotherapeutic drugs are of two varieties depending on the basis of their cell cycle specificity (Fig. 30.4) :

(a) Cell cycle specific agents which act on proliferating cells only (Table 30.4).

(b) Cell cycle non-specific agents which destroy both resting and cycling cells (Table 30.4).

It is observed that antitumour agents kill a **constant fraction** of cells (rather than a constant number) with each course of therapy. This is called **log kill hypothesis**. Intermittent courses of therapy are found useful to destroy more tumour cells. With this concept of cellular kinetics combination chemotherapy has been initiated.

Principles

(a) Rapidly growing tumours are more amenable than slow growing tumours.

(b) A constant fraction of neoplastic cells are killed with each dose of cytotoxic drug.

(c) Effect of drugs depends on :

- Tumour mass and growth rate.
- Sensitivity of resting phase cells.
- Immunocompetence of host cells.
- Type and dose schedule of agents.

(d) High dose intermittent course of chemotherapy may result in high cell kill and optimal destruction of the tumour (dose intensity).

(e) Combination agent chemotherapy is superior to single agent therapy for the treatment of most malignancies.

(f) Drugs combined, should have synergistic effect, different mechanism of action and different spectrum of toxicity. This will enhance the tumour cell kill and minimise the risk of drug resistance.

(g) Drug dose is adjusted according to the tolerance of the patient. Before starting any course of chemotherapy white blood cell count and platelet count (evidence of myelosuppression) is checked and the drug dose is tailored accordingly.

Single agent versus combination agents chemotherapy

- Combined chemotherapeutic agents attack different phases of cell cycle (synergistic effect), so reduces the tumour volume effectively.
- Use of combination (cell cycle specific and cell cycle non-specific) chemotherapy enhances tumour cell kill compared to single drug therapy.
- Because of toxicity, drug dose and duration of therapy cannot be increased when single agent chemotherapy is used.
- Emergence of drug resistance is more with single agent therapy.

DRUG RESISTANCE

Probable mechanisms

(i) Increased repair of DNA.
(ii) Decrease in cellular drug uptake.
(iii) Increased production of target enzyme to provide the cell with immunity to the drug.
(iv) Increase in drug degradation.
(v) Spontaneous mutations.

Combination chemotherapy

The following principles are to be maintained in selecting the combination of drugs :

- All drugs in the combination should have shown activity as single agents.
- Cell cycle specificity of the drugs should differ.
- Drugs with different mechanisms should be combined rather than drugs with similar action.

Classification of cytotoxic drugs in current use

Drugs used in cancer chemotherapy can be classified into the following groups.

These are principally based on structural similarity and mechanism of action.

(a) Alkylating agents

These drugs transfer their alkyl radical to nucleic acids. They prevent cell division by cross-linking the DNA strands. They produce single and double stranded DNA break. Cyclophosphamide inhibits DNA synthesis in addition. These are cell cycle non-specific agents (CCNS). These are most suitable for use in bulky slow growing tumours. These are often called radiomimetic drugs as they share some effects of radiation.

Examples : Cyclophosphamide (endoxan), Ifosfamide, Chlorambucil, Melphalan, Thiotepa.

(b) Antimetabolites

These are cell cycle specific agents. These agents impair intricate metabolic steps required for DNA and RNA synthesis by interacting with intracellular enzymes.

Examples :

- Methotrexate — Folic acid antagonist, prevents

Table 30.5

Toxic effects of the cytotoxic drugs and their management

Tissue or organ affected	Toxic effects	Management
Gastrointestinal	Nausea, vomiting, oral ulceration, stomatitis, necrotising enterocolitis, diarrhoea.	Antiemetics used for emetogenic chemotherapy • Dexamethasone 20 mg IV • Ondansetron 8 mg IV every 4 hrs. 2-3 doses • Metoclopramide 80-120 mg IV every 3-4 hours.
Hair roots	Alopecia (taxol, cyclophosphamide).	Generally reversible.
Haematological (bone-marrow)	Anaemia, granulocytopenia, thrombocytopenia. The danger level being : Hb% < 8 gm%, leucocyte count < 3,000/cumm and platelet count < 20,000/cumm (Paclitaxel, Etoposide, Carboplatin).	Blood transfusion, platelet transfusion, drug dose may be modified. Granulocyte colony-stimulating factor (G-CSF) and Granulocyte macrophase colony-stimulating factor (GM-CSF) have been used (250 µg/M^2, subcutaneously) for myelostimulation.
Skin	Dermatitis, pigmentation (bleomycin), extravasation, skin necrosis (Actinomycin D).	For extravasation and skin necrosis – removal of intravenous line, local infiltration of corticosteroids, ice pack therapy.
Cardiovascular	Toxic myocarditis (Doxorubicin), arrhythmias (Paclitaxel).	Discontinuation of drug, drug and dose modification, to consult cardiologist.
Liver	Hepatitis, elevated transaminases and bilirubin (Methotrexate).	Discontinuation of drug, drug and dose modification.
Lungs	Fibrosis (Bleomycin, Cyclophosphamide).	Pulmonary function tests, to consult physician.
Nervous system	Neurotoxicity, ototoxicity, peripheral neuropathy (Cisplatin, Ifosfamide)	Vitamin B complex, pyridoxin therapy, drug and dose modification.
Urinary system	Renal failure, azotemia (Cisplatin), haemorrhagic cystitis (Cyclophosphamide, Ifosfamide), red urine (Adriamycin).	Prehydration and mannitol induced diuresis before therapy, avoid simultaneous use of nephrotoxic drugs (aminoglycosides). **Mesna** is used for haemorrhagic cystitis due to cyclophosphamide or ifosfamide.
Immune system	Suppression of cellular and humoral immunity, loss of host defense mechanism.	Usually reversible.
Metabolic	Hyperkalaemia, hyperuricaemia, hypocalcaemia — due to rapid tumour lysis. Hyponatraemia — due to inappropriate ADH secretion.	Estimation of serum electrolytes and appropriate correction.
Surgical wound	Delayed healing.	
Gonads	Infertility, amenorrhoea.	Patient counselling.
Embryo	Teratogenic effect, congenital malformations.	Patient counselling, to assess risk and benefit.
Second malignancies	Due to mutagenic effect – leukaemia (melphalan).	

reduction of folic acid to folinic acid by inhibiting the enzyme dihydrofolate reductase.

- 5-Fluorouracil — Pyrimidine analogue, blocks thymidine synthesis and prevents DNA replication.
- 6-Mercaptopurine — Purine derivatives - competitive attachment to enzymatic catalytic site.

(c) Antibiotics

These are cell cycle non-specific agents. They prevent DNA replication, causes single and double stranded DNA break, e.g. actinomycin D, bleomycin, adriamycin, mitomycin.

(d) Plant alkaloids (natural products)

These are cell cycle specific agents. They act as spindle poison and cause arrest of mitosis at metaphase. Vincristine and vinblastin (from plant Vinca Rosea) bind to tubulin (intracellular microtubular protein) and prevents microtubule assembly.

Taxanes are the new class of cytotoxic drugs. Taxanes are obtained from the bark of pacific yew tree (Taxus brevifolia). Important members of this group are paclitaxel (taxol) and docitaxol (synthetic). Taxanes act by promoting microtubule assembly (polymerisation), and their stability. This results in 'meta-phase arrest' of the cell division. During this phase the cell becomes most sensitive to ionising radiation (radiosensitiser).

Other plant alkaloid — Etoposide.

(e) Hormones

The drugs induce regression of a hormone responsive tumour and also increase anabolic processes.

Progesterone preparations, e.g. hydroxyprogesterone caproate, medroxyprogesterone acetate, megestrol acetate.

Tamoxifen — an antioestrogen acts by competitive receptor binding — thus helpful in oestrogen dependent tumours.

(f) Miscellaneous

Platinum agents : Cisplatin, carboplatin — simulates alkylating agents (cross linking DNA).

Hexamethylamine — acts like antimetabolite.

Hydroxyurea — increases radiosensitivity of malignant tissue.

Gemcitabine (2', 2' – fluorodeoxy cytabidine) is a new agent used against ovarian, breast and cervical carcinoma.

(g) Biological

Interferon, Müllerian inhibiting factor — they act by improving the host immune defense.

Toxicity

The toxic reactions depend on the type of drug used, the method of administration, its dosage and general condition of the patient. The toxic reactions are tabulated in Table 30.5.

Route of administration

Oral — Alkylating drugs are mainly used orally. The intermittent therapy allows recovery of normal cells.

Parenteral — Administration (intravenous - commonly, intra-arterially) at interval of 1-4 weeks allows bone marrow to recover.

Intraperitoneal — Systemic administration is more effective. Drug penetration will be only 3-6 cells deep.

In cancer chemotherapy, single and multiple dose regimen with different permutations and combinations are being used, the details of which are beyond the scope of this book. But it is essential to understand the basic indications, limitations and complications of use of these drugs.

Pretreatment evaluation

Chemotherapeutic agents are highly toxic to the erythropoietic system, bone marrow in particular. The drugs are mostly metabolised in the liver and are excreted through the kidneys. The patients are also immunocompromised and as such, any source of infection is to be searched for, the organism isolated along with drug sensitivity. Pretreatment evaluation of all the important organ function is of paramount importance.

- Haematological — complete haemogram and platelet count.
- Serum — electrolytes.
- Renal functions — serum urea, uric acid, creatinine and creatinine clearance (specially when cisplatin is used).
- Liver functions — serum proteins, liver enzymes, bilirubin.
- Cardiac function — base line ECG and ventricular ejection fraction when cardiotoxic drug (doxorubicin) is used.
- Pulmonary function — when bleomycin is used.
- Throat swab, urine for culture and sensitivity.

Calculation of dose

The dose of a chemotherapeutic agent is usually calculated as square meter of body surface area. It provides a better measure of potential toxicity than

Table 30.6
Schematic presentation of commonly available agents, their average dosage schedule and route of administration

Cancerolytic drugs	Doses
A. Alkylating agent	
1. Cyclophosphamide (Endoxan)	750-1,000 mg/M² of body surface/IV. Single dose every 3 weeks. 50-110 mg/M² by mouth. Intracavitary – 1 gm in 10 ml of normal saline.
2. Ifosfamide (Ifex)	7-10 gm/M² IV over 3-5 days, to be repeated every 3-4 weeks.
3. Chlorambucil (Leukeran)	0.1-0.2 mg/kg of body weight orally/day for 4-6 weeks.
4. Thio-tepa	0.2-0.8 mg/kg/day IV – 5 days. Repeat after 4-6 weeks. Intracavitary 45-60 mg in 10 ml of normal saline.
5. Melphalan (Alkeran)	0.2 mg/kg/day orally × 5 days. Repeat after 4-6 weeks.
B. Antimetabolites	
1. Methotrexate	240 mg/M² IV with Leucovorin rescue. Oral 15-30 mg/day × 5 days.
2. 5-Fluorouracil (5-Fu)	10-15 mg/kg/day IV × 5 days. Repeat after 3-4 weeks. 10-15 mg/kg IV weekly, maximum up to 1 gm.
3. Hydroxy urea	1-2 gm/M²/day orally for 2-4 weeks.
4. Gencitabine	800-1000 mg/m² IV weekly every 3 weeks.
C. Antibiotics	
1. Actinomycin D	0.5 mg/M²/IV/weekly. Repeat 3-4 weeks *or* 0.5 mg/M²/IV/daily × 5 days
2. Doxorubicin (Adriamycin)	60-100 mg/M²/IV weekly. Repeat every 3-4 weeks
3. Bleomycin	10-20 mg/M²/IV/IM weekly
4. Mitomycin C	0.05 mg/kg/IV daily × 6 days, then on alternate days till 50 mg total dose.
D. Hormones	
1. 17–α-Hydroxyprogesterone caproate	1 gm IM twice a week for 1 year.
2. Medroxyprogesterone acetate (Depoprovera)	400-800 mg orally/IM weekly for 1 year.
3. Megestrol acetate (Megace)	40-120 mg tablet oral/day for 1 year.
E. Plant alkaloids	
1. Vincristine (Onvovin)	0.2-1.2 mg/M² IV weekly
2. Vinblastin (Velban)	5-6 mg/M² IV every 1-2 weeks
3. Etoposide (Epipodophyllotoxin)	100 mg/M² IV on days – 1, 3 and 5 repeat every 3-4 weeks
4. Paclitaxel (taxol)	135-250 mg/M² IV every 3-4 weeks
F. Miscellaneous drugs	
1. Cis-diaminedichloroplatinum (Cisplatin)	50-75 mg/M² IV every 1-3 weeks — usually 4-6 such
2. Carboplatin	300-400 mg/M² IV. Repeat every 3-4 weeks for 6 courses
3. Hexamethylamine	4-8 mg/kg/day orally for 14-21 days. Repeat every 6 weeks.
G. Anti-oestrogen	
1. Tamoxifen	10-20 mg twice daily orally
2. Leuprolide (Lupron)	1 mg daily orally or SC.

body weight. **The surface area closely reflects cardiac output and blood flow**. There is minimal change of surface area during entire course of therapy compared to body weight. Nomogram is used for calculating body surface area of adults (p. 626).

Use of drugs

A schematic presentation of commonly available agents and their average dosage schedule is made in Table 30.6. It should be realised that this schedule is flexible and treatment must be individualised according to need.

A scheme of use of chemotherapy in the management of different varieties of malignancy encountered in gynaecological practice is given in Table 30.8.

It is imperative that all cases undergoing chemotherapy should be monitored. This process should include recognition of evidences of retrogression of the disease by changes in clinical, biophysical and biochemical markers. Haematological profile must be checked at regular intervals (see above). The systemic changes should reach just short of irreversible toxicity for optimum benefit. Minor complications like nausea, vomiting, alopecia, glossitis should not preclude full treatment protocol. The benefits are to be weighed against toxic effects. Explaining the situation clearly helps in patient compliance and improves ultimate result.

Table 30.7
Formalities maintained in systemic chemotherapy

• Drugs used in combination should not be mixed together.
• The infusion set should be flushed with normal saline between the administration of each drug.
• To avoid sclerosis of the vein, the drugs should be washed through with normal saline.
• Extravasation should be avoided.
• Antiemetics should be given before start of therapy.

IMMUNOTHERAPY

The following considerations have led to the idea that host immune response can prevent tumour growth :

- Immune suppressed patients are more likely to develop malignant disease.
- Therapy with monoclonal antibodies is found to destroy tumour cells which is due to antibody dependent cellular cytotoxicity.
- Natural killer (NK) cells (lymphoid cells) with Interleukin-2 (IL-2), TNF can cause tumour cell lysis.
- Lymphokine-activated killer (LAK) cells together with IL-2 TNF, IFN can cause tumour cell destruction (adoptive immunotherapy).

Cytokines and cancer therapy

Cytokines are polypeptides secreted by different cells like, monocytes, macrophages, T cells and tumour cells. Cytokines are pleiotropic. Their functions include regulation of cell immune activity (interferons, interleukins), haematopoiesis (colony stimulating factor), and cytotoxic activity (interleukins and tumour necrosis factor). Due to this antitumour and immune stimulating effects, many of the cytokines are used currently in the therapy of cancer. But their exact role is not yet well-understood.

Principles of Immunotherapy

- Tumour mass must be reduced to a minimum by radial surgery, chemotherapy or radiation before immunotherapy.
- Immunotherapeutic approach should be a combined one.
- Any single agent therapy is often ineffective.
- Immunotherapy is more effective against tumours that are highly antigenic.

Augmentation of immune system

Approaches to augment the immune response to human tumour include :

Active immunotherapy (to induce host immune response).

- Biological immunostimulants — administration of BCG (*Bacille Calmette-Guérin), C. parvum (Corynebacterium parvum*).
- Chemical immunostimulants — levamisole, cimetidine.
- Cytokines — interferon (IFN), IL-2, tumour necrosis factor (TNF).
- Chemotherapeutic drugs — cisplatin, doxorubicin.

Passive immunotherapy (immunologically active substances are directly transferred to the host).

- Cytokines — interferon, TNF.
- LAK cells — together with IL-2.
- Monoclonal antibodies.
- Activated macrophages : Interferon.

Table 30.8
Chemotherapy in Gynaecology

Type of neoplasm	Indication (remarks)	Chemotherapy used
Squamous cell carcinoma of cervix	Very little scope except in stage IV or in recurrence as palliation	Various combinations are tried. • Bleomycin/Vincristine/Adriamycin/Vinblastine. • Cisplatin, Actinomycin D, Ifosfamide • Mitomycin, Hydroxyurea—to increase radio-sensitivity.
Squamous cell carcinoma of vulva and vagina	Rarely indicated except in advanced or recurrence as palliation	Topical 5-FU cream in vulval carcinoma has been tried. • Bleomycin
Endometrial carcinoma	As a routine or in late cases	Progestational agents, Ifosfamide, Doxorubicin, Cisplatin, Tamoxifen, Leuprolide
Endometrial sarcoma	Empirical	Adriamycin and Cyclophosphamide, VAC, Progesterone, Ifosfamide
Tubal carcinoma	Late cases	Adriamycin/Melphalan/Cyclophosphamide
Ovarian tumours : • Epithelial carcinoma	• Stage 1A May be used as a routine following surgery to improve the result • Advanced stage • Palliative chemotherapy • Gradually replacing radiotherapy	Single or multiple drug therapy : Cisplatin or Carboplatin (less toxic), Taxol, Melphalan, Thio-tepa, Chlorambucil, Hexamethyl melamine, Cyclophosphamide and Adriamycin/ (CAP or CP), Gemcitabine. Usually multiple drug therapy : • Taxol and Carboplatin • Adriamycin and Cyclophosphamide • Adriamycin, Cyclophosphamide and Cisplatin
Gonadal stromal tumour : • Granulosa cell tumour	Alternative to post-operative radiotherapy	• Vincristine + Adriamycin + Cyclophosphamide **(VAC)** • Bleomycin + Etoposite + Cisplatin **(BEP)**
• Secondary metastatic	—do—	Depends upon the primary lesion
Germ cell tumour : • Dysgerminoma	Radiotherapy preferred	Combination agents : Vinblastin, Bleomycin and Cisplatin **(VBP)** can be used for **successful treatment and preservation of fertility.**
• Endodermal sinus cell tumour, Embryonal carcinoma	• Highly malignant, • Chemotherapy preferred	Combination of drugs is used : • POMB-ACE = Vincristine, Methotrexate, Bleomycin, Cisplatin, Etoposide, Actinomycin D, Cyclophosphamide.
• Choriocarcinoma • Malignant immature teratoma, Polyembryoma	—do—	• VAC therapy/BEP therapy/VBP therapy. • Methotrexate/Actinomycin. • Vincristine/Adriamycin/Cyclophosphamide. • Cisplatin/Adriamycin/Cyclophosphamide.

Table 30.8 : Chemotherapy in Gynaecology *(contd. from previous page)*

Type of neoplasm	Indication (remarks)	Chemotherapy used
a. Hydatidiform mole	As a prophylactic therapy in selected cases.	• Methotrexate 5 days at every 14 days till β subunit becomes negative, thereafter 3 such. • Actinomycin D — 5 days every 14 days till β subunit becomes negative. • Three courses thereafter.
b. GTN	Mainstay in the management of GTN — non-metastatic and metastatic groups.	Described in Chapter 23. p. 351.
Chemotherapy for intraperitoneal small volume residual disease (<1-2 cm) and/or malignant effusions.		Intraperitoneal instillation of cisplatin, cyclophosphamide or taxol.

Immunotherapy has its limitations. Immune response enhancement leading to rejection of tumour can occur when the following conditions are fulfilled :

- Biological response modifiers are in direct contact with tumours.
- Tumour bulk is minimal.
- Blood supply is good.
- Combined with chemotherapeutic agents.

GENETICS AND GYNAECOLOGIC MALIGNANCY

Familial cancer of the breast, ovary, colon, endometrium and other sites have been observed in the female members of afflicted families. Well-defined cancer family syndromes with autosomal dominant inheritance pattern have been described (see p. 357). When life time risk of ovarian cancer in the population as a whole is 1.4 per cent, it is about 5 per cent when one first degree relative is affected and it rises to 7 per cent when two or more first degree relatives are affected.

Genetic basis of ovarian and breast malignancy have been explained with the mutation of the BRCA-1 gene on chromosome 17q and BRCA-2 gene on chromosome 13 q. Three types of genes (oncogenes, tumour suppressor genes and mutator genes) are involved with malignant change. Point mutation, deletion and insertion are the important changes observed in malignancy.

Oncogenes are dominant whereas **tumour suppressor genes (P53)** are recessive in function at cellular level. Oncogene activate cell proliferation to malignant behaviour whereas tumour suppressor genes (BRCA-1) restrain cell growth. However, majority of ovarian cancers are not associated with familial predisposition. Familial cancer account for less than 5 per cent of all cases of ovarian cancer. Familial cancers have an early age of onset.

Early detection of cancer may be possible by detecting mutated copies of a gene products (P53, HER-2/neu K-Jas), using polymerase or ligase chain reaction. Several oncogene products (her-2/neu, K-ras, C-myc, P21), tumour suppressor gene products (P53, P16, pRB) are currently being investigated as independent **prognostic markers.**

Oncogenes regulate cell growth in a positive fashion. Oncogenes include transforming genes of viruses and normal cellular genes that are activate by mutations to promote cell growth to a partly malignant behaviour. It needs one mutational events for its gain of function (Dominant).

Tumour suppressor gene (antioncogene)—Suppresses cellular growth, proliferation and malignant phenotype. It needs two mutational events (point mutation, deletions) for its loss of function (recessive).

Study for detection of gene mutation is at present restricted to research purpose only.

Gene therapy—The effects of **oncogene function** can be transformed by two approaches. One attempt is to remove the oncogene product or to block its function. Alternatively, one can use antisense oligonucleotides in an attempt to block the production of oncogene by preventing the transcription of chromosomal DNA to RNA. Antisense oligonucleotide can be administered systemically. Cytokine gene transfer to tumour cells stimulates a systemic immune response and destroy tumour cells. Cells are enginered to produce cytokines including interleukines 2,4,5 and 6, TNF and others. Clinical trials are in progress in patients with squamous cell carcinoma, ovarian epithelial cell carcinoma with this technology.

Tumour suppressor genes inhibit cell proliferation. Both

the copies of the gene must be inactivated (mutated) for neoplastic effect.

In cervical carcinoma, recurrent loss of heterozygosity (LOH) is identified is several chromosome regions (3 p 14-22, 4 p 15). Besides this, integration of viral (HPV 18, 16) DNA in chromosome (8, 12) is frequently observed.

Ovarian cancer — Point mutations of the p53 (17P) gene are the most frequent genetic alteration. Loss of heterozygosity (LOH) on chromosome 17q has been noted.

TUMOUR MARKERS

A tumour marker is a substance that is selectively produced by the neoplastic tissue. It is then released into the blood where from it can be detected.

Ideal tumour marker should fulfil the following criteria :

- It should be produced only by the tumour cells.
- It should be specific.
- Its measurement either in the blood or urine should be sensitive enough to detect microscopic or subclinical disease.
- Tumour markers are used to monitor the response of therapy. Ideally the antigen (tumour marker) level should represent the tumour volume correctly. Progressive rise in marker value indicates ineffective chemotherapy.
- The assay should be inexpensive and acceptable.

The tumour marker should not only indicate the presence but also the site of tumour origin.

Tumour marker is useful in screening, diagnosis and management of a case and for follow up. However, the detection of tumour marker is seldom made before the cell population becomes 10^{10}.

The role of serum CA–125 in the evaluation of disease (ovarian carcinoma) progression and regression is invaluable. Similarly, serum βhCG is useful in the diagnosis, management and follow up of cases with GTN. A list of tumour markers is given below (Table 30.9).

Table 30.9
Gynaecological tumour markers in common use

Marker	Tissue of origin of cancer
Human chorionic gonadotrophin (hCG)	Trophoblastic and some germ cell tumour (dysgerminoma).
Alpha fetoprotein (AFP)	Germ cell tumour (endodermal sinus tumour).
CA 125	Ovarian epithelial tumour, endometrial adenocarcinoma.
Carcinoembryonic antigen (CEA)	Ovarian (serous, endometrioid), cervical carcinoma (squamous cell).
Tumour associated glycoprotein – 72 (TAG-72)	Ovarian epithelial tumour.
Macrophage colony stimulating factor (M-CSF)	Ovarian epithelial tumour.
Squamous cell carcinoma antigen (SCC)	Carcinoma cervix, vulval and vaginal squamous cell carcinoma.
Lactic dehydrogenase (LDH)	Ovarian germ cell tumours.
CA 15–3 OVX 1, OVX 2 HER – 2/neu (oncogene product)	Ovarian epithelial carcinoma.
Galactosyltransferase associated with tumour (GAT)	To differentiate ovarian cancer from endometriosis.
Oestrogen Progesterone Testosterone	Gonadal stromal tumours.
Inhibin	Granulosa cell tumour.

KEY POINTS

- Marie Curie and Pierre Curie discovered the radioactivity of Radium in 1898.

  For therapeutic purpose, radium and caesium are commonly used.

  Effect of radiation at a point varies inversely as the square of the distance from the source (Inverse Square Law).

  Brachytherapy is the common form of radiation therapy specially when the tumour volume is small. After-loading technique is the modern development. Teletherapy is used to deliver to homogeneous radiation dose to a large volume of tumour.

  Rad is the absorbed dose. Recently, the unit gray (Joule/kg) is used. One centigray (cGy) is equivalent to one rad.

  Biological effects of radiation are due to fast electron, that ionises molecules to produce free radicals. Target for radiation injury is DNA. Tumour tissue recovers from radiation damage more slowly compared to normal tissue.

  Radiocurability of a tumour depends upon the biological behaviour of the cells. It is not identical to radiosensitivity which depends several factors (see p. 487).

  There may be localised or systemic radiation reactions for which appropriate therapy is needed. Early reaction is curable but the late reactions produce severe morbidity. Radiation reaction commonly affects GI tract, bone marrow and bladder (see p. 486).

- The cell replication cycle consists of M (mitosis), GI (RNA and protein synthesis), S (DNA synthesis) and G2 (RNA and protein synthesis) phases. Cells, not in the replication cycle are in G0 phase (p. 489).

  Diving tumour cells are most sensitive to cytotoxic agents. Radiation acts on cells primarily on M phase.

  Large tumours have smaller growth fractions and longer mass doubling time.

- The ideal chemotherapeutic drug which preferentially kills only the malignant cells is yet to be developed.

  The drugs are of two varieties — one acting on the proliferating cells only and the other one destroying both the resting and cycling cells. Rapidly growing tumours are more curable to treatment. Drugs used are alkylating agents, antimetabolites, antibiotics, plant alkaloids, hormones, etc. Toxic effects varies from slight to more severe one, even to the extent of death (p. 491).

  Cisplatin is more nephrotoxic and myelosuppressive compared to carboplatin. Doxorubicin is cardiotoxic. Bleomycin is associated with pulmonary toxicity. Vincristine and cisplatin cause peripheral neurotoxicity. Alopecia can occur with any chemotherapy. Taxol is a powerful antineoplastic agent that disrupts microtubule function (polymerisation) (p. 491).

  Combination therapy is preferred. It gives a synergistic effect by acting at different cell sites and reduces the development of drug resistance (p. 490).

  Pretreatment evaluation and proper monitoring during therapy are mandatory to prevent or minimise the toxicity (p. 492).

- Immunotherapy in malignancy — is being explored recently. Cytokines (polypeptes) have antitumour and immune stimulating effects. Augmentation of immune system is achieved by active (interferon, IL-2) and passive (LAK cells) immunotherapy.

- Tumour markers indicate the presence and also the site of tumour origin. It is useful in screening, diagnosis and management of cases and also for follow up. Gynaecological tumour markers in common use are — hCG in trophoblastic tumour, AFP in germ cell tumour, CA-125 in ovarian epithelial tumour and SCC in carcinoma cervix. HER-2/neu, a oncogene product is used for epithelial ovarian cancer (p. 497).

- Familial cancer (breast, ovary, colon) is explained on the basis of genes (oncogene, tumour suppressor gene and mutator gene). Point mutation, deletion and insertion are the important changes. Gene therapy to the tissues at risk by insertion of normal copies of genes is a way-forward.

Hormones in Gynaecological Practice

31

NOMENCLATURES

- **Hormones**
- **Factors**
- **Analogues**
- **Agonists**
- **Antagonists**

Hormones : Hormones are substances (either protein or steroid in nature), which are secreted by a gland and transported through the circulation to the target organs for their action.

Factors : Factors are substances that modulate cell function and proliferation by acting upon the cell membrane receptors. They act locally (unlike the hormones) by autocrine and paracrine mechanism.

Analogues : An analogue is a synthetic substance with a structure mostly similar to a natural one but differing from it in certain component. It may have agonist and/or antagonist function at the cellular level. GnRH analogue acts as an agonist initially but on chronic therapy it antagonises (down regulates) the pituitary GnRH receptors.

Agonists : Agonist is a substance that has increased affinity for cell receptors and it stimulates the cellular physiological response.

Antagonists : An antagonist tends to nullify the action of another substance binding on its receptor without eliciting a biological response. There is inhibition of receptor response.

Because of relative lack of receptor specificity, an antagonist for one class of hormone can have an antagonistic effect on another class of hormone.

Antagonists may have adverse effects apart from the intended use.

Cellular function

A cell function is modulated by any of the three ways.

Endocrine when a hormone in circulation (blood or lymph) regulates the function of a cell at a distant site.

Paracrine function is when a regulating substance diffuses from one cell to a contiguous cell (intercellular) and modulates the cell function. Insulin-like growth factor-II (IGF-II) is produced by the theca cells of ovary. It stimulates granulosa cell proliferation when it diffuses to it.

Autocrine function is explained when a regulating substance modulates the function of the same cell (intracellular). IGF-II is said to have autocrine function when it is produced by and acts on luteinised granulosa cells.

Introduction

Considerable advancement has been made in the understanding of chemistry and pharmacology of new compounds that modulate and influence the function of many endogenous hormones. Once the structure of natural hormones is defined, it becomes possible to synthesize not only the hormones themselves but also their agonists or antagonists. **These substances can be used** :

- To diagnose the functional integrity of endocrine control systems.
- To replace the hormone deficiency state.
- To modify the abnormal function of the endocrine system.
- To alter the normal function to gain objectives.

While, many natural hormones are not easily available in adequate quantities, with advanced technology, many such products are manufactured by synthetic, semisynthetic or hybridisation.

HYPOTHALAMIC HORMONES

GnRH (see p. 64)

- **Diagnostic** • **Therapeutic**

Diagnostic: The GnRH stimulation test is used to differentiate an amenorrhoea of pituitary or hypothalamic in origin (p. 449).

An intravenous dose of GnRH 50-100 μg is given to stimulate pituitary. The maximal response is observed at 15-30 minutes for LH and 30-60 minutes for FSH. **The absence of response usually denotes pituitary fault.** However, the result may not be unequivocal and as such, requires cautious interpretation.

Therapeutic:The pulsatile nature of hypothalamic GnRH in the control of gonadotrophin secretion affords a physiological basis for the activation of pituitary gonadal axis.

Induction of ovulation: **It is suitable in cases with** idiopathic hypogonadotrophic hypogonadism who have failed to respond to treatment with clomiphene. Pulsatile administration of GnRH 2.5-20 μg per pulse and the frequency ranged from once per 60 to once per 120 minutes induces satisfactory ovulation. Both subcutaneous and intravenous routes are employed. GnRH therapy results follicular growth and development similar to a normal cycle. In hypothalamic causes of anovulation GnRH is most effective. For intravenous route portable minipump is used. For subcutaneous route high dose (20 μg) is needed. **The main advantages of pulsatile administration are** lower incidence of hyperstimulation syndrome and multiple pregnancy when compared to hMG.

GnRH analogues

GnRH analogues (agonists and antagonists) have been synthesized by substitution of amino acids at different positions of GnRH molecule. This is done to overcome the short half life as well as to alter the functions of GnRH (see p. 64).

GnRH agonist is produced when there is substitution of amino acids at sixth and tenth positions (see Fig. 7.1A, p. 64). This makes GnRH more stable with increased receptor affinity.

Mode of action: Initially there is stimulation of anterior pituitary resulting in increased secretion of FSH and LH **(up regulation)**. This is called **flare effect**. After 1-3 weeks there is profound suppression of secretion **(down regulation)** due to loss of pituitary GnRH receptor sensitivity. This leads to a fall in pituitary gonadotrophic hormones — LH and FSH and consequently the gonadal secretion (hypogonadotrophic hypogonadal state). **The net effect is production of medical hypophysectomy.**

Mode of administration: It can be used by intranasal and subcutaneous route and the biodegradable implants last for a month (see Table 31.1).

Table 31.1
Common preparations available with their dose and route of administration

Preparation	*Dose*	*Route*
Buserelin (Superfact)	300-600 μg daily 200-500 μg daily	Intranasal subcutaneous
Nafarelin	400-800 μg daily	Intranasal
Goserelin (Zoladex)	3.6 mg every 28 days	Subcutaneous implant
Leuprorelin acetate	3.75 mg every 28 days	Subcutaneous or intramuscular
Triptorelin (Decapeptyl)	3 mg every 28 days	Intramuscular

Use of GnRH analogues

(1) **Controlled Ovarian Hyperstimulation in *in vitro fertilisation***

Suppression of endogenous pituitary gonadotrophin secretion by down regulation with GnRH analogues followed by administration of hMG or FSH allows good quality stimulation with superovulation. The problems of suboptimal response and premature luteinisation due to endogenous LH surge are thus avoided. This will allow significantly higher number of oocyte retrieval and significant improvement in pregnancy rate. This induction of ovulation protocol allows the clinicians to make convenient administration of hCG and oocyte collection. It is preferable to support the luteal phase with hCG.

Protocol: Two types of protocols are commonly used with probably of equal efficacy (p. 244).

Long protocol — The GnRH analogues are given from 21st day of previous cycle to desensitise the pituitary (LH level < 5 mIU/ml and E_2 < 50 pg/ml or when sonar fails to detect follicle) before the hMG or FSH is given. **The benefits include** less need of cycle monitoring, high pregnancy and live birth rates.

Short protocol — The hMG or FSH is given soon after

administration of GnRH agonists on day 2 and before the pituitary is desensitised. **The advantages of short protocol** are the economy and convenience, using for a short period of time.

Drug and Dose for pituitary desensitisation (see Table 31.1)

Buserelin :

- Intranasally—300 μg twice daily.
- Subcutaneously—200-400 μg daily.

(2) **Induction of ovulation with higher baseline LH in PCOS**

In refractory cases of ovulation induction, specially in patient with PCO, when the endogenous LH level is high, GnRH analogues offer a good success with long protocol regimen.

(3) **Endometriosis**—By producing medical hypophysectomy and thereby, a hypooestrogenic state, it produces atrophy of the ectopic endometrium.

Dose :

- Nafarelin nasal spray 200 μg twice daily is to be continued for about 6 months.
- Buserelin 300 μg (one 150 μg spray in each nostril) intranasally thrice daily or 200-400 μg by subcutaneous route daily for 6 months.
- Goserelin depot (3.6 mg) subcutaneously, in anterior abdominal wall.

(4) **Fibroid**—By producing hypooestrogenic state, they will produce shrinkage of the tumour by about 50 per cent. But the size comes back to previous state after the drug is withdrawn. The drug cannot replace surgery but may be advantageous when used prior to surgery (see p. 271).

(5) **Precocious puberty (p. 51)**—In only constitutional variety, to inhibit the premature activation of hypothalamopituitary gonadal axis, the analogues are highly effective. It also slows down the process of skeleton maturation and will stabilise or cause regression of the secondary sex characteristics.

Dose—100 μg intranasally twice daily for 6 months (see ch. 5).

(6) **Hirsutism**—In the idiopathic group, by suppressing the pituitary gonadal axis, the excess hair growth can be arrested with the use of GnRH analogues (see p. 548).

Dose—Nafarelin 100 μg per day subcutaneously will decrease the serum level of total and free testosterone and there is clinical improvement of hirsutism.

However, the improvement is only limited during the period of drug therapy and is in no way better than the use of 'pill'.

(7) **DUB**—During the time, the patient waiting for operation or during the period to improve the anaemic state (see p. 187).

(8) **Premenstrual syndrome (PMS)**

It is used for diagnostic as well as therapeutic purpose.

For diagnostic purpose, a depot preparation is administered for 3 months. Relief of symptoms confirm the diagnosis (see p. 179). For therapy, buserelin 400 μg is given intranasally daily or 50 μg/day subcutaneous injection up to 6 months.

(9) **Advanced breast carcinoma** in premenopausal women.

(10) **Contraception**—Trial is going on about its efficiency vis-a-vis hazards as contraceptives (see Chapter 29).

Used in male, GnRH analogues produce a decline in sperm density, sperm mobility and a decrease in testosterone level. The marked loss of libido makes it unacceptable. Currently use of GnRH antagonist along with testosterone (add-back therapy) is found to overcome the problem (see p. 481).

Used in female, GnRH analogues act by preventing the pituitary response to endogenous GnRH. Buserelin is given intranasally with daily doses of 300-600 μg over 3-6 months (see Table 31.1). **Add-back therapy** with conjugated oestrogen 0.625 daily and medroxyprogesterone 2.5 mg daily is effective to prevent the hypooestrogenic symptoms.

(11) **Endometrial resection/ablation**—Prior to endometrial resection, GnRH analogues are used to suppress the endometrial growth (see p. 589).

GnRH antagonists (see Table 31.2).

Hazards of GnRH analogues

Side effects are predominantly due to hypogonadotrophic and hypooestrogenic state. The important **side effects are** hot flushes, vaginal dryness, dyspareunia, headache and depression (menopause like symptoms, see ch. 6). Acne, muscle pain, back pain, dry skin are also noted. There is decrease in trabecular bone density (osteoporosis) when used for more than 6 months. They do not produce significant changes in lipid metabolism. For long-term use, GnRH analogues have been used with low dose oestrogen and progestin (**add-back therapy**) to minimise the side effects.

GnRH antagonist : Synthesised by modification of amino acids at positions 1, 2, 3, 6 and 10 (Ganirelix, Cetrorelix). **The important properties of GnRH agonist and antagonist are given below (Table 31.2).**

Table 31.2

GnRH Agonist	GnRH Antagonist
1. Suppression of endogenous LH surge	1. Suppression of endogenous LH surge
2. Initial flare effect	2. Immediate suppression of gonadotrophins
3. Pituitary function recovery—slow	3. Quick recovery following therapy
4. Risk of OHSS – present	4. Less OHSS (see p. 503)
5. Expensive	5. Less expensive

GONADOTROPHINS

The use of gonadotrophins in clinical use lies on the principle that gonadotrophic hormones act on the ovaries to induce ovulation. **The gonadotrophins, used widely today, are derived from urine obtained from postmenopausal women**. Human gonadotrophin can also be obtained from extract of cadaveric pituitary glands. Human pituitary gonadotrophin (hPG) is predominantly FSH. It is not easily available.

The most commonly used commercial preparation is human menopausal gonadotrophins (hMG). One ampoule of hMG (pergonal) contains LH activity of 75 IU and FSH activity of 75 IU. Purified FSH (Metrodin – 75 IU/ampoule) is available with minimum LH. Recently, a highly purified preparation of human FSH (Metrodin HP) has been made available (Serono). This is extracted from hMG using anti-hCG antibodies to cause absorption of LH on to gel columns. Metrodin HP can be administered subcutaneously. Recombinant FSH (Gonal F, Recagon) is now available. It is administered by subcutaneous route.

hCG (human chorionic gonadotrophin) is known to have a biological action like LH surge and is available in ampoules with 1000-5000 IU (pregnyl, profasi). **It is obtained from urine of pregnant women**. Recombinant hCG is now available.

Limitations

- It is expensive.
- It should only be used with back up facilities for monitoring the response by BBT, cervical mucus study, supplemented by serial serum oestradiol estimation and sonographic measurement of follicular enlargement (see ch. 16). As such, its use is limited only in women with ovarian reserve (p. 503).

Indications

- Anovulatory infertility where other factors (tubal, uterine, male) have been excluded.
- Induction of superovulation in assisted reproduction (see p. 244).
- hCG is administered for luteal phase support specially when GnRH agonist is used.
- Treatment of male infertility (hypogonadotrophic hypogonadism) (see p. 235).
- Treatment of cryptorchism.
- Hypogonadotrophic hypogonadism with or without amenorrhoea.
- Failed clomiphene induction specially in patients with polycystic ovaries (PCOS).

Contraindications

- High level of endogenous FSH, indicating ovarian failure (see p. 444, 449).
- Overt thyroid or adrenal dysfunction.
- Pituitary tumour.
- Indeterminate uterine bleeding.

Treatment protocol

The durg dose schedule should be individualised to get the best result. As a rule, a higher dose is required in cases of secondary amenorrhoea due to pituitary failure and a smaller dose may be required in ovulatory failure or corpus luteal insufficiency. Metrodin containing only FSH, is suitable in PCOS.

Treatment with hMG begins following spontaneous mens or induced withdrawal bleeding. A daily dose of 1-2 ampoules of hMG is given intramuscularly for at least 5 days and continued thereafter with the same dose or an increasing dose with cervical mucus study, E_2 estimation and sonographic (transvaginal) folliculometry at interval of 2-3 days or earlier until the preovulatory follicular diameter measures 18-20 mm (see p. 238). hMG is then discontinued and after 24 hours, hCG is given intramuscularly for ovulation. The dose of hCG is 5000 IU for induction of ovulation. The patient is advised to have sexual intercourse on a number of occasions over the next 36-72 hours.

In some cases, for adequate ovarian follicular growth, high doses of FSH (4-6 ampoules per day) may be needed.

High responders are those women who have exaggerated response in follicular development. The diagnostic features are : enlarged ovaries with large number of follicles, elevated serum oestradiol (> 3000 pg/ml).

Management options

(A) **Coasting** :

- To continue GnRH agonist.
- No gonadotrophin stimulation.
- To give hCG once oestradiol level is within the normal range (see above).

(B) **Oocyte retrieval and fertilisation** — freezing all embryos and no transfer to avoid ovarian hyperstimulation syndrome.

(C) **To delay** embryo transfer until the symptoms subside.

(D) **To cancel** the treatment cycle.

Poor responders are those women who develop fewer follicle (< 3) and have serum oestradiol < 500 pg/ml.

Management options :

- To use higher doses of gonadotrophin stimulation.
- To decrease the doses of GnRH agonist.
- To use GnRH antagonist instead of long acting agonist.

Results of gonadotrophin use : Pregnancy rate is 70-90 per cent after 6 cycles treatment. Spontaneous miscarriage rate is high (20%). Risk of ectopic pregnancy is high. Multiple pregnancy rate is between 10-30 per cent. Majority are twins. There is no increased incidence of congenital malformation of the fetus.

Ovarian reserve : Means the quantity as well as quality of follicles present in the ovary. The total number of oocytes declines with the age of a woman since her birth (see p. 79). Inhibin B secreted by the competent follicles exerts negative feedback on pituitary FSH secretion (see p. 72). With the progressive fall in follicle number as with age, inhibin B level is reduced. There is rise in FSH level even in the early follicular phase.

Tests for detection of reduced ovarian reserve : (i) Levels of cycle D3 serum FSH > 10–15 IU/L. (ii) Levels of D3 serum oestradiol > 75-80 pg/ml. (iii) Clomiphene citrate challenge test : Levels of D3 serum FSH and oestrdiol are measured. The women is given clomiphene citrate (100 mg daily from D5–D9). Serum levels of FSH is measured again on D10 and elevated values of serum FSH (more than 2 SD of the mean) are obtained. (iv) Levels of cycle D3 serum Anti-Müllerian Hormone (AMH) low (< 8.1 p mol/L). (v) Levels of basal serum inhibin B low (< 400 pg/ml). (vi) TVS : reduced antral follicles and mean ovarian volume. Poor ovarian reserve indicates poor outcome with IVF.

Hazards of ovulation induction (p. 247)

Ovarian hyperstimulation syndrome (OHSS)

OHSS is characterised by multiple follicular development and ovarian enlargement following hCG stimulation. It occurs mostly with the conception cycle. The clinical features appear about 3-6 days after the ovulating dose of hCG is administered. It is an iatrogenic and potentially a life threatening complication of superovulation.

Risk factors for OHSS are : Young age < 30 years, PCOS, Serum E_2 > 2500 pg/ml, Rapidly rising serum E_2 levels (> 75% rise from previous day), Ovarian 'necklace sign' on USG (multiple small follicles), hCG administration and multiple pregnancy.

Pathophysiology is poorly understood. Increased capillary permeability leads to leakage of fluid from the

Criteria for severity of OHSS

Severity	Clinical features
Mild (10–20%)	• Abdominal bloating, mild pain • Ovarian size < 8 cm
Moderate (5–10%)	• Nausea, vomiting, diarrhoea • USG evidence of ascites • Ovarian size 8–12 cm
Severe (1–2%)	• Clinical ascites, sometimes hydrothorax, • ARDS • Haemoconcentration (Haematocrit > 45%, WBC count > 15000/ml) • Oliguria with normal serum creatinine • Liver dysfunction • Anasarca • Ovarian size > 12 cm
Critical (rare)	• Tense ascities • Haematocrit > 55% • WBC count > 25000/ml • Oliguria with elevated serum creatinine • Renal failure • Thromboembolic phenomenon • Ovarian size > 12 cm.

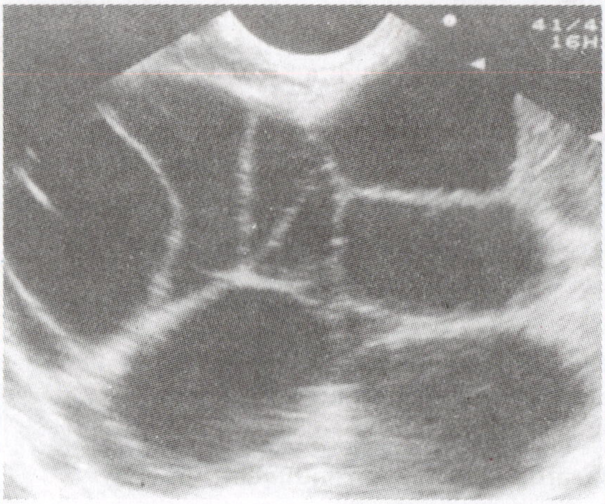

Fig. 31.1 : Ultrasonographic view of ovarian hyperstimulation syndrome. Enlargement of the ovary with multiple follicles

peritoneal and ovarian surfaces. Variety of chemical mediators like cytokines, vascular epidermal growth factor (VEGF), prorenin, renin and nitric oxide (NO) system are thought to be stimulated with hCG administration.

Prevention — Complete prevention may not be possible but severity can be reduced. The important steps to be taken are :

- Close monitoring of the superovulation cycles using TVS and serum oestradiol estimation (see p. 244).
- To withhold ovulatory dose of hCG in susceptible cases and to cancel the cycle or to delay the dose of hCG injection (coasting).
- Follicular aspiration after hCG administration and cryopreservation of oocytes or embryos for future use may reduce the severity of symptoms (coasting and cryopreservation).
- Aspiration of immature oocytes and *in vitro* maturation (IVM) are done. Subsequently ICSI is performed on IVM oocytes and embryos are transferred to the hormonally prepared uterus.
- Progesterone should be used for luteal phase support (see p. 245) instead of hCG.

Management of OHSS is mainly supportive.

Moderate and severe cases are to be admitted.

- To monitor complete haemogram, LFTs, RFTs, electrolytes, coagulation profile, ECG and urine output.
- Chest X-ray (shielding the pelvis), monitoring of O_2 saturation is needed when there is respiratory compromise.
- TVS is to be done to assess ovarian volume and ascites.
- Oral fluid is continued to prevent haemoconcentration and to maintain renal perfusion. Normal saline 150 ml/hr IV is given when haematocrit is > 45 per cent.
- To relieve respiratory distress, abdominal paracentesis may be done under USG guidance.
- Human albumin (50 mL of 25%) may be administered to correct hypovolaemia. It may be repeated.
- Pain is controlled with paracetamol or pethidine.
- Intensive care management is needed for specific complications like renal failure.
- Surgery is rarely indicated.

ANTI-GONADOTROPHINS

- **Danazol**
- **Gestrinone**

Danazol

Danazol is a derivative of 17-alpha ethinyl testosterone. It has got both androgenic and anabolic properties. **It is strictly anti-gonadotrophin but acts as an androgen agonist.**

Mode of action : The mechanism of action is complex and includes the following :

- Acting on the hypothalamo-pituitary gonadal axis → depression of frequency of GnRH pulses → suppression of pituitary FSH and LH surge. There is however, no change in the basal gonadotrophin level. Thus, it acts by producing "pseudomenopause" seems misnomer; while the oestrogen level is reduced but **unlike menopause, the gonadotrophins remain static in base levels.**
- Reduces the liver synthesis of SHBG and as such, free testosterone is increased which in turn has got direct action on endometrial atrophy.
- Acts directly on the ovaries, inhibiting the enzymes responsible for steroidogenesis.
- Able to bind with steroid receptors on the endometrium and endometrial implants.
- Immunologic effects of danazol include decrease in serum immunoglobulins, interleukin-1 and TNF production. This effect helps in the regression of endometriosis.

The net result is production of an hypo-oestrogenic state.

Precautions : It should be commenced in the early follicular phase of the menstrual cycle. **Barrier method of contraception** should be used to avoid being administered during early pregnancy following accidental ovulation. There is chance of virilisation of the female offspring. **It is contraindicated in liver disease.**

Dose : Depending upon the indication (Table 31.3) and response, the dose varies from 200-800 mg daily orally.

Table 31.3 : Indications of danazol

• Endometriosis	• Precocious puberty.
• DUB	• Premenstrual tension syndrome.
• Symptomatic fibroid	• Benign fibrocystic disease of the breasts (breast pain).
	• Prior to hysteroscopic endometrial ablation, to make the endometrium atrophic.

Side effects (Table 31.4)

The side effects are mostly related to hypo-oestrogenic and androgenic activity.

However, these effects revert back to normal soon following stoppage of the therapy.

It is recommended that the patient should discontinue the treatment, if they develop hirsutism or hoarseness of voice.

Gestrinone

Gestrinone is a derivative of 19-norethisterone. It is an androgen-agonist and progesterone agonist-antagonist. It markedly reduces SHBG levels and thus increases the free testosterone. It reduces the secretion of FSH and LH. It has a much longer half life and the dose required to produce equivalent results is much smaller than danazol.

Dose :

2.5 mg twice weekly starting on first day of cycle with second dose 3 days later, repeated on same two days preferably at same time each week.

Side effects are the same to those of danazol but usually less marked.

GONADAL HORMONES

There are three gonadal steroid hormones. These are oestrogen, progesterone and androgen.

Mechanism of action

Steroid sex hormones are well-absorbed through the skin and the gut. While most are subjected to extensive hepatic metabolic inactivation, there is some enterohepatic recirculation specially of oestrogens and this may be interrupted by diarrhoea to cause loss of efficacy. The sex hormones are transported in the blood non-specifically by albumin and specifically by SHBG.

Steroid hormone receptors are complex proteins inside the target cell. The steroid penetrates the cell membrane and mediates action via receptors within the nucleus (see Fig. 7.4).

OESTROGENS

Natural oestrogens are 18-carbon atom steroids. Oestradiol is the most active natural oestrogen in human uses.

Preparations available : • Natural • Synthetic

Natural : (a) It is available in the form of water soluble conjugated oestrogen as Premarin (Equine conjugated oestrogen). It is obtained from the urine of pregnant mares. It is available as tablets 0.625 mg and 1.25 mg and as injection of 20 mg ampoules for IM or IV injection. (b) Oestrogen valerate used for priming the endometrium in donor oocyte programme (vide Ch. 16).

Synthetic : Oral, Injectable, Cream/Gel, Pessary, Implant, Patch

Oral : This is the best route for synthetic preparations.

Table 31.4
Side effects of danazol

Hypooestrogenic	*Androgenic*	*Metabolic*
• Diminished breast size • Decreased libido • Atrophic vaginitis • Hot flushes	• Acne • Oily skin • Oedema • Weight gain • Hirsutism • Deepening of voice (irreversible)	• Elevation of LDL • Reduction of HDL • Decrease in TBG and total thyroxine level

- Ethinyl oestradiol (Lynoral) 0.01 mg and 0.05 mg daily is commonly used.
- Oestradiol valerate 1-2 mg.
- Mestranol — 0.05 mg.
- Oestriol succinate (Evalon) — 1-2 mg.

Injectable : • Oestradiol ester as progynon depot (Schering) – 10 mg ampoule. • Oestradiol benzoate or dipropionate – 1 mg and 5 mg ampoule.

Cream : • Vaginal cream–dienestrol (0.1 mg/gm), Oestriol (1 mg/gm). • Percutaneous cream — delivers 3 mg of oestradiol in each daily 5 gm applicator of cream.

Gel : • Oestradiol gel 1 mg to be applied once daily over the skin of the lower trunk.

Pessary :Dienestrol or diethyl stilboestrol pessary.

Implants : • Subcutaneous implants of 50 mg and 100 mg of 17β oestradiol effect lasts for 6 months.

Transdermal patch : It contains 3.2 mg of 17β oestradiol releasing about 50 μg of oestradiol in 24 hours. It should be applied below the waist line and changed twice a week.

Therapy

- **Replacement therapy** • **Pharmacotherapy**

Replacement therapy

Hypo-ovarian function : Oestrogen daily × 21 days followed by norethesterone or medroxyprogesterone 5 mg × last 10 days.

Menopausal symptoms

(a) Cyclic or continuous therapy in the form of oestradiol or conjugated oestrogens.

(b) Postmenopausal hormone replacement therapy (HRT) in otherwise symptom-free women.

- To reduce facial wrinkles.
- To prevent osteoporosis.
- To prevent cardiovascular disease.

It is administered either cyclic or continuous. Progestogen should be added to reduce endometrial carcinoma. However, in hysterectomised individuals, progestogen need not be added. **It is specially indicated** in premature ovarian failure, gonadal dysgenesis and in surgical menopause (details in ch. 5).

Pharmacotherapy : The oestrogen is most commonly used along with progestogen and as such, the use of the combined therapy is discussed later on. **The indications of only the oestrogen therapy are mentioned here**.

Oral contraception : While the combined oestrogen and progestogen preparations are widely used throughout the globe, oestrogen in isolation is only used as postcoital contraception (details in ch. 29).

Vaginitis : • Senile or atrophic vaginitis—either vaginal cream or oral oestrogens may be equally effective (see ch. 5).

• **Vulvovaginitis** in childhood, foreign body in the vagina or sexual assault—low dose of oral oestrogen or vaginal cream helps in increasing the vaginal defence and hastens recovery.

Intersex state : In Turner's syndrome (45, XO) or gonadal dysgenesis (46, XY), oestrogen therapy is helpful for the growth and development of the secondary sex characters (see ch. 27).

In androgen insensitivity syndrome (46, XY), after gonadectomy supplementary oestrogen therapy is indicated to prevent regression of the breast development, osteoporosis and cardiovascular complications (see ch. 27).

The oestrogen is used cyclically as ethinyl oestradiol 0.01 mg twice daily for 25 days. However, in prolonged use, progestogen in the form of medroxyprogesterone acetate 10 mg daily is added from day 16-25 to minimise the adverse effects of oestrogen. Alternatively, a combined oral 'pill' may be prescribed.

DUB : The oestrogen in pharmacological doses causes rapid growth of endometrium. As such, acute bleeding can be stopped by oral conjugated oestrogen in a dose of 10 mg a day. The bleeding usually stops within 24 hours. Alternatively, 25 mg may be given intravenously every 4 hours for 3 doses (see p. 52).

Delayed puberty : If the breast development fails to start even at the age of 14, 10 μg of oestrogen daily may be of help. In cases of irregular bleeding or when the breast development is well-advanced, progestogens may be added (ch. 5).

Cervical mucus hostility : To improve the quality of the cervical mucus in infertility, low dose of oestrogen (ethinyl oestradiol 0.01 mg) may be given cyclically, from day 1–14.

An adjunct with clomiphene therapy

In cases of hypo-oestrogenic state with hypomenorrhoea, small dose of oestrogen is of help to improve the quality of the cervical mucus.

Breast carcinoma in postmenopausal women particularly in tumours having oestrogen positive receptors.

Stress incontinence (GSI) in postmenopausal women to improve the tone of collagen tissue (see p. 386).

Comments : Oral route with preparations of ethinyl oestradiol is widely used because of its efficacy, low cost and minimal intolerance. Vaginal cream used in atrophic vaginitis has got its local and systemic effects.

Intramuscular administration of progynon depot 10 mg at interval of one month is helpful as a prophylaxis against postmenopausal symptoms, following hysterectomy with bilateral salpingo-oophorectomy in premenopausal women.

Table 31.5 Contraindications of oestrogen therapy
• History of venous thromboembolism. • Active liver disease. • Severe hypertension. • Organic heart disease. • Oestrogen dependent tumour such as breast adenoma.

Adverse effects

Minor ailments are :

- Nausea, vomiting
- Breast tenderness
- Breakthrough bleeding
- Weight gain

Major effects include :

- Increased incidence of endometrial carcinoma, thromboembolism, cerebral thrombosis and haemorrhage.

To minimise breakthrough bleeding and prevent endometrial carcinomas and vascular complications, progestogens should be combined with oestrogen therapy.

ANTI-OESTROGEN

- **Clomiphene** • **Letrozole** • **Tamoxifen**

Clomiphene

Clomiphene citrate is a non-steroid triphenylethylene compound with a structure similar to that of stilboestrol. The commercially available form is a mixture of two isomers, enclomiphene—a potent anti-oestrogen and zuclomiphene, a weak anti-oestrogen.

Mode of action

In the hypothalamus, clomiphene citrate binds to oestrogen receptors, occupies the nuclear site for a long time (weeks). The negative feedback of endogenous oestrogen is thus prevented. The frequency of pulsatile GnRH secretion is thereby increased which in turn results in rise of pulse frequency of both LH and FSH. Antioestrogenic effects are observed at the level of cervix and endometrium.

Indications :

- Anovulatory infertility where other factors have been excluded.
- Induction of ovulation — The ideal case is one of normogonadotrophic-normoprolactinaemic disorders of ovulation.
- Assisted reproductive techniques in producing superovulation.
- Male infertility with defective spermatogenesis due to hypogonadotrophic-hypogonadism.

Mode of administration : It is administered orally for 5 days starting between day 2 and day 5 of the cycle. The initial dose of 50 mg increasing in 50 mg steps to a maximum of 200 mg, if ovulation is not induced by the lower dose. Ovulation generally occurs 5-7 days after the last day of therapy. Patient is advised to have intercourse every other day for one week beginning 5 days after the last day of medication. Total treatment cycle should not exceed 6.

Adjuvant drugs : Adjuvant drugs are used when there is failure with clomiphene therapy (p. 237).

- GnRH agonist to eliminate endogenous high LH level (p. 238).
- Dopamine agonist (bromocriptine) when there is associated galactorrhoea or hyperprolactinaemia.
- Insulin sensitiser (metformin) in cases with hyperinsulinaemia.
- Oestrogen is given in the follicular phase to improve the quality of the cervical mucous.
- Other adjuvant drugs — see p. 237.

Contraindications :

- Patients who are hypogonadotrophic and hypooestrogenic.
- Presence of cystic ovaries.

Side effects : These include visual disturbances, headache, hot flushes, breast tenderness, abdominal discomfort, loss of hair, rashes and ovarian enlargement. Hyperstimulation syndrome (see p. 503) is less likely.

Results :While successful induction can be achieved by 80 per cent, pregnancy rate is about 50 per cent. The reduced pregnancy rate may be due to its anti-oestrogenic effect on endometrium cervical mucous and the oocyte. There may be the presence of other factors for infertility including luteal phase defect and LUF (see p. 230). Chance of multiple pregnancy ranges 0-5 per cent.

Letrozole

It inhibits the **enzyme aromatase** in the granulosa cells of ovarian follicles (p. 69). It suppresses oestrogen synthesis. Letrozole 2.5 mg given from D_3 to D_7 increases the release of gonadotrophins from the pituitary and stimulates development of ovarian follicle. Intraovarian androgens are increased which increase FSH sensitivity. As opposed to clomiphene it has no peripheral anti-oestrogenic effects on the endometrium and the cervical mucous. Half life of letrozole is 45 hours. Letrozole is used either as a first line therapy (alternative to clomiphene) or in clomiphene resistant women (p. 237) with anovulatory infertility. Pregnancy rates are comparable or better than that of clomiphene. Multiple pregnancy rates are low. No increased risk of fetal congenital malformations has been observed with letrozole.

Anastrozole, another aromatase inhibitor is found to be effective in reducing the growth of pelvic endometriosis and in pain relief.

Tamoxifen (SERMs) p. 59

Tamoxifen is similar to clomiphene both structurally and functionally. It has got both oestrogen antagonist and agonist effect.

- It is a competitive inhibitor to oestrogen at the receptor site. Antioestrogenic function of raloxifene is more selective in uterus and breasts.
- It decreases antithrombin III and increases the sex hormone binding globulin (SHBG) level (agonist action).
- It can be used for induction of ovulation in doses of 20 mg per day for 5 days, in cases of intolerance to clomiphene.
- It is widely used for the treatment of benign breast diseases.
- In postmenopausal breast carcinoma, it is given in doses of 10 mg twice daily for 2 years as an adjuvant therapy. It is effective both in oestrogen receptor positive and negative cases.
- In recurrent endometrial carcinoma, it inhibits the binding of oestradiol to the oestrogen receptor. Tamoxifen increases the progesterone receptors. A dose of 20-40 mg per day has been used. Low grade tumours and hormone receptor positive tumours have got better response.
- Raloxifene (p. 59) therapy is effective in regression of endometriosis.

PROGESTERONE

Progesterone is a natural hormone (C-21 steroid) produced mainly by the theca lutein cells of the corpus luteum. It is also secreted by the adrenal cortex in small amount. During pregnancy placenta is the main source. Progesterone produces secretory changes in an oestrogen primed endometrium. Natural progesterones are rapidly metabolised and inactivated when administered by the oral route and as such, it is to be used parenterally. During the last few decades, a number of compounds were sythesized having the properties of progesterone and could be given in tablet form. **These are called** progestational agents, gestagens, progestogens or progestins. Classification of progestogens and their grades of progestional activity are given in Tables 31.6 and 31.7.

Uses : • **Diagnostic** • **Therapeutic**

Diagnostic

Progesterone challenge test : In the investigation of pathological amenorrhoea, this test is employed. If withdrawal bleeding occurs, it proves (i) intact hypothalamo-pituitary ovarian axis, (ii) there is adequate endogenous oestrogen (> 40 pg/mL), (iii) the endometrium is responsive and (iv) the uterovaginal canal is patent. The individual is likely to respond to ovulation induction drugs (p. 449).

Dose : Medroxyprogesterone acetate 10 mg daily for 5 days is given orally.

Therapeutic indications

Contraception : Combined preparations of oestrogen and progestogen are widely used as contraceptive pill (see ch. 29). Uses of only progestogens as contraception are :

- Minipill (oral).
- Levonorgestrel :emergency contraception (p. 471).
- Depomedroxyprogesterone acetate (DMPA) (injectable).
- Norethisterone enanthate : NET-EN (injectable).

Table 31.6
CLASSIFICATION OF PROGESTOGENS

Progesterone Derivative	Progesterone Content
I. **Progesterone**	Natural progesterone
II. **Pregnane progestogens** They do not alter carbohydrate metabolism.	• 17α hydroxy progesterone caproate. • Medroxyprogesterone acetate. • Chlormanidone acetate. • Cyproterone acetate.
III. **Norpregnane progestogens.**	• Nomegestrol acetate. • Gestonorone caproate.
IV. **Stereoisomer of progesterone : Retroprogesterone.** They do not inhibit ovulation.	• Dydrogesterone.
V. **19 norprogesterone derivatives** (norpregnanes)	• Demegestone • Promegestone • Nestorone • Trimegestone
VI. **Alkyl derivatives of 19 nortestosterone**	
A. ***Oestrane steroids*** They alter carbohydrate metabolism slightly. Metabolically they are converted into norethisterone.	• Norethisterone • Norethisterone acetate • Norethynodrel • Ethynodiol diacetate • Lynestreno
B. ***Gonane steroids*** They have excellent contraceptive efficacy and cycle control. Side effects are less. They are more potent than the oestrane steroids.	• Norgestrel • Levonorgestrel • Desogestrel • Etonogestrel (3 ketodesogestrel) • Gestodine • Norgestimate • Norelgestromin • Dienogest
VII. **Spironolactone derivatives.**	• Drospirenone
VIII. **Unsaturated 19 norsteroid.**	• Gestrinone

Table 31.7
METABOLIC EFFECTS OF PROGESTOGENS AND THEIR GRADES OF PROGESTATIONAL ACTIVITY

Progestogens	Progestational activity	Androgenic activity	Anti-androgenic activity	Levels of SHBG↓
1. Progesterone	1	–	+	–
2. Cyproterone acetate	4	–	+++	–
3. Medroxy progesterone	4	+	–	+
4. Norethosterone	4	+	–	–
5. Norgestimate	4	+	–	–
6. Drospire none	4	–	+	–
7. Dienogest	4	–	+	–
8. Nomegestrol	5	–	+	–
9. Levonorgestrel	6	++	–	++
10. Desogestrel	8	+	–	–
11. Gestodene	9	+	–	+
12. Nestorone	10	–	–	–
13. Trimegestone	10	–	+	?

Progestational activity is graded 1-10; Considering progesterone as 1, 10 being the most potent.

SHBG = sex hormone binding globulin;

(–) = no effect

(+) = effect

(++) = strong effect

(+++) = very strong effect

- Implant (norplant subdermally) (p. 470).
- Vaginal ring containing levonorgestrel.
- LNG-IUS — containing L-norgestrel (p. 459).

Dysfunctional uterine bleeding (DUB)

Progestogen administration will cause secretory changes in the endometrium. Thus, it is very active in cases of anovulatory than in an ovulatory DUB. The therapy is ideal in puberty, adolescent and those approaching menopause.

To stop bleeding, norethisterone or norethisterone acetate 5 mg thrice daily is quite effective. To regulate the cycle, the same preparation is used from day 5 to day 25 or from day 15 to day 25 of cycle.

Mode of action : Progesterone decreases synthesis of oestrogen receptors in the endometrium.

- It converts oestradiol to less potent oestrone through enzymatic action.
- It inhibits mitotic activity of the endometrial cells.
- It induces the enzyme oestradiol dehydrogenase — which degrades oestradiol in the endometrium.
- Over all progesterone acts as an antioestrogen on the endometrium.

Endometriosis : The use of progestogens induces a hyperprogestogenic hypooestrogenic state. Progestogens cause decidualisation of endometrial tissue. There will be atrophy of the glands, fibrosis and atrophy of the ectopic endometrial tissues.

The drugs commonly used are medroxyprogesterone acetate or dydrogesterone or derivatives of 19-norethisterone.

Dose : Norethisterone 5 mg or medroxyprogesterone 10 mg twice or thrice daily and continued for 6-9 months. The patient remains amenorrhoeic.

Alternatively, intramuscular injection of medroxyprogesterone acetate 100 mg every 2 weeks for 4 doses and then 200 mg every month for 4 doses will produce amenorrhoea. This is suitable in cases of older women who have completed family.

Primary dysmenorrhoea : Dydrogesterone 5 mg starting from day 5 for 20 days, relieves dysmenorrhoea probably by inhibiting uterine contractions. The ovulation is not suppressed.

Luteal phase defect (LPD) (see p. 239) : In a proven case, daily intramuscular injection of 12.5 mg progesterone in oil, beginning on the day after the BBT shift until menstruation occurs or if conception has taken place until 10-12 weeks of gestation. Micronised progesterone 100 mg thrice daily can be administered either vaginally or orally. Vaginal suppositories 25 mg twice daily starting 2-3 days after the BBT rise is equally effective.

Endometrial hyperplasia and endometrial carcinoma

Its role in endometrial carcinoma depends on the number of steroid receptors on the tumour. **Well-differentiated grade I endometrial carcinoma has got the highest number of receptors.** These cases are suitable for progestogen therapy. Recurrent endometrial carcinoma having good steroid receptor status is also suitable.

Dose : 17 α hydroxyprogesterone caproate 1000 mg IM daily for 1 week, weekly for 3 months and thereafter at interval of 2 weeks for 1 year. Alternatively, medroxyprogesterone acetate 400 mg IM. weekly for 3 months and then every 2 weeks for 1 year.

Premenstrual syndrome (see p. 179) : On the hypothesis that progesterone deficiency may be the cause, progestogens have been tried to relieve the symptoms. Dydrogesterone 5 mg twice daily from day 5 for 20 days in each cycle for 3-6 cycles may be tried.

- **Luteal support** : It is usually given on the day after oocyte retrieval for ART (see p. 245). Progesterone is used in any of these forms. • Progesterone in oil 50 mg IM daily. • Vaginal suppository 200 mg

Table 31.8
Side effects of progestogens

- Nausea — subsides gradually
- Leg cramps
- Mastalgia
- Weight gain due to salt and water retention
- Acne
- Scanty periods
- Loss of libido
- Virilism

(Acne, scanty periods, loss of libido, virilism: due to androgenic progestins)

- Headaches — migraines should be excluded.
- Depression and mood changes — may be due to low level of pyridoxin as progestins alter the tryptophan metabolism.
- Lipid profile — increase in LDL and decrease in HDL level.

twice daily or • Micronised progesterone orally 200 mg twice daily. It is usually continued for about 14 days (see p. 246).

Postponement of menstruation : In order to postpone the menstruation, norethisterone preparation 5 mg tab thrice daily is to be taken at least 3 days prior to the expected date of menstruation. This should be continued till such time when the patient wishes to have her period. The period usually starts after 48-72 hours. **This should not be taken casually, as it may disturb the menstrual pattern.** There is no contraceptive protection during the period of intake of medicine.

Hormone replacement therapy (HRT): Progestins are combined with oestrogen as an HRT for postmenopausal woman whose uterus is present. This prevents endometrial hyperplasia. Progestins can be used cyclically for last 12-14 days of the cycle or continuously with oestrogen (see p. 60).

Combined preparations (Oestrogen and Progestogen)

• Diagnostic • Therapeutic

Diagnostic

The combined preparations may be used as oestrogen-progesterone challenge test in amenorrhoea to exclude uterine pathology. **If bleeding fails to occur, it suggests uterine synechae.**

Therapeutic

- Contraception — The commonest and widely use of combined preparations is in the field of fertility control (details in ch. 29).
- Dysfunctional uterine bleeding (p. 187)
- Endometriosis (p. 299)
- Dysmenorrhoea (p. 175)
- Postponement of period (p. 92)
- Premenstrual syndrome (p. 179)
- Idiopathic hirsutism — cyclic therapy of combined preparations containing 50 μg of ethinyl oestradiol together with new progestin is more effective (see p. 548).
- Hormone replacement therapy (HRT) see p. 60.

ANTI-PROGESTERONE

Mifepristone (RU 486)

It is a competitive antagonist of progesterone and glucocorticoid receptors. It is a derivative of 19-nortestosterone. It binds competitively to progesterone receptors and nullifies the effect of endogenous progesterone. As a result, there is increased release of prostaglandins from the endometrium, resulting in menstrual bleeding or termination of early pregnancy.

Three important biochemical characters of RU 486 are **high affinity for progesterone receptors, long half life and active metabolites**.

Uses: *Therapeutic abortion*

It is an effective abortifacient upto 7 weeks. Combination of prostaglandins as vaginal pessary 48 hours after RU 486, increases its efficacy.

Dose: Tab 600 mg (1 tab = 200 mg) orally, followed 48 hours later by misoprostol 400 μg (PGE_1) oral or vaginal pessary. Success rate is 95-100 per cent.

Postcoital contraception

A single dose of 600 mg (3 tabs) is to be taken on 27th day of the cycle irrespective of the day and number of intercourse. Pregnancy rate is 1.6 per cent.

Induction of labour — Mifepristone has been used recently for cervical ripening. It is given orally.

Uterine fibroids — Shrinkage of uterine leiomyoma has been observed following mifepristone therapy (see p. 270).

Ectopic pregnancy — Injection of mifepristone into the ectopic pregnancy (unruptured sac) is used as a medical management.

Cushing's syndrome — as it blocks the glucocorticoid receptors.

Side effects: Minor side effects are nausea, vomiting, headache and cramp. There is risk of ongoing pregnancy (failure of medical induction of abortion) in about 1 per cent of cases. Evacuation of the uterus should be done for such a failure.

Contraindications:

- Adrenal insufficiency.
- Corticosteroid therapy.
- Age > 35 years.
- Heavy smoker.

ANDROGENS

In a female, androgen sources are adrenal cortex (25%), ovaries (25%) and in adipose tissues from peripheral conversion (50%). Most of the androgens are metabolised in the liver and are excreted as 17 ketosteroid. About 80 per cent of circulating testosterone is bound to SHBG, 19 per cent to albumin and remaining 1 per cent is free. In adult female, blood testosterone level is less than 1 ng/ml. Testosterone is converted to dihydrotestosterone within the target cell by the action of 5 alpha reductase and then combines with the specific receptors and is transported to the nucleus.

Androgens are partly anabolic and effect sebum formation and are implicated in acne during adolescence. Testosterone particularly, influences the growth of hair on face and body. Androgens are transported in blood specially in combination with sex hormone binding globulin (SHBG). Oestrogen largely influences synthesis of this protein in the liver.

Therapeutic aspect

Androgens are not active by oral route. Methyl testosterone is used as sublingual tablets to bypass the enterohepatic circulation. **Its use in clinical practice is now a rarity**. In females, not more than 200 mg should be given in one cycle. In some sensitive women, even smaller doses may cause hirsutism and hoarseness of voice.

It may be used in cases of frigidity and premenstrual syndrome either orally or as an implant. In postmenopausal or perimenopausal woman androgens are combined with oestrogen to improve libido.

Its use in male infertility has been discussed in ch.16. Testosterone derivatives like danazol (isoxasole derivative of 17 α-ethinyl testosterone), gestrinone (19-nor testosterone derivative) are used in different clinical situations (see p. 300).

Anabolic hormones are androgenic steroids. These are of limited use for ill health and during convalescence. The preparations available are nonadrolone phenylproprionate (Durabolin) 25 mg IM per week or Decadurabolin 25 mg IM at interval of 3-4 weeks.

ANTI-ANDROGENS

- **Cyproterone acetate**
- **Spironolactone**
- **Flutamide**
- **Finasteride**

Cyproterone acetate

Cyproterone acetate is an anti-androgenic progestogen. **The compound blocks the hormone action at the receptor level**. It decreases 5 α reductase activity and reduces LH secretion. It induces hepatic enzymes and increases the metabolic clearance of plasma androgens. It also acts as a potent progestogen having agonist effects on progesterone receptors.

Use : It is used in idiopathic hirsutism or hyperandrogenic state (see p. 544).

Dose : 50-100 mg is taken daily for 10 days starting from 5th day of cycle. This is accompanied by 30 μg of ethinyloestradiol which is then continued alone for a further period of 11 days **(reverse sequential regimen)**. The next regimen is started after a gap of 7 days. This form maintains regular cycle without ovulation. Treatment is to be continued for 1 year. However, in patient wanting pregnancy, it should be limited in the first half of cycle without oestrogen.

Available preparation containing cyproterone acetate 2 mg and ethinyl oestradiol 35 μg (Dianette) may be given from day 5 for 21 days.

Side effects are— weight gain, loss of libido, mastalgia.

Spironolactone

It is an anti-aldosterone diuretic. It inhibits androgen biosynthesis from ovary and adrenal.

- Inhibits 5 α reductase activity.
- It competes with androgen at the receptor sites.

Dose : The dose varies from 25-150 mg per day. This may produce hyponatraemia and hyperkalaemia for which initial monitoring of serum potassium and creatinine is necessary at doses above 100 mg per day.

Important side effects are : menstrual irregularity, fatigue, diuresis and electrolyte imbalance.

Flutamide is a nonsteroidal anti-androgen. It blocks the androgen receptor sites. Dose of 250 mg daily for 6 months is optimum. Important side effects are dry skin, decreased libido and liver damage.

Finasteride inhibits 5 α reductase activity. A dose of 5 mg daily is effective for hirsutism without any side effects.

Ketoconazole inhibits the enzyme for androgen synthesis. A dose of 200 mg daily is adequate to reduce the level of androgens.

Dexamethasone and for other anti-androgens (see p. 548).

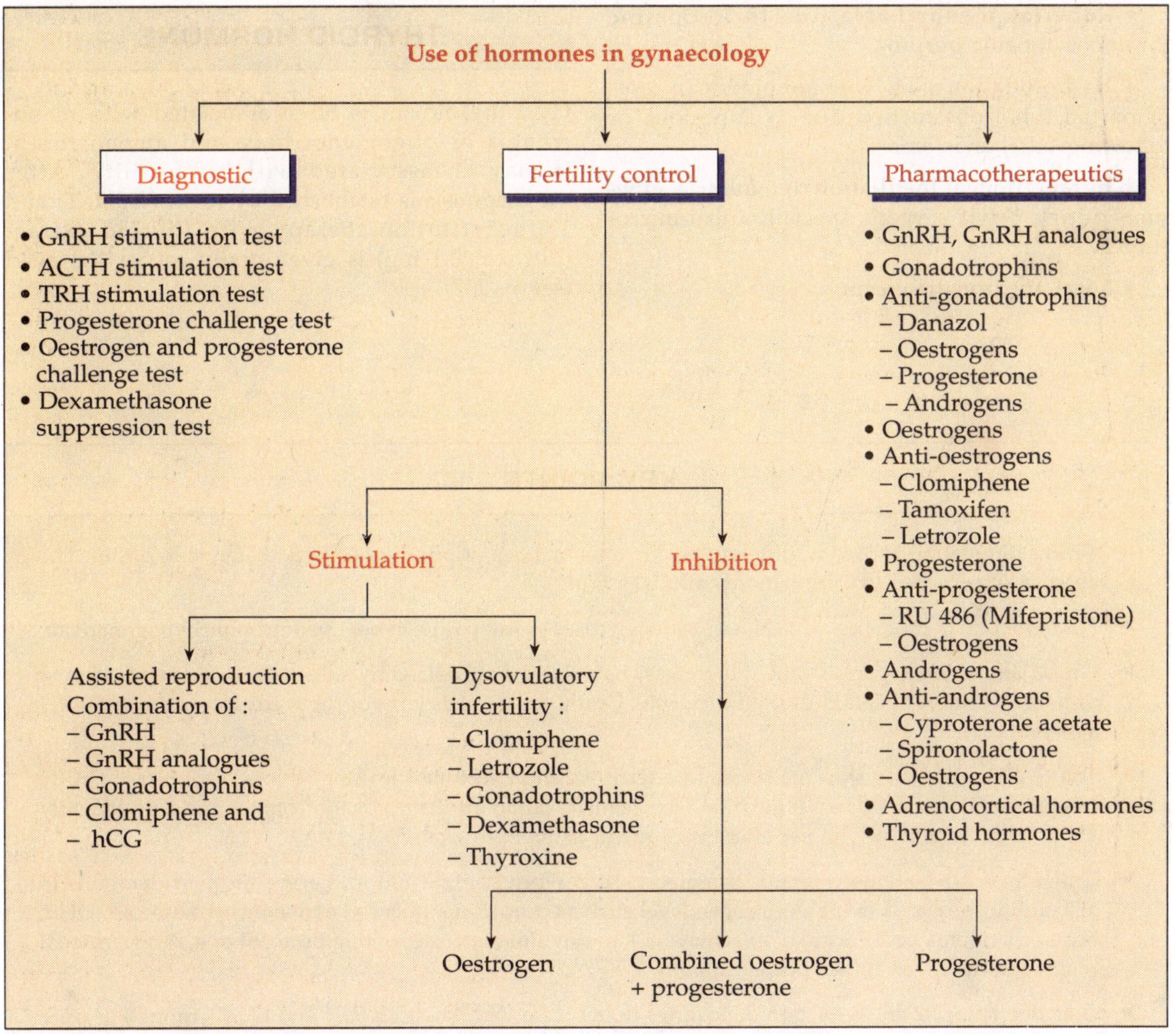

ADRENOCORTICAL HORMONES

• **Diagnostic** • **Therapeutic**

Diagnostic

Dexamethasone suppression test

A base level plasma cortisol is estimated at 8 a.m.

Dexamethasone 1 mg orally is given at 11 p.m.

Plasma cortisol level is estimated in the following morning at 8 a.m.

In normal individual, the cortisol levels are suppressed below 5 μg/100 ml but in Cushing's syndrome, the cortisol levels fall but do not go below 10 μg/100 ml.

Therapeutic

Dexamethasone is used mostly in hyperandrogenic state.

• **Hirsutism**—0.5-1 mg tab daily at midnight for a period of 6-12 months. It should be withheld in obese patient.

• **Adrenal hyperplasia**—Dexamethasone 0.5-0.75 mg in divided doses.

• **Polycystic ovary**—Along with combined oestrogen and progestogen preparations (oral pill), dexamethasone 0.25-0.5 mg is given at bed time.

• **As an adjuvant therapy** with clomiphene citrate in induction of ovulation with elevated LH.

- **Pubertal menorrhagia** due to idiopathic thrombocytopenic purpura.
- **Hydrotubation** along with antibiotics, in cases of partial tubal obstruction due to adhesions or following tubal anastomosis.
- **Intraperitoneal instillation** to minimise adhesions during pelvic surgery, specially tubal microsurgery.
- **Local antipruritic cream**.

THYROID HORMONE

Hypothyroidism is often associated with menorrhagia or oligomenorrhoea and amenorrhoea. It may be associated with subfertility. After the diagnosis is established by RIA of TSH, T_4 and T_3, substitution therapy with thyroid extract (Eltroxin 0.1 mg) is given orally as per the need (see p. 237).

KEY POINTS

- GnRH stimulation is used to differentiate an amenorrhoea of pituitary or hypothalamic in origin. The absence of response usually denotes pituitary fault.
- For induction of ovulation, GnRH is effective in cases of idiopathic hypogonadotrophic hypogonadism.
- **GnRH analogues** (agonists and antagonists) have been synthesized by substitution of amino acids at different position of GnRH molecule (p. 500). GnRH antagonists has got some advantages over GnRH agonist (Table 31.2).
- The GnRH analogues stop the normal pattern of GnRH secretion leading to loss of pituitary GnRH receptors and thereby down regulation. This leads to fall in pituitary gonadotrophins and consequently the gonadal secretion. The net effect is of medical hypophysectomy.
- GnRH analogues are used for superovulation in IVF programme and in therapeutic considerations to all conditions related to high oestrogen level such as precocious puberty, endometriosis, fibroid, DUB, breast carcinoma and the alike. In achieving superovulation, either a long protocol or a short protocol regimen is followed under proper monitoring.
- Gonadotrophic hormones act on the ovaries to induce ovulation. Both FSH and LH (Pergonal) or pure FSH (Metrodin) are available and are obtained from the urine of postmenopausal women. hCG is obtained from the urine of pregnant women.

  Gonadotrophins are expensive and require close monitoring not only for induction of ovulation but also to prevent hyperstimulation syndrome.

  The induction of ovulation with gonadotrophins is indicated in hypogonadotrophic hypogonadism with or without amenorrhoea and in failed clomiphene, in patients with PCOS.

  There is increased incidence of multiple pregnancy (20-30%) and hyperstimulation syndrome (1-20%).
- Ovarian hyperstimulation syndrome usually appears about 3-6 days after the ovulating dose of hCG.

  Increased vascular permeability due to VEGF and activation of NO system, leads to leakage of fluid from peritoneal and ovarian surfaces.

  OHSS may be mild (10-20%), moderate (5-10%) or severe (1-2%) (p. 503).

  In severe cases, correction of hypovolaemia, electrolyte imbalance, metabolic acidosis and blood coagulopathy have to be done. Intensive care monitoring may be needed for a few (p. 504).

KEY POINTS

- **Ovarian reserve** means the quantity as well as quality of the follicles present in the ovary. There are tests to determine the ovarian reserve. Poor ovarian reserve indicates poor outcome following stimulation of ovulation (p. 503).
- Danazol is strictly an anti-gonadotrophin but acts as an androgen agonist. Its use is wide like that of GnRH analogues.

  It should be started in the early follicular phase and barrier methods of contraception should be used.

  The side effects are due to hypo-oestrogenic, androgenic and metabolic changes (see Table 30.4). The drug should be discontinued, if the patient develops hirsutism or hoarseness of voice.
- Gestrinone is an androgen agonist and progesterone agonist-antagonist. The dose is 2.5 mg twice or thrice a week. Side effects are like those of danazol but less marked.
- The sex hormones are transported in the blood non-specifically by albumin and specifically by SHBG.

  Cell nucleus is the principle site of action of the steroids as opposed to the cell membranes of gonadotrophins.

  Oestrogens are used as replacement therapy (HRT) in postmenopausal women even in otherwise symptom-free cases to prevent osteoporosis and cardiovascular disease.
- Clomiphene is anti-oestrogenic. In the hypothalamus, it binds to the oestrogen receptors preventing the negative feedback effect of endogenous oestrogens to GnRH resulting in more synthesis of gonadotrophins.
- Tamoxifen is also an anti-oestrogen and is widely used in benign breast disease. Raloxifen is a more selective antioestrogen.
- **Letrozole** is a specific aromatase inhibitor. It inhibits the enzyme aromatase to suppress synthesis of oestrogen. It enhances the secretion of pituitary FSH for the growth and development of follicles. It is used for induction of ovulation in women with anovulatory infertility.
- **Progestogens** are classified according to their structural derivatives and progestogen content (Table 31.6). They are also classified according to their metabolic effects and also with the grades of progestational activity (Table 31.7).
- Progestogens are used as diagnostic test to evaluate the cause of amenorrhoea. In presence of withdrawal bleeding, it signifies intact hypothalamo-pituitary ovarian axis and there is endogenous oestrogen production.
- Combined oestrogen and progestogen preparations are commonly used as oral contraceptives.
- Ru 486 is anti-progesterone and is effective in termination of early pregnancy.
- The source of androgens in female are adrenal, ovary and peripheral adipose tissues. The blood level of testosterone in female is less than 1 ng/ml.
- Cyproterone, spironolactone, flutamide and finasteride are anti-androgens. These are used in idiopathic hirsutism and hyperandrogenic state (p. 548).
- Dexamethasone suppression test is of help in the diagnosis of Cushing's syndrome.

Gynaecologic Problems from Birth to Adolescence

32

Introduction

Those who are familiar with adult gynaecology are often confused and embarrassed to deal with gynaecologic problems of the young one. The problems are peculiar to a particular period. These are not common, mostly narrated by the parents and often present difficulty in examination. Thus, these not only pose a diagnostic problem but at times of therapy too.

For descriptive purpose, the entire span from birth to adolescence is arbitrarily divided into three phases. Each phase has got distinct problems of its own.

- Neonates, toddlers and infants < 5 yrs.
- Premenarchal 5–11 yrs.
- Perimenarchal to adolescence 12-18 yrs.

Gynaecologists need specific communication skill considering the psychological and developmental milestones of the girl child and the adolescent.

NEONATES, TODDLERS AND INFANTS

Clitoral enlargement

Causes: Not infrequently, female babies are born with slightly enlarged clitoris. There is usually no

Table 32.1
Common clinical problems in different periods

Period	*Common problems*
< 5 years (Neonates, toddlers and infants)	• Diagnosis of sex at birth (Clitoral enlargement) • Genital crisis • Labial adhesions • Imperforate hymen – Hydro or mucocolpos • Ectopic anus • Nipple discharge
5–11 years (Premenarchal)	• Vulvovaginitis in childhood • Abnormal vaginal discharge • Vaginal bleeding • Precocious puberty (see p. 49) • Trauma to the genital tract (Ch. 26) • White lesion of the vulva (Ch. 17) • Neoplasm (Ch. 23)
12–18 years (Perimenarchal to adolescence)	• Menstrual abnormalities (p. 52) • Delayed puberty (see p. 51) • Hirsutism (see p. 544) • Neoplasm (Ch. 23) • Primary amenorrhoea (p. 431) • Leucorrhoea (see p. 524) • Congenital anomalies of the vagina (vaginal anomalies (p. 40) and uterine anomalies (p. 43). • Intersex (see p. 420) • Miscellaneous problem

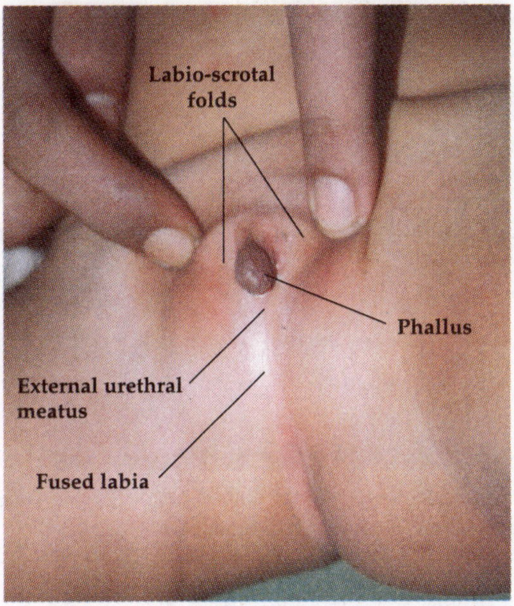

Fig. 32.1. Newborn baby with enlarged phallus due to adrenogenital syndrome causing confusion in the diagnosis of sex

evidence of intrauterine androgen stimulation of the child. Careful history taking reveals development of some degree of masculinising features of the mother during pregnancy, probably due to increased adrenocortical activity (Fig. 32.1).

Rarely, the enlargement may be one of the manifestations of intersexuality of type, female pseudohermaphrodite. This may cause confusion in the determination of sex at birth. The details have been mentioned in chapter 27 (Fig. 27.1).

Management

In the idiopathic group, no treatment is required. However, an apparently female child with enlarged phallus and impalpable gonads requires at least estimation of serum 17-OHP, urinary 17 ketosteroid and chromosomal analysis to rule out congenital adrenal hyperplasia (p. 421) Fig. 32.1.

Genital crisis

It includes spectrum of disorders noticed within few days of birth. It is due to the effect of passive oestrogenic stimulation which has passed across the placenta from the mother. The presence of the oestrogen so obtained produces changes in the endometrium and other target tissues such as breasts and cervical glands.

Bleeding per vaginam

It usually occurs within 10 days following birth; mostly blood stained but at times frank bleeding. This is due to decline in level of oestrogen which is unable to support the endometrium resulting in withdrawal bleeding. There is no cause for concern.

Enlarged breasts

Due to effect of maternal oestrogen and progesterone, there may be some development of duct and alveolar system of the breasts. Withdrawal of hormonal suppression of prolactin leads to discharge from the nipple called 'witch's milk'. No treatment is required; only assurance is enough.

Neonatal leucorrhoea

This is due to excessive secretion of cervical mucus from the hypertrophied cervical glands under the influence of oestrogen.

Labial Adhesion

Causes : Commonly, it is due to mild infection of the vulva which is favoured by lack of local defence due to absence of oestrogen. There is denudation of the surface epithelium of the labia minora → adhesions.

The adhesions of the labia minora start from behind forwards leaving a small opening at the foremost tip through which urine escapes out.

Rarely, it may be a manifestation of minor form of masculinisation following maternal intake of androgen during pregnancy.

Diagnosis

The condition usually appears within 2-3 years of birth. The mother usually, anxious about the entity, brings to the notice of the physician for not visualising the vaginal opening. The adhesions may cause difficulty in micturition or periodic attacks of urinary tract infection. There may be inflammation of the vestibule and vagina.

Examination reveals, adhesions of labia minora obliterating the vaginal opening and at times even the external urethral meatus (Fig. 32.2A).

Confusion arises with :

- Imperforate hymen.
- Agenesis of vagina.
- Intersex.

In imperforate hymen and agenesis of vagina, the labia minora and external urethral meatus are clearly

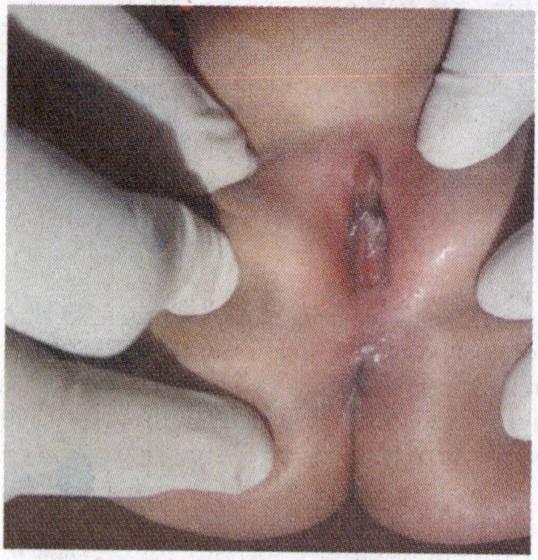

Fig. 32.2A. Labial adhesions in a 1 1/2 –year–old girl

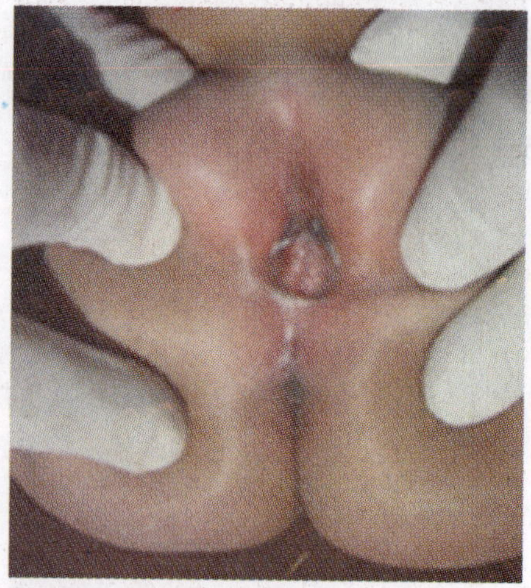

Fig. 32.2B. Separation of adhesions by fingers. Local application of oestrogen ointment is also helpful

visible. In intersexuality, there is usually associated clitoral enlargement (see p. 421).

Treatment : Separation of the adhesions using fingers or by a probe is almost always effective (Fig. 32.2B). The raw area is treated with topical application of oestrogen or any other antibiotic ointment to prevent reagglutination.

There is a tendency of recurrence. If it does, instead of repeated separations, it is better to await spontaneous cure at puberty because of high level endogenous oestrogen.

Muco or Hydrocolpos

Pathophysiology

There is imperforate hymen or a transverse vaginal septum just above the hymen. Due to excess oestrogen stimulation acquired *in utero* from the mother, there is increased secretion of mucus or watery discharge from the cervical and uterine glands. If a large quantity of fluid is collected in the vagina, it produces hydro or mucocolpos. It may rarely be big enough to produce an abdominal swelling.

This is rarely met beyond 1 year of age because the uterine and vaginal transudation is not produced in sufficient quantity beyond that age.

Later on, the candidate may be the subject of haematocolpos → haematometra.

Clinical features

There is usually some urinary problems to the extent of retention of urine. Variable degrees of pain in lower abdomen is a constant feature.

Abdominal examination reveals a lower abdominal lump. Distended bladder makes the lump apparently bigger.

Vulval inspection reveals a tense bulge of the obstructing membrane which looks shiny. Rectal examination confirms the vaginal bulge.

Treatment

Cruciate incision is enough to drain the pent up mucus. Antibiotic is given. Head end is to be raised.

Ovarian enlargement

After the withdrawal of maternal oestrogen, there is transient elevation of gonadotrophins in neonates. This influence of elevated gonadotrophins can stimulate to produce ovarian follicular cysts. These will regress spontaneously. As such, the cysts need no surgery unless complicated.

Ectopic anus

The anal canal may open either in the vestibule or in the vagina. The details have been described in chapter 4.

PREMENARCHAL

Vulvovaginitis

The premenarchal girls are specially vulnerable to vaginal infection because of —

- Lack of or very low level of circulatory oestrogen → lack of stratification of vaginal epithelium → lack of glycogen and absence of Doderlein's bacillus → no acid formation → vaginal pH remains high, around 7.

- Inadequate care of perineal hygiene.
- Lack of protective pubic hair and fatty pads of labia majora.

As the vaginal infection is almost always associated with vulvitis, the terminology of vulvovaginitis is appropriate.

Causes : The infection may be due to non-specific or specific organisms.

I. The non-specific organisms (common)

The infection is *polymicrobial in* nature and it is difficult to pinpoint any particular one responsible for infection. The organisms are however, of low virulence.

II. Specific

- Non-gonococcal (common)
  - *Streptococcus*
  - *Chlamydia trachomatis*
  - *Esch. coli*
  - *Gardnerella vaginalis*
  - *Candida albicans*
  - *Trichomonas vaginalis*
- Gonococcus

III. Foreign body

IV. Threadworm infestation

V. Following systemic illness

- Viral infection like measles, chickenpox.
- Juvenile diabetes.

VI. Following antibiotic therapy

Sources of infection

- Direct contact from infected person.
- Indirect from foreign body, infected towel or bath tub and intestinal infestation.
- Associated juvenile diabetes or antibiotic therapy favours monilial infection.

Symptoms

- Vaginal discharge which may be purulent or even blood stained in presence of foreign body.
- Pruritus or soreness in external genitalia.
- Painful urination.

Signs

Vulva becomes oedematous and red or even ulcerated. Vaginal inspection using aural speculum reveals congested epithelium with pent up discharge. The offending foreign body may be detected. The examination may be done under anaesthesia. It should be remembered that the vaginal epithelium in young girls looks red. **Rectal examination** is often helpful to detect the foreign body.

Investigations

- Examination under anaesthesia
- **Vaginoscopy** is needed to visualise the upper vagina for bleeding, foreign body or neoplasm. Specially designed speculum (Huffman Graves) is inserted into the vagina. For better visualisation water cystoscope (to wash away secretions, debris or blood) or laparoscope (8 mm) may be used.

Bacteriological examination of the discharge either by Gram stain or hanging drop preparation or culture, to identify the causative organism (see p. 160).

- Smear from the anal area for detection of pin or threadworm.
- Stool examination may reveal the threadworm.
- Blood examination for estimation of sugar in suspected cases of juvenile diabetes.
- Urine for protein, sugar and culture study.

Treatment : As the cause remains obscure in majority, the principles to be followed are :

- **Vulvar hygiene**—Proper wiping will reduce rectal flora in the vulvovaginal area.
  - Sitz baths are very helpful in relieving symptoms.
  - Scrubbing the vulvar area is avoided.
  - To keep the local area dry.
  - To wear cotton undergarments.

Medication

- To reduce the overgrowth of pathogenic bacteria, Amoxicillin 20-40 mg/kg/day in 3 divided doses is effective.
- In refractory cases, oestrogen locally as cream twice daily for 3 weeks is effective to improve the vaginal defence and to promote healing.

Specific therapy

- Trichomoniasis is treated by metronidazole (100 mg thrice daily for 10 days).

• Monilial infection is treated by local application of clotrimazole 1 per cent cream.

• For gonococcal vaginitis (see p. 143).

• Associated systemic illness should be treated by intramuscular antibiotic therapy.

• Foreign body is to be removed followed by use of oestrogen therapy.

• Helminth is eradicated by oral use of Albendazole.

Leucorrhoea (see p. 524)

As the puberty approaches, there may be excessive white discharge per vaginam. It is non-offensive and nonirritant. It is due to excessive production of mucus from the cervical glands and increased transudation from the vaginal epithelium.

Neoplasm

The neoplastic conditions encountered during this period are usually ovarian in origin and rarely from the cervix and vagina. The ovarian neoplasms (see p. 367) are malignant in about 25 per cent. Germ cell tumours are common (70%). Granulosa cell tumour is oestrogen producing tumour and may cause precocious puberty. Mixed germ cell tumour is highly malignant and dysgerminoma is intermediary in position, provided the capsule remains intact. The benign tumours are cystic teratoma (30%) and epithelial tumours (see p. 280, 367).

Sarcoma botryoides : It should be remembered that the entity is most often present as early as 2 years of age (see p. 355).

Vaginal bleeding — Common causes are :

- Precocious puberty.
- Foreign body in the vagina.
- Trauma.
- Sexual abuse.
- Neoplastic conditions (mentioned earlier).
- Leech bite.
- Prolapse of the urethral mucosa.

Leech bite : This is more prevalent in tropics where pond bath is quite common. The bleeding may at times be brisk and requires varying amount of blood transfusion. Bleeding usually stops spontaneously but may at times require haemostatic suture.

Prolapse of the urethral mucosa

It presents as a vascular swelling surrounding the external urethral meatus which bleeds easily. Treatment is by excision.

POSTMENARCHAL TO ADOLESCENCE

Adolescence

The period of life beginning with the appearance of secondary sex characters and terminating with cessation of somatic growth is described as adolescence. **The problems during the period are** :

- Menstrual disorders.
- Delayed puberty (p. 51).
- Delayed manifestations of intersex.
- Hirsutism.
- Leucorrhoea.
- Neoplasm.

MENSTRUAL DISORDERS

The neurohormonal mechanism essential for maintenance of normal menstruation takes some time (usually 2-3 years) to come to a normal balance. Till then, various types of menstrual abnormalities may occur causing concern to the young girls or their parents (see p. 52).

Common causes of menstrual irregularity

A. *Hypothalamic – Pituitary – Ovarian (HPO) axis dysfunction.*
   - Dysfunctional uterine bleeding (p. 52)
   - Stress (p.444)
   - Obesity (p. 546)

B. *Endocrinopathies*
   - Thyroid dysfunction (p. 448)
   - PCOS (p. 440)
   - Prolactinoma (p. 445)
   - CAH (p. 446)

C. *Others*
   - Pregnancy
   - Bleeding disorders (Idiopathic Thrombocytopenic Purpura p. 181).
   - Local — Polyps, neoplasms (p. 274).

Improvement of general health and assurance are enough in majority. It is expected that after a certain period of time, the menstrual cycles become normal with the onset of regular ovulation.

The unresponsive or problematic cases have been dealt with in appropriate chapters. These are cryptomenorrhoea (ch. 4), delayed puberty (ch. 5) or primary amenorrhoea, (ch. 28), puberty menorrhagia (ch. 5) and spasmodic dysmenorrhoea (ch. 13), CAH (p. 446) and PCOS (p. 440).

DELAYED MANIFESTATIONS OF INTERSEX

While majority of cases of intersex are diagnosed at birth, there are cases where the diagnosis is only revealed after puberty. These are :

- Mild degrees of congenital adrenal hyperplasia (p. 421) with late manifestations of postpubertal hyperandrogenism (Fig. 33.4).
- Gonadal dysgenesis (p. 422).
- Androgen insensitivity syndrome (p. 424).

HIRSUTISM

Hirsutism is one of the manifestation of hyperandrogenism and often causes problem to the young girls. One should not forget to elicit iatrogenic cause of hirsutism following intake of androgenic steroids, corticosteroid or synthetic progestogens. The causes and management of hirsutism are discussed in p. 544.

Leucorrhoea

Excessive normal vaginal secretion in this period may be due to :

- Relative hyperoestrogenic phase.
- Malnutrition and ill health.
- Congenital ectopy (erosion).
- Sexual excitement or masturbation.
- Vaginal adenosis.

VAGINAL ADENOSIS

Vaginal adenosis is present in about 30–50 per cent of the teenagers who had DES exposure *in utero*. This is a benign condition. The columnar epithelium of the endocervix extends onto the ectocervix and also variable part of the vaginal fornices. There is thus copious vaginal secretion from the columnar epithelium. The pathology regresses spontaneously in due course of time. Rarely, it may progress to clear cell carcinoma (p. 327).

Congenital ectopy producing copious discharge should be cauterised. In others, assurance and improvement of general condition cure the state.

Infective discharge during the period may be due to :

- Non-specific infection following unhygienic use of menstrual pads or foreign body in the vagina.
- Specific infections such as Trichomonas vaginalis or monilial infection.
- New growths from the vagina or cervix.

The investigations and management have been mentioned earlier in the chapter.

NEOPLASM

Ovarian—Functional cysts which are rare in premenarchal period are quite common during this period. They are usually 6–8 cm in diameters and usually regress within 3–6 months. These are usually follicular cysts.

Commonest neoplastic cyst during this period is cystic teratoma (dermoid cyst). The others, though rare are benign epithelial tumours, dysgerminoma, mixed germ cell tumour or androblastoma. **Germ cell tumours constitute 50-75 per cent of all ovarian neoplasms in this age group**.

The patients usually come late with symptoms. Common symptoms are lump in the lower abdomen, acute pain abdomen or at times with retention of urine.

Diagnosis

The diagnosis is made by abdominal, bimanual vaginal or rectal examination. Ultrasound is an invaluable tool in the diagnosis of ovarian mass.

Treatment

A suspected functional cyst (6–8 cm) may be observed for 3–6 months. Unilocular functional cysts usually resolve spontaneously. Surgical therapy is needed in cases where there are symptoms, masses that fails to resolve or masses with solid or multilocular appearance on ultrasound.

Laparoscopy is usually done when an adnexal mass appears to be benign. However, prompt laparotomy should be done when there are evidences of malignancy.

The surgery is usually conservative (ovariotomy or ovarian cystectomy) considering her future fertility and endocrine functions. **Unilateral salpingo-oophorectomy is justified for most young girl with stage I ovarian cancer.** Germ cell tumours are highly responsive to chemotherapy (p. 367). Well-capsulated unilateral dysgerminoma should be dealt with ovariotomy to be followed by chemotherapy or radiotherapy after shielding the contralateral ovary. However, if the capsule is ruptured radical surgery, i.e. total hysterectomy with bilateral salpingo-oophorectomy is to be done followed by radiotherapy or chemotherapy.

Table 32.2
Common causes of lump in lower abdomen

Age	Causes
< 5 years	— Hydro or mucocolpos
5-11 years	— Retention urine due to vulvovaginitis — Pelvic neoplasm
12-18 years	— Pregnancy — Retention of urine — Ovarian tumour — Haematometra — Encysted peritonitis

A problem may arise when an apparently cystic epithelial benign ovarian tumour is removed which ultimately proves malignant histologically. In such cases, in consultation with oncologist, chemotherapy followed by relaparotomy and removal of uterus with contralateral tube and ovary may be done. This should be followed by chemotherapy.

Alternatively, the patient may be treated with chemotherapy alone with follow-up.

Uterus—Sarcoma botryoides (see p. 355).

Vagina—Clear cell adenocarcinoma of the vagina (p. 327).

SEXUALLY TRANSMITTED DISEASES (STDs)

STDs are increasing among the adolescents. The younger the age of first intercourse, the higher the risk for STDs. Chlamydia infection though most common, other infections are : HPV (p. 312), HIV (p. 149), Gonorrhoea (p. 143), Hepatitis B, Syphilis (p. 144) and others (ch. 11). Impact on health due to STD complications include : cervical metaplasia, PID and its consequences (p. 128).

Major problems faced with the management of adolescent STDs are denial of history and symptoms. Fear and social embarrassment causes delay or at times incomplete treatment.

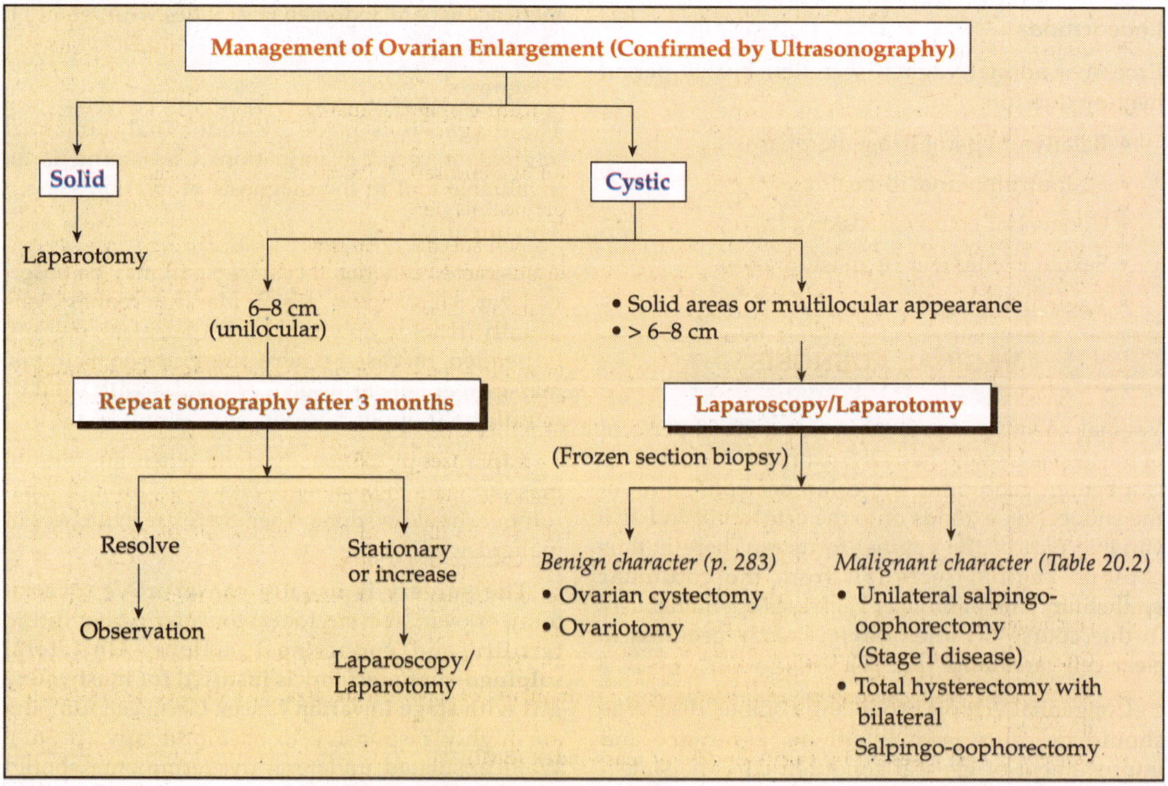

Treatment

Sex education among the adolescent girls, practice of safer sex and maintenance of perineal hygiene are essential. Proper use of condoms protect STDs. Treatment of STDs among adolescents is same to that of the adults (see p. 142).

MISCELLANEOUS PROBLEMS

Acne : This is of concern due to cosmetic reason. The cause is due to excess androgen secretion by the adrenals. Assurance is enough. No treatment is required. It passes off spontaneously.

Obesity : Obesity is best assessed by calculating body mass index (BMI). BMI is expressed (see p. 627) as weight (kg) divided by the height squared (M^2). Ideal BMI should be between 20 and 24. BMI 25 or more is called over weight. Whereas BMI 30 or more is considered obese. Obesity increases the risk of cardiovascular (e.g. hypertension) and metabolic (e.g. diabetes) diseases (see p. 546).

Usually, it is due to over-eating and constitutional. Rarely, it may be due to hypofunction of pituitary or manifestation of Cushing's syndrome or PCOS (see p. 440) even at a younger age.

Abnormal height : Apart from constitutional as found in premenarchal period, abnormal tallness is due to :

- Hypersecretion of the growth hormone from the anterior pituitary. This may be due to pituitary eosinophilic adenoma resulting in gigantism. The treatment is excision of the pituitary adenoma. If the features are well-established, it is however irreversible.
- Primary ovarian failure—There is lack of endogenous oestrogen → delayed closure of the epiphysis of long bones. There is associated unopposed action of the growth hormone from the anterior pituitary resulting in linear growth of the long bones (see p. 444).

KEY POINTS

- Undue clitoral enlargement seen at birth may be due to intersexuality. It requires at least estimation of 17 OHP, 17 ketosteroid and chromosomal analysis. Levels of 17 OHP > 800 ng/dL are virtually diagnostic of congenital adrenal hyperplasa (21-hydroxylase deficiency).
- Genital crisis is due to hyperoestrogenic state and includes bleeding per vaginam, enlarged breasts and neonatal leucorrhoea (p. 517).
- Labial fusion is commonly due to infection and rarely a feature of intersexuality. Separation of the adhesions is effective using fingers or a probe (p. 517).
- Muco or hydrocolpos is usually found within 1 year of age and results from imperforate hymen.
- The childhood vulvovaginitis is mainly due to poor perineal hygiene.
- Vulvovaginitis in premenarchal period is mostly due to non-specific organisms and occasionally to specific gonococcal infection. Bacteriological examination should be carried out from the discharge prior to therapy.
- Ovarian follicular cysts are common in adolescent girls and are usually self limiting. An ovarian enlargement more than 5 cm need to investigated.
- The neoplasm in premenarchal period is usually ovarian and in about 25 per cent, it is malignant. The common is germ cell tumour (benign cystic teratoma, dysgerminoma, mixed germ cell tumour). The others are granulosa cell tumour or epithelial tumours. The benign tumours are epithelial tumours.
- Sarcoma botryoides is most often observed before the age of 5 (see p. 355).
- In tall girl — to achieve arrest of bone growth, oestrogen therapy for 3-6 months may be effective.
- The menstrual disorders in adolescent period are usually self limiting and the hormones should not be used injudiciously. Assurance and improvement of health are enough in majority.
- Vaginal adenosis is present in about 30-50 per cent and is a benign lesion. Rarely, it progresses to clear cell carcinoma.
- Commonest ovarian neoplasm in adolescence is benign cystic teratoma (p. 283).
- STDs are increasing among the adolescents. Sex education, use of condoms and treatment of STDs are essential (p. 522).
- Obesity is best assessed by calculating body mass index (BMI).

Special Topics

33

ABNORMAL VAGINAL DISCHARGE

Introduction

Abnormal vaginal discharge is a frequent complaint of women seen in the gynaecologic clinic. The discharge may range from what is called excess of normal to one which is a part of wide spectrum of ailments. It may be blood-stained or contaminated with urine or stool, all of which are however excluded from the discussion made below.

Characteristics of normal vaginal fluid : It is watery, white in colour, nonodorous with pH around 4.0. Microscopically it contains squamous epithelial cells and a few bacteria. Lacto-bacilli (Doderlein bacilli, p. 7), few gram-negative bacteria and anaerobes are present without any white or red blood cells.

Causes of abnormal discharge are schematically presented below (Table 33.1) :

LEUC(K)ORRHOEA

Definition

Leucorrhoea is strictly defined as an excessive normal vaginal discharge. The symptom of excessive is a subjective one with individual variation, while to declare it to be normal and not an infective one, requires clinical and laboratory investigations.

The term leucorrhoea should fulfil the following criteria :

- The excess secretion is evident from persistent vulval moistness or staining of the undergarments (brownish yellow on drying) or need to wear a vulval pad.
- It is non-purulent and non-offensive.
- It is non-irritant and never causes pruritus.

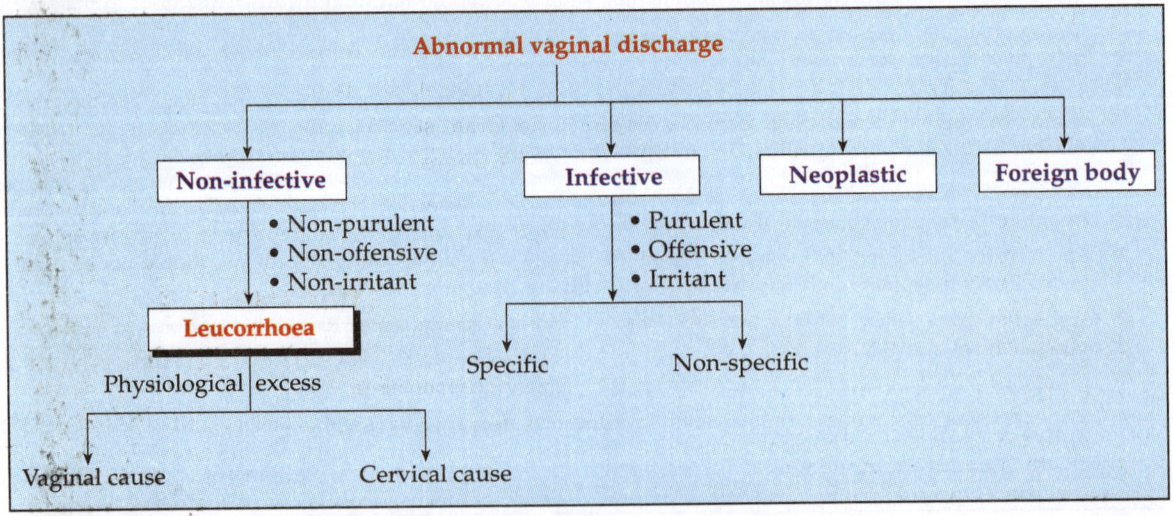

PATHOPHYSIOLOGY

Normal vaginal secretion

The origin and nature of the normal vaginal secretion during the reproductive period has been described in page 6. However, a short resume is presented here.

The physiologic basis involved in normal vaginal secretion is dependent on the endogenous oestrogen level. With the rising oestrogen level, there is abundant secretory activity of the endocervical glands and the superficial vaginal epithelium becomes rich in glycogen (see p. 7).

The mucoid secretion from the cervical glands is normally small in amount. The carbohydrate radicle of the glycoprotein mucin is split off and fermented into lactic acid. If however, the mucus is secreted in excess, it pours out at the vulva.

The excessive secretion is due to:

- Physiologic excess
- Cervical cause (cervical leucorrhoea)
- Vaginal cause (vaginal leucorrhoea)

Physiologic excess

The normal secretion is expected to increase in conditions when the oestrogen levels become high. Such conditions are :

During puberty—Increased levels of endogenous oestrogen lead to marked over-growth of the endocervical epithelium which may encroach onto the ectocervix producing congenital ectopy (erosion) → increased secretion.

During menstrual cycle

- Around ovulation—Peak rise of oestrogen → increase in secretory activity of the cervical glands.
- Premenstrual pelvic congestion and increased mucus secretion from the hypertrophied endometrial glands.

Pregnancy—There is hyperoestrinism with increased vascularity. This leads to increased vaginal transudate and cervical gland secretion.

During sexual excitement, when there is abundant secretion from the Bartholin's glands.

Cervical cause

Non-infective cervical lesion may produce excessive secretion which pours out at the vulva. Such lesions are — cervical ectopy, chronic cervicitis, mucous polyp and ectropion (cervical glands are exposed to the vagina).

Vaginal cause

Increased vaginal transudation occurs in conditions associated with increased pelvic congestion. The conditions are uterine prolapse, acquired retroverted uterus, chronic pelvic inflammation, 'pill' use and vaginal adenosis. Ill health is one of the important causes of excessive discharge. It produces excess exfoliation of the superficial cells.

DIAGNOSIS

- General examination may reveal ill health. The patient often states the discharge as the cause of ill health but in reality, the reverse is true; the ill health producing leucorrhoea.
- Vulval inspection reveals :
  - White or creamy discharge
  - No evidence of pruritus
- Bimanual including a speculum examination reveals :
  - Either a negative pathology
  - Associated pelvic lesions mentioned earlier causing cervical or vaginal leucorrhoea.
- To exclude the infective nature, the discharge is subjected to microscopic examination for detection of pus cells.

If the pus cell is not detected, it is considered as a case of true leucorrhoea. If however, pus cells are detected, further investigations are to be carried out to identify the organism from the discharge provided neoplasm and foreign body are excluded. These examinations include :

- Hanging drop preparation (see p. 160).
- Clue cells (p. 148).
- Gram stain.
- Culture.

The detection of the specific or non-specific organisms are dealt with in appropriate chapters.

TREATMENT

The following guidelines are prescribed to treat a case of leucorrhoea.

- Improvement of general health.
- Cervical factors require surgical treatment like electrocautery, cryosurgery or trachelorrhaphy.

Table 33.1
Life Table of Abnormal Vaginal Discharge

Period of life	*Associated symptoms*	*Probable diagnosis*
Early neonatal	Nil	Leucorrhoea
Period upto premenarchal	Nil Offensive Vulval itching	• Ill-health • Foreign body • Threadworm
Puberty	Nil	Leucorrhoea
Reproductive period		
Non-pregnant		
Related to menstrual cycle	Nil	Leucorrhoea
Pill users	• Nil • Pruritus	• Leucorrhoea • Moniliasis
Any time	• Nil • Pruritus • Offensive	• Ill health • Infective vaginitis • Neoplasm, foreign body
During antibiotic therapy	Pruritus	Moniliasis
Diabetes	Pruritus	Moniliasis
Pregnancy	• Nil • Pruritus	• Leucorrhoea • Vaginitis (Moniliasis)
Postmenopausal	• Nil • Pruritus/diabetic • Offensive	• Senile vaginitis • Moniliasis • Pyometra, neoplasm

- Pelvic lesions producing vaginal leucorrhoea require appropriate therapy for the pathology.
- Pill users may have to stop 'pill' temporarily, if the symptom is very much annoying.
- Above all, local hygiene has to be maintained meticulously.

PRURITUS VULVAE

About 10 per cent of patients attending the gynaecologic clinic complain of vulval itching.

Definition

Pruritus means sense of itching. When it is confined to the vulva, it is called pruritus vulvae.

It should not be confused with pain. The pain is almost always associated with tenderness. Pruritus does not produce pain nor there is any local tenderness or any detectable lesion.

Mechanisms of itching

The possible mechanisms of initiation of sensation of itching are mediated through the following :

- Special sensory innervation of the area.
- Underlying vascular instability (greatly influenced by emotion) results in production of histamine like substance → induction of itching.
- Aggravation at night because of :
  - Absence of distraction of mind.
  - Tired central nervous system.
  - Local warmth and lack of aeration.

Aetiology

Vaginal discharge — The commonest cause of pruritus vulvae is vaginal discharges either due to *Trichomonas vaginalis* or *Candida albicans* or both. It should be remembered that a purulent vaginal discharge produces pain and tenderness of the vulva rather than pruritus (see p. 155, 159).

Local skin lesions — The lesions may be either localised in the vulva or part of generalised lesions. Such lesions include — psoriasis, seborrhoeic dermatitis, intertrigo, etc.

Infections of the vulva

Fungal—Candida (p. 160).

Viral—herpes genitalis, genital warts (p. 148, 152).

Parasitic—threadworm may migrate to the area (specially in children), scabies, pediculosis (p. 153).

STD—gonorrhoea, Trichomoniasis (p. 143, 159)

Allergy or contact dermatitis — Use of nylon undergarments or washing those with certain soaps or detergents, idiosyncrasy to chemical contraceptives or condom is often related.

Non-neoplastic epithelial disorders of the vulva (p. 250)

- Squamous hyperplasia (p. 252).
- Lichen sclerosus (p. 250).

Neoplastic epithelial disorders

- VIN (see p. 307).
- Paget's disease (p. 308).
- Invasive carcinoma of the vulva (p. 321).

Pruritus vulvae due to some systemic diseases

A. **Medical disorders**: Glycosuria (diabetes mellitus) causes local changes in the skin (raw beef colour) and pruritus. It favours the growth of *Candida*. Others : Thyroid disorders, Chronic liver disease.

B. **Dermatological causes** : Contact dermatitis, drug allergy.

C. **Deficiency state**: Deficiencies of iron, folic acid, vitamin B_{12} and vitamin A are all implicated. Malabsorption syndrome along with chronic diarrhoea, hypochlorhydria with megaloblastic anaemia are often associated with pruritus.

D. **Psychosomatic causes**: When no cause is detected, psychic factor is to be excluded. Mental anxiety or sexual frustration may be responsible for scratching.

Investigations

It should be borne in mind that pruritus vulvae is a manifestation of some underlying pathology either located at the site or elsewhere in the body. **The investigations should include**:

Detailed history regarding — age of onset, intensity of itching, duration, associated vaginal discharge, contraceptive practice, relation with

Table 33.2
Common causes of vaginitis and abnormal vaginal discharge

	Cause	*Nature*
Infective	• Trichomonas vaginitis (p.159) • Monilial vaginitis (p.160) • Bacterial vaginosis (p.147) • Cervicitis	• Frothy yellow discharge • Curdy white in flakes, pruritic • Gray-white, fishy odour and non-pruritic • Mucoid discharge
Atrophic	Postmenopausal	• Discharge is not prominent • Irritation is prominent
Foreign body	• Forgotten pessary, tampoon • Mechanical irritation	Offensive, copious, purulent, often blood stained
Chemical	• Douches, Latex condoms, Deodorants • Chemical irritation or allergy	Soreness is pronounced than the discharge
Excretions	Contamination with urine or faeces producing secondary vaginitis	Offensive discharge with pruritus
Neoplasms	Fibroid polyp or genital malignancy	Serosanguinous, often offensive

psychologic upset or neurosis, allergy to nylon, soap or particular detergents.

General examination—Thorough systemic examination is needed. Features of malnutrition or anaemia, evidences of fungal infection in the interdigital folds of fingers and toes, scabies, leucodermic patches elsewhere in the body are to be looked for. Examination for diabetes mellitus, liver and thyroid disorders, haematological diseases are to be made.

Local examination—The extent of the lesion is to be noted. If the itching area is predominantly anal or intercrural, the cause is probably threadworm, tinea or intertrigo.

If itching is predominantly on the vulval area, one should think of :

- Infective causes (trichomoniasis, moniliasis or others).
- Local dermatological conditions.
- Glycosuria.
- Non-neoplastic and neoplastic epithelial disorders of the vulva.

Inspection of the area may reveal the pathology related to itching. Bimanual including speculum examination may reveal the nature of vaginitis.

Special investigations

- Microscopic examination of the vaginal discharge or vulval scraping to detect *Candida* or *Trichomonas vaginalis.*
- Urine for sugar, protein and pus cells.
- Blood—Haemoglobin estimation, postprandial glucose. Detailed haematological workup (polycythaemia, leukaemia), thyroid profile, liver function and renal function tests are carried out.
- Stool—Ova, parasites and cysts are to be looked for.
- In long-standing cases (more than one year) specially with vulval epithelial disorders, biopsy either random or toluidine blue or colposcopic directed, is to be taken to note the type of skin changes and exclude malignancy.

Treatment

General principles

- Appropriate local hygiene is to be taken care of. The area should not be washed with soap.
- Vulvovaginal douching is to be avoided.
- To use loose fitting undergarments preferably made of cotton to keep the area aerated.
- To prevent the vicious cycle of scratch-itch-scratch.

Local application of antibiotics or clobetasol propionate 0.05 per cent (p. 252) ointment may be helpful. Sedation at night is to be ensured. If the skin is atrophic, oestrogen or testosterone cream may be helpful.

- **To treat the specific aetiological factor** causing pruritus by appropriate therapy—local or systemic.

Surgery : If the biopsy reveals features of severe dysplasia or malignancy or in cases of unresponsive pruritus in menopause, even if the biopsy is negative—simple vulvectomy is justified. **It should be emphasised that simple vulvectomy is not the treatment of pruritus** and the recurrence rate after casual vulvectomy is to the extent of more than 50 per cent.

PELVIC PAIN

Pain is an unpleasant sensory and emotional experience associated with actual or potential tissue damage. Pelvic pain is a common symptom in gynaecology. It may be present in **acute form** or **in chronic form**. It should be remembered that the pain is just a symptom of an underlying disorder. Whereas, it is often easy to find out the underlying cause of acute pain, it is often difficult to find out the cause of chronic pelvic pain. **Sensation of pain is found to depend on many factors in an individual : e.g. emotional status, genetic factors, experience, gender, pain threshold, anxiety and expectations**.

Neurophysiology of pain

Impulse generated due to depolarisation of a peripheral nerve ending (Transduction) → Transmission of the nerve impulse → Modulation (control of impulse transmission to neurones by neurotransmitters) → perception of pain.

Unlike somatic structures which are well-represented in the cerebral cortex in terms of localisation, visceral structures are poorly localised in the cerebral cortex. Thus, the pain arising from the pelvic organs is often localised not to the organ but referred to the skin area supplied by the same spinal nerve. Various neuromodulators (prostaglandins, endorphins) and neurotransmitters (norepinephrine, serotonin) are involved to modify the pain sensation in the brain. Visceral pain may be due to distension, stretching, hypoxia, necrosis, chemical irritants or inflammation of the viscera. Pelvic pain may be splanchnic or referred.

Table 33.3
Localisation of referred pain

Organs	Site of referred pain
Body of uterus	Hypogastrium, anterior and medial aspect of thighs
Fallopian tubes and ovaries	Above the mid-inguinal point
Cervix	Upper sacral region
Uterosacral ligament	Lower sacral region

ACUTE PELVIC PAIN

Acute pain is of short duration and generally the symptoms are proportionate to the extent of tissue damage. In chronic pelvic pain the onset is insidious and the degree of pain is not proportionate to the extent of structural tissue damage.

Most often, the basic mechanism of acute pain is due to irritation of the peritoneum by either blood or infection. The causes of acute pelvic pain are given in the Table 33.4.

Table 33.4 : Causes of acute pelvic pain

Mechanism	Clinical conditions
Haemoperitoneum—peritoneal irritation	• Disturbed tubal pregnancy • Ruptured chocolate cyst • Ruptured corpus luteum or follicular cyst
Infection—peritoneal irritation	Acute PID
Chemical irritation	Following HSG
Uterine cramp	Abortion
Vascular complication with neurologic involvement	Axial rotation of ovarian tumour pedicle
Visceral distension	• Intracystic haemorrhage • Hyperstimulation syndrome • Haematometra or pyometra
Non-gynaecological	• Appendicitis • UTI • Intestinal obstruction • Rectus sheath haematoma • Mesenteric vein thrombosis • Pancreatitis

Diagnosis

A meticulous history taking and examinations—systemic, abdominal and pelvic, most often clinch the diagnosis.

Guidelines in clinical diagnosis :

- Pain of gynaecologic origin usually starts in the lower abdomen and then spreads to the entire abdomen.
- Pain preceded by amenorrhoea is usually obstetrically related—**disturbed ectopic pregnancy should be kept in mind.**
- Anorexia, nausea and vomiting are usually correlated well with gastrointestinal mischief.
- Frequency of micturition, dysuria with or without fever point to the diagnosis of urinary tract infection.
- Fever with chills and rigor is most often associated with acute PID.
- Pain with syncopal attacks with collapse suggests intraperitoneal haemorrhage.
- Abdominopelvic lump along with more or less stable vital signs points towards complicated pelvic tumour.

Investigations

Basic investigations to substantiate the clinical diagnosis as when indicated include :

Blood—Haemoglobin estimation, total and differential count of white blood cells and packed cell volume are essential. An increase in white cell count specially with a shift to left may indicate infection. Decreased haemoglobin level with low haematocrit value indicates hypovolaemia.

Midstream urine for microscopic examination and culture is to be done to diagnose UTI. Presence of pus cells, bacteria and red blood cells suggests UTI.

Urine for immunological test of pregnancy. A positive test needs to be followed with serial β subunit of hCG measurement, if the exact location of pregnancy is in doubt.

With these protocols, diagnosis is established in majority and for those remaining undiagnosed cases, the following are to be employed.

X-ray abdomen—(upright, supine and lateral decubitus film) is to be done to diagnose—intestinal obstruction or perforation. Perforation of air-filled viscus is evident by presence of free air under the diaphragm. Free fluid suggests ruptured cyst. Calculus can be evident from X-ray.

Sonography (transvaginal) is helpful to detect pelvic mass or pregnancy — uterine or tubal.

Laparoscopy is helpful to visualise the pelvic pathology. Surprisingly, laparoscopic examination confirms the provisional clinical diagnosis in only 25 per cent of the cases. In acute PID, aspiration of the tubal exudate is to be done for microbial study.

Management

The patients are most often critically ill. Intensive resuscitative or supportive measures are to be taken. The definitive treatment of some of the common events are formulated in the Table 33.5.

Table 33.5
Management protocol

Definite diagnosis	***Immediate laparotomy*** • Haemoperitoneum • Rupture tubo-ovarian abscess • Twisted ovarian cyst • Acute surgical condition ***Institution of medical therapy*** • Urinary tract infection • Pelvic inflammatory disease (see p. 124) • Gastroenteritis • Hyperstimulation syndrome (see p. 503)
Doubtful diagnosis	• To be subjected to diagnostic sonography or laparoscopy • Observation

CHRONIC PELVIC PAIN

Chronic pelvic pain (CPP) is defined as the pain (non-menstrual) of 6 months duration or more localised to the pelvis, anterior abdominal wall below the pelvis or lower back, severe enough to cause functional disability or require medical or surgical treatment.

CPP is a common problem (10%) seen in the gynaecologic outpatient. Approximately 20-30 per cent of laparoscopies and 10 per cent of all hysterectomies are done due to CPP.

Diagnosis

While it is comparatively easy to diagnose the cyclic chronic pelvic pain, but it is difficult at times to pinpoint the diagnosis of acyclic and the non-gynaecologic group. However, meticulous history taking and thorough clinical examinations — abdominal and vaginal with the possibility in mind, are often enough to clinch the diagnosis.

In confused state without any detectable pelvic pathology to account for CPP, **the following guidelines are of help to arrive at the diagnosis.**

Table 33.6
Common causes of chronic pelvic pain

Cyclic	Acyclic
• **Intermenstrual pain** (Mittelschmerz)	• Endometriosis, adenomyosis • PID
• **Dysmenorrhoea** – Spasmodic – Congestive	• **Uterine displacement** – Retroversion – Prolapse
• **Premenstrual syndrome**	• Uterine fibroid • Ovarian cyst – Functional – Neoplastic
• **Pelvic congestion syndrome** • **Endometriosis** • **Adenomyosis** • **Ovarian remnant syndrome**	• Pelvic adhesive disease secondary to PID, endometriosis or postsurgical. • IUD • Trapped or residual ovarian syndrome (see p. 532) • Idiopathic – Pelvic varicosities – Psychosomatic

Table 33.7
Common non-gynaecologic causes of chronic pelvic pain

Gastrointestinal	• Irritable bowel syndrome • Appendicitis • Constipation • Diverticulitis
Urological	• Interstitial cystitis (see p. 393) • Urethral syndrome (see p. 396) • Calculi.
Orthopaedic	Diseases of the bones, ligaments, muscles of the lumbosacral region
Neurological	Nerve entrapment or compression
Hernias	Inguinal, femoral, obturator

• **Nerve entrapment pain** is localised to a particular point of the lower abdominal wall. This may be due to entrapment of ilioinguinal, iliohypogastric or genitofemoral nerve. Local infiltration of bupivacaine 0.25 per cent and relief of pain is a confirmatory test. It is therapeutic also. Surgical exploration and excision of the nerve is also recommended.

• **Pessary test**—In mobile retroverted uterus or slight degree of uterine descent, a pessary test may be employed. The pessary is inserted and kept for 3 months. If the symptoms are relieved, the diagnosis is certain and surgical correction is advisable.

• **Combined oral contraceptive pills**—Cases with functional ovarian cyst producing CPP are given cyclic OC for 3 months. The functional cyst is likely to regress with the relief of symptoms. The same therapeutic test can be employed to relieve the midmenstrual pain or primary dysmenorrhoea by making the cycle anovular.

• **Patient having IUD** and pelvic pain should be cautiously interpreted. **The possibility of PID or ectopic pregnancy should be kept in mind.**

• **Non-gynaecological disorders** as cause of CPP should be kept in mind (table 33.7). These are mostly related with disorders of bowel (spastic colon, irritable bowel syndrome). Spasm or rigidity of muscles specially those of vertebral column suggests orthopaedic, neurologic or rheumatic lesion.

• **CPP without any organic lesion**—The women are usually parous and perimenopausal. Associated symptoms of vaginal discharge, menorrhagia, dyspareunia or bladder irritability are usually present. These cases may be attributed to pelvic congestion, or may be due to psychosomatic disturbances.

Pelvic congestion syndrome (Taylor syndrome) is characterised by chronic pelvic pain, dyspareunia, abnormal uterine bleeding along with pelvic venous congestion. Diagnosis can be made by transuterine venography, transvaginal colour Doppler sonography (TV-CDS) or by laparoscopy. Congested pelvic veins are seen. **Therapeutic options are**: Medroxyprogesterone acetate 50 mg daily is found to be effective. GnRH agonist with oestrogen add back therapy is also recommended. Hysterectomy and bilateral salpingo-oophorectomy is considered as the treatment of last resort for these who fail to respond with medical therapy.

Ancillary aids in diagnosis

• **Blood**—Total and differential count of white blood corpuscles and ESR are helpful in the diagnosis of infection.

• **Cervical and vaginal discharge** is subjected to hanging drop preparation, Gram stain and culture, both aerobic and anaerobic. This can give a clue in the diagnosis of PID.

• **Endometrial biopsy** should be subjected to histology and culture examination in suspected cases of genital tuberculosis.

• **Laparoscopy**—Laparoscopy is an invaluable diagnostic tool in the investigation of chronic pelvic pain. It has been found that in about 50 per cent of cases with normal clinical pelvic findings, have got detectable abnormality on laparoscopy. Conversely, one-third of women with detectable clinical pathology ultimately prove to be a normal pelvis on laparoscopy.

Its chief value is to detect minimal endometriosis and pelvic adhesions. The negative finding also have got value—assures the clinician that no abnormality exists. This can relieve the patient's psychosomatic factor related with CPP.

• **Sonography**—It is of value in diagnosis of tumour either fibroid or ovarian. Transvaginal sonography (TVS) can detect adenomyosis and ovarian enlargement due to cysts. Colour Doppler sonography (CDS) is helpful to detect ovarian torsion. Calculi in the urinary system can also be detected with sonography. It is also helpful in assessing the progress of the therapy in PID specially when laparoscopy is contraindicated or as an alternative to it.

• **X-ray** lumbosacral region and hip joints helps to detect orthopoedic lesions. CT scan or MRI have no place in the diagnosis of CPP except in malignant conditions.

Treatment

Principles

• To have a definite diagnosis of the underlying disorders.

• To establish the relationship between the pathology and the symptoms.

• To evaluate psychosomatic factors — cause or effect.

• **Multidisciplinary approach** involving a psychologist is ideal specially when no pathology could be detected.

In detectable pathology

• Conservative or radical surgery is to be done to remove the offending pathology. Hysterectomy is ideal for women with pelvic endometriosis or adenomyosis, when she has completed child-bearing.

Medical Management of Pain

• Assurance and sympathetic handling too often cure or ameliorate the pain.

• **NSAIDs** : Ibuprofen, Naproxen : COX-2 inhibitors (p.175) — Celecoxib, Ketorolac.

• **Neurolytic agents** : Tricyclic antidepressants — Amitriptyline, Imipramine, **Serotonin uptake inhibitors** Fluoxetine, Paroxetine, **Ion channel Blockers** : Gabapentin, Carbamazepine.

• **Narcotics (under supervision)** : Codeine, Methadone.

• **Others** : OC pills, progestogens, danazol or even GnRH analogues (see p. 500) is indicated in young patient with minimal endometriosis, spasmodic dysmenorrhoea or midmenstrual pain.

• **Minimal invasive surgery** includes laser therapy in pelvic endometriosis or laparoscopic adhesiolysis. **Laparoscopic** presacral neurectomy (PSN) and uterine nerve ablation (LUNA) is considered for midline dysmenorrhoea when conservative management has failed.

• **Surgery** like ventrosuspension, plication of round ligaments (p. 574) in deep dyspareunia or even presacral neurectomy may be employed.

• **Hysterectomy** should be contemplated judiciously in selected cases.

• Intractable pain of malignant origin — Apart from narcotic analgesics, PSN or LUNA may relieve pain for few months (see p. 340).

TRAPPED (RESIDUAL) OVARIAN SYNDROME

The syndrome is characterised by chronic pelvic pain, deep dyspareunia and a fixed tender ovary felt at the vault of the vagina.

It may appear in 1-3 per cent of all cases of hysterectomy with preservation of one or both the ovaries. **The pain is due to tension within the developing follicle of the ovary with periovarian adhesions. Pain may also be due to perioophoritis with a thickened ovarian capsule**. Ultrasonography (TVS) can detect characteristic ovarian enlargement.

The relief of pain may be achieved by ovarian suppression with hormones (high dose progestins, OC pills, danazol or GnRH agonists). Cure is by removal of the ovaries.

OVARIAN REMNANT SYNDROME

The syndrome is defined as the persistence of the ovarian function even after an apparently bilateral oophorectomy. Oophorectomy becomes technically difficult during hysterectomy in cases with extensive endometriosis or pelvic inflammatory disease. **Pain is due to the remnant of ovarian cortical tissue, left behind unintendedly following a difficult oophorectomy.**

The presenting complaints are chronic pelvic pain (cyclic), deep dyspareunia and persistence of symptoms of endometriosis. **Confirmation is done** by serum FSH levels in premenopausal range. Laparoscopic visualisation of the remnant ovarian tissue is difficult because of adhesions. Vaginal ultrasound and MRI are helpful to the diagnosis.

Ovarian suppression as mentioned above may be used for diagnosis. Cure is effective by surgical removal.

POSTMENOPAUSAL BLEEDING

Introduction

Bleeding per vagina following established menopause is called postmenopausal bleeding.

The significance of postmenopausal bleeding, whatever slight it may be, should not be underestimated. **As many as one-third of the cases are due to malignancy**. The same importance is also given to those cases where normal menstruation continues even beyond the age of 55.

Causes

The causes of postmenopausal bleeding are :

- Senile endometritis (p. 164).
- Atrophic endometrium.
- Endometrial hyperplasia (p. 317).
- Dysfunctional uterine bleeding.
- Genital malignancy.
  - Carcinoma of the cervix, endometrium, vagina, vulva and Fallopian tube.
  - Sarcoma uterus.
  - Granulosa cell tumour of the ovary.

- Uterine polyp.
- Tubercular endometritis.
- Cervical erosion and polyp.
- Senile vaginitis.
- Decubitus ulcer.
- Retained and forgotten foreign body such as pessary or IUCD.
- Withdrawal bleeding following oestrogen intake.
- Urethral caruncle, polyp, prolapse mucosa or carcinoma.
- Unknown is about 25 per cent. **The incidence however, decreases with wider use of hysteroscopy.**

Table 33.8
Common causes of postmenopausal bleeding

• Genital malignancy • DUB • Senile endometritis	• Decubitus ulcer • Urethral caruncle • Retained pessary or IUCD

Investigations

Initial step is to establish the fact that it is vaginal bleeding and not bleeding per rectum or haematuria.

Detailed history regarding

- Age of menopause.
- Menstrual pattern prior to menopause.
- Amount of bleeding, number of episodes.
- Sensation of something coming out of the introitus.
- Urinary problems like dysuria or frequency of urination.
- Intake of oestrogen—Even if the history of intake is present, full investigations should be carried out to exclude malignancy.
- Family history of endometrial and/or ovarian carcinoma (first degree relative).

General examination

Obesity and hypertension are often related to endometrial carcinoma.

Enlarged groin or supraclavicular lymph nodes may be palpated. Metastatic nodules in the anterior vaginal wall may be present. Breasts should be palpated because gynaecological symptoms may be related to breast cancer (p. 371).

Per abdomen

A lump in the lower abdomen may be due to pyometra or uterine sarcoma or adnexal mass.

Inspection of the perineum

- If the uterus is outside the introitus, a decubitus ulcer may be detected.
- Careful inspection of vulva may reveal a growth. If it is present, biopsy is to be taken.

Palpation

- Induration over the vulval area.
- To separate the labia for better inspection of the urethral meatus to find out any caruncle, polyp or mucosal prolapse.

Speculum examination

To note the condition of the cervix and the vault of the vagina.

- If a growth is found, punch biopsy is to be taken.
- If no growth is visible and the cervix looks apparently healthy :
  - Cervical smear along with endocervical sampling for cytologic examination for malignant cells.
  - Aspiration cytology — for endometrial carcinoma.

Pipelle endometrial sampling can be done with a long and narrow plastic cannula (Fig. 9.23). This is done as an OPD procedure during speculum examination. Adequate sample is obtained with this procedure and the tissue is subjected for histological examination.

Bimanual examination

- Uterus may be normal, atrophic or enlarged due to pyometra or sarcoma.
- Adnexal mass (infective or ovarian) may be palpable.

Special investigations

Ultrasonography transvaginal probe (TVS) is more accurate because of its proximity to the target tissue (endometrium). Endometrial thickness less than 5 mm indicates atrophy on the other hand thick polypoid endometrium (9-10 mm), irregular texture, fluid within the uterus require further evaluation (to exclude malignancy).

- **Saline Infusion Sonography** (SIS) (see p. 114).

• **Endometrial biopsy** may be done using the Sharman curette as an outpatient basis.

• **Fractional curettage**, if the cervical cytology becomes negative (p. 344).

• **Hysteroscopic** evaluation and directed biopsy.

• **Laparoscopy** in suspected cases of ovarian or adnexal mass.

• **CT and MRI** may be useful in selected cases of postmenopausal bleeding (p. 114).

Detection of a benign lesion should not prevent further detailed investigations to rule out malignancy.

Treatment

• **If the cause is found**, the treatment is directed to it.

• **If no cause is detected** and there is only minimal bleeding once or twice, careful observation is mandatory, if conservatism is desired.

• **In cases of recurrences or continued bleeding** whatever may be the amount, it is better to proceed for laparotomy and to perform hysterectomy with bilateral salpingo-oophorectomy. Unexpectedly, one may find a pathology either in the ovary or Fallopian tube or else, an uterine polyp — benign or malignant may be evident in the removed uterus.

LOW BACKACHE

Low backache is a frequent complaint of parous women in a gynaecologic clinic. It may be the part of the gynaecological complaints or the case may be referred by an orthopaedic surgeon to exclude the pelvic pathology to account for the low backache. **The reasons to refer are** :

• The low backache often dates back to childbirth process or gynaecological operation.

• The symptoms often aggravate in relation to period.

To establish a correlation between the low backache and gynaecologic pathology, **the following facts are to be remembered.**

• As the posterior peritoneum is poorly innervated, the pain is dull and diffuse.

• Backache of pelvic origin never reaches beyond the 4th lumbar vertebra.

• The pain pointed by finger tip is not of gynaecologic origin.

Causes : Common causes of backache of pelvic in origin are :

Uterine displacement

• Prolapse—Uterine prolapse produces backache due to stretching of the ligaments supporting the uterus in position. If the ligaments are atrophic, there will be no pain. **Vaginal prolapse does not cause backache.**

The pain in prolapse subsides when the patient is at rest and aggravates on standing.

• Retroversion—Retroverted uterus may produce backache only when it is fixed by inflammatory or endometriotic adhesions. **Mobile retroverted uterus does not produce backache.**

Chronic pelvic infection : Chronic PID producing adhesions and TO mass formation may be responsible for backache. There are associated menstrual abnormalities and dyspareunia. Chronic cervicitis produces backache by parametritis.

Endometriosis : Endometriosis involving the pelvic peritoneum, uterosacral ligament or rectovaginal septum produces backache and deep dyspareunia.

Neoplasm : Benign neoplasm like ovarian tumour or fibroid will not ordinarily produce backache. However, cervical or broad ligament fibroid by producing pressure on the nerve routes over the sacrum produces backache.

Pelvic malignancy produces backache by involving the nerve roots, metastasis in the vertebrae or involving the lateral pelvic wall.

BREAST IN GYNAECOLOGY

Breast is one of the target organs for the various hormones, of particular oestrogens, progesterone and prolactin. As such, many a breast related complaint or disease is associated with endocrine dysfunctions.

Development : The breast develops at 10-12 weeks from the "milk ridge" which is an **ectodermal thickening** that extends longitudinally from the axilla to groin. Pectoral part of the ridge persists and the rest regresses. In the 3rd month a depression called "mammary pocket" appears in the centre of the milk ridge. Solid buds grow from the mammary pocket into the underlying mesoderm at around the 5th month. During 7th to 9th month the solid buds degenerate and develop into acini. At birth the inverted nipples become everted by the growth of the underlying stroma. The connective tissue stroma is developed from the mesoderm.

At birth : There is only nipple with system of ducts without alveoli. Due to maternal oestrogen, the growth becomes exaggerated with occasional mucoid discharge (witch milk). The involution usually is completed by 1-2 weeks after birth.

Puberty changes (see p. 48) : The breast duct growth is primarily stimulated by oestrogen. The alveolar cells and sebaceous glands are stimulated by progesterone. The maturation of the breast components is accelerated by growth hormone, adrenal hormones, thyroid hormone, prolactin and insulin.

Anatomy of the adult breast

The breasts are bilateral glandular structures and in female, constitute accessory reproductive organs as the glands are concerned with lactation following childbirth.

The shape of the breast varies in women and also in different periods of life. But the size of the base of the breast is fairly constant. It usually extends from the second to sixth rib in the midclavicular line. It lies in the subcutaneous tissue over the fascia covering the pectoralis major or even beyond that to lie over the serratus anterior and external oblique. An axillary prolongation (axillary tail), if present, lies in the axillary fossa, sometimes deep to the deep fascia.

Structures (Non-lactating breasts)

The areola is placed about the centre of the breast and is pigmented. It is about 2.5 cm in diameter. There are numerous sebaceous glands over it. It contains few involuntary muscles. The nipple is a muscular projection covered by pigmented skin. It is vascular and surrounded by unstriped muscles which make it erectile. It accommodates about 15-20 lactiferous ducts and their openings. The whole breast is embedded in the subcutaneous fat. The fat is, however, absent beneath the nipple and areola. **The breast tissue consists of the following structures** (Fig. 33.1).

Each breast is divided into 15-20 lobes by fibrous tissue septa which radiate from the centre. Each lobe consists mainly of fibro-fatty tissue. The glandular tissue consists mainly of duct system in non-lactating breast. One lactiferous duct drains a lobe. The lining epithelium of the duct is cubical, becomes stratified squamous near the openings. Each duct divides and subdivides and ultimately ends in alveoli, the total number being 10-100. Each alveolus is lined by columnar epithelium where milk secretion occurs.

A network of branching longitudinal striated cells, called myoepithelial cells surround the alveoli and the

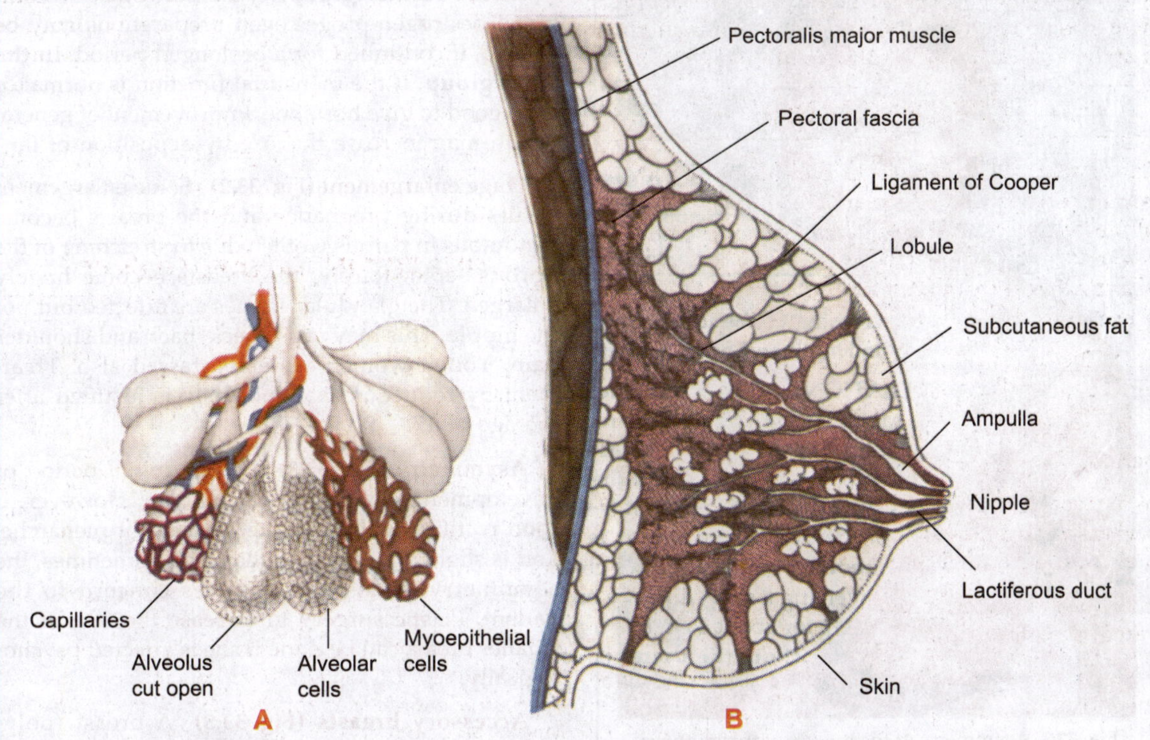

Fig. 33.1. (A) Structure of the basic unit of the mammary gland. (B) Structure of adult female breast

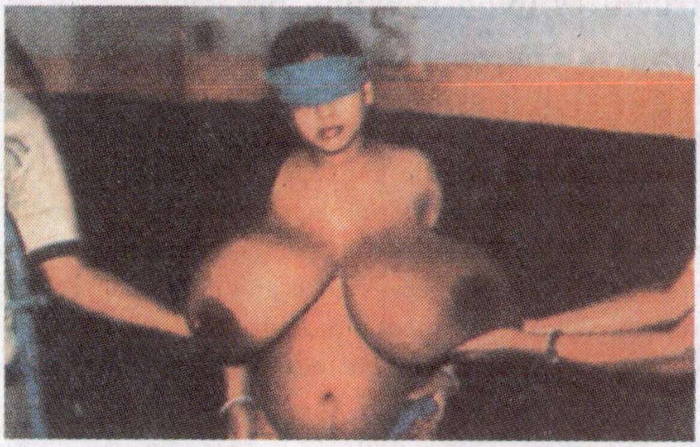

Fig. 33.2. Marked hypertrophy of the breasts *(By courtesy — Dr. N. Chowdhury)*

smaller ducts. There is a dense network of capillaries surrounding the alveoli. These are situated between the basement membrane and epithelial lining. Contraction of these cells squeezes the alveoli and ejects milk into the larger duct. Behind the nipple, the main duct (lactiferous) dilates to form ampulla where the milk is stored. At places, the fibrofatty connective tissue extends from the skin down to the deep fascia in between the lobes. These bands are called suspensory ligaments of Cooper.

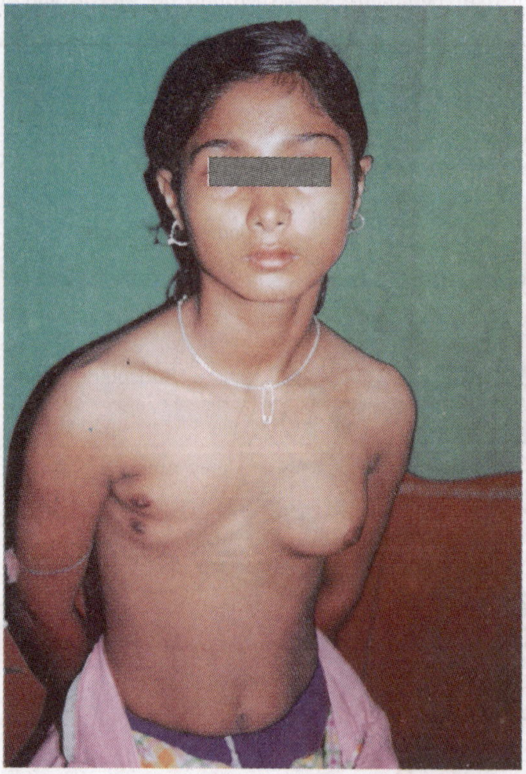

Fig. 33.3. Asymmetry of the breasts with polythelia (accessory nipple)

Blood supply : ***Arterial supply***

- Lateral thoracic — branches of the axillary artery.
- Internal mammary.
- Intercostal arteries.

Veins — The veins follow the courses of the arteries.

Lymphatics :

- Lateral hemisphere : Anterior axillary nodes.
- Upper convexity : Infraclavicular group.
- Medial convexity
  - Mediastinal glands (cross connection between the two breasts). There is no contralateral drainage of lymph, until and unless there is ipsilateral obstruction.
- Inferior convexity : Mediastinal glands.

Nerves — The nerve supply is from fourth, fifth and sixth intercostal nerves.

Anatomical defects : Small breasts

This may be due to :

- Non or under production of ovarian oestrogens.
- Developmental defect in the breasts.

In the former group, cyclic oestrogen or combined oestrogen-progestogen preparations may be of help, if continued for a prolonged period. **In the latter group**, if the menstrual function is normal, it is no good to give hormone. Improvement of general health may increase the size by deposition of fat.

Huge enlargement (Fig. 33.2) : Some enlargement occurs during pregnancy and the breasts become pendulous in parous women due to stretching of the fibrous septa. Rarely, the breasts become hugely enlarged. The glandular tissues are affected but not the nipple. This may cause neck, back and shoulder pain. Young women are embarrassed also. Treatment by reduction mammoplasty is justified after the age of 17.

Asymmetry (Fig. 33.3) : During initial period of development, asymmetry is common. However, it soon rectifies within couple of years of menarche. Left is slightly larger than the right. Sometimes, the asymmetry persists and causes concern to the patient. Plastic surgery to increase the size of the smaller breast can be done if she is affected psychologically.

Accessory breasts (Fig. 33.3) : A breast (polymastia) or a part or a nipple (polythelia) may develop and tends to grow anywhere along a line extending from the axilla to the groin (milkline). **The commonest site of extension is as a 'tail' into the axilla**. They can be the site of all diseases as found in a normal breast tissue. Excision may be needed because of discomfort, cosmesis or disease.

Diseases of the Breast

- Premenstrual mastalgia (see chapter 13).
- Fibrocystic changes.
- Infective (mastitis).
- Fibroadenoma.
- Carcinoma.

Fibrocystic breast disease

Fibrocystic breast disease is the most common benign lesion. It is generally observed between 20-50 years of age.

The aetiology is not known. It may be due to altered oestrogen : progesterone ratio or relative decrease in progesterone or else, the breast tissues are more sensitive to prolactin. Stress factor may at times be related.

Histologically a fibrocystic mass is characterised by adenosis, fibrosis, ductal epithelial proliferation and papillomatosis. Two types are observed : localised and diffuse. Vast majority (70%) are nonproliferative lesions. Of the proliferative lesions only Z few (4%) present with cellular atypia where the risk of breast cancer is high (five-fold). Risk factors are nulliparity and delayed menopause.

The patients are usually premenopausal. The patient complains of breast pain present throughout the cycle but aggravated premenstrually (cyclic). The pain is either dull continuous or intermittent and severe.

Examination reveals affection of both the breasts; one is more than the other. On palpation, coarsely nodular areas resembling ill-defined lumps either localised or diffused, are felt. These are prominent in premenstrual phase.

The patients become anxious of malignancy and the physicians too are confused to negate it. **Careful palpation, mammography, ultrasound and aspiration biopsy is helpful to exclude malignancy**.

Treatment

- Assurance and re-examination at intervals.
- To wear a well fitting brassier day and night.
- To prescribe diuretics and tranquilizers in the second half of the cycle.
- To reduce the intake of methylxanthines (coffee, tea, chocolates, caffeinated soda) and tobacco.
- Vitamin E 400 mg daily may be helpful.
- In refractory cases, any of the following may be tried :
  - Cyclic combined oestrogen-progestogen preparations.
  - Danazol 200 mg daily in divided doses.
  - Bromocriptine—2.5-5 mg daily at bed time.
  - Surgery—rarely indicated.

Fibroadenoma

This is the most common benign tumour of the breast occurring among the younger (20-35 years) women. It is symptomless being accidentally discovered by self palpation.

On palpation, an uniform, firm, mobile, painless and well-defined mass is felt. Commonly they are bilateral and 2-3 cm in diameter. Histologically they have an epithelial and a stromal component. A young patient however, may be reviewed **6 monthly** as the risk of malignancy is less than 0.2 per cent.

Surgical excision and biopsy is indicated only when the mass enlarges and or report of FNAB is inconclusive.

BREAST CARCINOMA

Breast cancer is the commonest (32%) of all cancers and is the second (next to lung cancer) common cause of cancer deaths in women. One out of 8 obstetric-gynaecologic patients is likely to develop breast carcinoma at sometime during her adult life in USA and Western countries.

Obstetricians-gynaecologists examine millions of patients on a regular basis. As such, they are expected to evaluate, screen, counsel and to formulate the treatment planning for breast diseases (table 33.11).

Screening for breast cancer

Breast carcinomas are generally without any symptoms to start with. Screening can detect breast cancer at an earlier stage (table 33.10). Ideally screening should be performed for all women from 40 years of age. Earlier detection improves the survival rate. 5–year survival is about 85 per cent when axillary lymph nodes are not involved.

Screening and diagnostic methods include :

- A complete breast examination by a physician
  - Inspection.
  - Palpation.
- Breast self examination.
- Breast imaging
  - Screening mammography.
  - Diagnostic mammography.
  - Ultrasonography.
  - Magnetic resonance imaging (MRI).
  - Digital mammography, Positron emission tomography.
- Breast biopsy
  - Fine needle aspiration biopsy (FNAB).
  - Stereotactic and ultrasound guided core biopsy.
  - Open biopsy : Excisional biopsy
    Incisional biopsy.

Inspection (see Fig. 9.1, chapter 9)

Inspection is performed while the patient is sitting with arms relaxed by her sides. Both the breasts are observed for contour, symmetry, nipple positions, and any skin changes. Patient is asked to press her hands on her hips so as to contract the pectoralis major muscles. Skin dimpling and nipple retraction if any, may be obvious with this method.

Palpation (See Fig. 9.1 p. 97)

Entire breast is palpated methodically by quadrant with the flat part of the fingers both in upright and in supine positions (see p. 97).

Generally a malignant mass is felt firm, non-tender, fixed with ill-defined borders. Entire axilla and the supraclavicular areas are palpated for any lymph nodes. Nipple is compressed for any discharge. Breast palpation is best done during the first half of the menstrual cycle.

Breast self examination

Breast self examination should be made into a habit, **certainly by the age of 20**. The examination should be made on a monthly basis following the menses as the breasts become less tender and less engorged.

The procedures (as described above) are demonstrated to the patient. Inspection should be done standing in front of a mirror in a well lit-room. The patient should palpate her breasts with the opposite hand both in sitting position and lying supine with a pillow beneath her back. Axillary and supraclavicular areas are to be palpated. The nipples should be compressed for any discharge. She is instructed to contact physician whenever there is any abnormal finding.

Table 33.9
High risk factors for breast carcinoma

- Early menarche
- Late menopause
- Obesity
- Nulliparity
- Late age of first birth (>35 years)
- Never breastfed
- Atypical lobular hyperplasia
- Nipple discharge other than milk
- High dose breast or chest irradiation
- High dietary fat intake
- Oestrogen replacement therapy
- Breast carcinoma in first degree relative (Mother, sister or daughter)
- Carcinoma in the other breast
- Previous cancer of endometrium, ovary, colon
- Inherited mutations of BRCA 1 and BRCA 2 genes.

Genetic predisposition—is high when there is mutation of the BRCA 1 (on chromosome 17 q) and or BRCA 2 (on chromosome 13 q) genes. BRCA 1 and BRCA 2 are the tumour suppressor genes. Hereditary breast cancer is seen in younger women and is often bilateral. Around 5% of breast cancers are familial.

Breast imaging

Mammography : Baseline mammogram should be done by the age of 40. Mammography in conjunction with physical examination for early detection is **to be done annually as a routine** :

- From 40 years of age for all women.
- From 35 years of age in 'high risk' group.
- At any age, if one breast is removed for cancer.

Mammography can detect nearly 30-50 per cent of early breast cancers that are not clinically palpable. Two views, one mediolateral side view and the other craniocaudal view are to be taken for each breast. **The characteristic features suggestive of malignancy on mammography are** : Spiculated microcalcifications, asymmetric soft tissue densities, skin thickening or nipple retraction. **Screening mammogram should be performed in all women by the age of 40 years.** Sensitivity of mammography is 60–90 per cent. It is most sensitive in older woman when compared to young women. It has reduced breast cancer mortality by about 33 per cent. In the presence of any suspicious mass, one should always perform biopsy, irrespective of the mammographic findings.

Ultrasonography is useful to differentiate a cystic lesion from a solid one. Solid masses with ill-defined borders and complex cystic lesions are considered suspicious. Ultrasound cannot detect microcalcifications and it is less accurate than mammography.

Magnetic resonance imaging (MRI) is an excellent method for screening and without any radiation risk. Contrast enhanced MRI are used at present. However it is not a substitute for conventional mammography and biopsy.

Positron emission tomography (PET) is used to detect occult breast carcinoma with positive axillary lymph nodes. It is expensive.

Breast biopsy is essential for the confirmation of diagnosis. Biopsy is generally done as an outpatient procedure.

Fine-needle aspiration biopsy (FNAB) is done for **cytologic evaluation** inserting a narrow gauge (22G) needle into a breast lesion. This is a simple and cheap procedure with no morbidity. Unfortunately false-negative diagnosis may be high (up to 10%) and it cannot differentiate a non-invasive carcinoma from an invasive one.

Stereotactic and ultrasound guided core biopsy is done using a large bore cutting needle (14G). In this method a core of tissue is obtained for histological examination. Both frozen and permanent sections can be done.

Table 33.10 : Clinical features of early malignancy

- Non-tender lump in the breast (mostly located in the upper and outer quadrant).
- Non-milky nipple discharge of any type, specially bloody.
- Retraction of the nipple (previously everted).
- Indrawing of the overlying skin.
- Localised oedema of the skin.
- Persistent erosion or crusting of the nipple (refractory to medication).

Open biopsy is performed either as a primary procedure or when the results of FNAB are inconclusive. With excisional biopsy the lesion is completely removed under local anaesthesia. Incisional biopsy is done where only a portion of the mass is excised for confirmation of diagnosis.

Nipple discharge

A nipple discharge when spontaneous, persistent and unrelated to lactation is considered abnormal. Any significant nipple discharge must be thoroughly evaluated with the following information :

- Nature of discharge (milky, serous or bloody).
- Unilateral or bilateral.
- From a single duct or multiple ducts.

Table 33.11 : Staging for Breast Cancer

(American Joint Commission on Cancer, American Cancer Society, American College of Surgeons Committee on Cancer)

Stage	*Tumour size (T)*	*Lymph node metastases (N)*	*Distant metastases (M)*
0	Carcinoma-*in-situ*	NIL (N_0)	M_0
I	T_1	NIL (N_0)	M_0
IIa	$T_0 - T_2$	Metastasis to ipsilateral axillary node(s) but mobile (N_1)	M_0
IIb	$T_2 - T_3$	As in stage IIa (N_1)	M_0
IIIa	$T_0 - T_3$	Metastasis to ipsilateral axillary lymph node(s) and fixed (N_2)	M_0
IIIb	T_4 – Any T	As stage IIIa and or metastasis to ipsilateral internal mammary lymph node(s) (N_3) or any N	M_0
IV	Any T	Distant metastasis (M) and any N	M_1

T = Primary tumour in greatest dimension; T_0 = no tumour; T_1 = Tomour ≤ 2 cm; T_2 = > 2 cm but ≤ 5 cm; T_3 = > 5 cm; T_4 = any T with extension to chest wall or skin; MO = No distant metastasis. M_1 = Distant metastasis (including ipsilateral supraclavicular lymph nodes).

- Association of any mass in the breast.
- History of any drug intake (phenothiazines or oral contraceptives).
- Premenopausal or post menopausal.

For common causes of nipple discharge — see Table 33.12.

Table 33.12
Common causes of nipple discharge

Colour	Probable diagnosis
Milky	• Physiologic (lactation) • Pregnancy • Oral contraceptives • Inappropriate (galactorrhoea see p. 548)
• Bloody • Sangui-neous	• Intraductal papilloma • Intraductal cancer • Malignancy • Duct ectasia • Fibrocystic disease
Clear watery	• Ductal cancer
Green, Yellow	• Ductal ectasia
Purulent	Infective
Serous or sticky	Fibrocystic disease

Except milky discharge, one should exclude malignancy by all means before concluding a benign lesion.

Treatment

The treatment of breast carcinoma is within the domain of general surgeon. As such, the interested readers are requested to consult Textbook of Surgery for therapeutic protocol of breast carcinoma.

PSYCHOSEXUAL PROBLEMS

Female sexual dysfunction includes the different disorders : Loss of sexual desire, disorders of arousal, or orgasm and also painful intercourse.

Loss of Libido is loss of sexual desire. Loss of libido may be due to depression or it may develop from a traumatic event (e.g. rape, sexual abuse or bereavement) in the past. Several drugs can cause disorders of desire (antipsychotics, lithium, antihypertensives, beta blockers, oral contraceptives, phenytoin sodium, etc.).

Treatment : Psychosexual therapy is essential to deal with the underlying psychologic problems. Psychiatric consultation is needed when there is depressive symptoms. Specialist Physicians are to be consulted when medications are responsible.

VAGINISMUS

Definition

Vaginismus is defined as the psychogenically mediated involuntary spasm of the vaginal muscles including the levator ani muscles and/or the thigh adductor muscles. This results in inability of penetrative sexual intercourse.

Aetiology : • Primary • Secondary

Primary : Nothing has entered into the woman's vagina ever. However, the vagina is normal anatomically and physiologically. The cause is mostly psychosexual in origin. There is often presence of a subconscious fear of sexual intercourse (sexual phobias).

Secondary : Vaginismus usually appear after childbirth or any other event in life. There is usually some local painful lesions. Such lesions include vulvitis, lacerations of the hymen, tender scar on the perineum or narrow vaginal introitus. The entity is usually transient and is relieved, when the cause is removed.

Clinical presentation : The woman with vaginismus avoids vaginal examination and smear. She might present with painful sexual intercourse or with infertility.

Diagnosis : While diagnosis of the secondary one is not so difficult but to find out the cause of the primary one, examination under anaesthesia may be required. If the two fingers can be easily introduced through the vaginal introitus, the calibre of the vagina is proved normal.

Treatment : • Primary • Secondary

Primary : The following guidelines are prescribed :

- **Psychodynamic therapy** : Main causes of fear are removed. To educate and to gain confidence of the husband and wife. This may take time.
- **Behavioural therapy** : Dilatation of the vaginal introitus digitally followed by introduction of gradually increasing size of the dilators is to be done. Plastic vaginal trainers (Pseudopenises) with graduated sizes can help her to remove her fear. This will gain her confidence that her vagina is anatomically of normal calibre.

• Daily introduction of the dilators (pseudopenises) for 1-2 weeks and to keep it inside for 10-15 minutes is enough before she is allowed to attempt coital act.

• Surgery is required, if the hymen is found tight — hymenectomy or Fenton's operation (operation to enlarge the introitus), if the introitus is narrow (see chapter 34, p. 562).

Secondary : The local lesion is to be treated medically or surgically.

DYSPAREUNIA

Definition

Dyspareunia means that the coital act is difficult and or painful. Apareunia is inability to practice coitus. The two are most often interchangeable. Dyspareunia is the most common sexual dysfunction.

Aetiology : • **Male** • **Female**

Male causes : The following male factors are responsible :

- Impotence.
- Premature ejaculation.
- Congenital anatomic defect of the penis.
- Lack of technique of coital act.

Female causes : Depending upon the site of pain, the dyspareunia may be either :

• **Superficial or entrance** • **Vaginal** • **Deep**

Superficial : Any lesion of the lower part of the labia minora or around the fourchette may be responsible.

These are :

- Narrow introitus.
- Tough hymen.
- Bartholin gland cysts.
- Tender perineal scar.
- Vulval infection.
- Urethral pathology.
- Vulvar vestibulitis syndrome (see p. 255).

Vaginal : Burning pain along the barrel of vagina either during or following intercourse is the presenting complaint. Common causes are :

- Vaginitis.
- Vaginal septum.
- Tender scar—following gynaecologic operation or delivery.
- Secondary vaginal atresia.
- Tumour.
- Vaginal atrophy (menopause).

Deep : The patient experiences pain while the penis penetrates deep into the vagina. As the vagina is insensitive to pain, deep dyspareunia usually results from pathology of paravaginal tissues or other pelvic organs. Such lesions are :

- Endometriosis, specially on rectovaginal septum.
- Chronic cervicitis.
- Chronic PID.
- Retroverted uterus — mostly acquired and fixed.
- Prolapsed ovary in the pouch of Douglas.

Treatment : Treatment depends upon the cause. Too often, sex education of both the partners relieves the symptom.

The infective lesions of the vulva and or vagina are to be treated. Tender scar on the perineum or the vagina is to be excised.

Retroverted uterus or prolapsed ovary may require surgical correction, if the symptom is not relieved even by changing the position of the coital act.

The treatment of vaginismus has been mentioned earlier.

Other relevant organic lesions are to be appropriately treated.

ABDOMINOPELVIC LUMP

Throughout the text, emphasis has been given in medical gynaecology. It has been mentioned earlier that in most of the cases, detailed history taking and physical examination, at best with vulval inspection can give a clue to the diagnosis. However, variable ancillary aids may be required at times to pinpoint the diagnosis.

But in spite of what has been mentioned in the text, too often the students and also the physicians are confused to arrive at a diagnosis of the nature of a lump in the lower abdomen. As such, it is prudent to formulate in the chapter the salient features of such lumps so as to minimise the mistakes.

Full bladder

It is an axiom that prior to gynaecologic examination, bladder must be kept empty. Not only full bladder may be confused with some abdominopelvic pathology but empty bladder ensures better evaluation of pelvic findings on bimanual examination.

Table 33.13
Common causes of lump in the lower abdomen

Toddlers (< 5 years)	• Ovarian tumour • Mucocolpos • Full bladder
5 years of age to puberty	• Ovarian tumour • Full bladder • Haematocolpos
Childbearing period	• Pregnancy • Full bladder • Ovarian tumour • Fibroid • Adenomyosis • Chocolate cyst • TO mass • Pelvic haematocele • Pelvic abscess • Encysted peritonitis • Pseudocyesis
Postmenopausal	• Ovarian tumour • Pyometra • Sarcoma uterus

Features of a full bladder

- Strictly suprapubic, may even reach upto the umbilicus.
- Cystic or tense cystic.
- Margins—ill-defined.
- Tendency of urge for micturition on pressure.
- Disappears after catheterisation.

Pregnancy

Pregnancy with an uterine size of 16-18 weeks is most confusing. The confusion is accentuated with a history of oligomenorrhoea, conception occurring during lactational amenorrhoea or illegal pregnancy.

In fact, amenorrhoea during childbearing period with a lump in the lower abdomen should be provisionally diagnosed as pregnancy unless proved otherwise.

Features are :

- Recent history (grows in weeks).
- History of amenorrhoea.
- Feel — soft elastic.
- Braxton-Hick's contractions — present.
- External ballottement — elicited.
- Internal examination reveals :
  - Swelling is uterine.
  - Cervix-soft.
  - Internal ballottement — elicited.
  - Sonography — foetal echo confirms the diagnosis.

Ovarian tumour (also see p. 280)

Features are :

- Slow growing (takes months to grow).
- Menstrual history — unaffected.
- Feel — cystic, tense cystic or solid.
- Margins — well-defined but lower pole may not be reached.
- Ascites — may be present.
- Internal examination reveals :
  - The swelling is separated from the uterus.
- Sonography (see p. 286).

Fibroid (see p. 262)

Features are :

- Slow growing (takes years to grow).
- Menstrual history—menorrhagia.
- Feel—firm, may be cystic in cystic degeneration.
- Surface—nodular.
- Pregnancy features—absent.
- Internal examination reveals :
  - Swelling is uterine in origin.
  - Cervix—feels firm.
- Sonography (see p. 268).

Adenomyosis (see p. 303)

- Usually associated with parous woman.
- Menorrhagia with increasing dysmenorrhoea—congestive and persists even after the period.
- Lump—rarely more than 14-16 weeks.
- Uniform with well-defined margins.
- Soft and tender.
- PV examination reveals :
  - Swelling is uterine.
  - Cervix-firm, uterus-tender.
  - Associated pelvic endometriosis may be present.
  - Sonography (see p. 304). (For Differentiation of Fibroid Uterus and Adenomyosis see p. 622).

Encysted peritonitis

- History of Koch's infection.
- Amenorrhoea of longer duration may be present.
- Swelling — ill-defined margins.
- Feel — cystic.
- Internal examination reveals :
  - Uterus is separated from the cystic mass.
- X-ray chest — A lesion may be found.
- Mantoux test — may be positive.
- Sonography.

Pseudocyesis

- Usually present in women having problem of infertility or approaching menopause with an intense desire to have a baby.
- History of amenorrhoea.
- Abdominal examination reveals absence of positive signs of pregnancy.
- EUA — uterus of normal size.
- Sonography — absence of fetal echo.

ADNEXAL MASS

An adnexal mass refers to any mass occupying the region of the uterine appendages (adnexa). Major concern is the ovarian neoplasm (malignancy).

COMMON ADNEXAL MASSES

Ovarian
- Ovarian neoplasm
- Ovarian cyst
- Endometriomas
- Tubo-ovarian mass

Uterine
- Myoma

Gastrointestinal
- Diverticulitis
- Appendicular mass (Right)

Tubal pathology
- Ectopic pregnancy
- Hydrosalpinx
- Tubal neoplasms

Genitourinary
- Pelvickidney

Evaluation of an adnexal mass

A. **Clinical—(Bimanual pelvic) Examination** for its size, shape, consistency, mobility and tenderness.

B. **Transvaginal ultrasonography**—Whether the cyst is simple or complex, internal echoes, nodularity. **Doppler ultrasound** to study blood flow and to measure R1 and P1.

C. **Computed tomography (CT)**—Contrast tomography can differentiate loop of bowel, dermoid cyst, myomas (Fig. 36.81B).

D. **Magnetic resonance imaging (MRI)** is also helpful and it has no risk of ionising radiation.

E. **Position emission tomography (PET)** is more sensitive in detecting metastatic disease.

F. **Tumour markers** — Numerous tumour markers have been studied for the detection and follow up of ovarian malignancy namely CA–125, CA–15-3, TAG-72 CA–19-9 (see p. 497).

Management of an Adnexal Mass

Whenever any adnexal mass is diagnosed the management will depend mainly on — (i) Nature of the mass. (ii) Age of the woman.

Ovarian Cysts in Postmenopausal women — Should be assessed for the risk of malignancy clinically and also using CA–125 and transvaginal sonography (TVS). **Important points on TVS for scoring are** : Multilocular cyst, presence of a solid areas; metastases; ascites and bilateral lesions (p. 283).

According to RMI (**Risk of Malignancy Index**) the women are triaged into **Low risk** : RMI < 25. **Moderate Risk** : RMI 25-250 and **High Risk** : RMI > 250 (see p. 363).

Actual management

Conservative management is ideal for a simple, unilateral unilocular ovarian cyst, ≤ 8 cm with low RMI. Such women are followed up with TVS at an interval of 4 months. 50 per cent of such cysts resolve spontaneously.

Surgical management: Besides those as described above, all need some form of surgical treatment (Cyst aspiration, Laparoscopy and Laparotomy).

Cyst aspiration for cytologic examination to differentiate benign from malignant tumours is done. But in a postmenopausal women it is not recommended.

Laparoscopic approach should only be made with moderate risk women (RMI : 25-250). **Cystectomy** for young women and oophorectomy for post-menopausal women is recommended. Such women should be counselled preoperatively that a full staging laparotomy may be needed if evidence of malignancy is seen.

Laparotomy—All ovarian cysts that are suspicious of malignancy specially in a postmenopausal women (RMI > 250), or with positive findings of laparoscopy, need a full staging laparotomy in a specialised centre. **Procedure includes** : Laparotomy (midline incision) → Peritoneal washings (for cytology) → Staging → Biopsies → TAH + BSO + Infracolic omentectomy (± selective pelvic and para-aortic lymphadenectomy). (RCOG Guideline : 34 : 2003).

HIRSUTISM

Nomenclature

Hirsutism : Hirsutism is the excessive growth of androgen dependent sexual hair (terminal hair) in facial and central part of the body that worries the patient (Fig. 33.4).

Hypertrichosis : Hypertrichosis connotes excessive growth of non-sexual (fetal lanugo type) hair.

Hyperandrogenism : Hyperandrogenism is a state of increased serum androgen level with or without any biological effect of hyperandrogenemia.

Virilism : Virilism is defined as the presence of any one or more of the following features—deepening of the voice, temporal balding, amenorrhoea, enlargement of clitoris (clitoromegaly) and breast atrophy. It is a more severe form of androgen excess.

Androgen sources in female

Testosterone is the second most potent androgen in circulation, the first one being dihydrotestosterone (DHT). The daily production rate of testosterone in normal female is 0.2-0.3 mg.

Approximately, 50 per cent of testosterone arises from peripheral conversion of prohormones, predominantly androstenedione. The principal sites of peripheral conversion are skin, muscle, fat, liver and lungs. The adrenal glands (z. reticularis and z. fasiculata) and ovaries (theca, stroma and granulosa) contribute approximately equal amounts (25%) to the circulatory levels of testosterone.

Dehydroepiandrosterone sulphate (DHEA-S) arises exclusively from the adrenal glands while about 90 per cent of DHEA is secreted from the adrenals.

Androstenedione arises from the adrenals and ovaries in equal amount.

The sources of androgens in normal female are schematically depicted below.

Most of testosterone (80%) in the circulation is bound to SHBG and is biologically inactive. About 19 per cent is bound loosely with albumin and **only 1 per cent, the testosterone remains free which is biologically active.**

To exert a biological effect, testosterone (T) is metabolically converted in target tissues to dihydrotestosterone (DHT) by the enzyme 5 α-reductase. DHT is the most potent androgen to stimulate the hair follicles and sebaceous glands (pilosebaceous unit). 3 α-androstanediol glucuronide (3 α-AG) is an important tissue metabolite of DHT. 3 α-AG is thought to reflect the activity of the enzyme 5 α-reductase at tissue level.

T → (5 α-reductase) → DHT → 3 α-androstanediol (3 α-A) → 3 α-androstanediol glucuronide (3 α-AG).

Therefore the biochemical marker for each androgen compartment *is different. For the ovary it is testosterone; for the adrenal gland it is DHEA–S and for the periphery it is 3 α–AG.*

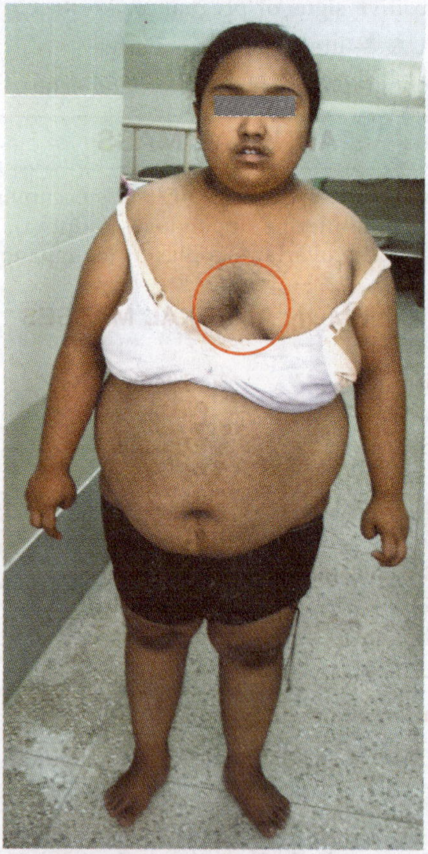

Fig. 33.4. 15 years, young obese (BMI : 34) girl with excessive growth of hair in a male distribution (face, chest and inter-mammary region)

Principal sources of androgen in normal female

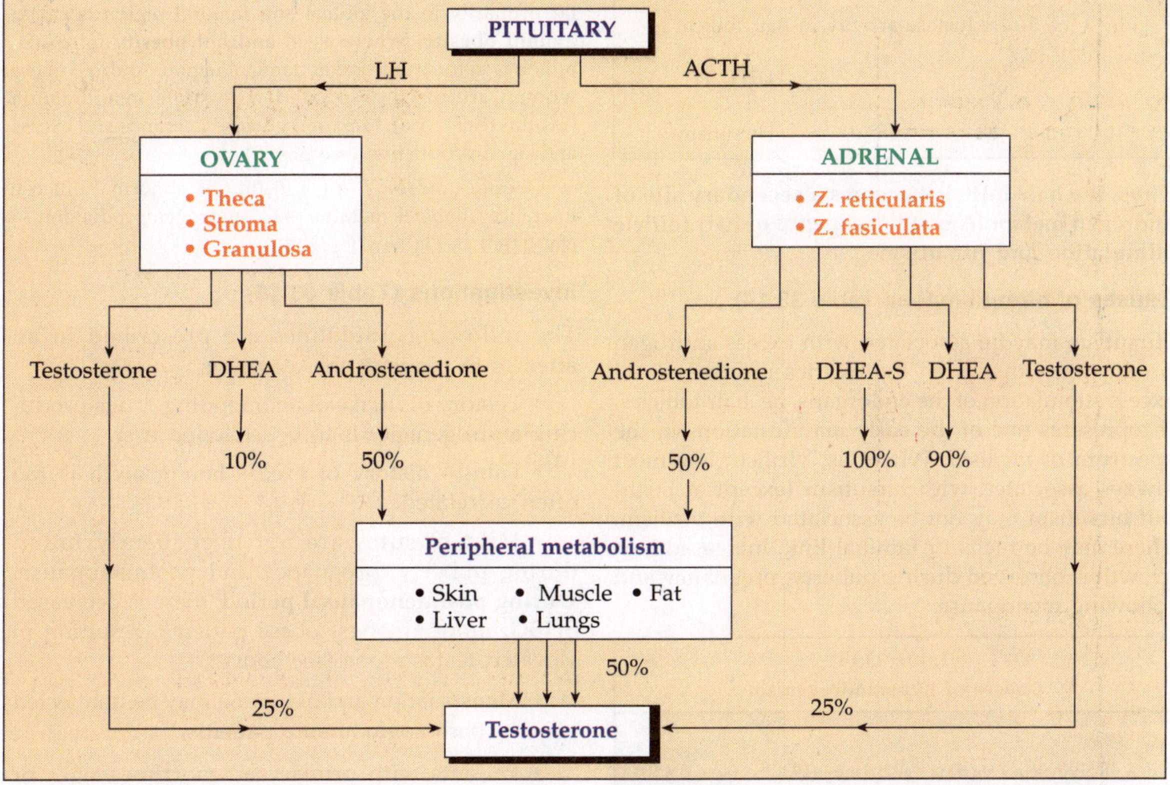

Androgens and pilosebaceous unit

The pilosebaceous unit consists of sebaceous glands and hair follicles. Both are sensitive to androgens. The sebaceous glands are more sensitive to androgens than the hair follicles. Hypestimulation of the sebaceous glands leads first to oily skin and subsequent infection results in acne.

The skin and hair follicle play an active role in serving as target organs for the androgens and also in producing androgens from circulatory prohormones.

Mechanism of excessive hair growth

The stimulus for the excessive hair growth is testosterone. Testosterone binds to the androgen receptors in the hair follicle. This is followed by activation of the enzyme 5 α-reductase. This will convert testosterone to most potent androgen—dihydrotestosterone (DHT) and androstenediol which stimulate proliferation and growth of terminal hair (anagen phase). Once the black terminal hair is produced, the changes persist even in the absence of a continuing androgen excess. Increased hair follicle stimulation and increased 5 α-reductase activity enable prohormones DHEA and androstenedione to be metabolised directly to DHT. This leads to further hair follicle growth. **This latter phenomenon explains continued growth even if the initiating testosterone source has been removed**.

Pathophysiology of hirsutism

It involves combination of the following :

- Increased concentration of serum androgens specially of testosterone.
- Decreased level of SHBG resulting increased free testosterone (testosterone itself reduces SHBG level).
- Increased responsiveness of the target organ (skin) to the normal circulating androgens. This may be related to ethnic background. Oriental women have less number of hair follicles per unit area of skin compared to a Caucasian woman.
- Increased activity of 5 α-reductase which converts testosterone to DHT in the skin and hair follicles.

T → Plasma T ↑ → SHBG ↓ → Free T ↑
↓
↑ ↑ 5 α-reductase activity in hair follicle
↓
DHT
↓
Hirsutism

Thus, the hair follicle becomes a secondary site of androgen metabolism at the expense of hair follicle stimulation and hirsutism.

Causes of hirsutism (see Table 33.14)

Hirsutism may be associated with excess androgen production either from the ovaries or adrenals or excess stimulation of the endorgans, i.e. hair follicles. It represents one of the early manifestations in the spectrum of virilism. Where as, virilism is almost always associated with hirsutism (except at birth) but hirsutism may not be associated with virilism. There may be racial or familial link. Increased hair growth is observed during puberty, pregnancy and following menopause.

Table 33.14
Causes of hyperandrogenism

- **Ovarian**
  - Polycystic ovarian syndrome (PCOS) (see p.440)
  - Sertoli-Leydig cell tumour (see p. 371)
  - Hilus cell tumour
  - Lipoid cell tumour
  - Hyperthecosis
  - Luteoma of pregnancy
- **Adrenal**
  - Adrenal hyperplasia (congenital or late onset) (see p. 445)
  - Cushing's syndrome (see p. 446)
  - Adrenal tumour
- **Obesity (android)**
  - Insulin resistance and androgen excess (p. 441)
- **Exogenous (drug therapy)**
  - Androgens, anabolics, oral contraceptives, synthetic progestogens, danazol, phenytoin, diazoxide, cortisone, etc.
- **Postmenopause**
- **Pituitary tumour** — secreting
  - Excess ACTH (Cushing's diseases)
  - Excess growth hormone (acromegaly)
- **Idiopathic**

Obesity (android) — Insulin resistance and androgen excess. Obesity (BMI > 25) associated with distribution of fat primarily in the gluteal and femoral region is called **gynoid obesity**. Where as in **android obesity** fat distribution is in the trunk and abdominal region. Android obese women are often associated with hyperinsulinaemia (insulin resistance), impaired glucose tolerance and excess androgen production (see p. 450).

Obesity (android) → (↑) insulin → abnormal glucose tolerance/diabetes mellitus → (↑) androgen production → (↓) SHBG → (↑) free T and E_2.

Investigations (Table 33.15)

The following guidelines are prescribed in an attempt to pinpoint the diagnosis.

- History of intake of an offending drugs producing androgenicity is to be excluded first.
- Family history of excess hair growth is too often correlated.
- Mild hirsutes are not infrequently found during puberty, pregnancy and postmenopause. **During postmenopausal period**, there is decreased SHBG, more amongst obese patients, resulting in elevated testosterone (see above).
- Menstruation and ovulation may be unaffected even in pathologic hirsute patients.
- Patients with primary amenorrhoea with or without virilism, require karyotyping to exclude 'Y' bearing dysgenetic gonads.
- Hirsutism of rapid onset irrespective of age, requires evaluation for adrenal or ovarian tumour.
- High serum level of testosterone (> 2ng/ml) raises the suspicion of an androgen producing tumour. Serum level of DHEA–S correlate well with daily urinary 17–KS secretion. Further evaluation should be done with ultrasonography, CT or MRI (see Table 33.14).
- Young age, insidious onset, unassociated with virilisation and having normal menstruation without any abnormal clinical finding usually point towards idiopathic or peripheral cause. This should be confirmed by at least 3 minimal hormone evaluations—serum testosterone (normal), DHEA-S (normal) and 3 α-AG (elevated). However, it is not necessary to measure 3 α-AG without elevated circulatory androgen levels, because the presence of hirsutism is itself an evidence of increased peripheral androgen activity.
- The diagnostic features of adrenal or ovarian causes are outlined in the Table 33.15.

Table 33.15 : Diagnostic features for adrenal or ovarian causes of hyperandrogenism

ADRENAL		OVARIAN	
Hyperplasia	**Tumour**	**Tumour**	**PCOS**
Prepuberty and young Insidious Hirsutes + Virilism ± MH – Amenorrhoea	Any age Rapid onset Hirsutes ++ Virilism + MH – Amenorrhoea	Any age Rapid Hirsutes ++ Virilism + MH – Amenorrhoea	Early reproductive Insidious Hirsutes ± Virilism — Nil MH – Oligomenorrhoea or amenorrhoea
Hormone status • 17 hydroxy progesterone ↑↑ (> 8 ng/ml) • DHEA-S ↑ • Testosterone (T) – Normal (< 0.8 ng/ml) • Dexamethasone suppression test — positive	**Hormone status** • DHEA-S ↑↑ (> 700 μg/100 ml) • T-normal or ↑ • Dexamethasone suppression test — negative • IVP • Sonography • CT scan • MRI	**Hormone status** • T ↑↑ (> 200 ng/100 ml) • DHEA–S Normal or ↑ • Sonography • Laparoscopy • Biopsy	**Hormone status** • LH : FSH-3 : 1 • T ↑ (> 150 ng/dl) • DHEA-S — may be ↑ • Insulin resistance (IR) : Raised fasting serum insulin ↑ (> 25 μ IU/ml) and levels of serum insulin response > 300 μ IU/ml at 2 hours post-glucose (75 gm) load. Sonography (see p. 440) Laparoscopy (see p. 441)

• In Cushing disease, because of increased ACTH secretion from the anterior pituitary, there is increased glucocorticoid and androgen secretion from the adrenals. The findings include hirsutism, menstrual abnormalities, centripetal obesity, abdominal striae, etc. If the plasma cortisol level is < 5 μg/ml after overnight 1 mg dexamethasone suppression, Cushing's syndrome can be ruled out.

• Late onset congenital adrenal hyperplasia is rarely associated with hirsutism. This is due to partial deficiency of 21-hydroxylase enzyme. Serum level of 17 α-hydroxy progesterone (17-OHP) is elevated both base line and after stimulation of ACTH.

Management

The principles of management are :

- To remove the source of excess androgen.
- To suppress or neutralise the action of androgen.
- To remove the excess hair.

Weight reduction—is an important step of management. Weight loss is associated with reduction of hyperinsulinaemia and androgen excess. Ideal body mass index (BMI) should not be more than 25 (see p. 546).

Removal of the source

- Adrenal or ovarian tumour should be surgically treated.
- Cushing's disease can be treated by adrenalectomy, radiation to the pituitary or removal of ACTH producing tumour by transsphenoidal surgery.
- In iatrogenic cases, the offending drug (see Table 33.14) should be stopped.

To suppress or neutralise the excess androgen action

The drugs used—depending upon the site of production of excess androgens are :

- Combined steroidal contraceptive pill.
- Dexamethasone.
- Antiandrogens.

Contraceptive pill

Mode of action

- Suppression of LH secretion from the pituitary (progestin effect).

- Anti-androgen at the level of hair follicle.
- Elevation of SHBG (oestrogen effect).
- Progestins in OC pills inhibits 5 α-reductase activity in the skin.
- Inhibits adrenal androgen secretion.

OC pills with **new progestins** (norgestimate, desogestrel, gestodine — see ch. 29) have very little androgenic effects. They increase the level of SHBG. They reduce free testosterone level significantly.

Case selection : Pill is suitable in cases of PCOS or idiopathic group specially in young and unmarried where only 'T' is elevated (Table 33.16).

Dexamethasone : It acts by suppressing pituitary – adrenal axis. It is used in adrenal or mixed adrenal and ovarian hyperandrogenism.

The dose varies from 0.25-1 mg daily at bed time.

GnRH agonists are used to suppress selectively ovarian steroid production by inhibiting LH secretion from the pituitary. This is used only when other anti-androgens have failed to give a response.

Anti-androgens : *Cyproterone acetate*—It inhibits gonadotrophin secretion and interferes with androgen action on the target organs by competing for the androgen receptors. It blocks the action of DHT and T at both the nucleus and cytosol receptor level.

It should be administered along with ethinyloestradiol to prevent menstrual irregularities and ovulation. 100 mg is given from day 5 to day 14 with ethinyloestradiol 30 μg, from day 5 to day 25 (reversed sequential regimen).

Improvement of hirsutism is observed after 3 months of therapy. This regimen gives contraceptive benefit also. Important side effect are : nausea, fatigue, weight gain, loss of libido and mastalgia.

Spironolactone — 100-200 mg daily, maintenance dose is 25-50 mg daily. It is an aldosterone antagonist and acts as a potassium sparing diuretic.

Anti-androgen effects of spironolactone are :

- It inhibits ovarian and adrenal androgen biosynthesis.
- It competes for the androgen receptors in the hair follicle.
- It inhibits 5 α-reductase activity directly.

Important side effects are : menstrual irregularity, hyperkalaemia.

Flutamide—100-200 mg daily. It is a nonsteroidal anti-androgen. It blocks the androgen receptors as well as it inhibits testosterone biosynthesis. Results are observed after 3 months of therapy. Side effects are : nausea, dry skin, headache and hepatotoxicity.

Finasteride—5 mg daily. It inhibits 5 α-reductase activity. It improves hirsutism significantly without any side effects.

Ketoconazole — see p. 512.

Duration of therapy : All the drugs should be continued for at least 6 months. Anti-androgens inhibit the growth of new hair follicle but fails to remove the hair that is already present.

Removal of hair : The excess hair is to be removed by bleaching, twitching, epilation, waxing, lasers, shaving or electrolysis. In electrolysis individual hair follicle is destroyed. Side effects are pain, scarring and pigmentation.

Table 33.16
Hormone profile and drug therapy

Hormone profile	Drugs
Elevated T	• Oral contraceptives (OC) • GnRH agonist
Normal T and DHEA-S 3 α-AG ↑ (idiopathic)	Anti-androgens
DHEA-S ↑, normal T	Dexamethasone
DHEA-S ↑, T ↑	OC + dexamethasone

GALACTORRHOEA

Definition

Secretion of milk looking discharge from one or both breasts unrelated to childbirth is called **galactorrhoea** (inappropriate lactation). **The secretion contains fat globules** when examined under microscope and is confirmatory for milk. A high prolactin level is encountered in one-third of cases with idiopathic amenorrhoea.

Prolactin (PRL) is the most important hormone involved in the **pathophysiology of galactorrhoea**. Prolactin is under tonic hypothalamic inhibitory control of prolactin inhibitory factor (PIF).

Prolactin inhibits GnRH pulse secretion. Gonadotrophin levels are suppressed. Hyperprolactinaemia inhibits ovarian steroidogenesis.

Prolactinoma is present in about 50 per cent of women with hyperprolactinaemia. Serum prolactin level when raised on repeat assay beyond 20 ng/mL, suggests evaluation of sella turcica (see p. 445). Level beyond 100 ng/ml is associated with high incidence of prolactinoma. Most of the prolactinomas are microadenomas. High prolactin levels are associated with amenorrhoea with or without galactorrhoea. **About 30 per cent of women with high prolactin levels, have galactorrhoea**. However galactorrhoea can be seen in women with normal serum prolactin. About 30 per cent of women with galactorrhoea have normal menses.

Table 33.17 : Indications of prolactin assay

- Amenorrhoea with or without galactorrhoea
- Galactorrhoea with or without amenorrhoea
- Oligomenorrhoea
- Corpus luteum insufficiency
- Unruptured luteinised follicle
- Delayed puberty

For causes, diagnosis (Table 33.17) and management of hyperprolactinemia (see p. 445, 450, ch.28).

KEY POINTS

- Leucorrhoea defines strictly as an excessive normal vaginal discharge which stains the undergarment. It is nonpurulent, non-offensive and never causes pruritus.

  The excess normal secretion occurs during puberty, menstrual cycle (around ovulation and premenstrual), pregnancy and sexual excitement. Abnormal vaginal discharge is mainly infective in origin (see Table 33.2).

  Improvement of general health, sympathetic attitude towards ailments, local hygiene and appropriate therapy for the local ailments are enough to cure the state.

- Pruritus means sense of itching. It does not produce pain nor there is any local tenderness.

  Local skin lesions, vaginal discharge, allergy, intestinal worms or diabetes are some of the important causes.

  Appropriate therapy is to be instituted depending upon the factors involved. Vulvectomy is not the treatment to cure pruritus.

- The significance of postmenopausal bleeding should not be underestimated. About one-third of the cases are due to pelvic malignancy, the commonest being uterine (Table 33.8).

  Apart from routine use of gynaecological examination, the special investigations include cytology, transvaginal sonography, fractional curettage, hysteroscopic evaluation and/or laparoscopy.

  Even if no cause is detected, recurrence or persistent uterine bleeding dictates hysterectomy with bilateral salpingo-oophorectomy.

- Pain arising from the pelvic organs is often localised not to the organ but referred to the skin area supplied by the same spinal nerve (Table 33.3).

  The basic mechanism of acute pain is due to irritation of the peritoneum by either blood or infection.

  Apart from history and clinical examination, the investigations to pinpoint the diagnosis of acute pelvic pain include — examination of blood for haematocrit, midstream urine examination for UTI and urine for immunological test for pregnancy (Table 33.4). The diagnosis is established in most cases.

  Management in cases of definite diagnosis includes either immediate laparotomy or institution of medical therapy. In doubtful cases, diagnostic laparoscopy and observation are of help (Table 33.5).

KEY POINTS

Chronic pelvic pain (CPP) is defined as six months or more of constant or intermittent pain (non-menstrual pain) localised in the pelvis or lower back severe enough to cause functional disability or require medical or surgical treatment. CPP is often without any visible pathology (Table 33.6). Incidental detection of pathology may not be the cause of pain. Laparoscopy is done both for diagnostic and therapeutic purposes as "one-stop" procedure. In the absence of definite pathology medical management of pain should be tried first.

Medical treatment includes — analgesics, prostaglandin synthetase inhibitors, OC pills, progestogens, danazol or even GnRH analogues. Minimal surgery includes laser therapy in pelvic endometriosis and adhesiolysis endoscopically. Hysterectomy should be contemplated judiciously.

- Trapped or residual ovarian syndrome is manifested with chronic pelvic pain. The pain arises from the ovaries (preserved during hysterectomy) due to tension within the growing follicle or due to periovarian adhesions. The chronic pelvic pain in ovarian remnant syndrome is due to the remnant of ovarian cortical tissue, left behind unintendedly following a difficult oophorectomy.
- The backache pointed by finger tip is not of gynaecologic in origin. The pain in prolapse subsides when the patient is at rest and aggravates on standing. Mobile retroverted uterus does not produce backache.
- Breast carcinoma is one the leading cause of death amongst female malignancies.

  The screening includes — breast self-examination, routine physical examination, imaging studies and breast biopsy (see p. 539). Base line mammogram is to be done at 40 years. Mammography along with physical examination is to be done annually from the age of 40 and earlier in high risk group.

  Irrespective of mammographic findings, presence of any suspicious mass suggests biopsy.

  FNAB is a rapid diagnostic method with high degree of accuracy. Ultrasound guided procedure allows the needle tip at the exact site.

  High risk factors for breast carcinoma are many (Table 33.9). Mutations in BRCA-1 and BRCA-2 genes (tumour suppressor genes) account for familial breast cancer (5%), which has an early age onset.

  Causes of bloody nipple discharge are (Table 33.12) malignancy, intraductal papilloma, fibrocystic disease and duct ectasia. Purulent discharge is due to infection and serous or sticky discharge is due to fibrocystic disease.
- Female sexual dysfunction includes different disorders (p. 540). Dyspareunia means that the coital act is difficult and or painful. Apareunia is inability to practice coitus. Causes of deep dyspareunia are pelvic endometriosis, chronic cervicitis, chronic PID, fixed retroverted uterus or prolapsed ovary in the pouch of Douglas.
- Prior to gynaecological examination, bladder must be kept empty. Full bladder should be excluded first in the differential diagnosis of abdominopelvic lump; similarly, pregnancy has to be excluded in childbearing period irrespective of the status of the women (Table 33.13) — married, unmarried, widow, divorced or separated.
- The principal sources of androgen in female are peripheral (50%), ovaries and adrenals (p. 545 – flow chart).

  Most of the testosterone (80%) in the circulation is bound to SHBG; 19 per cent is bound with albumin and 1 per cent remains free which is biologically active.

  In the pilosebaceous unit, the testosterone is converted into potent dihydrotestosterone by the enzyme 5 α reductase. Hirsutism may be associated with excess androgen production either form the ovaries or adrenals or excess stimulation of the hair follicles. Virilism is almost always associated with hirsutism except at birth but hirsutism may not be associated with virilism.

KEY POINTS

Causes of hirsutism may be in the adrenals, ovaries, exogenous drug therapy or idiopathic (Table 33.14).

In adrenal hyperplasia, 17-hydroxyprogesterone is elevated; in adrenal tumour DHEA-5 is elevated; in ovarian tumour, testosterone is elevated and in PCOS, LH : FSH ratio is increased. Dexamethasone suppression test is positive in adrenal hyperplasia but not in tumour. Sonography, CT scan, MRI, IVP and laparoscopy may be extended to exclude organic lesion (see Table 33.15).

- For each major compartment of androgen source, one biochemical marker is used. Testosterone reflects ovarian, DHEA-S reflects adrenal gland and 3 α–AG reflects peripheral tissue source (p. 546).
- Increased 5 α-reductase activity is seen in idiopathic hirsutism.
- Women with PCOS often suffer from android obesity (BMI > 25). Biochemical abnormalities observed in women with PCOS are : elevated levels of biologically active LH, hyperinsulinaemia (insulin resistance), impaired glucose tolerance and excess circulating androgen (see Ch. 28).
- Treatment of hirsutism depends on the source of excess androgen (see Table 33.15). Oral contraceptive therapy is instituted when serum testosterone is elevated (ovarian androgen). Dexamethasone is the drug of choice when DHEA-S is elevated (adrenal androgen). Antiandrogens (see p. 548) are used when neither is elevated (peripheral androgen).
- Anti-androgens should be continued for a minimum of 3 months before any response is observed. This is due to the length of hair growth cycle. While the antiandrogen inhibits the growth of new hair follicle, it fails to remove the hair that is already present.
- Source of excess androgen may have to be removed surgically (see Table 33.14). Removal of hair is done by bleaching, twitching, epilation or electrolysis.
- Prolactin is the most important hormone, involved in the pathophysiology of galactorrhoea.

  Common causes are pituitary microadenoma (smaller than 10 mm), hypothalamic, drug therapy (reserpine, OC, psychotrophic agents, methyldopa, etc.) and primary hypothyroidism (see ch. 28). Serum prolactin level of > 100 ng/ml is too often associated with tumour (prolactinoma).

  Bromocriptine is the drug of choice. Pergolide and carbergoline have less side effects (see p. 450). Pregnancy following bromocriptine have got no teratogenic effect on the offspring. There is no increased incidence of multiple pregnancy. In unresponsive cases of microadenoma, surgery (transnasal-transsphenoidal excision) is done.
- An adnexal mass needs to be critically evaluated to formulate the management. Clinical examination, imaging studies, tumour markers and the genetic markers (p. 543) are helpful to distinguish a benign from a malignant tumour. An adnexal mass may be followed up or may need medical or surgical intervention depending upon its nature (benign or malignant), size and the patient's age.

Operative Gynaecology

34

Introduction

Perioperative management encompasses the care in the pre, intra and postoperative periods. The decision to operate and whether it should be emergently or electively is also important.

The prime objective of this chapter is to make the readers familiar with the basic information about different aspects of practical gynaecology. While the technical details may only concern the specialists, **the beginners should be familiar with the basic principles of operative gynaecology**. The interested readers may go through the available textbooks of operative gynaecology for further details.

PREOPERATIVE PREPARATIONS

The ultimate objective of surgery is to cure the ailments and or to arrive at a diagnosis, if it is done for diagnostic purpose.

Preoperative evaluation should include a detailed history (general, medical and surgical), a complete physical examination and laboratory investigations. BMI (see chapter 9) is recorded for assessment of nutritional status. Past records of illness or surgery should be evaluated. An anaesthesiologists should see the patient preoperatively. A physician or other specialists may be involved depending upon the patient's need. For any elective (planned) operation, the general condition of the patient must be improved, prior to operation any systemic disorder including anaemia must be corrected.

Investigations

The objectives of preoperative investigations are :

- To evaluate the health status of an individual who may be otherwise healthy.
- To provide a base line information in the event of any postoperative complication.
- To assess the severity of a pre-existing medical disorder that needs further attention.

The investigations should preferably be done prior to admission.

Rationale for preoperative investigations

Any major gynaecological surgery involves anaesthesia, blood loss and disturbances in major organ function like cardiovascular and respiratory. The purpose of preoperative investigations is to assess the individual's physiological reserve and the ability to withstand the surgical stress.

Routine investigations for major surgery

Blood—Estimation of haemoglobin, haematocrit, total and differential leucocyte count, platelet count, blood group and cross matching are done. ***Other blood tests*** : Liver function, renal function, serum electrolytes, blood sugar in aged women or in complicated cases.

Urine—Routine and microscopic analysis includes examination for protein, sugar, casts and pus cells. If the pus cells are more than 5 per high power field, culture sensitivity is required.

Chest X-ray (CXR) and ECG—For an otherwise healthy individual below the age of 40, these are not essential. But women above 40 years of age should preferably have CXR, ECG and serum electrolytes analysis.

If there is any history of systemic disease, relevant investigations should be carried out accordingly. Relevant investigations (e.g. echocardiography, coagulation profile) should be done as indicated. Special investigations appropriate to some lesions such as VVF, malignancy have been mentioned in the concerned chapters.

To protect the surgical staff, screening for hepatitis B virus in high risk group is necessary. The screening for HIV antibodies should be done following patient counselling and permission (see p. 149).

To make the patient fit for surgery

In elective (cold) surgery, every attempt should be made to correct anaemia by haematinics or blood transfusion. Eradication of septic foci, control of hypertension or diabetes is also needed.

Admission : The patient is to be admitted on the day or 1-2 days prior to operation. Special cases need earlier admission. During this period, re-evaluation of the case and examination by anaesthetist should be done.

Preoperative work up

Enquiry should be made about :

- Drug allergy.
- Continued medication for any ailments particularly, monoamino-oxidase inhibitors, insulin or antihypertensive drugs. These may help the anaesthetist to modify the drug and dose of anaesthetic agents.
- History of corticosteroid therapy in recent past.
- False tooth.

PREOPERATIVE COUNSELLING AND INFORMED CONSENT

Preoperative discussion between a doctor and a patient or guardian in case of minor, should be in general terms. It should remove patient's anxiety and fear for operation. The following should be explained to her :

- Diagnosis of the abnormality, the nature of the operation and its modifications depending on the findings during operation.
- The likelihood of successful outcome following surgery.
- The potential risks and complications of surgery.
- Alternative forms of treatment available.
- An informed consent must be in writing and in a prescribed proforma.
- All consent must be voluntary and without coercion.
- Consent form must be signed by the patient and the physician.

Diet : Light diet is given in the previous evening and nothing in the morning of the day of operation. Nothing by mouth for at least 8 hours before the operation is ideal so that the stomach is empty at the time of anaesthesia.

Preparation of the bowel : A cleansing enema is commonly given in the evening before the operation day. Rigorous bowel preparation is not routinely required unless bowel surgery is expected. However, in cases where satisfactory bowel preparation is needed, osmotic oral purgation using polyethylene glycol solution (Macrogols) are used. Patient is asked to drink 1-2 litres of such mixtures. To avoid dehydration intravenous fluids may be needed.

Night sedation : To ensure good sleep at night prior to the day of operation, either diazepam 5-10 mg or alprazolam 0.25–0.5 mg tab is given at bed time.

Local antiseptic care : ***Abdominal preparation***—Routine shaving of the operative area before surgery is not recommended. Hair clipping reduces the rate of wound infection. Cleaning of the operative area with soap and water is generally done by the patient. The surgically prepared area should extend from the inferior rib cage to the midthigh. The abdomen is cleaned with a five minute scrub using povidone iodine solution before surgery.

Vaginal operation—The vaginal preparations include clipping of the pubic hair and up to middle of both the thighs. Presence of active vaginal or cervical infection requires eradication prior to surgery. Routine douching is not preferred.

The perineum and the vulva are cleaned with Savlon using a sponge held in a sponge forceps (Fig. 36.15). The vagina is cleaned with povidone iodine solution. This solution is then flushed away with sterile water poured into the vagina. Then a sterile sponge on a sponge forceps is used to clean the vagina.

Morning medication : In consultation with anaesthetist, sedative like diazepam 5–10 mg orally, is given about two hours prior to sending the patient to the operation theatre. Inj. atropine sulphate 0.6 mg is usually (not as a routine) administered in the operation theatre intravenously by the anaesthetist.

Other medications : The patient is generally advised to take all regular medications on the morning of surgery with sips of water, unless contraindicated.

Prophylactic antibiotics

Prophylactic use of antibiotics during the peri-operative period significantly reduce the risk of infection following all major gynaecological surgery. A broad spectrum antibiotic is selected to cover the common gram-positive, gram-negative and the anaerobic organisms.

Generally a third generation cephalosporin (ceftriaxone 1 gm) is given by slow intravenous route on induction of anaesthesia. Second dose is repeated after 12 hours.

Preoperative work up in the operation table

IV infusion—An infusion of Ringer's solution drip is started.

Anaesthesia—Local, regional or general anaesthesia is administered with sole discretion of the anaesthetist.

Position of the patient—In abdominal operation, the position is dorsal, whereas in vaginal operation, it is lithotomy.

Antiseptic dressings : **Bladder preparations** : For minor operations the patient voids before being taken to the operating room. For major operations, soft rubber catheter or Foley's catheter is inserted in operating table. In **vaginal operation**, metal catheter is used after draping and Foley's catheter is introduced at the end of the operation and (see Fig. 36.6).

Draping—Proper draping is done prior to surgery using sterile linen, towel and leggings (in vaginal operation). Towel clips are used (see Fig. 36.40).

Formalities in minor vaginal operations

- Examination of the cardiovascular system.
- Blood examination for haemoglobin estimation and total and differential count.
- Urine examination for protein, sugar and pus cells.
- The patient is to be admitted in the morning of the day of operation.
- Oral feeding is to be withheld for at least 8 hours prior to surgery.
- Vulval cleaning is only done.
- The patient is asked to pass urine before entering the operation theatre.
- Anaesthesia.
- Lithotomy position.
- Antiseptic painting of the vulva and vagina.
- Draping.
- Examination under anaesthesia.

Day care surgery includes selected surgical procedures where patients are admitted, operated and discharged **on the same day**. The operation should not be unduly complex or time consuming. Patients are screened before hand (see above). **Benefits of day care surgery are** : (i) increased patient turn over, (ii) reduced hospital stay, (iii) reduced inpatient work load and (iv) reduced concomitant cost.

Assessment of suitability for day care surgery is important. After operation the patient should be seen both by the patient and the anaesthetist. Before the discharge, follow up procedures, analgesia and availability of emergency services are explained to the patient.

Common gynaecological operations for day care surgery are :

- Dilatation and curettage
- Termination of pregnancy (D and E)
- Biopsy procedures
- Examination under anaesthesia
- Endoscopic procedures like (see ch. 35) :
  - Diagnostic hysteroscopy, laparoscopy (p.117)
  - Laparoscopic sterilisation operation (p. 476)
  - Ovarian diathermy (p.450)
  - Transcervical resection/ablation of endometrium (p.189).

INTRAOPERATIVE CARE

Incisions

Most of the gynaecological operations are done though transverse incisions **Pfannenstiel incision** (muscle separating) is commonly used. **The main advantages of transverse incision are**—(i) Rapid wound healing, (ii) Better postoperative convalescence, (iii) Superior cosmetic result, (iv) Good access to pelvic organs. Less incidence of postoperative (v) wound dehiscence and (vi) incisional hernia.

Disadvantages are —

Incision is difficult to extend when exploration of the upper abdomen is needed. Other transverse incisions are :

Cherney incision : The rectus muscle is dissected from its insertion at the symphysis. During closure the rectus tendons are united to inferior portion of the rectus seath with interrupted sutures.

Maylard incision is a true transverse muscle cutting incision. The inferior epigastric vessels are ligated before incising the rectus. The muscles are approximated during closure.

Vertical (Median or Paramedian) incisions give good access to whole of abdomen with excellent exposure. It spares all major nerves, vessels and muscles, as opposed to the transverse incision. It gives rapid entry to the abdominal cavity.

Disadvantages : It lacks all the advantages of transverse incision.

Drains are used to prevent any accumulation of blood, pus, or intestinal secretion. They are less commonly used in gynaecological surgery.

Closure of peritoneum : Traditionally closure of the pelvic and parietal peritoneum is done at the end of the operation to decrease adhesions. However, the current studies have shown that such closure increases adhesions (RCOG—1998). Peritoneum rapidly spreads across any raw areas left after surgery and there is no need of peritoneal closure.

POSTOPERATIVE CARE

Return from operation theatre

Immediate postoperative care—On return from the theatre the patient is taken to the recovery room or ward which is usually placed adjacent to the operation suite. Patient is accompanied by a responsible person—doctor or nursing staff. **The prerequisites prior to shifting are** :

- Vital signs such as pulse, respiration and blood pressure become steady.
- Patient recovers from anaesthesia and fully conscious.
- Anaesthetist's consent should be available.
- Fluid balance and any bleeding from the surgical site is checked.

In the ward

First 24 hours

Placement in the bed : The patient is gently placed on her side in the bed. This reduces the risk of inhalation of vomitus or mucous. If spinal anaesthesia is given, the foot end is raised for about 12 hours.

Observation : The observation of the vital signs such as pulse, respiration and blood pressure is made half hourly in the initial period. The interval is gradually increased if these are found steady. Attention should be paid for any bleeding from the operated site.

Fluid replacement : Following any major operation fluid is replaced intravenously. The amount of fluid to be replaced is decided upon the following factors : intraoperative blood loss, operating time, urine output and the volume of fluid already replaced.

Blood transfusion, if needed is given during operation and soon after. **Blood transfusion should not be given unnecessarily**. Urine output of at least 30 ml/hour indicates adequate fluid replacement. On an average, after replacement of the fluid loss at operation, additional 2-2.5 litres of fluid are infused. As there is sodium retention following major surgery, the replacement is by 5 per cent dextrose in water along with 0.5 to 1 litre of Ringer's solution.

Pain control : Liberal analgesics should be given to relieve pain and to ensure sleep. A sedative is prescribed at night. For this purpose, intramuscular injection of pethidine hydrochloride 100 mg or morphine sulphate 10 mg is administered at an interval of 6-8 hours. Adequate pain control ensures deep breathing, adequate oxygenation, early mobilisation and reduced hospital stay. Non-steroidal anti-inflammatory agents (Ketorolac) are also effective analgesics. In some centres, **patient controlled analgesia (PCA)** infusion pumps are used. Patient is instructed to use a preset dose of morphine without any overdosage. Nausea or vomiting may be prevented by simultaneous administration of metoclopramide 10 mg or ondansetron 4 mg IM/IV.

Antibiotics : Perioperative prophylactic antibiotics as mentioned in preoperative care are to be considered. Alternatively, routine postoperative antibiotics are prescribed. This should be administered parenterally for 48 hours followed by oral route for another 3 days.

Bladder care : The patient is encouraged to pass urine at least 6-8 hours after operation. If she fails, catheterisation should be done taking aseptic precautions with 'no touch' technique. If repeat catheterisation is required, it is better to leave behind an indwelling catheter for 24-48 hours. The catheter is attached to a sterile bag for closed drainage of urine.

General : The patient should be encouraged to move freely in bed and to lie in any posture comfortable to her. Deep breathing and movements of the legs and arms are encouraged to minimise leg vein thrombosis and pulmonary embolism. It is advantageous to allow the patient to sit or to stand by the side of the bed on the first day. The patient can have sips of water to relieve the thirst.

Second day

General care : The patient is expected to look better and fresh. Vital signs are noted at least twice daily. Abdominal auscultation is done for appearance of peristaltic sounds. Enquiry is to be made about the escape of flatus. Vaginal plug (if any) is to be removed early in the morning. The patient is encouraged to walk few steps by the side of the bed and to sit on the bedside or on a chair. Deep breathing exercises and leg and arm movements while on bed are encouraged.

Diet : Oral feeding in the form of plain or electrolyte water is given in small but frequent intervals. With the appearance of bowel sounds or passage of flatus, full liquid diet is prescribed.

Antibiotics (as discussed above).

Sedative and analgesics : Parenteral analgesics during day time and a sedative at bed time are usually needed.

Third day

- The patient is expected to feel comfortable and look fresh.
- She can move around in the room and go to the toilet.
- Light solid diet of patient's choice is given.
- Although, analgesics may not be required but a sedative at bed time is given.
- The self retaining catheter if present, is removed with or without prior periodic clamping.

Fourth and fifth day

- Daily observation of vital signs twice daily is to be done as a routine.
- The diet is gradually brought to her normal.
- The bowels usually move normally, otherwise low enema or suppository may be given.

Sixth or seventh day

The abdominal stitches are usually removed on the 6th day in transverse incision and on 7th day in vertical incision. **The stitches are to be removed in early morning with the patient in empty stomach.** The precaution is taken so that emergency repair of the wound can be done, if burst abdomen occurs.

Care of the perineum : Following vaginal plastic operation, the perineal wound is dressed at least twice daily or following each act of micturition and defaecation. The dressing is done with spirit and antibiotic powder or ointment. Local pain and oedema may be relieved by hot compress with magnesium sulphate or infra red rays.

Discharge

There is a trend towards shorter hospital stay these days. But complete recovery of all organ functions is needed before discharge. It may take 5-7 days when she is fit for discharge. **Written information** is given to the patient as regard the operative procedures.

While an uniform guideline is difficult to formulate, in an otherwise uneventful postoperative recovery, the patient may be discharged by 5-7 days following hysterectomy.

Examination prior to discharge

Abdominal operation

- Abdominal wound is to be thoroughly checked for evidences of sepsis, haematoma or dehiscence.
- Vaginal discharge if any, is to be noted. If the discharge is offensive, gentle vaginal exploration by a finger should be done to exclude a foreign body (gauze piece).

Vaginal operation

- Perineal wound is checked to assess the state of healing.
- Vaginal exploration with a finger is useful to detect accidentally a retained and forgotten gauze piece.

Advices given on discharge

Rest : Light household work can be resumed after 3 weeks and outside or office works to be resumed after 6 weeks. However, there may be variation of the period of rest. While some resume their work earlier comfortably, others may find it difficult.

Coitus: There is no fixed time bar. As soon as she is physically and psychologically fit, intercourse is permissible. However, it should not be resumed prior to the postoperative check up (i.e. 6 weeks) specially following vaginal plastic operation and hysterectomy.

Special instructions are mentioned in appropriate chapters.

Follow-up is usually after 6 weeks or earlier if some complications occur.

GYNAECOLOGICAL OPERATIONS

As mentioned in the introduction, the technical details of the operation while concern to the specialists but **the students should be acquainted with the principles involved**. Some considerations are however given in cases of minor operations. Such operations are common and some may have to do it following graduation during house officer job.

DILATATION OF CERVIX

This is an operation to dilate the cervix. While in some cases, dilatation of the external os is enough but in majority, the entire canal including the internal os is to be dilated.

The dilatation is done by graduated cervical dilators.When the internal os is to be dilated, prior introduction of uterine sound is mandatory to confirm the position of the uterus.

Indications

The indications of only dilatation are:

- Prior to amputation of cervix (see p. 210).
- Prior to hysteroscopy.
- Pyometra or haematometra (see p. 165).
- Prior to introduction of uterine curette and insertion of IUD, radium or laminaria tent.
- Spasmodic dysmenorrhoea (see p. 174).

DILATATION AND CURETTAGE

This is an operative procedure whereby dilatation of the cervical canal followed by uterine curettage is done. This is the commonest gynaecological operation performed both in the hospital and in the office.

Indications

The indications are grouped into:	
Diagnostic	• Infertility • DUB • Pathologic amenorrhoea • Endometrial tuberculosis • Endometrial carcinoma • Postmenopausal bleeding • Chorionepithelioma
Therapeutic	• DUB • Endometrial polyp • Removal of IUD • Incomplete abortion
Combined	• DUB • Endometrial polyp

Steps of operation

- The patient is to empty the bladder prior to operation.
- The operation is done under general anaesthesia or under diazepam sedation with or without paracervical block.
- She is placed in lithotomy position.
- Local antiseptic cleaning and draping done.
- Bimanual examination is performed.
- Posterior vaginal speculum is introduced.
- The anterior lip of the cervix is held with an Allis tissue forceps.
- An uterine sound is introduced to confirm the position and to note the length of the uterine cavity.
- Cervical canal is dilated with graduated dilators.

Hawkin-Ambler dilator should be held in such a way that the knob is inside the palm and the index finger rests on the body of the instrument. The tip of the finger should be placed at a distance of about 3 cm (slightly more than the length of the cervical canal) from the tip of the instrument. The finger tip acts as a guard. The tip of the instrument should pass beyond the internal os evidenced by the fact that it is grasped by it and does not fall even when the support of the instrument is withdrawn. The tip of the dilator should be directed anteriorly or posteriorly according to the position of the uterus.

- When the dilator is introduced, the cervix is made steady by traction of the vulsellum.
- After the desired dilatation, the uterine cavity is curetted by an uterine curette either in clockwise or anticlockwise direction starting from the fundus down to internal os.

In benign lesion, sharp curette and in suspected malignancy, blunt curette is used.

The curette should be gentle but thorough. Vigorous curettage may damage the basal layer of the endometrium and uterine muscle.

- Vulsellum and the speculum are removed.
- The curetted material is **preserved in 10 per cent formol-saline (normal saline in suspected tubercular endometritis), labelled properly and sent for histological examination.** Short history of the case and **first day of last menstrual period** specially in infertility cases and DUB should be positively mentioned.

Discharge

After a short period of observation (say 3-4 hours) with passing off of the anaesthetic effect, the patient may go home.

Complications

- Immediate
- Remote

Immediate : Although it is a minor operation, but complications do occur. Such complications are :

- Injury to the cervix
- Uterine perforation
- Injury to the gut
- Infection

Injury to the cervix : **The injury to the lip of cervix is caused by** vulsellum bite or lateral tear by dilator. The bleeding from the vulsellum site is usually slight and stopped by gauze pressure or at best by a haemostatic suture.

Management of lateral tear : If slight, haemostasis is effective by intracervical or vaginal gauze plugging. The brisk haemorrhage is likely due to injury of the descending cervical artery and requires haemostatic sutures taking deep bite of the cervical tissue on the same side. If however, the tear extends upwards to involve the uterine artery, laparotomy has to be done along with resuscitative measures. Haemostasis is achieved by opening the anterior leaf of the broad ligament failing which ligation of the anterior division of the internal iliac artery may have to be done, if the uterus is to be preserved.

Uterine perforation : Uterus is perforated by uterine sound, or dilator or uterine curette. The perforation is more common in pregnant rather than non-pregnant uterus.

Diagnosis is made by :

- Sudden loss of resistance.
- Passage of the instrument more than the length of the uterine cavity.
- Undue mobility of the instrument.
- Vaginal bleeding.

Management

Attempt to confirm the perforation by reintroducing the instrument is to be condemned. Once perforation is suspected, following guidelines are to be followed :

- To stop the operative procedure.
- To watch the pulse and blood pressure and vaginal bleeding.
- To formulate the definitive treatment.

Non-infective/Non-malignant uterus

- Small perforation by sound or small dilator
  - To watch the vital signs.
  - To administer antibiotics.
  - To discharge the patient after 24-48 hours, if abdomen is soft, vital signs (pulse, BP) are stable and no untowards effects are noticed.
- Perforation by large dilator or curette.

Usually the perforation is large and associated with varying degrees of internal haemorrhage. The gut may also be injured. As such laparotomy is justified. Repair of the rent or hysterectomy as the case may be is to be done. Associated gut injury is to be looked for and if found, to be tackled accordingly — repair or resection.

If laparoscopy facilities are available, it can be employed in all cases at the earliest. This will help to complete the operative process under its guidance if the perforation is small, to minimise the period of observation and to guide the urgency of laparotomy.

Infective/Malignant uterus : In suspected malignancy or in pyometra, prompt laparotomy is justified. This is to be followed by definitive surgery. However, if perforation occurs in potentially infected uterus of young woman, conservative treatment with antibiotics is justified and to watch for evidences of peritonitis.

Remote complications :

- Cervical incompetence due to injury to internal os resulting in midtrimester abortion.
- Uterine synechiae due to injury to uterine muscle resulting in secondary amenorrhoea.

DILATATION AND INSUFFLATION (D + I)

This is an operation of dilatation of the cervix and introduction of air or CO_2 into the uterine cavity to know the patency of the Fallopian tubes. It is also known as **Rubin test**.

Indications

To note the tubal patency in :

- Investigation for infertility
- Following tuboplasty operation

It should be done in the first half of the cycle (between 8-12th day) and **should not be done** in the presence of pelvic infection (see p. 128).

Steps

- The steps up to cervical dilatation are similar to D + C operation.
- After the desired dilatation of the cervix, the insufflation cannula fitted with a 'Y' rubber tube is introduced into the cervical canal (chapter 35).
- Although CO_2 is better but air is usually introduced. The pressure in the manometer is raised gradually by an assistant by pressing the rubber bulb. The rise of pressure in the manometer is watched by the operator. The assistant auscultates over the flanks for any hissing sound.

A positive test is evidenced by :

- A hissing sound is audible on the flank due to exit of air through the abdominal ostium.
- Drop in the manometer reading from 80-120 mm Hg.
- Patient complains of shoulder pain on sitting (due to irritation of the diaphragm by air and the pain sensation is carried by phrenic nerve).

If the test is negative :

- Air pressure can be raised gradually to a maximum 180 mm Hg without a fall.
- There is no hissing sound audible on the flanks.

If the test is negative, it may be repeated in the same sitting (thrice).

False-positive may be due to instrumental leakage or uterine perforation.

False-negative is due to uterotubal spasm which may be overcome with general anaesthesia or amyl nitrate inhalation.

- After the test is completed, the cannula, vulsellum and the speculum are taken off.

Complications : • Immediate • Remote

Immediate : The complications due to the use of uterine sound and cervical dilators are those of D + C operation. **Special complications related to the operation include** :

- **Air embolism**—About 7-10 ml of air is enough to produce embolism. Chance of air embolism is abolished with the use of CO_2.
- **Rupture of the tube**—If the tube is blocked and the pressure is raised beyond 200 mm Hg.
- **Flaring up of the pre-existing pelvic infection.**

Remote : • Pelvic endometriosis

HYSTEROSALPINGOGRAPHY (HSG)

HSG is an operative procedure used to assess the **interior anatomy of the uterus and tube including tubal patency**. It is a radiographic study and a contrast media is used.

Indications

- To note the tubal patency in the investigation of infertility or following tuboplasty operation (p. 230).
- To detect uterine malformation in recurrent midtrimester abortion (p. 45).
- To diagnose cervical incompetency (p. 45).
- To identify the translocated IUD whether lying inside or outside the uterine cavity (p. 462).
- To diagnose uterine synechiae (p. 438).
- To confirm the diagnosis of secondary abdominal pregnancy.

Incidental diagnosis of submucous fibroid or an uterine polyp or hydrosalpinx or nodular tube is an additional gain.

Steps

The operation is done in the radiology department and without anaesthesia.

- Patient is to empty her bladder.
- She is placed in dorsal position with the buttocks on the edge.
- Internal examination is done.
- Posterior vaginal speculum is introduced; the anterior lip of the cervix is held by Allis forceps and an uterine sound is passed.
- Hysterosalpingographic cannula is fitted with a syringe containing radio-opaque dye—either water soluble contrast medium, meglumine diatrizoate (Renografin-60) or a low viscosity oil-based dye, ethiodized oil (Ethidol). The dye is introduced slowly. About 5-10 ml of the solution is introduced. The passage of the dye into the interior may be observed by using a X-ray image intensifier and a video display unit.
- The speculum and the Allis forceps are removed but not the cannula.

• Two radiographic views are generally taken. The first one to show the filling of uterine cavity and the other at the completion of the procedure (after 10-15 minutes) showing tubal findings. The tubal patency is evidenced by peritoneal spillage (see Fig. 36.67).

Advantages of watery medium over oil-based solution

• Permits rapid absorption.

• Eliminates granuloma formation.

• Negligible peritoneal irritation.

• No risk of embolism when extravasated.

• Wider margin of safety.

Advantages of oil based medium over the watery contrast medium

• Better resolution of tubal architecture

• Less uterine cramping pain

• Higher subsequent pregnancy rate (better flushing of tubes).

Advantages over D+ I

• Lesser false-negative report (Cornual spasm can be overcome by prior IM injection of atropine sulphate 0.6 mg or prompt IV glucagon 1 mg).

• Precise identification of the side and site of obstruction.

• Identification of uterine cavity abnormality.

• Flimsy intraluminal adhesions may be broken, as such chance of conception within 3-4 months is more.

Timings : HSG is done between D6 and D10 of the cycle. Antibiotic prophylaxis should be given. Doxycycline 100 mg P.O. twice daily is given, beginning the day before HSG and continuing for 5 days.

Complications

Apart from the inherent complications of the uterine sound (uterine perforation) haemorrhage, HSG has got the following complications even with the use of watery solution.

• Peritoneal irritation and pelvic pain.

• Vasovagal attack.

• Intravasation of dye within the venous or lymphatic channels (common in tubercular endometritis) (see Fig. 10.6).

• Flaring up of pelvic infection (1-3%).

Contraindications to HSG : (i) Pelvic infection. (ii) Women known to have hydrosalpinges (Fig. 36.77). (iii) Presence of adnexal mass (PID). (iv) Pelvic tenderness on bimanual examination.

CERVICAL BIOPSY

This is the common diagnostic procedure carried out both in the hospital and in the office.

Types

- **Surface (ch. 9)**
- **Punch**
- **Wedge**
- **Ring**
- **Cone**

Punch biopsy : Punch biopsy is done in the outpatient or as an office procedure, without anaesthesia.

Using Cusco's bivalve speculum, biopsy is taken from the suspected area or a four quadrant using punch biopsy forceps. Alternatively, the biopsy may be taken from the unstained area (white) when the cervix is painted with Schiller's iodine or colposcopic directed. Haemostasis is usually achieved by pressure with a gauze piece.

Wedge biopsy : This is done when a definite growth is visible. Necrotic area is to be avoided. **An area nearer the edge is the ideal site.**

• Posterior vaginal speculum is introduced.

• Anterior or posterior lip of the cervix is to be held by Allis forceps.

• With a scalpel, a wedge of tissue is cut from the edge of the lesion **including adjacent healthy tissue for comparative histologic study**.

• Haemostasis may be achieved by gauze packing or by sutures.

Ring biopsy : Whole of the squamocolumnar area of the cervix is excised with a special knife. The tissue is subjected to serial section to detect CIN or early invasive carcinoma. This is almost replaced by directed biopsy either Schiller or colposcopy.

Cone biopsy (conisation) : The operation involves removal of cone of the cervix which includes entire squamocolumnar junction, stroma with glands and endocervical mucous membrane.

Indications : Conisation is done as **diagnostic and therapeutic purpose in CIN**. With the advent of colposcopy and identification of the extent of the lesion, a diagnostic conisation can be effective for the therapeutic purpose as well. **Cases of CIN suitable for conisation are** (see p. 314 — Table 22.3) :

• Unsatisfactory colposcopic findings. The entire margins of the lesion are not visualised.

- Inconsistent findings—Colposcopic, cytology and directed biopsy.
- Positive endocervical curettage.
- When biopsy cannot rule out invasive cancer from CIS or microinvasion.

Procedures (Fig. 34.1)

The procedure is usually done with conventional knife (cold knife cone). Currently, it is being done with the help of CO_2 laser used as scalpel under colposcopic guidance with advantages.

Table 34.1 Advantages of laser over cold knife conisation
• Can be done in the outpatient under local anaesthesia.
• Less tissue damage and less blood loss.
• Postoperative pain and discharge (morbidity) — less.
• Regeneration of epithelium occurs earlier (3-4 weeks).
• All types of CIN can be treated.
• Fertility and pregnancy outcome are not affected adversely.

Principal steps (Cold Knife)

- The operation is done under general anaesthesia.
- Blood loss is minimised with prior haemostatic sutures at 3 and 9 O'Clock positions on the cervix by ligating the descending cervical branches.
- The cone is cut so as to keep the apex below the internal os (Fig. 34.1).
- After the cone is removed, a margin suture is placed at 12 O'Clock position for identification of the cone.
- Routine endocervical curette above the apex of the cone is performed and uterine curettage is done, if indicated.
- Cone margins are repaired by haemostatic sutures. Sturmdorff haemostatic suture should not be used as it interferes with future colposcopic examination.

The excised cervical tissue is sent for histological examination (serial section – minimum 6). **If the margins of the cone are involved in neoplasia**, hysterectomy should be seriously considered either within 48 hours or at a later date (6 weeks) to avoid infection.

Complications

The complications include (p. 563)

- Secondary haemorrhage.
- Cervical stenosis leading to haematometra.

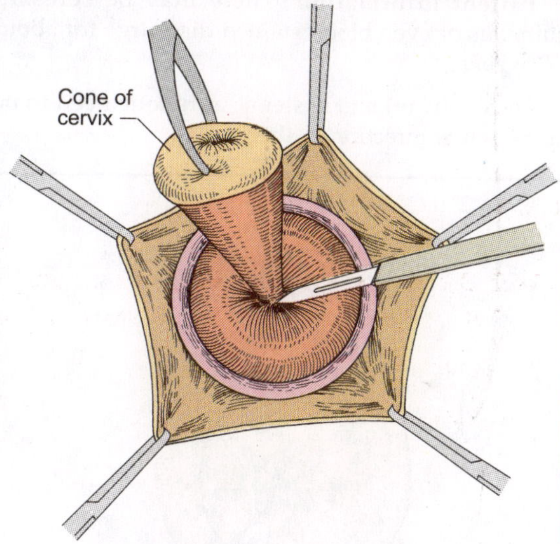

Fig. 34.1. Cone biopsy (knife)

- Infertility.
- Diminished cervical mucus.
- Cervical incompetence leading to adverse pregnancy outcome.
- Midtrimester abortion or preterm labour.

THERMAL CAUTERISATION

This is an operation whereby the eroded area of the cervix is destroyed either by thermocoagulation or red hot cauterisation.

Indication : Cervical ectopy with troublesome discharge. Prior cervical smear or biopsy if necessary, should be undertaken.

Procedures (Fig. 34.2) : While the superficial cauterisation can be done without anaesthesia as an outdoor procedure but where extensive cauterisation is required, it should be done under general anaesthesia.

- Lower part of the cervical canal is dilated by one or two small dilators.
- The whole eroded area is cauterised by cautery point (see Fig. 36.42) giving **linear radial strokes starting from inside the cervical canal to over the eroded area. The strokes should be made about 2 mm deep and at a distance of 1 cm.**
- The area is smeared with antibiotic ointment.

Healing : It takes about 2-3 weeks for sloughing of the burn area. Complete epithelialisation by squamous epithelium occurs by 6-8 weeks.

Patient information: There may be serosanguineous or even blood stained discharge for about 2-3 weeks.

Local (cream) and systemic antibiotic need to be given when infection is there.

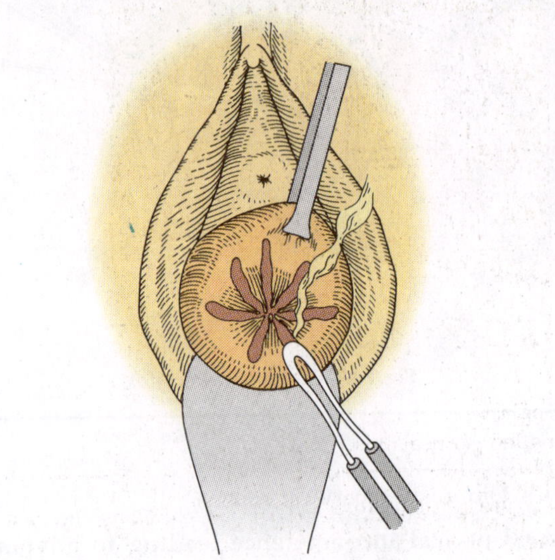

Fig. 34.2. Procedure of thermal cauterisation

CRYOSURGERY

This is a procedure whereby destruction of the tissue is effective by freezing.

Indications

- Benign cervical lesions—such as CIN, condyloma accuminata, leucoplakia, etc.
- Condyloma accuminata of vulva and VIN diagnosed colposcopically and not more than 2 cm in size.
- VAIN, condyloma accuminata or vault granulation tissue following hysterectomy.
- As a palliative measure to arrest bleeding in carcinoma cervix or large fungating recurrent vulval carcinoma.

Principle

It consists of a 'probe', the tip of which is cooled to a temperature below freezing point (– 60°C). **Freezing produces cellular dehydration by crystallisation of intracellular water and ultimately death of cells.** This is effective by rapid expansion of gas which is passed through it. Carbon dioxide is widely used while nitrous oxide and liquid nitrogen are also used.

Procedures

This is an outpatient procedure and is done without anaesthesia. Commonly used technique is freeze-thaw-freeze.

A probe that adequately covers the lesion is selected. The probe tip is lightly covered with water-soluble jelly to provide good thermal contact with the cervix.

The appropriate cryosurgery probe is applied to the cervix and the freezing activated. When a good iceball extending 4-5 mm beyond the edge of the probe is obtained, the freezing is stopped; the probe thawed (to raise the temperature above freezing point) and removed. The probe which adhered to the tissue should not be pulled out until the temperature rises again. Usually $1^1/_2$ - 3 minutes are required to obtain a satisfactory freeze. If necessary, a second time freezing technique may be employed to get a good result.

The application to the cervix freezes the tissue to a depth of about 3 mm.

Advantages over thermal cautery

- Anaesthesia is not required.
- Precise destruction of tissue.
- There is no secondary haemorrhage.
- Cervical stenosis is rare.

Drawbacks

There is excessive discharge for about 2-3 weeks.

Healing is complete in 6 to 10 weeks.

PERINEOPLASTY

Perineoplasty is the reconstruction of the narrow vaginal introitus to make it adequate for sexual function (Fig. 34.3).

Indications are :

(a) Congenitally small introitus.
(b) Rigid perineal body.
(c) Rigid hymeneal ring.
(d) Narrowed introitus following overzealous perineorrhaphy or episiotomy repair.

Principal steps

- A longitudinal incision is made in the mid line from above (2 cm) the fourchette to the skin of the perineum below (2 cm). See Fig. 34.3(A).
- The incision is deepened through the vaginal mucosa, skin and the perineal body.

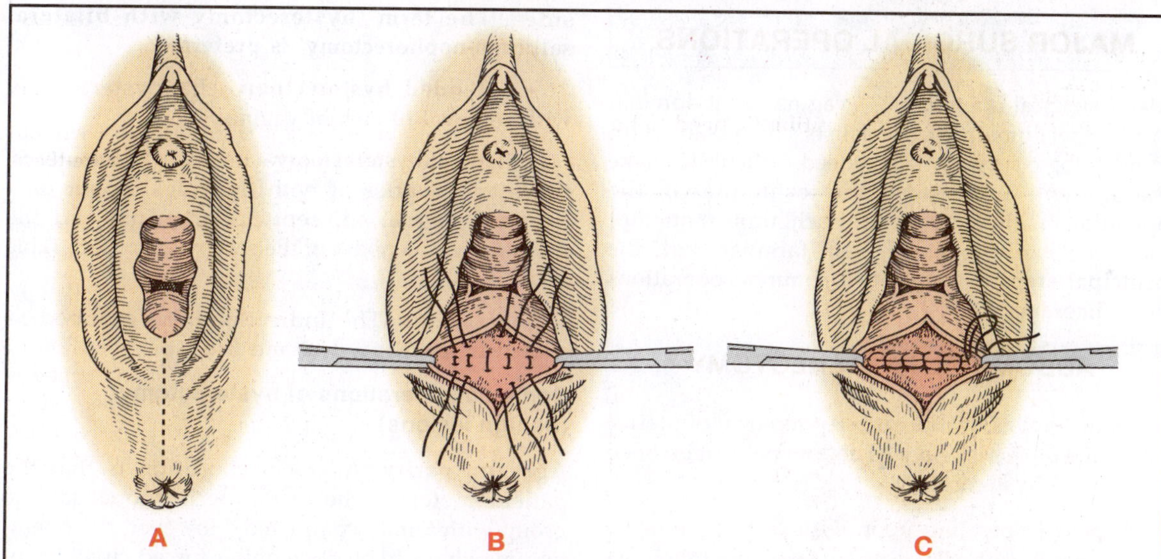

Fig. 34.3. Perineoplasty
A : Longitudinal incision on the perineum. B and C : Divided perineal muscles are sutured transversely

- Mobilisation of the vaginal mucosa and perineal skin is done.
- Two gloves are worn on the left hand. Left index finger in passed into the rectum and it is hooked upwards and outwards, while the superficial perineal muscles are divided.
- Finally the wound is sutured in layers transversely by using interrupted sutures [Fig. 34.3 (B and C)].

[In **Fenton's method** a transverse incision is made along the fourchette].

Repair of complete perineal tear (see p. 414).

AMPUTATION OF CERVIX

Amputation is an operative procedure whereby a part of the lower cervix is excised.

Indications

- Congenital elongation
- Chronic cervicitis with hypertrophied cervix not relieved by conventional therapy.
- As a component part of Fothergill's operation to rectify the supravaginal elongation.

Guidelines

The following practical guidelines are formulated :

- Except in congenital elongation, prior exclusion of malignancy should be done.
- High amputation is to be avoided in cases where future childbirth prospect is retained. High amputation may produce cervical incompetency.

Amputation of cervix

Principal steps

Initial steps are same as that of cold knife cone biopsy (see p. 560).

- A circumferential incision is made around the cervix and vaginal mucosa is separated from the stroma of the cervix.
- A cone–shaped amputation is done and the cut margins are repaired with haemostatic mattress sutures.
- Raw surfaces of the cervix are covered by the Bonney-Sturmdorf suture using a cutting needle (see Fig. 15.18).

Complications

Immediate complications include :

- Haemorrhage—both primary and secondary.
- Sepsis.

Remote complications include :

- Cervical stenosis leading to haematometra.
- Cervical incompetency leading to midtrimester abortion.
- Secondary cervical dystocia during labour.

MAJOR SURGICAL OPERATIONS

Major surgical operations — vaginal or abdominal are in the domain of specialists conversant with gynaecologic surgery. It is indeed difficult to make the students understand the techniques of the operations with language. As such, utmost attempt has been made to make them familiar with the **principal steps** of some such common operations with diagrams.

ABDOMINAL HYSTERECTOMY

Hysterectomy is the operation of removal of uterus. When the uterus is removed abdominally, it is called abdominal hysterectomy.

Types: Depending upon the extent of removal of the uterus and adjacent structures, the following types are described.

- **Total hysterectomy**—Removal of the entire uterus.
- **Subtotal**—Removal of the body or corpus leaving behind the cervix.
- **Panhysterectomy** — Removal of the uterus along with removal of tubes and ovaries of both sides. **The term 'hysterectomy with bilateral salpingo-oophorectomy' is preferred.**
- **Extended hysterectomy**—Panhysterectomy with removal of cuff of vagina.
- **Radical hysterectomy**—Removal of the uterus, tubes and ovaries of both the sides, upper one-third of vagina, adjacent parametrium and the draining lymph nodes of the cervix (see p. 338, Table 23.11).

Table 34.2 : Indications

Benign lesions	• Dysfunctional uterine bleeding • Fibroid uterus • Tubo-ovarian mass • Endometriosis • Adenomyosis • CIN • Endometrial hyperplasia • Benign ovarian tumour in perimenopausal age
Malignancy	• Carcinoma cervix • Carcinoma ovary • Carcinoma endometrium • Uterine sarcoma • Choriocarcinoma
Traumatic	• Uterine perforation • Cervical tear • Rupture uterus
Obstetrical	• Atonic PPH • Morbid adherent placenta • Hydatidiform mole > 35 yrs. • Septic abortion

Indications: The indications are grouped as shown in the Table 34.2 and 34.3.

Some considerations of hysterectomy (benign lesions)

Age and parity: An ideal condition is that the patient preferably be in the perimenopausal age group with family completed. However, the operation may have to be done under forced circumstances even in comparatively young age group or unmarried or nulliparous women. (Example—Contemplating myomectomy).

Total or subtotal: The preferred surgery is always a total hysterectomy unless there is sufficient reason to leave behind the cervix. **The indications of subtotal (supracervical) hysterectomy are**:

- Difficult tubo-ovarian mass with obliteration of the anterior and posterior pouches.
- Pelvic endometriosis particularly involving the rectovaginal septum.
- Emergency hysterectomy (caesarean hysterectomy).

Advantages of subtotal (supracervical) hysterectomy

Controversy exists as regard the usefulness of subtotal hysterectomy. **The benefits mentioned are**: reduced operative and postoperative morbidity, reduced vaginal shortening and vault prolapse and increased sexual satisfaction. Hospital stay is shorter. Papanicolaou cervical smear must be normal before contemplating supracervical hysterectomy. It should be maintained as a routine follow up (see Table 9.1).

The risks of the cervical stump left behind are:

- Cervicitis with abnormal vaginal discharge.
- Stump carcinoma may develop (1%).

Preservation of ovaries: Amidst controversy, it seems rational to preserve the ovaries in premenopausal women if they are found healthy. Some

Benefits and Risks of Ovarian Conservation During Hysterectomy

Benefits	Risks
1. Ovarian functions continues till the expected time of spontaneous menopause.	1. Risks of developing ovarian neoplasms (Benign or malignant). Relative risk (R.R.) of ovarian cancer is 0.6 even 10 years after hysterectomy.
2. Menopausal symptoms appear late and the severity is less.	2. Residual ovarian syndrome occurs in 1-3 per cent of cases due to multiple cystic follicles and/or periovarian adhesions (p. 553).
3. Decreased incidence of vasomotor symptoms, osteoporosis and atherosclerotic changes (see p. 55).	3. Chronic pelvic pain and dyspareunia.
	4. Risk of relaparotomy in 3-5 per cent.

however, remove the ovaries beyond 45 years and preserve the same before that age, if found healthy.

Special considerations for removal of ovaries

- If the ovaries are diseased in inflammatory process or involved in neoplastic conditions with the patient around the age of 40 or older.
- Hysterectomy done in a woman of any age who has a history of ovarian or breast cancer in first degree relative.
- Postmenopausal women as a routine.

Hormone replacement therapy is to be considered when ovaries are removed (see p. 55).

Removal of Fallopian tubes

The uterine tubes are removed :

- When the ovaries are removed (salpingo-oophorectomy).
- When the tubes are diseased but ovaries are conserved (salpingectomy) due to young age.

Steps of operation (Benign lesion)

Preoperative workup (see p. 552)

Actual steps (Fig. 34.4)

- Abdomen is opened either by a infraumbilical paramedian or midline or low transverse incision.
- The uterus is drawn out of the wound.
- Doyen's retractor is placed in position.
- The patient is placed in Trendelenburg position.
- The guts and omentum are packed off from the operative area.
- The pelvic organs are examined. The decision of preserving or removing the adnexae is made.
- The traction of the uterus is given by either using vulsellum or placing long artery forceps on either side of the uterine cornu (myoma screw is used in fibroid). The uterus is pulled to one side while clamps are placed on the contralateral side.
- **If the ovaries are to be removed**, paired clamps (two long straight artery forceps) are placed in the infundibulo-pelvic ligament [Fig. 34.4(1)].

The tissues in between are cut and replaced by transfixation sutures (Vicryl No. '0' or chromic catgut No. '1'). **If the ovaries are to be preserved**, the paired clamps are placed near the cornu of the uterus to include Fallopian tube, mesosalpinx containing uterine vessels and ovarian ligament. The structures are cut in between the clamps and replaced by transfixation sutures (Vicryl No. '0' or chromic catgut No. '1') [Fig. 34.4(2)].

- Paired clamps are placed on the round ligament, cut and replaced by sutures (Vicryl No. '0' or chromic catgut No. '1') [Fig. 34.3(3)].
- Similar procedures up to this stage are followed on the other side.
- Loose peritoneum of the uterovesical fold [Fig. 34.4 (13)] is cut and extended from one divided round ligament to the other. The bladder is pushed down and out with gauze added with scissors stripping till the anterior vaginal wall is reached. **This will minimise injury to the bladder and ureters in subsequent steps of operation** [Figs 34.4(4) and (5)].
- Paired clamps are placed on the parametrium containing ascending branch of the uterine artery, close to the uterus at the level of internal os. The tissues in between are cut with the scalpel and replaced by ligature (Vicryl No. '0' or catgut No. '1'). Similar step is followed on the other side [Fig. 34.4(6)].
- The uterus is now pulled forwards to make the uterosacral ligaments prominent. Clamps are placed over the uterosacral ligaments as close to the cervix. The

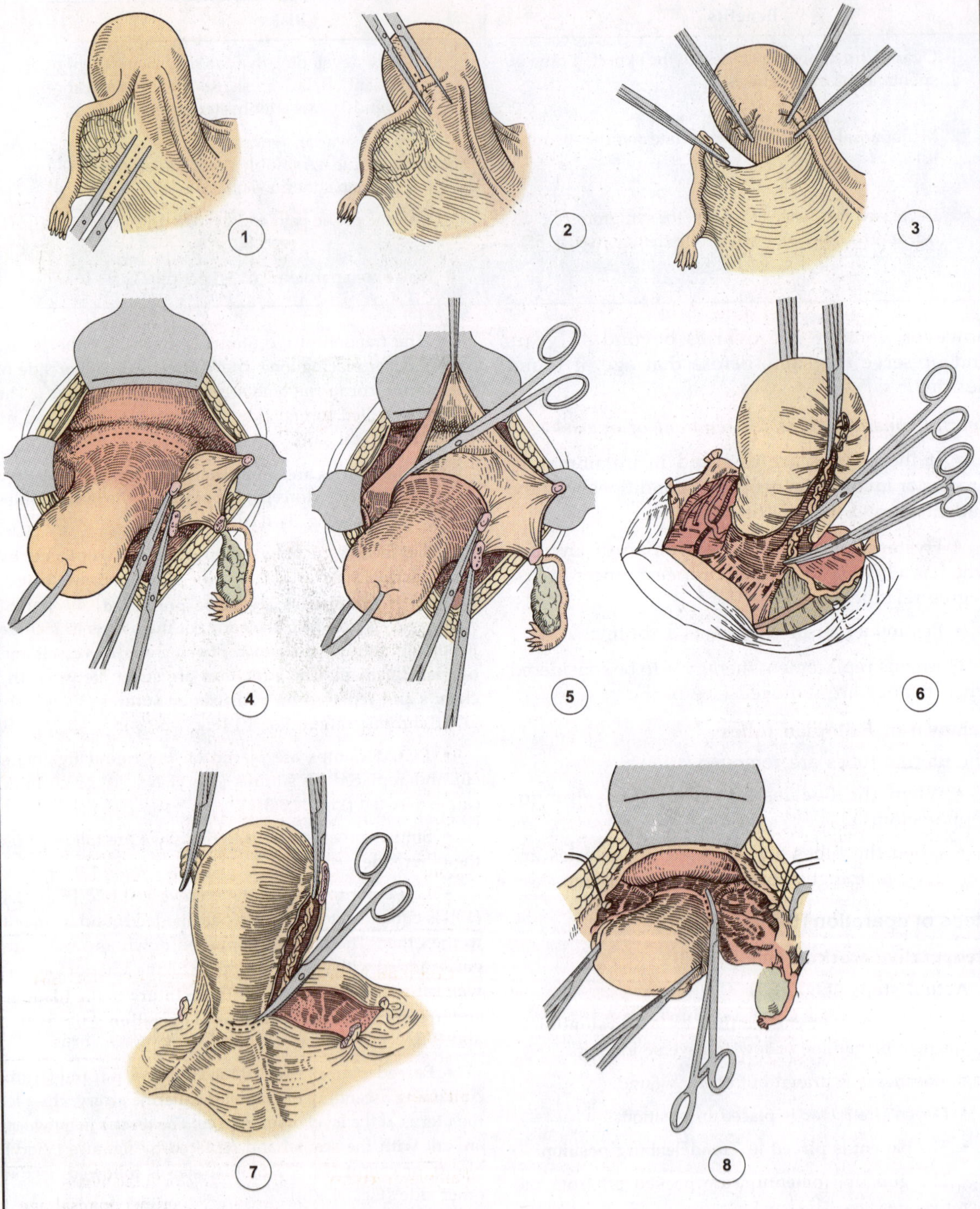

Fig. 34.4. Principal steps of abdominal hysterectomy

Fig. 34.4 (contd.) next page

Fig. 34.4. (contd.) from previous page

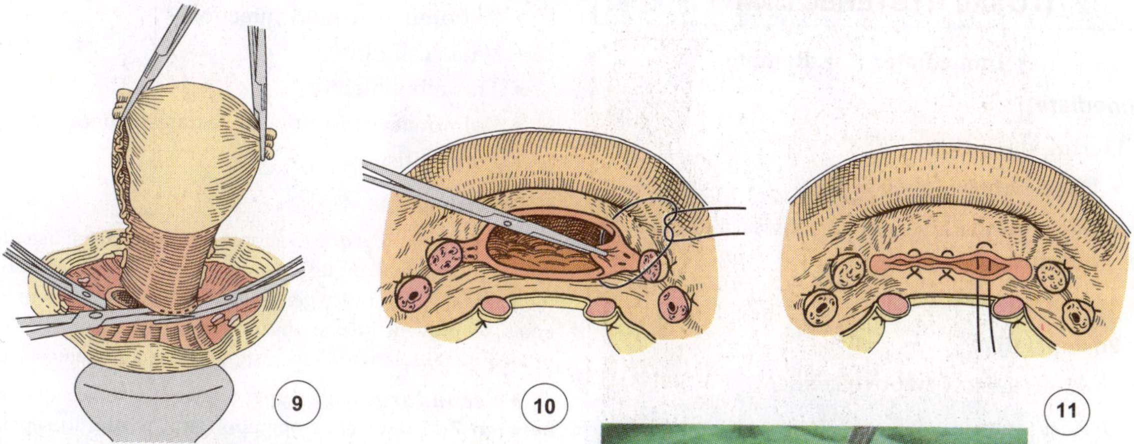

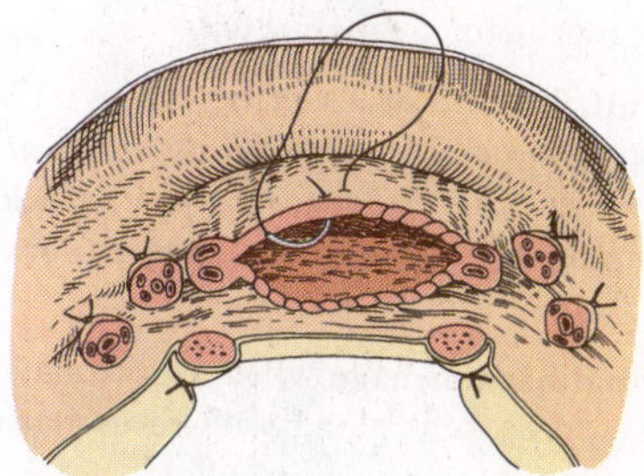

Fig. 34.4. Principal steps of abdominal hysterectomy

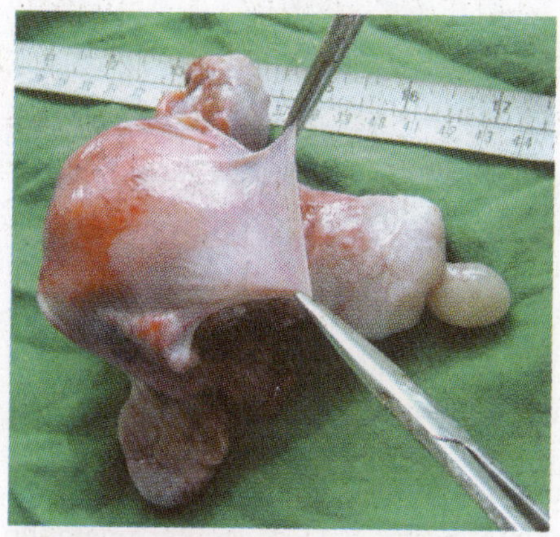

Uterovesical fold of peritoneum dissected out during hysterectomy

ligaments are cut. The peritoneum in between the ligaments is dissected down with scissors and finger. The clamps are replaced by sutures (same suture material) [Fig. 34.4(7)].

• Clamps are placed close to the cervix on the paracervical tissue (Mackenrodt's) containing descending cervical artery, cut and replaced by ligature (same suture material). Similar step is followed to the other side [Fig. 34.4(8)].

• Vault of the vagina is opened by a stab incision with a scalpel at the cervicovaginal junction. The remaining vault of the vagina is cut while traction is given with a single toothed vulsellum on the cervix [Fig. 34.4(9)].

• The edges of the cut vaginal vault are held by Allis forceps [Fig. 34.4(10)].

• Lateral vaginal angles are closed by transfixation suture (Fig. 34.4(10)].

• Vault is closed by interrupted sutures [Fig. 34.4(11)] or the free vaginal margin is reefed with a continuous locking suture (Fig. 34.4(12)].

• Pelvic peritonisation may be done (optional) by running sutures using catgut No.'0'.

• Abdominal packs are removed; peritoneal toileting is done.

• Abdomen is closed in layers.

Table 34.3
Common indications of abdominal hysterectomy

Total	• DUB • Uterine fibroid • TO mass • Endometriosis
Subtotal	• Difficult TO mass • Endometriosis (rectovaginal septum) • Obstetric causes
Panhysterectomy	• Indications for total hysterectomy in perimenopausal age
Extended	• Carcinoma endometrium
Radical	• Carcinoma cervix-stage I and II

COMPLICATIONS (TOTAL HYSTERECTOMY)

- Immediate
- Remote

Immediate

During operation

- Haemorrhage.
- Injury to the adjacent structures like bladder, intestine or ureter.
- Anaesthetic hazards.

Postoperative

Shock — usually hypovolaemic.

Urinary —

- Retention
- Cystitis
- Anuria — It is predominantly due to inadvertent ligature of the ureters.
- Incontinence
  - Overflow due to prolonged overdistension of the bladder.
  - Stress due to prolonged catheterisation.
  - True—If occurs immediately after operation, it is caused by injury to the bladder or ureter. If occurs 7-14 days after operation, it is due to sloughing necrosis either of the bladder or ureter.

Pyrexia—fever may be due to :

- Cystitis
- Abdominal wound infection
- Vault cellulitis
- Thrombophlebitis
- Pulmonary infection, atelectasis, pneumonia
- Peritonitis.

Haemorrhage

- ***Primary*** : It is due to slipping of the ligature usually that of the vaginal angle. Haemostasis can be achieved by the vaginal route under general anaesthesia. Care is to be taken to prevent bite of the ureter in the suture. If the procedure fails, laparotomy has to be done for haemostasis.

- ***Secondary*** : This type of haemorrhage occurs between 7-14 days after operation and is due to sepsis. Bleeding source may be from the vault or internally (rare) from the sloughing uterine or ovarian artery.

If from the vault, haemostasis can be achieved by interrupted or mattress suture using 'Vicryl' under general anaesthesia. In cases of recurrences, one may have to tackle the situation through abdominal route as mentioned below.

In cases of internal haemorrhage which is fortunately rare, laparotomy has to be done along with resuscitative procedures. If the uterine artery is involved, anterior division of the internal iliac artery has to be tied to secure haemostasis.

Haematomas—In the pelvis or rectus sheath may cause low grade temperature. Large haematomas should be drained.

Table 34.4
Postoperative bowel dysfunction : Ileus versus obstruction

Ileus	Obstruction
Distension — Present	Present
Pain — Mild due to distension	Progressively severe due to cramps
Bowel sounds — Absent	Peristaltic rushes
Vomiting — Present	Present
Onset — Within 48-72 hours of surgery	Delayed 5-7 days postoperative
X-ray — Loops of small and large bowel distended with gas	Distended bowel loops with air-fluid level
Treatment — Conservative : nasogastric suction, intravenous fluids, enemas, correction of electrolyte imbalance and control of infection	Initial conservative may need surgical intervention

Wound dehiscence is seen commonly with vertical incision. Patients with infection, malnutrition and malignancy are at high risk.

Paralytic ileus and intestinal obstruction—Postoperative bowel dysfunction may be due to ileus or obstruction (Table 34.4).

Phlebitis—Intravenous cannula related phlebitis causes pain, redness and fever. Venous cannula should be removed and antibiotic should be continued.

Deep vein thrombosis (DVT)—is not an uncommon problem. Calf veins are commonly affected. It is associated with low grade fever, pain and swelling of the affected cuff. B-mode ultrasound can detect an intramural clot. Heparin is administered intravenously (30,000-40,000 units/24 hours) once the diagnosis is confirmed. Activated partial thromboplastin time (APTT) is maintained at 1.5-2.5 times the control. Heparin is replaced by warfarin orally after 5 days and it is continued for 4-6 weeks. Low molecular weight heparin (Fragmin) 2500U S.C. every 24 hours or low dose heparin 5000U S.C. every 12 hours, starting 1-2 hours before surgery, for 5-7 days is recommended as a preventive measure against venous thromboembolism.

Pulmonary embolism is a rare but fatal complication. Patient commonly presents with sudden onset of chest pain, dyspnoea, tachycardia, tachypnoea and haemoptysis. Arterial blood gas analysis, ventilation/perfusion scan and pulmonary angiography are the diagnostic aids. Ventilation-perfusion scan reveals areas with decreased perfusion but adequate ventilation. Heparin is the drug of choice. Thrombolytic therapy (recombinant human plasminogen activator) clear the emboli more rapidly when infused IV. Pulmonary artery embolectomy or inferior vena cava filter placement may have to be considered for massive pulmonary embolus. Warfarin should be started orally after 2-3 days of heparinisation. Heparin is withdrawn once the therapeutic level of warfarin is obtained. Dose of warfarin is aimed to prolong the prothrombin time. International normalised ratio (INR) is maintained at 2.0 to 3.0.

ABDOMINAL HYSTERECTOMY

Advantages	Disadvantages
1. Scope of wide exploration of the abdominal and pelvic organs (ovaries, appendix, gallbladder, etc.). 2. Tubo-ovarian pathology can be tackled effectively and simultaneously. 3. Concurrent surgical procedures (appendicectomy) may be performed when needed. 4. Operation can be done by a relatively less experienced surgeon.	1. Difficult to perform in too obese patients. 2. Postoperative complications are slightly high. There is increased incidence of peritonitis, fever, pulmonary and vascular complications. 3. More postoperative pain and more need of analgesia. 4. More hospital stay. 5. Delayed resumption in day-to-day activities. 6. Morbidity and mortality are more compared to a vaginal hysterectomy. 7. Presence of abdominal scar.

VAGINAL HYSTERECTOMY (See ch. 15 p. 211)

Advantages	Disadvantages
1. Can be effectively done in obese patients. 2. Postoperative complications are less. 3. Less morbidity and mortality. 4. Less postoperative pain and less need of analgesia. 5. Less hospital stay. 6. Early resumption of day-to-day activities. 7. No abdominal incision and scar.	1. More skill and experience are needed on the part of the surgeon. 2. Exploration of abdominal and pelvic organs cannot be done. 3. Tubo-ovarian pathology when detected is difficult to tackle. 4. Limitation in cases with : uterus > 12 weeks of size, presence of pelvic adhesions or, previous history of laparotomy with adhesions.

Remote complications

- Vault granulation—It is more with catgut and less with Vicryl.
- Vault prolapse—less compared to vaginal.
- Incisional hernia—more with mid-line vertical incision than with low transverse one.
- Prolapse of the Fallopian tube through the vault.

Comments

Vaginal hysterectomy is the ideal method if not contraindicated. In the hands of an expert conversant with vaginal hysterectomy even in undescended uterus, vaginal hysterectomy is the method of choice. This route still offers benefits.

Complications of Vaginal Hysterectomy : See p. 208, 209.

Laparoscopic assisted vaginal hysterectomy (LAVH) (see p. 561), does not have any superiority over traditional vaginal hysterectomy even in an undescended uterus. The cost of the former is very high where as perioperative morbidity is the same (for details see p. 585).

Pelvic floor repair (PFR)—see p. 210.

Fothergill's or Manchester Operation—see p 210.

Operations for vault prolapse—see p. 214.

Cervicopexy (Sling or Purandare's Operation)—see p. 215.

Complications of vaginal operations—see p. 216.

OPERATIONS ON THE OVARY

Ovarian cystectomy (Fig. 34.5)

Removal of the ovarian tumour leaving behind the healthy ovarian tissue is called ovarian cystectomy.

It is the operation of choice specially when both the ovaries are involved with benign neoplasm in young women.

Principal steps

- Incision (elliptical) is made with a scalpel through the ovarian cortex at the base of the ovarian cyst [Fig. 34.5(1)].
- The cyst wall is separated gently, using the handle of the scalpel or by scissors and the cyst is shelled out without rupture [Fig. 34.5(2)].
- The dead space is obliterated using (4-0) absorbable suture. Ovarian surface is approximated using very fine interrupted sutures [Fig. 34.5(3)].

Ovariotomy (Fig. 34.6) : Removal of the tumour along with healthy ovarian tissue is called ovariotomy. The term is better replaced by oophorectomy. This is indicated when the tumour is big or complicated by torsion or haemorrhage and the other ovary is healthy.

Principal steps

- Paired clamps are placed laterally over the infundibulopelvic fold of peritoneum with its contents (see p. 293). Medial pair of clamps are applied on the side of uterus to include the ovarian ligament and the Fallopian tube [Fig. 34.6(1)].

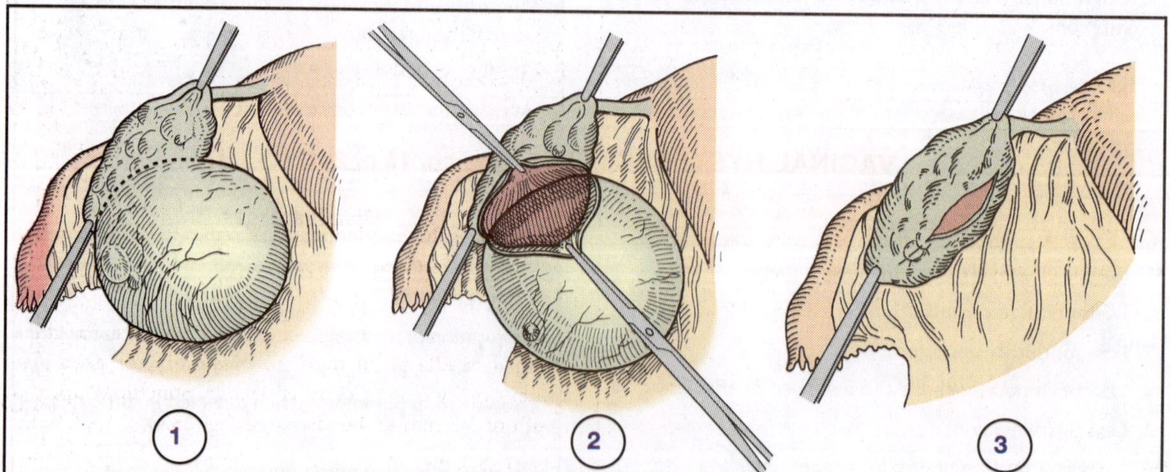

Fig. 34.5. Steps of ovarian cystectomy
(1) Line of incision (2) Enucleation of the tumour (3) Closure of the ovarian incision

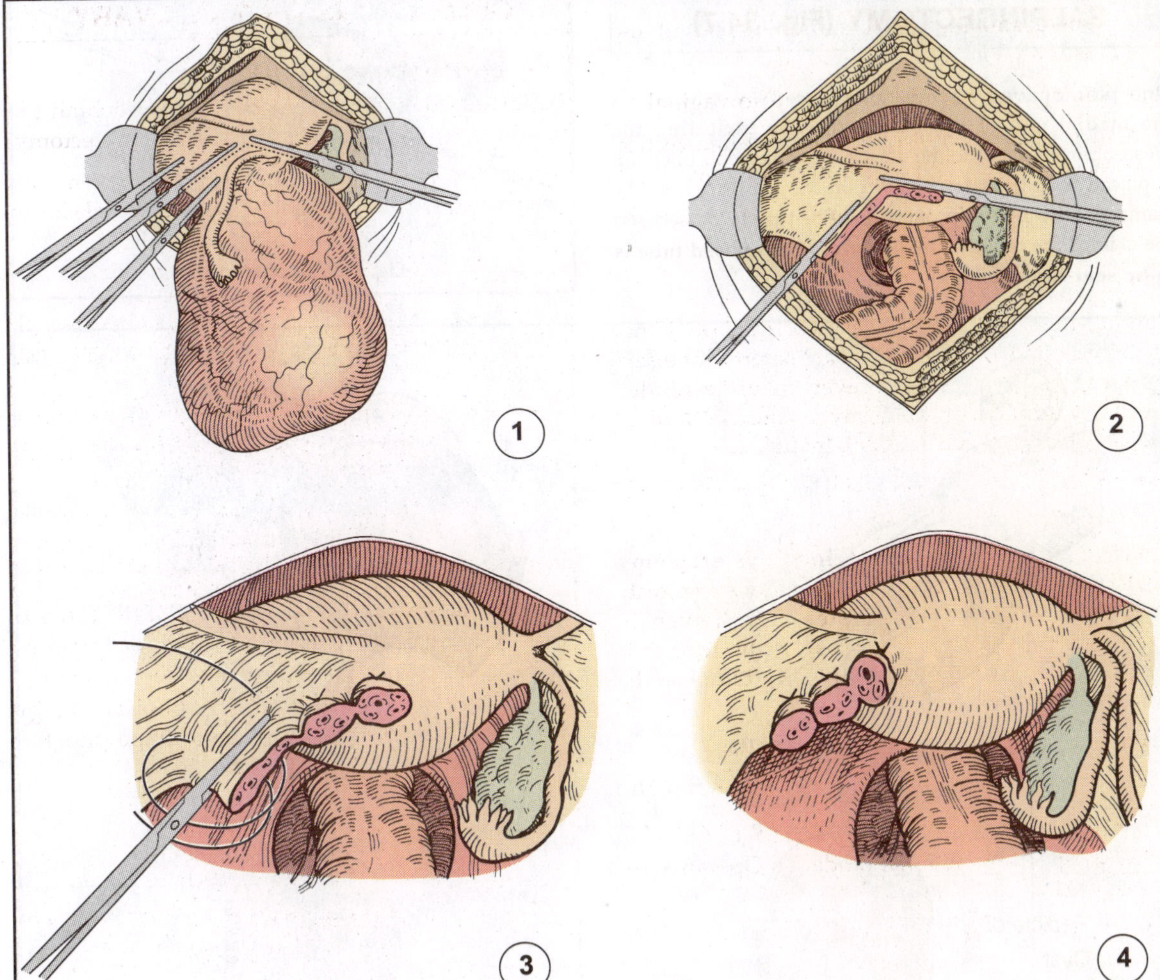

Fig. 34.6. Steps of ovariotomy — 1. Clamps are placed on either side of the ovarian pedicle. 2. Removal of tumour with the clamps placed over the pedicle. 3. The clamps are replaced by sutures, the lateral one by transfixing. (4) Look at the operation site.

- Pedicles are cut in between and the tumour is removed [Fig. 34.6(2)].
- Clamps are replaced by transfixing ligatures [Fig. 34.6(3)].
- Pedicles are checked carefully for haemostasis [Fig. 34.6(4)].

Wedge resection

A wedge of ovarian tissue with the base on the surface and the apex extending to medulla is removed in PCOS when medical treatment fails to induce ovulation. About one-third of the ovarian tissue is removed by the wedge method.

Laparoscopic ovarian drilling is more commonly done than ovarian wedge resection (see p. 239). It can be done using a needle point monopolar cautery, or a bipolar cautery or by laser. Cortex is usually punctured up to a depth of 3-5 mm at 4-6 sites (see Fig. 35.4).

Ovarian biopsy

This is indicated to differentiate premature ovarian failure from resistant ovarian syndrome or for the problem of intersexuality.

SALPINGECTOMY (Fig. 34.7)

One pair of long haemostatic forceps is placed on the medial end of the Fallopian tube including the mesosalpinx as close to the uterus. A second pair of clamp is placed from the lateral aspect on the mesosalpinx. The clamp tips are to be approximated. The tube is excised and the clamps are replaced by ligatures. **The excised tube is to be sent for histology**.

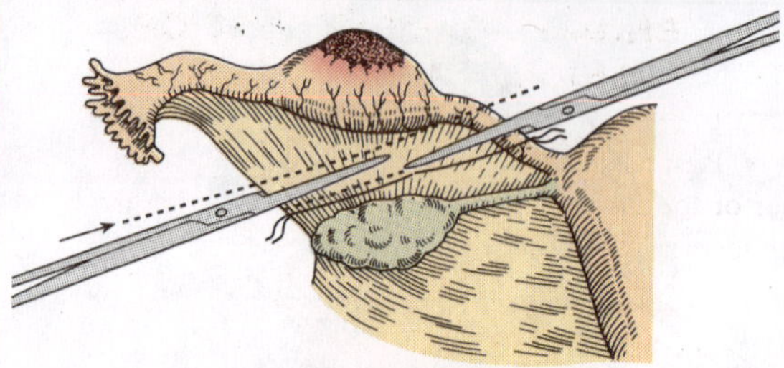

Fig. 34.7. Salpingectomy

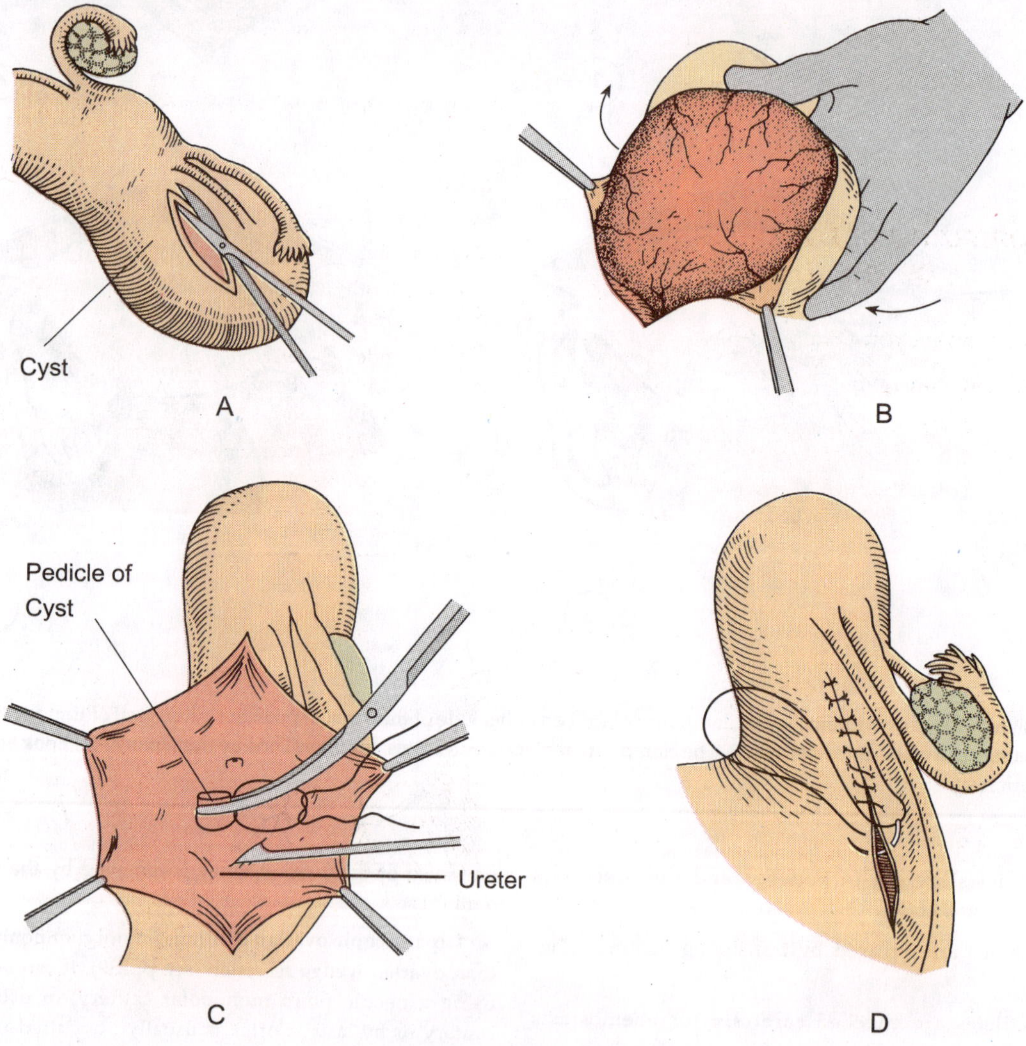

Fig. 34.8. Broad ligament cyst

A. Post box incision on the anterior leaf of broad ligament parallel to the round ligament. B. Enucleation of the cyst. C. Haemostatic suture placed on the pedicle on the cyst. Note the position of the ureter. D. Closure of the peritoneum

BROAD LIGAMENT CYST OR LEIOMYOMA (Fig. 34.8)

- Post box incision is made with a knife on the anterior leaf of the broad ligament making parallel to the round ligament [Fig. 34.8(A)].
- Fingers are used to separate the tumour from the leaves of broad ligament up to the base [Fig. 34.8(B)]. In a case of fibroid, the capsule is incised and the myoma is enucleated from its bed by sharp and blunt dissection.
- Position of the ureter is checked and a clamp is placed on the tumour pedicle.
- The pedicle is cut and the clamp is replaced by a ligature [Fig. 34.8(C)].
- The leaves of broad ligament are closed with a continuous suture [Fig. 34.8(D)].

OPERATIONS FOR INVERSION OF THE UTERUS

Haultain's operation (Fig. 34.9A)

Principle of the operation

This is done abdominally. Correction of inversion is done after cutting the posterior rim of the cup-like depression (see Fig. 34.9A).

Actual steps

- Antiseptic cleaning of the vagina is done preoperatively.
- Abdomen is opened with the patient in Trendelenburg position.
- The ring of tissue is grasped by Allis forceps. A vertical incision is made on the midline at the posterior rim.
- A finger is passed through the incision and the inverted fundus is pushed up. An assistant may also push up inverted fundus through the vagina.
- Uterine incision is repaired with chromic catgut sutures in two layers.

Kustner's operation (Fig. 34.9B and C)

This is a vaginal procedure.

Actual steps

- Uterus is drawn upwards and forwards by a single tooth vulsellum holding at the fundus.
- Pouch of Douglas is opened by a transverse incision made on the posterior vaginal wall.
- Left index finger is introduced along the hollow of the inverted uterus. Posterior uterine wall is cut through by a scalpel from fundus to the external os (Fig. 34.9B).
- The inverted uterus is then turned inside out and inversion is corrected.

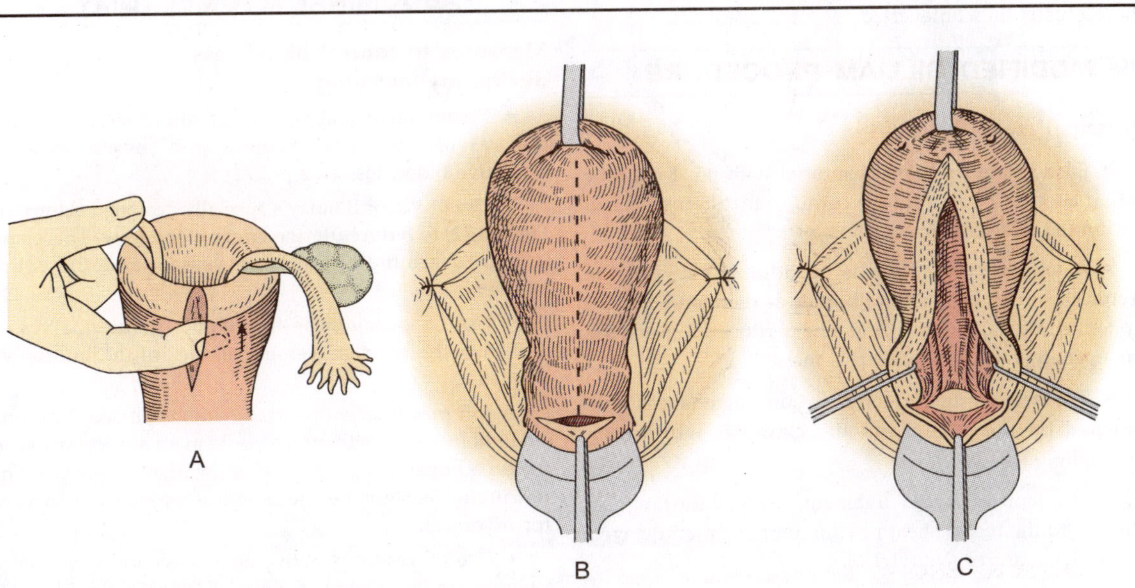

Fig. 34.9. Operations for inversion of the uterus. A : Haultain's operation. B and C : Kustner's operation

• Repair of the incised uterine wall is done with chromic catgut sutures in two layers.

• Repair of the pouch of Douglas and posterior vaginal wall is done.

Spinelli's operation is a vaginal procedure and principle is the same as that of Kustner. Here uterovesical pouch is opened and uterine incision is made on the anterior wall.

VENTROSUSPENSION OPERATION

This operation is less commonly performed these days. Common indications of this operation in relation to retroversion of uterus have been mentioned before (see p. 190). Other indications are to prevent adhesions over the posterior uterine surface following (i) myomectomy operation (ii) operation for endometriosis, where the uterus is bulky.

It may be done by (i) plication of the round ligaments (ii) Modified Gilliam procedure or by (iii) Laparoscopic suspension operation.

Actual steps : Abdomen is opened by suprapubic transverse incision.

Plication of the round ligaments

Reefing suture is passed through the substance of the round ligaments extending from the internal abdominal ring up to the myometrium at the cornu of the uterus. Suture material used is either chromic catgut or Vicryl. The suture is tied firmly at the end. Similar procedure is done on the other side. The round ligaments are shortened and the uterus is thus anteverted.

MODIFIED GILLIAM PROCEDURE

Principal steps (Fig. 34.10)

• Each round ligament is sutured with no. 1 chromic catgut about 3-4 cm. from the cornu of the uterus. This is left untied and used for traction.

• A long curved clamp is introduced between the rectus sheath and the lateral border of the rectus muscle up to the internal inguinal ring. The peritoneum overlying the opened jaws of the clamp is incised.

• The traction ligature on the round ligament is now grasped by the clamp and the clamp is withdrawn gradually.

• The loop of round ligament, such withdrawn, is sutured to the rectus sheath by three interrupted delayed absorbable sutures (Vicryl 1-0).

• Similar procedure is repeated on the other side.

• Abdomen is closed in layers.

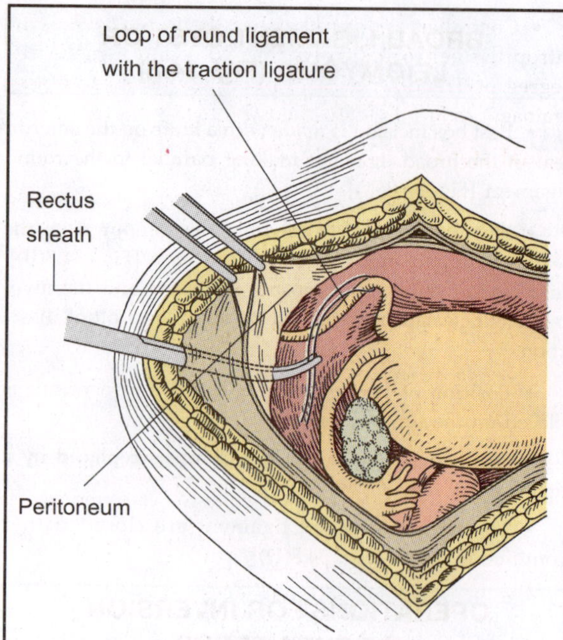

Fig. 34.10. Modified Gilliam procedure

Complication of ventrosuspension operation

• Pain — when there is excessive stretching of the round ligaments.

• Avulsion of the round ligament and bleeding — rare.

ABDOMINAL MYOMECTOMY

Measures to control blood loss during myomectomy

• Preoperative treatment with GnRH analogue reduces the vascularity of the tumour and thereby reduces operative blood loss (see p. 271).

• Use of Victor Bonney's specially designed clamp (see Fig. 36.22) to reduce uterine artery blood flow. This clamp is placed around the uterine vessels and the round ligament.

• Use of tourniquets—to occlude the uterine vessels and also the ovarian vessels at the infundibulopelvic ligament.

A soft plastic tube (less traumatic) is passed through a small hole one on either side made in an avascular part of the broad ligament at the level of the uterine isthmus. This tourniquet is tightened just before making the incision for myomectomy.

• Use of vasoconstrictive agents—commonly used is vasopressin (Synthetic). 20 units of vasopressin diluted in 20 ml of normal saline is injected into the myometrium overlying the myoma.

• Controlled hypotensive anaesthesia (using sodium nitroprusside) to reduce venous tone and a moderate degree of Trendelenburg position (to enhance venous drainage) reduce operative blood loss.

Actual steps

• Uterine incision — a single incision (linear or elliptical) in the midline on the anterior wall of the uterus is preferred.

This has the following advantages :

- Avoids any injury to the tube and ovary
- Lateral fibroids are removed by tunnelling without any additional scar on the uterine surface.
- Fibroids from the cavity or posterior wall can be removed by transcavity approach. This avoids scar on the posterior wall and adhesion formation.

• Incision is deepened through the myometrium and the (pseudo) capsule, till the myoma is reached.

• The myoma is grasped with a single toothed vulsellum and dissection is continued in the plane between the myoma and the capsule (to minimise blood loss). Myoma is enucleated (intracapsular) from its bed by sharp (scissors) and blunt (knife handle) dissection.

• The myoma bed (deep space) is obliterated by interrupted mattress or figure-of-eight sutures. Sometimes layers of sutures (tire stitch) may be required to approximate the myometrium (Fig. 34.11).

• **Bonney's hood operation** — is done to remove a large fundal myoma. A low transverse incision is made on the myoma over the anterior uterine surface. After enucleation of the myoma, the capsule is trimmed and is sewn over the anterior uterine wall. This minimises adhesion formation (see Fig. 34.12).

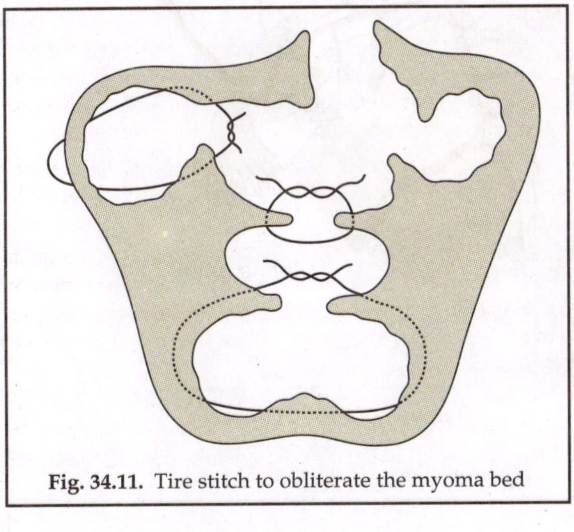

Fig. 34.11. Tire stitch to obliterate the myoma bed

• The serous coat of the uterus is approximated with a thin absorbable suture. To prevent adhesion over the incision site, interceed (oxidised cellulose) or Gore-text (surgical membrane) can be used.

Cervical myoma

• *Anterior cervical myoma*—can be approached by making a transverse incision over the uterovesical peritoneum. Bladder is dissected down before the incision over the capsule of the fibroid is made. Fibroid is then enucleated (intracapsular).

• *Posterior cervical myoma*—approach is made by low posterior incision on the uterine surface through the pouch of Douglas.

• *Central cervical myoma*—The peritoneum of the uterovesical pouch is incised transversely and the bladder is dissected down. Hemisection of the uterus is done from above downwards to reach the myoma which is then enucleated (intracapsular). The dead space is obliterated without closure of the cervical canal. The bisected uterus is then repaired.

Broad ligament myoma (see p. 573).

COMPLICATIONS OF MYOMECTOMY

General complications of any abdominal procedure has been discussed (see p. 568). The specific complications are :

Immediate

• Haemorrhage—intraperitoneal from the uterine wound. This may occur when haemostasis during operation is imperfect.

• Injury to bladder and ureter—specially with cervical and broad ligament myomas.

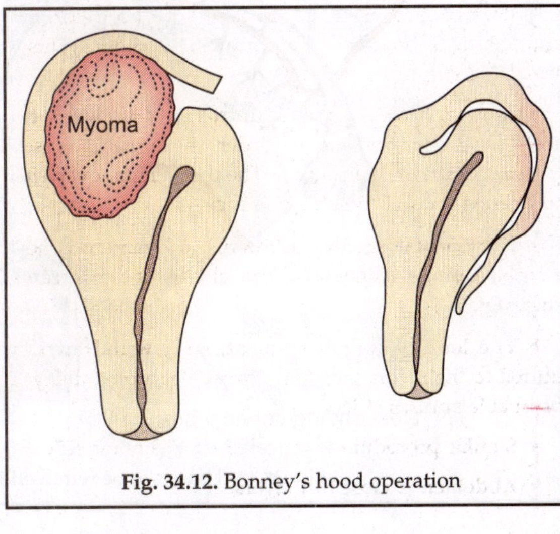

Fig. 34.12. Bonney's hood operation

• Injury to the Fallopian tubes—interstitial portion is commonly damaged during incision and suturing.

• Injury to bowel.

• Febrile morbidity—due to tissue reaction or infection.

Remote — (see ch. 19, Table 19.9).

RADICAL HYSTERECTOMY (see p. 338)
(Syn : Class IV radical hysterectomy)

Wertheim's original operation was less extensive. With this procedure only a selective group of lymph nodes (e.g. enlarged and palpable) and only the medial half of the cardinal and uterosacral ligaments were removed.

The classic radical hysterectomy (Type IV) which is performed in most centres these days, includes wide resection of the parametrium, periureteral tissue, superior vesical artery, cardinal and uterosacral ligaments, upper three-fourth of vagina and thorough pelvic lymphadenectomy (see Fig. 34.13).

Steps of operation

Preoperative work up (see p. 337, Tables 23.7 and 23.9)

- Continuous bladder drainage by Foley catheter.
- Vaginal packing under anaesthesia.

Actual steps

• Abdomen is opened by low mid-line or transverse incision.

• Abdominal and pelvic exploration is done to detect any metastatic disease.

• Liver, under surface of the diaphragm, kidneys, para-aortic lymph nodes, stomach, omentum and ovaries are examined thoroughly.

• Traction of the uterus is given by long artery forceps, placed one on either side of the uterine cornu.

• The round ligament is clamped, cut and ligated near the pelvic side wall. The infundibulopelvic ligament is also clamped, cut and transfixed at this juncture (when ovaries are to be removed).

In some doubtful cases, opening up of the peritoneum of the uterovesical pouch is done first. The cervix is then palpated for evidence of tumour extension. The operation is abandoned in favour of concurrent chemo and radiotherapy, if bladder is found involved with the tumour.

• The broad ligament leaves are opened up and the paravesical and pararectal spaces are explored.

Paravesical space is bounded anteriorly by the symphysis pubis, medially by the bladder, laterally by the obturator muscle and the pelvic side wall and posteriorly by the cardinal ligament.

Pararectal space is bounded anteriorly by the cardinal ligament, posteriorly by the sacrum, medially by the

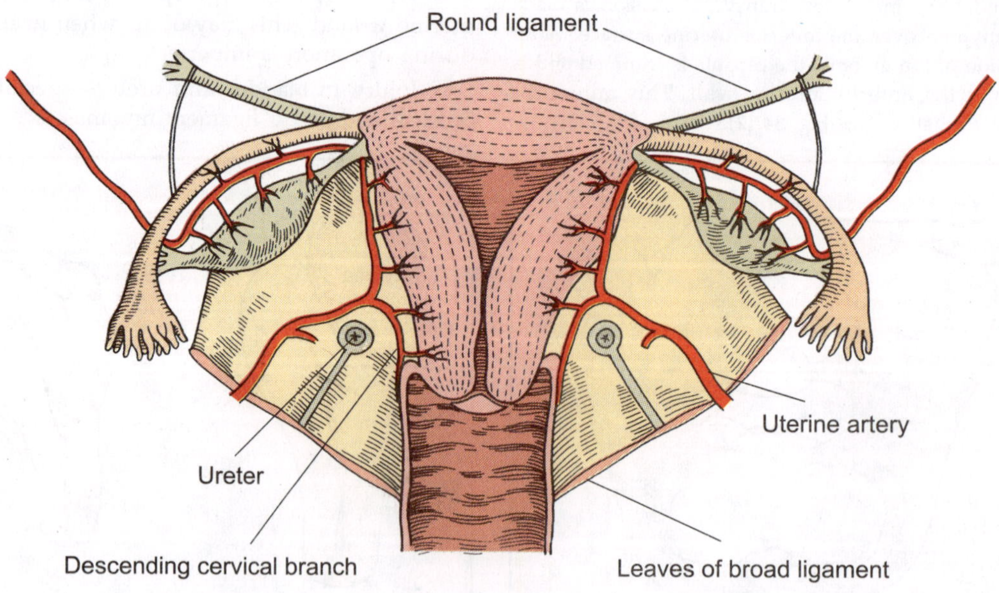

Fig. 34.13. Tissues to be removed in radical hysterectomy (*Diagrammatic*)

rectum and the uterosacral ligament and laterally by the hypogastric vessels.

• **The uterine artery** is identified and dissected out. It is then clamped cut and ligated at its origin from the anterior division of internal iliac artery. Some prefer to ligate the anterior division of internal iliac artery just distal to its posterior division.

• **On the medial flap of peritoneum, the ureter is identified** and is dissected free from the parametrial tissue. Great care is taken when the ureter is dissected from the tunnel of the cardinal ligament (base of broad ligament). Damage to the adventitia and the muscular coat of the ureter should be avoided. Ureter can be retracted, when required, with an umbilical tape.

• **Bladder** is reflected off the cervix and the upper vagina and the vesicocervical and vesicovaginal space is created.

• The peritoneum of the pouch of Douglas is incised to expose the uterosacral ligaments. The rectum is rolled free and the rectovaginal space is created by sharp and blunt dissection.

• **The uterosacral ligament** is clamped close to the sacrum, cut and ligated (with no.1 delayed absorbable suture). The cardinal ligament and paravaginal tissues are clamped close to the lateral pelvic wall, cut and ligated.

• **The vaginal pack** is pulled out. Long right angled clamps are applied one on either side of vagina, low down to remove upper 3 cm of the vagina. The specimen is removed by cutting below the clamps (to avoid tumour spillage). The edges of the vagina are grasped with long Allis forceps.

• **The vaginal margins** are sutured if it is left open for drainage. Some prefer to close the vagina by interrupted sutures so that postoperative suction (vacuum) drainage can be used.

• **Thorough pelvic lymphadenectomy** is done (external iliac, internal iliac, common iliac, obturator). Para-aortic lymph nodes are evaluated and sampling is done if found enlarged.

• Haemostasis is checked. Pelvic peritonisation may be done. Abdominal packs are removed.

• Abdomen is closed in layers. Continuous bladder drainage is maintained for 7-10 days.

(Surgical steps are described for one side and similar steps are repeated on the other side).

Laparoscopic Radical Hysterectomy is currently being evaluated for the management of early stage cervical carcinoma. **The laparoscopic procedures used are**:

A. **Laparoscopic surgical staging only**: (i) Transperitoneally or (ii) Retroperitoneally.

B. **Laparoscopically Assisted Radical Vaginal Hysterectomy (LARVH) with pelvic and aortic lymphadenectomy.** The abdominal part of the procedure includes division of (i) ovarian vessels (ii) round ligaments. (iii) Uterine artery by opening up of the pararectal and paravesical spaces and (iv) pelvic and aortic lymphadenectomy (see p. 585).

C. **Laparoscopic Radical Hysterectomy with pelvic and aortic lymphadenectomy.**

D. **Laparoscopically Assisted Radical Vaginal Trachelectomy (LARVT) with pelvic and aortic lymph adenectomy**—done in (i) selected young women (ii) early stage disease (stage IA_2 or $IB_1 \leq 2$ cm) and (iii) to preserve the reproductive function. This procedure includes (i) Laparoscopic pelvic and aortic lymph node dissection and (ii) vaginal radical trachelectomy if only there is no lymph node metastasis (see p. 339).

Involvement of para-aortic nodes without involvement of the pelvic nodes is extremely rare. If para-aortic nodes are found to be involved with metastatic tumour on frozen section biopsy in the beginning, the procedure of radical hysterectomy is abandoned. Concurrent chemotherapy and radiotherapy are then considered.

Other indications of Radical Abdominal Hysterectomy

- Endometrial carcinoma : Stage IIB (see p. 346).
- Vaginal carcinoma : Stage I-II (Limited to upper one third vagina).
- Recurrence of cervical cancer after radiotherapy : Growth limited to cervix and upper vagina.

Complications of radical hysterectomy

(see p. 336).

OPERATIONS ON THE VULVA

Simple vulvectomy

Preoperative work up (see p. 552).

Actual steps

• Lithotomy position.

• Outer incision—an elliptical incision is made commencing anteriorly on the mons pubis → encircling laterally along the medial side of labiocrural fold → posteriorly across the mid-line of perineum (Fig. 34.4).

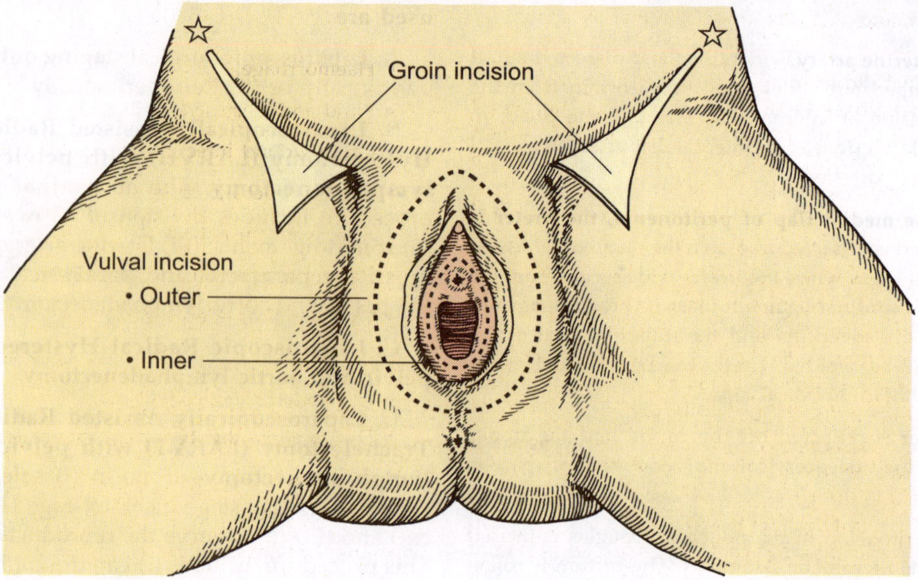

Fig. 34.14. Radical vulvectomy with bilateral inguinofemoral lymphadenectomy (three incision technique)

• Inner incision — Passes around the introitus and anterior to urethra (see Fig. 34.14).

Vulval skin (not deeper tissues) is removed. Bleeding vessels (branches of internal pudendal artery) are ligated separately.

• Apposition of the skin edges is done (interrupted sutures) without tension.

• Continuous bladder drainage is maintained with a Foley's catheter for 3-4 days.

Tissues removed are—mons pubis, clitoris, labia majora and minora.

Radical vulvectomy with bilateral inguinofemoral lymphadenectomy (Figs 34.14 and 34.15)

No single operation technique is standard. En bloc dissection of the groin nodes in continuity with vulvectomy is done only for large vulval lesion. Modifications has been made using three separate incisions to reduce the considerable morbidity of en bloc procedure (see p. 324).

Actual steps

Three incision technique is preferred in most centres. These are—(i) vulval incision. (ii) Groin incision one on either side (see Fig. 34.14).

• Vulval incisions are same as described in simple vulvectomy. Special points to note are :

– Wide tumour free margin (at least 1 cm) is essential. If the tumour is close to urethra or vagina, lower 2 cm of urethra and lower vagina may be sacrificed.

– Dissection must be done down to the deep fascia.

Inguinofemoral lymphadenectomy

• Dissection is carried out down to external oblique fascia and fascia overlying the sartorius muscle.

• At the caudal end of femoral triangle—the long saphenous vein is dissected and doubly ligated with 2-0 silk.

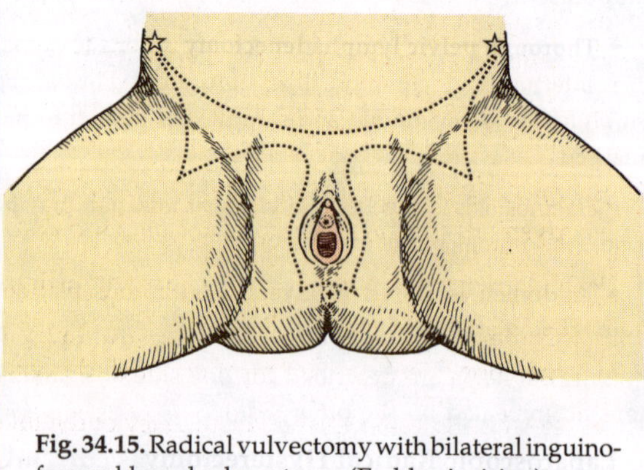

Fig. 34.15. Radical vulvectomy with bilateral inguinofemoral lymphadenectomy (En bloc incision)

- The lymph nodes, lateral and medial to femoral artery and vein are dissected out by sharp dissection.
- Inguinal and femoral lymph nodes are removed and sent for frozen section biopsy. The Cloquet lymph node at the femoral canal may be absent in more than 50 per cent cases. If these nodes are positive, ipsilateral retroperitoneal pelvic lymphadenectomy can be performed.
- **Lymphatic drainage** occurs in a stepwise fashion. The sentinel lymph node when negative for tumour metastasis, it is rare for the other nodes to be involved. Identification of the sentinel lymph node can therefore guide the extent of surgery and also the surgical lymph node dissection. This can reduce the risk of surgical morbidity and mortality.

  Sentinel node biopsy (p. 328) is done using either blue dye or radio colloid. Methylene blue dye is injected at the periphery of the tumour → the blue dyed lymphatics are followed → dyed nodes are then removed and subjected to frozen section biopsy. Otherwise **technetium-99m** is injected into the tumour and the radioactive tracer uptake in the regional lymph nodes is then identified by a hand-held gamma camera.
- However radiation therapy is preferred to surgery for pelvic node dissection (see p. 324).
- Closed system suction drains are placed in the groin area. Groin incision is closed by interrupted sutures.

Complications of radical vulvectomy

***Early*:**

- Haemorrhage.
- Fluid and electrolyte imbalance.
- Groin wound infection, necrosis and dehiscence.
- Urinary tract infection.
- Deep vein thrombosis.
- Pulmonary embolism (see p. 569).
- Psychological—depression.

***Late*:**

- Leg oedema, leg cellulitis.
- Dyspareunia due to introital stenosis.
- Femoral hernia.
- Osteitis pubis.
- Loss of body image.
- Recurrence.

Operations for urinary incontinence (see p. 387).

Repair of vesicovaginal fistula (see p. 401).

Repair of ureteric injuries (see p. 408).

Vaginal reconstruction operation (vaginoplasty) (see p. 437).

KEY POINTS

- Preoperative investigations should preferably be done prior to admission in hospital.
- In elective operations, the patient should be made fit for surgery prior-hand.
- Even in minor surgery, examination of the cardiovascular system, complete haemogram and complete urine examination should be done.
- For any operation, preoperative counselling and informed consent are essential (p. 553).
- Day care surgery has many benefits. Here the patients are admitted, operated and discharged on the same day (p. 554). Patients are screened before hand.
- Postoperative care should include record of vital signs, fluid replacement, adequate pain control, antibiotic therapy and vigilance to the close system suction drains.
- Only dilatation of the cervix is indicated in—prior to amputation of the cervix, spasmodic dysmenorrhoea, pyometra or haematometra.
- Common indications of D + C are infertility, DUB, incomplete abortion and endometrial pathology.

  Common complications of D + C are injury to the cervix, uterine perforation, injury to the gut and infection. Remote complications include cervical incompetence and uterine synechiae.
- D + I is indicated to note the patency of the tubes in cases of infertility or following tuboplasty operation.
- HSG is done in the radiology department without anaesthesia (p. 559).

KEY POINTS

- Types of cervical biopsy include—surface, punch, wedge, ring and cone type (see p. 560).
- Destruction of the benign pathological cervical lesions can be done by thermal cauterisation, cryosurgery or laser (see p. 561).
- Complications of cervical conisation or amputation include postoperative haemorrhage and cervical stenosis or cervical incompetence (see p. 216; Table 15.3).
- Common indications of total hysterectomy for benign lesions are DUB, fibroid, TO mass and endometriosis (see p. 564, Table 34.2).
- Common indications of subtotal hysterectomy are difficult TO mass, endometriosis of rectovaginal septum and sudden deterioration of the general health while contemplating total hysterectomy.

  Premenopausal ovaries are better to be preserved, if not pathological.
- Conisation of the cervix is done either as a diagnostic or therapeutic procedure in CIN or in microinvasive carcinoma. Laser cone has got distinct advantages over the cold knife cone (see Table 34.1).
- Perineoplasty is the reconstruction of the narrow vaginal introitus to make it adequate for sexual function.
- Complications of abdominal hysterectomy are many (see p. 568). Postoperative bowel dysfunction (ileus and obstruction) need to be differentiated (see Table 34.4).
- Hysterectomy can be abdominal, vaginal, laparoscopic or laparoscopic assisted vaginal. Each method has got advantages and disadvantages (see p. 569, 586). Each case needs to be individualised for any particular method.
- Laparoscopic ovarian drilling is more commonly done compared to wedge resection in the management of PCOS cases (see p. 450).
- Operations for chronic inversion of the uterus may be abdominal (Haultain) or vaginal (Kustner or Spinelli).
- Ventrosuspension operations are less commonly done these days. Plication of the round ligaments, modified Gilliam procedure or laparoscopic suspension operation are the different methods (see p. 574).
- Abdominal myomectomy could be done either by open surgery or laparoscopically. Control of operative blood loss is an important step (see p. 574). A single incision on the anterior wall is preferred.
- Radical hysterectomy (Type IV) is the operation of choice for invasive carcinoma of the cervix (see p. 338 and p. 576).
- Laparoscopic radical hysterectomy is currently being done (p. 577). Laparoscopically assisted radical vaginal trachelectomy (LARVT) is a fertility sparing surgery done for early stage (IA_2 or $IB_1 \leq 2$ cm) diseses.
- Radical vulvectomy with bilateral inguinofemoral lymphadenectomy could be done either by en bloc procedure (butterfly horned incision) or by three incision technique (preferred).
- Node of Cloquet or Rosenmüller (deep femoral mode) may be absent in more than 50 per cent cases.
- Pelvic node metastases are rare unless inguinofemoral nodes are involved. However, radiation therapy is preferred to surgery for pelvic node dissection (see p. 325).

  Complications of radical vulvectomy may be early or late (p. 579) and increases the morbidity.

Endoscopic Surgery in Gynaecology

(Syn:Minimally invasive surgery, Minimal access surgery)

35

History

First description of endoscopy is recorded by Phillip Bozzini in 1805. He used a simple tube and candle light to visualise the interior of the urethra. Pantaleoni of Ireland first used a cystoscope in 1869 as an hysteroscope to diagnose a case of irregular vaginal bleeding. Jacobaeus of Sweden in 1910 first introduced a cystoscope in the peritoneal cavity and coined the term laparoscopy. In 1938, Veress first reported the spring loaded needle for introducing pneumothorax in patients with tuberculosis. In 1967 Steptoe of England first published the monograph "Laparoscopy in Gynaecology" in english language. First laparoscopic hysterectomy was reported by Reich *et. al.* in 1989.

The range of surgical procedures in gynaecology, performed with the use of either a laparoscope or a hysteroscope is designated as **endoscopic surgery**. With very fast technological advancement, as much as 80 per cent of gynaecological operations can be performed endoscopically.

Advantages

When compared to conventional open surgery it has the following advantages :

- Rapid postoperative recovery.
- Less postoperative pain and reduced need of postoperative analgesia.
- Shorter hospital stay and reduced concomitant cost.
- Quicker resumption of day-to-day activity.
- Less adhesion formation.
- Minimal abdominal scars (cosmetic value).

Disadvantages

Disadvantages are mainly related to case selection and experience of the surgeon :

- Operation time—may be longer.
- Risk of iatrogenic complications (see p. 590).
- High initial expenditure (instruments are expensive).

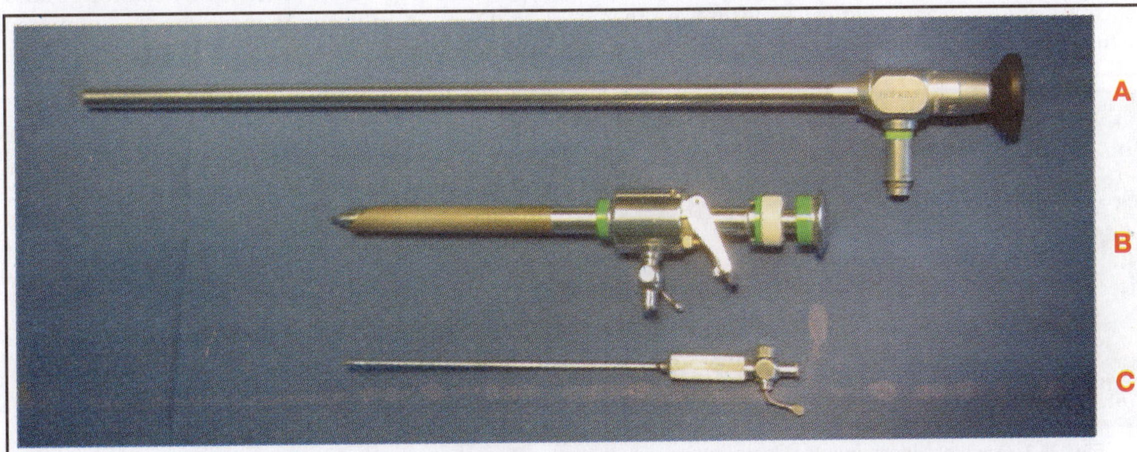

Fig. 35.1. Laparoscopic instruments : (A) Telescope (B) Trocar and cannula (C) Veress needle

- Surgeon skilled at open surgery must be specially trained.

Basic instruments and electrosurgical units for laparoscopic surgery (Fig. 35.1)

Telescope—Caliber varies from 4-12 mm with rod lens system. Angle of view may be either straight forward (0°) or fore oblique (30°).

Veress needle—It is used for creating pneumoperitoneum by carbon dioxide. It is spring loaded to prevent visceral injury. The blunt tip point springs out when it enters the peritoneal cavity.

Trocar and cannula—is inserted through the abdominal wall following pneumoperitoneum. The trocar is removed and the telescope is introduced through the cannula (sleeve). Disposable trocar and veress needles are available.

Light source—High intensity light (xenon or halogen source) beam (cold light) is transmitted to the telescope for excellent visualisation. Fibre optic cables are used to transmit the cold light from source to the telescope.

Insufflator—is used to create controlled pneumoperitoneum as there is some amount of gas (CO_2) leak through the different ports. Either low flow rate (0.5-1L/min) or high flow rate is used depending on the need.

Cameras—The telescope is connected with the camera lens and pictures are obtained from the monitor (television) screen.

Ancillary instruments (Fig. 35.2)

Scissors — of different sizes and designs are used for dissection and to cut tissue.

Grasping forceps — of different designs are used to hold tissue without any trauma.

Probes — Blunt probe is used for manipulation of visceras (e.g. intestines and ovaries) to visualise other structures.

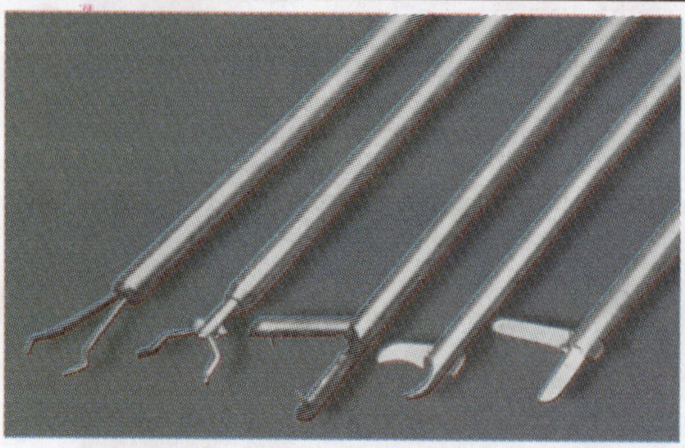

Fig. 35.2. Ancillary instruments : Coagulators, graspers, scissors

Aspirator and irrigator — Blunt and sharp aspirators are used for aspiration of fluid from the peritoneal cavity or ovarian cysts. **Irrigation** is done for washing the peritoneal cavity with normal saline at the end of a surgical procedure.

Morcellator — is needed when a large piece of tissue (myoma) is morcellated into small pieces so as to be removed through the laparoscopic sleeve.

Uterine manipulator — is used for adequate visualisation of the uterus and adnexae during operation.

Haemostasis during laparoscopic surgery

Perfect haemostasis is mandatory at the end of any endoscopic surgery.

Electrosurgical units are used for cutting and coagulation of biological tissues. **Cutting mode** provides high voltage to vaporise tissue and **coagulation mode** creates an initial high voltage to dessicate the outer layer of tissue. In **blended mode** cutting and coagulation currents are combined creating alternate high and low voltage current.

Monopolar electrosurgery

The current (electrons) is pushed from the generator through the active electrode to the contact tissue. The current returns back to generator through the neutral electrode after it has passed through the patient.

Depending upon the size of the electrodes (current density) and voltage used, unwanted burns may be produced due to stray current flow.

Bipolar electrosurgery

Here the current flows from the generator between the two jaws of the forceps or scissors, holding the target tissue (Fig. 35.5). There is no need for ground plate. Damage to tissue is more precise compared to unipolar mode.

Laser (see p. 119)

Lasers used in gynaecological surgery are CO_2, 532-nm potassium-titanyl phosphate (KTP-532) and neodymium : yttrium-aluminium-garnate (Nd : YAG) lasers. For effective cutting, vaporisation and coagulation of tissue, power density is an important factor. The depth of tissue penetration depends on the type of laser used, e.g. for CO_2 (most commonly used) 0.1 mm, KTP-532-0.4-0.8 mm and Nd : YAG is 0.6-4.2 mm.

Sutures

Like an open surgery sutures can be used to ligate blood vessels and to secure vascular pedicles. Different methods of suturing and knot tying are

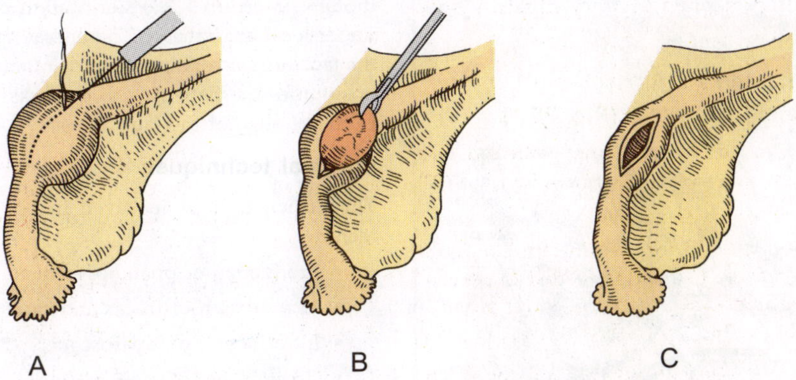

Fig. 35.3. Laparoscopic linear salpingotomy for unruptured tubal pregnancy

used : (a) intra-corporeal knot tying, (b) extra-corporeal knot tying or (c) endoloops pretied ligature (Roeder loops).

Mechanical clips and staples

Titanium clips and staples are used for haemostasis by securing blood vessels. Disposable stapling cartridge with a self contained knife blade (Endo GIA 30) is used for laparoscopic hysterectomy producing quick cut and haemostasis.

Indications of laparoscopic surgery

Advances in electrosurgical units, optics and technology, have widened the area of endoscopic surgery day by day. The laparoscopic surgical procedures are graded according to the extent of surgery and also to the competence of the surgeon. They are labelled as follows :

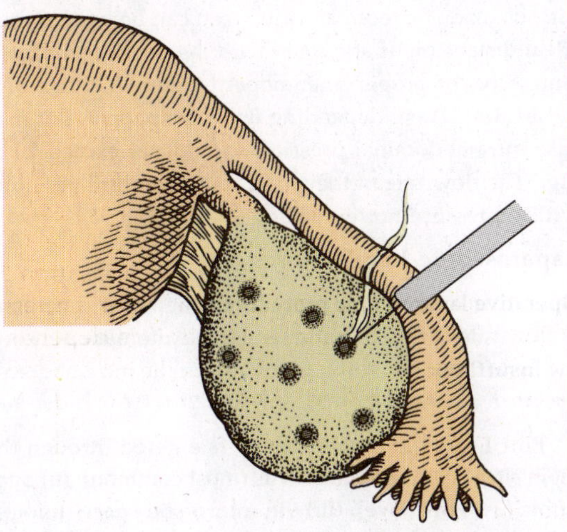

Fig. 35.4. Surgical treatment of PCOS by laser drilling

A. Diagnostic laparoscopy (see p. 117)

B. Therapeutic laparoscopy

Minor procedures

- Tubal sterilisation (p. 476).
- Adhesiolysis (without bowel involvement) (Fig. 35.5).
- Aspiration of simple ovarian cysts.
- Ovarian biopsy.

Moderate procedures (Fig. 35.3)

Ectopic pregnancy :

- Salpingostomy.
- Segmental resection.
- Salpingectomy.
- Salpingo-oophorectomy.

Endometriosis : Ablation by diathermy or laser.

Ovary (Fig. 35.4)

- Diathermy for PCOS.
- Drainage of endometriomas.
- Ovarian cystectomy.
- Salpingo-ovariolysis.

Uterus

- Myomectomy.
- Laparoscopic assisted vaginal hysterectomy (LAVH).
- Adhesiolysis – including bowel involvement (Fig. 35.5).

Extensive procedures

- Major endometriosis.
- Myomectomy.
- Pelvic lymphadenectomy.
- Urinary incontinence.

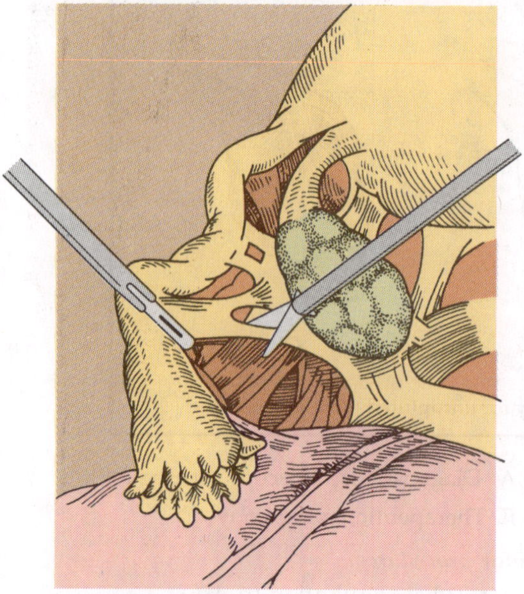

Fig. 35.5. Laparoscopic adhesiolysis (salpingolysis and ovariolysis)

Contraindications (Table 35.1)

With experience, the contraindications, to the procedure have been reduced. One should be familiar with the contraindications to maximise the patient safety and minimise the procedure related morbidity.

Table 35.1
Contraindications of Laparoscopy

- Severe cardiopulmonary disease.
- Patient haemodynamically unstable.
- Generalised peritonitis.
- Significant haemoperitoneum.
- Intestinal obstruction.
- Extensive peritoneal adhesion.
- Large pelvic tumour.
- Pregnancy > 16 weeks.
- Previous periumbilical surgery (relative).
- Extreme obesity.

Operative procedures for laparoscopy

Preoperative screening is essential and contraindications are excluded (see Table 35.1). Informed consent is taken and it should include the permission for open surgery if necessity arises. **General anaesthesia** is generally preferred though procedures like sterilisation could be performed under local anaesthesia. The operating table should have the facilities for rotating at different angles. Low lithotomy position of the patient with buttocks protruding slightly from the edge of the table is used.

Surgical techniques

The principal steps involved in operative laparoscopy include :

- Production of pneumoperitoneum.
- Introduction of trocar and cannula.
- Introduction of laparoscope.
- Creation of accessory ports.
- Surgical techniques employed through laparoscope.
- Deflation of the peritoneal gas.
- Closure of the parietal wound.

Position of patient : The patient is placed in lithotomy position. The operating table is tilted to approximately 15-30 degrees of Trendelenburg position. For good view and hand-eye coordination, both for the surgeon and the assistants the video monitor is placed at the foot end of the table. The electrosurgical unit and the suction irrigator should be placed behind the surgeon or assistant. The bladder is emptied by a Foley's catheter. Pelvic examination is done methodically. An uterine manipulator is introduced through the cervical canal for manipulation to visualise the tubes and uterus at a later step.

Pneumoperitoneum : A small skin incision (1.25 cm) is made just below the umbilicus. The veress needle is introduced through the incision with 45° angulation into the peritoneal cavity. The abdomen is inflated with about 1L-4L of gas (carbon dioxide). But for diagnostic purposes nitrous oxide or room air or oxygen can be used. Symmetrical distension of abdomen with loss of liver dullness is suggestive of proper pneumoperitoneum. Volume of gas varies from 1L-4L depending upon the patient. But in any case intra-abdominal pressure should not exceed 20 mm Hg. The flow rate of the gas is about one litre per minute with a pressure not exceeding 20 mm Hg.

Laparoscopic Insufflator

Operative laparoscopic procedures, high flow is necessary. A flow rate of 10-20 L/min is used. Automatic sensors of the **insufflator** shut off gas flow when the intra-abdominal pressure reaches 15 to 20 mm Hg.

Port Entry : Peritoneal cavity is entered through three main sites : (i) At the umbilicus (most common). (ii) Suprapubic (2-4 cm above). (iii) 9th intercostal space (midclavicular line) on the left (Palmer's point). In obese patients the needle is inserted more vertically.

Introduction of trocar and cannula

The abdominal wall is elevated and the trocar with cannula is inserted through the same incision. The angle of insertion is similar to that of the veress needle, directing towards the hollow of the sacrum. There is escape of gas when the trocar is within the peritoneal cavity. The trocar is removed and the laparoscope is then introduced. **Open laparoscopy** was introduced (Hasson-1971) to reduce the risk of blind insertion of the veress needles and trocars. Peritoneal cavity is opened through a small incision (1 cm) at the umbilicus pneumoperitoneum is done through a special cannula inserted in the incision. The laparoscope is then introduced.

Secondary trocar insertion is needed for both the diagnostic and operative procedures. Sites selected are either on the flank (3-4 cm lateral to the median umbilical ligament) or lateral to the lateral margin of rectus abdominis muscle or on the suprapubic region. This is done under direct vision with illumination to avoid trauma to abdominal organs and the inferior epigastric vessels.

Laparoscopic procedures of tissue dissection are several : (i) Blunt dissection. (ii) Sharp dissection (using scissors). If it bleeds when cut, bipolar diathermy is used for haemostasis. (iii) Aqua dissection hydraulic pressure is used to create tissue planes. (iv) **Electrodissection** using unipolar or bipolar diathermy for dissection and coagulation. (v) Laser dissection (see p. 119).

Methods of haemostasis in laparoscopic surgery are : Electrocoagulation (unipolar and bipolar), laser coagulation, extracorporeal ligatures, sutures (extra corporeal or endocorporeal) and clips.

Removal of specimens : Large volume of tissues after laparoscope could be removed by any of these methods : (i) Morcellation. (ii) By enlarging any of the suprapubic trocar incision site. (iii) Through the colpotomy incision. The specimen is put in a Endo-Catch bag and is taken out without spilling.

Examination of the pelvis

After introduction of the laparoscope, a systematic inspection of the pelvic and abdominal organs is done. The patient is put to Trendelenburg position for proper visualisation of the pelvic organs.

Visualisation

Diagnostic procedures may be performed with direct optical visualisation. Operative procedures are carried out with video camera (Fig. 35.9). Video camera with single or triple chip is attached to the eyepiece of the laparoscope. Depending on the light sensitivity and resolution power of the camera, the images are processed and transferred to a monitor.

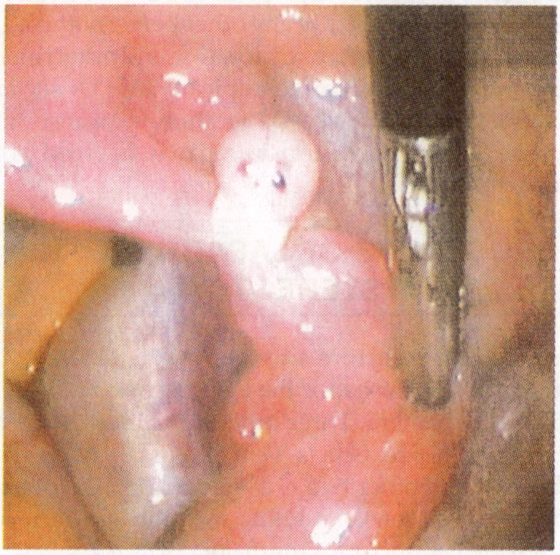

Fig. 35.6. Laparoscopic view showing tubal sterilisation with silastic rings

Monitor is a television set with same resolution as that of the video camera for producing images with excellent quality.

Video cassette recorder is used for the purpose of teaching and documentation.

OPERATIVE LAPAROSCOPY

Tubal sterilisation with single puncture technique : The various operative techniques of laparoscopic procedures are beyond the scope of the book. As the laparoscopic sterilisation is commonly done, this procedure is described in p. 476 (see Fig. 35.6).

Laparoscopic Hysterectomy and Laparoscopic Assisted Vaginal Hysterectomy (LAVH)

Laparoscopic Hysterectomy (LH) : Uterus is freed of all its attachment laparoscopically. The uterus is removed either vaginally or abdominally following morcellation. Vagina is closed with sutures laparoscopically LH is not a substitute of abdominal hysterectomy and also not for vaginal hysterectomy.

Laparoscopic Assisted Vaginal Hysterectomy

Laparoscopy is done to get some benefits during vaginal hysterectomy. A major advantage of using LAVH is the avoidance of abdominal incision which is a significant cause of morbidity and longer hospital stay with abdominal hysterectomy.

Benefits of laparoscopy prior to vaginal hysterectomy are : (i) Diagnosis of any other pelvic pathology. (ii) Adhesiolysis or excision of endometriosis. (iii) Adnexae is freed laparoscopically. (iv) Dissection of bladder from uterus. (v) Desiccation and transection of uterine artery (vi) Entire uterus may be freed from its attachments.

PROCEDURE OF LAPAROSCOPIC HYSTERECTOMY

Three or four puncture sites are made. One 10 mm umbilical port is used for the laparoscope, connected to the video camera. Three other punctures are made each of 5 mm size. One is 3 cm above the symphysis pubis, and the other two are 4-5 cm laterally, one on each side (between the midline and epigastric artery). The left lower puncture is the major portal for operative manipulation. The right is used for retraction with atraumatic grasping forceps.

Bipolar coagulation and transection are used to transect pelvic ligaments and to achieve haemostasis. Bipolar coagulation desiccates the blood vessels. Scissors are used to transect the pedicles following coagulation. The round ligament, infundibulopelvic ligament are similarly coagulated and transected. Sutures, staples or clips can also be used instead of bipolar cautery but are expensive. The leaves of the broad ligament are opened up with the scissors. The peritoneum of the vesicouterine pouch is dissected with the scissors. Hydrodissection is used to develop the space.

For LAVH, the laparoscopic procedure is stopped at this point. The rest of the operation is completed vaginally. This is exactly the same as that of vaginal hysterectomy (see p. 211).

For total hysterectomy (LH)

Hydrodissection is also used to expose the uterine vessels. After careful identification of the uterine vessels and the ureter, the uterine vessels are desiccated using bipolar cautery and then cut.

Uterus is then freed from the rest of attachment. The cardinal ligaments on each side are divided. Circumferential culdotomy (division of cervicovaginal attachments) is done. Bipolar cautery is used for haemostasis. Vaginal vault is closed. Extra corporeal sutures may be used.

After completion of the procedure, laparoscope is used to check the pelvis for haemostasis. Peritoneal cavity is irrigated with Ringer's lactate solution and suctioned until clear fluid is obtained. Bleeding vessels are coagulated. 500 ml of Ringer's solution are left in the peritoneal cavity. The laparoscopic instruments are then removed and the pneumoperitoneum is deflated. The trocar incisions (ports) are closed.

Complications:Similar for hysterectomy in general (p. 568) including injury to ureters (p. 408), bladder, rectum and infection at vaginal vault (see below).

COMPLICATIONS OF LAPAROSCOPY

Complications are grouped into : (i) specific to laparoscopy itself, (ii) due to anaesthesia, (iii) common to any surgical procedures.

Complications due to laparoscopy itself :

(i) Extraperitoneal insufflation — surgical emphysema.

(ii) Omental emphysema.

(iii) Cardiac arrhythmia.

(iv) Injury to blood vessels—mesenteric, omental, injury to major pelvic or abdominal artery or vein. Inferior epigastric vessels may be injured during insertion of accessory trocars.

(v) Injury to bowel — with veress needle or trocar specially when there is adhesions.

(vi) Injury to organs like bowel, bladder or ureter. Damage may be mechanical during dissection or thermal by electrical or laser energy.

(vii) Electrosurgical complications — causing thermal injury (electrode burns, insulation defects).

(viii) Gas (carbon dioxide) embolism — resulting in hypotension, cardiac arrhythmia.

Anaesthetic complications peculiar to laparoscopy are :

(i) Hypoventilation (pneumoperitoneum and Trendelenburg position lead to basal lung compression and reduced diaphragmatic excursion).

(ii) Hypercarbia and metabolic acidosis (when CO_2 is used for pneumoperitoneum).

(iii) Basal lung atelectasis.

(iv) Others — oesophageal intubation, aspiration and cardiac arrest.

Complications common to any surgical procedure

(i) Haemorrhage, (ii) Infection,
(iii) Wound dehiscence, (iv) Port site hernia.

Death rate in diagnostic laparoscopy is about 5/100,000 procedures. With experience, the fatality is markedly reduced to even zero. **Causes of death are** : cardiac arrest, gas embolism and consequences of intestinal injury.

HYSTEROSCOPY

Hysteroscopy is a procedure that allows direct visualisation inside the uterus (see Fig. 35.7). It can be used for diagnostic as well as therapeutic purposes (Fig. 35.9).

Basic instruments and electrosurgical units for hysteroscopic surgery (Fig. 35.8)

Telescope — Rigid telescopes are commonly used. The telescope may be either straight on (forward view) (0°) or fore oblique view 30°, 70° or 90°.

Flexible telescopes — The tip of the hysteroscope can bend upto 110°. It has the advantage of easy uterine entry through the angle between cervix and uterus. It helps easy aligning the catheter for tubal cannulation (see Fig. 35.7).

Microhysteroscope acts as a high powered microscope by switching the lens to 150X. Light contact with the mucous membrane is needed.

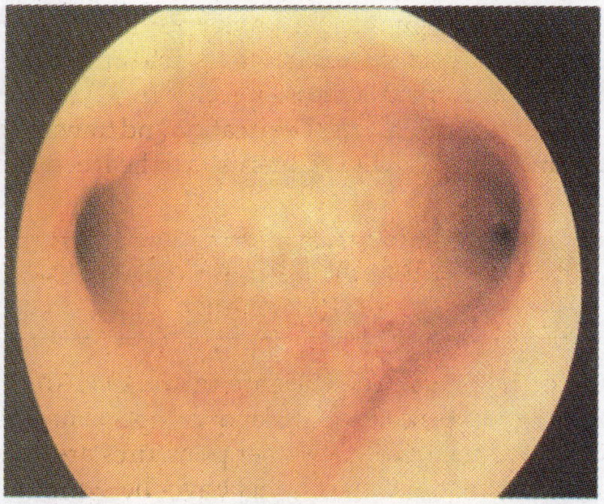

Fig. 35.7. Panoramic view of the uterine cavity with a hysteroscope. Tubal ostium is seen one on either side

The inflow sheath carries the distension medium to the tip of the telescope, from where it is withdrawn via the outer sheath. This helps to maintain the clear view.

Distending media — The uterine cavity is distended with a media to separate the uterine walls and to have a panoramic view. The media used could be either a gas or a liquid.

Carbon dioxide (CO_2) — is commonly used for diagnostic purposes. It is soluble in blood and is safe.

Hysteroflator provides gas flow rate of maximum 100 ml per minute and a maximum pressure of 100 mm Hg.

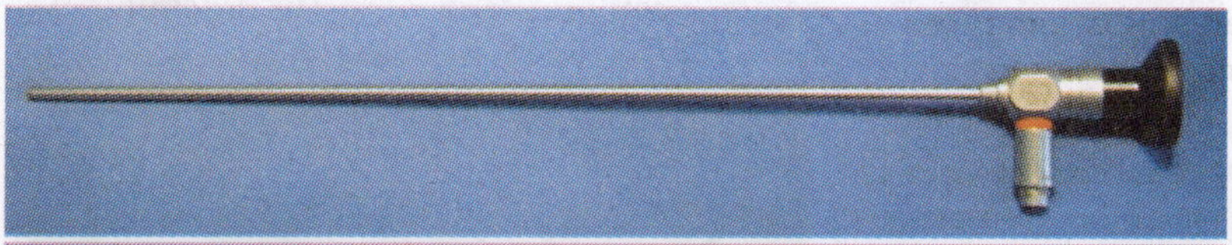

A

Fig. 35.8A. Hysteroscope

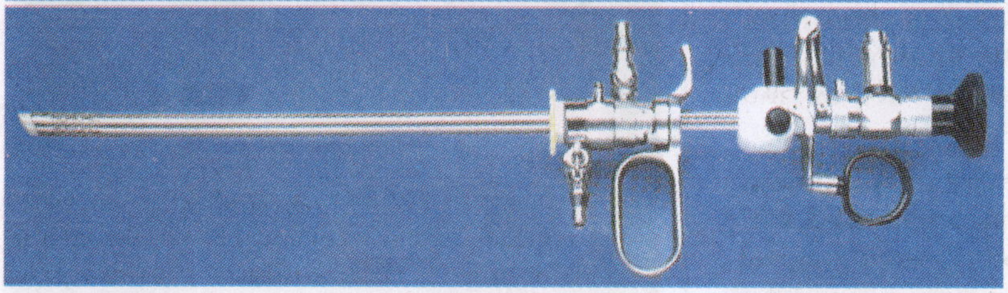

B

Fig.35.8B. Hysteroscope with working element for operative interventions (outer diameter : 8 mm)

Telescope sheath — A sheath is required to introduce the telescope. Sheath used for diagnostic purposes are smaller (5 mm) than that for operative sheath (7-10 mm). Operative instruments are introduced through the sheath. Operative hysteroscopy needs separate inflow and outflow sheaths.

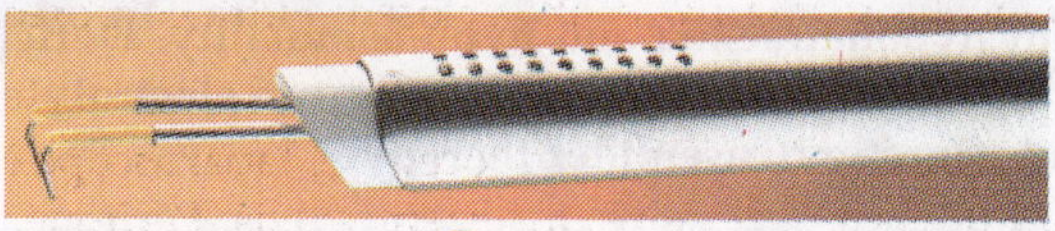

C

Fig. 35.8C. Resectoscope (with an angled cutting loop)

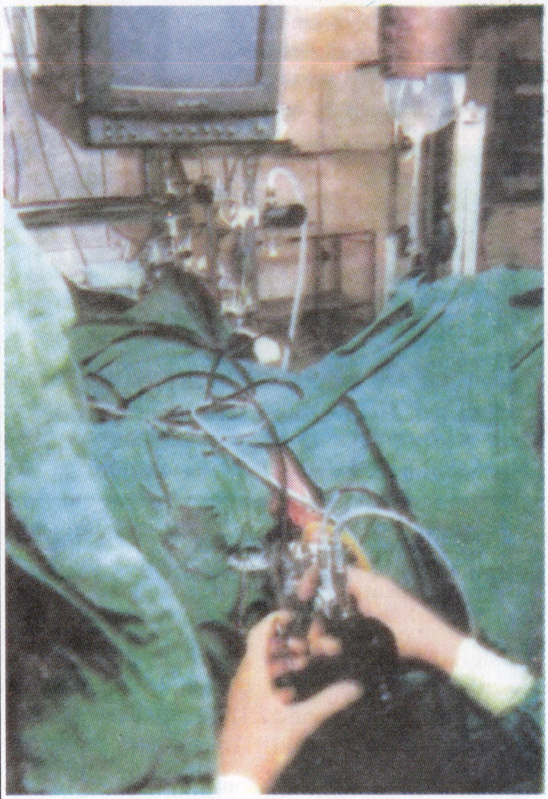

Fig. 35.9. Hysteroscopic procedures in progress

Liquid media is used for operative procedures.

Normal saline can be used safely. Constant flow is to be maintained to flush the operative area.

Glycine 1.5 per cent is used in many centres for excellent visualisation. It is hypo-osmolar. Resectoscope (monopolar electrosurgery) can be used as it does not conduct electricity. Fluid can be pressurized via a roller pump or by a pressure infusion bag cuff system with a maximum flow rate of 100 ml/min and maximum pressure of 100 mm Hg.

Mannitol (5%) and Glycine (2.2%) are Iso-osmolar, so can be used safely. They can be used with electrosurgical devices also.

A fluid deficit of (≥ 500 ml is alarming to prevent hyponatraemia and hypo-osmolality. Deficit of ≥ 1L require measurement of serum electrolytes and diuretic (frusemide) therapy.

A pressure of about 45 mm Hg is required for adequate distention of the uterine cavity. This pressure should not exceed the mean arterial pressure to avoid extravasation.

Image-recorder — recorded images are useful as teaching aids to the trainees. They can also be used as an evidence (in defense) for medicolegal purpose.

Camera : The hysteroscopic image is visualised on the monitor with the help of a camera. The camera used for laparoscopy can also be used. The monitor is checked before hand for visualisation of appropriate image. A high resolution camera and colour monitor is required for both the surgeon and the assistants.

Light source : Xenon or mercury halide can provide high intensity light sources for excellent illumination.

Anaesthesia

Diagnostic procedures — are carried out under paracervical block with 1 per cent xylocaine (10-15 ml).

Operative procedures — are carried out under general anaesthesia or regional anaesthesia (spinal or epidural).

INDICATIONS OF DIAGNOSTIC HYSTEROSCOPY

(a) **Abnormal uterine bleeding** :

- Menorrhagia (Fig. 35.10).
- Postmenopausal bleeding (see p. 532).

(b) **Infertility** — when associated with abnormal hysterosalpingogram (filling defect, synechiae).

(c) **Müllerian anomalies** like arcuate, subseptate, septate, bicornate uterus or uterus didelphys can be

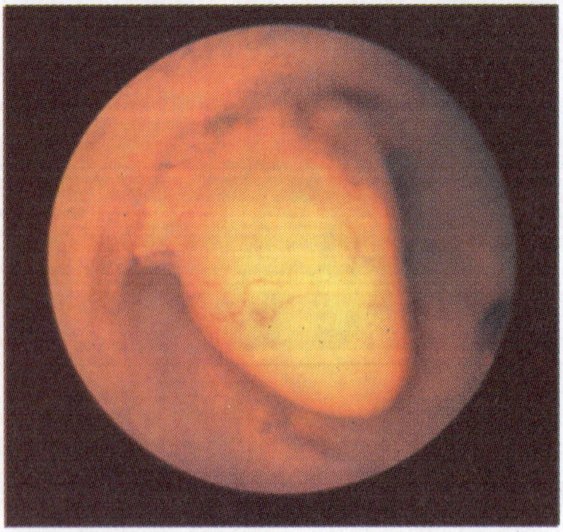

Fig. 35.10. Hysteroscopic view of a submucous fibroid

diagnosed with hysteroscopy. The procedure is combined with laparoscopy for confirmation.

(d) **Recurrent miscarriage**: Intrauterine pathology such as fibroids, polyps, Asherman's syndrome (Fig. 36.73) can be diagnosed and treated.

(e) **Misplaced IUD** (Fig. 29.6).

(f) **Chronic pelvic pain** due to obstructive uterine anomaly, fibroids, bicornuate uterus may be diagnosed. Laparoscopy is done to exclude other pelvic pathologies.

(g) **Transformation zone** (p. 310) could be visualised with colpomicrohysteroscopy.

INDICATIONS OF OPERATIVE HYSTEROSCOPY

(a) Polypectomy and myomectomy.

(b) Lysis of intrauterine adhesions (synaecolysis).

(c) Endometrial ablation (laser or roller ball) for patients suffering from DUB (see p. 189).

(d) Endometrial resection — where endometrium is excised using a resectoscope (Fig. 14.4) for patients with DUB.

(e) Metroplasty (resection of uterine septum).

(f) Removal of foreign body or IUD, when the thread is missing.

(g) Biopsy of suspected endometrium under direct vision.

(h) Tubal cannulation—under hysteroscopic guidance can release any proximal tubal obstruction (due to mucous plugs or spasm). A special catheter is passed through the tubal ostium upto the interstitial part of the tube.

(i) Sterilisation—by destroying the interstitial portion of the tubes using Nd-YAG laser or electrocoagulation or for insertion of Essure (p. 481).

When to be done? Hysteroscopy should be done in the postmenstrual period or in the midproliferative phase. The endometrium is thin which facilitates intracavity viewing. Bleeding is absent or less and there is no chance of conception at that phase.

Pretreatment evaluation and protocol

- The operation should preferably be limited to women with normal sized uterus.
- Should be preceded by diagnostic hysteroscopy.
- Pretreatment with danazol, GnRH analogue or progestogen for 4-6 weeks to make the endometrium thin prior to endometrial ablation/resection.

CONTRAINDICATIONS OF HYSTEROSCOPY

Pelvic infection: Hysteroscopy can cause spread of infection. The distension media flowing through the tube spreads the infection in the peritoneal cavity.

Pregnancy: However, hysteroscopy can be done to remove an IUCD when the threads are missing.

Cervical cancer: Trauma to the friable cervix can cause excessive bleeding.

Cardiopulmonary disorders are at higher risk of anaesthesia as hysteroscopy carries its own risk of gas embolism, fluid over load and pulmonary oedema (see p. 590).

Cervical stenosis: Can cause cervical trauma. PGE_2 gel inserted 2 hours before surgery, softens the cervix and help easy dilatation.

OPERATIVE HYSTEROSCOPY

Transcervical resection of endometrium (TCRE) or laser ablation of endometrium (LAE) is done as an alternative to hysterectomy for dysfunctional uterine bleeding. Hysterectomy is a major surgical procedure which has got known risks of operative morbidity and mortality. TCRE or LAE is completed by about 30 minutes time and patient can go home on the same day. Provided the procedure is done by an expert, it is simple and safe.

The principle of this operation is to destroy the endometrium up to a depth of 3–5 mm. There would be no further regeneration of endometrium as the basal layer of endometrium as well as the basal and spiral arterioles are destroyed.

Total resection or ablation of endometrium should result in amenorrhoea. **Selection of the patient** is very important. Uterus should be normal in size and there should not any other pelvic pathology. Presence of pelvic pain is a contraindication. Before TCRE or LAE, endometrium is suppressed using danazol or GnRH analogue for 4-6 weeks (see p. 511). Therapeutic response following TCRE or LAE has been observed in 80-85 per cent of cases (see p. 189).

HYSTEROSCOPIC MYOMECTOMY

It is done for submucous myomas as an alternative to hysterectomy or laparotomic myomectomy for a patient with intractable symptoms.

Indications : (i) Infertility (ii) Menorrhagia.

Classification of intrauterine myomas (European Society of Hysteroscopy)		
Grade (G)	:	Degree of intramural development of myoma.
G_0	:	Myoma, limited to uterine cavity (pedunculated).
G_1	:	Myoma, endocavitary component > 50%.
G_2	:	Myoma, endocavitary component < 50%.

Surgical technique : Pre-operative GnRH agonist therapy is used (p. 501). Resectoscope is normally used for myoma resection. Electro surgical working element with 90° cutting loop (Fig. 35.8) is usually used to shave off any submucous leiomyoma (Fig. 19.8). Myometrium is desiccated through contact coagulation for 30-40 seconds to control bleeding.

Common complications are : Uterine perforation and haemorrhage (see below).

COMPLICATIONS OF HYSTEROSCOPY

Complications may arise from any o f these following sources :

(a) **Distension media** :
- Fluid overload.
- Pulmonary oedema, cerebral oedema.
- Hyponatraemia.
- Neurological symptoms.
- Ammonia-toxicity due to excess glycine absorption.
- Embolism (CO_2).

(b) **Operative procedures**
- Uterine perforation.
- Haemorrhage—intraoperative or postoperative.
- Injury to intra-abdominal organs.

(c) **Electrosurgical** — Thermal injury to intra-abdominal organs due to laser or electricity.

(d) **Others** — Infection, anaesthetic complications and treatment failure.

KEY POINTS

- Endoscopy is the procedure to visualise the interior of a viscus or space with the use of a telescope. In gynaecology as much as 80 per cent of operations can be performed endoscopically with the use of either a laparoscope or a hysteroscope.
- During laparoscopy, the magnification of the object depends upon the distance of the laparoscope from the object. With 'Storz' it is nearly 10 times when working distance is 3 mm and is 1 when the distance is 30 mm.
- Laparoscopic surgery could be diagnostic (p. 117) or therapeutic (see p. 583). Before any procedure is undertaken, contraindications must be carefully excluded (Table 35.1). Informed consent should include the permission for open surgery if necessity arises.
- Haemostasis during laparoscopic surgery can be achieved using electrosurgical units (p. 582) or by using mechanical clips and staples (p. 583) or by ligatures (p. 585).
- Thermal damage caused by electro-surgery or laser depends on the degree of heat applied to the tissues. Tissue damage with heat is as follows : 45°C = Tissue death; 70°C = Coagulation; ≥ 90°C = Desiccation; ≥ 100°C = Vaporisation; ≥ 200°C = Carbonisation (charring).
- Laparoscopic tubal sterilisation is the commonest surgical procedure. In LAVH the uterine arteries are clamped and secured through vaginal route.
- Complications of laparoscopy may be due to the procedure itself or due to anaesthesia (see p. 586).
- The distending media commonly used in hysteroscopy is normal saline or glycine (1.5%).
- The contraindications (p. 589) of hysteroscopy are pelvic infection, pregnancy and active uterine bleeding. Complications include fluid overload, pulmonary oedema, and injury to genital or abdominal organs or electrosurgical injuries (p. 590).
- Hysteroscopic surgery should be done in the postmenstrual phase. Pretreatment with danazol or GnRH analogue for 4-6 weeks facilitate endometrial ablation or resection.

Practical Gynaecology

• Instruments
• Specimens
• Imaging studies : (X-ray, USG, CT, MRI plates)

36

INSTRUMENTS

Spatula and Cytobrush (Fig. 36.1)

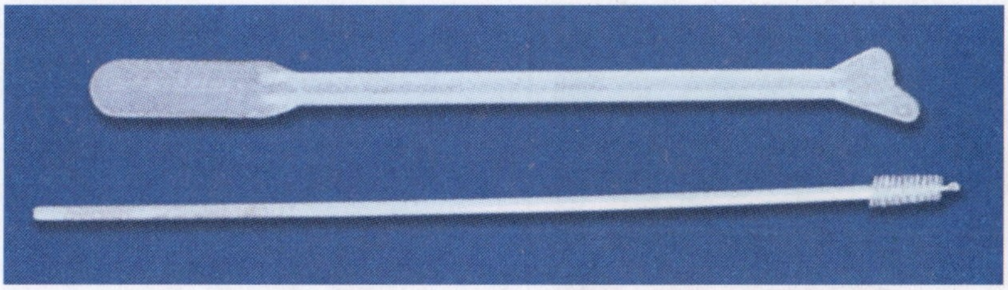

Fig. 36.1. Spatula (top) and Cytobrush (bottom)

Ayre's spatula (wooden or plastic) and the endocervical brush are used for collection of cells for cytology screening.

Uses

- For cervical cells — Projected end of the spatula goes within the external os. The spatula is rotated 360° to collect cells from the entire ectocervix [see Fig. 9.16(ii)].
- For endocervical cells — the cytobrush goes within the cervical canal and is rotated to collect cells [Fig. 9.16(iii)].
- For cytohormonal study (p. 107), the rounded end of the spatula is used [Fig. 9.16(i)].

Self-assessment : Methods of slide preparation and fixation : The material so collected is immediately spread over a slide. Fixative (95% ethyl alcohol) is spread over it. Once dried up, the slide is then stained (in the laboratory) either with Papanicolaou or Sorr's method. It is examined under the microscope by a cytopathologist.

Q. Who are the women (at risk), that they need cervical cytology screening?

Ans. • Any sexually active women over 18 years and upto 70 years of age.

• Others : (see p. 107).

Q. What is the grading of Papanicolaou's smear?

Ans. Gradings are total five : Normal, infective, suspicious, few malignant cells and plenty of malignant cells (p. 109).

Q. What is a dyskaryotic smear? What are the different types of dyskaryotic smear?

Ans. Dyskaryosis is the morphological abnormalities of the nucleus. Abnormalities may be nuclear enlargement in size and shape, irregularity in outline, multinucleation and hyperchromasia. Dyskaryotic smear may be : (i) Mild, (ii) Moderate and, (iii) Severe (p. 108).

Q. What is Koilocytosis?

Ans. It is the nuclear abnormalities observed in HPV infection. The typical changes are : Perinuclear halo, nuclear irregularity, hyperchromasia and multinucleation (Fig. 22.4).

Q. What is CIN? How do you diagnose CIN?

Ans. It is the histological observation where part or whole of thickness of cervical squamous epithelium is replaced by cells with varying degree of atypia. Basement membrane remains intact. Diagnosis of CIN is made by :

(i) Cytology, (ii) VIA, (iii) Colposcopy, (iv) Cervicography, (v) Biopsy and, (vi) Conisation of cervix (p. 312).

Q. How do you manage a case of CIN?

Ans. (a) Local ablative methods. (b) Excisional methods or by (c) Hysterectomy (p. 315, scheme 3).

Q. How to take cervical smear?

Ans. Cervix is exposed with a Cusco's bivalve speculum without any lubricant. Prior bimanual examination should not be done. Rest see p. 107.

Q. How HPV infection and CIN are related and how it could be prevented? **Ans.** p. 312, 315.

Sims' double bladed posterior vaginal speculum (Fig. 36.2)

The instrument was designed by Marion Sims. The blades are of unequal breadth. The use of one is dependent on the calibre of the vagina. It may be single bladed.

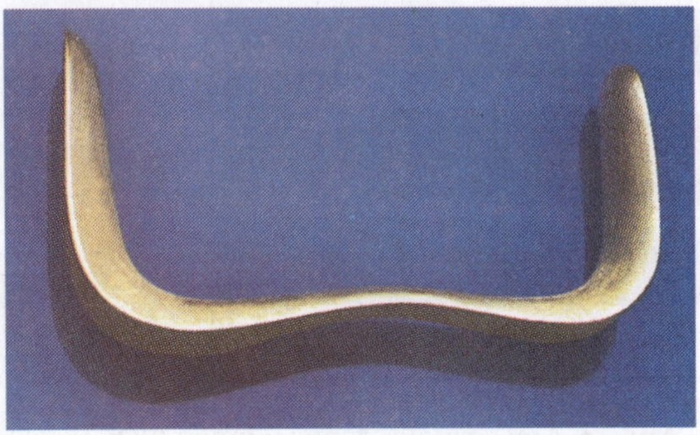

Fig. 36.2. Sims' speculum

Uses

- It is commonly used in vaginal operations such as D + C, D + E, anterior colporrhaphy, vaginal hysterectomy, etc. to retract the posterior vaginal wall.
- To visualise the cervix and inspect the abnormalities in the anterior vaginal wall like cystocele, VVF or Gartner's cyst after placing the patient in Sims' position.
- To collect the materials from the vaginal pool for cytology or Gram stain and culture.

Self–assessment

- Sims' position (p. 99).
- Sims' triad (p. 406).
- Introduction of Sims' speculum (p. 100).
- Why the blades are of unequal sizes?
- Lesions in the anterior vaginal wall.
- Indications of D + C (p. 557).
- Steps of D + C (p. 557).

Cusco's bivalve self-retaining vaginal speculum (Fig. 36.3)

The valves are to retract the anterior and posterior vaginal wall so as to have a good look to the cervix.

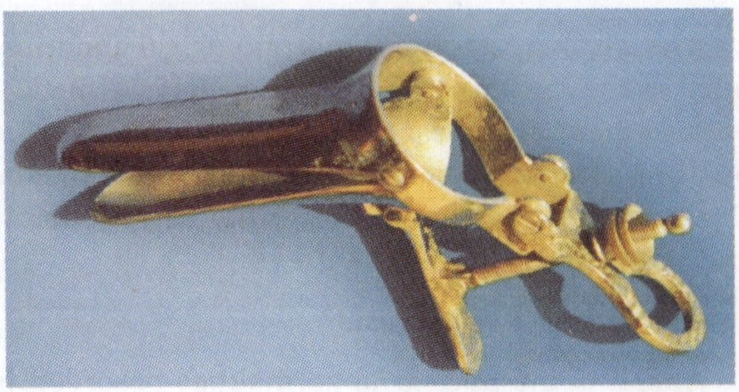

Fig. 36.3. Cusco's speculum

A light source from behind is essential. It is commonly used in the OPD.

Uses

- To visualise the cervix and vaginal fornices.
- To collect vaginal pool materials and cervical smear for cytologic screening (p. 101).
- To have cervicovaginal swabs for Gram stain and culture.
- To insert or to remove IUCD or to check the threads.
- To perform minor operations like punch biopsy, surface cauterisation or snipping a small polyp.

Self–assessment

- Use of two blades (see above).

- Lesions in the cervix (p. 163, 257, 309, 327).
- Ectopy (erosion) cervix (p. 257)
- Procedures to take materials for Pap stain (p. 106).
- Pap's gradings (p. 109).
- Polyps (p. 280).

Q. *What is cervical ectopy?*

Ans. It is the replacement of squamous epithelium of the ectocervix by columnar epithelium of endocervix by the process of metaplasia. (See p. 257).

Q. *What are the different types of Polyps?*

Ans. Polyps may be Benign (Mucous, Fibroid or Placental) or Malignant. It may be sessile or pedunculated. See p. 274.

Auvard's self-retaining posterior vaginal speculum (Fig. 36.4)

Uses

- It is used as posterior vaginal wall retractor in operations like anterior colporrhaphy, vaginal hysterectomy, etc.
- It should be used only when the operation is done under general or regional anaesthesia as the instrument is heavy. It requires no assistant.
  (Prolonged use may cause perineal pain in the postoperative period).

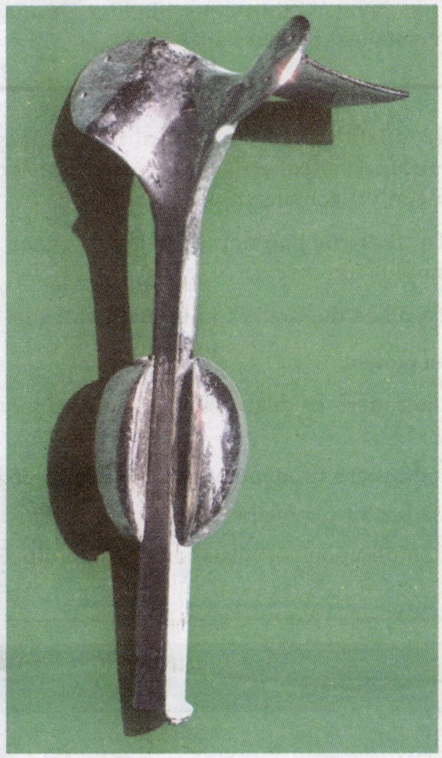

Fig. 36.4. Auvard's speculum

Female rubber catheter (Fig. 36.5)

Uses

- To empty the bladder in retention of urine.
- To administer oxygen.
- To use as a tourniquet in myomectomy operation as an alternative to myomectomy clamp.

Self-assessment

- Causes of retention of urine (p. 393).
- Procedures of catheterisation (p. 105).

Q. *What are the causes of acute and chronic retention of urine?*

Ans. (i) Postoperative (common), (ii) Obstructive, (iii) Failure of detrusor contraction, (iv) External sphincter spasm and, (v) Others (see p. 393).

Q. *What are the different causes of urinary incontinence?* **Ans.** See page 382.

Q. *What are the different menstrual abnormalities that can manifest with retention of urine? See p. 394 Table 24.8.*

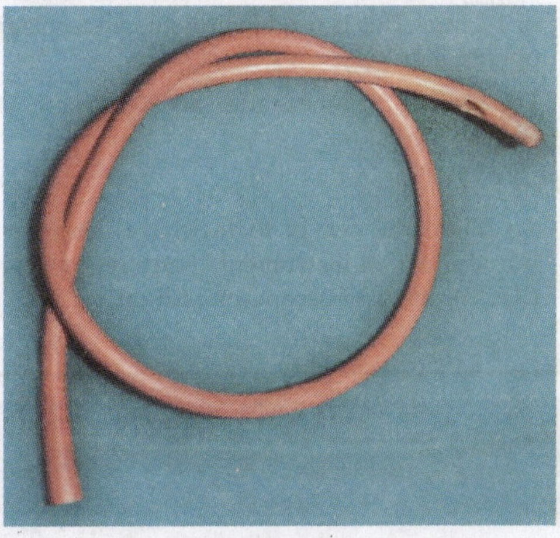

Fig. 36.5. Female rubber catheter

Ans. (i) Primary amenorrhoea (cryptomenorrhoea) → Haematocolpos (see p. 431).

(ii) Secondary amenorrhoea → Retroverted gravid uterus (see p. 394).

(iii) Menorrhagia → Impacted uterine fibroid in the POD (see p. 267).

(iv) Irregular bleeding and pain → pelvic haematocele, pelvic abscess (see p. 171).

(v) No menstrual abnormality → Impacted ovarian tumour, cervical fibroid or ovarian mass.

Female metal catheter (Fig. 36.6)

Uses

- To empty the bladder prior to major vaginal operations. Not only it facilitates the operation but minimises the injury to the bladder.
- To confirm the diagnosis of Gartner's cyst from cystocele (see p. 196).
- It is not used in obstetrics to avoid trauma.

Use in PFR (see p. 210)

- To empty the bladder prior to the operation.
- To note the lower limit of the bladder before making the incision on the vagina.
- Prior to cutting the vesicocervical ligament.
- At the end of the operation to make sure about absence of any injury.

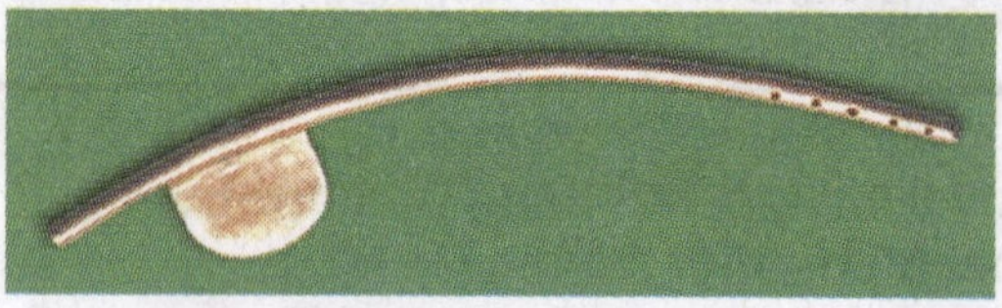

Fig. 36.6. Female metal catheter

Self-assessment

- Length of female urethra (see p. 13).
- Differentiation of Gartner's cyst from cystocele (p. 204).
- Management of injury to bladder during operation : Bladder mucosa is apposed with 3-0 delayed absorbable suture (Vicryl) as a continuous layer. A second layer of (musculofascial) suture with the same material is used to reinforce the first layer. Continuous bladder drainage is maintained for ten days.

Cervical dilators (Figs. 36.7 and 36.8)

Varieties

- Hawkin–Ambler — There are 16 sets starting from 3/6 and ends with 18/21 (Fig. 36.7).
- Hegar's — There are 12 sets, the smallest one is of 1-2 mm. This is used mainly in gynaecological operations.
- Das's dilator (named after Sir Kedarnath Das) (Fig. 36.8).

Uses

- To dilate the cervix to facilitate intrauterine introduction of instruments (curette) or devices (IUCD) or hysteroscope or radium.
- To dilate the cervix to facilitate drainage of intrauterine collection — pyometra, haematometra or lochiometra (p. 165, 431).
- To confirm patency of cervical canal after amputation cervix.
- To dilate the urethra in urethral stricture.

Self-assessment

- Indications of dilatation of the cervix only (p. 557).
- Indications of amputation of cervix (p. 563).
- Causes of pyometra (p. 165).
- Complications of dilatation operation (p. 558).

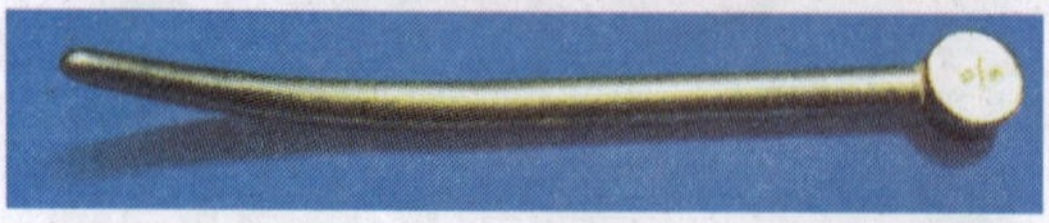

Fig. 36.7. Hawkin–Ambler dilator

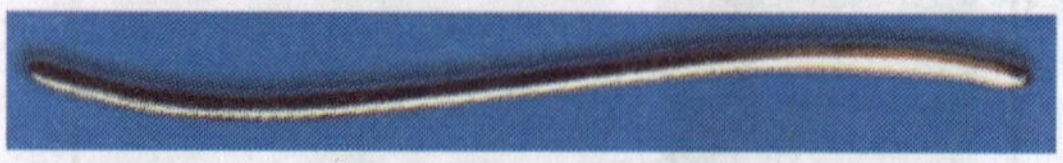

Fig. 36.8. Das's dilator

Multiple toothed vulsellum (Fig. 36.9)

Uses

- To hold the parous cervical lip in operations like D + C, anterior colporrhaphy or vaginal hysterectomy.

Its function is to make the cervix steady by traction.

- To remove a polyp by twisting as an alternative to Lane's tissue forceps
- To hold the fundus of the uterus and to give traction while the clamps are placed in operation of total abdominal hysterectomy for benign lesion.

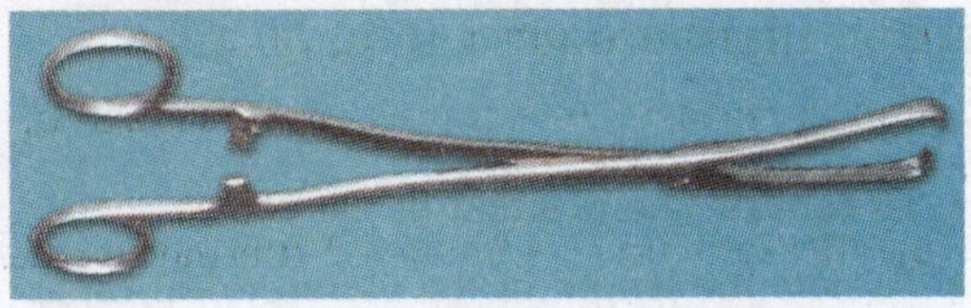

Fig. 36.9. Multiple toothed vulsellum

Cervical lip to be held

Usually the anterior lip is held but in some conditions, the posterior lip is to be held. Such conditions are :

- In amputation cervix or vaginal hysterectomy when the posterior cervicovaginal mucous membrane is cut. (see p. 211, 563)
- Posterior colpotomy for drainage of pus or vaginal ligation (p. 172).
- Growth in the anterior lip.
- Culdocentesis (p. 116).

Single toothed vulsellum (Fig. 36.10)

Uses

- To hold the cervix after opening the vault of vagina and to give traction while the remaining vault is being cut in total abdominal hysterectomy (p. 567).
- To hold the new cervical stump after amputation of the cervix and Fothergill's operation (p. 210, 563).
- To hold the cervical stump left after subtotal hysterectomy (p. 564).
- Sometimes to hold the anterior lip of nulliparous cervix in operation of D + C. (Allis' tissue forceps preferred).

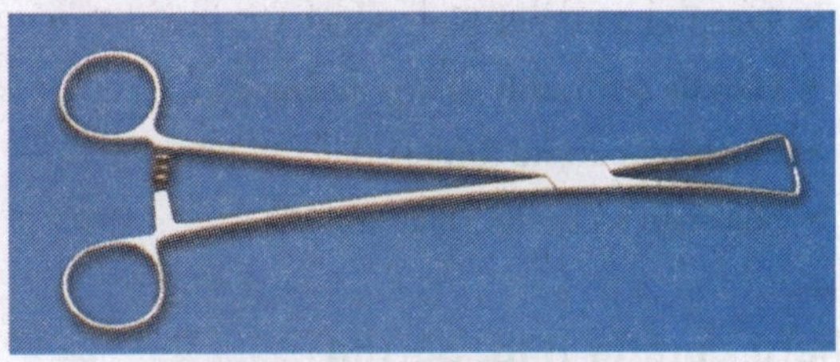

Fig. 36.10. Single toothed vulsellum

Self-assessment

- Indications of amputation cervix (p. 563).
- Indications of subtotal hysterectomy (p. 564).
- Common indications of abdominal hysterectomy (p. 564).
- Indications of vaginal hysterectomy (p. 211).
- Indications of Fothergill's operation (p. 210).
- Principal steps of Fothergill's operation (p. 210).
- Complications of Fothergill's operation (p. 216, Table 15.3).
- Causes of pelvic abscess (p. 171)

Anterior vaginal wall retractor (Fig. 36.11)

Use

- To retract the sagging anterior vaginal wall to have a good look on the cervix while retracting the posterior vaginal wall by the Sims' speculum.

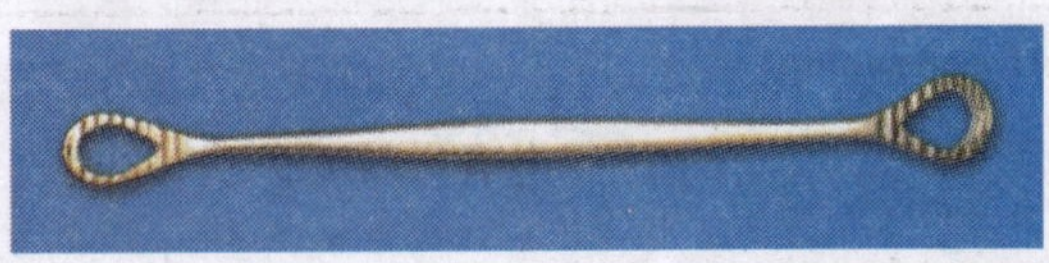

Fig. 36.11. Anterior vaginal wall retractor

Olive pointed malleable graduated metallic uterine sound (Fig. 36.12)

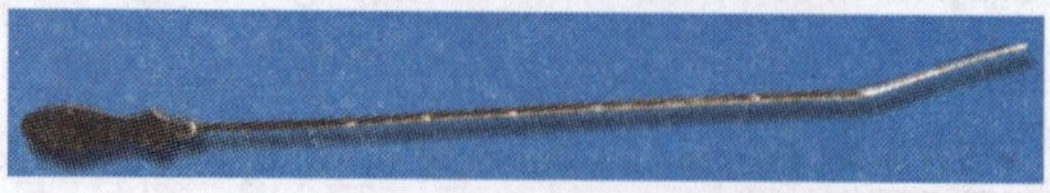

Fig. 36.12. Olive pointed malleable graduated metallic uterine sound

Uses

- To confirm the position of the uterus.
- To note the length of the uterocervical canal.
- It acts as a first dilator.
- To sound the uterine cavity in a case of IUCD with missing threads.
- To differentiate a polyp from inversion.

Self-assessment

- Normal position of the uterus and length of the uterocervical canal (p. 7).
- Conditions where the length of the uterocervical canal is increased : Fibroid uterus, elongation of cervix, endometrial carcinoma.
- Causes of elongation of the cervix (p. 260).
- Management of uterine perforation (p. 558).

Uterine curette (Fig. 36.13)

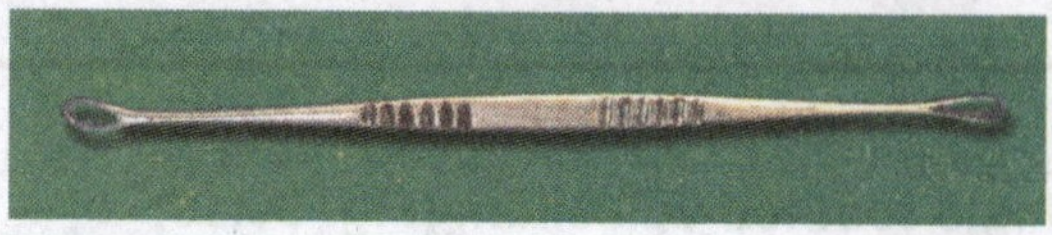

Fig. 36.13A. Sharp at one end, blunt at the other end

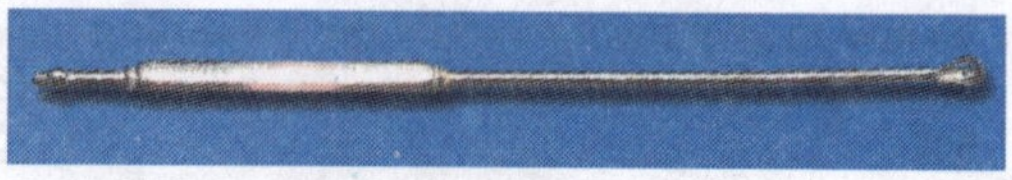

Fig. 36.13B. Flushing curette

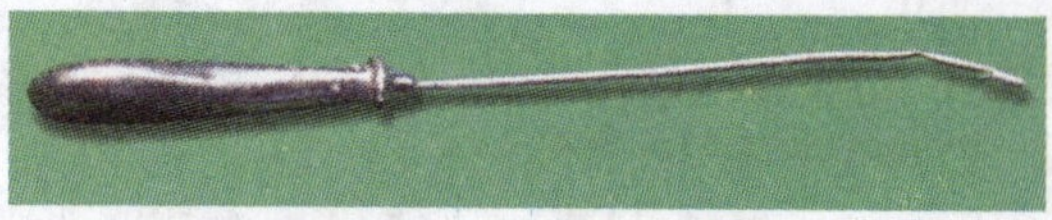

Fig. 36.13C. Sharman's curette

Fig. 36.13. Uterine curette

Types

- Sharp at one end, blunt at the other (Fig. 36.13A).
- Sharp or blunt at both ends.
- Handle with only sharp at one end.
- Flushing curette (blunt) (Fig. 36.13B).
- Sharman's curette (Fig. 36.13C).

Uses

Sharp curette (Fig. 36.13A)

- Infertility (p. 229).
- DUB (p. 183).
- TB endometritis (p. 135).

Blunt curette

- Suspected choriocarcinoma (p. 349).
- Suspected endometrial carcinoma (p. 344).

Flushing curette (Fig. 36.13B)

- Following D + E.

Sharman's curette (Fig. 36.13C)

- Infertility work up, where only a strip of endometrium is enough to study the hormonal reflection. It is done as an outpatient procedure and without anaesthesia.

Self-assessment

Q. *What is the purpose of doing endometrial biopsy in a woman with infertility?*

Ans. To detect evidence of ovulation — by seeing the secretary changes in the endometrium (see p. 87).

Q. *Which day of the menstrual cycle endometrial biopsy is usually done?*

Ans. Biopsy should be done on D21-D23 when the cycle is regular. When the cycles are irregular, it is done within 24 hours of the mens.

Q. *In the endometrial biopsy, what is the earliest evidence of ovulation?*

Ans. Subnuclear vacuolation is the earliest evidence appearing within 36-48 hours of ovulation (see page 88).

Q. What are the other methods of diagnosis of ovulation?

Ans. BBT, cervical mucous study, vaginal cytology, serum progesterone, serum LH and oestradiol, sonography and laparoscopy (see p. 228).

Q. What are the ovarian causes of infertility? See p. 222.

Ans. Anovulation, LPD and LUF.

Uterine dressing forceps (Fig. 36.14)

The instrument is often confused with laminaria tent introducing forceps. The blades are transversely serrated while in the latter, there is a groove on either blade.

Uses

- To swab the uterine cavity following D+E operation with a small gauze piece.
- To dilate the cervix in lochiometra or pyometra.
- To plug the uterine cavity with gauze twigs in continued bleeding after removal of polyp.

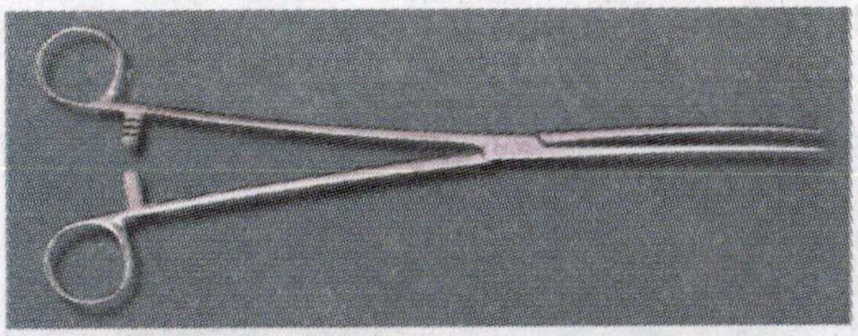

Fig. 36.14. Uterine dressing forceps

Self-assessment

- Causes of pyometra (p. 165).
- Polyps (p. 274).

Sponge holding forceps (Fig. 36.15)

Uses

- Antiseptic dressing before any abdominal or vaginal operation.
- To clean the vagina with gauze pieces before and after vaginal operations.
- To hold the cervix in circlage operation during pregnancy.

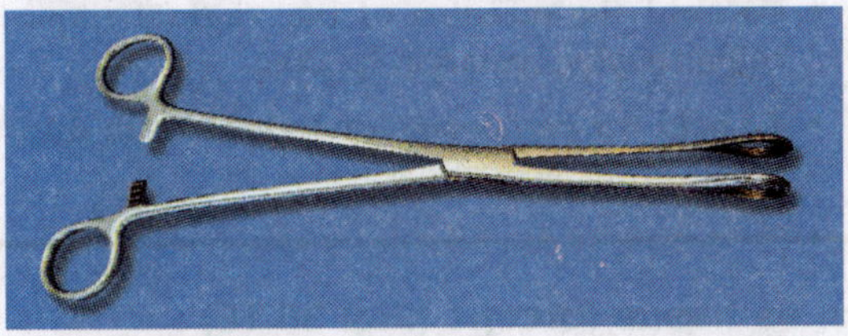

Fig. 36.15. Sponge holding forceps

Self-assessment

Q. Name a few common abdominal operations.

Ans. Abdominal hysterectomy (p. 564), myomectomy (p. 574), ovariotomy (p. 570).

Q. Name a few common vaginal operations.

Ans. PFR (p. 210), vaginal hysterectomy (p. 211), Fothergill's operation (p. 210).

Ovum forceps (Fig. 36.16)

It is often confused with sponge holding forceps but it has no catch. As such, it minimises trauma to the uterine wall if accidentally caught and also it has got no crushing effect on the conceptus.

Uses

- To remove the products of conception in D and E after its separation partially or completely.
- To remove molar tissue in hydatidiform mole.
- To remove uterine polyp (small).

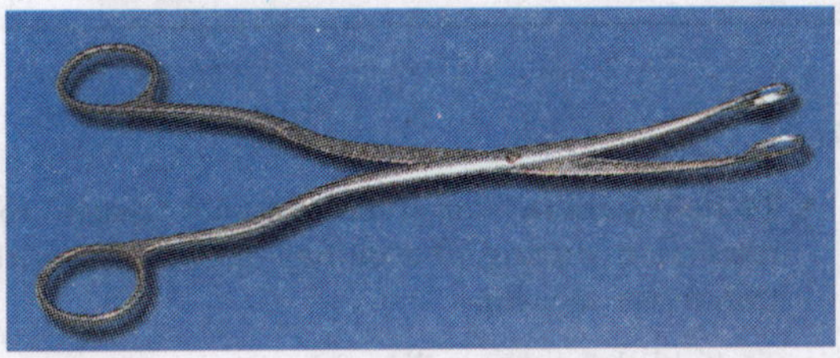

Fig. 36.16. Ovum forceps

Methods

The cervical canal is dilated first. The instrument is introduced with the blades closed and opened inside the cavity. The products are caught and then with twisting movements and simultaneous traction, the products are removed.

Dangers

It may produce injury to the uterine wall to the extent of even perforation. Not infrequently, a segment of intestine or omentum may even be pulled out through the rent.

Allis tissue forceps (Fig. 36.17)

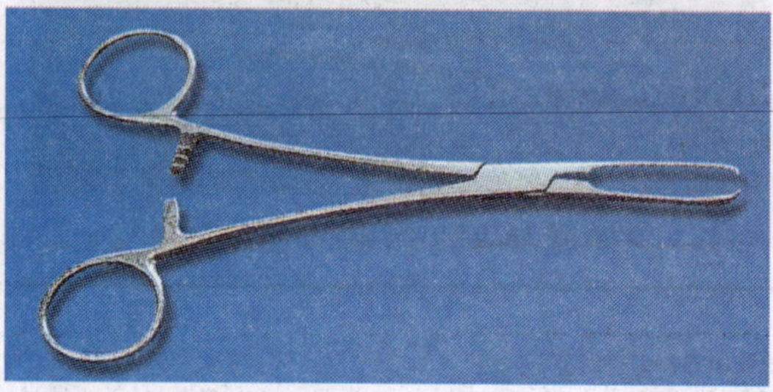

Fig. 36.17. Allis tissue forceps

Uses

- To hold the margins of the vaginal flaps in colporrhaphy operation (p. 206).
- To hold the peritoneum or rectus sheath during repair of the abdominal wall.
- To hold the margins of the vagina in abdominal hysterectomy (p. 564).
- To hold the anterior lip of the cervix in D and C operation (p. 557).
- To catch the torn ends of the sphincter ani externus in CPT repair (p. 413).
- To remove a small polyp.
- To take out the tissue in wedge biopsy (p. 560).
- **Q.** ***What are the common symptoms associated with genital prolapse?***

Ans. Woman may remain asymptomatic if the prolapse is mild. The common symptoms are : genital organs protruding out of the vaginal opening, difficulties in walking, sitting, urination or defecation. Prolapse may interfere with sexual intercourse or may cause vaginal bleeding due to ulceration of mucosa. It may cause incontinence of urine, pelvic pressure or backache (p. 202).

Lanes tissue forceps (Fig. 36.18)

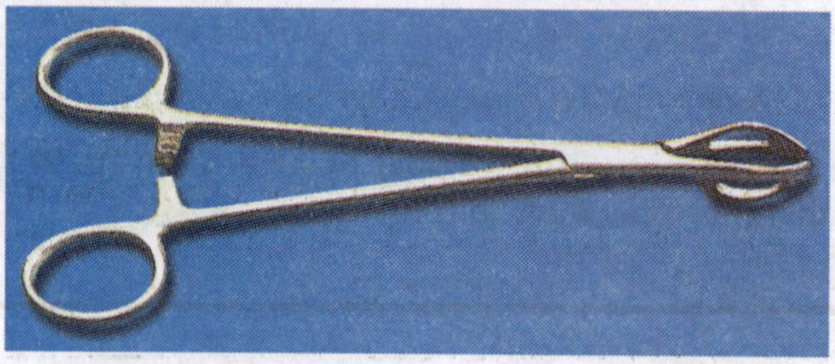

Fig. 36.18. Lanes tissue forceps

Uses

- To hold parietal wall (bulk of tough tissues) for retraction during abdominal operations with transverse incision.
- To hold the polyp or fibroid in polypectomy or myomectomy operation.
- To hold the towel during draping.

Uterus holding forceps (Fig. 36.19)

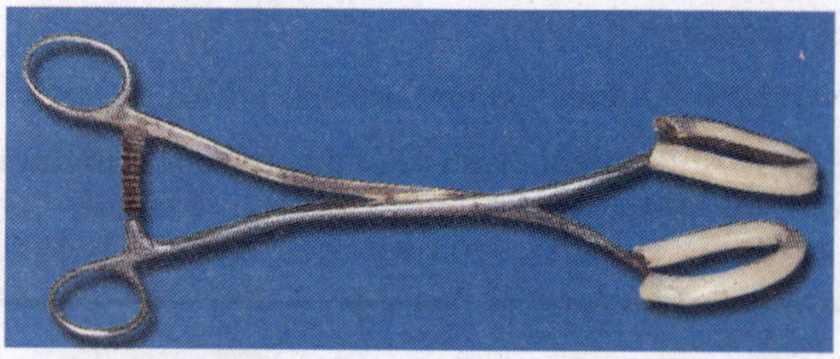

Fig. 36.19. Uterus holding forceps

The blades are protected with rubber tubes to minimise trauma to the uterus.

Uses

- To fix and steady the uterus when conservative surgery is done on the adnexae (tuboplasty page 240).
- What are the different surgical procedures for proximal and distal tubal disease? p. 240.

Cervical occlusion clamp (Fig. 36.20)

The blades are guarded with rubber tubes to avoid trauma to tissues.

Uses

Evaluation of tubal patency during laparotomy (following tuboplasty). Cervix is occluded with the instrument and methylene blue dye is injected into the uterine cavity through the fundus using a syringe and a needle.

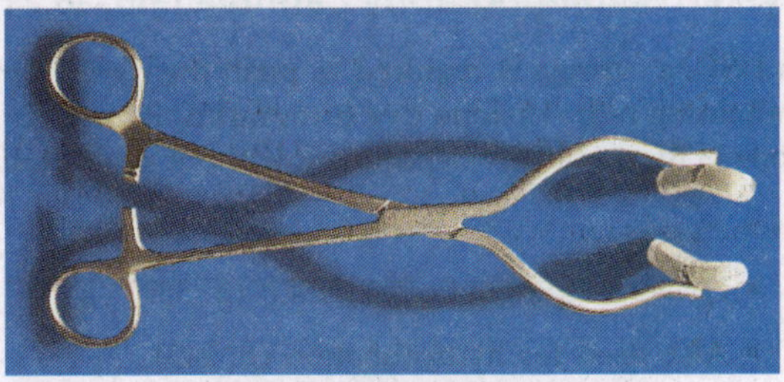

Fig. 36.20. Cervical occlusion clamp

Self-assessment

- Different methods to assess tubal patency (p. 230).
- Different types of tubal reconstructive surgery (p. 240)

Myoma screw (Fig. 36.21)

Uses

- To fix the myoma after the capsule is cut open and to give traction while the myoma is enucleated out of its bed (myomectomy).
- To give traction in a big uterus (multiple fibroid) requiring hysterectomy while the clamps are placed.

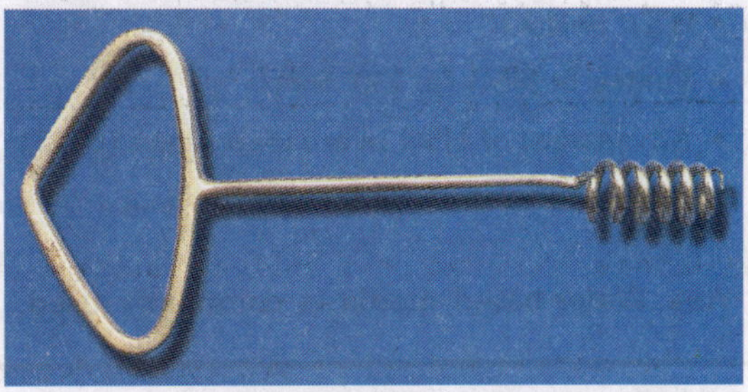

Fig. 36.21. Myoma screw

Self-assessment

- Steps of myomectomy (p. 574)
- Complications of myomectomy (p. 575)
- Important considerations before myomectomy (p. 272)

Bonney's myomectomy clamp (Fig. 36.22)

Uses

- The clamp is used in myomectomy operation. It curtails the blood supply to the uterus temporarily, thereby minimising the blood loss during operation. Simultaneous, bilateral clamping of the infundibulopelvic ligaments by rubber guarded sponge holding forceps may be employed.
- The instrument is placed at the level of internal os with the concavity fitting with the convexity of the symphysis pubis. The round ligaments of both sides are included inside the clamp to prevent slipping of the instrument and preventing the uterus from falling back. The clamp is removed after suturing the myoma bed but before closing the peritoneal layers.
- It is seldom used nowadays and is being replaced by preoperative use of GnRH analogue (p. 500), and/or intraoperative use of tourniquates (p. 574), vasoconstrictive agents (vasopressin) (p. 574) and others (p. 574).

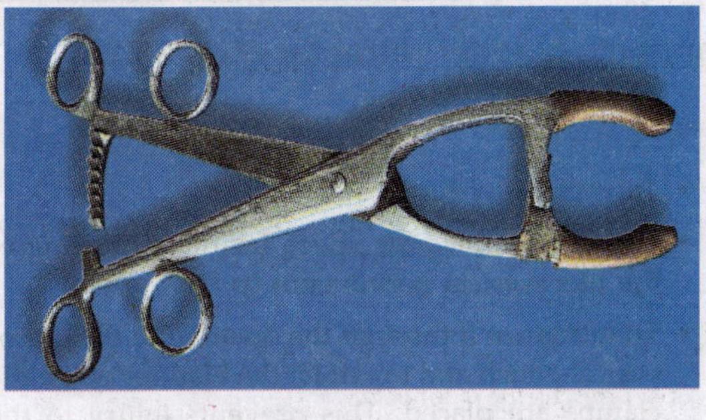

Fig. 36.22. Bonney's myomectomy clamp

Hysterosalpingography cannula (Fig. 36.23)

In HSG, a syringe is required to push the dye. Iodine containing radio-opaque dye (urograffin) is used. It is done in the radiology department without anaesthesia.

Uses

- Hysterosalpingography (HSG) (p. 559).
- Also used for hydrotubation (p. 243).

Hydrotubation — Medicated solution is pushed transcervically in conditions such as following tuboplasty operation or suspected flimsy fimbrial adhesions. The drugs instilled are dexamethasone 4 mg with gentamicin 80 mg in 10 ml normal saline. It should be instilled in the proliferative phase for at least 3 cycles (see p. 243).

Self-assessment

- What is HSG?
- Timing of HSG (p. 230, 560).
- Advantages of HSG over laparoscopy (p. 231).

Q. *How do you compare the oil-based versus water-based media used in HSG?*

Ans. Water-based media is commonly used. It causes less cramping pain and discomfort. Oil-based media gives better image and has higher pregnancy rates. Granuloma is more with oil-based media. Embolisation is minimal with either media (p. 560).

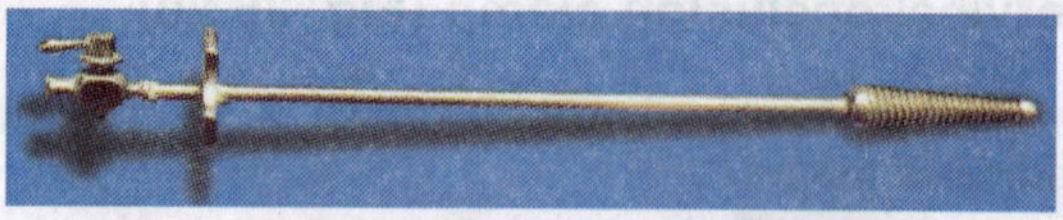

Fig. 36.23. Hysterosalpingographic cannula

Q. *What are the indications of HSG?*

Ans. See p. 559.

Q. *Advantages of laparoscopy over HSG.*

Ans. See p. 231.

Q. *What are the complication of HSG?*

Ans. See p. 560.

Q. *What are the other alternatives to HSG?* (p. 234).

Diagnostic laparoscopy and dye test; sonohysterosalpingography and insufflation test (p. 230 and p. 560).

Q. *What is sonohysterosalpingography?*

Ans. See p. 231.

Kocher's artery forceps (Fig. 36.24)

Use

- To use as a clamp in hysterectomy operation.

Self-assessment

- What added advantage it has got?

  Due to the presence of tooth, it gives a firm grip to the pedicle hold.
- Indications abdominal of hysterectomy (p. 564).
- Mention the different sites where the clamps are placed in total abdominal hysterectomy (p. 565).

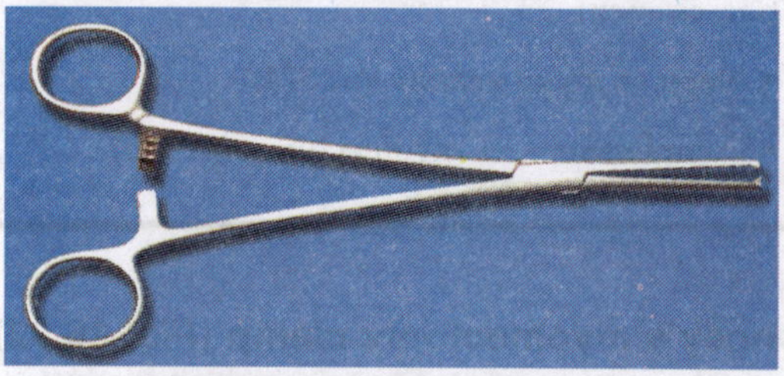

Fig. 36.24. Kocher's artery forceps

- Principal steps of Fothergill's operation (p. 210).
- Complications of Fothergill's (p. 216, Table 15.3).

Landon's bladder retractor (Fig. 36.25)

Uses

- In vaginal hysterectomy.
- To keep the bladder up, to facilitate opening of the uterovesical peritoneum (p. 207).
- To introduce it through the opening of the uterovesical pouch and to retract the bladder while the clamps are placed. This prevents injury to the bladder (p. 211).

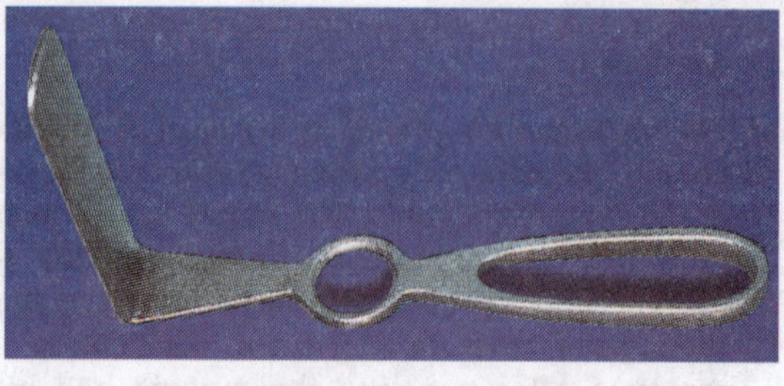

Fig. 36.25. Landon's retractor

- To inspect the suture lines after completion of vaginal plastic operations by retracting the anterior or posterior vaginal wall.
- Intravaginal plugging can be done under its guidance.
- To use as lateral vaginal wall retractor.

Self-assessment

- What are the non-surgical treatments of prolapse?

Ans. Conservative treatments include : (i) to avoid aggravating factors (obesity, chronic cough, constipation) p. 198. (ii) Pelvic floor exercise. (iii) Oestrogen replacement therapy. (iv) Pessary in some cases (p. 205).

- Mention the different sites where the clamps placed during vaginal hysterectomy (p. 210).
- Important postoperative complications following vaginal hysterectomy with PFR (p. 216).

Insufflation cannula (Fig. 36.26)

The instrument is not complete. It requires a 'Y' rubber tube. The one end is attached to a bulb and the other end to a manometer.

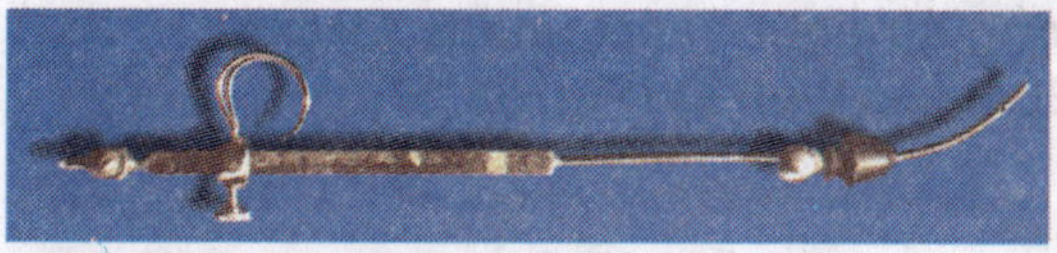

Fig. 36.26. Insufflation cannula

Use

- To know the patency of the tube in infertility investigation or following tuboplasty.

Self-assessment

- Ideal time of operation (p. 230).
- Complications (p. 559).
- Advantages of HSG over D and I (p. 560).

Abdominal retractors (Figs. 36.27A to C)

Retractors are used to retract tissues out of the operative field. This is needed for better exposure during surgery. Retractors are held in place either by an assistant (manual retractor) or by counter pressure with some device (self-retaining retractor). Manual retractor can be used alone or in combination with a self-retaining retractor.

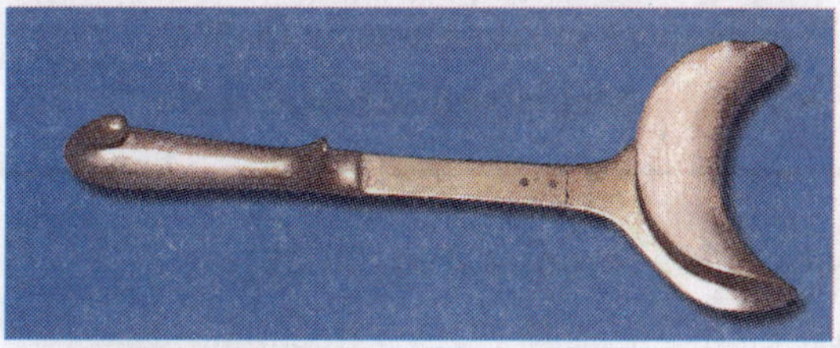

Fig. 36.27A. Doyen's retractor

Doyen's retractor (Fig. 36.27A)

Use

- To retract the abdominal wall in abdominal pelvic surgery to expose the field of operation.
- As an alternative, self-retaining retractor may be used.

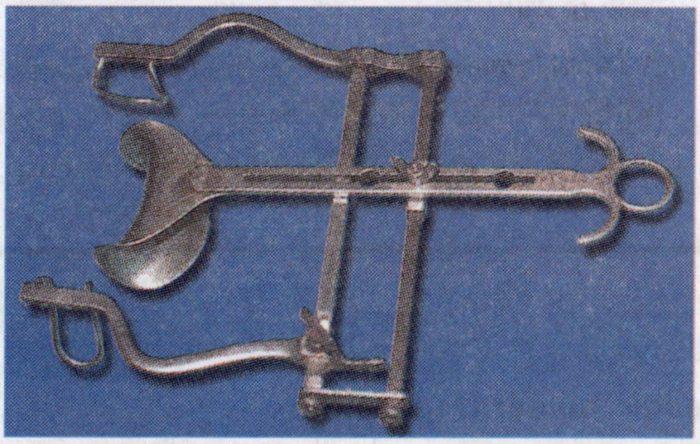

Fig. 36.27B. Balfour self-retaining retractor

Balfour self-retaining retractor (Fig. 36.27B)

Two lateral blades and an additional (third) blade. All the blades are detachable and may be of different sizes.

Use

- To retract the abdominal wall all around.
- To expose the field of operation widely (No assistant is needed for manual retraction).

Deaver's retractor (Fig. 36.27C)

It is a manual retractor either used alone or in combination with a self-retaining one. It has got different sizes.

Uses

- It is used in abdominal operation to retract the viscera as and when required in order to facilitate the operative procedures like abdominal hysterectomy. For that purpose, it may also be used as a lateral retractor.
- To retract the parietal wall during abdomino-pelvic surgery (hysterectomy).
- To retract the bladder and intestines during the surgery.

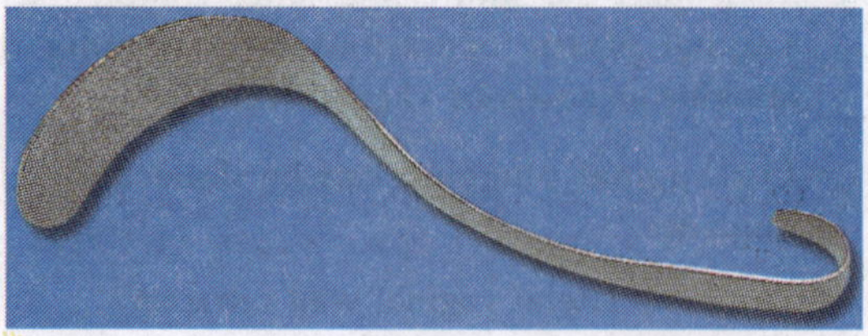

Fig. 36.27C. Deaver's retractor

Long straight haemostatic forceps (Spencer Well's) (Fig. 36.28)

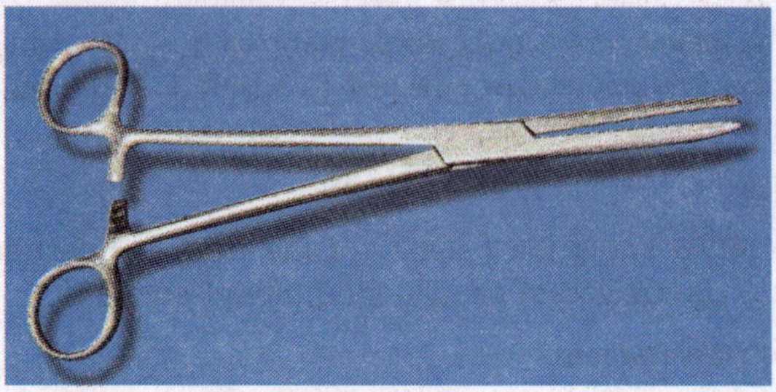

Fig. 36.28. Long straight haemostatic forceps

Uses

- It is used as a clamp in hysterectomy, salpingectomy or salpingo-oophorectomy operation.
- To catch a bleeding vessel for haemostasis deep into the pelvis.

Self-assessment

- Pedicles hold in total abdominal hysterectomy.
- Indications of salpingectomy (p. 572).
- Pedicles hold in vaginal hysterectomy.
- Pedicles hold during salpingo-oophorectomy (p. 565). [Fig. 34.4(1), p. 566].
- Complications of abdominal hysterectomy (p.568).

Babcock's forceps (Fig. 36.29)

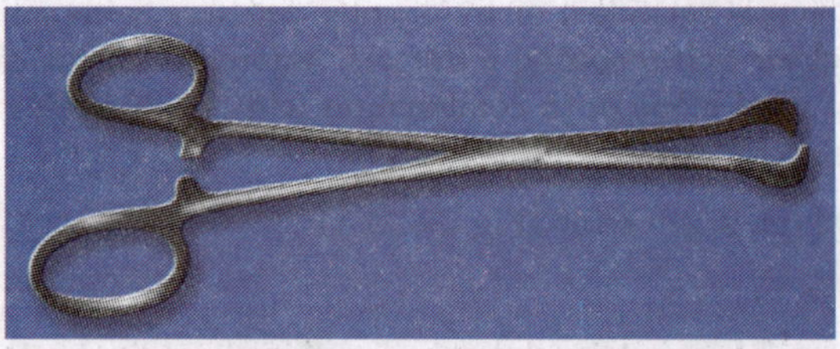

Fig. 36.29. Babcock's forceps

Uses

- To hold the Fallopian tube in tuboplasty operation (see p. 240).
- To hold lymph glands during dissection in radical hysterectomy (lymphadenectomy p. 576).
- To hold the appendix during appendicectomy.

Needle holder (Fig. 36.30)

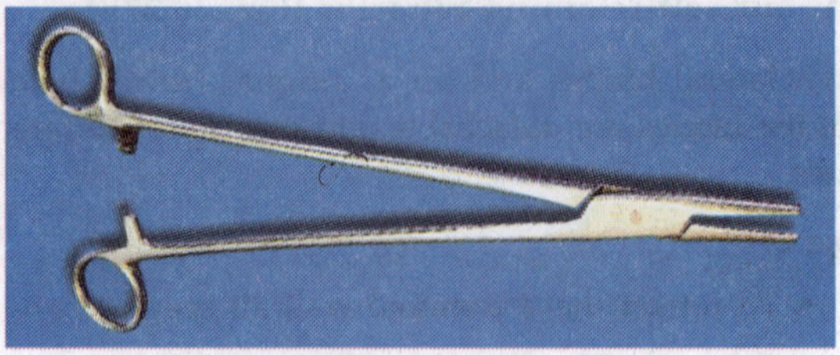

Fig. 36.30. Needle holder

Uses

- It may be straight or curved.
- To catch-hold the needle. The needle should be caught at the junction of anterior 2/3rd and posterior 1/3rd.

Barkelay Bonney vaginal clamp (Fig. 36.31)

Use

- To occlude the vaginal canal prior to cutting the vagina in Wertheim's hysterectomy (p. 576).

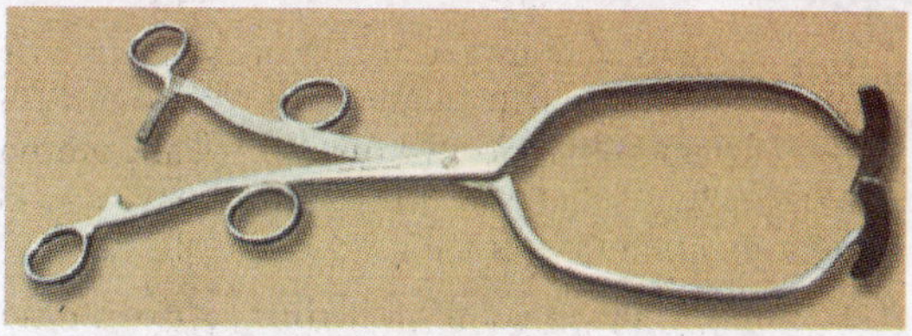

Fig. 36.31. Barkelay Bonney vaginal clamp

Punch biopsy forceps (Fig. 36.32)

Uses

- To take biopsy from the cervix.
- The biopsy is taken as an outdoor procedure without anaesthesia. The site of biopsy is either from the suspected area or Schiller's iodine or colposcopic directed.

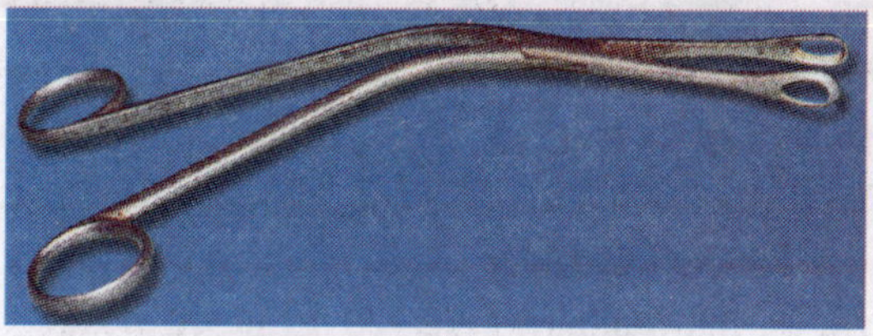

Fig. 36.32. Punch biopsy forceps

Self-assessment

- Mention the different types of cervical biopsy (p. 560).
- Procedure of sending the material for histology (p. 561).
- Schiller's test (p. 314).
- VIA (p. 313).
- Histology of carcinoma cervix (p. 328).
- Early diagnosis of carcinoma cervix (p. 331).
- Complications of cervical biopsy (p. 561).
- Complications of cone biopsy (p. 561).

Dissecting forceps (Figs 36.33 and 36.34)

Toothed

Use

- To hold tough structures like rectus sheath, cut margins of vaginal vault or margins of vaginal flaps in PFR or the skin margins during suturing.

Plain or non-toothed

Use

- To hold soft tissues like peritoneal margins during suturing.

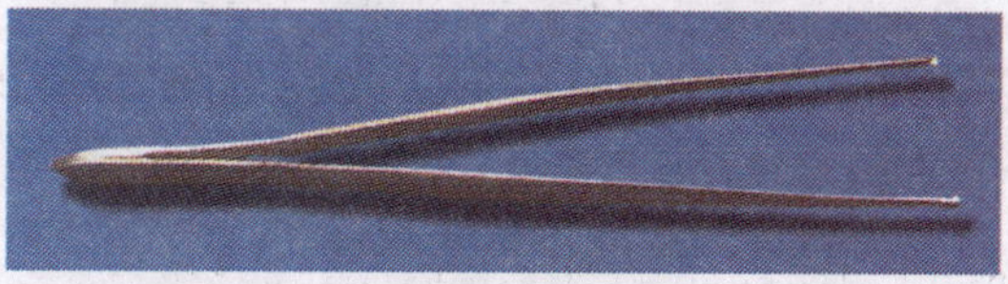

Fig. 36.33. Toothed dissecting forceps

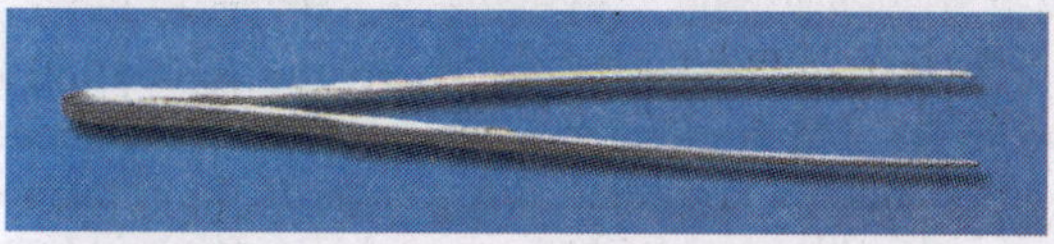

Fig. 36.34. Non-toothed dissecting forceps

Scalpel (Fig. 36.35)

The instrument is detachable — handle and blade.

Uses

- To cut the abdominal wall — skin, subcutaneous tissue, rectus sheath and opening the peritoneum.
- To cut the mucous coat in vaginal plastic operation and to cut tissues during surgery.
- To cut pedicles during hysterectomy.

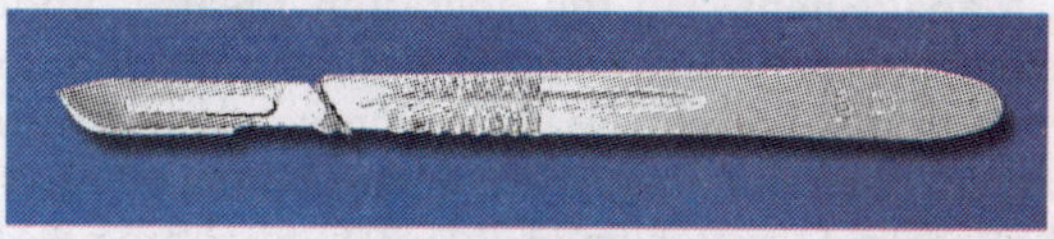

Fig. 36.35. Scalpel

Needles

Round bodied (curved)

It is used while suturing soft structures like :

- Peritonisation, suturing muscles.
- Suturing the pedicles in hysterectomy.
- Suturing the pubocervical fascia.
- Tubectomy or salpingectomy.

Cutting (Curved)

It is used while suturing tough structures like :

- Suturing the vaginal margins in PFR (p. 207).
- Closure of the vaginal vault in abdominal hysterectomy (p. 567).
- Repair of the rectus sheath.
- Suturing the skin.

Scissors (Figs 36.36 to 36.39)

Mayo's type — (Fig. 36.36)

This is used in almost every operation requiring tissue dissection and excision.

Bent on flat (Bonney) type — (Fig. 36.37)

This is used conveniently in anterior colporrhaphy to dissect the vesicovaginal space and also for tissue dissection.

Metzenbaum — (Fig. 36.38)

This is used for tissue dissection.

Perineorrhaphy — (Fig. 36.39)

It is comfortably used in perineorrhaphy operation; also used in episiotomy.

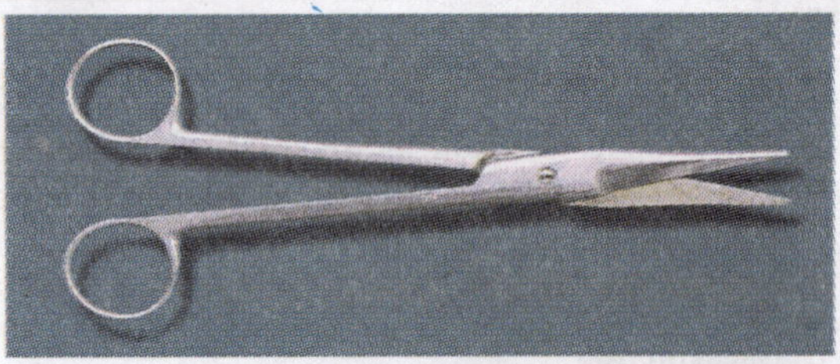

Fig. 36.36. Scissors (Mayo's type)

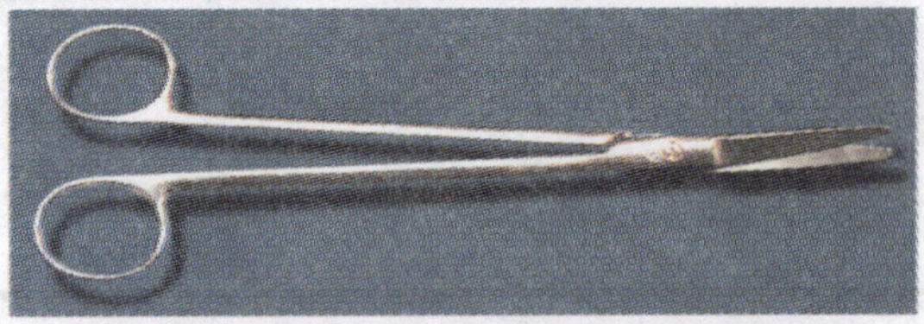

Fig. 36.37. Scissors (Bonney) — bent on flat type

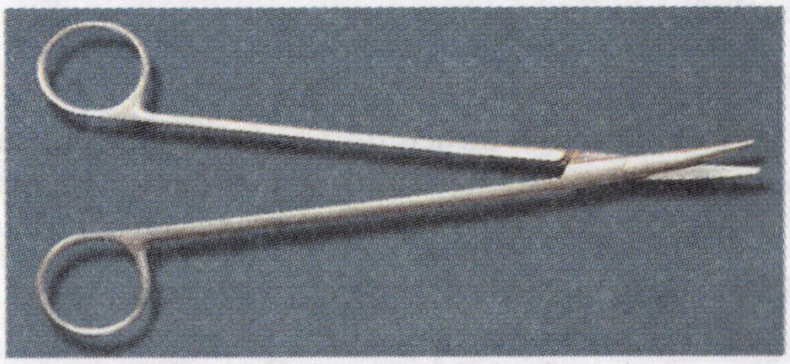

Fig. 36.38. Scissors (Metzenbaum)

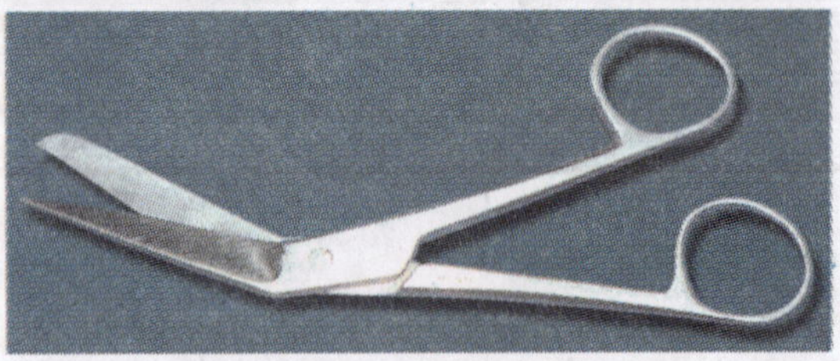

Fig. 36.39. Scissors (Perineorrhaphy)

Self-assessment :

- Indications of perineorrhaphy (p. 205).
- Indications of PFR (p. 205).
- Complications of PFR (p. 216).
- Principal steps of perineorrhaphy, PFR, CPT repair (p. 210, 413).
- Complications in abdominal wound (p. 568).

Ans. Wound dehiscence : When the separation of the layers of abdominal wound is upto the peritoneum — it is called a complete dehiscence. If the intestines come out of the wound, it is called **evisceration or burst abdomen**.

Burst abdomen usually occurs between seven and ten days of the operation. Predisposing factors are malnutrition, infection, cough due to chronic lung disease or abdominal distension.

Management : In the operation theatre, under general anaesthesia, necrotic tissues and clots are removed. The bowel is cleansed thoroughly with warm normal saline and placed back in the abdominal cavity. Through and through nylon (No. 2) sutures are passed 2 cm apart and about 3 cm from the skin margins to close the wound. Sutures are left in place for three weeks. Antibiotic (broad spectrum) is started and modified according to the culture and sensitivity report. Predisposing factors are to be taken care of.

Towel clips (Fig. 36.40)

Use

- These are used in draping the operative area—abdominal or vaginal. The towels or sheets are fixed to the skin and each other with these clips.

Self-assessment :

- Antiseptic preparations in abdominal or vaginal operation in operation table prior to draping.

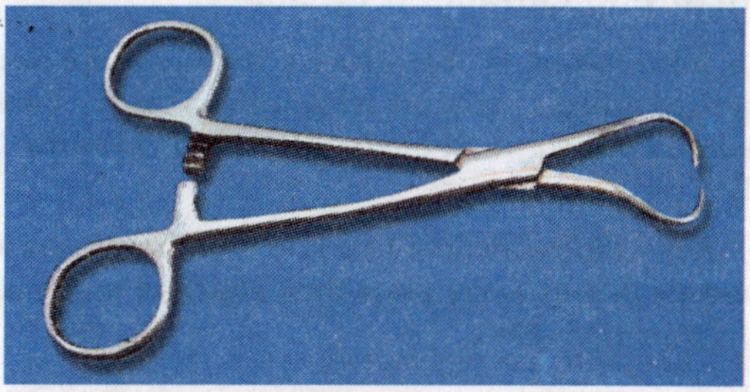

Fig. 36.40. Towel clip

Loop hook (Fig. 36.41)

Use : To remove IUCD from the uterine cavity when the threads are missing (see p. 462).

Method of use : The cervical canal is dilated if needed (p. 557). The hook is introduced within the uterine cavity. The IUCD is felt and is grasped within the hook. It is then pulled out.

Precautions : Location of the IUCD within the uterine cavity must be confirmed. Trauma (perforation) to the uterus is to be avoided. Hysteroscopic removal can also be done.

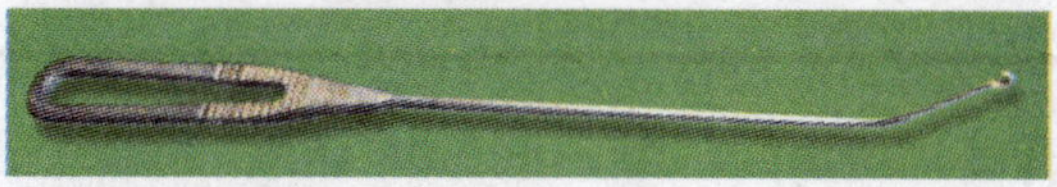

Fig. 36.41. Loop hook

Electrocautery (Fig. 36.42)

Use : Thermal cauterisation of the cervix for cervical ectopy (p. 561).

Self-assessment :

- Steps of thermal cauterisation (p. 561).
- How tissue healing occurs? (p. 561).
- How the patient is counselled for the postoperative care? (p. 562).
- Complication of the procedure (p. 562).

Ans. Excessive vaginal discharge, slight vaginal bleeding and pelvic pain (see p. 562).

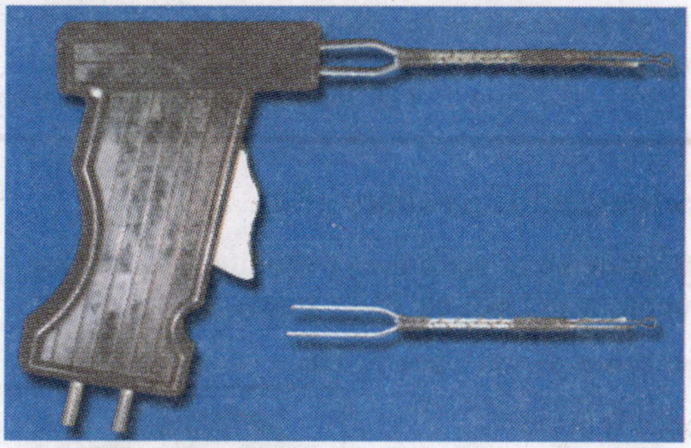

Fig. 36.42. Electrocautery (*inset — the cautery probe)*

Laparoscopic instruments (Fig. 36.43)

A. Telescope (p. 582).

B. Trocar and cannula (p. 582).

C. Veress needle (p. 582).

The veress needle consists of a spring loaded blunt perforated trocar within a sharp cannula. Resistance allows the sharp cannula to protrude but when the resistance disappears, the blunt trocar protrudes out. This prevents injury to the viscera.

Use : It is used in laparoscopy operation to produce pneumoperitoneum. The common site of puncture is through a small incision made in the lower rim of the umbilicus (see p. 585).

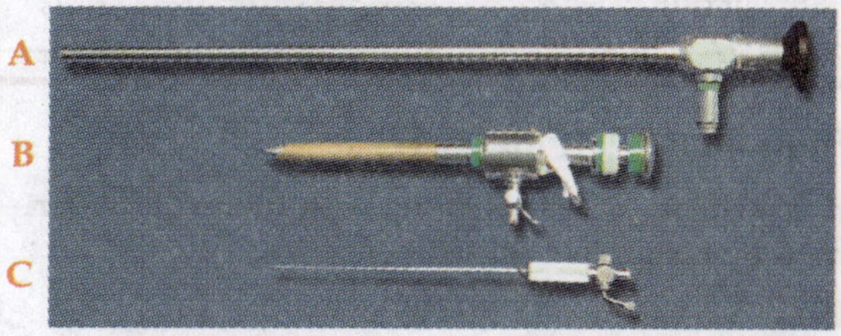

Fig. 36.43. Telescope, trocar and cannula and veress needle

Trocar and cannula (Fig. 36.44)

The instrument is introduced through the same infraumbilical incision through which veress needle is passed at an angulation of 45° towards the pelvis.

After its introduction, trocar is withdrawn and the telescope is introduced. It is then attached to the cold light source (p. 588).

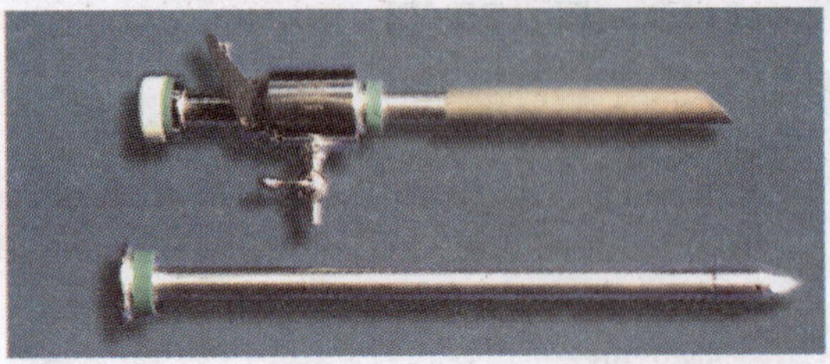

Fig. 36.44. Cannula and trocar — separated

Self-assessment :

- Indications of laparoscopy (p. 117 and 583).
- Complications (p. 586).
- Distension media used (p. 584).
- Advantages and disadvantages of laparoscopic sterilisation operation over conventional methods (p. 474).

Hysteroscopic Instruments (Fig. 36.45)

A. Telescope (p. 587)

B. Telescope with working element (p. 587)

C. Electrodes (coagulating roller ball electrode)

Self-assessment

- Indications of hysteroscopy (p. 588)
- Distension media used (p. 587)
- Complications (p. 590)

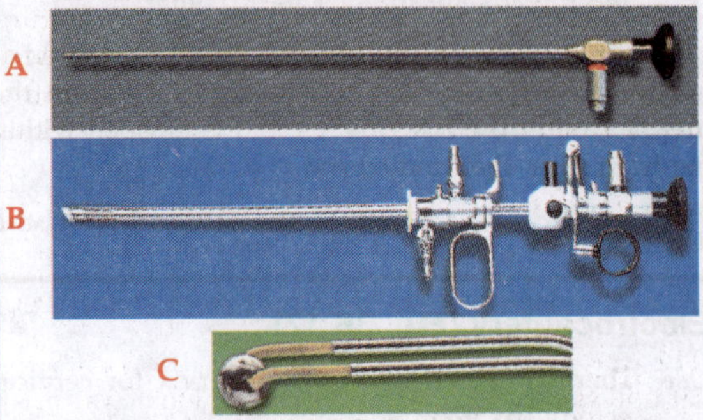

Fig. 36.45. Hysteroscopic instruments

Hodge-Smith pessary (Fig. 36.46)

It is made up of volcanite or ebonite. It is sterilised by keeping it in lysol for 24-48 hours.

Indication of use : See p. 196.

Contraindications

- **Fixed R. V. uterus**
- **Presence of infection**

Self-assessment : How to determine the size of a pessary? See p. 196.

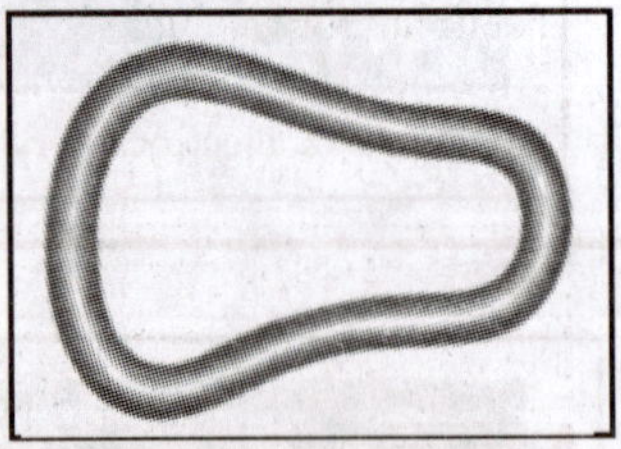

Method of insertion : The patient lies in dorsal position with an empty bladder. The pessary is hold collapsed or folded to make the insertion easy. A lubricant may be used. It is introduced inside the vagina and is pushed high. The broad end lies in the posterior fornix, the narrow end behind the symphysis pubis and the concavity is directed upwards.

Instructions to the patient

- To have vaginal douche at least twice a week.
- To check after 1 month.
- To be removed or reintroduced after 3 months.

Fig. 36.46. Hodge-Smith pessary

Ring pessary (Fig. 36.47)

It is made up of watch-spring with rubber. It is sterilised by boiling for half an hour.

Uses : See Chapter 15 (p. 205).

Contraindications of use

- Presence of sepsis.
- Gross relaxation of pelvic floor muscles.

Measurements : As in Hodge-Smith pessary.

Instructions : As in Hodge-Smith pessary.

Self-assessment :

- Indications of pessary (p. 205).
- Mechanism of action (p. 196).

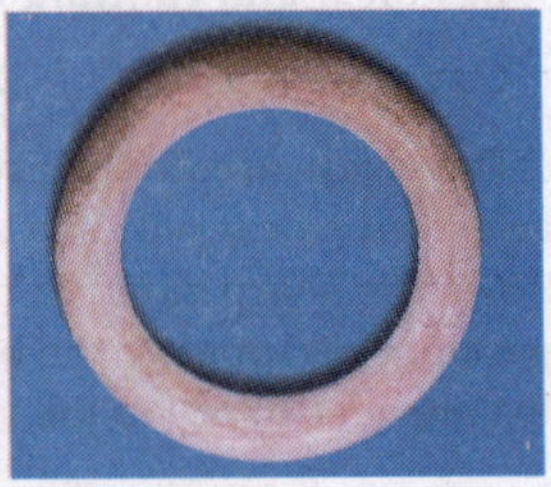

Fig. 36.47. Ring pessary

STERILISATION OF INSTRUMENTS

Blunt instruments

All blunt instruments are sterilised either by boiling for half an hour or in an autoclave for 20 minutes with 20 lbs pressure at 120°C.

Sharp instruments

Sharp instruments like knife, needle, etc. are sterilised by keeping in lysol for 24 hours.

SUTURES

The suture materials used in a particular surgical step depend on the strength of the tissues to be sutured and the time required for the wound to regain its strength. Depending on diameter, sutures are categorised into no. 0, 1, 2, etc. Sutures when smaller than no. 0, are indicated as 1-0, 2-0 and so forth. Due considerations also to be given on tensile strength of the suture, the rate at which the suture material loses its strength *in vivo* and the interaction expected between suture and tissues.

Classification

The suture materials may be classified either as absorbable or non-absorbable. Their biological origin or synthetic preparations are mentioned briefly.

- **Absorbable**
- **Non-absorbable**

Absorbable

- **Biological**
- **Synthetic**

Biological

- **Catgut and Collagen**

The catgut (derived from the word *kitgut* — strings of a musical instrument known as kit) is obtained from the submucosa of sheep or ox intestines. Collagen is derived from ox Achilles tendon. Both are available in plain and chromic form. Treatment with chromic sulphate produces chromic catgut and the untreated material produces plain catgut. Chromic catgut is degraded by proteolytic enzymes of white blood cells (inflammatory cells) slowly. Chromic catgut loses half of its tensile strength by 10 days and maintains some strength upto *21 days*. Plain catgut loses 70 per cent of its tensile strength by *7 days*.

Synthetic

- ***Dexon***

Dexon (polyglycolic acid) is a copolymer of glycolic acid and is degraded by hydrolysis with minimal inflammation. It loses half of its tensile strength in *15 days* and is absorbed in *4 months*.

- ***Vicryl (coated)***

Vicryl (polyglactin) is a copolymer of lactide and glycolide. It loses its tensile strength in *30 days*. It is absorbed by *70 days*. It produces less tissue reaction than catgut.

Vicryl rapide (coated) : It is also a polyglactin suture. It is similar to plain catgut. Absorption is rapid with minimal tissue inflammation. 70 per cent of its tensile strength is lost by 7 days. It is used for soft tissues, episiotomy repair and skin.

The tensile strength of the above sutures is much greater than that of catgut. But these sutures need more throws to secure knots compared to catgut.

- ***Polydioxanone suture (PDS)*** is a pliable monofilament made of polydioxanone. It loses half of its tensile strength in *28 days*. Tissue inflammation is minimal. Monofilament sutures have no interstices to lodge any bacteria. So infections are rare. **Polyglyconate sutures** have got similar properties. These are used for fascial closure.

Sutures

Nature	Type	Tissue where used
Absorbable	• Plain catgut • Chromic catgut	• Subcutaneous tissue • Pedicle, vaginal wall, rectus sheath, etc.
Delayed absorbable	• Dexon • Vicryl • PDS	• Subcuticular • Fascial structure • Skin • Microsurgery • Vaginal vault • Rectus sheath
Non-absorbable	• Nylon • Prolene • Silk • Dacron	• Skin • Rectus sheath • Skin of the abdomen

All the synthetic absorbable materials are sterilised by ethylene oxide.

Non-absorbable :

- **Biological** • **Synthetic**

Biological

- **Silk** suture can be handled and tied easily. It has excellent knot security. It is sterilised by gamma radiation. It is a foreign protein and initiates strong inflammatory response and loses half of its tensile strength by one year. It should not be used in contaminated or infected tissue.
- **Cotton** is the weakest non-absorbable suture. It loses 50 per cent of the tensile strength by 6 months. Wet cotton is stronger (10%) than dry cotton. It is rarely used now.

Synthetic

- **Terelene or Dacron** — These are extruded from a homopolymer.
- **Polyamide (Nylon)** — is a man made monofilament or multifilament. It is very much non-reactive in tissues. Monofilament nylon has greater tensile strength, incites less tissue reaction and is less prone to infection than braided nylon.
- **Polypropylene (Prolene)** is a hydrocarbon polymer and is monofilament. It has least tissue reaction. Knot security is greater. It is sterilised by ethylene oxide.
- **Steel** suture is non-reactive and has highest tensile strength. It is not commonly used now.

Non-absorbable sutures maintain their tensile strength for a long time. However, there may be suture related pain or rarely sinus formation.

SPECIMENS

Description

The description of a specimen includes :

- Identification of the organ/organs.
- To describe the pathology as seen on naked eye examination.

Identification of the organ

Uterus

The uterus is identified by :

- Pear-shaped structure
- Adnexal attachment
- Cervical opening
  - Circular in nulliparous
  - Transverse slit in parous

Anterior surface is identified by :

- Attachment of round ligament
- Loose attachment of uterovesical peritoneum [Fig. 34.4(13)] p. 567.

Posterior surface is identified by :

- Attachment of ovarian ligament with or without ovary.
- Cut margin of the posterior peritoneum which is densely attached and placed at a lower level than the cut edge of the anterior peritoneum.

Uterine tubes

Tubular structures with abdominal ostium surrounded by fimbriae and mesosalpinx.

Ovary

Fallopian tube is usually attached to the ovarian specimen. If the uterine tube is not mounted, even then the specimen is likely to be ovarian as there is no other pelvic organs resembling it, exception being a parovarian cyst (Fig. 36.64).

SPECIMEN — 1 and 2

Description (Figs. 36.48 and 36.49)

This is a specimen of uterus with tubes and ovaries of both the sides (Fig. 36.48).

There is alteration in the size (enlarged) and shape (irregular) of the uterus due to multiple fibroids. The fibroids are of different sizes. Some are cut open to show whorled appearance (Fig. 36.49B). A capsule is seen surrounding it (interstitial fibroid) or part of the tumour is covered by endometrium (sub-mucous fibroid Fig. 36.49A) or a part is covered by serous coat (subserous fibroid Fig. 36.49B). One subserous fibroid has got a pedicle (Fig. 36.49B) — pedunculated.

The tubes and the ovaries are looking normal.

Operation done :

Total hysterectomy with bilateral salpingo-oophorectomy.

Diagnosis : Multiple fibroids of the body of the uterus.

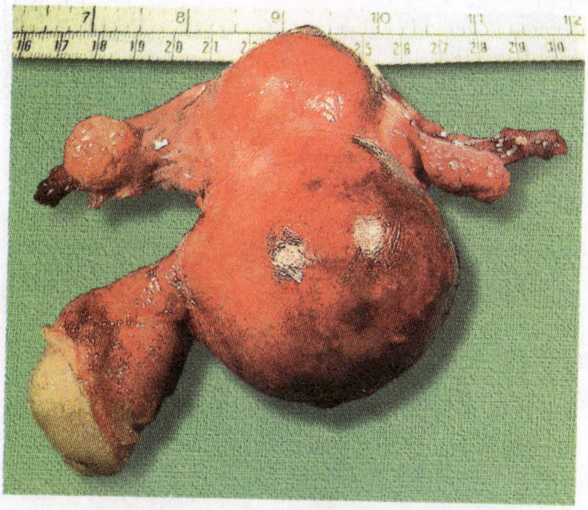

Fig. 36.48. Multiple fibroid uterus

Self-assessment

- What are the different types of uterine fibroid (p. 263).
- Causes of menorrhagia (p. 266).
- Causes of infertility (p. 267).
- Causes of pelvic pain (p. 267).
- How to differentiate a fibroid from an ovarian tumour on clinical examination (p. 103, 268).
- Place of medical management (p. 269).
- Different types of surgical management available (p. 271).

Q. ***What could be the presentation of the woman in the clinic?*** **P. 266.**

N.B. As with these specimens with total hysterectomy, the women are unlikely to suffer from infertility and as bilateral oophorectomy had been done, their probable age would be ≥ 45 years.

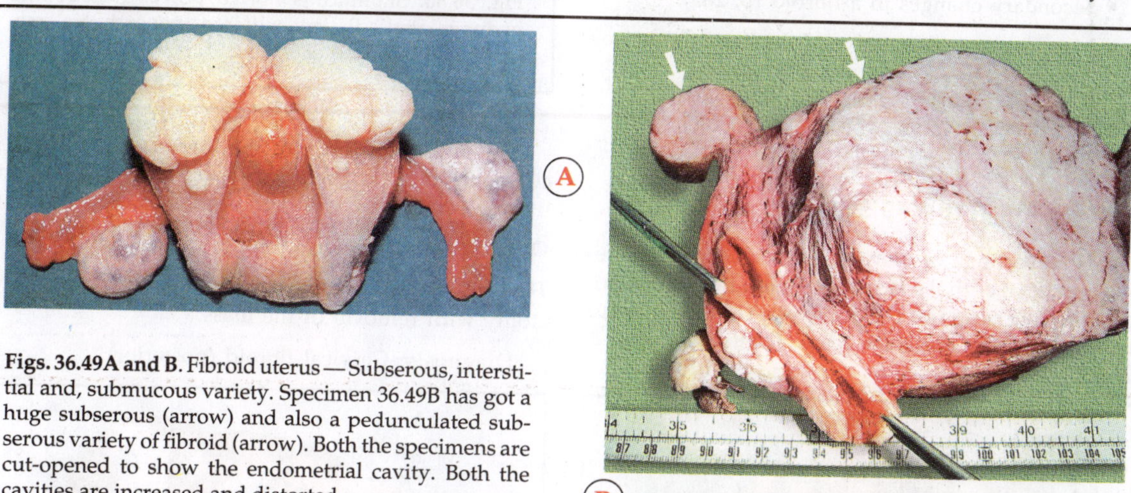

Figs. 36.49A and B. Fibroid uterus—Subserous, interstitial and, submucous variety. Specimen 36.49B has got a huge subserous (arrow) and also a pedunculated subserous variety of fibroid (arrow). Both the specimens are cut-opened to show the endometrial cavity. Both the cavities are increased and distorted

(B) Uterine cavity is shown with Allis tissue forceps

Q. ***What are the indications, conditions to be fulfilled before myomectomy? What are the contraindications?*** **Ans.** See p. 272.

Q. ***What are the different treatment options available for fibroids?*** **(p. 271).**

Ans. A. Surgery — (a) Hysterectomy, (b) Myomectomy : (i) Laparotomy, (ii) Laparoscopy, (iii) Hysteroscopy (see p. 271). (c) Myolysis.

B. Medical therapy (p. 269).

C. Interventional radiology — uterine artery embolisation (p. 273).

Q. ***How do you differentiate fibroid uterus from adenomyosis?*** **Ans.** See p. 269, 622.

SPECIMEN—3

Description (Fig. 36.50)

This is a specimen of uterus, with tubes and ovaries of both the sides.

Anterior surface of the uterus is cut open to show a mass arising from the fundus protruding into the uterine cavity. Another mass is seen to come out of the uterus through the cervical canal with a long pedicle.

Operation done : Total hysterectomy with bilateral salpingo-oophorectomy.

Diagnosis : Submucous fibroid polyps — Sessile and pedunculated.

Self-assessment

- Clinical presentation of such a case (p. 275).
- Confirmation of diagnosis (p. 277).

Q.When do myomas require to be removed (indications of myomectomy)?

Ans. (i) Any myoma growing during the follow up period. (ii) Menorrhagia not responding to medical therapy. (iii) Excessive pain or pressure symptoms. (iv) Woman with infertility or recurrent miscarriage when no cause other than fibroid is present (see text p. 272).

- Secondary changes in a fibroid (p. 265).
- Management alternative to hysterectomy (see p. 269 and 271).

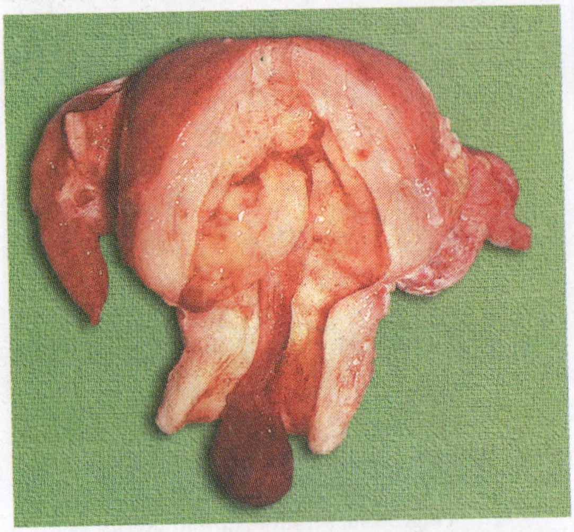

Fig. 36.50. Submucous fibroid polyps (sessile and pedunculated). Patient suffered menorrhagia, metrorrhagia and dysmenorrhoea

SPECIMEN—4

Description (Figs 36.51A and B)

This is a specimen of uterus (Fig. 36.51A) with tubes and ovaries of both the sides. There is a huge mass arising from the posterior cervical wall. The small uterus sits on the top of the huge mass. (*Lantern on dome of St. Paul's*).

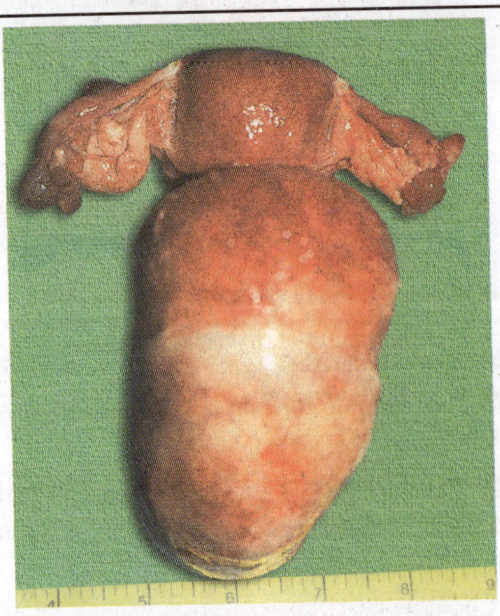

Fig. 36.51(A). A huge posterior cervical fibroid

The anterior surface of the uterus (Fig. 36.51B) is cut open to show the anterior cervical wall and the uterine cavity.

Operation done :

Total hysterectomy with bilateral salpingo-oophorectomy with removal of the mass.

Diagnosis : Cervical fibroid (posterior).

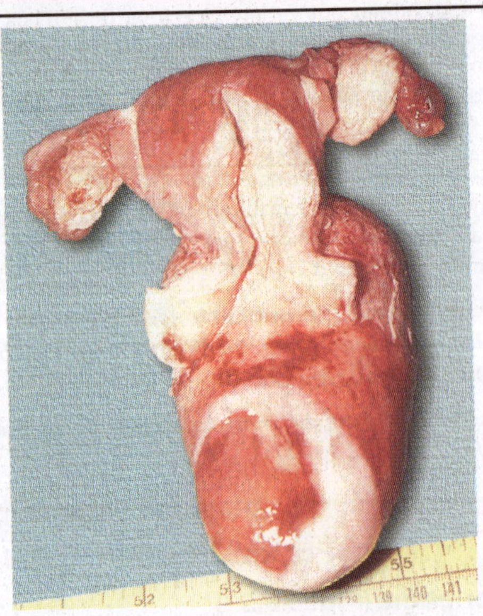

Fig. 36.51(B). Same specimen as in 36.51(A), is seen from the anterior surface

Self-assessment :

- Types of cervical fibroid (p. 274).
- Modes of presentation in a case with cervical fibroid (p. 273).
- Approach for surgical removal of cervical myoma (p. 575).
- Displacements of the ureter and risks of ureteric injury (p. 408).
- Common gynaecological pathologies where ureteric injury is more likely (p. 408).

SPECIMEN—5

Description (Figs. 36.52A and B)

This is a specimen of the uterus and the tubes and ovaries of both the sides. The uterus is enlarged and is cut open to show a diffuse growth located at one wall. The growth presents a striated appearance with scattered dark haemorrhagic spots. It has got no capsule. (c.f. — fibroid — whorlled appearance and a capsule).

Operation done — Total hysterectomy with bilateral salpingo-oophorectomy.

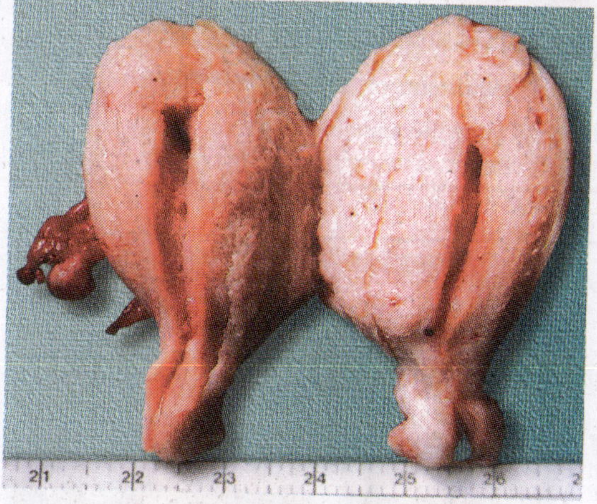

Fig. 36.52A. Specimen of adenomyosis

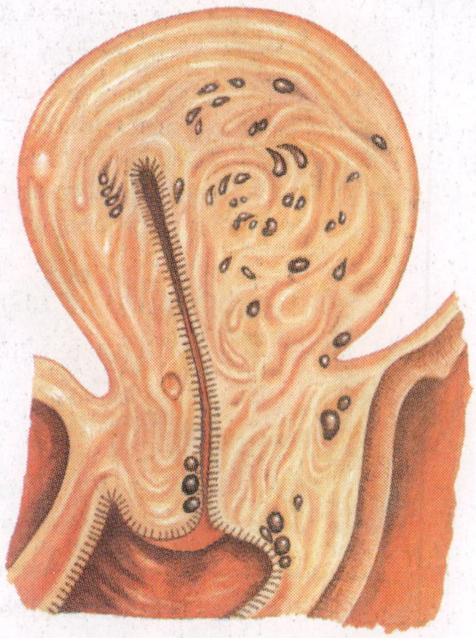

Fig. 36.52B. Adenomyosis *(Diagrammatic)*

Diagnosis : Adenomyosis.

Self-assessment :

- Clinical features of pelvic endometriosis (p. 296).
- Causes of infertility in endometriosis (p. 224).
- Clinical features of adenomyosis (p. 303)
- Histological picture of adenomyosis (p. 303).
- Treatment for pelvic endometriosis (p. 298).
- Treatment for adenomyosis (p.304).

SPECIMEN—6

Description (Fig. 36.53)

This is a specimen of the uterus with tubes and ovaries of both the sides. The ovaries are hugely enlarged, lobulated with a yellowish tinge. The uterus is also enlarged. Vesicular mass is seen protruding out through the incised uterus.

Operation done — Total hysterectomy with bilateral salpingo-oophorectomy.

Diagnosis : Hydatidiform mole with large theca lutein cysts of both the ovaries.

Self–assessment

- High-risk factors for gestational trophoblastic neoplasia (GTN) (p. 348).
- Clinical features of GTN (p. 350).
- Management of GTN (p. 351).
- Place of uterine curettage in GTN (p. 350).

- **Management of theca lutein cysts** : once hydatidiform mole or GTN is treated, spontaneous regression (within a few months) of the cysts are observed. Rarely they are removed when complications like torsion or intracystic haemorrhage occur.

Q. *What are the common sites of Metastasis?*

Ans. See p. 350.

Q. *What is the place of prophylactic chemotherapy and what are its limitations?*

Ans. See p. 351.

Q. *WHO scoring system for risk assessment.* **Ans.** See p. 351.

Q. *Reproductive behaviour of women following treatment of GTN.* **Ans.** See p. 353.

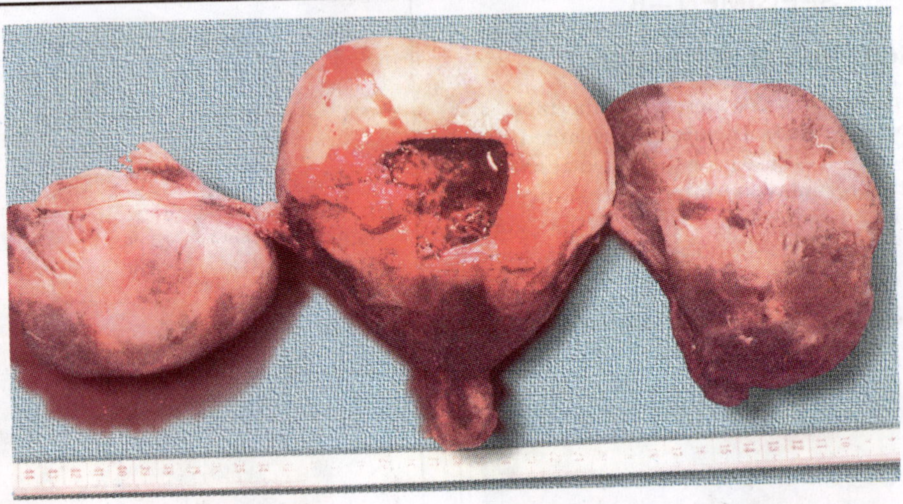

Fig. 36.53. Hydatidiform mole with bilateral large theca lutein cysts

SPECIMEN—7

Description (Fig. 36.54)

This is the specimen of a uterus with the tubes and ovaries. The uterus is enlarged. The anterior surface of the uterus is cut open to show a purplish growth invading the myometrium. The tube and the ovary are looking healthy.

This 37 years old parous lady was admitted with irregular bleeding P/V following a miscarriage. She underwent D/C thrice. Her serum β hCG level was 96,000 mIU/ml. Following courses of chemotherapy the serum hCG level remained persistently elevated.

Operation done : Total hysterectomy with bilateral salpingo-oophorectomy. Histology confirmed choriocarcinoma.

Diagnosis : Choriocarcinoma of the uterus.

Self-assessment

Q. *How the selection of chemotherapy regimen is done?* **Ans.** See p. 352.

- Place of hysterectomy in GTN (p. 353).

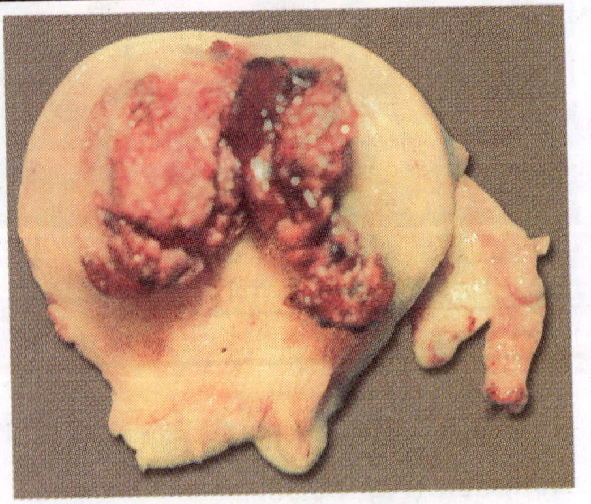

Fig. 36.54. Resistant choriocarcinoma. Lesion is seen in the wall of the uterus

- Prognosis of GTN following treatment and the risk of recurrence (p. 353).
- Place of other type of surgery (p. 353).
- Follow up following treatment (p. 353).

SPECIMEN—8

Description (Fig. 36.55)

This is a specimen of uterus, tubes and ovaries of both the sides. The left tube is markedly enlarged specially towards the outer half. The shape looks like a 'retort'. The inside fluid appears to be clear.

Diagnosis : Hydrosalpinx of the left tube.

Self-assessment

- Pathogenesis of hydrosalpinx (p. 167).
- Organisms involved in pathology (p. 167).
- Mode of affection in gonococcal infection (p. 123).
- Cause of the 'retort' shape (p. 167).
- Steps of salpingectomy (p. 572).

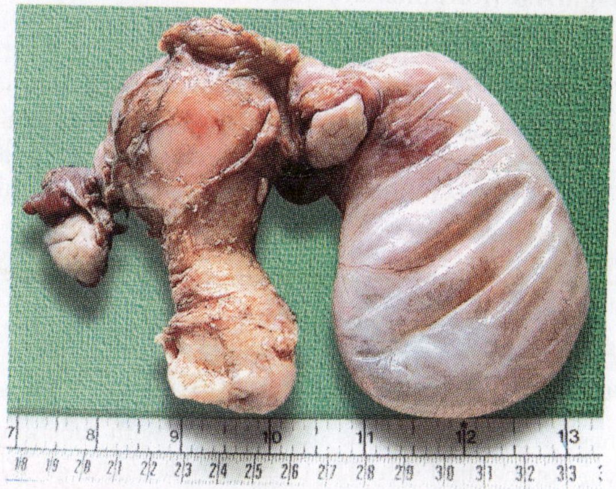

Fig. 36.55. Specimen of total hysterectomy with bilateral salpingo-oophorectomy showing a large hydrosalpinx (retort-shaped) of the left tube.

SPECIMEN—9

Description (Fig. 36.56)

This is a specimen of the uterus, tubes and ovaries of both the sides. The tubes of both sides are hugely dilated, coiled, wall is thickened and matted with the ovaries. There are evidences of adhesions over the surfaces of the tubes and uterus. Pus is coming out of through the fimbrial end of the tube.

Diagnosis : Bilateral pyosalpinx.

Self-assessment

- Pathogenesis (p. 168).
- Causes of bilateral tubal infection (p. 165).
- Clinical features (p. 126).
- Mode of spread of infection in tubercular, pyogenic and other infections (p. 123, 134).

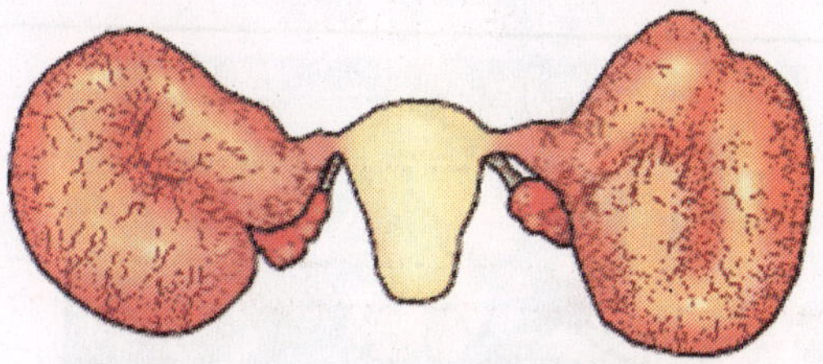

Fig. 36.56. Specimen of bilateral pyosalpinx

- Mention the clinical diagnostic criteria of PID (p. 126).
- How infertility and menstrual abnormalities could be explained with genital tuberculosis? (p. 136).
- Mention the complications of acute PID and its late sequelae (p. 128).
- What are the features of the tube on HSG when infected with tuberculosis? (p. 137).

SPECIMEN—10

Description (Fig. 36.57)

This is a specimen of a non-communicating horn of a bicornuate uterus (cut-opened) with the tube. The tube is elongated, sausage shaped and purplish in colour. The cut-open uterus shows the cavity which was filled with blood. The tube is filled with blood.

Operation done : Excission of the non-communicating horn and salpingectomy.

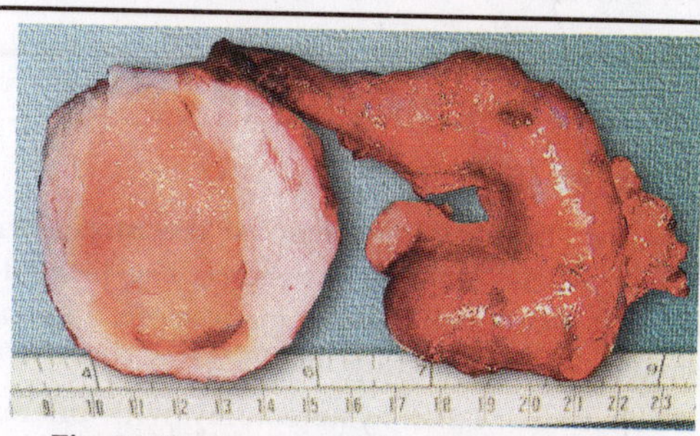

Fig. 36.57. Haematosalpinx of the right tube

Diagnosis : Rudimentary horn of the uterus with haematosalpinx.

Self-assessment

- Causes of haematosalpinx : tubal ectopic pregnancy, endometriosis, cryptomenorrhoea (p. 431) and rarely primary tubal carcinoma (0.3% of all genital malignancies).
- Causes of cryptomenorrhoea (p. 431).
- Clinical presentation of a tubal carcinoma : triad of lower abdominal pain (colicky), profuse watery discharge (hydrops tubaeprofluens) and vaginal bleeding (p. 356). Preoperative diagnosis is rare and often mistaken as an ovarian tumour (p. 356).

SPECIMEN—11

Description (Figs. 36.58A and B)

These are the specimens of the uterus with tube and ovary of the right side. The ovarian cysts (right) are cut open to show inspissated sebaceous material, hair and other mature (mesenchymal) tissues. Teeth is present in about a third (see Figs. 36.58A and 36.82A and B).

Operation done : Total hysterectomy with bilateral salpingo-oophorectomy.

Diagnosis : Dermoid cyst of the right ovary.

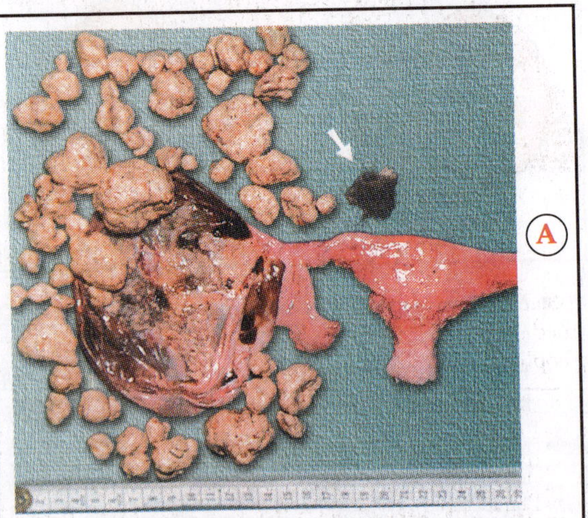

Fig. 36.58A. Gross appearance of a dermoid cyst of the ovary showing hair, teeth (arrow) and butter balls (sebum aggregated to form spherules)

Self-assessment

- Name the tissues arising from the three germ cell layers (p. 284).
- Frequency of bilaterality and association with pregnancy (p. 283).
- Common complications (p. 288).
- Management in a young patient (p. 291).
- Risk of malignant change (p. 283).
- What are strumal carcinoids? (p. 284).

Q. *How carcinoid tumours of the ovary are treated?*

Ans. Excision of the tumour (ovariotomy) causes rapid fall in the serum level of serotonin and disappearance of 5-hydroxy indole acetic acid in the urine. There is rapid remission of symptoms.

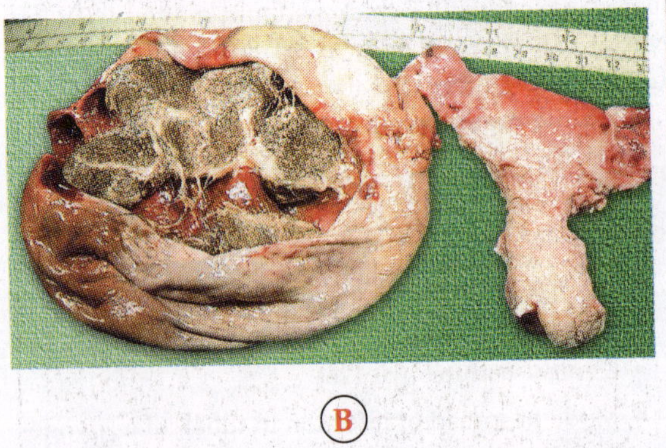

Fig. 36.58B. Gross appearance of dermoid cyst of the ovary with hair and sebaceous material (cut section)

SPECIMEN—12

Description (Fig. 36.59)

Description : This is a specimen of the uterus with tubes and ovaries of both the sides. The left sided ovarian cyst is cut open to show many septa. There are few smaller cysts projecting inside.

Operation done : Total hysterectomy with bilateral salpingo-oophorectomy.

Diagnosis : Mucinous cyst adenoma.

Self-assessment

- Common epithelial tumours of the ovary (p. 281).
- Discuss the differential diagnosis of a pelvic abdominal lump? (p. 287).
- Clinical presentation of a benign ovarian tumour (p. 284).

- Features of a functional cyst (p. 279).
- How a benign ovarian tumour could be differentiated from a malignant one clinically? (p. 283).
- How laparotomy findings could be helpful to differentiate a benign tumour from a malignant one? (p. 283).
- What are Psammoma bodies? (p. 283).
- What are the complications of a benign ovarian tumour? (p. 288).
- Management of a benign ovarian tumour (p. 290).
- Structures forming the ovarian pedicle (Table 20.3, p. 288).

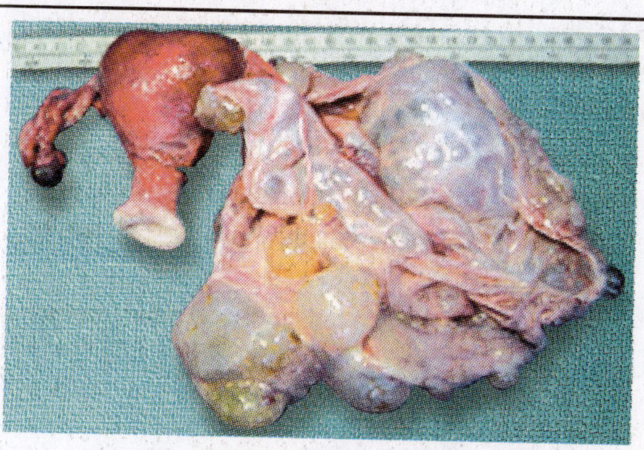

Fig. 36.59. Left sided mucinous cyst adenoma *(gross appearance on cut specimen)*

SPECIMEN—13

Description (Fig. 36.60)

This is a pathological specimen of the uterus and both the ovaries. The ovaries are enlarged lobulated with the walls irregular and shaggy. Cut section shows solid areas with haemorrhage and necrosis at places.

Diagnosis : Most likely malignant ovarian tumours.

Self-assessment

- Clinical features of a malignant ovarian tumour (p. 360).
- What are the common malignant ovarian tumours? (page 358, Table 23.22).
- How omentectomy is helpful in the management of ovarian malignancies? (see p. 364).
- Is epithelial ovarian cancer hereditary?

  Ans. About 5-10 per cent of all epithelial ovarian cancers are familial. There are three different syndromes of hereditary ovarian cancer : (i) Breast/ovarian familial cancer (75-90%). (ii) Site specific ovarian cancer (5%) and (iii) Lynch II syndrome (2%) — see p. 357.
- Preventive measures against ovarian malignancy (p. 362).
- Mention the high-risk factors as well as the protective factors for ovarian malignancy (p. 363).

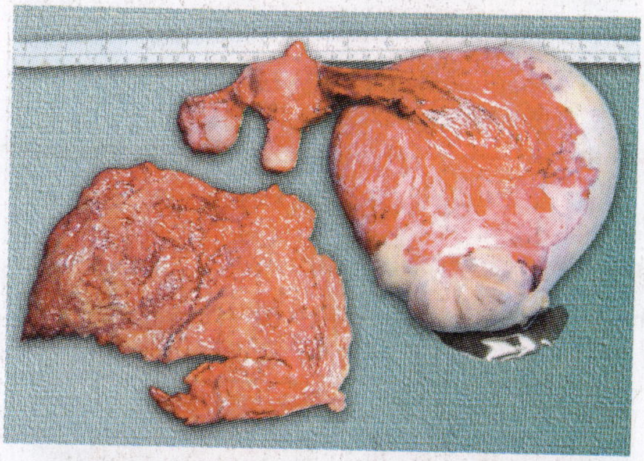

Fig. 36.60. Bilateral mucinous cyst adenocarcinoma (confirmed on histology). Total hysterectomy, bilateral salpingo-oophorectomy with infracolic omentectomy done.

- Principles of surgical approach (guidelines) in a malignant ovarian tumour (p. 364).
- Place of prophylactic oophorectomy during hysterectomy (p. 362).
- ***How serum CA–125 measurement is helpful*?**

  Ans. It is helpful with a known case of ovarian cancer : (i) To know the response of treatment. (ii) To know tumour resistance to chemotherapy. (iii) Early detection of tumour recurrence (p. 363).

SPECIMEN—14

Description (Fig. 36.61)

This is a specimen of uterus with tubes and ovaries of both the sides. The right ovary is hugely enlarged and cut opened to show its solid texture and a yellowish hue. The surface of the tumour is bosselated and glistening.

Operation done : Total hysterectomy with bilateral salpingo-oophorectomy.

Diagnosis : Solid ovarian tumour.

Self-assessment

- Common solid tumours of the ovary.

Benign : Fibroma, thecoma, Brenner tumour (p. 283, 370).

Malignant : Primary ovarian carcinoma, dysgerminoma, Immature teratoma, mesonephroma (p. 356, 367).

- ***What is Meig's syndrome* (p. 285)?**

Ans. It is a triad of findings including ascites, pleural effusion and benign ovarian fibroma. The cause is unknown. The ascites and pleural effusion resolve spontaneously when the ovarian tumour is removed.

- Hormone producing tumours of the ovary.
  - Feminising tumours : Granulosa cell and theca cell (p. 370).
  - Masculinising tumours : Sertoli-Leydig cell and Hilus cell (p. 371).

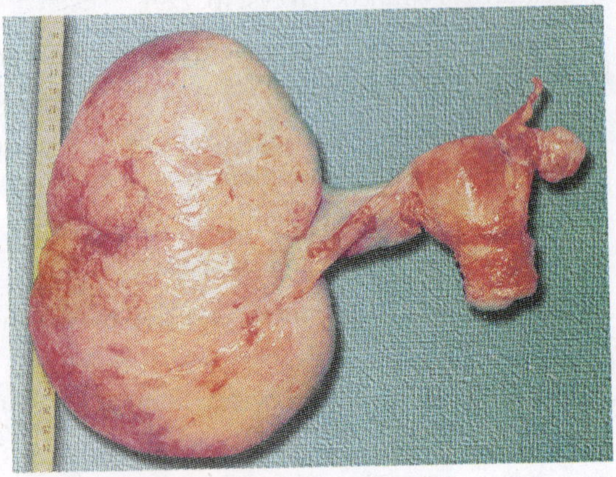

Fig. 36.61. Gross appearance of a solid ovarian tumour (right)

  - Others : Struma ovarii (thyroid hormones) (Carcinoids are rare specialised germ cell ovarian tumours that secrete 5-HT (p. 284).
- Germ cell tumours of the ovary (p. 367).

SPECIMEN—15

Description (Fig. 36.62)

This is a specimen of the uterus with tubes and ovaries of both the sides. The ovaries are enlarged with capsules ruptured. There is exophytic papillary growth on the surface and the growth infringes the surrounding organs. The cut surfaces show solid texture, extensive areas of haemorrhage and necrosis.

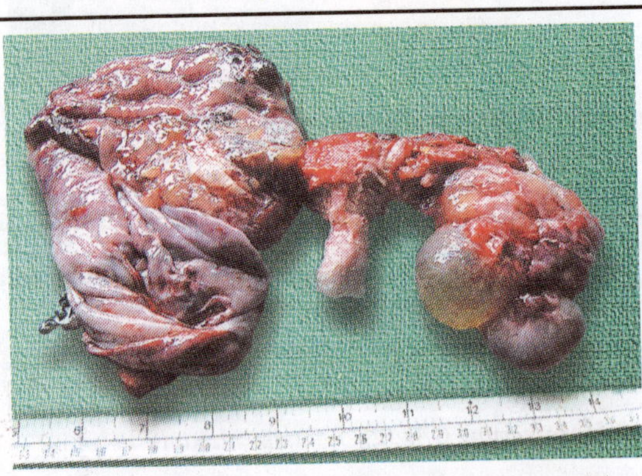

Fig. 36.62. Bilateral mucinous adenocarcinoma of the ovaries (gross appearance on cut specimen)

Operation done : Total hysterectomy with bilateral salpingo-oophorectomy.

Diagnosis

Bilateral ovarian carcinoma (papillary serous cyst adenocarcinoma).

Self-assessment

- Reasons for difficulties in the management of ovarian cancers (p. 366).
- Place of adjuvant chemotherapy for ovarian malignancy (p. 364).
- Methods of spread in a case of ovarian malignancy (p. 359).
- Place of second look surgery (p. 366).
- Prognostic factors in ovarian malignancy (p. 366).

SPECIMEN—16

Description (Fig. 36.63)

This is a specimen of the uterus with tubes and ovaries of both the sides. The ovaries are found enlarged with lobulated appearance and are free of adhesions. The shape of the ovary is maintained. The colour is pinkish with smooth surfaces. Uterus and tubes are found normal.

Operation done : Total hysterectomy with bilateral salpingo-oophorectomy.

Diagnosis

Probably Krukenberg's tumour.

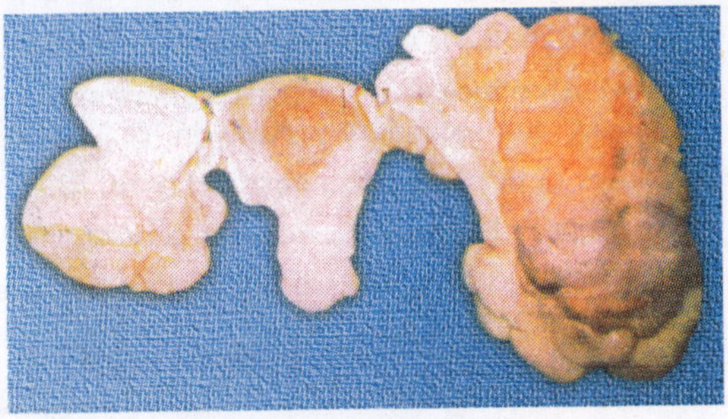

Fig. 36.63. Krukenberg tumour

Self-assessment

- ***What is a Krukenberg tumour?***

  Ans. This is a metastatic adenocarcinoma of the ovary. Almost all metastasize from the stomach. Few arise in the breast, colon or biliary tract.
- Suggestive appearance for diagnosis (p. 372).
- Primary sites (p. 371).
- Mode of spread to the ovaries (p. 372).
- Histological picture (p. 372).
- Prognosis (p. 372).
- Survival rate (p. 372).

SPECIMEN—17

Description (Fig. 36.64)

This is a specimen of the uterus with the tubes and ovaries. A hugely enlarged cyst is attached to the fimbrial end of the left tube which is stretched out. Left ovary is seen clearly (*see arrow*) behind the tube.

Operation done : Total hysterectomy with bilateral salpingo-oophorectomy with removal of the cyst is done.

Diagnosis : Parovarian cyst (Left).

Self-assessment

- Diagnosis of a parovarian cyst (p. 291).
- Embryological origin of the cyst : From the remnant of the Wolffian body situated in the mesosalpinx.
- Usually the cyst is unilocular, has a thin wall and is filled with a clear fluid.

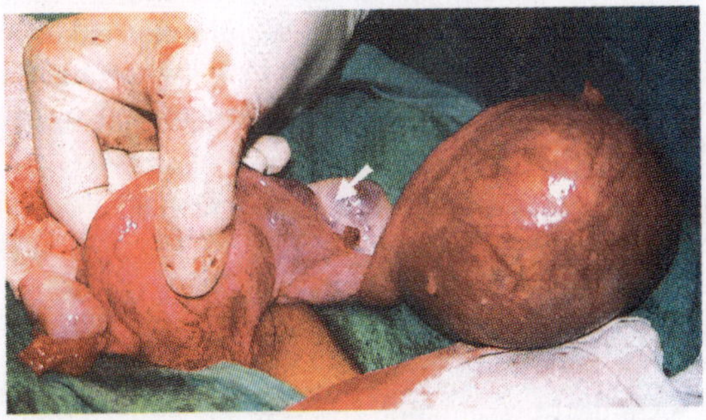

Fig. 36.64. At a glance, it seems to be ovarian but careful inspection reveals the ovary is separated from the cyst

- Clinical features and management : Same as ovarian tumour (p. 284).
- Management : Excision of the cyst.
- Risk of malignancy — rare.

SPECIMEN—18

Description (Fig. 36.65)

This is a pathological specimen of the uterus, tubes and ovaries of both the sides with upper vagina and parametrium of both the sides. The uterus is cut open to show a nodular growth on the ectocervix.

Operation done : Radical hysterectomy for carcinoma cervix.

Diagnosis : Carcinoma cervix.

Self-assessment

- Histological types (p. 328).
- Diagnosis of early carcinoma (p. 331).
- Lymphatic drainage of the cervix (p. 29).

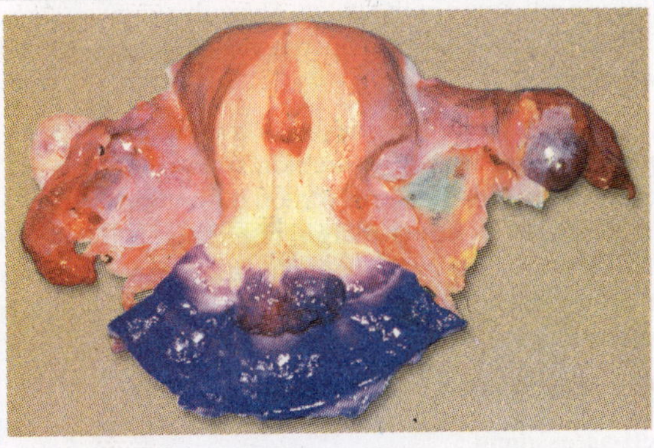

Fig. 36.65. A nodular growth (squamous cell carcinoma) occupies the posterior lip of the cervix in this specimen—radical hysterectomy done

- Management of CIS, microinvasive and early stage carcinoma (p. 314, 338).
- Advantages and disadvantages of radiotherapy (p. 336, 337).
- Principal steps of radical hysterectomy (p. 576).
- Tissues removed in radical hysterectomy (p. 335, 576).
- Significance of sentinel node biopsy (p. 328, 579).
- Staging procedures allowed by FIGO (p. 329).
- Complications of radical hysterectomy (p. 336).
- Preventive measures for carcinoma cervix — Primary and secondary prevention (p. 333).
- Causes of death in carcinoma cervix (p. 333).
- Differential diagnosis of carcinoma cervix (p. 333).
- Place of laparoscopic assisted vaginal trachelectomy (p. 339, 577).

SPECIMEN—19

Description (Fig. 36.66)

This is a specimen of the uterus with tubes and ovaries of both the sides. The uterus is uniformly enlarged. The anterior surface is cut open to show a fungating growth confined to the body. The tubes and ovaries are healthy.

Operation done : Total hysterectomy with bilateral salpingo-oophorectomy.

Diagnosis : Endometrial carcinoma.

Self-assessment

- Clinical presentation (p. 343).
- Methods of diagnosis (p. 344).
- Histological types of endometrial carcinoma (p. 342).
- Lymphatic drainage of body of the uterus (p. 28, 342).

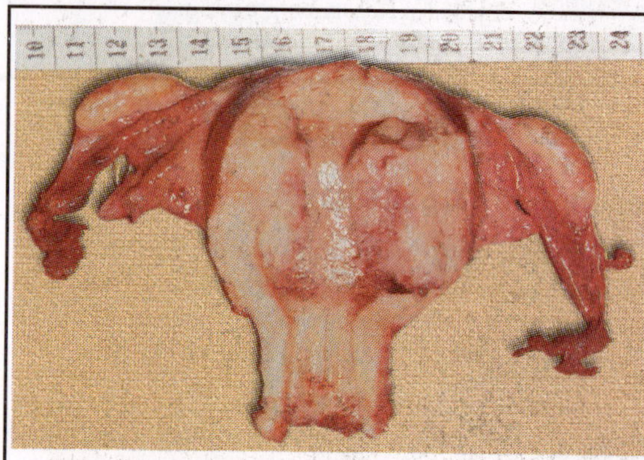

Fig. 36.66. The uterus is cut open to show a diffuse and partly necrotic growth of adenocarcinoma filling the uterine cavity

- High-risk women (p. 345).
- Surgical procedures in the management (p. 345).
- Place of chemotherapy and radiotherapy (p. 346).

SPECIMEN - 20

Description (Fig. 36.67)

This is a specimen of the vulva. The vulva shows a large exophytic growth and biopsy revealed squamous cell carcinoma.

Operation done : Radical vulvectomy. Vulvectomy specimen is obtained by the skin sparing "long horn" incisions. Tips of the horns rest on the anterior superior iliac spines. The upper margin of incision is interspinous, the lower margin is along the inguinal skin creases and the labiocrural folds. Three incision technique is currently used in most of the centres (p. 578).

Diagnosis : Carcinoma of the vulva.

Self-assessment :

- Common sites of vulval malignancy (p. 322).
- Different histological types (p. 322).
- Clinical presentation (p. 323).
- Types of vulvectomy (see p. 577).
- Complications of radical vulvectomy (see p. 579).
- Lymphatic drainage of the vulva and its clinical significance (see p. 29, 323).
- Significance of a sentinel node (p. 328, 579).
- Prognostic factors for vulval carcinoma (see p. 325).

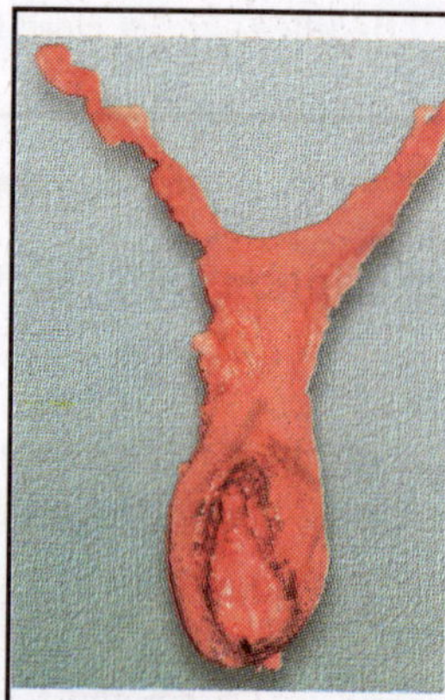

Fig. 36.67. Carcinoma of the vulva—radical vulvectomy done using "long horn" incisions

IMAGING STUDIES IN GYNAECOLOGY

PLATES: X-RAY, ULTRASONOGRAPHY, COMPUTED TOMOGRAPHY, AND MAGNETIC RESONANCE IMAGING

HYSTEROSALPINGOGRAM (HSG)

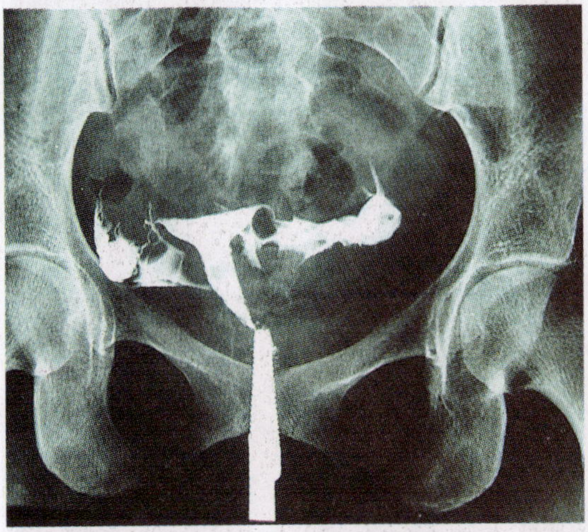

Fig. 36.68. Hysterosalpingogram with bilateral peritoneal spillage

ONE (Fig. 36.68)

Hysterosalpingogram showing radio-opaque shadow demarcating the uterine cavity. The radio-opaque dye is visible in the lumen of both the tubes. There is peritoneal spillage on both sides.

Diagnosis

Normal hysterosalpingogram (normal cavity) with bilateral patent tubes (free peritoneal spill).

Self-assessment

- Indications and contraindications of HSG (p. 559)
- Timing of HSG (p. 560)
- Steps of operation (p. 559)
- Complications (p. 560)
- Prospect of fertility in this case : As the tubes are patent, the couple should be investigated to assess the ovarian and male factors for infertility (ch. 16).
- Other methods for assessment of tubal patency (p. 230).

TWO (Fig. 36.69)

Hysterosalpingogram showing radio-opaque shadow demarcating the uterine cavity. No radio-opaque shadow is visible on either tube.

Diagnosis : Hysterosalpingogram showing bilateral cornual block.

Self-assessment

- Causes of cornual block (p. 138).
- Alternative investigations (p. 230).
- Management if tubes are damaged (p. 243).
- Results of tuboplasty (p. 241).
- Different methods of ART (Table 16.13, p. 243).

Management if tubes are normal :

- To assess the male factors and ovarian factors for infertility.

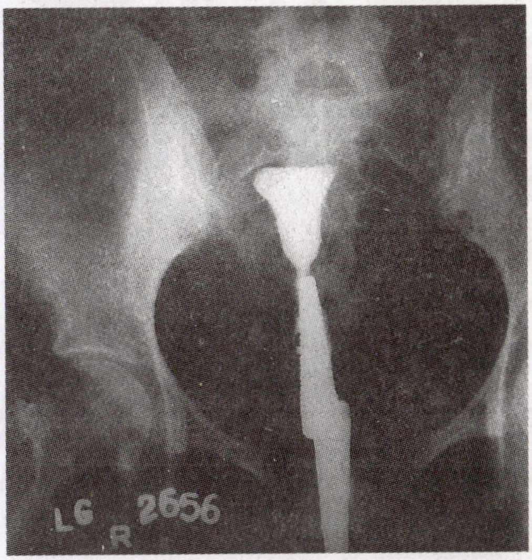

Fig. 36.69. Hysterosalpingogram showing bilateral cornual block. She had a history of MTP

- What other information can be obtained from HSG? p. 559.
- What are the causes of tubal block?

Ans. Salpingitis, salpingitis isthmica nodosa, benign polyps within the tubal lumen, tubal endometriosis, tubal spasm and intratubal mucous debris.

THREE (Fig. 36.70)

Hysterosalpingogram showing radio-opaque shadow filling the uterine cavity. The tubes of both sides are distended with the radio-opaque dye. There is no evidence of peritoneal spillage.

Diagnosis : Bilateral hydrosalpinx (fimbrial block).

Self-assessment

- Causes of bilateral fimbrial block (p. 166).
- Management for distal and proximal tubal block (p. 240).
- ***What is the appearance of the tube on HSG when infected with tuberculosis?*** (p. 137).
- ***What is the reproductive outcome in a woman with pelvic tuberculosis?*** (p. 139).
- Indications of IVF–ET (p. 244).
- Does the presence of hydrosalpinx impair the result of IVF?

Ans. Hydrosalpinges reduce the pregnancy rates of IVF by about 50 per cent. Endometrial receptivity is reduced resulting in implantation failure. Salpingectomy improves the outcome.

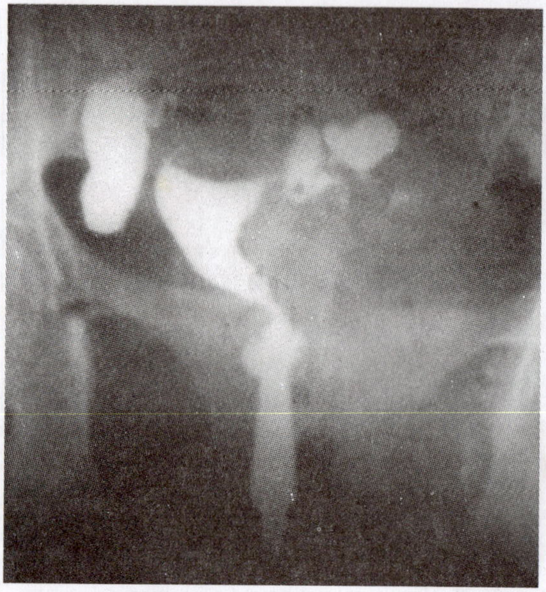

Fig. 36.70. Hysterosalpingogram showing bilateral hydrosalpinx (fimbrial block). Bilateral salpingostomy was done. Thereafter, she had an ectopic pregnancy

FOUR (Fig. 36.71)

Hysterosalpingogram showing a radio-opaque shadow filling both the horns of the uterus. The radio-opaque dye is visible within the tubes. There is peritoneal spillage on both the sides (Fig. 36.71).

Diagnosis

It seems to be a case of bicornuate uterus with bilateral patent tubes.

Self-assessment

- Confirmation of bicornuate from septate uterus (p. 45).
- Management of a septate uterus in recurrent miscarriage (p. 45).
- Gynaecological symptoms in bicornuate uterus (p. 45).
- Management of a bicornuate uterus is difficult. Metroplasty or unification (Strassman or Tompkins) operation has been recommended (p. 45).
- Reproductive behaviour in a woman with uterine anomalies (p. 45).

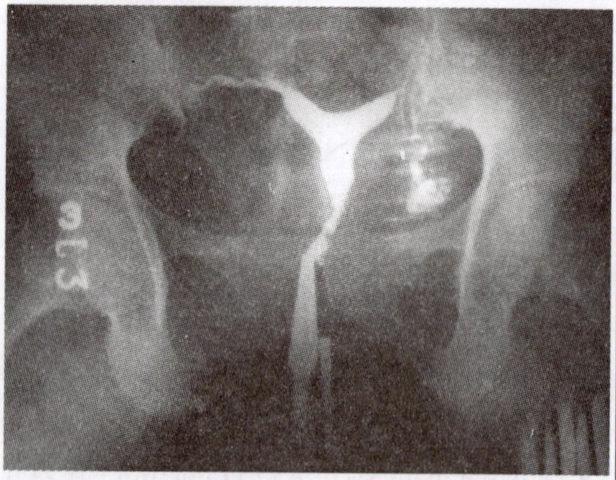

Fig. 36.71. Hysterosalpingogram showing bicornuate uterus. Metroplasty was done for recurrent midtrimester miscarriage. Subsequently, she had a live birth at term, delivered by LSCS

FIVE (Fig. 36.72)

Hysterosalpingogram showing a radio-opaque shadow filling a single horn of the uterus. There is peritoneal spillage from the tube.

Diagnosis

It seems to be a case of unicornuate uterus with patent tube.

Self-assessment

- Confirmation of diagnosis (p. 45).
- Types of Müllerian anomalies (p. 43).
- Reproductive outcome in a case with unicornuate uterus : poor — due to reduced uterine capacity, less muscle mass and inability to expand (p. 45).

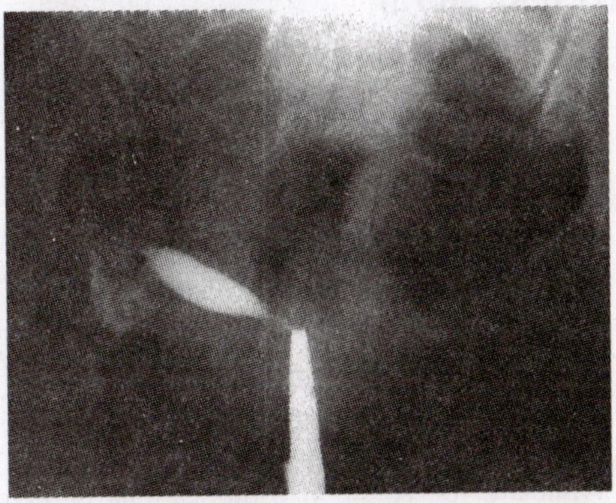

Fig. 36.72. Hysterosalpingogram showing a unicornuate uterus

SIX (Fig. 36.73)

Hysterosalpingogram showing irregular filling of radio-opaque dye without any outline of uterine tubes.

Diagnosis : Uterine synechiae (Asherman's syndrome).

Self-assessment

- Common causes of uterine synechiae (p. 438).
- Other methods of diagnosis (p. 449).
- Management of uterine synechiae (p. 449 & 451).
- Uterine causes of amenorrhoea (p. 438).
- ***In what conditions of amenorrhoea karyotyping is needed?***

Ans. (i) Patients with uterus but no breasts and high FSH level–Gonadal failure (p. 433). (ii) Patients with no uterus but breasts present – Androgen insensitivity syndrome (p. 424). (iii) Premature ovarian failure if < 30 years of age (p. 444). (iv) Short stature (< 60") with Turner Stigmata – Turner's syndrome (p.422).

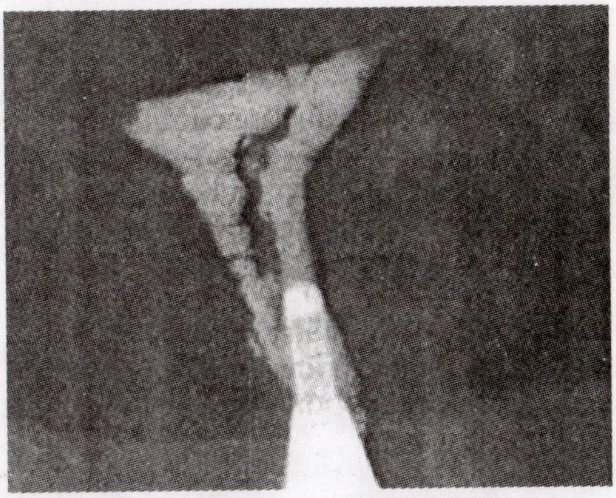

Fig. 36.73. Hysterosalpingogram showing intrauterine adhesion

SEVEN (Fig. 36.74)

Ultrasonographic view of a septate uterus.

Self-assessment

- What are the different types of uterine abnormalities? (p. 43).
- What may be the clinical presentation of such a case? (p. 45).
- What are the different obstetric complications? (p. 45).
- What are the different modes of diagnosis? (p. 45).
- What are the treatment options available? (p. 45).

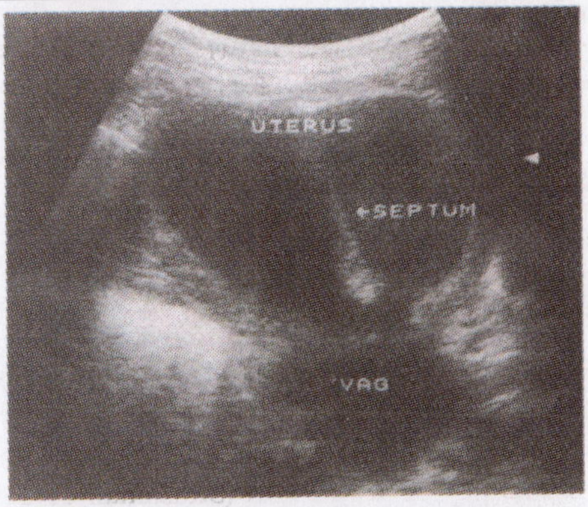

Fig. 36.74. Ultrasonographic view of a septate uterus

EIGHT (Fig. 36.75)

Self-assessment

- Cause of symmetrical enlargement of the uterus (p. 268, Table 19.5)
- How a couple should be counselled before proceeding to myomectomy? (p. 271).
- What are the principal steps of myomectomy? (p. 575).
- What are the measures that can be adopted to minimise blood loss in myomectomy operation? (p. 574).
- What are the different types of surgery for myomectomy? (p. 271).
- What are the common complications of myomectomy? (p. 575).
- What are the long-term results of myomectomy in respect of recurrence and others? (See page 271).

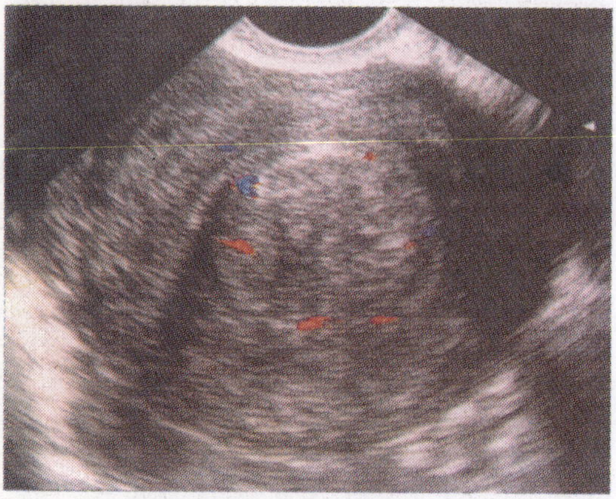

Fig. 36.75. Ultrasonographic (TV) view of a leiomyoma

NINE (Fig. 36.76)

Self-assessment

- Different modalities of treatment options for pelvic endometriosis (p. 299).
- ***What are the common sites of pelvic endometriosis?*** (p. 294).
- Mention the indications and the different types of surgery that can be done for endometriosis (p. 301).
- How do you manage a case of chocolate cyst (ovarian endometrioma) of the ovary? (p. 301).
- What are the different hormones used in the management of endometriosis? (p. 299).
- Treatment of scar endometriosis (p. 302).
- How fibroid uterus could be differentiated from adenomyosis ? (see Table below).

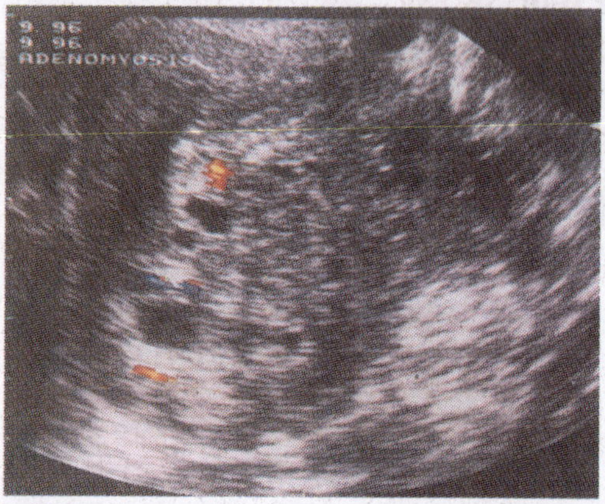

Fig. 36.76. Sonographic view of adenomyosis showing diffusedly enlarged uterus with cystic spaces

Differentiating features of Fibroid uterus and Adenomyosis

	Fibroid uterus (Fig. 36.75)	Adenomyosis (Fig. 36.76)
Age	• Usually observed in the **reproductive age**.	• Commonly seen in women **older than 40 years**.
Pathology	• It is the benign neoplasia of the smooth muscle and fibrous tissue of the uterus.	• It is due to the presence of functioning endometrium within the muscle layers of the uterus.
Uterus	• Irregularly enlarged depending upon the site, size and number of myomas. It is firm and non-tender (unless degeneration).	• Diffusely enlarged due to myohyperplasia. Uterus is soft and tender.
Symptoms	• Menorrhagia and dysmenorrhoea — often present.	• Menorrhagia—present. Dysmenorrhoea often begins a week before and it continues even after the period is over.
Diagnosis	• **Sonography (TVS)** — Homogeneous echogenic area over the fibroid.	• Cystic spaces within the myometrium.
	• **Cut section** : *Capsule* present, smooth and whitish surface with whorled appearance.	• *Capsule* absent. Diffuse trabeculated appearance, cystic spaces with haemorrhagic spots.
	• **Histology** : Proliferation of smooth muscle and fibrous tissue (p. 265).	• Proliferation of endometrial glands and stroma. Phagocytic cells laden with haemosiderin pigment are present (p. 296, 303).

TEN (Fig. 36.77)

Ultrasonographic view of Cu T inside the uterine cavity. Thread was missing in this case.

Self-assessment

- What are the possible causes of missing thread ? (p. 462).
- How do you investigate such a case with missing thread? (p. 462).
- What are the indications of removal of IUDs? (p. 462).
- What are the complications of IUD use? (p. 461).
- What are the specific advantages of the third generation of IUDs over the others? (p. 463).

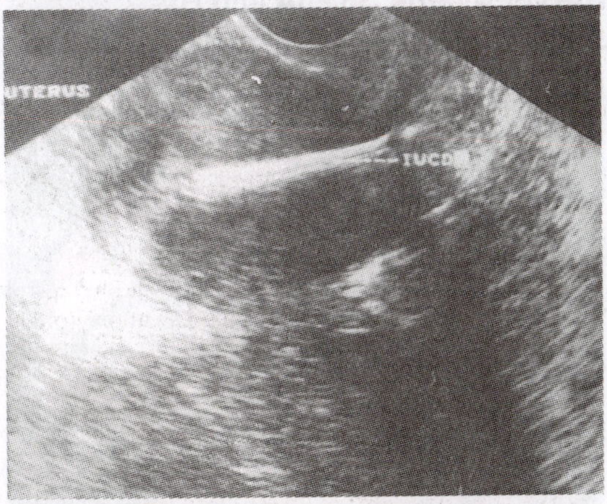

Fig. 36.77. Ultrasonographic view of a Cu T inside the uterine cavity, in a case of missing thread

ELEVEN (Fig. 36.78)

Hysterosalpingogram showing markedly dilated tube with retention of dye (right).

Diagnosis : Hydrosalpinx of the right tube.

Self-assessment

- ***What are the other methods of diagnosis?***
  Ans. USG, laparoscopy.
- Dangers of HSG in such a case (p. 560).
- What are the common types of tubal reconstructive surgery? (p. 240).
- What factors are related to the success of tuboplasty? (p. 241).
- What are the guidelines for tubal surgery? (p. 240).

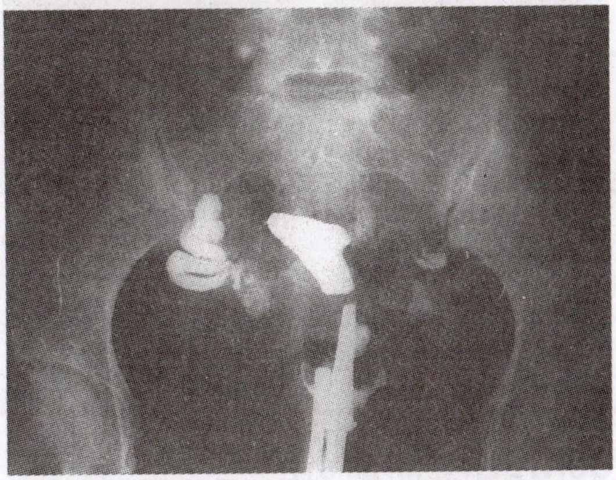

Fig. 36.78. Hysterosalpingogram showing markedly dilated tube with retention of dye (*right*)

TWELVE (Fig. 36.79)

Ultrasonographic view of an ovarian hyperstimulation syndrome (OHSS). Multiple follicles are seen.

Self-assessment

- What are the different grades and the clinical features of OHSS? (p. 503).
- How could this problem be prevented? (p. 504).
- Indications of use of gonadotrophins in infertility (p. 502).
- What is ovarian reserve? (p. 503).
- Who are the high responders (p. 503).
- What is coasting? (p. 503).
- How do you manage a case of OHSS? (p. 504).

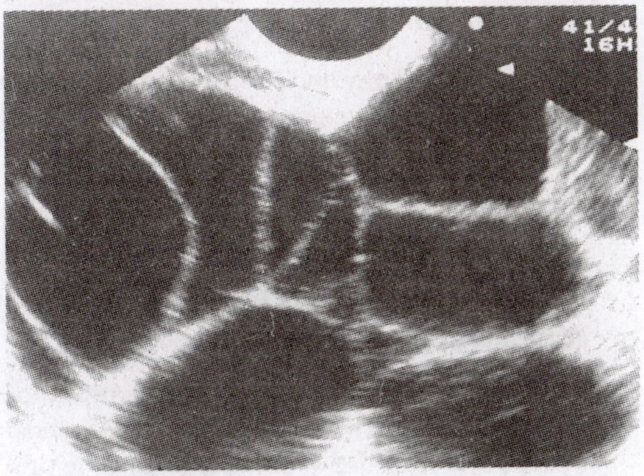

Fig. 36.79. Sonographic view of OHSS

THIRTEEN (Figs. 36.80A and B)

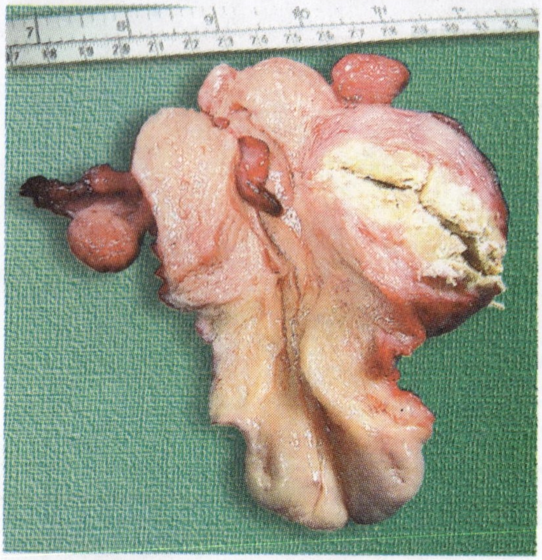

Fig. 36.80A. Specimen of a uterus, tubes and ovaries cut opened to show multiple fibroids of the uterus. The uterine cavity is enlarged. The fibroid is cut to show the calcific degeneration ("womb stone") within it.

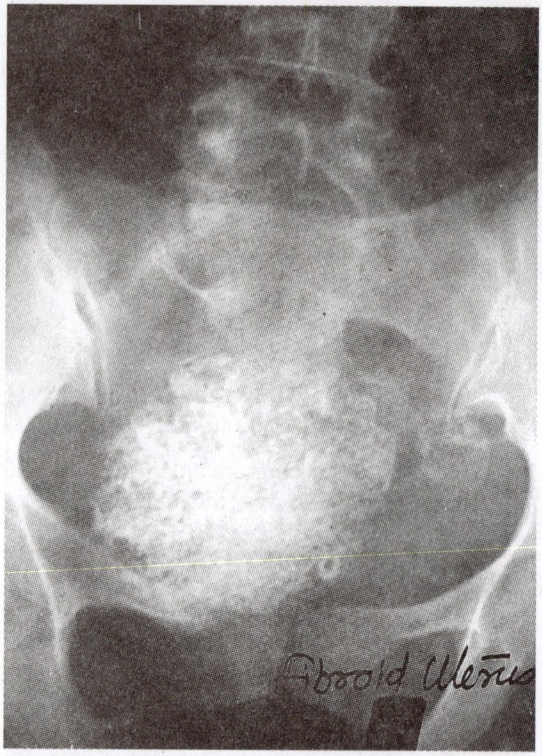

Fig. 36.80B. Plain X-ray of the pelvis and lower abdomen showing the calcific degeneration of a fibroid (popcorn appearance) [*By courtesy : Dr. P. Panigrahi, Senior Consultant Gynaecologist, JLN Hospital, Bhillai*]

Self-assessment

- Secondary changes in a fibroid (p. 265).
- Degenerations in fibroid (p. 265).

FOURTEEN (Fig. 36.81)

Computed tomographic view of an ovarian tumour.

Self-assessment

- What special advantages CT has got in gynaecology? (See p. 114 and p. 361).
- Place of sonography and Positron Emission Tomography (PET) in the management of ovarian malignancy (p. 361).
- As a diagnostic aid how magnetic resonance imaging (MRI) is useful in gynaecology? (p. 115 and 361).
- ***What is the value of CT in the evaluation of pelvic or periaortic lymph node metastasis?***

  Ans. For most pelvic malignancies lymph nodes more than 8 mm in maximum short-axis dimension (MSAD) are regarded as abnormal. CT is helpful to detect retroperitoneal metastatic nodes. However, results may be false-negative due to micrometastasis or false-positive due to lymphadenitis or reactive hyperplasia.

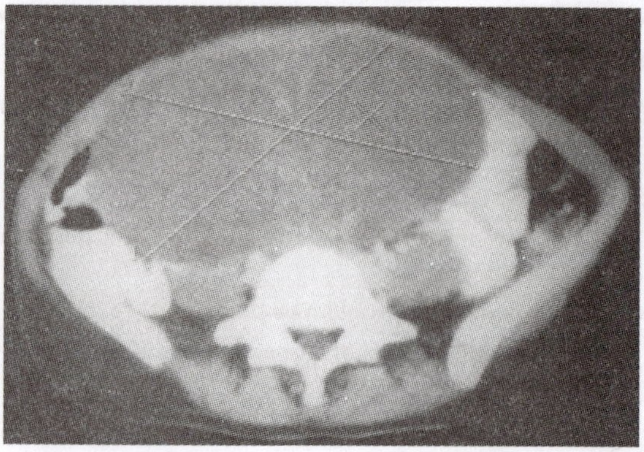

Fig. 36.81. Computed tomographic (CT) view of an ovarian tumour

FIFTEEN (Figs 36.82A and B)

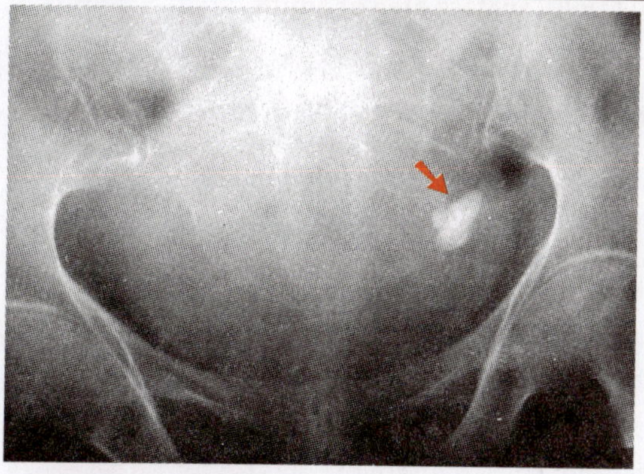

Fig. 36.82A. Straight X-ray of the abdomen pelvis with an ovarian tumour showing (arrow) the shadow of a tooth (Dermoid cyst)

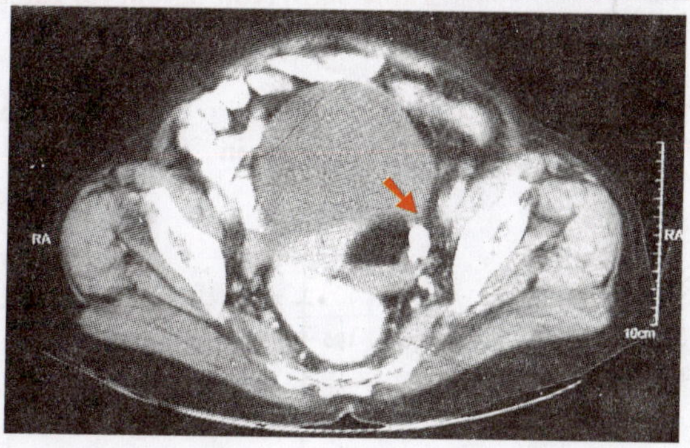

Fig. 36.82B. Computed tomographic view of the abdomen and pelvis of the same woman as in Figure 36.82A) showing the tooth (Dermoid cyst of the ovary)

Self-assessment

- Describe the cut section of an ovarian dermoid cyst (p. 283).
- Typical findings of an ovarian dermoid cyst in CT.

Ans. Characteristics of a dermoid cyst in CT include the mixture of low density areas due to fat, high density areas from dental elements or calcification (arrow) and a fat-fluid level.

- ***What is the limitation of USG?***

Ans. Compared to CT or MRI, USG is not sufficient for accurate staging of any pelvic malignancy.

SIXTEEN (Fig. 36.83)

Self-assessment

- ***How normal endometrium and myometrium could be studied with MRI?***

Ans. With MRI endometrium is shown as the inner zone of high-signal-intensity stripe. The deeper myometrium is recognised as a very-low-signal intensity zone. The junctional zone demarcates the two (Fig. 36.83). The myometrium appears as the intermediate signal-intensity zone. In postmenopausal women, the contrast between the junctional zone and the myometrium decreases.

- ***What special advantages MRI has got in gynaecology?***

Ans. 1. MRI offers multiplaner images.

2. Gadolinium enhanced T_2-weighted images can determine.

(i) Depth of myometrial invasion and that of pelvic and periaortic (retroperitoneal) nodal metastasis in endometrial carcinoma. (ii) Invasion of malignant process in the cervix accurately (p. 115). (iii) It can detect recurrence of pelvic tumour. (iv) It is superior to CT in detecting metastatic nodes (p. 115).

3. MRI is safe in pregnancy.

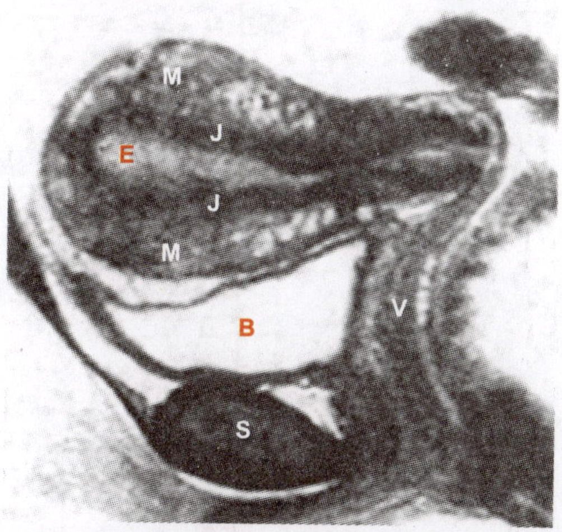

Fig. 36.83. MRI plate of a normal uterus on a sagital T_2-weighted spin-echo image showing endometrium (E), the junctional zone (J), the myometrium (M), urinary bladder (B) and the vagina (V).

Table 36.1 : Nomogram for calculating body surface area of adults

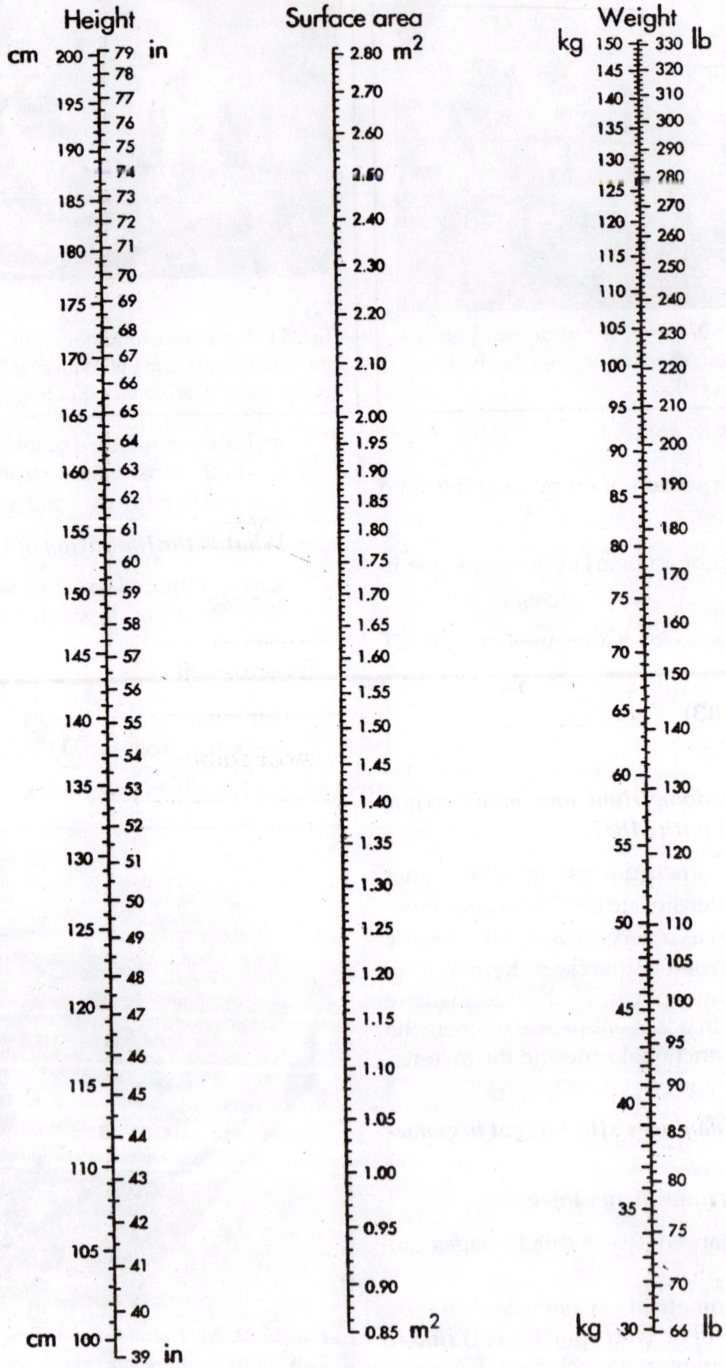

Table 36.2 : Body mass Index (see p. 546)

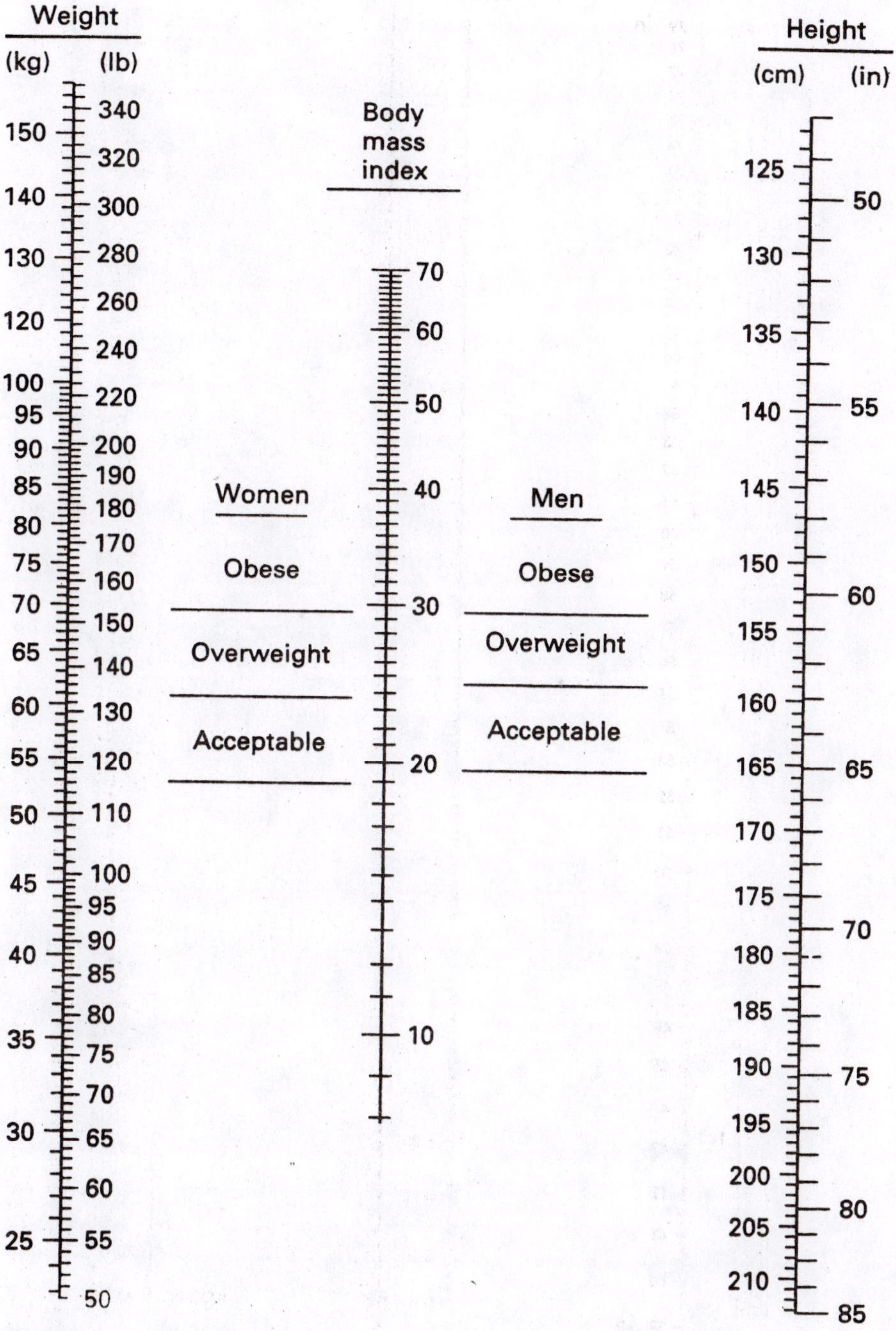

INDEX

A

C

G

M

P

Q

R

S

T

W

X

Y

Z

U

V

Critical Theories in Dark Tourism

Issues, Complexities and Future Directions

Edited by
Nitasha Sharma, Annaclaudia Martini and Dallen J. Timothy

DE GRUYTER

ISBN 978-3-11-079203-4
e-ISBN (PDF) 978-3-11-079207-2
e-ISBN (EPUB) 978-3-11-079210-2
ISSN 2570-1657
e-ISSN 2570-1665

Library of Congress Control Number: 2024940915

Bibliographic information published by the Deutsche Nationalbibliothek
The Deutsche Nationalbibliothek lists this publication in the Deutsche Nationalbibliografie; detailed bibliographic data are available on the Internet at http://dnb.dnb.de.

Typesetting: Integra Software Services Pvt. Ltd.
Printing and binding: CPI books GmbH, Leck

www.degruyter.com

Acknowledgements

The editors would like to thank all the authors who contributed their wonderful work to this edited book. All the contributors come from diverse disciplinary backgrounds and this book would not have been possible without their enthusiasm, patience and positivity.

We are grateful to De Gruyter for their patience as we navigated through the challenges that came along the way in editing this book. A special thanks to Jillian Rickly, the Series Editor of the De Gruyter Studies in Tourism, who encouraged envisioning this project on dark tourism and Professor Duncan Light, for graciously agreeing to write a foreword despite his busy schedule.

While critical theory as a paradigm has its limitations, the broad rubric of critical theories, unlike more conventional models and paradigms has seen several onto-epistemological changes in recent times with dark tourism scholarship standing to benefit from them. As scholars interested in dark tourism and critical theories, our objective for this book is to open a line of dialogue and deliberation that has not been considered earlier in dark tourism studies. While fulfilling this objective, we acknowledge the plethora of knowledge and rich academic literature that exists because of the hard work of academic scholars, some of them our friends and colleagues, who have diligently contributed to it over the past years. Having said this, Dallen J. Timothy also wishes to acknowledge those who have gone before us, especially those whose suffering and demise have sparked a sense of marvel and awe in the collective human psyche. May their afflictions have been brief, may they rest in peace, and may they never be forgotten.

https://doi.org/10.1515/9783110792072-202

Contents

Duncan Light

Foreword

Dark tourism has enjoyed quite an unexpected popularity over the past 25 years. When the concept was originally proposed (along with thanatourism) it appeared as a rather off-beat curiosity that looked likely to remain at the margins of tourism studies. This was far from being the case! Instead, dark tourism has established itself as a core theme within contemporary tourism research. It also grabs the attention of our students in ways which few other topics seem to. Furthermore, dark tourism is a concept that has been enthusiastically embraced by the media and is rapidly establishing itself within popular culture. Curiously, only the tourism industry largely eschews the term.

From the early 2000s onwards, researchers set out with enthusiasm to examine the concepts of dark tourism and thanatourism in more detail. This first stage of research focused on identifying examples of this apparently new form of tourism, developing typologies of 'dark' resources, identifying sub-forms of such tourism, and considering the ethical implications. This produced numerous case studies, mostly focused on supply perspectives. At this stage, the conceptualization of dark tourism was framed around fairly crude (and not always convincing) binaries (Golańska, 2015), dark versus light, authenticity versus commodification, education versus entertainment, respectful versus kitsch, serious visitors versus tourists. Without doubt, this early stage of research was important in generating a more detailed picture of what dark tourism involved, but the endeavour was stronger at telling us about 'what' rather than 'why' (Ashworth, 2002). Furthermore, beyond some engagement with postmodernism, much of this early research shunned theorization (perhaps not surprisingly given the challenge involved). Consequently, after a decade of research, Richard Sharpley identified dark tourism as being "theoretically fragile" (2005, p. 216). The largely atheoretical nature of dark tourism meant that the concept was not taken particularly seriously by other disciplines and fields concerned with death, even where the inclusion of a tourism perspective had a potentially important contribution to make.

Nevertheless, some scholars sought to give dark tourism a stronger theoretical foundation. One notable example was the theory of mortality mediation (Stone & Sharpley, 2008; Stone, 2012) which explicitly drew on thanatology and the sociology of death in seeking to understand the experiences of the people who visited sites of dark tourism. This proposed that, in a societal context where death was largely sequestered, dark tourism was a means through which the living could engage with, and understand, death. Other researchers later developed these ideas, bringing in perspectives from terror management theory and, increasingly, mortality salience. But these are challenging theories to work through and apply, and many researchers have found it easier to avoid them altogether. However, it seems surprising that theories specifically about

https://doi.org/10.1515/9783110792072-001

how individuals and societies deal with death and dying should have received such limited attention among those seeking to understand dark tourism.

Over time, new researchers approaching dark tourism showed a willingness to engage with theory, particularly for understanding the experience of visiting places of death and suffering. There were two broad perspectives. One strand adopted a social science approach and applied a diverse range of theoretical perspectives for understanding dark tourism. These included issues that were already well-established within tourism studies (such as authenticity and identity), but other researchers looked further afield. For example, some drew on developments in memory studies to engage critically with issues of individual and collective remembering. More innovative approaches attempted to understand dark tourism consumption through the lens of performance, deviance, heterotopia or psychoanalysis. More recently, there has been an increased focus on affect and the affective dimensions of visiting places of death and suffering, reflecting the growing influence of more-than-representational theories in the social sciences.

Another group of researchers approached dark tourism from the broad perspective of consumer behaviour and drew on an eclectic range of theories of human behaviour to better understand the dark tourist as a consumer. This approach was often underpinned by a positivist approach (and use of the increasingly ubiquitous structural equation modelling). The broad focus was motivations and experiences, and researchers sought to tease out the inter-relationships between (for example) satisfaction, benefits, emotions, past experiences, and repeat visit intentions. This body of research gave us a fuller understanding of dark tourism consumption in specific contexts but, on the other hand, its contribution to understanding the 'dark tourist' (if such a person actually exists) is more limited. One curious feature about this strand of research is that the significance of death (and an encounter with the dead) is often marginal or overlooked completely; instead, a visit to a place of death or suffering is treated as more or less like any other form of tourist consumption.

Nevertheless, after 25 years of research, dark tourism is nowhere near as theoretically fragile as Sharpley identified in the mid-2000s. But there is still plenty more to be done; as a recent review paper has noted, theory in dark tourism research remains underdeveloped (Rajasekaram, Hewege & Perera, 2022). Given the growing body of critical research within tourism studies, dark tourism has lagged behind. For example, critical tourism researchers have been examining postcolonialism for two decades, but dark tourism research has only sporadically engaged with this topic. Similarly, the issue of gender has been curiously neglected within dark tourism (Stone & Morton, 2022) beyond identifying gender differences in the behaviour of consumers. In addition, dark tourism research has tended to shy away from the 'big' challenges facing contemporary societies. As Sharma and Martini (2024, p. 5) have argued, the majority of dark tourism scholarship has "maintained a distant and reluctant relationship with real and pragmatic issues of contemporary social, political and environmental importance". In short, there are many more aspects of the interplay between tourism and death which await fuller scrutiny and theorization (Pratt, Tolkach & Kirillova, 2019).

This is where this book makes an important contribution. Through its engagement with a range of critical theories this volume addresses gaps in the existing dark tourism literature, but also moves the debate forward in exciting new directions. Some of the chapters add innovative perspectives to existing strands of dark tourism research. For example, there are new considerations of tourists' emotional and affective experiences at places of death and suffering. A number of the chapters examine issues of memory, trauma and violence, in hitherto unexamined settings and contexts (including digital environments). The volume also takes forward the previously limited engagement with postcolonial theory to consider the challenges of addressing the trauma of colonial eras within the practices of tourism. Other chapters focus on issues which have been largely neglected by dark tourism researchers. One example is atmosphere (see Martini & Buda, 2020), something which seems such an obvious aspect of a place of death or suffering that it is astonishing that it has received so little attention. A number of the contributors move the focus of dark tourism beyond human deaths, whether in the case of animals, or the slow death of the natural environment. Others put the representations of women (and associated issues of misogyny) within dark tourism under critical scrutiny. We also hear the perspectives of the people who work at dark tourism places and the role of emotional labor within their employment.

In short, this volume brings a welcome critical perspective to dark tourism research. It highlights the ways in which dark tourism can engage with broader social, cultural and political issues and challenges, thereby providing a more nuanced (and culturally sensitive) interpretation of what dark tourism means for the various (not exclusively human) actors involved and implicated in it. By moving away from a positivist and masculine gaze towards a realist approach, the contributors to this volume bring to the fore places, people, experiences, and voices that, up to now, have been frequently overlooked or even dismissed within dark tourism research. This volume is well-placed to demonstrate to other disciplines and fields that dark tourism research can be critical, theoretically grounded, and transformative.

References

Ashworth, G.J. (2002). Review of *Dark tourism: the attraction of death and disaster* by J. Lennon and M. Foley (London: Continuum). *Tourism Management*, 23, 190–191.

Golańska, D. (2015). Affective spaces, sensuous engagements: In quest of a synaesthetic approach to 'dark memorials'. *International Journal of Heritage Studies*, 21(8), 773–790.

Martini, A. & Buda, D.M. (2020). Dark tourism and affect: framing places of death and disaster. *Current Issues in Tourism*, 23(6), 679–692.

Pratt, S., Tolkach, D. & Kirollova, K. (2019). Tourism & death. *Annals of Tourism Research*, 78, 102758.

Rajasekaram, K., Hewege, C.R. & Perera, C. R. (2022). "Tourists' experience" in dark tourism: a systematic literature review and future research directions. *Asia Pacific Journal of Tourism Research*, 27(2), 206–224.

Sharma, N. & Martini, A. (2024). Dark tourism geographies: ontological, epistemological and axiological perspectives. *Tourism Geographies* (published online), DOI: 10.1080/14616688.2024.2319103

Sharpley, R. (2005). Travels to the edge of darkness: Towards a typology of "dark tourism". In Ryan, C., Page, S. & Aitken, M. (eds) *Taking Tourism to the Limits: Issues, Concepts and Managerial Perspectives*, pp. 215–226. Oxford: Elsevier.

Stone, P.R. (2012) Dark tourism and significant other death: Towards a model of mortality mediation. *Annals of Tourism Research*, 39(3), 1565–1587.

Stone, P.D. & Morton, C. (2022). Portrayal of the female dead in dark tourism. *Annals of Tourism Research*, 97, 103506.

Stone, P. & Sharpley, R. (2008). Consuming dark tourism: a thanatological perspective. *Annals of Tourism Research*, 35(2), 574–595.

Nitasha Sharma, Annaclaudia Martini & Dallen J. Timothy

1 Dark tourism: The need for a critical approach

The power wielded by the tourism industry, and its increasing global reach and economic power in recent decades has produced ambivalent and contradictory outcomes. This has generated new opportunities and tourism niches but also important critical reflections on how tourism changes and influences the places and communities where it is embedded, especially in times of ecological and sociopolitical instability (see for example Gibson, 2021; Morgan et al., 2018; Timothy, 2022). It has also shed light on how tourism can be utilized to critically approach pressing issues in our times, such as climate change (Kajan & Saarinen, 2013; Scott, 2011), ethics and morality (Caton, 2011; Fennell, 2018), postcoloniality (Carrigan, 2014), eurocentrism and non-western perspectives (Chang, 2015), feminism (Cole, 2018; Figueroa-Domecq et al., 2015; Pritchard, 2014), as well as broader processes of globalization, commodification, and the economic and political underpinnings of leisure and recreative activities (Ateljevic, 2011; Bianchi, 2018; Bramwell, 2011; Cole, 2012; Duffy, 2013; Timothy, 2019).

Dark tourism refers to visiting places of death, disasters, atrocities and other manifestations of human suffering (Foley & Lennon, 1996; Hartmann, 2014). In the first twenty years since its formalization as a sub-field of tourism studies, dark tourism scholarship has mostly focused on establishing itself and setting its boundaries, defining the phenomenon, establishing positivistic taxonomies, classifications and lists, as well as providing insight into the management and planning of tourism sites related to death and atrocities. The locution itself has been deemed controversial (Wight, 2006), and a considerable number of sub-groups and alternatives have been proposed (for an exhaustive list, see Light, 2017). Alternative terms for this phenomenon have not found currency in broader academia, with the exception of the term 'thanatourism', coined by Seaton (1996) to emphasize the touristic consumption of death and spaces of death. Thanatourism is used especially in heritage-oriented papers as a more neutral (or sometimes extreme) alternative to other definitions of dark tourism. However, the two terms are not superimposable, as they illustrate two different temporal arcs for the phenomenon. While dark tourism refers specifically to tourism in a postmodern era (Foley & Lennon, 1996; Lennon & Foley, 2000), thanatourism, based on thanatopsis, actual or imagined encounters with death (Stone, 2012), extends to a much broader temporality dating back to the Roman games in the Colosseum. Other concerns pertaining to earlier dark tourism scholarship include inventories of dark places and their characteristics, lists of motivations and behaviours, "dark" suppliers, and types of experience possible in such places, and integrated supply-demand frames (see Biran et al., 2014; Dann, 1998; Hartmann, 2014; Miles, 2002; Seaton, 1996; Stone, 2006; Stone & Sharpley, 2008; Strange & Kempa, 2003; Timothy, 2018).

https://doi.org/10.1515/9783110792072-002

Academic interest in dark tourism gained momentum in the mid-2000s, with different trajectories appearing in relation to approaches and methodologies. Some of the trajectories were predominantly positivist and stood in opposition to the ethos of poststructuralist epistemologies that encouraged treating tourism as a crucial social, political and cultural practice (Buda, 2015; Tucker, 2016). Sharma and Martini (2024) point out that a major critique of dark tourism and thanatourism in the past has been the gap between theory and praxis and, as rightly pointed out by Light (2017), little engagement with broader themes in critical social science. Biran and Hyde (2013) noted that dark tourism discourse has moved beyond classifications and definitions, now being recognised for the complex and subjective social phenomenon it is. Biran and Hyde argue that for the development of a greater body of knowledge surrounding dark tourism, there must be a move from the descriptive to the experiential and the critical. Roberts (2018) points out the potential capacity of dark tourism to inform and reflect contemporary interpretive and pedagogic theory and praxis.

Although more recently tourism scholars and other social scientists have re-evaluated dark tourism as a field of knowledge that can tell us more about the world where we live, this relatively new sub-field of tourism is still incipient when it comes to critical analysis. Most early studies leaned towards positivist modes of inquiry, tourist-centric approaches, binary constructions, uncritically accepted power hierarchies, researchers' unconscious biases, and dominant ideologies that influence narratives of place and neo-colonial representations. While these earlier perspectives on dark tourism were significant and useful, they lacked a degree of critical engagement with socially relevant issues such as migration, colonialism, inclusivity, social and environmental justice, indigenous rights, power relations, feminism, human and animal rights, disabilities, climate change and sustainability. This lack of critical engagement in dark tourism is noteworthy because dark tourism research exposes spatial inequalities, racial hierarchies, dissonant heritages, geopolitical friction, indigenous inequities, and the ignoring of other historically marginalized communities, the study of which, in most cases, remains limited and underexplored. Such issues require an approach that is sensitive, reflective and emancipatory. It also requires an approach that challenges and critiques society's conflicts, contradictions, taboos, power structures, ideological forces and oppressive hierarchies. Delanty (2020) argues that a critical theory perspective can offer much-needed insight into the pressing socio-political challenges of our time.

The need for dark tourism, as a field of study, to interrogate itself, and move on from positivistic approaches and into a more positioned, reflexive posture, is slowly being recognized (Sharma & Martini, 2024). Sharma and Martini note that only in recent years has a line of inquiry emerged, stemming from geographical critical theories and new materialism, utilizing dark tourism as a case study with its own specificities and debates analysed using broader social sciences paradigms. Scholars have begun to understand the potential of dark tourism as a framing tool for contemporary issues and debates, such as the role of women, children, and indigenous groups in dark tourism;

animal and plant studies within debates on posthumanism; multispecies research; crime and social justice; the Anthropocene and climate change; debates on postcolonialism and trauma; feminism; and intersectionality, morality and ethics, using geographical, biopolitical and thanatological perspectives along with non-human and posthuman trajectories.

Further, critical studies of tourism have provided an impetus to the field of dark tourism, engendering a series of reflections and questions regarding its intersection with critical theory. Some of the questions that have emerged are: What role does dark tourism play in reinforcing or renegotiating issues of postcoloniality, decolonization, gender, intersectionality, and trauma? How, for instance, does dark tourism analysis reflect on the role of globalization and its economic and political influences in places and communities? What is the role of post-disaster and death-related heritage in shaping our collective national histories and our prospective futures? And finally, how does dark tourism scholarship inform and offer us a lens through which to interpret the impacts of the Anthropocene, the age we live in, and all the issues and challenges it brings forth? An attempt to find answers to these questions will require adopting a positioned and reflexive attitude and a recognition that dark tourism can be a useful context and crucible for investigating those issues that are central to our social, cultural and political environment.

Although several psychological theories have been used in dark tourism such as mortality salience, terror management theory, etc., most of these theories largely ignore complex social issues such as institutional racism, postcolonialism, gender, and deficits in social justice for minority groups and therefore, cannot be included under the broad rubric of critical theory. This book contributes a deeper investigation of some of the gaps in the dark tourism literature, navigating through some onto-epistemological issues, possibilities, and interconnections of dark tourism with critical theoretical approaches. In doing so, it advances the need to connect critical theory, pragmatism and contemporary issues of relevance.

Critical approaches in dark tourism: Past, present and future possibilities

The polysemantic nature of the term 'critical theory' and the ensuing debates, has been widely recognized. Bohman (2005) mentions how 'Critical Theory' (capitalised) and 'critical theories' (not capitalised) are often used interchangeably in academic discourse, with Critical Theory (capitalised) referring to the range of different theories and approaches driven by Idealist and Marxist stances, developed by social theorists at the Institute for Social Research, an independent research centre established in 1923 in Frankfurt, Germany, with Critical Theory broadly referring to theories focusing on different power structures and aiming at human emancipation without belonging to, or being loosely associated with, the Frankfurt School and its followers (Bohman, 2002). Critical theory, first defined by Max Horkheimer in his 1937 essay 'Traditional and Critical Theory', emerged as an "ideologically oriented inquiry" (Guba, 1990, p. 23) in opposition to positivist social science, the non-interactive and distant relationship between researcher and participant, and the pursuit of knowledge separate from its origins, values and contexts (Guba, 1990). Critical theory involves collaborative inquiry, embracing alternative ideological approaches, capturing the lived experiences of the participants, identifying the 'oppressive constraints' and including the voices of participants (Doucet et al., 2010) while doing research. Kellner, (1990) mentions that as critical theory continued to evolve over the years, it strived to provide both a substantive social theory of the present age and a meta-theory of its theoretical presuppositions and method. Although in the context of tourism, the term 'critical tourism studies' has no formal definition, Morgan, et. al. (2023, p. 1) state that critical tourism researchers strive for "transformation of the way of seeing, being, doing, and relating in tourism worlds, and for the creation of a more equal, sustainable planet through action-oriented, participant/researcher-driven learnings and acts". This often involves disrupting hegemonic discourses and practices in tourism through research and action (Ateljevic, Pritchard & Morgan, 2013; Boluk, Cavaliere & Duffy, 2019; Devine & Ojeda, 2017).

Within dark tourism, Sharma and Martini (2024) point out that while early works do not demonstrate a close engagement with the Frankfurt School critical theorists, barring a few exceptions (see Fisher & Schoemann, 2018; Goatcher & Brunsden, 2011), a range of theoretical approaches under the broad rubric of 'critical' have been adopted where authors have called for further investigations on the intersections between dark tourism places and postcolonialism (Carrigan, 2014), feminism (Stone & Morton, 2022), deconstruction (Lennon, 2017), queer theory (Nicholls, 2018), affect (Biscaia & Marques, 2022), race (Alderman, 2017), spectrality (Tiberghien et al., 2023) and psychoanalysis (Buda & McIntosh, 2013). They further add that "apart from those belonging to the Frankfurt School such as Walter Benjamin and Theodor Adorno, ideas of other theorists such as Derrida (hauntology), Foucault (biopolitics), Bourdieu (symbolic violence), Deleuze (aesthetics), Kant (sublime) and Žižek have also been briefly mentioned or partially used" (Sharma & Martini, 2024, p. 5).

It is, however, important to note that the usage of the word 'critical' moves beyond the aims of the Frankfurt School of Critical Theory, and embraces contemporary critical, interpretative and deconstructive perspectives founded on inclusivity to create more room for non-Western epistemologies and strive for de-centring Western expertise and knowledge production in dark tourism. The word 'critical' in the context of this book must be treated as a broad set of ideas and orientations that attend to the engagement of dark tourism with broader sociocultural and political contexts and issues calling for an inquiry and re-examination of long-standing conceptual ideas and generalisations, recognising and questioning the status-quo and the dominant ideologies and assumptions, binaries, power asymmetries, privileges and inequities in knowledge production, and other normative, exclusive and centred elements in dark tourism.

We, therefore, use 'critical' as an umbrella term for perspectives that encompass – critical reflection (examination of existing beliefs), critical evaluation (approach to evaluation that values data transparency and inclusivity) and critical consciousness (a critically reflective understanding of oneself, others and the world; values reflexivity and positionality). Amidst the vast rage of critical theories and approaches often used in tourism studies, this book aims to highlight some major ones that have been used in dark tourism scholarship and in doing so, generate an overall consciousness about the culturally and socially constructed nature of knowledge, the various underlying philosophical influences, the limitations of traditional approaches and the diversity in ideological views that can enrich our understanding of dark tourism.

New materialist approaches

Critical theory has often been criticized for holding anthropocentric conceptions of nature and rationalist ideas of society. However, recent developments within critical theory and new materialism point to a potential convergence between these two intellectual currents, despite their internal dissensions and different origins (Rosa et. al, 2021), the point of convergence being the move beyond anthropocentric rationalism. Although the two schools of thought, the Frankfurt School of Critical Theory and new materialism differ from each other, we have included new materialism under the broad rubric of critical inquiry as it involves questioning the fundamental distinction between matter and life by proposing a 'critical vitalist' perspective (Bennett, 2010) and questioning the boundaries between biological and symbolical life (Grosz, 2011). Further, growing research in dark tourism on virtual tours and 'edutainment' using sound branding (SB), virtual reality (VR), augmented reality (AR) and artificial intelligence (AI) techniques, calls for an approach that taps into post-humanist potential. Earlier publications on virtual dark tourism are Handayani and Korstanje (2020), McDaniel (2018), Nicholls (2018), Fisher and Schoemann (2018) and Kaelber (2007).

The term 'new materialism' was coined in the 1990s to describe a theoretical turn away from the persistent dualisms in modern and humanist traditions whose influences are present in much of cultural theory (Tuin and Dolphijn, 2012). New materialist approaches call for a view that transcends the duality between ontology and epistemology, between nature and culture and focuses on cross-disciplinary efforts to challenge assumptions about humans and the non-human or other-than-human world (Sharma & Martini, 2024). Sharma and Martini point out the growing use of new materialist perspectives in dark tourism and how it demonstrates the potential for an interdisciplinary and changing assemblage within the field that goes beyond traditional anthropocentric views of place.

New materialism approaches involve ideas around more-than-human worlds, human-nonhuman assemblages, the vitality and vibrancy of things, sensory encounters, posthumanist performativity, identifying entanglements and shared agency, identifying exclusions, respectful engagements with disciplinary differences, the micropolitics of relations and affects, embodied habits, emotions, animacies and post-Anthropocene politics, posthuman environmental ethics, affective atmospheres and non-representational methodologies (Lupton, 2018). Some key theorists of new materialist approaches include Spinoza, Deleuze, Guattari, Barad, Braidotti, Latour, Foucault, Haraway and Thrift.

This book contains several chapters that adopt new materialist perspectives. In the following sections, we provide an overview of some selected critical theoretical approaches in dark tourism.

Critical memory – traumascapes and dystopia

A body of work that deserves special attention in the context of dark tourism is 'critical memory studies'. Kaplan (2023) notes that memory studies examine how memorialization can happen, what shapes it takes, and what it means. There have been several studies in dark tourism that have addressed how memory comes to be expressed and known, but critical memory studies go a step further in opening up a wide spectrum of new approaches to memory in culture besides addressing issues of relevance such as race. Memory, environment and the threat of a dying planet in the Anthropocene (also referred to as environmental memory) and counter monumental memory "insists on reflection and resists the easy dismissal of a sort of 'been-there-done-that' temptation viewers may experience in more monumental forms of memorialization" (Kaplan 2023, p. 5). Although exploring the politics of memory in dark tourism is not new, the relatively new approach known as 'critical memory studies' has recently come to the fore especially due to its attunement to contemporary new technologies and media. 'Critical memory studies' has opened up new perspectives in tourism studies generally but may also be particularly effective and relevant in the context of dark tourism, as it can help reframe memories of death and disaster in a way that accounts for the traumas still embedded in the physical and emotional landscape of those who were subject to the dark event. It can also serve as a useful tool to explore commemorative events, death-related events and funeral rites, post-disaster spaces and dark exhibits.

From trauma and environmental studies and memory to digital memory in a virtual context and memory associated with monuments, memorials, and museums, 'critical memory studies' demonstrates strong potential to foster "dialogue between (inter) media, visual studies and critical/cultural theory with an awareness of acquired knowledge from past critical thinking as well as our current Zeitgeist (i.e. posthumanism)" (Ionescu, Milesi and Herbrechter, 2023). Brunow (2015) states how critical memory studies can help in understanding what role immersive media may play in the production, circulation and transformation of cultural memory. The importance of critical memory studies has grown as it is believed to carry the potential to shed light on how digital/virtual media technologies, and processes (re)shape cultural and aesthetic objects, generating new memorial practices, which is becoming increasingly relevant in dark tourism contexts.

Sharma and Martini (2024) note that the values attached to memories or forgotten pasts will always remain a concern when dark tourism engages with memory studies in contexts associated with violence, trauma, suppression of voices and acts of destruction and erasure. The complex relationship between dark tourism and memory deserves critical theoretical investigation, with ideas such as 'hauntology' and 'spectrality' being potential theories that can be used particularly in the context of digital and environmental memories. Two chapters in this book deal with these two types of memories – one in the context of virtual tourism (video games) and another in the context of disappearing Arctic cryospheres.

Over the past few years, there has been an increase in research examining the role of memory in imagination and future thinking or simulating the future using artificial intelligence. This creation of imaginary memories and liminal, futuristic scenarios that provide us a peek into how any kind of crises can come and go or come and stay and how our lives may be altered, is given meaning through dystopian literature. Dystopias, their pervasiveness in our lives and their historical alignments can be analyzed using critical theories such as the case where the works of Theodor Adorno, a leading member of the Frankfurt School of Critical Theory, have been used (McManus, 2022). Several studies around the concept of dystopia in dark tourism have come up in the last decade. In relation to consumption behavior, Podoshen et. al (2014) conceptualize dystopia as a collective vision for a future, alternate society. Other similar studies include Podoshen et. al (2015), Pimentel Biscaia et al. (2022), Khader (2019), Farkic (2020) and Bergman (2018).

Another field that has emerged in close partnership, its boundaries almost indistinguishable from critical memory studies, is trauma studies. The conventional theory of trauma developed in Holocaust and trauma studies, has been used, with only limited attempts to develop alternative conceptualizations applicable to localized, culturally specific representations of suffering (Traverso & Broderick, 2010). With reference to trauma studies and representation of traumatic memory, Traverso and Broderick (2010, p. 4) add that while "the application of the notion of trauma to the analysis of history, culture and politics is widespread, the methodological distinction between this term's original psychological denotation and its analogical use in relation to the socio-cultural realm is often ambiguous if not altogether obscure". In dark tourism, the intensity and complexity of that traumatic memory and its cultural and political expressions can be understood through critical, self-reflexive and interdisciplinary approaches. The consumption of trauma at sites of dark tourism has been addressed by a few studies such as Carrabine (2017), Lischer (2019), and Korstanje and George (2017).

Biopolitical approaches

The concept of biopolitics entered the public debate in 1976 with the publication of Michel Foucault's *The Will to Knowledge: History of Sexuality Volume I*, and *Society Must Be Defended* (1976), in which the philosopher outlines how human populations are managed and controlled through the institutional exercise of power. According to Foucault, biopolitics relates not just to the management of populations' lives, but also to their mortality. In *Society Must Be Defended*, he asks: "How can the power of death, the function of death, be exercised in a political system centered upon biopower?" (1976, p. 254). Biopolitics can be understood as a political rationality that takes the administration of life and populations as its subject: 'to ensure, sustain, and multiply life, to put this life in order'. Biopower thus names the way in which biopolitics is put to work in society (Adams, 2017).

The nexus between tourism and biopolitics has been analysed in tourism studies (Lisle, 2016; Roelofsen & Minca, 2018; Rutherford, 2013; Simpson, 2015), with a special focus on the concept of the tourism enclave as 'camp' (see for example Ek & Tesfahuney, 2019, 2021; Minca, 2009), which allows the definition of issues related to territorialization, postcolonialism, subjectivity, and of the enclave as critically representative of a neoliberal capitalistic world order (Saarinen, 2019). In critical tourism studies, biopolitics has been used to look into the commodification of the labour force in tourism, and the processes of disciplining the bodies of both tourism workers and tourists (Tzanelli, 2022), as sovereign power makes and breaks ontological distinctions which are located in the liminal space between law and outlaw, life and death.

Dark tourism has just now started to incorporate a biopolitical lens to critically assess contexts of death, disaster and atrocities. As biopolitics refers to the control and management of populations – their life, but also their death in Mbembe's (2006) necropolitical perspective – the two topics find strong points of convergence and can constitute a critical nexus for future research. One trajectory relates to negative biopolitics, or thanatopolitics (Esposito, 2011; Lynch, 2019). As thanatopolitics is defined as the sovereign control on who or what is allowed to live, dark tourism experiences in places of atrocities, murder and other death represent a heritage and historical perspective that reframes thanatopolitical processes and histories as neoliberal commodities, thus harnessing and sedating their negativity in a way that affirms the life of the tourist itself.

As Minca and Ong (2016, p. 38) explain, indeed "carceral spaces often become converted into sites of leisure and tourism". The commodification of sites of death and pain can open the possibility to analyses that consider processes of commodification in relation not just to place, but to broader temporal perspectives in which traces of past violence, forced control or repression of bodies are exhibited through present forms of dark (but also educational) tourism. Moreover, the biopolitical turn can be applied to dark tourism to "reveal the technological construction of many of the foundational categories sustaining the colonial imaginary" (Lisle, 2015, p. 2) in tourism as well as dark tourism places, governing and subverting the governance of the neoliberal bodies of tourists, labourers, and local residents alike.

Affect, atmospheres and emotions

Death, disaster, and atrocities are highly emotional events, which can elicit strong and violent emotions. Dark tourism encapsulates the same potential for emotional and affective expressions, as emotional and affective engagement help visitors to generate meaning through their dark tourism experiences (Sigala & Steriopoulos, 2021). However, a critical approach to the fields of emotions and affect has developed just recently in dark tourism studies, in response to a broadening of work on the marketing perspectives of dark tourism, in which emotions and affects have been treated uncritically and in positivistic ways. In much work on dark tourism, indeed, taxonomies of emotions appear, often collected through quantitative data such as surveys or multiple-choice questionnaires. More recently, academics have recognized and investigated the emotional, subjective and specific value of these sites, both for tourists and locals (Amujo & Otubanjo, 2012; Ashworth & Isaac, 2015; Mair, Ritchie, & Walters, 2016; Martini & Buda, 2020; Tucker et. al, 2017; Wright & Sharpley, 2018).

Affects can be defined as intensities, other-than-conscious potential for feelings that can surface (see Massumi, 2002; Thrift, 2004, 2008), an intensity that can increase and become perceivable and expressed as emotion (Ngai, 2005). Approaching emotions and affects utilising critical theory offers dark tourism scholarship the opportunity to broaden its scope, and recognise the lived, vital role of our inner worlds in shaping the dark tourism experience. Indeed, the seemingly paradoxical departure point of dark tourism is that it is a form of tourism based on the desire of tourists to experience negative feelings. Nonetheless, when looking at emotions and affect critically, we see that negative feelings may even be a magnet for visitors (Nawijn & Fricke, 2015; Oren, Shani & Poria, 2021), as they can produce profound positive transformative and enlightening experiences for tourists (Martini & Sharma, 2022) and for locals (Martini & Minca, 2021).

Places where dark tourism is practised and dark heritage is exhibited cannot be considered solely in relation to their connection to death and disaster, as this would diminish the importance of the spatial characteristics of the place and agency of the tourist (Bowman & Pezzullo, 2009). Dark heritage, in particular, is often affectively entrenched with broader management issues related to culture and politics and national identity (Wang et al. 2021), education and nostalgia (Martini & Buda, 2020). Highlighting the dark element of a place of heritage, or conversely suppressing it, is a form of engineering of tourism places that is markedly political and connects to the manipulation of emotions and affects to propose specific messages and perspectives on history (Duff, 2010), whether it is an expression of active management or passive constitution (Wetherell, 2015).

In our globalized and interconnected society, as dark places are in most cases first apprehended through media, scholars have also reflected on the affective role the media has in shaping the flows of affect that contribute to the image and imaginary connected to dark tourism places (Andén-Papadopoulos, 2009; Lisle, 2007; Tzanelli, 2013), creating familiarity with places of death and disaster, and the communities which experienced the tragic event (Buda & McIntosh, 2013) but also producing a numbing effect on the spectator (Pile, 2011). Work on dark tourism in connection to emotions and affect has a long way to go, and multiple compelling trajectories to follow. Animals in dark tourism, dark tourism and climate change, biopolitics and geopolitics in connection to dark tourism, all present strong affective and emotional elements, which should be further unearthed in dark tourism critical research (Kline & Rickly, 2021; Mahoney, 2020; Varnajot & Salim, in press; Zhang et al., 2023).

Atmospheres, a term closely connected to affect studies and often used in the context of memory and the spectral, has recently garnered attention in dark tourism. According to d'Hauteserre (2015, p. 80), "atmospheres signify bodies affecting other bodies and the spaces in which they perform". In dark tourism, the role of atmosphere, or the concept of atmospherics, has considerable potential in not only understanding both the production and consumption of the tourist encounter but also creating the planning, designing and architecture of dark tourism places that are likely to influence tourist experiences, emotional engagement, perceptions of authenticity, and transformative changes and behaviors. There are relatively few studies that have provided insights into atmospheric conflicts, a gap that is addressed in Chapter 2 of this book. Using an atmospheric approach in dark tourism, one can learn a lot about sensitive issues like atmospheric conflicts and negotiation, harmonization and exclusion, particularly as it pertains to war and conflict-ridden dark tourism places. The designing and creation of atmospheres at dark tourism festivals and events such as the Bram Stoker Festival and the Salem Festival of the Dead, as well as other virtual tours, are useful in understanding both digital and in-person tourist experiences. Since atmospheric encounters are connected with bodily encounters, sensuous experiences, rituals and performative enactments, the politics behind the construction and its commodification merits critical inquiry (See Duncombe, 2007). Within the context of dark tourism, affective atmospheres have been largely ignored, with Goulding and Pressey's (2023) study being an exception. They explore the nature and meaning of felt atmospheres at a former concentration camp by using the concept of the palimpsest (a metaphorization of memory and a process of historical layering) as an enabling framework. Other studies that have covered this concept are Martini and Buda (2020), Sun and Lv (2021), and Martini and Minca (2021).

Postcolonial and decolonial approaches

Tourist negotiations with places associated with power differences and hierarchies, suffering, trauma and dark histories have yet to be critically analysed. Few dark tourism scholars have acknowledged the importance of cultural differences and alternative forms of knowledge in the treatment of death, interactions involving the subaltern, any agency on the part of the colonized, and the concept (and process) of othering in dark tourism practices.

Sharma and Martini (2024) point out the absence of cultural humility in dark tourism discourse and discuss the dominance of Western scholars in shaping dark tourism theory with the creation of classification systems and frameworks that are often acontextual, geographically and culturally non-inclusive, and have little or no room for non-Western interpretations and representation of death. This is a prominent problem in the area of heritage with its meanings, values and tourism use. The colonial and Eurocentric view of heritage often varies considerably from how traditional societies see the relics and performances they inherit from the past. For example, Western perspectives emphasize excavating, restoring and preserving as a means to learn about the past. In many traditional societies, however, ancestral ruins should remain undisturbed and certainly not placed in a museum! Instead, their past is learned through oral traditions, performances and legends, and the archaeological remains should be left undisturbed because they belong to the ancients, not to their descendants. Such 'colonialist' differences have caused considerable conflicts in heritage management circles in postcolonial societies, especially when native relics have been removed to the colonial metropoles for display in museums and royal collections (Timothy, 2023). Likewise, from a dark tourism perspective, in some non-Western cultures, consuming spaces and events associated with death and suffering is abhorrent, taboo and even antithetical to respecting the dead. In societies where even mentioning the deceased is offensive or off-limits, commercializing trauma, suffering and death may be entirely unacceptable (Timothy, 2024).

Globalized Eurocentric discourses of history have been criticized by scholars in the past (e.g., Chakravarty, 1992) and dark tourism scholarship is not untainted, especially in terms of knowledge production and applicability of concepts. Light (2017) points out the lack of studies addressing the critical intersections between dark tourism and post-colonial scholarship. Skinner (2010) brought forth the idea of performativity to the analysis and representation of travel practices and points out the failure in understanding the Other and its representations. Within the context of dark tourism, the use of frameworks, models and spectrums to index the cultural complexity of trauma has been criticized by many, including Clarke, Dutton, & Johnston. (2014). (2018) and Bowman and Pezzullo (2009).

While discussing postcolonial travel writing, Clarke (2018, p. 50) noted that "travellers are inevitably caught up in a consumerist culture that exploits the exotic aura of the past", and dark tourist sites exemplify how the violence and trauma of the colonial past is mediated through the narratives and representations of history and memory. He refers to postcolonizing cultures as those "'aftermath' cultures acting out and working through the legacies of their violent pasts" (Clarke, Dutton and Johnston, p. 222). In terms of postcolonial travel practices, he added that while some of them could be "considered continuous with a colonial heritage, others can be interpreted as oppositional and ameliorative" (p. 222) and based on one's negotiation with colonial discourses and power, travelling subjects can be crudely distinguished between two kinds: metropolitan and subaltern travellers.

Carrigan (2014, p. 239) stresses the fact that "much of the initial work in dark tourism studies has been shaped by a sociological sensibility that tends to subdue cultural or anthropological difference, accounting quite generally and at times ethnocentrically for issues like fascination with death and engaging with moral quandaries for the purpose of better anticipating supply and demand concerns". He argues for a greater focus on the perspectives and voices of indigenous communities and mentions how non-Western dark tourism sites often tend to "pander to western sensibilities and ignore culpability of western governments in generating conflicts and disasters" (Lennon and Foley, 2000, p. 163) and how (Western) scholars in the field do not always pay heed to such complexities associated with the production and consumption of dark tourism attractions. In remediating this, he discussed the importance of a postcolonial approach in dark tourism studies which holds the potential to form part of a 'transformative' praxis striving towards social, cultural and economic empowerment. Ravi (2014) also highlights the usefulness of postcolonial approaches in enhancing our understanding of experiential and affective dimensions of dark tourism.

Postcolonial studies have widely challenged the hegemonic discourse on globalization, neoliberal economic and development policies (Krishna, 2018), climate change negotiations (Saran, 2015) and refugee and migration policies (Bilgic, 2018). Challenging the dominant discourses has empowered several social movements and research directions in tourism studies related to colonialism, race, and genocide.

Postcolonial approaches are not only useful in critically analysing places with dark historical pasts marked by national conflicts, colonial oppression and injustice but also critically understanding the inequalities of contemporary tourism practices reflected in the way different places of death and suffering are treated and commoditized. However, it is essential to note that postcolonial scholarship, has faced its share of criticism (Spivak, 1985) and has moved from the analysis of postcolonial discourses to the exploration of alternative epistemologies (Ling, 2014; Shahi & Ascione, 2016), particularly the decolonization of "our minds and our world politics" (Ling, 2014, p. 582). Decolonial theory (often considered more radical than postcolonial theories) emerged in the early 2000s, influenced by the Latin American and Caribbean scholars in the Modernity/Coloniality group and their ideas related to Latin American Marxism, world systems theory, and indigenous political struggles.

When applied to dark tourism scholarship, these approaches indicate how its production and consumption have been highly Eurocentric with knowledge production and academic discourse shaped through a Western gaze. Chambers and Buzinde (2015) note that, while postcolonial and related critical theoretical perspectives have furthered our understanding of colonialism's consequences, they have failed to provide an epistemological perspective of tourism that legitimises the cosmologies of, and actively empowers traditionally marginalised groupings. In response to this reality, they argue that epistemological decolonisation can provide an 'other' way of thinking, being and knowing about tourism as the idea of decolonization is founded on multiple and relational identities (Bhabha, 1994).

Within dark tourism, this does not mean rejecting all previous Eurocentric notions and theories but essentially enabling spaces to open up for other ways of thinking and new epistemological approaches. For example, how does one analyze Black travel at slavery heritage sites? Here, decolonization does not challenge the soundness of previously established knowledge but seeks to broaden knowledge trajectories and discourses based on context, historicity, positionality, reflexivity and an acknowledgement of power relations between the researcher and the researched. It will enable diversification of the tourist gaze and allow spaces for subaltern perspectives and intersectional experiences in dark tourism. Therefore, such an approach can be particularly useful for critically analysing the potential of dark tourism in promoting reparation, peace, reconciliation and repatriation – at sites that involve indigenous or other marginalized communities or refugee camps and war-torn areas that have transformed into dark tourism destinations.

Gender-based perspectives

The importance of gender perspectives in tourism has been highlighted by many scholars since the 1990s. Gender perspectives have been used in consumer behavior research, tourism development, relationships between residents and tourists, and the design of tourist destinations (Apostolopoulos et al., 2001; Swain, 1995). Kinnaird et al. (1994) discussed the interconnections of gender with the hierarchical and unequal social realities and relationships including age, race, religion or class, that how gender relations are often shaped by economic, political, social, cultural and environmental factors of societies in which tourism is carried out. The contributions to Apostolopoulos et al.'s (2001) volume address the politics of gender in the production and consumption of tourism in the Global South, highlighting the significant imbalances and disparities between the 'haves' (those who travel) and the 'have-nots' (those who are visited and gazed upon by travellers.

Figueroa-Domecq et al. (2015, p. 87) stress that, despite years of research and volumes of publications, "tourism gender research remains marginal to tourism enquiry, disarticulated from wider feminist and gender-aware initiatives". They argue that "any critical accounting of tourism gender research must scrutinize the systems of knowledge production, which shape the broader tourism field. The idea of academic 'gatekeepers' and questioning "who controls what, how hierarchies are built, maintained and changed and how equity occurs" have also been noted by Hall et al. (2014, p. 10) and Swain (2004, p. 102). Moreover, considering more seriously the gender gaze in tourism research may reveal new scenarios and a greater understanding of reality. A recently published article by Stone and Morton (2022) used this perspective to critically analyze how the female dead are portrayed in dark tourism and in doing so, they discuss erased identities, eroticization and beautification, Othering, misogyny, sexual grotesquery, as well as the sense of empowerment. This led them to call for an empathetic and empowering curation of the female dead at sites of public exhibition and consumption.

Within the broader domain of gender studies, feminist theory as an expression of critical theory has significant potential in tourism inquiry as a set of complex and heterogeneous ideologies that combine theory and activism for emancipation and transformation. Feminist theory allows the reinterpretation of existing theories, provides insights into the social production of complex hierarchies of difference, paves the way for new lines of inquiry (Fox-Keller, 1995), and challenges how we think about gender and society and the traditional epistemological and methodological foundations that have historically influenced what and how we research (Wylie, 2007). Critical feminist theories can be useful in tourism studies not just because they critique the masculine gaze and gender subordination and oppression, but also because of their intersections with other forms of subordination such as racism, heterosexism, and class oppression. Its broad envisioning prospects for emancipation and individual and collective resistance to hierarchies of difference, privilege, and power, can be particularly useful in understanding the construction and production of identity, ideologies, and assumptions about people and places along with the everyday experiences of men and women in the tourism industry.

Figueroa-Domecq & Segovia-Perez (2020, p. 264) note that "power distribution, labor division, the construction of the tourist landscape (natural, historical, cultural or artistic), the social perception of the 'other,' and the realities of the experiences of tourists and residents are impossible to analyze and evaluate without taking into account the importance of gender in the construction of every one of these variables". Sharma (2020) writes how the 'Otherness' of dark tourism is universal since every culture has its own way of handling the topic of death. Roberts (2018) also argues how site interpretation within dark tourism is important in encouraging understanding and awareness of the 'Other' and, thus, helping them become less othered. Seaton (2009) argues that the Otherness of death is the central, distinctive and compelling element in thanatourism. The theoretical conceptualization of Othering and the production and consumption of the exotic and erotic Other is often informed by feminist analyses (de Beauvoir, 1949; Clifford & Marcus, 1986; Fowler & Hardesty, 1994; Said, 1978; Wilkinson & Kitzinger, 1995), especially poststructural and postcolonial feminism. In fact, McClintock (1995) notes how postcolonial feminism has challenged postcolonial theory and its lack of engagement with the dynamics of gendered power in colonial and imperial contexts. Needless to say, gendered power relations play an important role in the cultural construction of places and people.

Feminist approaches have been influenced by phenomenology, radical feminism, critical race, Marxist socialism, intersectionality, post-structuralism, postcolonialism and decolonial theory. Although all of these are applicable in the context of dark tourism knowledge production, the contextual and sensitive intersectional lens is particularly useful. Intersectionality, a term first introduced by Black civil rights activist and lawyer Kimberlé Crenshaw (See Crenshaw, 1989), can help researchers explore the dynamic effects of 'difference' in more than one dimension across a variety of contexts (Mooney, 2018). Despite its pragmatic nature, the intersectional research design process can be quite complex and challenging. Intersectional approaches are particularly useful in studying marginalized communities, indigenous peoples, persons with disabilities, women and children. In dark tourism, such approaches are highly applicable in analysing sensitive, traumatic and complex issues such as the heritages associated with slavery, witch hunts, indigenous battle sites, and dark events and festivals that perpetuate the male gaze and masculine spaces.

Munar et al. (2017, p. 587) highlight that feminist perspectives propose an alternative way of doing research that includes engagement with the "principles of reflexivity, positionality and reciprocity . . ., emotional commitment . . ., democratic discussion" and mixed methods, considering possible subjective biases. Bakas (2017), Narayan (1997) and Intemann (2011) provide extended commentaries on these subjects. Reflexivity in dark tourism research has not been addressed adequately commensurate with its importance and potential contribution (Sharma & Rickly, 2018; Sigala & Steriopoulos, 2022; Stone, 2012). The same holds true for positionality and reciprocity. Although a few recent studies in dark tourism have adopted a gender-based lens (e.g., Cifci et al. 2023; Ibsen & Papadopoulou, 2021), the potential of gender-aware/feminist perspectives in constructing knowledge that is holistic, inclusive, meaningful, deep and transformative, is underutilised.

Human-animal studies in dark tourism

Critical animal studies can provide a fresh perspective on the various ways animals are perceived and utilized as part of the touristic experience (Fennell, 2024; Kline & Rickly, 2021; López López et al., 2023; Markwell, 2015). A recent perspective in dark tourism has been the growing concern for the ethics of human engagements with animals in the tourism industry (Fennell, 2024). Panko and George (2018) explore animal sexual abuse and the darkness of touristic immorality by highlighting a serious problem: human-animal pornography. López López and Venegas (2021) criticize scientific humanism and discuss animal-based dark tourism through the example of bullfighting in Mexico, raising the question why the death of non-human animals is absent in the ethical reflections of dark tourism. In their critical work, López López and Venegas' (2021) use a post-humanist ethics perspective to analyze the work of bulls in their fighting capacity, which ultimately ends in their demise, much to the delight of tourists and other onlookers in the bullfighting arena. The animals' own death is therefore the climax of the entire event and the pinnacle of the observers' experience. In his most recent work, David Fennell (2024) highlights the ethical implications of animal use in dark tourism settings.

Human-animal studies in dark tourism emphasize animal sentience, agency and welfare (Carr & Broom, 2018; Carr & Young, 2018; Fennell, 2013) using theoretical frameworks such as posthumanism. Fennell (2015) identifies five distinct theoretical approaches to animal ethics that have important implications for human-animal interactions in tourism: welfarist, animal rights, utilitarianism, ecocentrism, and ecofeminism. Posthumanist frameworks focus on the experiences of nonhuman animals that are intentionally killed, die or otherwise suffer as tourism objects (Cohen, 2019; Doyle, 2017). According to Phillips (2008), 120 billion animals live in captivity, either in zoos or as work/entertainment animals. The animal-based tourism industry contains many violent and dark elements that qualify it as a form of dark tourism if we apply the definition of dark tourism to a context that moves beyond the traditional human-focused perspective. Several scholars (e.g., Fennell & Sheppard, 2021; Yerbury et al., 2021; Wichert & Nussbaum, 2021) have discussed the need for the ethical consideration of rights and justice for powerless non-humans who serve the tourism industry, often forced into captivity, suffering physically and psychologically, enduring varying levels violence, and suffering illness and often premature death.

This book contains a chapter on the convergence of dark tourism and animal ethics in the form of a post-humanist prototype for understanding and categorizing dark human-animal tourism entanglements that aims to shift away from anthropocentrism and humanism. The three main categories include the characteristics of animal suffering and death, the subjective nature of the human-animal relationship and tourism supply and demand. As Sharma and Martini (2024) point out, a discussion on the ethical implications of dark tourism in the context of non-human animals, challenges anthropocentric and hierarchical narratives of human exceptionalism and the limitations of critical theory in addressing the ecological crisis, non-human justice and the binaries of nature/culture and human/non-human.

Structure of the book

The theoretical underpinnings of the chapters in this book range from early critical theory to emerging new materialist theories around affect. Given the breadth and diversity of critical theories, this book seeks to be suggestive rather than exhaustive. It covers useful and timely chapters that can provoke further research and debate in dark tourism studies. The chapters have been categorized according to the different critical theoretical perspectives they adopt.

Part 1, 'Dark Tourism, Affect and Emotions', contains two chapters that demonstrate glimpses of new materialism for studying tourist experiences in dark tourism. In Chapter 2, Ethan Bottone, Derek Alderman, Stefanie Benjamin and Sarah Frankel draw upon atmospheric studies to critically examine how competing atmospheres may manifest and are negotiated within the same touristic space. They do this by using a case study of the multiple affective atmospheres constructed in and through the Titanic Museum Attraction (TMA) in Pigeon Forge, Tennessee, USA. In Chapter 3, Rami Isaac uses an experiential perspective based on emotions theory and affect to investigate tourist experiences, particularly the tangible and intangible attributes that could trigger emotions at Chernobyl.

The chapters in Part 2 explore the intersections between dark tourism and critical animal studies. Chapter 4, which is a re-published work by David A. Fennell, Bastian Thomsen and Samuel R. Fennell, presents a novel framework based on the confluence of dark tourism and animal ethics literature providing avenues for thinking about future research in the field of animal dark tourism. This is followed by José-Carlos García-Rosell and Philip Hancock's work (Chapter 5), which adopts a critical animal studies perspective to evaluate dark tourism and its tendency to marginalise the death and suffering of animals as a worthy subject of either tourist or academic moral consideration. They argue that the exploitation of animals, or more accurately the death of animals in a farm tourism context, constitutes an object of dark tourism.

Part 3 delves into critical memory studies and contains five chapters that revolve around the politics of memoryscapes or traumascapes. Chapter 6 by Alexis Whitacre examines refugee camp tourism as a form of dark tourism and how the human suffering of the camps becomes a spectacle for tourists' consumption. Based on her fieldwork at Palestinian refugee camps and drawing upon critical memory studies and authenticity literature, she explores the social construction of refugee suffering as a form of 'authenticity' for tourists and examines the role social media plays in mediating suffering during political conflict. Magdalena Banaszkiewicz and Jonathan Skinner (Chapter 7) present two case studies – the Chornóbyl Exclusion Zone (CEZ) and the Montserrat Volcano Exclusion Zone (MEZ) – to examine 'exclusion' as a dark tourism concept associated with apocalyptic separation from everyday living. In Chapter 8, Alix Varnajot, Margaréta Pintér, Vesa-Pekka Herva, Albina Pashkevich and Thora Hermann highlight dark tourism practices associated with other-than-human deaths by investigating the conceptual intersections between dark tourism and Arctic traumascapes in the Anthropocene raised by the shrinking cryosphere in Finnish Lapland. Chapter 9 by Alena Pirok critically investigates the origin of dark tourism in the case of Colonial Williamsburg's 1993 slave auction. By focusing on public history professionals' motives and the concept of emotional labor, she argues that, in the world of educational institutions, dark tourism is more of a professional fear, than a reality. In Chapter 10, Florence Smith Nicholls discusses virtual dark tourism, particularly the video game Disco Elysium, using Derrida's concept of hauntology. She concludes that the game can be understood as haunted on various levels: with reference to the video game medium itself, in terms of its post-revolution fantasy-realism setting, and as a product of the alleged toxic work environment that the game was produced under.

Part 4 is titled 'Dark Tourism, Power and Identity' and contains four chapters that challenge power differences, hegemonic discourses, dominant ideological forces and oppressive hierarchies. Maximiliano E. Korstanje (Chapter 11) critically investigates the contributions and limitations of dark tourism theory in a post-colonial context. He explores the political nature of dark tourism, as well as its intricacies in the configuration of (neo)colonial cosmologies through the bloody legacy of trauma and violence in former colonies. Korstanje also discusses the extent to which dark tourism heals or affirms the dominant discourses forged during colonial rule. In Chapter 12, Sarike van Slooten uses a postcolonial approach to explore how the legacies of colonialism are experienced by visitors through museum exhibitions in various colonial geographies and how museums can connect better to contemporary debates of colonialism. This is particularly relevant in the context of dark tourism that often deals with legacies of colonial trauma, including slavery, genocide and human oppression. Chapter 13 by Cecilia de Bernardi, Bailey Ashton Adie, and Esther Snell discusses the representations of crime in state-run police museums that function as an expression of official narratives of justice, control, and state-sanctioned morality, all of which come in the guise of edutainment. Their approach is a critical stance on ideologies, hegemony, and power. Lastly, Chapter 14 by Rebecca Finkel and Katherine Dashper, uses a feminist lens in dark tourism to examine how witches, and related dark histories of misogyny and violence, are represented in witch tours in Britain.

This introductory chapter has provided a conceptual foundation for the chapters that follow. The contributors to this volume have adopted many critical theory perspectives on a wide range of dark tourism contexts and cases. The importance of moving beyond normative positivistic approaches to dark tourism (and other forms of tourism) to embrace a deeper understanding of the human and non-human experience with spaces and events of trauma and death could not be clearer. This sort of profound assessment is warranted as tourism continues to grow, more places are affected by it, and it continues to raise salient challenges to fundamental ethics, moralities, equality and justice in the human and non-human natural realms.

References

Adams, R. (2017). Michel Foucault: Biopolitics and Biopower. *Critical Legal Thinking*, 10.

Alderman, D. H. (2017). Tiya miles. Tales from the haunted south: Dark tourism and memories of slavery. *African American Review, 50*(1), 87–89.

Amujo, O. C., & Otubanjo, O. (2012). Leveraging rebranding of 'unattractive'nation brands to stimulate post-disaster tourism. *Tourist Studies*, 12(1), 87–105.

Andén-Papadopoulos, K. (2009). US soldiers imaging the Iraq War on YouTube. *Popular Communication*, 7(1), 17–27.

Apostolopoulos, Y., Sönmez, S., & Timothy, D.J. (Eds.) (2001). *Women as Producers and Consumers of Tourism in Developing Regions*. Westport, CT: Praeger.

Ashworth, G. J., & Isaac, R. K. (2015). Have we illuminated the dark? Shifting perspectives on 'dark'tourism. *Tourism Recreation Research*, 40(3), 316–325.

Ateljevic, I., Morgan, N., & Pritchard, A. (Eds.). (2011). *The critical turn in tourism studies: Creating an academy of hope* (Vol. 22). Routledge.

Bakas, F. E. (2017). 'A beautiful mess': Reciprocity and positionality in gender and tourism research. *Journal of Hospitality and Tourism Management*, *33*, 126–133.

Bennett, J. (2010). *Vibrant matter: A political ecology of things*. Duke University Press.

Bergman, K. (2018). Fukushima Daiichi as a heterotopia: *Dark tourism in dystopian places*.

Bhabha, H.K. (1994). The Location of Culture (2nd ed.). Routledge.

Bergman, K. (2018). *Fukushima Daiichi as a heterotopia: Dark tourism in dystopian places*. [Master's Thesis, Lund University] http://lup.lub.lu.se/student-papers/record/9023543

Bianchi, R. (2018). The political economy of tourism development: A critical review. *Annals of tourism research*, 70, 88–102.

Bilgic, A. (2018). Migrant encounters with neo-colonial masculinity: Producing European sovereignty through emotions. *International feminist journal of politics*, *20*(4), 542–562.

Biran, A., & Hyde, K. F. (2013). New perspectives on dark tourism. *International Journal of Culture, Tourism and Hospitality Research*, 7(3), 191–198

Biran, A., Liu, W., Li, G., & Eichhorn, V. (2014). Consuming post-disaster destinations: The case of Sichuan, China. *Annals of Tourism Research*, 47, 1–17.

Pimentel Biscaia, M. S., & Marques, L. (2022). Dystopian dark tourism: affective experiences in Dismaland. *Tourism Geographies*, *24*(2–3), 306–325.

Bohman, J. (2002). How to make a social science practical: pragmatism, critical social science and multiperspectival theory. *Millennium*, *31*(3), 499–524.

Bohman, J. (2008). Critical theory as practical knowledge: Participants, observers, and critics. In S. P. Turner & P. A. Roth (Eds.), *The Blackwell guide to the philosophy of the social sciences* (pp. 91–109). Blackwell.

Boluk, K. A., Cavaliere, C. T., & Duffy, L. N. (2021). A pedagogical framework for the development of the critical tourism citizen. In Boluk, K. A., Cavaliere, C. T., Higgins-Desbiolles. *Activating Critical Thinking to Advance the Sustainable Development Goals in Tourism Systems* (pp. 19–35). Routledge.

Bowman, M. S., & Pezzullo, P. C. (2009). What's so 'dark' about 'dark tourism'?: Death, tours, and performance. *Tourist Studies*, *9*(3), 187–202.

Bramwell, B. (2011). Governance, the state and sustainable tourism: A political economy approach. *Journal of sustainable tourism*, 19(4–5), 459–477.

Brunow, D. (2015). *Remediating transcultural memory: Documentary filmmaking as archival intervention* (Vol. 23). Walter de Gruyter GmbH & Co KG.

Buda, D. M., & McIntosh, A. J. (2013). Dark tourism and voyeurism: Tourist arrested for "spying" in Iran. *International Journal of Culture, Tourism and Hospitality Research*, *7*(3), 214–226.

Buda, D. M. (2015). *Affective tourism: Dark routes in conflict*. Routledge.

Carr, N., & Broom, D. M. (2018). *Tourism and animal welfare*. CABI.

Carr, N., & Young, J. (Eds.). (2018). *Wild animals and leisure: Rights and wellbeing*. Routledge.

Carrabine, E. (2017). Iconic power, dark tourism, and the spectacle of suffering. In *The Palgrave handbook of prison tourism* (pp. 13–36). London: Palgrave Macmillan UK.

Carrigan, A. (2014). Dark tourism and postcolonial studies: Critical intersections. *Postcolonial Studies*, *17*(3), 236–250.

Caton, K. (2012). Taking the moral turn in tourism studies. *Annals of Tourism Research*, 39(4), 1906–1928.

Chambers, D., & Buzinde, C. (2015). Tourism and decolonisation: Locating research and self. *Annals of Tourism Research*, *51*, 1–16.
Chang, T. C. (2015). The Asian wave and critical tourism scholarship. *International Journal of Asia-Pacific Studies*, 11.
Chakrabarty, D. (1992). Postcoloniality and the artifice of history: who speaks for" Indian" pasts?. *Representations*, (37), 1–26.
Cifci, I., Rather, R. A., Taspinar, O., & Altunel, G. K. (2023). Demystifying destination attachment, self-congruity and revisiting intention in dark tourism destinations through the gender-based lens. *Tourism Recreation Research*, 1–17.
Clarke, R., Dutton, J., & Johnston, A. (2014). Shadow zones: dark travel and postcolonial cultures. *Postcolonial Studies*, *17*(3), 221–235.
Clarke, R. (2018). History, memory, and trauma in postcolonial travel writing. *The Cambridge Companion to Postcolonial Travel Writing*, 49–62.
Clifford, J., & Marcus, G. E. (Eds.). (2023). *Writing culture: The poetics and politics of ethnography*. Univ of California Press.
Cohen, E. (2019). Posthumanism and tourism. *Tourism Review*, *74*(3), 416–427.
Cole, S. (2012). A political ecology of water equity and tourism: A case study from Bali. *Annals of tourism Research*, 39(2), 1221–1241
Cole, S. (Ed.). (2018). Gender equality and tourism: Beyond empowerment. CABI
Crenshaw, K. (1989). Demarginalizing the Intersection of Race and Sex: A Black Feminist Critique of Antidiscrimination Doctrine, Feminist Theory and Antiracist Politics. In *University of Chicago Legal Forum* (Vol. 1989, No. 1, p. 8).
Dann, G. (1998). The pomo promo of tourism. *Tourism Culture & Communication*, 1(1), 1–16.
De Beauvoir, S. (1949) *The Second Sex*. Harmondsworth: Penguin.
Devine, J., & Ojeda, D. (2017). Violence and dispossession in tourism development: A critical geographical approach. *Journal of Sustainable Tourism*, *25*(5), 605–617.
d'Hauteserre, A-M. (2015). Affect theory and the attractivity of destinations. *Annals of Tourism Research*, 55, 77–89.
Doucet, S. A., Letourneau, N. L., & Stoppard, J. M. (2010). Contemporary paradigms for research related to women's mental health. *Health care for women international*, *31*(4), 296–312.
Doyle, C. (2017). Captive wildlife sanctuaries: definition, ethical considerations and public perception. *Animal Studies Journal*, *6*(2), 55–85.
Duff, C. (2010). On the role of affect and practice in the production of place. *Environment and planning D: Society and Space*, 28(5), 881–895.
Duffy, R. (2015). Nature-based tourism and neoliberalism: Concealing contradictions. *Tourism Geographies*, 17(4), 529–543.
Duncombe, S. (2007). *Dream: Re-imagining Progressive Politics in an Age of Fantasy*. The New Press.
Ek, R., & Tesfahuney, M. (2019). Topologies of tourism enclaves. *Tourism Geographies*, 21(5), 864–880.
Ek, R., & Tesfahuney, M. (2021). Open Access: Topologies of tourism enclaves. In *Tourism Enclaves* (pp. 126–142). Routledge.
Esposito, R. (2011). *Immunitas: The protection and negation of life*. Polity.
Farkic, J. (2020). Consuming dystopic places: What answers are we looking for?. *Tourism Management Perspectives*, 33, 100633.
Fennell, D. A. (2013). Tourism and animal welfare. *Tourism Recreation Research*, *38*(3), 325–340.
Fennell, D. A. (2015). Akrasia and tourism: why we sometimes act against our better judgement?. *Tourism Recreation Research*, *40*(1), 95–106.
Fennell, D. A. (2018). *Tourism ethics*, 2nd Edn . Bristol: Channel View Publications.
Fennell, D. A. (2019). Sustainability ethics in tourism: The imperative next imperative. *Tourism Recreation Research*, 44(1), 117–130.

Fennell, D. A. (2024). *Tourism and animal ethics*, 2nd Edn . London: Routledge.

Fennell, D. A., & Sheppard, V. (2021). Tourism, animals and the scales of justice. In *Justice and Tourism* (pp. 172–193). Routledge.

Figueroa-Domecq, C., Pritchard, A., Segovia-Pérez, M., Morgan, N., & Villacé-Molinero, T. (2015). Tourism gender research: A critical accounting. *Annals of Tourism Research, 52*, 87–103.

Figueroa-Domecq, C., & Segovia-Perez, M. (2020). Application of a gender perspective in tourism research: A theoretical and practical approach. *Journal of Tourism Analysis: Revista de Análisis Turístico, 27*(2), 251–270.

Fisher, J. A., & Schoemann, S. (2018). Toward an ethics of interactive storytelling at dark tourism sites in virtual reality. In *Interactive Storytelling: 11th International Conference on Interactive Digital Storytelling, ICIDS 2018, Dublin, Ireland, December 5–8, 2018, Proceedings 11* (pp. 577–590). Springer International Publishing.

Foley, M., & Lennon, J. J. (1996). JFK and dark tourism: A fascination with assassination. *International Journal of Heritage Studies*, 2(4), 198–211.

Fowler, D.D. & D.L. Hardesty (1994) *Others Knowing Others: Perspectives on Ethnographic Careers*. Washington, DC: Smithsonian Institute Press.

Foucault, M. (1976*). The history of sexuality (The will to knowledge: History of sexuality vol. 1).* London: Allen Lane.

Fox-Keller, E. (1995). *Reflections on gender and science*. London: Yale University Press.

Gibson, C. (2021). Theorising tourism in crisis: Writing and relating in place. *Tourist Studies*, 21(1), 84–95.

Goatcher, J., & Brunsden, V. (2011). Chernobyl and the sublime tourist. *Tourist Studies, 11*(2), 115–137.

Goulding, C., & Pressey, A. (2023). A palimpsestic analysis of atmospheres at dark tourism. *Annals of Tourism Research*, 101, 103577.

Grosz, E. (2011). *Becoming undone: Darwinian reflections on life, politics, and art*. Duke University Press.

Guba, E. G. (1990). *The paradigm dialog*. Sage.

Hall, C. M., Williams, A. M., & Lew, A. A. (2014). Tourism: conceptualizations, disciplinarity, institutions and issues. In A. Lew, C. M. Hall, & A. Williams (Eds.), *A tourism companion* (2nd ed., pp. 3–24). Oxford: Blackwell.

Handayani, B., & Korstanje, M. E. (2020). Virtual dark tourism: The role of sound branding and augmented reality for death sites. In *Destination management and marketing: Breakthroughs in research and practice* (pp. 183–203). IGI Global.

Hartmann, R. (2014). Dark tourism, thanatourism, and dissonance in heritage tourism management: New directions in contemporary tourism research. *Journal of Heritage Tourism, 9*(2), 166–182.

Intemann, K. (2011). Diversity and dissent in science: does democracy always serve feminist aims?. In Anderson E. (Ed.). *Feminist Epistemology and Philosophy of Science*. (pp. 111–132). Springer: Dordrecht

Ibsen, K., & Papadopoulou, E. D. (2021). *Dark tourism experiences: The case of witch tourism* (Doctoral dissertation, Doctoral dissertation, Copenhagen Business School. (CBCMO1001E)-Contract).

Ionescu, A., Milesi, L. and Herbrechter, S. (2023, December 13) Critical Memory Studies for the Posthumanist Age. *Genealogy of the Posthuman*. https://criticalposthumanism.net/critical-memory-studies-for-the-posthumanist-age/.

Kaelber, L. (2007). A memorial as virtual traumascape: Darkest tourism in 3D and cyber-space to the gas chambers of Auschwitz. *E-Review of Tourism Research, 5*(2), 24–33.

Kaján, E., & Saarinen, J. (2013). Tourism, climate change and adaptation: A review. *Current Issues in Tourism*, 16(2), 167–195.

Kaplan, B. A. (Ed.). (2023). *Critical memory studies: new approaches*. Bloomsbury Publishing.

Kellner, D. (1990). Critical theory and the crisis of social theory. *Sociological Perspectives, 33*(1), 11–33.

Khader, J. (2019). Dystopian dark tourism, fan subculture and the Ongoing Nakba in Banksy's Walled Off heterotopia. In Isaac, R., Çakmak, E. and Butler, R. (Eds). *Tourism and hospitality in conflict-ridden destinations* (pp. 137–152). Routledge.

Kinnaird, V., Kothari, U. and Hall, D. (1994) Tourism: Gender perspectives. In V. Kinnaird and D. Hall (Eds) *Tourism: A Gender Analysis* (pp.1 33). Chichester: John Wiley and Sons.

Kline, C., & Rickly, J. M. (Eds.) (2021). *From Beasts of Burden to K9 Security: The Working Animals of the Tourism Industry*. Berlin: de Gruyter.

Korstanje, M., & George, B. (Eds.). (2017). *Virtual traumascapes and exploring the roots of dark tourism*. IGI global.

Krishna, S. (2018). Postcolonialism and its relevance for international relations in a globalized world. In *Race, Gender, and Culture in International Relations* (pp. 19–34). Routledge.

Lennon, J.J., & Foley, M. (2000). *Dark Tourism: The attraction of death and disaster*. London: Continuum

Lennon, J. (2017). *Dark Tourism*. Oxford Research Encyclopedia of Criminology and Criminal Justice. https://doi.org/10.1093/acrefore/9780190264079.013.212

Light, D. (2017). Progress in dark tourism and thanatourism research: An uneasy relationship with heritage tourism. *Tourism management, 61*, 275–301.

Ling, L. H. (2014). Decolonizing the international: Towards multiple emotional worlds. *International Theory, 6*(3), 579–583.

Lischer, S. K. (2019). Narrating atrocity: Genocide memorials, dark tourism, and the politics of memory. *Review of International Studies, 45*(5), 805–827.

Lisle, D. (2007). Defending voyeurism: Dark tourism and the problem of global security. In *Tourism and politics* (pp. 333–345). Routledge.

Lisle, D. (2016). Exotic endurance: Tourism, fitness and the Marathon des Sables. *Environment and Planning D: Society and Space*, 34(2), 263–281.

López López, Á., Quintero Venegas, G.J., & Kline, C. (Eds.) (2023). *Tourism, heritage and commodification of non-human animals: A post-humanist reflection*. Wallingford: CABI.

Lupton, D. (2018) *New materialism: key approaches*. Available online at https://simplysociology.wordpress.com/2018/01/15/new-materialisms-key-approaches/

Lynch, H. (2019). Esposito's affirmative biopolitics in multispecies homes. *European Journal of Social Theory*, 22(3), 364–381.

Mair, J., Ritchie, B. W., & Walters, G. (2016). Towards a research agenda for post-disaster and post-crisis recovery strategies for tourist destinations: A narrative review. *Current issues in tourism*, 19(1), 1–26.

Mahoney, P. (2020). Behold, the horror of man: Dark tourism in the anthropocene. *Journal of Tourism and Leisure Studies*, 5(2), 1.

Martini, A., & Buda, D. M. (2020). Dark tourism and affect: Framing places of death and disaster. *Current Issues in Tourism*, 23(6), 679–692.

Martini, A., & Minca, C. (2021). Affective dark tourism encounters: Rikuzentakata after the 2011 great East Japan disaster. *Social & Cultural Geography*, 22(1), 33–57.

Martini, A., & Sharma, N. (2022). Framing the sublime as affect in post-disaster tourism. *Annals of Tourism Research*, 97, 103473.

Massumi, B. (2002). *Movement, affect, sensation*. Duke University Press

McClintock, A. (2013). *Imperial leather: Race, gender, and sexuality in the colonial contest*. Routledge.

McManus, P. (2022). *Critical theory and dystopia*. Manchester University Press.

Markwell, K. (Ed.) (2015). *Animals and tourism: Understanding diverse relationships*. Bristol: Channel View Publications.

Mbembe, A. (2006). Nécropolitique 1. *Raisons politiques*, (1), 29–60

McDaniel, K. N. (Ed.). (2018). *Virtual dark tourism: Ghost roads*. Springer.

Miles, W. F. (2002). Auschwitz: Museum interpretation and darker tourism. *Annals of tourism research*, 29(4), 1175–1178.

Minca, C. (2009). The island: Work, tourism and the biopolitical. *Tourist Studies*, 9(2), 88–108.

Minca, C., & Ong, C. E. (2016). The power of space: The biopolitics of custody and care at the Lloyd Hotel, Amsterdam. *Political Geography*, 52, 34–46.

Mooney, S. (2018). Illuminating intersectionality for tourism researchers. *Annals of Tourism Research, 72*(C), 175–176.

Morgan, N., Pritchard, A., Causevic, S., & Minnaert, L. (2018). Ten years of critical tourism studies: Reflections on the road less traveled. *Tourism Analysis*, 23(2), 183–187.

Morgan, N., Pritchard, A., & Munar, A.M. (2023). Critical tourism studies. In: Jafari, J., Xiao, H. (eds) *Encyclopedia of Tourism*. Springer, Cham. https://doi.org/10.1007/978-3-319-01669-6_41-2

Munar, A. M., Khoo-Lattimore, C., Chambers, D., & Biran, A. (2017). The academia we have and the one we want: on the centrality of gender equality. *Anatolia, 28*(4), 582–591.

Narayan, U. (2013). *Dislocating cultures: Identities, traditions, and third world feminism*. Routledge.

Nawijn, J., & Fricke, M. C. (2015). Visitor emotions and behavioral intentions: The case of concentration camp memorial Neuengamme. *International Journal of Tourism Research*, 17(3), 221–228.

Ngai, S. (2005). *Ugly feelings*. Harvard University Press.

Nicholls, F. S. (2018). Virtual dark tourism in The Town of Light. In *The phenomenology of real and virtual places* (pp. 223–236). Routledge.

Oren, G., Shani, A., & Poria, Y. (2021). Dialectical emotions in a dark heritage site: A study at the Auschwitz Death Camp. *Tourism Management*, 82, 104194.

Panko, T. R., & George, B. P. (2018). Animal sexual abuse and the darkness of touristic immorality. In *Virtual traumascapes and exploring the roots of dark tourism* (pp. 175–189). IGI Global.

Phillips, C. (2008). *The welfare of animals: the silent majority* (Vol. 8). Springer Science & Business Media.

Pile, S. (2011). For a geographical understanding of affect and emotions. *Transactions of the Institute of British Geographers*, 36(4), 603–606.

Pimentel Biscaia, M. S., & Marques, L. (2022). Dystopian dark tourism: affective experiences in Dismaland. *Tourism Geographies*, *24*(2–3), 306–325.

Podoshen, J. S., Venkatesh, V., & Jin, Z. (2014). Theoretical reflections on dystopian consumer culture: Black metal. *Marketing Theory*, *14*(2), 207–227.

Podoshen, J. S., Venkatesh, V., Wallin, J., Andrzejewski, S. A., & Jin, Z. (2015). *Dystopian dark tourism: An exploratory examination. Tourism Management*, 51, 316–328.

Pritchard, A. (2014). Gender and feminist perspectives in tourism research. *The Wiley Blackwell companion to tourism*, 314–324.

Ravi, S. (2014). Home and the 'failed' city in postcolonial narratives of 'dark return'. *Postcolonial Studies*, *17*(3), 296–306.

Roberts, C. (2018). Educating the (dark) masses: Dark tourism and sensemaking. In Stone, P.R., Hartmann, R., Seaton, T., Sharpley, R., White, L. (Eds.) *The Palgrave handbook of dark tourism studies*, 603–637.

Roelofsen, M., & Minca, C. (2018). The Superhost. Biopolitics, home and community in the Airbnb dream-world of global hospitality. *Geoforum*, 91, 170–181.

Rosa, H., Henning, C., & Bueno, A. (Eds.). (2021). *Critical theory and new materialisms*. London: Routledge.

Rutherford, S., & Rutherford, P. (2013). Geography and biopolitics. *Geography Compass*, 7(6), 423–434.

Said, E. W. (1978). *Orientalism*. New York: Penguin.

Saran, S. (2015). *New Room to Manoeuvre: An Indian Approach to Climate Change*. Observer Research Foundation.

Saarinen, J., & Wall-Reinius, S. (2019). Enclaves in tourism: producing and governing exclusive spaces for tourism. *Tourism Geographies*, 21(5), 739–748.

Scott, D. (2011). Why sustainable tourism must address climate change. *Journal of Sustainable Tourism*, 19(1), 17–34.

Seaton, A. V. (1996). Guided by the dark: From thanatopsis to thanatourism. *International journal of heritage studies*, *2*(4), 234–244.

Seaton, T. (2009). Purposeful otherness: Approaches to the management of thanatourism. In R. Sharpley & P. R. Stone (Eds.), *The darker side of travel: The theory and practice of dark tourism* (pp. 75–108). Bristol: Channel View.

Shahi, D., & Ascione, G. (2016). Rethinking the absence of post-Western International Relations theory in India: 'Advaitic monism' as an alternative epistemological resource. *European Journal of International Relations*, *22*(2), 313–334.

Sharma, N., & Martini, A. (2024). Dark tourism geographies: ontological, epistemological and axiological perspectives. *Tourism Geographies*, 1–10

Sharma, N., & Rickly, J. M. (2018). Self-care for the researcher: dark tourism in Varanasi, India. *Journal of Teaching in Travel & Tourism*, *18*(1), 41–57.

Sigala, M., & Steriopoulos, E. (2022). Does emotional engagement matter in dark tourism? Implications drawn from a reflective approach. In Isaac, R. (Ed.) *Dark Tourism Studies* (pp. 54–74). Routledge.

Simpson, T. (2015), "Tourist utopias: biopolitics and the genealogy of the post-world tourist city", *Current Issues in Tourism*, 19(1), pp. 27–59.

Skinner, J. (2010). Introduction: Writings on the dark side of travel. *Journeys*, *11*(1), 1–29.

Spivak, G. C. (1999). *A critique of postcolonial reason: Toward a history of the vanishing present.* Harvard University Press.

Stone, P. R. (2006). A dark tourism spectrum: Towards a typology of death and macabre related tourist sites, attractions and exhibitions. *Tourism: An International Interdisciplinary Journal*, 54(2), 145–160.

Stone, P., & Sharpley, R. (2008). Consuming dark tourism: A thanatological perspective. *Annals of tourism Research*, 35(2), 574–595.

Stone, P. R. (2012). Dark tourism and significant other death: Towards a model of mortality mediation. *Annals of tourism research*, *39*(3), 1565–1587.

Stone, P. R., & Morton, C. (2022). Portrayal of the female dead in dark tourism. *Annals of Tourism Research*, *97*, 103506.

Strange, C., & Kempa, M. (2003). Shades of dark tourism: Alcatraz and Robben Island. *Annals of tourism research*, 30(2), 386–405.

Swain, M. B. (1995). Gender in tourism. *Annals of tourism research*, *22*(2), 247–266.

Swain, M. (2004). (Dis)embodied experience and power dynamics in tourism research. In J. Phillimore & L. Goodson (Eds.), *Qualitative research in tourism: Ontologies, epistemologies and methodologies* (pp. 102–118). London: Routledge.

Sun, J., & Lv, X. (2021). Feeling dark, seeing dark: Mind–body in dark tourism. *Annals of Tourism Research*, *86*, 103087.

Thrift, N. (2004). Intensities of feeling: Towards a spatial politics of affect. *Geografiska Annaler: Series B, Human Geography*, 86(1), 57–78.

Thrift, N. (2008). *Non-representational theory: Space, politics, affect.* Routledge.

Tiberghien, G., Mukhamedjanova, R., & Xie, P. F. (2023). Authenticity and spectrality of space heritage: Baikonur Cosmodrome, Kazakhstan. *Tourism Geographies*, *25*(5), 1445–1464.

Timothy, D.J. (2018). Sites of suffering, tourism and the heritage of darkness: Illustrations from the United States of America. In P. Stone, R. Hartmann, A. Seaton, R. Sharpley, & L. White (Eds.) *The Palgrave Handbook of Dark Tourism Studies*, pp. 381–398. Basingstoke: Palgrave Macmillan.

Timothy, D.J. (ed.) (2019). *Handbook of Globalisation and Tourism*. Cheltenham: Edward Elgar.

Timothy, D.J. (2022). Geopolitics in the Himalaya: Territorial conflict, political instability, uprisings, and tourism. In G.P. Nyaupane, & D.T. Timothy (Eds.) *Tourism and Development in the Himalaya: Social, Environmental, and Economic Forces*, pp. 94–110. London: Routledge.

Timothy, D.J. (2023). Heritage tourism in Africa: Where do we go from here? In D.J. Timothy (Ed.) *Cultural Heritage and Tourism in Africa*, pp. 304–321. London: Routledge.

Timothy, D.J. (2024). Ghost towns, landscapes of abandonment and journeys forward. In S. Brunn (Ed.) *Geography of Time, Place, Movement and Networks: Mapping Heritage Journeys and Sameness*. Cham, Switzerland: Springer.

Traverso, A., & Broderick, M. (2010). Interrogating trauma: Towards a critical trauma studies. *Continuum*, 24(1), 3–15.

Tucker, H. (2016). Empathy and tourism: Limits and possibilities. *Annals of tourism research*, 57, 31–43.

Tucker, H., Shelton, E. J., & Bae, H. (2017). Post-disaster tourism: Towards a tourism of transition. *Tourist studies*, 17(3), 306–327.

Tuin, I. V. D., & Dolphijn, R. (2012). *New materialism: Interviews & cartographies*. Open humanities press.

Tzanelli, R. (2013). *Heritage in the digital era: Cinematic tourism and the activist cause*. Routledge.

Tzanelli, R. (2022). Biopolitics in critical tourism theory: A radical critique of critique. Via. *Tourism Review*, (21).

Varnajot, A., & Salim, E. (in press). The hauntology of climate change: Glacier retreat and dark tourism. *Tourism Geographies*, 1–18.

Wang, E., Shen, C., Zheng, J., Wu, D., & Cao, N. (2021). The antecedents and consequences of awe in dark tourism. *Current Issues in Tourism*, *24*(8), 1169–1183.

Wetherell, M. (2015). Trends in the turn to affect: A social psychological critique. *Body & Society*, 21(2), 139–166.

Wichert, R. N., & Nussbaum, M. C. (2021). Can There Be Friendship Between Human Beings and Wild Animals?. *Journal of Human Development and Capabilities*, *22*(1), 87–107.

Wight, A. C. (2006). Philosophical and methodological praxes in dark tourism: Controversy, contention and the evolving paradigm. *Journal of Vacation Marketing*, 12(2), 119–129.

Wilkinson, S. E., & Kitzinger, C. E. (1995). *Feminism and discourse: Psychological perspectives*. Sage Publications, Inc.

Wright, D., & Sharpley, R. (2018). Local community perceptions of disaster tourism: the case of L'Aquila, Italy. *Current Issues in Tourism*, 21(14), 1569–1585.

Wylie, A. (2007). Doing archaeology as a feminist: introduction. *Journal of archaeological method and theory*, *14*, 209–216.

Yerbury, R., Boyd, W., & Weiler, B. (2021). Encounters with wild, ecotour, and captive marine mammals: what do they tell us about human well-being and environmental behavior?. *Tourism in Marine Environments*, *16*(1), 1–19.

Zhang, Y., Moyle, B., Lohmann, G., de Oliveira, R. P., Chang, L., & Weaver, D. (2023). A social identity perspective on dark tourism impacts. *Annals of Tourism Research*, *103*, 103669

Part I: **Dark tourism, affect and emotions**

Ethan Bottone, Derek Alderman, Stefanie Benjamin, Sarah Frankel

2 Atmospheric instability in dark tourism: Spatial construction of conflicting affective atmospheres at the Titanic Museum & Attraction, Pigeon Forge, Tennessee (USA)

Abstract: The relationship between tourism spaces and atmosphere, a concept that seeks to capture the relational interplay between the bodily/sensorial experiences of the visitor and the material setting of the destination, has become a topic of increasing interest for dark tourism scholars. Despite the rise of atmospheric studies, few have explored the topic through a critical lens to understand how competing atmospheres may manifest and are negotiated within the same touristic space. In order to provide more understanding on atmospheric conflicts within dark tourism spaces, we provide a case study of the multiple affective atmospheres constructed in and through the Titanic Museum Attraction (TMA) in Pigeon Forge, Tennessee, USA. Located on the strip of "tourist traps" leading to Great Smoky Mountains National Park, the Titanic Museum Attraction attempts to tell and memorialize the highly emotional and tragic story of the famed ocean liner's sinking, while also providing a space where children and adults alike can find amusement through games and activities. These competing missions require the TMA to engineer different atmospheres or distinct moods of experience for visitors. Emerging is the potential for "atmospheric instability" that permeates the spaces where visitors seek to learn about this dark event, while also reveling in the entertainment provided by the attraction. As such, visitors to the Titanic Museum Attraction are faced with a conflicting experience that influences their perceptions of both the historical event that the attraction is based upon and the present site itself. The authors carry out a collaborative autoethnography of their experiences visiting the TMA to reflect on the conflicting atmospheres constructed through the museum and how this atmospheric instability can create differing visitor experiences at one of Pigeon Forge's most unique dark tourism destinations while exposing the potential dissonances accompanying the operation of "edutainment" at many dark tourism sites. While analysis rests largely with author observations, these impressions are put in conversation with other visitor comments, particularly in the chapter's concluding section.

Keywords: dark tourism, atmosphere, affect, edutainment, Titanic, autoethnography

https://doi.org/10.1515/9783110792072-003

Introduction

> Boarding the Titanic is a crowded experience, much like what the first passengers must have encountered. After parking, we make our way to the entrance and are directed into a winding gated pathway, which quickly fills with other visitors. We are directed towards a TV screen above, and a cartoonish Officer Buster (clothed like a Titanic officer, but with Harry Potter glasses and a stylish hairdo) explains that photography is not allowed in the museum until you reach the grand staircase. I quickly realize that this will be unlike any museum experience I've had before. -Quote from Ethan's field notes

Along Pigeon Forge's tourist trap-lined Parkway is a giant ship-shaped building, "docked" between the Hatfield & McCoy Dinner Show and the Hollywood Wax Museum (Figure 2.1). Opened in April 2010 by John Joslyn, an entertainment mogul, the Titanic Museum Attraction (TMA) is located in the tourism hotspot of Pigeon Forge, Tennessee, USA, at the gateway to the Smoky Mountains. The first TMA location was opened in 2006 in Branson, Missouri, another tourism mecca. Both Branson and Pigeon Forge represent highly popular regional tourism destinations for working and middle-class families who are enticed by the hyper-real and often highly fragmented geographic and temporal experiences offered by each city's attractions – with the TMA especially demonstrative of this dynamic (Fletchall, 2013). Since its opening, the Titanic Museum Attraction has educated thousands of visitors about the 1912 sinking of the RMS *Titanic*, one of the most famous (and deadliest) shipwrecks in world history. Constructed as a half-scale replica of the ship's front half, the site bills itself as the "World's Largest Museum Attraction," claiming to feature over 400 artifacts salvaged from the ship, both immediately after its wreck and from later dives led by the museum attraction's owner (About Titanic, 2022). The mission of the site is to let visitors, described as "passengers," "learn what it was like on the RMS *Titanic* by experiencing it first-hand" (About Titanic, 2022). The TMA's website describes the experience as a "celebration of the ship, passengers and crew," stating that the "best way to respect and honor those who gave their lives is to simply tell their stories" (About Titanic, 2022).

But is it that simple, especially in the context of the spaces designed and managed within the museum and Pigeon Forge at large? Ann Fletchall (2013, p. 119), writing on Pigeon Forge's tourist strip, posits that the TMA, "arguably the most educational of the area's attractions, is firmly ensconced in upbeat hyperreality," promoting an inauthentic and irrational understanding of the mighty ship's legacy. It is this perceived irrationality of the TMA, as well as its immense popularity with tourists, that attracted our group to the site. In an effort to better understand how the TMA presents the story of the vessel, and how sites of dark tourism may more generally deal with the juxtaposition of education and entertainment, we conducted an autoethnographic study of the Titanic Museum Attraction. Through two separate visits to the TMA, our team of geographers and tourism scholars experienced the site as both tourist and researcher to take account of how the mission of "edutainment" – the complex and often uncomfortable mixing of education and entertainment – shapes the narratives and material spaces of

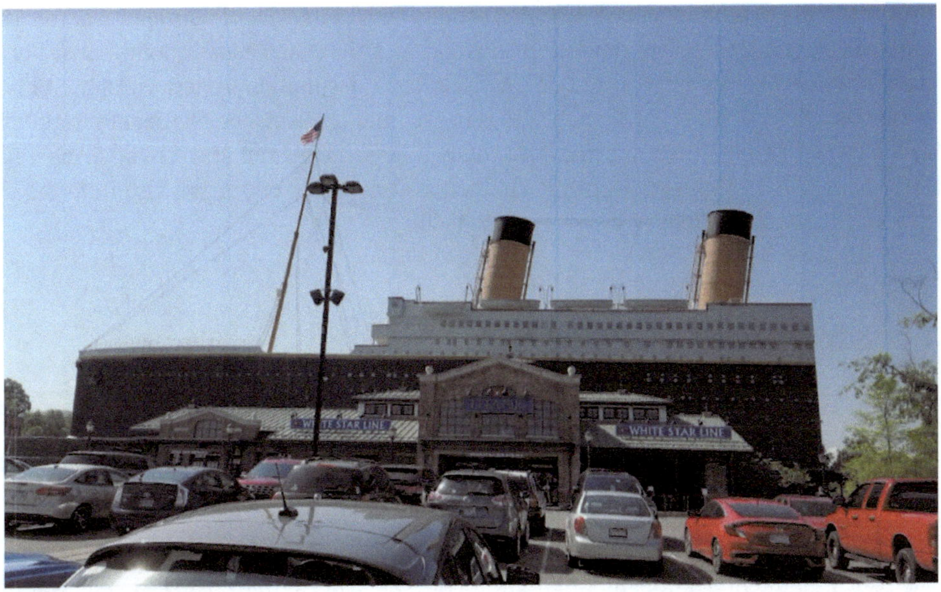

Figure 2.1: The Titanic Museum Attraction in Pigeon Forge, Tennessee, USA. (Source: Ethan Bottone).

the museum attraction (Potter et al., 2020). Our interpretations of the TMA are unavoidably subjective and influenced by our respective positionalities and the varying material-affective relations formed between our bodies and museum environments. That such relations vary and differently affect the visitor experience is indicative of the always emerging and indeterminate nature of atmosphere – even as that atmosphere is engineered. In the words of Anderson (2009, p. 79), atmospheres "are always being taken up and reworked in lived experience – becoming part of feelings and emotions that may themselves become elements within other atmospheres".

Notwithstanding the fluid and diverse impact of affective atmospheres for different visitors and visitor groups internalizing museums, the authors' tourist experiences raise questions regarding how the uneasy balance between education and entertainment at similar sites of dark tourism may lead to museum spaces being designed, operated, and experienced by tourists in ways that can produce competing atmospheres, or senses of place and the past, that work against each other – creating what we call "atmospheric instability." On the one hand, the TMA seeks to create a space where somber atmospheres can assist in telling the highly emotional and tragic story of the famed ocean liner's sinking. Meanwhile, the museum engineers decidedly differentiate affective atmospheres by providing spaces where children and adults alike can find amusement through games and activities. The atmospheric instability and affective dissonance experienced during our visits are presented below in short quotes and vignettes and help to raise critical questions concerning the ethical implications of edutainment carried out at many dark tourism attractions. Finally, at key places in our analysis, and especially so in the chapter's concluding section, the authors' impressions about atmospheric instability at the Titanic Museum Attraction are put in conversation with the stated expectations and evaluations of other visitors as reported on TripAdvisor, a destination review website. While these posts are not ideal barometers, they suggest that these visitors sense an instability in the Pigeon Forge Museum attraction's competing purposes and affective atmospheres. They react to this instability in highly charged discussions of ethics, but also in terms of more ordinary discussions of visitor dissatisfaction.

Constructing the Titanic

Before we present our descriptions of the atmospheres experienced at the TMA, we need to better understand how museums and atmospheres are constructed. Museums, as one example of a tourist landscape, have caught the attention of scholars from a multitude of disciplines. Used to present historical artifacts and narratives of the past, while simultaneously attracting paying customers, museums form an integral part of the educational-entertainment, or edutainment, tourism complex. However, such edutainment sites have been criticized, as doing justice to difficult social histories and creating moments of deep reflection can be compromised by creating an amusement experience for the visitor (Balloffet et al., 2014; Potter et al., 2020). As constructed landscapes, developed by those in power, museums are not immune from the politics of discourses and narratives (Hoelscher & Alderman, 2004; Foote & Azaryahu, 2007). For instance, Inwood (2009) details how the Martin Luther King, Jr. National Historic Site only presents certain aspects of King's life, excluding radical beliefs the pastor held in his later life. This manufactured absence reproduces hegemonic narratives of the civil rights movement and undercuts important histories of resistance that were key in obtaining social justice advances for marginalized peoples. In the specific case of the RMS *Titanic*, divisive memories of Belfast's turbulent past are left out of exhibits at the recently constructed Titanic Belfast museum (Johnson, 2014). Segregation along religious lines and sectarian violence between Catholics and Protestants are excluded from the museum's narrative, largely as a strategy to diffuse lingering tensions from "The Troubles." However, as other scholars have argued, Johnson (2014, p. 256) describes this absence as "an opportunity missed" to reconcile Ireland's colonial past with the history of Belfast and the Titanic.

While the contents of museums have received much scrutiny, the production of space within museums has been given less attention. Just like how certain narratives are included in museums and historic sites because of active decision-making, the spatial arrangement of these narratives is a (re)presentation and (re)production of hegemonic discourses (Crang, 1994; Hetherington, 1997; Smith & Foote, 2017; Hanna et al., 2019). Using the History Colorado Center as a case study, Smith and Foote (2017, p. 135) demonstrate how the "spatial positioning of text, artifacts, maps, photos, and multimedia are all part of the storytelling process". These strategies allow the creators of the museum landscape to shape how the stories of Colorado are told and how visitors will experience them. However, Azaryahu and Foote (2008, p. 191) identify that, despite spaces being designed to tell a story in a specific sequence, there is "no assumption that the [visitor] will start at a given place, follow a path in a predetermined order, or travel a route from its beginning to end". Despite the agency of visitors, the fact remains that museums are spatially constructed to portray a specific story in a specific way.

One set of concepts developed to critically question museum spaces is particularly important for enlightening the production of space: affect and atmosphere. Defined as an "other-than-conscious potentiality that can be brought [to] the surface," affect is a part of the more-than-representational turn in place studies (Martini & Buda, 2020, p. 680). The potentiality of affect can be apprehended as an "intensity, a mood, that permeates a place or event and creates a resonance, an attunement between the feeling bodies" (Martini & Buda, 2020, p. 683). In studying the relationships between passengers on public transit, Bissell (2010, p. 272) notes that "many geographers . . . have highlighted the transverse qualities of affect in that it travels *between* things" (emphasis in original). Therefore, the flow of affect between bodies, objects, environments, and other non-human representations works to develop experiences in and with places that may or may not be perceptible to the individuals embedded in the affective field (Conradson & Latham, 2007; Bissell 2010; Anderson, 2014). Working hand-in-hand with affect, atmospheres are the "[qualities] of environmental immersion that [register] in and through sensing bodies while also remaining diffuse, in the air, ethereal" (McCormack, 2008, p. 413). As this definition identifies, as well as arguments by scholars like Edensor and Sumartojo (2015, p. 253), atmospheres require the interaction between a subject and a space: "Designers set the conditions in which the atmosphere appears, creating tuned spaces with tones, hues, and shapes," but the atmosphere does not emerge until a subject interacts with the space. Therefore, atmospheres exist at the intersection between designers and visitors, meaning "it is also essential to take account of the social, historical, cultural and political contexts in which atmospheres emerge and dissipate" (Edensor & Sumartojo, 2015, p. 252). Some designers may try to influence atmospheric creation to drive home certain narratives, while visitors may enter a designed space primed with certain preconceptions that may color the atmospheres that emerge during their visit. For example, Waterton and Dittmer (2014) demonstrate how specific atmospheres are created through design features at the Australian War Memorial in Canberra, such as lighting changes, video and radio excerpts, wax mannequins, as well as the actions of the visitors. One visceral episode recounted in their vignettes included a group of high school students who accidentally watched a program more violent than they expected. After viewing the program, the atmosphere noticeably changed as the students left "far more muted . . . than they were when they entered" (Waterton & Dittmer, 2014, p. 130).

Using the context of atmospheres explored above, this chapter seeks to understand the atmospheres constructed at the Titanic Museum Attraction in Pigeon Forge, Tennessee. The TMA is an important site to understand given its status as a major tourism destination in Pigeon Forge, as well as its claim to be the largest museum attraction in the world. Further, the event itself commemorated by the museum attraction, the sinking of the RMS *Titanic*, makes it notable to investigate given its continued place in public consciousness, as recently evidenced during the June 2023 search for a private submersible lost while visiting the shipwrecked remains (Helmore & Cecco, 2023). The phenomenon of dark tourism, the presentation and consumption by tourists of real and commodified sites of death and disaster (Stone & Sharpley, 2008), has rapidly developed as a major form of touristic consumption. Debates around how sites of tragedies should be marketed and developed have raged through the dark tourism literature for several decades, particularly in regards to how places associated with death can be commodified, or even if they should be (Stone, 2020; Stone & Grebenar, 2022). Understandings of dark tourism have evolved to identify a broad range of reasons for both operating and consuming touristic sites of death and destruction, including political relationships (Lischer, 2019), psychological reflections on mortality (Stone & Sharpley, 2008), and even souvenir collecting (Potts, 2012). Informing our analysis of the TMA is a point made by Morris and Arford (2019, p. 423), who argue that the simulation of painful pasts through tourism are not "apolitical platform[s] for entertainment". Rather, these dark simulations produce a set of historical narratives, material spaces, and embodied experiences that perpetuate a selective remembering of and ethical engagement with that painful past for the visitor.

Despite the rise in interest in dark tourism, discussions of the atmospheres produced at such museums have remained relatively limited (for recent examples, see Turner & Peters, 2015; Sun & Lv, 2021). Given the emotions and sensitivities surrounding death, as well as the increasing commodification of death, dark tourism atmospheres are particularly significant for understanding how designers and visitors come together to produce atmospheres. These issues of dark tourism intersect at the TMA, especially as the site squarely sits at the junction of entertainment and education. While not located at the specific location of the tragedy, the TMA was constructed to be a site that remembers and commemorates the sinking of the RMS *Titanic* in 1912, which caused the death of 1,517 passengers. Perhaps one of the most well-known shipwrecks in popular memory, buoyed by the numerous films, plays, and songs written about the loss of the "unsinkable" ship, the TMA uses artifacts, audio-visual displays, and other interactive exhibits to tell the story of the ship's demise. Costumed docents, dressed like ship's officers and maids that would have served passengers, lead tours and await to answer questions for those wandering through on their own. Visitors exit through a gift shop, full of Titanic-branded merchandise and souvenirs. The TMA is designed to both commemorate and commodify, putting spaces inside the site within potential conflict as they were constructed to fulfill different missions. Our chapter asks, then, what atmospheres are produced at the TMA, and how the atmospheres within the museum attraction interact.

Experiencing the Titanic

To answer these questions, our interdisciplinary team, made up of scholars from geography and tourism and hospitality studies, conducted a collaborative autoethnographic study of the TMA. This form of autoethnography, itself a method of data collection that calls for the researcher to collect data via self-reflection through lived experience, uses multiple authors to co-produce a description of some ethnographic process or situation (Chang et al., 2013). When conducting autoethnographic studies, "personal experience must be used deliberately and for the purpose of offering unique insights about social life about a specified topic," necessitating the inclusion of one's "expression and experience of emotion" (Adams & Herrmann, 2023, p. 2) In collaborative autoethnography, multiple expressions and experiences of emotion are brought together in one piece, creating nuance and expanded understandings of a place or event. Particularly important for this style of research, though, is the acceptance that "emotional and reflexive embodied performances" are described "without recourse to claims to objectivity or neutrality" (Waterton et al., 2019, p. 88). Autoethnographers are expected to be subjective, occupying both the role of researcher and participant. As such, the collaborative autoethnographic method is exceptionally suitable for the research at hand, given that atmospheres emerge through bodily interactions between guests and their surroundings. Each tourist entering a space may have differing responses, depending on identity and lived experience. Therefore, the collaborative autoethnography allowed us as researchers and tourists to begin to understand the atmospheres permeating the TMA. Previous studies investigating museum atmospheres have used this method, intentionally engaging with the site "to access and consume the managed and engineered atmospheres (co)produced by the . . . museum curators and tourists as users of the space" (Turner & Peters, 2015, p. 315). Collaborative autoethnography has also been particularly useful for questioning contested spaces of tourism, "precisely because of the conflictual perceptions of the meaning of space" (Shepherd et al., 2020, p. 2).

Therefore, we visited the TMA to interact with the museum attraction, viewing its spaces through the lens of tourists, coupled with our respective research and lived identities: Ethan, an early career scholar in geography; Stefanie, a mid-career researcher in tourism studies; and Sarah, an early career scholar in tourism and retail studies. Between the multiple members of our team, two trips were taken to the TMA in Pigeon Forge, in May 2018 (Ethan, Stefanie, and Sarah) and in July 2022 (Ethan).[1] Despite the temporal distance between these two trips, very few changes were noted in the design of the museum, with the only difference being the "iceberg" that visitors could touch, which was removed in 2021 after three visitors were injured when it col-

1 One member of our research team (Derek) did not visit the TMA but substantively contributed to the conceptualizing and writing of this manuscript. Derek is a senior academic in geography who has grown up, lived, and worked mostly in the Southeastern United States.

lapsed (Belam, 2021). During our site visits, we took notes on what we each personally saw, felt, and experienced, and we later debriefed as a group regarding our observations. These visits and debriefing sessions contributed to our understandings regarding the atmospheres that emerged during our time at the TMA. In the following sections, we provide quotes and short vignettes that demonstrate our perceived experiences at the museum attraction. While not all authors provide examples for each section, our collaborative discussions contributed to collective narratives that arose and which are presented below. Overall, our visits to the TMA in Pigeon Forge yielded a shared perception that numerous affective atmospheres are co-constructed within the site, yet these atmospheres at times conflict and become "unstable," muddling the message conveyed by the attraction.

"Home Port"

> I have lived near the Titanic museum for several years and have not had an interest to visit it. Even when there were billboards on I-40, I did not feel that it was an authentic or credible attraction simply because of the location. I love history and enjoy visiting museums . . . Maybe because of the location, I put more emphasis on the attraction part than the museum part . . . As a local, I do not feel that a museum in the area is going to educate me. -Quote from Sarah's field notes

Understanding Pigeon Forge, Tennessee, is essential for understanding the Titanic Museum Attraction. The city's economy became oriented towards tourism in the 1950s, with the growing popularity of Great Smoky Mountains National Park, the most visited national park in the United States. However, Pigeon Forge itself became a destination for tourists with the 1986 opening of Dollywood, an amusement park themed around country music star Dolly Parton and the region's Appalachian culture (Martin, 2007). In the last three decades, Pigeon Forge has developed a tourism landscape that has been compared to the Las Vegas strip, albeit in lesser terms (Fletchall, 2013). Tourism continues to grow too, as in 2021 4.7 million visitors spent over 2.1 billion dollars in Pigeon Forge, both annual records for the city (Pigeon Forge Department of Tourism, 2022).

The tourism landscape of Pigeon Forge has been described as a "postmodern pastiche," a phrase that captures the hyper-realistic and ostentatious nature of many of the city's attractions (Fletchall, 2013, p. 107). These attractions "present a sanitized, idealized, fetishized version of nature, the past, the world," as "in our postmodern hyperreal condition, the fake is preferred to the real" (Fletchall, 2013, p. 104). Up and down Pigeon Forge's strip one can find portrayals of Appalachian and/or Southern life, such as Dolly Parton's Stampede and the Hatfield & McCoy Dinner Show. Each of these attractions presents a representation of what visitors expect to find, even if expectations do not align with reality. Visitors to these locations are "well-aware of the fake and [take] pleasure in the games the multiplicity of texts provide" (Fletchall 2013, p. 109). It is important to note that the abundance of Southern-themed attractions, particularly those associated with the American Civil War, is likely the result of rural Southern towns being the main source of visitors to Pigeon Forge (Martin, 2007; Fletchall, 2013). As a result of this pattern, tourism developers constructed spaces that were familiar and welcoming to these visitors, creating a landscape infused with a romanticized version of the American South.

It is within this postmodern hyper-realistic context that the TMA is situated. Far away from its home port of Belfast, the TMA is nestled between over-the-top representations of hillbilly feuds and Civil War battles. The nearest water body is the west prong of the Little Pigeon River, a small stream that drains parts of Great Smoky Mountains National Park. The TMA is effectively "docked" in a mountainous region of a landlocked state, 1,800 miles from the location of the RMS *Titanic*'s resting place in the North Atlantic. It is out of place, yet within the postmodern pastiche of Pigeon Forge, it is a unique addition. The TMA is an "unsunk" version of one of the grandest ships ever built, and thousands of visitors "board" this simulated representation every year. Postmodern tourists, or "post-tourists," "adopt a stance that conveys recognition, even celebration, of the artificiality of the performance" (Wood, 2005, pp. 321–322). The fact that a building designed to imitate the front half of a ship exists in a landlocked location is part of the draw for tourists, attracting them through the artificiality of the space.

As the entire landscape of Pigeon Forge is constructed in such a hyper-realistic manner, visitors are surrounded by a mélange of spaces designed to imitate locations far from the city, creating an artificiality that permeates the city. As noted by Sarah, a local to the region, in this section's introductory quote, Pigeon Forge can be interpreted as an inauthentic location, which influences how spaces within the destination are perceived. This perception prevented Sarah from visiting the TMA until our research trip. Other "passengers" at the TMA may likely have preconceived notions of what to expect from previous visits to Pigeon Forge, or even from just driving down the main highway through town. For instance, phrases like "pleasantly surprised" appear often in online reviews from visitors who expected an inauthentic tourist attraction, but were treated to an informational and educational experience (Titanic Museum Attraction, 2023). Through this atmospheric co-construction between the city of Pigeon Forge, the visitors, and the TMA itself, the museum attraction is (re)made as an edutainment space where visitors both learn about and experience amusement from the RMS *Titanic*'s story.

All aboard!

When I first enter the line to "board" the Titanic, a costumed employee hands me a large paper card, on which is the name and story of a passenger who sailed with the ship during its first and only voyage. [During my first visit in 2018, I was assigned the identity of William Carter, a first-class passenger from Philadelphia. In 2022, I was assigned Olaus Abelseth, a third-class passenger from South Dakota, who had previously migrated to the US from Norway.] Each card contains a backstory about the passenger, told in the first-person, including information about what hap-

> pened on the night of the sinking. Each card also ends with a mysterious question, asking whether the individual survived the sinking. Visitors are told to hold on to this card for the duration of their tour, at the end of which we find out if our assigned identity survived or not. A wall containing the names of all the surviving passengers reveals the fate of each, and visitors to the museum must find the correct name to discover how their journey ends. When I received my cards, I was excited to read and learn more about my character, but I was also put off a little by the storytelling nature of the narrative. I believe this is a product of my standpoint, as before I first visited the site, I was expecting more of a serious museum (though I may have been naïve in this respect). While reading the card, I stood in a snaking line that let visitors into the museum, group by group. Halfway through the line, there was an opportunity to take a postcard-like group photo that you could purchase once you leave the museum. I did not participate. As I got closer to the front of the line, the Office Buster video played, telling me the rules of passage (this is the second time I've heard the video). Finally, I reached the front and was greeted with a chain blocking my entrance until the group ahead of me boarded. I felt like I was at an amusement park ride. -Quote from Ethan's field notes

This vignette describes the entrance to the TMA, which is a heavily regulated and designed space that interacts with guests, leading to emergence of affective atmospheres. The passenger cards are one of the first direct interactions visitors have with the site and helps prepare the visitors to engage with the spaces of the museum attraction (Figure 2.2). The cards prime visitors before they even enter the site, conditioning them to think along certain lines. As Ethan's vignette demonstrates, the characters assigned to visitors "boarding" the TMA changed the way he thought about the museum attraction as a tourist, bringing the "attraction" side of the site to the forefront. The cards also serve to potentially gamify the visitor experience, placing the guests within a win/loss binary (survive or die) that could overshadow educational efforts within the site. Gamification, or the process of applying game-like mechanisms to non-game scenarios, has been increasingly studied within the tourism literature, with most researchers taking an optimistic viewpoint towards the concept (Negruşa et al., 2015; Xu et al., 2017; Abou-Shouk & Soliman, 2021). However, in the context of the TMA, it appears that the gamified experience presented by the passenger cards distracts from the educational mission of the site, capturing the atmospheric instability inherent in the dark tourism edutainment complex. The characters assigned to passengers follow the mission of the Titanic Museum Attraction, to "learn what it was like on the RMS *Titanic* by experiencing it first-hand" ("About Titanic," 2022), but they also appear to produce unintended side-effects that influence the way the site is experienced. These thoughts on gamification were voiced by both researchers in our group and online reviewers. For instance, a tourist who visited and reviewed the site in October 2017 stated they "felt like [the TMA] treat the deaths as part of a game . . . So, the whole visit, you have holding over you to find out at the end whether you (your character who was a real person, not a game element) lives or dies . . . Historically accurate, but something gloomy that sticks with you to flavor your vacation" (Titanic Museum Attraction, 2023).

Alongside the passenger cards, designers of the TMA use television characters, chained guide rails, and stationed employees that reify the attraction-like atmosphere of the site. These features work to create a space more akin to an amusement park than an educational museum. The movements and actions of visitors are regulated, being guided through a snaking line like one would find at Disney World or Dollywood. Visitors are also asked to take a group photo while waiting in line (which they can purchase after the tour in the gift shop). Combined with the assigned passenger identities, an amusement-like atmosphere emerges before visitors even enter the museum space. In fact, many visitors are "pleasantly surprised" when they discover that the first three rooms of the "ship" are educational in nature, telling the story of the RMS *Titanic*'s con-

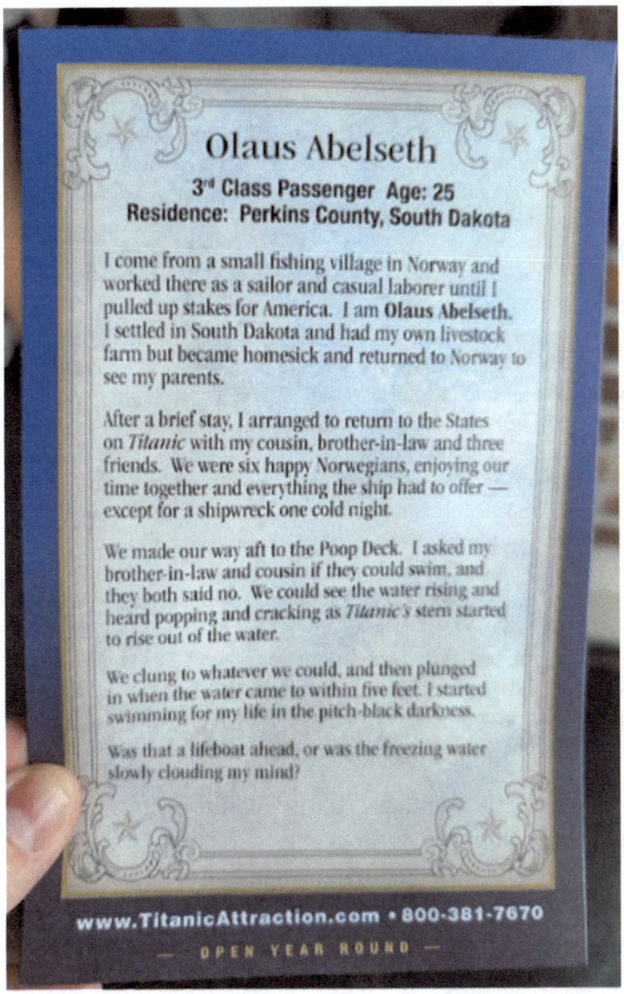

Figure 2.2: Example of passenger card given out at the TMA entrance. (Source: Ethan Bottone).

struction in Belfast and the beginning of its maiden voyage. The atmosphere of the first three rooms is quite dissonant with Office Buster and the amusement-like atmosphere of the boarding area. Atmospheric instability is seen from the very moment visitors step through the doors, potentially influencing how visitors understand and engage with the tragic and emotional story they are about to experience.

Iceberg right ahead

> Now I am seeing the sign, the iceberg right ahead, the tour continues. As I walk, it is becoming colder. Darker. Now . . . oh wow. That is why it is colder and quieter. Because in this room, we are outside. It is dark. I am next to a giant freaking iceberg. I put my hand against the iceberg and my knee-jerk reaction was "oh god, it just got real." It is definitely overwhelming in here. In this area, it is really dark, it is cold, [and] we are encouraged to touch 28-degree water. There is no pleasant music . . . It is dark. This is the first time it really starts to sink in. The fear. I am getting back to that again, the realness of it. It is so dark it is scary. It is cold. There is no happy music, the people walking into this room are quiet. Before everyone was really talking and hustling, [but now] they are walking in being really quiet. And slow moving. Some realizations are hitting. I am really scared. -Quote from Sarah's field notes

> As I begin to exit the theater, I start to hear a low rumble, with sounds of people talking loudly filtering into the corridor leading to the next part of the tour. Almost immediately after exiting the darkened corridor, I enter a large open room where the loud noises are emanating from. The room has a hodgepodge of tables and exhibits that draw visitors to various parts: to my immediate right are a set of ramps, made up to imitate the stern section of the Titanic, sloping at various degrees to represent the sinking of the ship. Teenagers are playing on the ramps, jumping from one to the next to try to beat their friends by getting farther up. Next to the ramps is an imitation lifeboat, cut in half down the center with seats inside. Each seat is connected to a speaker that tells the story of a Titanic passenger, if pushed by the occupant. I watch the lifeboat, where one person listens, but others sit and rest on the benches. Further down the room there's kiosks where visitors can play computerized programs to send S.O.S. telegrams and dive to the sunken ship to see its present-day condition. There's a knot-tying station, and a children's play-area for those 10 and under (called Tot-Titanic). As I look around the room, I am struck with many thoughts and feelings: "I gotta try the ramps," "What the hell is this place?" I feel defeated, because what is the point of having this playroom, especially after such a somber part of the tour? Is it to decompress? Is this a space for reflection? Is this merely the tourist-trap that I thought it was when I first pulled into the parking lot? -Quote from Ethan's field notes

On the second floor of the museum attraction (after ascending the recreated grand staircase and are told pictures are now allowed), visitors enter a recreation of the captain's wheelhouse. Through the wheelhouse, "passengers" are directed towards a door labeled "Iceberg Right Ahead!", which leads to an almost pitch-black room containing a tank of water chilled to 28 degrees Fahrenheit. Visitors are encouraged to stick their hand in the water tank, so as to experience what the passengers of the RMS *Titanic* experienced on that cold, dark April night in 1912. In this room is also a recreated iceberg, standing in the cold-water tank (though the physical iceberg had been replaced with a virtual iceberg projected onto a screen behind the tank before our visit in 2022). This space is designed to pull forth affective atmospheres through the interactions between visiting bodies, the objects (iceberg, cold water), and the conditions (ominous music, lack of lighting) in the room. The almost complete immersion into the experience passengers had to endure once the ship began sinking transforms the feelings, emotions, and perceptions that visitors encountered in previous spaces of the museum attraction. Before the iceberg room, visitors are led through a maze of rooms that tell the story of the ship through interpretive signs and artifacts behind glass, but upon entering the darkened space visitors are asked to explicitly feel and sense through various means. As Sarah notes in the introductory quote, a different affective atmosphere than previously experienced flows from this space's assemblage, producing feelings of solemnity, authenticity, and even fear. Sarah also takes stock of fellow visitors' reactions, sensing that "some realizations are hitting" as people enter the room and interact with the various elements. These reactions from visitors, combined with the engineered design of the iceberg room, allow an affective atmosphere to emerge that influences what and how the museum attraction's narrative is received. The sobering experience continues after the iceberg room, as visitors exit into a theater showing a short film that tells the story of Addergoole, a small town in Ireland that lost 11 of the 14 residents sailing on the ship when it sank. While not as central to the RMS *Titanic*'s story as the iceberg, the film allows the affective atmosphere to flow along with the movement of visitors between spaces, connecting spaces designed to highlight the suffering and loss experienced by those on or connected to the RMS *Titanic*.

Yet, as the second vignette in this section describes, upon exiting the theater and adjacent rooms the atmosphere as related through Ethan's experience suddenly shifts. Immediately beyond these solemn spaces is an arcade-like space full of activities and exhibits that visitors can interact with. Perhaps most notable of these activities are the three ramps that represent the increasing slope of the RMS *Titanic*'s deck as the ship slowly sank beneath the water (Figure 2.3). As observed during our time in this space, visitors, particularly children but also adults, flocked to these activities and vigorously enjoyed them. Visitors were seen climbing over the railings of the ramps, taking selfies in the replica lifeboat, and spelling their names in Morse code on the wireless set. In this space, our affective experience again returned to that similar to an amusement park or a carnival, like encountered at the entrance to the TMA. Design aspects, such as the openness of the room, the children's play area, and the video games, appeared to signal to visitors that the purpose of the space had changed, providing "passengers" the license to act differently than in the rooms they just left. In relation to these design aspects, visitors behave differently as well, expressing amusement and joy after leaving a space full of death and suffering.

The sudden change in spatial and narrative design seen between the iceberg room/theater and the playroom, and the experiences of the visitors in these spaces, exemplifies the atmospheric instability that permeates the TMA. The rapid shift between affective atmospheres related through visitors in adjacent parts of the museum attraction becomes so great that it has the potential to cause conflicts in the meaning or message of the site. The message emerging from the assemblage of the iceberg room/theater is one of tragedy, of great loss, of reverence even. The message imbued by the playroom may contain hints of this, but the affective atmosphere enveloping the space through the interaction of visitors with material objects produces a message of merriment, of touristic bliss, of a loss that may not matter. Leaving the playroom, visitors descend the grand staircase and enter the gift shop, where this message becomes further blurred by the merchandise sold. Some souvenirs are serious and educational, such as the numerous books sold, while others make light of one of the largest tragedies to ever strike the high seas, like the "Teatanic," a ship shaped tea infuser. Others, such as the heart-shaped blue diamond necklace, reference the 1997 blockbuster movie *Titanic*, which furthers the dissonance between education and entertainment at the TMA. In fact, it is the gift shop area that receives the largest amount of complaints by reviewers on TripAdvisor, with words like "concerning," "morbid," and "disrespectful" used to describe the commodification of tragedy found here (Titanic Museum Attraction, 2023). Just as the engineered exhibit spaces within the TMA emanate an affective atmosphere through interactions with material objects, the gift shop does so with "kitschy" souvenirs, generating atmospheric instability between spaces and visitors within the site.

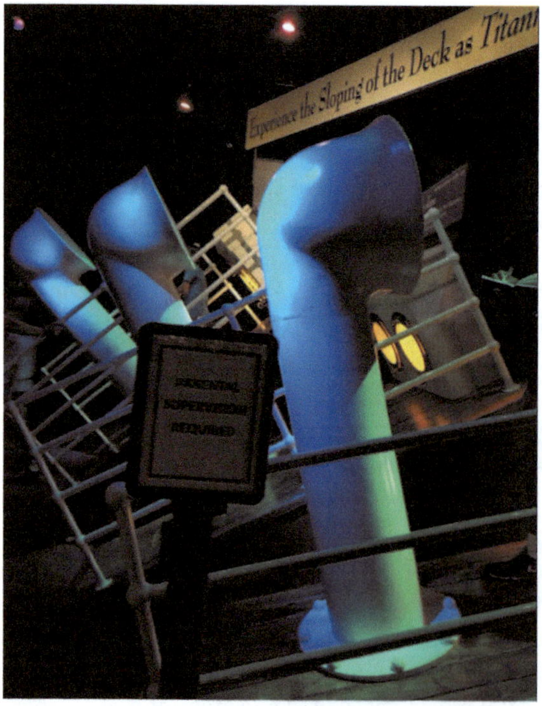

Figure 2.3: Sloping deck ramps located in the playroom of the TMA. (Source: Ethan Bottone).

If the attraction designers intended for there to be a space of reflection, our collective experiences at the site did not notice one. Nowhere was there a space to sit and take all the information in about the tragedy of the RMS *Titanic*. Visitors were shunted along a fast-paced tour leading from one room to the next, bombarded with exhibits, artifacts, and interactive activities from all sides. This lack of reflecting space was especially notable in the iceberg room/theater-to-playroom/gift shop transition, where we felt atmospheric instability at its greatest. Dark tourism scholars have noted the importance of emotional engagement in creating meaning and understanding of tragic events (Sigala & Steriopoulos, 2021). However, there was not a space to stop and reflect on any emotional engagements made, especially after those emotions had been brought to the fore by the affective atmospheres encountered. Any emotional engagements created by the iceberg room and theater seem to become entwined or overshadowed by the amusement experienced in the playroom and gift shop. A final note made by Sarah after exiting the TMA revealed the confusion over the message conveyed by the museum attraction: "But why do I feel like I didn't go to a Titanic museum as much as I feel like I went to a historical attraction?"

Conclusion

Like many tourism spaces, including those associated with dark tourism, the Titanic Museum Attraction is split between competing needs: to entertain and to educate. This split is particularly apparent in the atmospheres that emerge between the interactions with exhibits and the visitors touring the site. As the collective experiences described in our collaborative autoethnography relate, an atmospheric instability permeates the site, seemingly confusing the message and purpose of the TMA. In the context of dark tourism, this instability may obscure emotional engagements with suffering and death, as well as lessons learned from the tragedy itself. Given the sensitive nature of dark tourism matters, these instabilities are vitally important for understanding how visitors interact with sites. Given our positionalities as scholars of tourism and the subjectivity of our experiences shared in this autoethnographic exercise, gathering the views of visitors by talking to and listening closely to them is the logical step forward in recognizing how others experience the TMA. As a brief illustration, though, of what could be, our research team conducted some loose observation of TripAdvisor reviews posted by visitors to the Pigeon Forge location. This cursory analysis is of course not fully suitable for understanding the dynamics encountered by others, considering the self-selecting nature of those who post reviews and the relational nature of affective atmospheres. Nonetheless, these posts allow us to see potentialities of atmospheres emerging from guest interactions with the site and their own individual life stories and situations.

Several TripAdvisor posts revealed some evidence of the atmospheric instability experienced during our own time at the TMA. One such review from November 2017, entitled “A Wonderful Museum About Titanic,” describes similar feelings and confusions about the site that are relayed in the quotes and vignettes included in this chapter. For example, the author of the review states “I felt emotional looking at all the pictures and hearing the stories of the people on board. I thought the rooms that were designed to be just like the rooms on the ship were a nice touch, as well as feeling how cold it would’ve been on the night near the iceberg.” Yet, the reviewer also expresses disappointment towards parts of the tour that they believed were at odds with the educational mission of the site: “I was disappointed that there’s a photo [opportunity] within. I felt it was a little on the tacky side.” Similarly, the author states “I was both thrilled and disappointed in the gift shop. I enjoyed (and bought) a lot of things in the gift shop, but others left me angry. Like the magnet with water inside and a ship and an iceberg so you have to shake it around to get the ship to hit the iceberg . . . They were pretty tasteless I [thought] and incredibly disrespectful.” Finally, the author goes through a similar realization regarding other guests visiting the TMA: “It sounded as though a lot of people treated it [as] an experience based on a movie rather than an educational experience about an actual disaster that people lost their lives in, which is a shame” (Titanic Museum Attraction, 2023).

Other TripAdvisor posts recognize the dissonance between the emotions and senses evoked by different spaces within the TMA. One such review from December 2014 takes specific aim at the juxtaposition of the gift shop with the rest of the tour: “At the end of this very solemn and thought-provoking attraction, they immediately dump you off into a very tacky gift shop. We found this extremely tacky and quite offensive” (Titanic Museum Attraction, 2023). Another review from July 2016 took exception to the way certain artifacts were presented within the museum, posting “I found the mentions of items’ monetary worth to be disrespectful given the subject matter, especially the 3rd class items where a massive percentage of people died because of their marked lack of money” (Titanic Museum Attraction, 2023). While the reviews that explicitly referred to the affective instabilities created by their interactions with the museum attraction were relatively rare, a number of posts mentioned more seemingly mundane issues experienced while at the TMA. One recent example, from June 2023, complained about long queues, lamenting that “This is the worst museum experience we had . . . it was more frustrating than being trapped in a Disney line . . . you are forced to listen to the preshow at least 3 times” (Titanic Museum Attraction, 2023). Other negative reviews reference crowded conditions in front of exhibits, the darkness of certain rooms, and the amount of reading along the tour. While these complaints may seem banal and could apply to many attractions around the world, they nevertheless speak to a sense of instability present within the TMA. They demonstrate the constantly flowing, relational, and emerging nature of affective atmospheres, and in particular the sense that visitors want to have a fun experience, but one different than what the museum attraction supplies.

A final observation made during the investigation of the TMA’s TripAdvisor page reveals another way that atmospheric instability is produced through the tourist site.

In response to several negative reviews, members of the TMA's management have replied and provided justifications for the design and operating decisions that some guests have taken offense to. Replying to one review regarding the gift shop and its "tacky" souvenirs, an account signing as "Titanic Owner" replied: "As far as the retail shop, on the *Titanic*, the ship offered merchandise as a way for their passengers to remember their trip. That is the intent of our retail shop. Sorry you felt this left a sour-note to your total experience" (Titanic Museum Attraction, 2023). Responding to a review describing negative feelings of gamification, an account signing as "Titanic Crew" defended their choices, citing that "We have had over 300 *Titanic* descendants visit our ships, and each one makes the same comment, 'Thank you for sharing our family story.' Our answer: 'It is our honor.'" (Titanic Museum Attraction, 2023). The fact that descendants have praised the way the museum attraction handles the story of the ship is repeated multiple times in responses to complaints, putting TMA management in direct opposition to visitors who may feel differently. When confronted with visitor experiences that suggest the attraction puts entertainment over education, operators of the TMA appear to fall back on the memory work function of the site, discrediting the opinions of those who disagree. These management decisions are a part of the TMA assemblage that works to produce affective atmospheres that interact with guests touring the site. Their repeated commitment to the idea that the TMA is respecting the memory of the disaster's victims further contributes to the atmospheric instability of the attraction, particularly for visitors who may share a different lived experience.

While the brief analysis of TripAdvisor postings reviewing the TMA does not serve as a complete testament to the experiences of visitors, it does provide a glimpse beyond what our autoethnographic exercise presents. A number of reviews appear to capture elements of atmospheric instability, though each instance is colored by the positionality and situatedness of the author. The relationality of affective atmospheres to individual experiences with a larger assemblage of objects, emotions, conditions, and other bodies demonstrates their fluidity and their constantly emerging nature. Further, they show that atmospheric instability is also fluid and constantly emerging, generating instances where visitors to the same site may encounter vastly differing experiences, including conflict and confusion. Overall, our collaborative autoethnography raises questions about dark tourism sites partaking in edutainment, as it appears conflicts exist in presenting messages and delivering entertainment. Importantly, these conflicts extend beyond the explicit interpretation of history to include atmospheric and affective qualities that are often overlooked. We suggest that future research should further elucidate how visitors co-produce atmospheres within dark tourism sites, particularly those focusing on the dual mission of education and entertainment. It is necessary to understand how visitors to sites partaking in edutainment ultimately make meaning from tragedy and difficult histories.

References

Abou-Shouk, M., & Soliman, M. (2021). The Impact of Gamification Adoption Intention on Brand Awareness and Loyalty in Tourism: The Mediating Effect of Customer Engagement. *Journal of Destination Marketing & Management* 20: 1–10.

"About Titanic." (2022) *Titanic Pigeon Forge*. Accessed October 19th, 2022. Retrieved from https://titanicpigeonforge.com/about-titanic/.

Adams, T.E., & Herrmann, A.F. (2023). Good Autoethnography. *Journal of Autoethnography* 4 (1): 1–9.

Anderson, B. (2009). Affective Atmospheres. *Emotion, Space and Society* 2 (2): 77–81).

Anderson, B. (2014). *Encountering Affect: Capacities, Apparatuses, Conditions*. Surrey: Ashgate.

Azaryahu, M., & Foote, K.E. (2008). Historical Space as Narrative Medium: On the Configuration of Spatial Narratives of Time at Historical Sites. *GeoJournal* 73: 179–194.

Balloffet, P., Courvoisier, F.H., & Lagier, J. (2014). From Museum to Amusement Park: The Opportunities and Risks of Edutainment. *International Journal of Arts Management* 16 (2): 4–18.

Belam, M. (2021, August 4). Visitors to US Titanic Museum Injured by Replica Iceberg. *The Guardian*. Accessed October 20th, 2022. Retrieved from: https://www.theguardian.com/uk-news/2021/aug/04/three-injured-as-iceberg-wall-collapses-at-us-titanic-museum.

Bissell, D. (2010). Passenger Mobilities: Affective Atmospheres and the Sociality of Public Transport. *Environment and Planning D: Society and Space* 28 (2): 270–289.

Chang, H., Ngunjiri, F.W., & Hernandez, K.C. (2013). *Collaborative Autoethnography*. Walnut Creek: Left Coast Press.

Conradson, D., & Latham, A. (2007). The Affective Possibilities of London: Antipodean Transnationals and the Overseas Experience. *Mobilities* 2 (2): 231–254.

Crang, M. (1994). Spacing Times, Telling Times and Narrating the Past. *Time & Society* 3: 29–45.

Edensor, T., & Sumartojo, S. (2015). Designing Atmospheres: Introduction to Special Issue. *Visual Communication* 14 (3): 251–265.

Fletchall, A. (2013). Making Sense of the Strip: The Postmodern Pastiche of Pigeon Forge, Tennessee. *Southeastern Geographer* 53 (1): 102–122.

Foote, K.E., & Azaryahu, M. (2007). Toward a Geography of Memory: Geographical Dimensions of Public Memory and Commemoration. *Journal of Political and Military Sociology* 35 (1): 125–144.

Hanna, S.P., Carter, P.L., Potter, A.E., Forbes Bright, C., Alderman, D.H., Modlin, E.A., & Butler, D.L. (2019). Following the Story: Narrative Mapping as a Mobile Method for Tracking and Interrogating Spatial Narratives. *Journal of Heritage Tourism* 14 (1): 49–66.

Helmore, E., & Cecco, L. (2023, June 20). Titanic Tourist Submersible: Desperate Search for Sub Missing with Five Onboard. *The Guardian*. Accessed June 30th, 2023. Retrieved from: https://www.theguardian.com/uk-news/2023/jun/19/titanic-tourist-submarine-missing-north-atlantic.

Hetherington, K. (1997). Museum Topology and the Will to Connect. *Journal of Material Culture* 2: 199–218.

Hoelscher, S., & Alderman, D.H. (2004). Memory and Place: Geographies of a Critical Relationship. *Social & Cultural Geography* 5 (3): 347–355.

Inwood, J.F.J. (2009). Contested Memory in the Birthplace of a King: A Case Study of Auburn Avenue and the Martin Luther King Jr. National Park. *Cultural Geographies* 16 (1): 87–109.

Johnson, N.C. (2014). Exhibiting Maritime Histories: Titanic Belfast in the Post-Conflict City. *Historical Geography* 42: 242–259.

Lischer, S.K. (2019). Narrating Atrocity: Genocide Memorials, Dark Tourism, and the Politics of Memory. *Review of International Studies* 45 (5): 805–827.

Martin, C.B. (2007). *Tourism in the Mountain South: A Double-Edged Sword*. Knoxville: The University of Tennessee Press.

Morris, P., & Arford, T. (2019). "Sweat a Little Water, Sweat a Little Blood": A Spectacle of Convict Labor at an American Amusement Park. *Crime, Media, Culture* 15 (3): 423–446.

Martini, A., & Buda, D.M. (2020). Dark Tourism and Affect: Framing Places of Death and Disaster. *Current Issues in Tourism* 23 (6): 679–692.

McCormack, D.P. (2008). Engineering Affective Atmospheres on the Moving Geographies of the 1897 Andrée Expedition. *Cultural Geographies* 15 (4): 413–430.

Morris, P., & Arford, T. "Sweat a Little Water, Sweat a Little Blood": A Spectacle of Convict Labor at an American Amusement Park. *Crime Media Culture* 15 (3): 423–446.

Negruşa, A.L., Toader, V., Soficâ, A., Tutunea, M.F., & Rus, R.V. (2015). Exploring Gamification Techniques and Applications for Sustainable Tourism. *Sustainability* 7 (8): 11160-11189.

Pigeon Forge Department of Tourism. (2022). City Profile. *Annual Department of Tourism Report.* Retrieved from: https://pigeonforgedevelopment.com/.

Potter, A.E., Hanna, S.P., Carter, P.L., & Modlin, E.A. (2020). "Give Them More and More for Their Dollar:" Searching for Slavery Amongst the Plantation Edutainment Complex. In J. Micieli-Voutsinas & A.M. Person (eds.), *Affective Architectures: More-Than-Representational Geographies of Heritage*, London: Routledge, pp.19–39.

Potts, T.J. (2012). 'Dark Tourism' and the 'Kitschification' of 9/11. *Tourist Studies* 12 (3): 232–249.

Shepherd, J., Laven, D., & Shamma, L. (2020). Autoethnographic Journeys through Contested Spaces. *Annals of Tourism Research* 84: 1–13.

Sigala, M., & Steriopoulos, E. (2021). Does Emotional Engagement Matter in Dark Tourism? Implications Drawn from a Reflective Approach. *Journal of Heritage Tourism* 16 (4): 412–432.

Smith, S.A., & Foote, K.E. (2017). Museum/Space/Discourse: Analyzing Discourse in Three Dimensions in Denver's History Colorado Center. *Cultural Geographies* 24 (1): 131–148.

Stone, P.R. (2020). Dark Tourism and 'Spectacular Death': Towards a Conceptual Framework. *Annals of Tourism Research* 83: 1–4.

Stone, P.R., & Grebenar, A. (2022). 'Making Tragic Places': Dark Tourism, Kitsch and the Commodification of Atrocity. *Journal of Tourism and Cultural Change* 20 (4): 457–474.

Stone, P., & Sharpley, R. (2008). Consuming Dark Tourism: A Thanatological Perspective. *Annals of Tourism Research* 35 (2): 574–595.

Sun, J., & Lv, X. (2021). Feeling Dark, Seeing Dark: Mind-Body in Dark Tourism. *Annals of Tourism Research* 86: 1–14.

"Titanic Museum Attraction." (2023). *Tripadvisor*. Accessed June 30th, 2023. Retrieved from https://www.tripadvisor.com/Attraction_Review-g55270-d1649446-Reviews-Titanic_Museum_Attraction-Pigeon_Forge_Tennessee.html.

Turner, J., & Peters, K. (2015). Unlocking Carceral Atmospheres: Designing Visual/Material Encounters at the Prison Museum. *Visual Communication* 14 (3): 309–330.

Waterton, E., & Dittmer, J. (2014). The Museum as Assemblage: Bringing Forth Affect at the Australian War Memorial. *Museum Management and Curatorship* 29 (2): 122–139.

Waterton, E., Staiff, R., Bushell, R., & Burns, E. (2019). Monster Mines, Dugouts, and Abandoned Villages: A Composite Narrative of Burra's Heritage. *Journal of Heritage Tourism* 14 (2): 85–100.

Wood, A.F. (2005). "What Happens [in Vegas]": Performing the Post-Tourist *Flâneur* in "New York" and "Paris." *Text and Performance Quarterly* 25 (4): 315–333.

Xu, F., Buhalis, D., & Weber, J. (2017). Serious Games and the Gamification of Tourism. *Tourism Management* 60: 244–256.

Rami K. Isaac

3 Understanding the emotions of visitors to Chernobyl

Abstract: Few studies have focused on the case of Chernobyl as a dark tourism site. The conceptualization of dark tourism still needs to be broadened and is nowadays shifting towards a focus on the experience rather than the sites. This chapter investigates the emotions elicited by the Chernobyl tourist experience by studying Chernobyl visitors' internet publications (blogs). Data were collected from popular travel blog sites, which include online posts about Chernobyl and its visitors' emotions. Five emotions were deduced from the blogs, including surprise/amazement, awe, fear/apprehension, interest/anticipation, and disgust. Additionally, this chapter also shows that both tangible and intangible attributes of the experience could trigger these emotions. The study offers implications for enhancing tourists' experience at Chernobyl which could be adopted for other dark destinations.

Keywords: Chernobyl, emotions theory, experience, dark tourism, content analysis, semantic analysis

Introduction

Over the past few decades, scholars have demonstrated an increased interest in dark tourism, which has become a globally recognized term and tourism phenomenon (Stone, 2018). Stone (2018) states that consuming dark tourism in this day and age can help change our perspectives on interpreting tragic events and ensure room for remembrance and commemoration. However, conceptualizations of dark tourism have been shifting (Ashworth & Isaac, 2015). Whereas past literature focused primarily on dark tourism sites, there is now a shift in focus toward the experience (Ashworth & Isaac, 2015).

Dark tourism was previously only seen as a means to commemorate past events; nowadays, it also allows for a connection with the future. It is no longer viewed solely as a means to learn and enjoy but as a way of engaging with our present world (Podoshen, 2018). Biran and Buda (2018) suggest that motivations are one of many areas of interest in dark tourism studies, and we now see an emerging shift towards considering the drive, the emotional experiences, and the benefits of dark experiences. Stone (2011) believes that visiting a dark tourism destination can stimulate people to contemplate their own mortality by experiencing the significance of the death of others. Ashworth and Isaac (2015) argue that to understand the tourist experience, one must focus on emotions because of the difficulty in measuring one's subjective

https://doi.org/10.1515/9783110792072-004

experience. The importance of the role of emotion triggered by encounters with dark places has also been highlighted by several authors (i.e., Buda et al., 2014; Oren et al., 2021). Until now, only a small handful of tourism studies have been undertaken at Chernobyl (e.g., Bakota et al., 2020; Rush-Cooper, 2020; Yankovska & Hannam, 2014), and the only one to focus on visitors' experiences depended on the tour guides' interpretation (Yankovska & Hannan, 2014). To the best of this author's knowledge, no study has been published about critically analysing visitors' emotions at Chernobyl using online travel blogs. Based on critical theories of emotion, this research aims to fill a gap in the literature and provide essential data regarding the feelings of Chernobyl tourists as a result of their visit.

Dark tourism and emotional experiences

In literature, the term 'dark tourism' was first introduced by John Lennon and Malcolm Foley as they explored visits to sites related to the life and death of former US president John F. Kennedy (Foley & Lennon, 1996). That same year, the concept of 'thanatourism' was introduced by Tony Seaton, which deals more directly with the death element of dark tourism (Seaton, 1996). Visits to sites of death and suffering go by many different names, including visiting black spots (Rojek, 1993), dark tourism (Foley & Lennon, 1996; Sharpley & Stone, 2009), thanatourism (Seaton, 1996), morbid tourism (Blom, 2007), grief tourism, disaster tourism, atrocities tourism (Ashworth & Hartmann, 2005), and visiting 'sites associated with death and disaster' (Isaac & Cakmak, 2014). All of these categories refer to people visiting sites associated with death, suffering, and tragedy. For example, Seaton (1996, p. 240) has defined thanatourism as an interest in the representation, symbolization, and material evidence of death. It is travel to a locale wholly or partially motivated by a desire for actual or symbolic encounters with death, particularly, but not exclusively, violent, which may, to varying degrees, be activated by the person-specific features of those whose death are the focal point.

Dark tourism research focuses on three main perspectives: the demand side (experiences and expected outcomes), the supply side of dark tourism (locations and dark phenomena), or a more holistic view that studies both demand and supply. Until now, most dark tourism research has comprised primarily descriptive accounts of the dark tourism supply (Sharpley, 2009; Isaac, 2022). Indeed, recent studies have accounted for the diversity and variety of dark sites, focusing on defining and classifying them based on their specific attributes (Kang et al., 2012). Consequently, Miles (2002) distinguishes between dark, darker, and darkest sites, and Stone's (2006) 'dark tourism spectrum' offers a conceptual framing of visitor sites that range from lightest to darkest, referring to their intensity or depth of suffering and tragedy (Timothy, 2021).

This approach has been criticized for ignoring the diversity of experiences and arbitrarily treating them all as homogeneous encounters (Sharpley, 2009). As such, a supply-side-only perspective raises questions about whether it is justifiable or appropriate to classify all dark tourism experiences collectively at themed attractions, such as the London Dungeon, alongside experiences at genocide camps, and whether the concept of dark tourism is indeed helpful at all for broader tourism research (Biran & Hyde, 2013). That said, given the dynamic, diverse, and sophisticated nature of dark tourism experiences, its global reach, and therefore, the ever-increasing role of darkness in the current tourism marketplace, the 'experience economy' within dark tourism is yet to be developed as an important area of scholarly exploration (Stone, 2018, p. 510).

Emotional experiences

The study of emotions plays a pivotal role in tourists' cognitive evaluations and behavioral responses, and dark tourism studies can benefit from a deeper understanding of emotions and their interplay with experiences. Volo (2021, p.1) states, "in a study of affect and emotion in dark tourism, a geographical perspective offers more food for thought regarding disciplines used to investigate emotion and related constructs" (see also Martini & Buda, 2020). This research approach could help progress the study of death and the emotions that arise during a visit. As a result, it is proposed here that this technique for evaluating emotions at dark tourism locations is required to comprehend the visitor experience and how these emotions elicit certain experiences. Ashworth and Isaac (2015, p. 320) claim that, despite the variability of the classification of emotions, there is an inefficient prelude to answering important questions like 'What human emotions are evoked'? 'Which of those are often classified as dark or light'? Because emotions are a part of any tourist experience, dark tourism is not distinct based solely on emotions. However, Nawijn et al. (2016) propose that the nature of emotions differs between darker forms of dark tourism and other types of tourism. Dark tourism is regarded as emotionally laden (Nawijn & Fricke, 2015), with subjective and personal implications (Martini & Buda, 2019, 2020), as well as both positive and negative outcomes (Iliev, 2020; Sharma & Nayak, 2019).

Podoshen (2013) claims that the focus of dark tourism is not always the story of the sites themselves but rather the influence they have on the visitor. Understanding emotions is important, as they influence visitors' behaviour and the meanings ascribed to the place (Nawijn, Isaac, van Liempt, & Gridnevskiy, 2016). Transferred emotions are likely a mix of both positive and negative emotions, but even with regard to negative emotions, people can still benefit from the experience. According to Nawijn and Biran (2019), negative emotions are essential in the experience of dark tourism (see also Oren et al., 2022). Thus, in some situations, meaningful experiences are only stimulated by adverse sensations, contributing to a sense of coherence, which tries to make sense of life. Moreover, these sensations can give life purpose or significance, which can add meaning to the dark tourism experience.

Emotions are felt, short-lived responses to external stimuli (Reeve, 2015). Like motivations, different types of visitors might have different emotional reactions to an experience. Emotional responses are highly personal. Ashworth and Isaac (2015) illustrate that even for a site such as Auschwitz-Birkenau, the experience can differ from person to person. Some might see it as a personal heritage experience, while for others it may be mainly an educational visit.

So far, few empirical studies have examined the emotions triggered by dark experiences. In research at the Tuol Sleng Genocide Museum in Phnom Penh, Cambodia, Isaac and Çakmak (2016) identified both positive and negative emotions. Visitors' positive emotions include adjectives and statements such as "intense", "powerful", "eye-opener", "unforgettable", and "glad I visited". Expressed negative emotions include horrific, scary, depressing, shocking, and disturbing. Research at concentration camp memorials shows what kind of emotions play a role in people's visits. These emotions are clustered into three main categories: misery, sympathy, and positivity (Nawijn, Isaac, van Liempt, & Gridnevskiy, 2016). Within the misery category, there are five sub-emotions: afraid, fear, despair, shame, and contempt. Within the sympathy type, four main emotions exist, including compassion, sadness, disgust, and awe. Positivity embraces gratitude, pride, hope, and fascination. No single set of emotions triggered by dark experiences has been identified. Therefore, more empirical research is required at different sites to understand this topic better.

Positive emotions (Best, 2007; Biran et al., 2014; Nawijn & Fricke, 2015; Thurnell-Read, 2009) and negative emotions (Austin, 2002; Miles, 2002; Nawijn & Biran, 2019) have been studied in dark tourism by a wide range of scholars. Cave and Buda (2018, pp. 707–726) refer to it as the "emotional souvenir process". Zhang et al. (2016) recognize five affective experiences, including fear, sorrow, shock, appreciation, and depression, while Zheng et al. (2019) concluded that dark tourism experiences elicit diverse and often undecided emotions.

Sadness, sorrow, grief, anger, and horror are emotions commonly found in the literature (e.g., Austin, 2002; Brown, 2016; Dunkely et al., 2011; Isaac & Cakmak, 2016; Kidron, 2013; Mowatt & Chancellor, 2011; Zhang et al., 2016). Other scholars have reported anger (Mowatt & Chancellor, 2011), disappointment (Podoshen, 2013), shock and fear (Buda et al., 2014; Zheng et al., 2017), and a sense of hope (Koleth, 2014). The work of Podoshen et al. (2015) reveals that some visitors also experienced repulsion and disgust.

One could think that dark sites trigger only negative emotions in visitors, but as noted previously, that is not true; some dark sites can evoke both positive and negative emotions (Nawijn et al., 2016). Oren et al. (2021) argue that negative feelings inspire people to visit and that even tourists' unfavourable emotions are an essential part of the experience. Other positive emotions include a sense of hope and pride (Cheal & Griffin, 2013; Koleth, 2014; Sharpley, 2012). Emotional reactions to the visit are essential in influencing tourists' satisfaction and behavioural intentions in dark tourism (Hosany & Prayag, 2013).

Light (2017, p. 288) argues that "visiting a dark site is a profoundly emotional experience". Most of the time, this experience is characterized by a variety of emotions, as visiting a place of darkness is more than simply sightseeing or superficial voyeurism (Light, 2017, p. 288; Nawijn et al., 2015). Dark visits can even be transformative as thanatouristic sites offer visitors an opportunity for connecting, engaging, and understanding (Cohen, 2011; Dunkley et al., 2011; Koleth, 2014; Light, 2017; Robert & Stone, 2014). According to Nawijn and Fricke (2015, p. 222), "existing empirical studies on emotional responses at sites associated with death and suffering are somewhat limited, as experience at dark sites cannot be overlooked".

When attempting to conceptualize emotions triggered by dark experiences, it is also essential to look at the attributes of the experience, for the connection between attributes and motivations is vital (Isaac & Çakmak, 2014). Eventually, these links influence the emotions triggered by the experience, so not only is it essential to understand what emotions are triggered, but an extra step is required to identify what attributes cause these emotions.

Only a small number of studies have focused on the affective dimensions of dark tourism (Buda, 2015a, 2015b; Buda et al., 2014; Light, 2017). There remain many gaps in the literature related to this phenomenon, and there have been many calls for additional research to build our knowledge on the subject (Lagos, Harris & Sigala, 2015; Hede & Hall, 2012; Prayag et al., 2017; Straker & Wringley, 2016). Hope, love, pride, fascination, and interest are additional emotional experiences that can also be segmented into tourists' affective experiences (Iliev, 2020).

Martini and Buda (2020) use affect theory to conceptualize dark tourists' experiences and to propose methods in which the ambiance of dark tourism destinations can stimulate affective reactions that tourists are attuned to and negotiate through their emotional responses. The turn towards affect in the social sciences, including tourism studies (Tucker & Shelton, 2018; Wetherell, 2015), particularly in social psychology, focuses on attempts to comprehend embodied emotional experiences. Tourists' affective responses to mortality might create moments of such intensity in their engagement with dark spaces that these engagements are perceptible.

Academics have generated a lot of work on the intricate links between dark experiences and emotional responses despite the challenge of clearly separating affect and emotion. Some scholars believe a distinction is not possible nor beneficial (e.g., Ahmed, 2004). Nevertheless, other authors have attempted to structure the interdependence of emotions and affects, defining emotions as personal and social projections of an individual's feelings (Davidson & Bondi, 2004), conscious, experienced, and articulated (Anderson, 2006). On the other hand, affect is unconscious, occurring under or beyond consciousness. Martini and Buda (2020) suggest that a proposed alternative is to define affect as a vibration rather than a structure that differs from emotion in degrees of intensity (Ngai, 2005). When an affect is felt so intensely that it becomes consciously perceptible, it becomes an emotion. Dark tourism sites are often purposefully constructed and presented to provoke such reactions (Martini & Buda,

2020). However, whether emotions and affects can be considered autonomous, they are always experienced relationally and in connection to the body and its responses (Martini & Buda, 2020). The psychoanalytical notions of voyeurism (Buda & McIntosh, 2013), as well as the concepts of the death drive (Buda, 2015b) and desire, have been applied to understand the affective experiences of visitors at dark tourism sites (Buda & Shim, 2015). Buda and her colleagues emphasize the importance of conceptualizing dark tourism in terms of subjective and emotive experiences rather than identifiable attractions to convey the intricacies of the dark tourism phenomenon.

Affect is a politically important subject for comprehending socio-spatial processes (Ansaloni & Tedeschi, 2016). Tourists at dark places make meaning of challenging and often contentious situations through the fluid relations between their bodies, whereas emotions affect thoughts and social, cultural, and spatial interactions (Martini & Buda, 2020). Affects can be regulated and assembled at levels other than conscious awareness, and they are also influenced by agency, expectations, habits, goals, and social ties (Barnett, 2008; Duff, 2010). Dark sites can thus be programmed to serve specific political objectives and messages. Political decision-making is, in and of itself, geared at generating intensities (Thrift, 2004, p. 58). It generates affect flows beyond simple categorization as an expression of active management or passive construction (Wetherell, 2015). In dark tourism landscapes, this means that narratives of death and tragedy coexist or override pre-existing narratives (Ness, 2005), to cater to tourists seeking a thrill, hope, terror, catharsis, interest, fascination, empathy, or any other affect. Tourism, in this respect, causes a dislocation that affects places and intentions (Ness, 2005) since the presence of tourists has the potential to shape and transform the geography, meaning, patterns of belonging, and inclusion and exclusion from national stories (Martini & Buda, 2020; Wetherell, 2015).

Tourism at Chernobyl

In 2006, some 2,000 people visited the Chernobyl Exclusion Zone around the former nuclear power plant. These visitors were mainly foreign journalists, public organizations, and tourists who traveled with one of only a few tour operators allowed to enter the zone (Kyiv Post, 2006). These trips, however, are recognized as tourism, and the area was officially branded a tourist destination in Ukraine in 2011. There has been a boost in visitation since HBO aired its series about the Chernobyl disaster (Hunder, 2019). Tour operators indicate that sales of Chernobyl tours increased by 30–40% after the series aired. Kyiv's tourism board saw 70,000 visitors in 2018 and was estimated to have 100,000 by the end of 2019 (Mitra, 2019).

The largest share of visitors (30%) in 2017 was Ukrainians. Other nationalities represented were Poles (9.6%), British (9.3%), Americans (5.8%), Germans (5.4%), Czechs (4%), Dutch (3%) and Swedes (2.3%). Residents of these countries comprised 70% of the total number of tourists at Chernobyl in 2017 (Scholts, 2018), although these numbers changed after the international success of the HBO series *Chernobyl*.

Methods

Based on similar methodological approaches used in other studies (Jani & Hwang, 2011; Pan et al., 2007), this study applied qualitative analysis to gain insight into the relationship between travel blogs and the site under examination. Netnography was first introduced by Kozinets (1999) and is best described as an ethnographic study of online communities. This method is considered more natural and less intrusive than other ethnographic methods (Whalen, 2018). Tourism researchers have used this method widely to understand better the perspectives of tourists (Tavakoli & Wijesinghe, 2019). This chapter uses netnography in three ways: word frequency analysis, semantic analysis, and content analysis. The word frequency analysis and semantic analysis provided quantitative data. A structure representing information as a pattern of interconnected nodes and arcs is a semantic network (Sowa, 2014), where nodes represent a particular aspect of a topic and arcs show the connection between the nodes. Different associations can be paired within the texts based on shared meaning (Doerfel, 1998). In addition, critical content analysis allows for a qualitative investigation into tourists' experiences at Chernobyl.

Data collection and analysis

Tavakoli and Wijesinghe (2019) found that the most common platforms used for netnographic analysis in tourism research were blog entries, TripAdvisor, and forums/discussion boards. A simple Google search of different combinations of terms like 'Chernobyl' or 'Chornobyl (the Ukrainian name),' 'travel,' 'blog,' 'wanderlust,' and 'Pripyat' (an abandoned city in the exclusion zone) results in many hits on travel blogs. By filtering between entries of travellers on travel blogs and blogs of travel agencies or tour operators that promote specific tours, a total of 116 separate travel blog entries were assessed. Initial data analysis provides an overview of the blogs used for this study, including demographic information and information about when the blogs were written. These insights can be used to compare emotions between different groups within the sample group.

Finding

The blog samples

To understand the results, we first take a closer look at the blogs used for this study. Table 3.1 provides an overview of the bloggers' countries of origin. The authors were 57% male and 43% female. The national origin of three bloggers could not be identified. Most authors live in the UK and the USA, though there is also a substantial share of Ukrainian bloggers. Most of the rest are Europeans and from sundry other countries.

Table 3.1: Blogs examined by country of origin.

Blogs per country of origin of the authors			
United Kingdom	29	Netherlands	2
United States of America	24	Armenia	1
Ukraine	11	Belarus	1
Canada	8	Belgium	1
Italy	5	Chile	1
Australia	4	Japan	1
Ireland	4	Norway	1
New Zealand	3	Philippines	1
Not Specified	3	Portugal	1
Poland	3	Puerto Rico	1
Denmark	2	Singapore	1
France	2	Spain	1
Germany	2	Sweden	1
Latvia	2	Thailand	1

This global diversity is also a logical explanation for the large number of blog entries in recent years. The most prominent peak was in 2019, which seems to correspond to the launch of HBO's tv show *Chernobyl* (Hunder, 2019). Figure 3.1 also shows the visitations to Chenobyle by bloggers per year.

Frequencies

Coding software can generate a quick overview of the most common blog topics. It proved useful in this exercise, and the findings are presented in this section. First, an overview is created of what these codes entail, followed by an analysis of the frequencies of those codes. The frequency of the codes indicates the most discussed topics in the blogs; these frequencies are used later for more thorough content analysis.

Table 3.2 shows the most common interest codes extracted from the blog entries. Different terms were put together in a single code to create a clear overview of the most popular topics discussed in the blog entries. This sometimes consists of singular and plu-

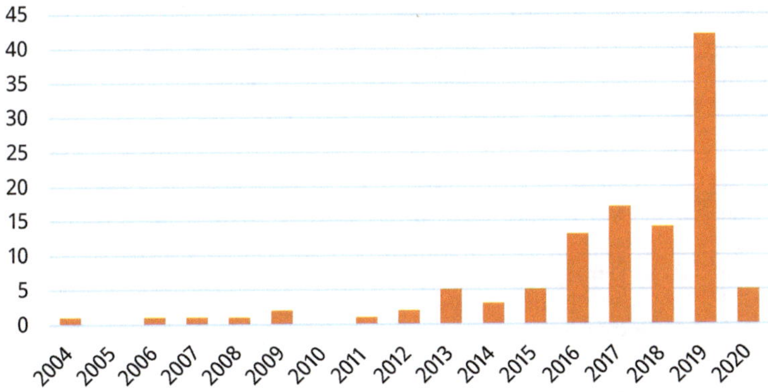

Figure 3.1: Blogger visitations per year.

Table 3.2: Scope of codes.

Code	Includes
Amazing	Amazing, Amazingly, Amazed
Beauty	Beauty, Beautiful, Beautifully
Chernobyl	Chernobyl, Chornobyl
Disaster	Disaster, Catastrophe, Accident
Eerie	Eerie, Eeriest, Ghost, Ghostly
Exclusion Zone	Exclusion Zone
Fascination	Fascinate, Fascination, Fascinated, Fascinates, Fascinating
Feelings	Feel, Feels, Feeling, Feelings, felt,
Feelings of Danger	Dangerous, Danger, Dangers, Dangerously, Unsafe
Feelings of Safety	Safe, Safety, Safely, Safer, Safest
History	History, Historic, Historical
Horror	Horror, Horrific
Incredible	Incredible, Incredibly
Interest	Interest, Interesting, Interested
Learning	Learn, Learning, Learnt, Learned, Learns
Memory	Memory, Remember, Remembered, Remembrance
Pripyat	Pripyat, Prypiat, Prypyat, Prypjat
Radioactivity	Radioactive, Radioactivity, Radio Active

ral forms, past and present-tense verbs, and a few different terms with the same meaning. Incidentally, not all codes are represented in the table, just those containing unique and individual elements. The codes in this table are listed alphabetically.

The software automatically coded these terms but they were manually checked for relevance. In some cases, the words were used in a different context, making them less interesting to consider here. For example, the word ‘incredible’; it can be used to describe the experience, but in many blogs, it was also used in links to other posts.

Table 3.3: Code frequencies.

Code	Count	Code	Count
Chernobyl	3183	Memory	163
Radioactivity	1260	Danger	149
Pripyat	1151	Nature	106
Disaster	1150	Fascination	90
Exclusion Zone	631	Beauty	75
Safety	395	Creepy	66
Abandoned	373	Learning	65
Eerie	330	Incredible	63
Interest	287	Amazing	62
Feelings	286	Horror	56
History	164	Scary	31

Therefore, it was essential to check each code thoroughly. Table 3.3 shows how many times the coded elements appeared in the blogs.

Semantic networks analysis

After identifying theme frequency in the blogs, the relation between different topics was examined. These networks are related to the destination and the tourist experience. This blog entry's five most common codes are all related to the destination. Figure 3.2 shows

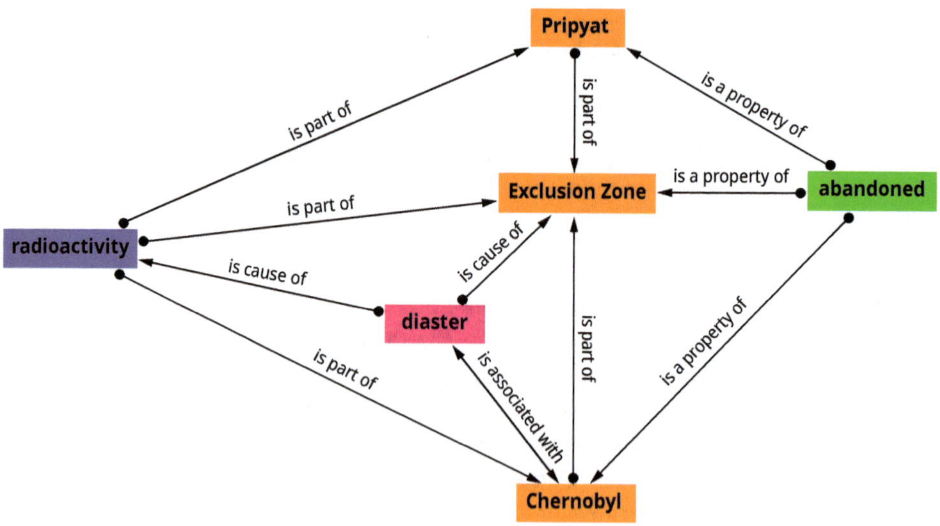

Figure 3.2: Destination network.

a network that explores the relationships between these codes. With this network, it is clear why these are the most common themes discussed. Within the dark Chernobyl experience, three parts relate directly to the destination. Chernobyl relates to the nuclear power plant, Pripyat (now a ghost town) is the city that housed the workers for the power plant, and the exclusion zone encompasses both. The disaster happened at Chernobyl, which resulted in radioactive contamination and the creation of the exclusion zone. This heightened radioactivity danger is now in all parts of the exclusion zone. Abandoned is one of the standard codes, which currently is a characteristic of the exclusion zone, including Pripyat and Chernobyl.

The second category of codes relates more to the tourist and, in light of the aim of this chapter, is even more interesting. It specifically relates to the emotional response to the tourist experience of Chernobyl. However, emotions are complex and not directly described by blog authors. Therefore, we first need to look at feelings because they are described more often. This is because emotions are often unconscious, but feelings are conscious interpretations of emotions (Wake Forest University, 2020). There is a distinction between positive emotions on the left side and negative emotions on the right side (Figure 3.3). There is an apparent contradiction between feelings of safety and danger, and because the code 'beauty' occurred together with 'eerie' in the blogs, there is a connection between these two. This will be further analysed in the content analysis section.

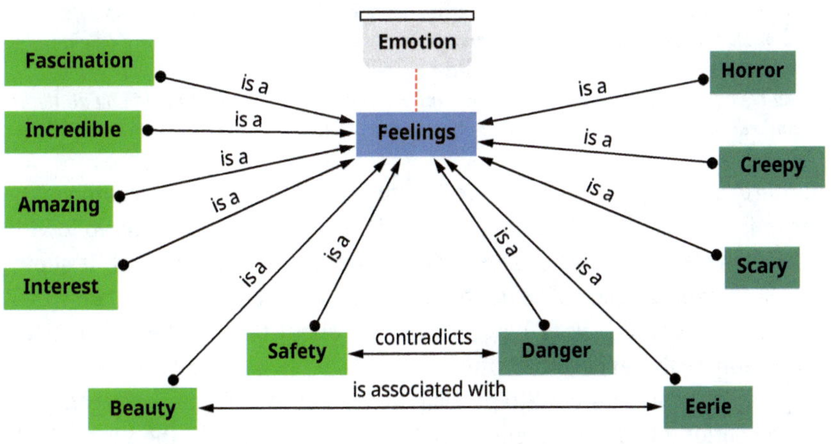

Figure 3.3: Visitor emotions.

So far, the frequency analysis and the semantic networks have provided an overview of the topics that often occur in blogs. There is a distinction between topics related directly to the destination and the felt emotion in the tourist experience. With this information, it is possible to do a content analysis of the topics highlighted before.

Content analysis

Following the overview of topics discussed in the blogs, a more thorough content analysis explores what these codes mean. To do this, blog quotations were used to explain specific topics. First, visitors' emotions experienced at Chernobyl are examined.

Emotion triggered by the tourist experience

Feelings of danger or safety

One topic that is frequently discussed is whether visiting Chernobyl is safe or not. The first thing usually mentioned is the level of radiation one might be exposed to while visiting the exclusion zone. However, most authors consider the level of exposure to radiation almost negligible. The most common concerns for safety are typically not related to radiation but the physical state of the abandoned place where structures may now be unstable and in derelict conditions. For example,

> *Dismissing safety concerns was easy – airport scans have probably exposed me to more radiation than remains in the Chernobyl exclusion zone. – Emilia Morano-Williams, Travelettes*

> *The first question most people ask when considering a trip to Chernobyl is whether it is safe. Ironically, the most significant danger in the Chernobyl exclusion zone is not radiation poisoning but other less invisible hazards. This is an area in decay, where the elements wreak havoc on structures already ravaged by intensive decontamination. However, if you read and abide by all the instructions and rules of your guide, you will be fine. – Anne Miles, From Miles to Smiles*

Even though there is still a degree of danger, visitors continue to go to Chernobyl. The sense of danger is, in fact, one of the appealing elements of the visit. The following quote critically reflects on its author's experience of danger at Chernobyl. It shows that tour operators selling Chernobyl deliberately use the element of danger to sell their products. Contrary to a lack of bloggers writing about thrill-seeking as motivation, the description of the experience often reveals that this is an essential part of Chernobyl's appeal. Visitors still tend to participate even if specific aspects need to fit their ethical conception of the experience. This is well illustrated in the blog Middle World Adventures.

> *However, Chernobyl has yet to find an appropriate tone for its tourism. The potential danger is almost commodified as a feature of the visit. We wore the suits and waved the Geiger counters not because we needed to but because those who brought us there sensed that we wanted to feel close to danger. – Ashlyn, Middle World Adventures*

Fear is the underlying emotion related to the sensation of danger and, thus, the thrill. According to Buckley (2016), the emotion of fear precedes the sensation of thrill, relief, or triumph.

Fascination

The line between fear and fascination is thin. Risk seekers are less affected negatively by terrifying experiences and are more easily fascinated with them (van den Berg & ter Heijne, 2005). For this reason, it is no surprise that 'fascination' is also one of the most frequent codes identified. It is usually paired with either an obsession with remnants of something that has been, or something that could be. This means that visitors can look at the history of the places they visit to get a sense of what life was like at an earlier time. This is related to the emotion of anticipation. Chernobyl is also viewed as a foreshadowing of an apocalyptic scenario humanity could face in the future, again showing a certain level of fear experienced among visitors.

Interest

Similar to fascination, interest is another recurring code. Most of the time interest occurs in combination with specific sites or places. Visitors have specific reasons for thinking places are interesting, but one that is common among authors is the human element. Places become of interest when there is a story about the human side of the catastrophe.

> *Our next stop was the hospital. This is one of the most exciting buildings in Pripyat because it housed the firefighters that battled the flames from nuclear reactor #4. – Johnny Chen, Johnny Africa*

Besides an interest in places, there are other connections with 'interest'. First, the impact of nature and its overgrowth on places suddenly undisturbed by humans is of interest. Secondly, there is also evidence that the history of Chernobyl is of interest.

Amazing

Another positive emotion used to describe the emotion experienced at Chernobyl is amazement. Three main aspects of Chernobyl were found to be amazing.

> *The Earth without man would have been quite a busy place, and the Chernobyl zone, particularly the Pripyat River, is an interesting object for such studies. – Sergei Rzhevsky, Chernobyl Travel Blog*

> *Seeing the iconic place known from the news and many stories was so interesting. – Kami, My Wanderlust.*

First, the area provides insight into everyday life during the Soviet era. Because it was suddenly abandoned, and in a sense 'frozen in time', visitors get a glimpse of what life was like during Soviet times. Second, the impact of nature (overgrowth) amazes many who visit the urban areas that have been overtaken by vegetation, a sort of unintentional rewilding. A third aspect that amazes visitors is the human story behind the whole experience, especially stories about real people who lived through the ordeal. These experiences are impactful.

> *However, we can understand better what living in the USSR was like visiting Pripyat. Moreover, that is amazing in my book of things! – Constanza Fernández, Experiencing the Globe*

> *The country needs the outside world to visit and not only meet the amazing Ukrainian population, find out their personal experiences, and visit places such as the Chernobyl museum, but learn about their Soviet past and learn from the people who are there and also visit a truly amazing country in its own right, live among the people and be friends with them – Joan Torres, Against the Compass*

Incredible

The blogs that describe aspects of the tour as 'incredible' do so mainly with reference to two aspects of the place. The first aspect related to incredibleness is the massive structures they encountered. Not only the ones at the actual nuclear power plant, like the sarcophagus placed over the remains of reactor number four, but the DUGA radar station also receives a good share of attention. Many are surprised by its massive size and the fact that the area used to be hidden from the public. Secondly, the term incredible also relates to the overgrowth of nature, and the rewilding of place, as noted previously in other contexts. Claudia provides examples of this.

> *One of the most incredible sights in the Chernobyl Exclusion Zone is that of the DUGA. It is 500 meters long and 90 meters high, and you will see that it is hardly possible to catch it on camera upon visiting. – Claudia Tavani, My Adventures Across the World*

The fact that authors describe this as incredible, or in other words impossible to believe, shows that surprise is again an essential emotion in the experience of Chernobyl.

Eerie and beauty

Certain aspects of the tour are often described as eerie or ghostly. Usually, if something is described as eerie, it stimulates feelings of fear because it is otherworldly, unknown, or strange. However, in the case of Chernobyl, the eerie atmosphere is ascribed a certain level of beauty too. This is also the result of the way nature is reclaiming the area. Buildings are becoming increasingly overgrown, and certain species of animals now thrive in the area. Beauty is also experienced by enjoying certain architectural features or memorials built for those who took care of the aftermath of the disaster.

> *This modern-day ghost town is a symbol of despair and hopelessness. – Anne Miles, From Miles to Smiles*

> *Pripyat was quiet. There was not a single person in sight. The atmosphere was eerie; the buildings were merely ghostly remains. The odd bird flew by. However, Pripyat was not just a desolate, decaying wasteland. What I saw was nature taking back what man had ruined. – Miriam Risager, Adventurous Miriam*

With the terms eerie and beauty, the relationship between positive and negative emotions becomes intertwined. Eerie relates to experiencing apprehension, while beauty is more related to serenity. In this case, the two terms appear to be experienced only together.

Creepy

Another term to describe the unpleasantness of visiting Chernobyl that is used often is 'creepy'. Whereas 'eerie' focuses on strangeness as the leading factor to induce apprehension, creepy is used for more general aspects that create feelings of fear. In other words, the cause of eerie feelings cannot be directly explained, while creepy is more concrete.

Horror

Chernobyl has also been compared to visiting a horror movie set, which can imply several things. One observation suggests that horror usually invokes feelings of fear and disgust. Secondly, the fact that Chernobyl is compared to a movie set shows that it is experienced as something unreal. This could also be an effect of the commodification of the place.

> *It encompasses all the horrific D-words you can think of: dull, dark, desolate, deserted, dreary, drab, doomed, dead, deadly, devilish, and I could go on – Jonny Blair, Do Not Stop Living*

Emotions related to attributes of the experience

The content analysis identified six attributes that reoccur when investigating emotions. This section explores those attributes and provides an overview of the links between those attributes and the emotions that arose before. First, it is crucial to see what attributes of the experience trigger emotions.

First are the human aspects of the story. This category relates to the Chernobyl stories about the people who experienced the catastrophe first-hand. Visitors are emotionally triggered by learning about the first responders who gave their lives to battle the initial fires, the hospital staff caring for those affected by radiation, and the large number of citizens who suddenly had to leave their homes forever. Secondly, the impact of nature's reclaiming a place that was suddenly abandoned triggers many different types of emotions. A third attribute is the architectural elements in the exclusion zone, from the abandoned Soviet-style city of Pripyat to the little villages in the woods, as well as the large sarcophagus covering reactor number four to the massive DUGA radar station. Thusly, Chernobyl as experienced by blogger-visitors resembles a post-apocalyptic world. It is not only the current situation that triggers emotions but also the Soviet history of the place, including aspects of daily life in the Soviet Union and the political history that impacted how the situation was handled.

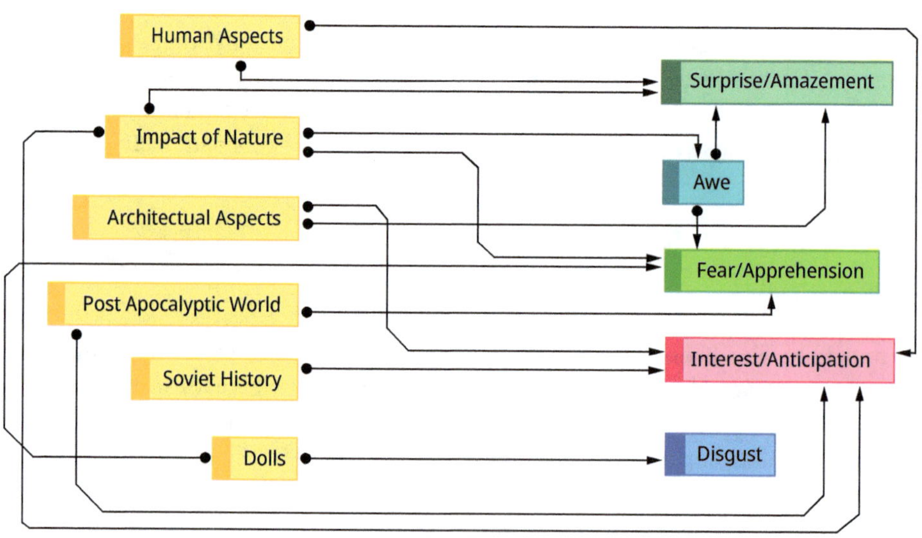

Figure 3.4: Emotions related to the attributes of the experience.

Figure 3.4 shows the relationship between the tourist experience's different attributes and the emotions deduced from the content analysis. On the left side are the reoccurring attributes, while the right side shows the different types of emotion. These attributes can be physical objects found at the site and/or intangible elements of Chernobyl.

This web shows that multiple aspects can trigger an emotion, and a specific aspect can trigger multiple emotions.

Discussion and implications

So far there has been no single view of emotions triggered by dark experiences. The emotion of fear is a constant. First described conceptually by Ashworth and Isaac (2015), later followed by appearances in empirical studies by Isaac and Çakmak (2016) and Nawijn, Isaac, van Liempt and Gridnevskiy (2016), Zhang et al. (2016), Podoshen (2013) and eventually, of course, this study. Whether it is about slight apprehension or downright terror, fear stimulates visitors in all types of dark experiences. Isaac and Çakmak (2016) also identified an emotion that they defined as an 'eye-opener', which indicates a certain level of surprise. In Plutchik's (1980) view, the combination of surprise and fear is awe, which Nawijn et al. (2016) also identified. Disgust as an emotional response to a dark experience was evident in this study and the study by Nawijn et al. (2016).

The findings showed that for some, Chernobyl turned out to be everything they had expected and even more. This is in line with Chang's (2014) statement that defined motivations translate into satisfactory experiences. However, this does not apply to all blog authors. Some reflect on their experience at Chernobyl with a more critical eye and realize that human interference at Chernobyl has already tampered with the authenticity of the place. Horror was discovered in the content analysis, which is consistent with Brown's findings (2016). Fascination and interest were also consistent with the findings of Nawijn et al. (2016) and Iliev (2020).

This study has important academic and management implications. From a theoretical point of view, leveraging a multimethod approach, this specific research has brought a clearer view of post-visit emotions about a tourism site and the use of visitors' blogs. Although qualitative methods have been increasingly recognized and employed to operationalize the constructs of emotions, they still tend to be an accompaniment to quantitative studies. However, quantitative and qualitative multimethod lines can disclose better holistic and psychological impressions associated with a site, which are not easily captured by structured quantitative methods alone. Moreover, analysing travel blogs can expose detailed and in-depth information that cannot be collected from a scalar measurement on visitor surveys.

From a managerial perspective, the fact that Ukraine's president Zelensky recognized the importance of Chernobyl in the tourism potential of his country and the locality's continued importance as a tourist destination (even during the current war) indicates the need for a proper site management. Since Zelensky wants to change the site's narrative to honour those who dealt with the aftermath of the disaster, it is first essential to consider how Chernobyl is experienced now. It is up to the Tourist Association of Ukraine to provide clear guidelines for operators to realize desirable approaches to tourism development. Thereafter, Chernobyl site managers can start implementing changes that are in line with the intended experience.

First, site managers must differentiate between diverse visitors and their motives for visiting Chernobyl. By understanding why visitors come to Chernobyl, it is possible either to reinforce visitors' experiences by providing ways to meet their expectations or provide them with something extra, different from the initial reason for visiting. Moreover, it is crucial to realize the differences in emotions triggered by the experience and the relation between the attributes and these emotions. Storytelling would be an exciting way to do this since we have seen that the human aspect of Chernobyl is often a trigger for different emotions. When looking at visitors motivated by a thrill, it would be interesting to see if this technique can add value. When expectations are met, but different emotions like surprise are triggered, it could add to the overall experience of Chernobyl.

Conclusion

To conclude, this study highlights the most frequently occurring themes within a sample of bloggers who have visited Chernobyl. These themes relate to the attributes of the destination and the tourist experience, visualized by the semantic networks. The analysis also shows that the geographical area where the blogger originates influences how Chernobyl is experienced, and this is something that requires further investigation.

By looking at the feelings described in the blogs, it was possible to deduce the underlying emotional response to the experience. For this, a closer look was taken at feelings of safety/danger, fascination, interest, amazing, incredible, eerie, beauty, creepy, and horror. The underlying emotions were analysed and finally divided into five main categories. These include disgust, interest/anticipation, fear/apprehension, surprise/amazement, and awe, in which awe combines surprise and fear.

It is also clear that there is a strong relationship between the attributes of the experience and visitors' emotional responses. A combination of tangible and intangible attributes of the experience often triggers emotions. At Chernobyl, these attributes include the human story, the impact of nature's power in vegetative overgrowth, the architectural aspects of Pripyat and other areas in the exclusion zone, a feeling of a post-apocalyptic world, and a better understanding of Soviet history.

References

Ahmed, S. (2004). *The cultural politics of emotion*. Edinburgh: Edinburgh University Press.

Anderson, B. (2006) Becoming and being hopeful: Towards a theory of affect. *Environment and Planning D: Society and Space*, 24, 733–752

Austin, N. (2002). Managing heritage attractions: Marketing challenges at sensitive historical sites. *International Journal of Tourism Research*, 4(6), 447–457.

Ansaloni, F., & Tedeschi, M. (2016). Understanding space ethically through affect and emotion: From uneasiness to fear and rage in the city. *Emotion, Space and Society*, 21, 15–22

Ashworth, G. J., & Hartmann, R. (2005). *Horror and human tragedy revisited: The management of sites of atrocities for tourism*. New York: Cognizant.

Ashworth, G. J., & Isaac, R. K. (2015). Have we illuminated the dark? Shifting perspectives on 'dark' tourism. *Tourism Recreation Research*, 40, 316–325.

Bakota, D., Machowski, R., Płomiński, A., Ramanchuk, A., Rzętała, M., & Zastavetska, L. (2020). The disaster as a factor in the development of modern tourism: A study case based on the Chernobyl nuclear power plant. *Journal of Environmental Management & Tourism*, 11(7), 1729–1741.

Barnett, C. (2008). Political affects in public space: Normative blind spots in non-representational ontologies. *Transactions of the Institute of British Geographers*, 33(2), 186–200

Best, M. (2007). Norfolk islands: Thanatourism, history, and visitor emotions. *Shima: The International Journal of Research into Island Cultures*, 1(2), 30–48.

Biran, A., & Buda, D. M. (2018). Unraveling Fear of Death Motives in Dark Tourism. In P. R. Stone, R. Hartmann, T. Seaton, R. Sharpley, & L. White, *The Palgrave Handbook of Dark Tourism Studies* (pp. 515–528). London: Macmillan.

Biran, A. & Hyde, K. (2013). Guest editorial: New perspective on dark tourism. *International Journal of Culture, Tourism, and Hospitality*, 7(3), 191–198.

Biran, A., Wei, L., Li, G., & Eichhorn, V. (2014). Consuming post-disaster destinations: The case of Sichuan, China. *Annals of Tourism Research*.14, 1–17.

Blom, T. (2007). Morbid tourism: The case of Diana princess of Wales and Althorp house. In P. Long and N. J. Palmer (Eds.), Royal tourism: Excursions around Monarchy (pp. 142–158). Clevedon, UK: Channel View Publications.

Brown, L. (2016). Tourism and pilgrimage: Paying homage to literary heroes. *International Journal of Tourism Research*, 18(2), 167–175

Buckley, R. C. (2016). Qualitative Analysis of Emotions: Fear and Thrill. *Frontiers in Psychology* 7, 1187.

Buda, D.M. (2015a). *Affective tourism: Dark routes in conflict*. New York: Routledge.

Buda, D.M. (2015b). The death drive in tourism studies. *Annals of Tourism Research*, 50, 39–51.

Buda, D. M., d'Hauteserre, A-M., & Johnston, L. (2014). Feeling and tourism studies. *Annals of Tourism Research*. 46, 102–114.

Buda, D. M., & McIntosh, A. J. (2013). Dark tourism and voyeurism: Tourist arrested for 'spying' in Iran. *International Journal of Culture, Tourism and Hospitality Research*, 7(3), 214–226.

Buda, D. M., & Shim, D. (2015). Desiring the dark: 'A taste for the unusual' in North Korean tourism? *Current Issues in Tourism*, 18(1), 1–6.

Cave, J., & Buda, D. (2018). Souvenirs in dark tourism: Emotions and symbols. In R. Stone, R. Hartmann, T. Seaton, R. Sharpley, & L. White (Eds.), *The Palgrave handbook of dark tourism studies* (pp. 707–726). Basingstoke: Palgrave Macmillan.

Chang, T.-Y. (2014). The Effects of Motivation and Environmental Attitudes on the Benefits of Experience. *Revista Internacional de Sociología* (RIS) 72, 69–86.

Cheal, F., & Griffin, T. (2013). Pilgrims and patriots: Australian tourist experiences at Gallipoli. *International Journal of Culture, Tourism, and Hospitality Research*, 7(3), 227–241.

Chernobyl Tour Operator Association. (2020, March 23). *Opgehaald van АСОЦІАЦІЯ ТУРОПЕРАТОРІВ ЧОРНОБИЛЯ*: http://chtoa.org/en/

Cohen, E. H. (2011). Educational dark tourism at an in populo site: The Holocaust Museum in Jerusalem. *Annals of Tourism Research*, 38(1), 193–209.

Contests on the River Kwai: How a wartime tragedy became a recreational, commercial and nationalistic plaything. (2010). *Current Issues in Tourism*, 13, 311–332.

Davidson, J. & Bondi, L. (2004). Spatialising affects; affecting space: An introduction. Gender, Place and Culture: *A Journal of Feminist Geography*, 11(3), 373–374

Doerfel, M. L. (1998). What Constitutes Semantic Network Analysis? A Comparison of Research and Methodologies. *Connections*, 21, 16–26.

Duff, C. (2010). On the role of affect and practice in the production of place. *Environment and Planning D: Society and Space*, 28, 881–895.

Dunkley, R., Morgan, N., & Westwood, S. (2011). Visiting the trenches: Exploring meanings and motivations in battlefield tourism. *Tourism Management*, 32(4), 860–868.

Foley, M., & Lennon, J. J. (1996). JFK and dark tourism: A fascination with assassination. *International Journal of Heritage Studies*, 4, 198 –211.

Hede, A.-M., & Hall, J. (2012). Evoked Emotions: Textual analysis within the context of pilgrimage tourism to Gallipoli. *Advances in Culture, Tourism and Hospitality Research*, 6, 45–60.

Hosany, S., & Prayag, G. (2013). Patterns of tourists' emotional responses, satisfaction, and intention to recommend. *Journal of Business Research*, 66(6), 730–737.

Hunder, M. (2019, June 14). *HBO show success drives chernobyl tourism boom*. Opgehaald van Reuters: https://www.reuters.com/article/us-ukraine-chernobyl-tourism/hbo-show-success-drives-chernobyl-tourism-boom-idUSKCN1T51MF

Iliev, D. (2020). Consumption, motivation, and experience in dark tourism: A conceptual and critical analysis. *Tourism Geographies*, 1–22.

Isaac, R. K., & Çakmak, E. (2014). Understanding visitor's motivation at sites of death and disaster: The case of former transit Camp Westerbork, the Netherlands. *Current Issues in Tourism*, 17, 164–179.

Isaac, R. K., & Çakmak, E. (2016). Understanding the motivations and emotions of visitors at Tuol Sleng Genocide Prison Museum (S-21) in Phnom Penh, Cambodia. *International Journal of Tourism Cities*, 2, 232–247.

Isaac, R., & Budryte-Ausiejiene, L. (2015). Interpreting visitors' emotions: A study of visitor comment books at the Grutas Park Museum, Lithuania. *Scandinavian Journal of Hospitality and Tourism*, 15, 400–424.

Isaac, R.K. (2022). (ed) *Dark Tourism Studies*. Oxon: Routledge.

Jani, D., & Hwang, Y. H. (2011). User-generated destination image through weblogs: A comparison of pre- and post-visit images. Asia Pacific Journal of Tourism Research, 16(3), 339–356.

Kang, E. J., Scott, N., Lee, T. J., & Ballantyne, R. (2012). Benefits of visiting a 'dark tourism' site: The case of the Jeju April 3rd Peace Park, Korea. *Tourism Management*, 33, 257–265.

Kidron, C. (2013). Being there together: Dark family tourism and the emotive experience of co-presence in the Holocaust past. *Annals of Tourism Research*, 41, 175–194.

Koleth, M. (2014). Hope in the dark: Geographies of volunteer and dark tourism in Cambodia. *Cultural Geographies*, 21(4), 681–694.

Kozinets, R. V. (1999). E-tribalized marketing?: the strategic implications of virtual communities of consumption. *European Management Journal*, 17, 252–264.

Kyiv Post. (2006, April 26). *Travel agencies cashing in on trips to Chornobyl*. Opgehaald van Kyiv Post: https://www.kyivpost.com/article/content/ukraine-politics/travel-agencies-cashing-in-on-trips-to-chornobyl-24356.html?cn-reloaded=1

Lagos, E., Harris, A., & Sigala, M. (2015). Emotional language for image formation and market segmentation in dark tourism destinations: Findings from tour operators' websites promoting Gallipoli. *Tourismos*, 10(2), 153–170.

Light, D. (2017). Progress in dark tourism and thanatourism research: An uneasy relationship with heritage tourism. *Tourism Management*, 61, 275–301.

Martini, A., & Buda, D. M. (2019). Analyzing affects and emotions in tourist e-mail interviews: A case in post-disaster Tohoku, Japan. *Current Issues in Tourism*, 22(19), 2353–2364.

Martini, A. & Buda, D.M. (2020). Dark tourism and affect: Framing places of death and disaster *Current Issues in Tourism*, 23 (6), 679–692

Miles, W. F. (2002). Auschwitz: Museum Interpretation and Darker Tourism. *Annals of Tourism Research*, 29, 1175–1178.

Mitra, M. (2019, June 15). *Pop culture is changing the tourism industry – the proof is in Chernobyl.* Opgehaald van CNBC: https://www.cnbc.com/2019/06/14/chernobyl-sees-a-spike-in-visitors-as-pop-culture-influences-tourism.html

Mowatt, R. A., & Chancellor, C. H. (2011). Visiting death and life: Dark tourism and slave castles. *Annals of Tourism Research*, 38(4), 1410–1434.

Nawijn, J., & Biran, A. (2019). Negative emotions in tourism: a meaningful analysis. *Current Issues in Tourism*, 22, 2386–2398.

Nawijn, J., & Fricke, M-C. (2015). Visitor emotions and behavioral intentions: The case of Concentration Camp Memorial Neuengamme. *International Journal of Tourism Research*, 17(3), 221–228.

Nawijn, J., Isaac, R. K., Gridnevskiy, K., & van Liempt, A. (2015). Holocaust concentration camp memorial sites: An exploratory study into an expected emotional response. *Current Issues in Tourism*, 21(2), 175–190.

Nawijn, J., Isaac, R. K., van Liempt, A., & Gridnevskiy, K. (2016). Emotion clusters for concentration camp memorials. *Annals of Tourism Research*, 61, 244–247.

Ness, S. A. (2005). Tourism–terrorism: The landscaping of consumption and the darker side of place. *American Ethnologist*, 32(1), 118–140.

Ngai, S. (2005). *Minor affects.* Cambridge, MA: Harvard University Press.

Oren, G., Shani, A. and Poria, Y. (2021). Dialectical emotions in a dark heritage site: A study at the Auschwitz Death Camp. *Tourism Management*, 82, 104194.

Pan, B., MacLaurin, T., & Crotts, J. C. (2007). Travel blogs and the implications for destination marketing. Journal of travel research, 46(1), 35–45.

Plutchik, R. (1980). *The Emotions.* Lanham: University Press of America.

Podoshen, J. S. (2013). Dark tourism motivations: Simulation, emotional contagion, and topographic comparison. *Tourism Management*, 35, 263–271.

Podoshen, J. S., Andrzejewski, S. A., Venkatesh, V., & Wallin, J. (2015). New approaches to dark tourism inquiry: A response to Isaac. *Tourism Management*, 51, 331–334.

Podoshen, J. S. (2018). Dark Tourism in an Increasingly Violent World. In P. R. Stone, R. Hartmann, T. Seaton, R. Sharpley, & L. White, *The Palgrave Handbook of Dark Tourism Studies* (pp. 173–182). London: Palgrave Macmillan.

Prayag, G., Hosany, S., Muskat, B., & Del Chiappa, G. (2017). Understanding the relationships between tourists' emotional experiences, perceived overall image, satisfaction, and intention to recommend. *Journal of Travel Research*, 56(1), 41–54.

Reeve, J. (2015). *Understanding Motivation and Emotion.* Hoboken: Wiley.

Roberts, C., & Stone, P. (2014). Dark tourism and dark heritage: Emergent themes, issues, and consequences. In I. Convery, G. Corsane, & P. Davies (Eds.), *Displaced heritage: Responses to disaster, trauma, and loss* (pp. 9–18). Woodbridge: Boydell Press.

Rojek, C. (1993). Ways of escape: Modern transformations in leisure and travel. Springer.

Rush-Cooper, N. (2020). Nuclear landscape: Tourism, embodiment and exposure in the Chernobyl Zone. *Cultural Geographies*, 27(2), 217–235.

Scholts, K. (2018). *The Development of Chernobyl as a Tourism Destination.* Breda: NHTV.

Seaton, A. V. (1996). Guided by the dark: From thanatopsis to thanatourism. International *Journal of Heritage Studies*, 2, p234 -244.

Sharma, P., & Nayak, J. (2019). Examining experience quality as the determinant of tourist behavior in niche tourism: An analytical approach. *Journal of Heritage Tourism*, 15(1), 76–92.

Sharpley, R. (2012). Towards an understanding of 'genocide tourism': An analysis of visitors' accounts of their experience of recent genocide sites. In R. Sharpley, & P. R. Stone (Eds.), *Contemporary tourist experience: Concepts and consequences* (pp. 95–109). London: Routledge

Sharpley, R., & Stone, P. R. (2009). *The darker side of travel: the theory and practice of dark tourism.* Bristol: Channel View.

Sharpley, R. (2009). Shedding light on dark tourism: An introduction. The darker side of travel: The theory and practice of dark tourism, 3–22.

Sowa, J. F. (2014). *Principles of Semantic Networks: Explorations in the Representation of Knowledge*. Burlington: Morgan Kaufmann.

Straker, K., & Wrigley, C. (2016). Translating emotional insights into digital channel designs. *Journal of Hospitality and Tourism Technology*, 7(2), 135–157.

Stone, P. (2006). A dark tourism spectrum: Towards a typology of death and macabre related tourist sites, attractions, and exhibitions. *`Tourism*, 54(2), 145–160.

Stone, P. (2011). Dark tourism experiences: mediating between life and death. In P. Stone, & R. Sharpley, (Eds.) *Tourist experience: contemporary perspectives* (pp. p32–36). London: Routledge.

Stone, P. (2013). Dark tourism, heterotopias, and post-apocalyptic places. In the case of Chernobyl. In L. White, & E. Frew, *Dark tourism and place identity. Managing and interpreting dark places* (pp. p79–93). New York: Routledge.

Stone, P. (2018). *The Palgrave Handbook of Dark Tourism Studies*. London: Palgrave Macmillan.

Tavakoli, R., & Wijesinghe, S. N. (2019). The evolution of the web and netnography in tourism: A systematic review. *Tourism Management Perspectives*, 29, 48–55.

Thrift, N. (2004). Intensities of feeling: Towards a spatial politics of affect. *Geografiska Annaler*, 86B, 57–78.

Thurnell-Read, T. (2009). Engaging Auschwitz: An analysis of young travelers' experiences of Holocaust tourism. *Journal of Tourism Consumption and Practice*, 1(1), 26–52.

Timothy, D.J. (2021). *Cultural Heritage and Tourism: An Introduction*, 2nd Edn. Bristol: Channel View Publications.

Tucker, H. & Shelton, E. (2018) Tourism, mood and affect: Narratives of loss and hope. Annals of Tourism Research, 70, 66–75.

van den Berg, A., & ter Heijne, M. (2005). Fear versus fascination: An exploration of emotional responses to natural threats. *Journal of Environmental Psychology*, 261–272.

Volo, S. (2021). The experience of emotion: Directions for tourism design. *Annals of Tourism Research*, 86, 103097

Wake Forest University (2020). *The Difference Between Feelings and Emotions*. Opgehaald van Wake Forest University: https://counseling.online.wfu.edu/blog/difference-feelings-emotions/

Wetherell, M. (2015). Trends in the turn to affect A social psychological critique. *Body and Society*, 21(2), 139–166

Whalen, E. A. (2018). Understanding a shifting methodology: A content analysis of the use of netnography in hospitality and tourism research. *International Journal of Contemporary Hospitality Management*, 30, 3423–3441.

Yankovska, G., & Hannan, K. (2014). Dark and toxic tourism in the Chernobyl exclusion zone. *Current Issues in Tourism*, 17, 929–939.

Zhang, H., Yang, Y., Zheng, C., & Zhang, J. (2016). Too dark to revisit? The role of past experiences and intrapersonal constraints. *Tourism Management*, 54, 452–464.

Zheng, C., Zhang, J., Zhang, H., & Qian, L. (2017). Exploring sub-dimensions of intrapersonal constraints to visiting "dark tourism" sites: A comparison of participants and non-participants. Asia Pacific Journal of Tourism Research, 22(1), 21–33.

Zheng, C., Zhang, J., Qiu, M., Guo, Y., & Zhang, H. (2019). From mixed emotional experience to spiritual meaning: Learning in dark tourism places. *Tourism Geographies*, 22(1), 105–126.

Part II: **Dark tourism and critical animal studies**

David A. Fennell, Bastian Thomsen, Samuel R. Fennell

4 Animals as dark tourism attractions: A prototype

Almost two decades ago, the primary author became interested in a no-longer-existent website showcasing hundreds of animal skulls in the American Museum of Natural History as part of a program of emerging research on animal ethics in tourism. It was this captivating display of death for tourism purposes that triggered reference to a previously observed display of the Rwanda genocide (April and July of 1994), that tourism scholars categorize as "dark tourism."

Dark tourism (DT), sometimes referred to as thanatourism, is a complex subset of the tourism industry, which capitalizes on human death and suffering from human and environmentally induced events. It is defined as "visitations to places where tragedies or historically noteworthy death has occurred and that continue to impact our lives" (Tarlow 2005, 48), or "a quest to experience a disaster from a safe place" (Martini and Buda 2020, 684). The allure of DT stems from its ability, indeed, its modus operandi, of exposing particularities of people, place, and culture to reveal ontological anxieties about the past and the future (Stone 2013). As such, it allows tourists who visit sites of natural disasters, tragedies, massacres, executions, or other eccentricities that took place in the past (Kulcsar and Simon 2015) to reflect on their mortality in the context of modern society's penchant for keeping death "sequestered" (Stone and Sharpley 2008) and sheltered from the realities of life.

Recent work now confirms the link between animals, tourists, and the darker side of the tourism industry (López López and Quintero Venegas 2021). We seek to amplify tourism and animal studies literature through the development of a novel typology, or "proto typology," designed to classify animals as dark tourism attractions. Dark tourism has been applied almost entirely in a human context, with several well-developed definitions, frameworks and empirical studies. However, given how rapidly animal studies research is advancing within tourism studies, our attempt at a classification represents a natural progression of thought on animals as entangled, active agents (Alaimo and Hekman 2008) in tourism.

Note: This article was first published on November 9, 2021, in EuropeNow an online journal published by the Council for European Studies (CES). It is being republished as a chapter in this book with the authors' permission.

https://doi.org/10.1515/9783110792072-005

Supply and consumption of dark tourism

Typologies of dark tourism supply have been developed before. Stone's (2006, 152–157) "Seven Dark Suppliers" of dark tourism products provides a good understanding of their range:

- *Dark fun factories* include attractions that have a high degree of infrastructure and entertainment value with a robust commercial ethic, and that offer real or fictional death and macabre events (e.g., the London Dungeon, or the Dracula Park in Romania);
- *Dark exhibitions* propose product designs that reflect education and potential learning opportunities (e.g., 9/11 terrorist attack artifacts at the Smithsonian);
- *Dark dungeons* represent attractions related to bygone penal and justice codes (e.g., the Old Melbourne Gaol in Australia);
- *Dark resting places* are cemetery sites where history-centric, conservational, and commemorative ethics intervene (e.g., the Père-Lachaise cemetery in Paris);
- *Dark shrines* constitute informal attractions close to death sites within a short time period of the death (e.g., the temporary shrine constructed at the gates of Kensington Palace after the death of Princess Diana, later moved to Althorp House);
- *Dark conflict areas* (e.g., battlefields, war-related attractions) are history-centric, war related, educational, and commemorative sites that are becoming more commercialized with increasing tourism infrastructure (e.g., Ypres and the Somme);
- *Dark camps of genocide* that stand as the darkest edge of the dark tourism spectrum, as their central thanatological themes are based on genocide, atrocity, and catastrophe (e.g., Auschwitz-Birkenau). Noteworthy in the provision of dark tourism attractions is authenticity. Those sites that possess a higher degree of locational authenticity are viewed as "darker" (Miles 2002).

Considerable attention has been placed on the psychology of consumers of dark tourism experiences. The list of motivations for visiting DT sites includes curiosity, entertainment, empathetic identification, compassion, nationalism, pilgrimage, event validation, remembrance, identity-seeking (family connection), honoring ancestors, education, social responsibility or moral duty, and the desire for contact and connection to death, black events, and violence (Ashworth 2004; Farmaki 2013; Light 2017; Seaton 1996; Tarlow 2005; Dunkley, Morgan, and Westwood 2011; Biran, Poria, and Oren 2011). Dark tourism sites generate a wide range of emotional states (Nawjin, Isaac, van Leimpt, and Gridnevskiy 2016), including anger (Israfilova and Khoo-Lattimore 2019; Timothy and Teye, 2004), disgust (Podoshen et al. 2015), shock and fear (Buda 2015), hope (Koleth 2014), denial (Stone 2013), and pride (Cheal and Griffin 2013). They also induce empathy based on the ability to connect the atrocities that took place there with the degree of suffering experienced by individuals and groups (Ashworth 2004).

Animals as dark tourism attractions

The present study aims to push the animal ethics literature in a new direction by presenting a novel framework based on the confluence of dark tourism and animal ethics literature. The tourism and animal ethics sub-field is relatively new (Fennell 2000) but has advanced steadily as a flurry of recent studies have attempted to define it (Fennell 2012; Markwell 2015; Carr and Broom 2018; Kline 2018; Rickly and Kline 2021). Some studies have also defined the conditions around the engagement of animals and the tourism industry based on setting, mode of engagement, animals' state, and mediators (Cohen 2009); and others have modelled how suffering could be eliminated in tourism (Fennell and Thomsen, 2021). Studies are also closing the gap between industry and research by providing tourists with the ability to measure animal welfare, governance, and conservation through a rating of whether care to animals is "deep," "intermediate," "shallow" or "just" (Fennell et.al, 2024).

The prototype includes three main categories and nine sub-categories, designed to incorporate a broad spectrum of factors that define the relationship between humans and animals in tourism.

Animal dark tourism proto typology (prototype):

A. Characteristics of animal suffering and death

Status & Setting
- Dead animals in built environments (e.g. museums)
- Captive live animals in built environments
- Animal representation in built settings (in story or fable)
- Dead animals in semi-built settings
- Live animals in semi-built settings
- Animal representation in semi-built settings
- Dead animals in wild settings
- Wild animals in wild settings
- Animal representation in wild settings
- Combination of above

Sources of suffering/death
- Human-induced: Humans are directly/indirectly responsible for death or suffering.
- Environmentally induced: The natural environment is directly/indirectly responsible for death or suffering.
- Both: Death or suffering a result of both humans and the environment.
- Natural causes: Animals suffer or die from natural causes.
- Unknown: Unknown reason for suffering or death.

Role of animal(s)
- Part of nature/pest: Free-living in nature or viewed as a detriment to social and commercial existence.
- Worker: Working in agriculture, porters, lifesavers, etc.
- Sport and subsistence: Hunted, fished, trapped for recreation and food.
- Competitor: Forced to compete against other animals or humans.
- Entertainment: Used primarily as entertainers for the pleasure and profit of humans.
- Education: Used primarily for educational purposes.
- Science and research: Used for science, research, or conservation.
- Spirituality: Used for spiritual celebrations or remembrance.
- Companionship: Used in building a cognitive/emotional/wellness bond with human(s) or other companion animals.
- Other: Other types of service to the tourism industry.

Temporal period
- Prehistoric: Animals referenced in prehistoric times.
- Historic: Animals referenced in historic times.
- Contemporary: Animals referenced in the present day.
- Combination: One or more periods of time.

The scale of suffering/death
- Individual animal: A single animal that dies/suffers through an intervention.
- Population (one species): More than one animal of the same species suffers or dies through an intervention.
- Community (more than one species): More than one species suffers or dies through an intervention.
- Ecosystem: Entire ecosystems decimated from the actions of humans or the natural world.

B. Subjective/normative nature of animal-human relationship leading to suffering or death

The negative-positive emotional state of handlers
- Misothery: Emotions or attitudes of hatred, fear or disgust of animals as pests, threats, or other.
- Indifference: Neutral emotions and attitudes to the animal(s) part of the attraction.
- Theriophily: Emotions/attitudes of love or reverence for an animal/animal, including iconic or heroic animals
- Unknown: The status of the relationship is unknown.

Animal ethics theories describing how animals were/are used

- Anthropocentric: Primary moral value rests in the interests of human beings over all other aspects of the natural world.
- Contractarianism: Only rational beings (humans) can enter into contracts to maximise self-interest via cooperation; animals not rational.
- Ecocentrism: Value is placed on whole systems, not individual animals.
- Welfare: Animals can be used as long as mental and physical needs are a priority.
- Utilitarianism: Equal consideration of interests. The suffering of a being is counted equally with the like suffering of other beings.
- Ecofeminism/Care ethics: Value is placed on an ethic of responsibility/care, emphasising compassion, equity and need.
- Rights: Individuals (human and non-human) have inherent value as subjects-of-a-life.
- Posthumanism: Animals seen as active, entangled agents alongside humans and deserving of the same justice and rights.

C. Tourism industry demand and supply

Attitudes of tourists towards animals (Kellert 1984)

- Naturalistic: A primary interest in and affection for wildlife and the outdoors.
- Ecologistic: A primary concern for interrelationships between wildlife species and natural habitats.
- Humanistic: A primary interest in and strong affection for individual animals, principally pets.
- Moralistic: The right and wrong treatment of animals, with strong opposition to animal exploitation and cruelty.
- Scientistic: The physical attributes and biological functioning of animals.
- Aesthetic: A primary interest in the artistic and symbolic characteristics of animals.
- Utilitarian: A primary concern for the practical and material value of animals.
- Dominionistic: Primary satisfactions derived from mastery and control over animals, typically in sporting situations.
- Negativistic: Active avoidance of animals due to dislike or fear.
- Neutralistic: Passive avoidance of animals due to indifference and lack of interest.
- Varied: Tourists holding different attitudes; cognitive dissonance.

Dark tourism products/supply (Stone 2006)

- Dark fun factories: A high degree of infrastructure & entertainment with a robust commercial ethic, presenting real or fictional events.
- Dark exhibitions: Product designs that reflect education and potential learning opportunities.
- Dark dungeons: Attractions related to bygone penal and justice codes.

- Dark resting places: Include cemetery sites based on history-centric, conservational and commemorative ethics.
- Dark shrines: Informal attractions close to the site of death and within a short period of the death occurring.
- Dark conflict areas: Sites (e.g., battlefields) that are history-centric, war-related, educational, commemorative, & commercialised.
- Dark camps of genocide: The darkest edge of dark tourism based on genocide, atrocity and catastrophe as the central thanatological theme.

The first domain, "Characteristics of animal suffering and death," incorporates five sub-categories that define basic features of how animals have been (or are being) used. These include the status and setting of animals killed or that suffer; the source of suffering or death; the role of animals; temporal period of use; and the scale of suffering or death. The second domain provides context around the subjective and normative (including cultural) dimensions of events that lead to suffering or death. Such includes the negative-positive emotional state of handlers, which range from hatred and fear of animals (misothery) to love and reverence (theriophily). A sub-category on animal ethics theories follows to describe how animals were (or are) being used to provide a theoretical lens to situate the human-animal relationship further. The third domain connects with aspects of demand and supply through reference to research by Kellert (1984) on attitudes of society towards animals, as well as the dark tourism product/supply typology developed by Stone (2006). Kellert (1984) acts as a proxy because, unlike the conventional research on dark tourism motivations, no such data currently exists for animals as dark tourism attractions.

Example of animal dark tourism: Head-Smashed-In Buffalo Jump

Head-Smashed-In Buffalo Jump is a World Heritage Site and provincial park in Alberta, Canada. The park documents how indigenous people over several centuries used group hunting techniques to channel buffalo in a manner that forced them to plummet over a cliff that is 11m high and 300m long. Members of the tribe waited at the bottom and used clubs and spears to kill the buffalos since their broken legs prevented them from getting away. While this human story has been told, it is also possible to view this attraction through an animal dark tourism lens. According to our classification, buffalos died in a wild setting; death was human-induced; the role of animals was for subsistence (now educational); the event took place during prehistoric times; and suffering/death of buffalos occurred at the population (species) scale. Furthermore, there is a tradition in indigenous culture to respect the animal as it gives its life for human sustenance. As such, theriophily (reverence for animals) is suggested, although the primary animal ethical focus would still be anthropocentric given the nature of the animal-human relationship. The relationship is ecocentric if indigenous people actively practiced conservation of the buffalo population. Tourists might view this practice as "varied", experiencing cognitive dissonance along moralistic, utilitarian, or dominionistic lines. Finally, this type of dark tourism attraction corresponds to Stone's (2006) dark resting places, likened to a cemetery or a site of commemorative ethics.

Along these lines, Table 4.1 classifies other animal dark tourism examples. These include museums of natural history, zones of war and human conflict, European animal extinctions, bullfighting in Spain, and zoos and aquaria with a focus on Marius the giraffe in Copenhagen. All examples have been selected to represent most of Stone's (2006) dark tourism spectrum. The only type of dark tourism attraction not included in Table 4.1 is dark dungeons (see Rollin 2012, who discusses, in general, the site where Descartes conducted vivisections on dogs and other animals).

Table 4.1: Animal dark tourism examples.

Categories of Animal Dark Tourism	Museums of natural history, or "Dead zoos" (Barrington, 2021)	Japanese animal shrines (Nara Park (2019)	Zones of war and human conflict (Wise, 2021)
Status & setting	Dead animals; built site	Dead animals; wild site	Dead & alive; combined settings
Source of death/ suffering	Unknown	Unknown	Human-induced
Role of animals	Education; Science & Research	Spirituality	Part of nature; *Educator*
Temporal period	Contemporary	Historical	Contemporary
The scale of death/ suffering	Community-level	individual animal	Community
Negative-positive emotive state of handlers	Unknown	Theriophily	Indifference
Primary theory of ethics	Ecocentrism	Care ethics	Anthropocentric
Tourist attitudes of animals	Scientistic	Humanistic	Moralistic
Dark tourism products/supply	Dark exhibitions	Dark shrines	Dark conflict zones

Table 4.1 (continued)

Categories of Animal Dark Tourism	European animal extinctions (e.g., Caspian tiger) (IUCN, 2015–2016)	Bullfighting in Spain (Oakley, 2016)	Zoos and aquaria (e.g., Marius the giraffe, Copenhagen) (Cohen and Fennell, 2016; Howley, 2015)
Status and setting	Dead; wild setting	Alive – Dead; built setting	Live animals; built site
Source of death/ suffering	Human-induced	Human-induced	Human-induced
Role of animals	Competitor; *Spirituality*	Competitors	Mainly as entertainer
Temporal period	Historical	Contemporary	Contemporary
The scale of death/ suffering	Population	Population	Individual animal
Negative-positive emotive state of handlers	Misothery	Indifference	Indifference
Primary theory of ethics	Anthropocentric	Contractarianism	Ecocentrism
Tourist attitudes of animals	Ecologistic	Dominionistic	Varied: scientistic to moralistic
Dark tourism products/supply	Dark camps of genocide	Dark fun factories	Dark exhibitions

Conclusion: Emerging from the dark

The prototype developed in this article assumes that animal dark tourism will become a realistic option for the industry in the future. There is little doubt that events, places, or situations where animals have been abused stir human emotion. Since animal ethics considerations have been quickly absorbed into the tourism studies literature, we believe that our prototype is likely to elicit scholarly interest. However, acceptance in the industry will most certainly depend on whether there is demand for such attractions.

Our typology provides avenues for thinking about future research in the field of animal dark tourism. Future work should seek to investigate both supply and demand in dark tourism to determine whether the suffering or death of animals can be considered "legitimate" sites of dark tourism. Moreover, classifying animal dark tourism attractions along "lightest" to "darkest" lines would also be useful to both scholars and practitioners, and researchers might also survey dark tourism scholars (through Delphi or other techniques) to analyze how they react to pictures and descriptions of animal sites when re-defining the borders of dark tourism. Such an approach would be helpful in refining the categories and sub-categories of animal dark tourism we propose. In agreement with López López and Quintero Venegas (2021), our research adopts a posthumanist perspective that moves us away from humanism and anthropocentrism (and the Cartesian dualisms inherent within it). Instead, we operate a paradigm shift towards a breaking down of barriers between humans and animals (Cohen 2019; Thomsen 2021) and new ways of doing/being/knowing (ethico-onto-epistemology) (Kuby 2017) that envisage humans and animals as entangled agents (Alaimo and Hekman 2008) in the complex world of tourism.

References

Alaimo, S., & Hekman, S. J. (Eds.). (2008). *Material feminisms*. Indiana University Press.

Ashworth, G. J. (2004). Tourism and the heritage of atrocity: managing the heritage of South African apartheid for entertainment. In *New horizons in tourism: Strange experiences and stranger practices*. pp. 95–108. Wallingford UK: Cabi Publishing.

Barrington, K. (2021). *Museum Dublin: The Dead Zoo*. Retrieved at https://dublin.ie/live/stories/museum-dublin-the-dead-zoo/

Biran, A., Poria, Y. and Oren, G. (2011). Sought Experiences at Dark Heritage Sites. *Annals of Tourism Research* 38 (3): 820–841.

Buda, D. M. (2015). *Affective Tourism: Dark Routes in Conflict*. New York: Routledge.

Carr, N., & Broom, D. M. (2018). Tourism and animal welfare. CABI.

Cheal, F., and Griffin, T. (2013). Pilgrims and Patriots: Australian Tourist Experiences at Gallipoli. *International Journal of Culture, Tourism and Hospitality Research* 7 (3): 227–241.

Cohen, E. (2009). The Wild and the Humanized: Animals in Thai Tourism. *Anatolia* 20 (1): 100–118.

Cohen, E. (2019). Posthumanism and tourism. *Tourism Review* 74 (3): 416–427.

Cohen, E. and Fennell, D. A. (2016). The Elimination of Marius, the Giraffe: Humanitarian Act or Callous Management Decision?. *Tourism Recreation Research* 41 (2): 168–176,

Dunkley, R., Morgan, N., and Westwood, S. (2011). Visiting the Trenches: Exploring Meanings and Motivations in Battlefield Tourism. *Tourism Management* 32 (4): 860–868.

Farmaki, A. (2013). Dark Tourism Revisited: A Supply/demand Conceptualisation. *International Journal of Culture, Tourism and Hospitality Research* 7

Fennell, D.A. (2000). "Tourism and Applied Ethics." *Tourism Recreation Research* 25 *(1)*: 59–70.

Fennell, D. A. (2012). *Tourism and Animal Ethics*. London: Routledge.

Fennell, D. A., Moorhouse, T. P., & Macdonald, D. W. (2024). Towards a model for the assessment of conservation, welfare, and governance in wildlife tourism attractions. *Journal of Ecotourism*, *23*(2), 166–193.

Fennell, D. A., & Thomsen, B. (2021). Tourism & animal suffering: Mapping the future. *Annals of Tourism Research*, *91*, 103317.

Hester, J.J. (1967). The agency of man in animal extinctions. In Martin, P.S. and Wright, H.E. (Eds) *Pleistocene Extinctions: The Search for a Cause*. pp. 169–192. Yale University Press.

Kellert, S.R. (1984). American attitudes toward and knowledge of animals: An update. In Fox, M.W. and Mickley, L.D. (Eds.) *Advances in Animal Welfare Science 1984/85*, pp. 177–213. Washington, DC: The Humane Society of the United States.

Kline, C. (2018). *Animals, Food, and Tourism*. London: Routledge.

Kuby, C. R. (2017). "Why a Paradigm Shift of 'More Than Human Ontologies' is Needed: Putting to Work Poststructural and Posthuman Theories in Writers' Studio." *International Journal of Qualitative Studies in Education* 30 (9), 877–896.

Howley, K. (2015). What We Mourned When We Mourned Cecil. Retrieved at https://www.newyorker.com/books/page-turner/what-we-mourned-when-we-mourned-cecil

Israfilova, F., & Khoo-Lattimore, C. (2019). Sad and Violent but I Enjoy It: Children's Engagement with Dark Tourism as an Educational Tool. *Tourism and Hospitality Research* 19 (4): 478–487.

IUCN. (2015–2016). Caspian Tiger. Retrieved at https://endangeredlist.org/animal/caspian-tiger/

Koleth, M. (2014). Hope in the Dark: Geographies of Volunteer and Dark Tourism in Cambodia. *Cultural Geographies* 21 (4): 681–694.

Kulcsár, E. and Simon, R.Z. (2015). The Magic of Dark Tourism. *Management & Marketing XIII* (1): 124–136.

Light, D. (2017). Progress in Dark Tourism and Thanatourism Research: An Uneasy Relationship with Heritage Tourism. *Tourism Management* 61 (C), 275–301.

López- López, Á. and Quintero Venegas, G. J. (2021). Animal Dark Tourism in Mexico: Bulls Performing Their Own Slaughter. In Rickly, J. and Kline, C. (Eds.) *Exploring Non-human Work in Tourism: From Beasts of Burden to Animal Ambassadors*, C, pp. 69–82. Berlin: De Gruyter.

Markwell, K. (2015). *Birds, Beasts and Tourists: Human-Animal Relations in Tourism*. Clevedon, UK: Channel View.

Miles, W. (2002). Auschwitz: Museum Interpretation and Darker Tourism. *Annals of Tourism Research* 29 (4): 1175–1178.

Martini, A. & Buda, D. M. (2020). Dark Tourism and Affect: Framing Places of Death and Disaster. *Current Issues in Tourism* 23 (6): 679–692.

Nara Park (2019). Temples and shrines for animal lovers. Retrieved at https://www.visitnara.jp/lists-and-stories/story/temples-and-shrines-for-animal-lovers/

Nawijn, J., Isaac, R., van Liempt, A., Gridnevskiy, K. (2016). Emotion Clusters for Concentration Camp Memorials. *Annals of Tourism Research*. 61: 244–247.

Oakley, N. (2016). Why people want "cruel" and "barbaric" bullfighting banned – and it's nothing to do with a matador's death. Retrieved at https://www.mirror.co.uk/news/world-news/people-want-cruel-barbaric-bullfighting-8397382

Podoshen, J., Venkatesh, V., Wallin, J., Andrzejewski, S., & Jin, Z. (2015). Dystopian Dark Tourism: An Exploratory Examination. *Tourism Management* 51: 316–328.

Rickly, J and Kline, C. (2021). *Exploring Non-human Work in Tourism: From Beasts of Burden to Animal Ambassadors*. Berlin: De Gruyter

Rollin, B. (2012). Do animals feel pain? Retrieved at https://youtu.be/zZc1HnOCtSk

Seaton, A. (1996). Guided by the Dark: From Thanatopsis to Thanatourism. *International Journal of Heritage Studies* 2 (4): 234–244.

Sharpley, R. (2005). Travels to the Edge of Darkness: Towards a Typology of 'Dark Tourism.' In Ryan, C., Page, S.J., and Aicken, M. (Eds.) *Taking Tourism to the Limits: Issues, Concepts and Management Perspectives*, pp. 215–226. London: Taylor & Francis.

Stone, P. (2006). A Dark Tourism Spectrum: Towards a Typology of Death and Macabre Related Tourist Sites, Attractions and Exhibitions. *Tourism: An International Interdisciplinary Journal* 54 (2): 145–160.

Stone, P., & Sharpley, R. (2008). Consuming Dark Tourism: A Thanatological Perspective. *Annals of Tourism Research* 35 (2): 574–595.

Stone, P. (2013). Dark tourism scholarship: a critical review. *International Journal of Culture, Tourism and Hospitality Research* 7 (3): 307–318.

Tarlow, P. (2005). Dark Tourism: The Appealing 'Dark' Side of Tourism and More. In Novelli, M. (Ed.) *Niche Tourism: Contemporary Issues, Trends and Cases*, pp. 47–57. Oxford: Elsevier.

Thomsen, B. (2021). Wolf Ecotourism: A Posthumanist Approach to Wildlife Ecotourism. In Fennell, D.A. (Ed.). Routledge Handbook of Ecotourism, pp. 1–26. London: Routledge.

Timothy, Dallen J. and Victor B. Teye. (2004). American children of the African diaspora: Journeys to the motherland. In Coles, T. and Timothy, D.J. (Eds.) *Tourism, Diasporas and Space*, pp. 111–123. London: Routledge.

Wise, N. (2021). The Humanitarian Economy: Animals Caught in the Crossfire. In Fennell, D.A. (Ed.) *Routledge Handbook of Ecotourism*, 1–26. London: Routledge.

José-Carlos García-Rosell and Philip Hancock

5 Meet, greet and eat: Farmed animals as dark tourism attractions

Abstract: The growing popularity of the countryside as a place of consumption and recreation has contributed to the diversification of farming into tourism and the commodification of farm animals for touristic use. For example, in the UK, a number of livestock farms have opened their premises to the public, configuring and promoting them as tourism attractions whereby visitors can experience the immediacy and vitality of animal life often portrayed as unfettered and joyful. At the same time, they have also responded to concerns around the negative impact on health and sustainability of conventional farming systems by opening farm shops that offer, amongst other things, their own fresh farm reared meat direct to the consumer. Drawing upon the concept of embodied ethics in organizational studies (Hancock, 2008) and embodiment in tourism research (Baerenholdt et al., 2004, Veijola & Valtonen, 2007), we problematize this idyllic view of farming and farm animals as a curious form of dark tourism whereby non-human animal life and death become intimately entwined as objects of profoundly embodied consumption practices. Gaze, touch, and practices of embodied incorporation are all combined as the living are looked upon, petted and often internalised as anthropomorphic friends and companions, while the dead are equally evaluated by eye and hand and, ultimately, both ingested and excreted. Therefore, by paying particular attention to embodied engagement between people and farm animals, we take an ethical perspective that is sensitive to the embodied and situated nature of animal dark tourism.

Keywords: dark tourism, non-human, human-animal interactions, embodiment, ethics

Introduction

In July 2022, UK celebrity chef and restaurateur Gordon Ramsey upset the world of social media by posting a TikTok video of him entering a farm enclosure full of initially inquisitive lambs while singing 'yummy yum yum I'm going to eat you!' and asking, 'which one's going in the oven first?' (Atkinson, 2022). While nothing entirely new in itself – for example, seafood connoisseurs have long chosen their living lobsters from a tank before condemning them to death and ingestion – the post received many critical comments from people who, while not adverse to eating meat, felt that Ramsey had gone too far and that his commentary was distasteful if not somewhat disturbing. Whatever one's reaction to Ramsey's actions, they reflect a broader question about the extent to which people can engage with livestock in what appears, at

https://doi.org/10.1515/9783110792072-006

first sight, a contradictory manner, both as living creatures and dead foodstuffs within a relatively bounded space and time, particularly with reference to the emergence and growth in farm tourism.

A response to both the increasing economic pressures faced by rural farming communities, alongside a growing public interest in the sourcing, reliability, and, most importantly, the safety of everyday foodstuffs, farm tourism has become very popular across Europe. While originating in mainland Europe over a century ago (Phelan & Sharpley, 2011), it has, since the 1980s, become the focus of both state and local promotion, often based on the principle that farms can provide for the accommodation and catering needs of groups of tourists, especially those who wish to experience the calmness of country life at a relatively low cost and often not too far from home (Frater, 1983; Nilsson, 2002). And while the UK has been something of a slow starter compared to mainland Europe, its popularity is clearly on the rise with a 200% year-on-year increase in traffic being reported in 2020 (Paterson, 2022). As with all sectors, however, the farm tourism market is a clearly differentiated one with some operators offering full accommodations, and even opportunities to experience work on the farms in question, while others position themselves as tourist attractions suitable for no more than a day trip (Nickerson et al., 2001; Sayre & Henderson, 2018).

In this chapter, we focus primarily on the latter type of tourist operation, namely small farms in the UK that cater primarily to day-trippers, offering a largely petting zoo-type experience. In doing so, they offer their patrons an opportunity to meet and greet predominantly, although not exclusively, farmed animals and experience the conditions under which they are raised. As we argue, however, such tourist attractions also have a decidedly darker aspect to them. While the immediate attraction offered to visitors is the experience of encountering calves and lambs nuzzling their mothers, chickens pecking freely, and other farmyard creatures living their best lives, there is another side to these venues, namely the almost ubiquitous farm shop and restaurant where if not these exact animals, then certainly their near relatives and possible playmates, are dismembered and served up both cold and hot as objects of gastronomical approval and consumption. In this chapter, we use the term animal in reference to nonhuman animals exclusively. We also use the term "farmed animal" instead of "farm animal" to acknowledge that farming is something done to these animals against their will, not something inherent to their nature (Freeman, 2009).

Taking a critical animal studies perspective (Best, 2009; Matsuoka & Sorenson, 2018), we argue that such attractions, rather than just promoting an idyllic view of farming and farmed animals, represent a curious form of dark tourism in which animal life and death become intimately entwined as objects of profoundly embodied consumption practices (cf. López-López & Quintero Venegas, 2021). Critical animal studies allow us to challenge the anthropocentric nature of dark tourism as a field of research and, thus, to extend the moral debate surrounding the commodification and commercialization of death and suffering beyond humans to include animals (see Matsuoka & Sorenson, 2018). As the attraction discussed in this chapter reflects, gaze, touch, and practices of embodied incorporation are all combined as the living are looked upon, petted, and often internalised as anthropomorphic friends and companions, while the dead are equally evaluated by eye and hand and, ultimately, both ingested and excreted (see Tully & Carr, 2021). In doing so we also reflect on some of the possible ethical implications of such practices and the forms of tourism they promote.

The chapter proceeds with a critical evaluation of the concept of dark tourism, noting its predominantly anthropocentric focus and, therefore, its tendency to marginalise the death and suffering of animals as a worthy subject of either tourist or academic moral consideration. It then considers the historical importance of animals to many tourist destinations and, in particular, the role they play in underpinning the appeal of forms of farm tourism and the atmospheric qualities of such attractions.

Moving beyond their importance as living signifiers of the attractions and benefits of a natural environment, the following section then considers the parallel rise of a secondary discourse surrounding such animals, namely that of Happy Meat and the benefits of eating organically and free-range raised animals and how this has also bolstered the tourist farm cause. The final sections offer up an illustrative discussion of such tourist attractions, drawing primarily from online publicity material and an observational visit to one such farm in the UK[1] before considering the implications for how we conceptualise dark tourism within the field, as well as reflecting on the ethical questions such a reformulation of activities might generate. The chapter concludes with some final reflections and a discussion of the importance of approaching farm tourism through a dark tourism lens. It also draws attention to potential avenues for future research.

Dark tourism beyond anthropocentrism

While contested and complex in nature (Light, 2017; Stone, 2013), and despite numerous conceptual and empirical studies contributing to a growing body of scholarship, dark tourism (or thanatourism) remains a largely anthropocentric concept (Fennell et al., 2021) that continues to privilege a human-animal dualism in which animals are considered lesser species (Freeman, 2009; Weitzenfeld & Joy, 2014). As an academic field, it has focused predominantly on exploring the commodification and commercialization of significant human suffering and is most widely used with reference to the act of visiting and experiencing deathscapes; that is, places where tragedies, disasters or historically noteworthy human deaths have occurred and continue to affect the lives of other human beings (Martini & Buda 2020; Stone, 2013; Tarlow, 2005). From this perspective, the ethical dimension of dark tourism has been discussed in relation to how places associated with human death are presented to visitors (Sharma, 2020) and their potential

1 The names of these farms have been changed to ensure anonymity.

impact on those who experience them. Even where dark tourism may occasionally refer to animals, their role is circumstantial as simple objects for human purposes or accompanying human death and suffering (Fennell et al., 2021; López López & Quintero Venegas, 2021).

Nevertheless, if we consider the growing public and interdisciplinary academic interest in human-animal relationships (Coulter, 2016; Irvine, 2008; Matsuoka & Sorenson, 2018; Räsänen & Syrjämaa, 2017; Tallberg & Hamilton, 2022; Thomas, 2022), including tourism (Fennell, D. 2011; Giampiccoli et al., 2020; Markwell, 2015; Rickly & Kline, 2021), then it may be time to move beyond limited discussions of dark tourism as pertaining exclusively to humans. This should not only be considered an ontological issue, but should also be thought of, in our view, as a profoundly ethical matter, given that the lack of a non-anthropocentric perspective on dark tourism contributes to reifying tourism practices that position humans above animals, thus reproducing a worldview in which animals are denied subjectivity and agency (see Äijälä, 2021; Colling, 2018; Dashper, 2019; Fennell, 2022; Haanpää et al., 2019; Tallberg et al., 2022). This is problematic as it contributes to speciesism and, thus, the legitimization of a social order that supports exploitation, prejudices, and discrimination towards animals (Matsuoka & Sorenson, 2018; Schneeberger, 2022; Taylor & Twine, 2014).

As such, dark tourism not only reinforces the human-animal divide in the realm of death and suffering but also reaffirms the anthropocentric line of thinking in tourism, where animals are considered only insofar as commodities for the tourist experience (see Colling, 2018; Derrida, 2008). Indeed, although the modus operandi of killing and inflicting pain on animals and humans is very much the same (Pedersen, 2011), it is only the commodification of human death and suffering that is given moral consideration. By limiting the notion of thanatourism to an anthropocentric worldview, dark tourism scholars construct a body of knowledge in which the exploitation, suffering, and killing of animals are normalized and rendered completely neutral. While death is at the core of dark tourism (Hartmann et al. 2018), a critical animal studies perspective on dark tourism draws attention not only to the killing but also to the breeding and management of animals for the sake of human entertainment (see Pedersen, 2011). An extension of dark tourism to include animals contributes to promoting compassion and empathy towards the suffering of both other species and human beings (see Aaltola, 2022; García-Rosell & Hancock, 2022). Some headway in this direction has already been made, of course (e.g., Fennell et al., 2021; López López & Quintero Venegas, 2021). Take, for example, bullfighting, where a matador kills a bull in an arena in the presence of domestic visitors and foreign tourists. This has been identified as one example of dark tourism that seemingly requires the human-induced suffering, dying and death of animals (Fennell et al., 2021; Lopez-Lopez & Quintero-Venegas, 2021). According to López-López and Quintero-Venegas (2021), this slaughtering of bulls in the arena is an anthropocentric action that reinforces not only patriarchal thinking but also the treatment of animals as resources to be exploited and merchandised. Other animal-based tourism attractions that have also been classified as objects of a dark form of tourism are museums of natural history, European animal extinctions, and zoos and aquaria where dead animals are dissected and necropsied in public events (see Fennell et al., 2021).

A non-anthropocentric perspective on dark tourism contributes not only to making visible the death and suffering of animals as part of tourism attractions but also to understanding how aesthetic and affective socio-spatial encounters shape the human-animal relationships connected to death and its representation (see Martini & Buda, 2020). Moreover, if dark tourism provides liminal spaces for reflexivity on the ethics of contemporary consumption, as some scholars have argued (Sharma, 2020; Stone, 2009), then a critical animal studies lens offers an opportunity to use dark tourism as a means for reassessing our relationship and moral reasoning towards animals more widely. It is within such liminal spaces that we can critically examine the use of animals not only through rational deontological judgments (rights and justice) but also in terms of affectual relations, compassion, or any forms of feeling experienced through the body (Aaltola, 2022; Hancock, 2008; Pullen & Rhodes, 2015; Tallberg et al., 2022).

In the next section of this chapter, we draw attention to animals as objects that are exploited for the creation of farm tourist experiences. In so doing, we also consider the importance of animals to the positioning and aesthetics of tourist destinations, particularly in the area of agricultural and animal husbandry and the growth of animal and farm tourism in the UK, and beyond.

Farmed animals as objects of consumption

Animals play a significant role in the tourism industry, both as primary attractions and as contributors to the overall destination atmosphere. Tourist destinations worldwide capitalize on the appeal of animal encounters to attract visitors and create desirable experiences (Fennell, 2011; Kline, 2018; Markwell, 2015; Rickly & Kline, 2021). In some instances, animals are the central focus of tourist activities. For example, African wildlife safaris allow visitors to observe and interact with iconic species such as elephants, lions, and zebras. Similarly, Australasian diving expeditions enable tourists to encounter tropical marine life, while Arctic excursions often revolve around the quest to spot polar bears, reindeer, and other Arctic wildlife. These animal encounters are regarded as primary objects or resources of the tourist experience. Visitors directly engage with animals, creating value through close interactions, observation, and sometimes even participation in conservation efforts. These encounters are often the main reason tourists choose specific destinations, shaping their expectations and defining their experiences.

Animals can also contribute, however, to the more general ambience of a destination, even if they are not the main attraction. They become part of the destination's atmosphere, adding to the overall appeal and creating a sense of place. For instance, a coastal town may have seagulls and other seabirds that enhance the seaside experience. In such cases, animals are not the primary focus of the tourist experience, but they play a crucial role in creating the destination's atmosphere. Not that these two roles are mutually exclusive. Many destinations incorporate both primary and secondary animal experiences. For example, a safari may include encounters with a variety of wildlife while incorporating the natural sounds and presence of animals in the surrounding environment, thereby contributing to the overall atmospherics of the destination (Äijälä, 2022; Burns, 2015; Kline, 2018; Mkono & Holder, 2019).

A field of interest in which the role and importance of animals have grown in recent years is that of farm tourism, which refers to tourism activities within a farm setting (e.g., Cassel & Petersson, 2015; Nickerson et al., 2001; Sayre & Henderson, 2018; Sharpley & Vass, 2006). Opening up a new space for tourist activities in which embodied encounters with animals has become both the aim and the backdrop, it has brought into sharp relief both our aesthetic and our ethical relationship to these creatures (Bertella, 2021; Tully & Carr, 2021). Unlike traditional zoos, these encounters take place on what remain working livestock farms whereby visitors are able to enjoy close contact with both recognised farmed animals as well as more atypical or even exotic species usually brought in to directly attract further visitors (Tully & Carr, 2021).

Such farms promote themselves, therefore, as tourist attractions that not only offer an opportunity for visitors to be immersed in a healthy rural environment (Nilsson, 2002; Sayre & Henderson, 2018) but also to experience an atmosphere that exudes fun, sentimentality, and the immediacy and vitality of embodied spontaneity as living animals are seen, heard, petted, and even befriended (Tully & Carr, 2021). Roaming, if not always freely, then usually in large pens and fields, they bring to the tourist experience a sense of vitality and the natural spontaneity of life, something perhaps most evident in the spring when the noises, sights, and sounds of lambing and the birth of other farmed animals reverberate around the fields and pens, often combining with the delighted squeals of visiting children and the hustle and bustle of farm workers. It is through these human-animal relations and the pseudo-human status assigned to animals through anthropomorphic symbols such as names and the attribution of human traits that the mythical rural idyll and authentic farm experience are created (see Tully & Carr, 2021). Even though the naming of animals and the acknowledgement of their subjectivity may bring them closer to the realm of moral subjects, the anthropocentric nature of food production and consumption systems continues to make humans morally indifferent to farm practices leading to the exploitation, manipulation and slaughtering of animals (see Clarke & Knights, 2021; Freeman, 2009; Pedersen, 2022). Indeed, as Pedersen (2022) argues, the implementation of animal-friendly farming models works as a form of disciplinary power that makes the breeding, managing, and slaughter of animals morally acceptable in the eyes of the public.

While these animals are integral to that constellation of factors that attributes to the atmospheric attraction and appeal of such tourist spaces, their presence is also entwined within a darker story. While profoundly embodied in character, this is a story in which they are largely stripped of their anthropomorphic status and personalities and reduced to mere objects with nothing more than their flesh, and perhaps heritage, to speak for them (Bertella, 2021). This is a story of their appearance as reformulated and repackaged commodities of consumption in the various farm shops and outlets that are often integral to the economic sustainability of such attractions. At this point, these animals are not appreciated anymore for their personalities but for their flesh and meat, which is described as tasty, superb and of excellent quality (Sayre & Henderson, 2018).

In the next section, we consider some of these issues in greater depth, drawing on research into both the self-presentation of such farms alongside other similar tourist environments and attractions. In doing so, we describe and reflect on the empirical manifestations and processes of this transformation before then moving on to consider not only the aesthetic but ethical implications for the animal-tourist relationship.

Welfare, happy farms and happy meat

Farm tourism is not an entirely new phenomenon (Frater, 1983). Originally a response to a need amongst many farmers to diversify income streams and contribute more widely to local economies (Busby & Rendle, 2000; Sharpley & Vass, 2006), it has grown globally as tourists seek out both new and often locally accessible short holiday or day-trip destinations. More recently, it has also been buoyed by a public increasingly interested in both the healthy production of human foodstuffs and, when it comes to questioning the rearing of livestock, the animal welfare conditions under which animals are bred and kept. In the UK, for instance, incidents such as the outbreak of bovine spongiform encephalopathy (BSE or 'mad cow disease') during the 1980s and 1990s, brought together these two concerns as animal and human welfare were increasingly viewed as interrelated (Mayfield et al, 2007). This interest, and the market it has created, has led to the formation of the UK's *National Farm Attractions Network*, and around 400 farm and rural attractions that receive around 25 million visitors annually.[2]

While such attractions can feature numerous activities ranging from adventure playgrounds and treasure hunts to seasonal events such as haunted pumpkin fields at Halloween, and Christmas markets in the winter, perhaps two of their staples are the opportunity to meet and greet farmed animals, and to enjoy fresh farm produce, including animals either purchased and cooked in the farm restaurant or café or processed in the farm shop for home preparation and consumption. For farm owners

2 https://www.farmattractions.net/about-the-national-farm-attraction-network/farm-attraction-tourism-industry/

themselves and, they would argue, the consuming public at large, such a combination of ethical and therefore tourist friendly animal farming practices, and the commercial activity of direct selling to the public makes sense for all parties concerned, including the farm's animals. For the farmer, it provides a source of direct income stripped of many of the overheads commonly associated with the shipping and marketing of animal-based products (Sharpley & Vass, 2006). For the consumer, it provides what is deemed to be better quality meat due to the lack of stress placed upon the animals during their lifetime, as well as a leisure opportunity that itself doubles up as a form of self-assurance as to the quality of both the lives and arguably the deaths of the creatures they are about to consume (see Sayre & Henderson, 2018).

Interestingly, the term that has increasingly come to identify animal-based products – albeit not exclusively – reared at such tourist-orientated farms is that of 'Happy Meat'. While aiming to appeal to several concerns, including human health and environmental spoilage, one of the primary selling points when it comes to marketing Happy Meat products is a commitment by those rearing such livestock to ensure that animals experience a high quality of life, one usually characterised by them living and eating in a natural, free-range environment, and dying in a gentle and managed way (Clarke & Knights, 2021; Renton, 2007). As such, Happy Meat is considered to be an antidote to intensive factory farming, something that is often characterised by cramped living conditions, livestock growth and development regulated by drug use, genetic modification, and mechanised forms of slaughter amongst other things. It is also widely argued that Happy Meat, while representing an improvement in the quality of life for farmed animals, also constitutes a better end product for the consumer. Meat is presented as both organic in nature and, as such, healthier as well as tastier. Beef is, for example, often described as richer and better marbled coming from such animals (Renton, 2007), due to these animals experiencing less stress and enjoying better diets.

While practices associated with the production of Happy Meat may indeed be considered an improvement on those associated with intensive animal rearing, it has also encouraged many critical voices to be raised. Many of these have come from those associated with the cause of animal welfare, as well as vegetarianism and veganism. In their 2013 book, *The Ultimate Betrayal: Is There Happy Meat?*, Bohanec and Bohanec (2013) argue that the very concept of Happy Meat is built on a betrayal of the animals that are one moment seemingly cared for and the next slaughtered or butchered by those very same carers, one that defiles both the animals and humans involved. Similarly, Vinding (2014) objects to what he considers to be the deception behind Happy Meat in that it is posited as an ethical alternative to mass farming when in fact, to take the life of any sentient creature, however they have been raised, is profoundly unethical. From a more academic perspective, several studies draw on the Foucauldian concept of biopower to offer a further critical analysis of Happy Meat and its legitimating discursive formations (e.g., Cole, 2011; Pedersen, 2022). In essence, Cole (2011) argues that attempts to position farmed animals as happy via the introduction of animal welfare initiatives represent a discursive shift towards a form of pastoral power that, once again, deceives all parties concerned as to the nature of the exploitive and ultimately murderous relationship between farmer and farmed. As Cole (2011: 96 *original emphasis*) himself puts it:

> Happy meat discourse then, represents the 'popular' expression of pastoral power relations manifested in 'animal centred' welfare discourse. It facilitates adoption of the benevolent role of pastor in place of the disciplinary role of gaoler. It reassures consumers that they *know* the needs and desires of 'farmed animals', and that those needs and desires are being fulfilled precisely *because* they eat the flesh of those animals.

Beyond the intractable contradiction of such a position what most, if not all critics of the Happy Meat idea and other animal-friendly farming models point to, is the fact that first and foremost it represents an attempt to market the flesh of animals to an increasingly concerned, or is that squeamish and ultimately self-interested, market. And even if one were to consider such meat to be a path to a better future for such creatures, one in which those who care are not also those who ultimately slaughter, as it stands, it appears to reproduce little more than a form of PR razzle-dazzle (LaVeck, 2006), one that obscures the real relations of death and exploitation that underpin the global meat producing industry (Hamilton & McCabe, 2016). It may well be true that such animals are treated relatively better or more humane than other creatures that find their way into the global meat industry. Yet, this interpretation fails to address the underlying repression of these farmed animals and thus, making their exploitation to look less painful and more acceptable (see Gunderson, 2014).

In this chapter, however, the concern is less with the activities of a global meat industry and more with, as noted above, those small farm producers that have decided to turn to the virtues associated with animal welfare and Happy Meat to not simply sell chopped and sliced flesh, but equally to share and sell the very happiness of these animals itself, whereby as consumers we are invited to now consume the lives, as well as the fruits of the deaths, of these creatures.

Life and death down on jollity farm

In this section, our aim is to demonstrate the presence of these farms and how they operate by examining a few illustrative instances located in the UK. Methodologically, the information collected has been drawn predominantly from relevant public-access websites and supplemented by informal visits to such establishments designed to confirm first-hand what was claimed for them. While the ambition of this chapter is not to criticise or evaluate the actual businesses and tourist attractions discussed but to protect all parties involved, pseudonyms have been used when referring to particular examples of such farms. In doing so, we hope to illustrate how such tourist attractions seek to manufacture, both discursively and materially, a series of conditions under which they can reconcile a conception of such attractions as both live(ly) and happy places while, at the same time reconciling visitors with the far darker role they play as purveyors of both death and flesh, integral to the experience they offer.

Perhaps nowhere is this better illustrated than *Davidsons Farm and Zoo*, based in the southeast of England. Combining a working farm and zoo, with the latter featuring in particular various species of reptile, *Davidsons* pitches itself as an educational and recreational tourist destination. The website, in particular, stresses its passion for ensuring education and fun for all the family by providing admission to both the farm and zoo for visitors to understand how animals are farmed and ranched, as well as their importance to the environment.[3] In particular, its website prides itself on its zoological attractions, which include reptiles such as alligators and snakes, and a host of exotic creatures such as wallabies, meerkats, and buffalo, amongst others, plus other attractions such as a small adventure playground. Equally integral to the attraction, however, is the attached farm shop that, while selling most of the usual goods associated with such outlets, including beers, cheeses, vegetables, and preserves, features, perhaps above all else, an impressive butchers counter. The framing of the farm and zoo attraction in terms of education and entertainment indicates how the commodification of animal life and death can be justified and made morally permissible or even neutral (see Christien, 2023; Pedersen, 2022). In doing so, the farm and zoo reinforces the position of humans as privileged and superior beings who can legitimately breed, manage, and kill animals so long as they do so humanely (Best, 2009).

Here the flesh of those animals that the visitor had only moments ago cooed over or admired is presented in a very different form. Boned, splayed, and displayed in large, refrigerated cabinets, they are both abject and yet compelling in that they demand not only a cognitive repositioning as what was perhaps only moments and meters ago witnessed to be vital and alive is now transposed into what is both dead and dismembered, but also scrutiny and discussion as they are presented up as choice objects of consumption. Here these animals enter into a new embodied relationship with visitors whereby they are still subject to forms of evaluation based on the eye, touch, and possibly ear of the visitor, but now the criteria are less of, say, 'cuteness', 'adorability' or 'liveliness' and rather the colour of their stripped flesh and the amount of fat, or rather a lack of it (see Sayre & Henderson, 2018).

Curiously, it is not only those animals that might be accepted as traditional farmed animals and, therefore, perhaps considered destined for such public display and consumption post-mortem that is presented here. Many of those animals that are exhibited in the zoo share the same status as their farmyard brethren, such as crocodiles, wallabies, and emus, amongst others, and are both regarded as attractions as

3 Across all the farm's publicity, terms such as sustainability, conservation and carbon neutrality all feature prominently as key descriptors of the owner's values and priorities.

well as sold and consumed as dead flesh. Not only do they share the same temporal and spatial environment, but they are also, in many instances, destined to share the same premature demise. While the zoo is both a site of carnivalesque spectacle and zoological exhibition based on the construction of wild animals as the unknowable other and, thereby, thrilling to its visitors (Christien, 2023), it is this otherness that turns these wild animals into exotic objects to be eaten and digested (Molz, 2007).

It could, of course, be argued that to conceptualise such attractions and activities as sites of dark tourism misunderstands the concept in that it is almost exclusively associated with visiting places of human death and suffering (Light, 2017). As we have already noted, this is the kind of anthropocentric understanding we are seeking to rethink as it overlooks the kind of anthropomorphic representations deployed across many such venues to profoundly humanise their farmed animals for the benefit of visitors (Tully & Carr, 2021). Take, for example, *Green Leaf Farm* in East Anglia. Focusing solely on the rearing of traditional farmed animals, *Green Leaf Farm* offers a regional tourist attraction that combines the opportunity to meet and greet a range of animals, including pigs, cows, and chickens, with a range of predominantly children's attractions including playground rides and farmyard equipment. Again, it stresses its ambition to address the needs of wildlife and conservation while being a working farm and a 'great day out'.

Yet these are no ordinary farmed animals, simple objects to be exhibited and consumed. They are anthropomorphised and accredited with personality characteristics that give them, if albeit illusionary, the quality of voice and even imputed autonomy on par with their human carers. As such, visitors are invited to 'meet' everyone 'from cheeky goats and happy pigs to clucking chickens and thoughtful cows'.[4] Or one can always say hi to one of the farm's 'friendly alpacas' who enjoy a good 'nuzzle and scratch'.[5] These are, therefore, animals that one can get to know, that one can come back to see time after time, and even possibly build relationships with, sharing and celebrating their cheeky and thoughtful lives (see Fudge, 2008; Tully & Carr, 2021).

Where life is enjoyed and celebrated, death, however, is once again not far away. While animals are not slaughtered on the premises, with the proud addition of its butchery a decade ago, Green Leaf Farm celebrates its ability to provide 'home-grown and freshly butchered meat' to its visitors through its shop and café. The website and the attraction are replete with images of freshly carved, processed, or packaged flesh, both raw and cooked. Alongside images of calving mothers, snuffling piglets, and gambolling lambs, we see whole chickens, slices of cured pig and fillets of cow flesh ready to be examined, chosen, and consumed by tourists who still consider them to be cheeky, happy, or indeed thoughtful.

---

4 https://www.hollowtrees.co.uk/meet-the-animals/

5 Nuzzle and scratch alludes to a British children's television series that featured two puppet alpacas who work for a job agency. It is a comic show in which these two personable characters frequently get into trouble due to their regular incompetence – https://www.bbc.co.uk/programmes/b00d9g0h.

However, not all farms operate in this manner. A few, such as *Water Farm* in the northwest of England, present themselves first and foremost as a provider of reared and butchered meat, with animal encounters carefully choreographed and predominately informative (with lamb feeding to one side) rather than sentimental. At the same time, a few visitor farms deliberately choose not to sell livestock meat directly from the premises or online in order to maintain a clear distinction between the living and the dead, the cared for and the consumed and, as such, avoid any scrutiny. Neither is this unique to the activities associated with farm tourism. These choices can be seen as strategies to hide or reduce the caring-killing paradox, that is, the emotional contradiction of first caring and then killing animals (Tallberg & Jordan, 2022). While this paradox is largely hidden from those who are not directly involved in the killing, the slaughtering of animals and the selling of butchered meat can contribute to negative emotional experiences among workers and visitors in a farm tourism context.

A similar relationship between life and death, light and dark, can also often be found where animals are a key ingredient in the production of atmospheric tourist destinations. As we have observed elsewhere (García-Rosell & Hancock, 2022), the role played by reindeer across Christmas tourist resorts in Finnish Lapland reflects this bifurcation in which they are encountered and consumed as both living if not supernatural embodiments of the festive spirit and seasonal atmosphere, and dead if still embodied signifiers of a hearty winter's meal in the form of poronkäristys (sautéed reindeer), or a holiday well-enjoyed as their flesh, skin and bone are sold as tourist souvenirs, especially in the form of the ubiquitous 'reindeer pelt'. Indeed, it is not unusual to witness visiting tourists board their homeward-bound flights with young children carrying plush 'Rudolph' souvenir toys and wearing their 'I Met Santa's Reindeer' t-shirts while accompanied by parents or guardians carrying the skins, and even the consumable flesh, of these creatures alongside them.

The difference here is that, unlike farm tourism, the animals here are not in themselves the primary attraction for tourists despite playing an integral role in the atmospherics and, indeed, the mythology of the destination. Nor is their eventual slaughter and consumption the primary function of the destination in question or part of the attraction as per the ability of farms to also offer customers meat that is purportedly organic and happy. Nonetheless, what they do share in common is how they constitute such playful destinations as places of death, dismemberment and, ultimately, the ingestion of those creatures that are equally charged while living with the responsibility of bringing life, fun, and playfulness into the lives of those tourists who visit them. This is an interesting paradox which needs serious contemplation within a non-anthropocentric dark tourism perspective.

Discussion and conclusion

In this chapter, we have aimed to make a case for recognising that the exploitation of animals, or more accurately the death of animals in a farm tourism context, constitutes an object of dark tourism. Unlike established, anthropocentric examples of this phenomenon, however, a major distinction is that in the majority of cases, the kinds of farms we have discussed above are not visited primarily because they are places associated with death and disaster (Foley & Lennon, 1996). Rather, it is important to highlight that these farms often go to great lengths to embrace and showcase their commitment to the well-being, vitality, and joy of the animals under their care. Marketing themselves as anthropomorphised attractions whereby visitors can experience the immediacy and vitality of animal life often portrayed as unfettered and joyful, death, or any hint of death, is largely excluded from how they present themselves to the outside world (Sayre & Henderson, 2018; Tully & Carr, 2021). The exclusion of death from the farm tourism context contributes to hiding any form of animal experiences related to pain and suffering (see Bertella, 2021).

At the same time, such attractions have also responded to concerns about the negative impact on health and sustainability of conventional farming systems by opening farm shops that offer, amongst other things, fresh farm-reared meat direct to the consumer. Often promoted as integral to the production of 'happy meat' (Renton, 2007), they celebrate the adoption of a more pastoral conception of animal husbandry (Cole, 2011) in which death and butchery are excluded in favour of a discourse of quality, health, and a life well lived. However, this is not the case. Such venues rely not only on an idyllic representation of life but also, economically at the very least, the reality of death, as the dismembered and packaged flesh of these creatures exposes their true status as livestock or farmed animals, an asset to be slaughtered and realised in the market for prime organic meat (see Tully & Carr, 2021). As we have observed, visitors, in most instances, initially fascinated by the environmentally attuned atmospherics of such tourist attractions and the promise of interaction with live animals, are quickly drawn into a new relationship with such creatures. This relationship is not only born of their presence as tourists or sightseers but also extends their engagement with the primary objects of their interest and as lifeless commodities that remain evaluated by eye and hand if albeit now as carriers of taste and nourishment.

As we indicated earlier, it is not the desire for contact and connection with the death of animals that attracts visitors to farm tourism attractions, despite death being an intrinsic part of a farm's daily life. Rather, it is the promise of a rural idyll where farmers care for their domesticated animals in the quietness and greenery of the countryside (Sayre & Henderson, 2018; Tully & Carr, 2021). But the question remains: why do we approach this type of tourist attraction as a form of dark tourism? In essence, our ambition is primarily a sensitising one in that it exposes the essentially anthropocentric values and practices that legitimize the operation of such tourist attractions, as well as bringing to the fore a similar problem within the current dark tourism literature. In the case of the former, we believe that a critical animal studies perspective on dark tourism offers a powerful lens through which farm tourism can be critically examined as a site of objectification, exploitation and death, a relationship often little thought about by those patrons who frequent such attractions. In doing so, by approaching the farm tourism in such a manner, we might shed light on how society perceives and deals with the life and death of animals and how it legitimizes the fact that billions of animals are exploited and slaughtered annually for food and other commercial purposes (see Clarke & Knights, 2021; Hamilton & McCabe, 2016).

Moreover, by exploring such a relationship, we also challenge the underlying anthropocentric binaries that underpin the concept of dark tourism itself, one that continues to predominantly conceptualize the death and suffering that defines the field in terms of that directly consequential to human life. This being so, dark tourism emerges as a space for compassion, empathy and the mutual recognition of both animal and human suffering as the basis for responsible behaviour and moral action (see Aaltola, 2022; García-Rosell & Hancock, 2022. By answering the call to apply dark tourism theorizing to an animal context (Fennell et al., 2021), our chapter contributes to paving the way for future research taking a non-anthropocentric perspective on dark tourism whereby future studies can focus on gaining further insights into the human-animal relations, values, feelings, and emotions whereby death is an intrinsic aspect of both the animal and tourist experience. Exploring attractions such as zoos (live animals), museums (dead animals) and so-called sports such as steeplechase racing or bullfighting (live/dead animals), taking a dark tourism perspective on animal attractions can promote an acknowledgement of such animals as sentient, suffering beings rather than simply as objects of consumption. Such recognition is needed to change the system that exploits, enslaves, and kills animals in tourism and society in general. It does so by creating opportunities for re-imagining multispecies tourism organizations and developing more sustainable spaces for humans and animals to respectfully coexist (see Coulter, 2022).

References

Aaltola, E. (2022). Empathy and inclusion: A philosophical reading of the ethics of nonhuman animals in organizations. In L. Tallberg, & L. Hamilton (Eds). *The Oxford handbook of organization studies* (pp. 331–345). Oxford: Oxford University Press.

Äijälä, M. (2021). Mobile video ethnography for evoking animals in tourism. *Annals of Tourism Research*, 89, 103203.

Äijälä, M. (2022). *Tourist landscapes as multispecies trails: Storying a mushing landscape through mobile video ethnography*. Rovaniemi: University of Lapland.

Atkinson, E. (2022). 'Yummy yum': Gordon Ramsay upsets TikTok viewers after picking lamb to eat. Independent, July. Available at, https://www.independent.co.uk/life-style/gordon-ramsay-tiktok-lamb-b2134641.html

Bertella, G. (2021). Animal-based experiences and animal experiences: Farm animals' perspective on human leisure in rural settings. *Annals of Leisure Research*, 24(5), 631–645.

Best, S. (2009). The rise of critical animal studies: Putting theory into action and animal liberation into higher education. *Journal for Critical Animal Studies*, 7(1), 9–52.

Bohanec, H., & Bohanec, C. (2013). *The Ultimate betrayal: Is there happy meat?* Bloomington: iUniverse.

Burns, G. L. (2015). Animals as tourism objects: Ethically refocusing relationships between tourists and wildlife. In K. Markwell (Ed.), *Animals and tourism* (pp. 44–59). Bristol: Channel View Publications.

Busby, G. & S. Rendle (2000). The transition from tourism on farms to farm tourism. *Tourism Management*, 21(6), 635–642.

Cassel, S. H. & K. Pettersson (2015). Performing gender and rurality in Swedish farm tourism. *Scandinavian Journal of Hospitality and Tourism*, 15(1–2), 138–151.

Clarke, C., & D. Knights (2021). Milking it for all it's worth: Unpalatable practices, dairy cows and veterinary work? *Journal of Business Ethics*, 176(4), 673–678.

Cole, M. (2011). From "animal machines" to "happy meat"? Foucault's ideas of disciplinary and pastoral power applied to 'animal-centred' welfare discourse. *Animals*, 1(1), 83–101.

Colling, S. (2018). Animal Agency, Resistance, and Escape. In A. Matsuoka & J. Sorenson (Eds.), *Critical animal studies: Towards trans-species social justice* (pp. 21–44). London: Rowman & Littlefield International.

Coulter, K. (2016). *Animals, work, and the promise of interspecies solidarity*. New York: Palgrave Macmillan.

Coulter, K. (2022). From interesting to influential: Looking forward with multispecies organization studies. In L. Tallberg & L. Hamilton (Eds.), *The Oxford handbook of animal organization studies* (pp. 18–27). Oxford: Oxford University Press.

Christien, L. (2023). Why write about animals? Organization and the Daily Occurrences of London Zoo. *Culture and Organization*, 29(4), 356–373.

Dashper, K. (2019). Moving beyond anthropocentrism in leisure research: multispecies perspectives. *Annals of Leisure Research*, 22(2), 133–139.

Derrida, J. (2008). The animal that therefore I am. New York: Fordham University Press. Edited by Marie-Louise Mallet.

Fennell, D., B. Thomsen, & S. R. Fennell (2021). Animals as Dark Tourism Attractions: A Prototype. alencia: EuropeNow, p. 45. Available online at: https://www.europenowjournal.org/2021/11/07/animals-as-dark-tourism-attractions-a-prototype/

Fennell, D. (2022). Animal-informed consent: Sled dog tours as asymmetric agential events. *Tourism Management*, 93, 104584.

Foley, M. & J. Lennon (1996). JFK and Dark tourism: A fascination with assassination. *International Journal of Heritage Studies*, 2(4), 198–211.

Frater, J. M. (1983). Farm Tourism in England: Planning, funding, promotion and some lessons from Europe. *Tourism Management*, 4(3), 167–179.

Freeman, C. P. (2009). This little piggy went to press: The American news media's construction of animals in agriculture. *The Communication Review*, 12(1), 78–103.

Fudge, E. (2008). *Pets*. New York: Routledge

García-Rosell, J. C. & P. Hancock (2022). Animals and Business Ethics. In N. Thomas (Eds.), *Animals and Business Ethics* (pp. 91–110). Cham: Palgrave Macmillan.

Giampiccoli, A., O. Mtapuri, & S. Jugmohan (2020). Community-based tourism and animals: Theorising the relationship. *Cogent Social Sciences*, 6(1), 1–11.

Gunderson, R. (2014). The first-generation Frankfurt School on the animal question: Foundations for a normative sociological animal studies. *Sociological Perspectives*, 57(3,: 285–300.

Haanpää, M., T. Salmela, J. C. García-Rosell, & M. Äijälä (2019). The disruptive 'other'? Exploring human-animal relations in tourism through videography. *Tourism Geographies*, 23(1–2), 97–117.

Hamilton, L. & D. McCabe (2016). 'It's just a job': Understanding emotion work, de-animalization and the compartmentalization of organized animal slaughter. *Organization*, 23(3), 330–350.

Hancock, P. (2008). Embodied generosity and an ethics of organization. *Organization Studies*, 29(10), 1357–1373.

Hartmann, R., J. Lennon, D. P. Reynolds., A. Rice., A. T. Rosenbaum, & Stone, P. R. (2018). The history of dark tourism. Journal of Tourism History, 10(3), 269–295.

Irvine, L. (2008). Animals and Sociology. *Sociology Compass*, 2(6), 1954–1971.

Kline, C. (2018) (Ed.). *Tourism experiences and animal consumption*. London: Routledge.

LaVeck, J. (2006) Compassion for sale? Doublethink meets doublefeel as happy meat comes of age. *Satya*, September. Available at, http://www.satyamag.com/sept06/laveck.html.

Light, D. (2017). Progress in dark tourism and thanatourism research: An uneasy relationship with heritage tourism. *Tourism Management*, 61, 276–300.

López-López, A. & G. J. Quintero Venegas (2021). Animal dark tourism: Bulls performing their own slaughter. In J. M. Rickly & C. Kline (Eds.), *Exploring non-human work in tourism: From beasts of burden to animal ambassadors* (pp. 69–82). Berlin: De Gruyter.

Markwell, K. (Ed.) (2015). *Animals and tourism*. Bristol: Channel View Publications.

Martini, A. & D. Buda (2020). Dark tourism and affect: Framing places of death and disaster. *Current Issues in Tourism*, 23(6), 679–692.

Matsuoka, A. & J. Sorenson (2018) (Eds.) *Critical animal studies: Towards trans-species social justice*. London: Rowman & Littlefield.

Mayfield, L. E., R. Bennett, R. Tranter, & M. J. Wooldridge (2007). Consumption of welfare friendly food products in Great Britain, Italy and Sweden, and how it may be influenced by consumer attitudes to, and behaviour towards, animal welfare attributes. *International Journal of Sociology of Food and Agriculture*, 15(3), 59–73.

Mkono, M. & A. Holder (2019). The future of animals in tourism recreation: Social media as spaces of collective moral reflexivity. *Tourism Management Perspectives*, 29, 1–8.

Molz, G. J. (2007). Eating difference. The cosmopolitan mobilities of culinary tourism. *Space and Culture*, 10(1), 77–93.

Nickerson, N. P., R. J. Black, & S. F. McCool (2001). Agritourism: Motivations behind Farm/Ranch Business Diversification. *Journal of Travel Research*, 40(1), 19–26

Nilsson, P. Å. (2002). Staying on Farms: An ideological background. *Annals of Tourism Research*, 29(1), 7–24.

Räsänen T. & T. Syrjämaa (2017). *Shared lives of humans and animals: Animal agency in the global north*. London: Routledge.

Renton, A. (2007). 'Happy Meat'. *The Guardian*, October 19th. Available at, https://www.theguardian.com/lifeandstyle/wordofmouth/2007/oct/19/happymeat.

Rickly, J. M. & C. Kline (Eds.) (2021). *Exploring non-human work in tourism: From beasts of burden to animal ambassadors*. Berlin: De Gruyter.

Sayre, R. & K. Henderson (2018). Farm animal and tourist interactions on Long Island's North Fork. In Kline, C. (Ed.). *Animals, Food, and Tourism* (pp. 82–95). London: Routledge.

Schneeberger, D. (2022). How can we reduce speciesism? A psychological approach to a social problem. In L. Tallberg & L. Hamilton (Eds). *The Oxford handbook of organization studies* (pp. 241–257). Oxford: Oxford University Press.

Sharma, N. (2020). Dark tourism and moral disengagement in liminal spaces. *Tourism Geographies*, 22(2), 273–297.

Sharpley, R. & A. Vass (2006). Tourism, farming and diversification: An attitudinal study. *Tourism Management*, 27(5), 1040–1052.

Stone, P. (2013). Dark tourism scholarship: A critical review. *International Journal of Culture, Tourism and Hospitality Research*, 7(3), 307–318.

Stone, P. R. (2009). Dark tourism: Morality and new moral spaces. In R. Sharpley & P. R. Stone (Eds). *The darker side of travel: The theory and practice of dark tourism* (pp. 56–72). Bristol: Channel View Publications.

Paterson, R. (2022). Heading for the farm: Why more and more people are taking working holidays. *Country Life*, August 20th. Available at, https://www.countrylife.co.uk/travel/heading-for-the-farm-why-more-and-more-people-are-taking-working-holidays-246392.

Pedersen, H. (2011). Release the moths: Critical animal studies and the posthumanist impulse. *Culture, Theory and Critique*, 52(1), 65–81.

Pedersen, H. (2022). Organizing a real that is yet to come: A critical inquiry of education in animal organization studies. In L. Tallberg & L. Hamilton (Eds). *The Oxford handbook of organization studies* (pp. 73–84). Oxford: Oxford University Press.

Phelan, C. & R. Sharpley (2011). Exploring agritourism entrepreneurship in the UK. *Tourism Planning & Development*, 8(2), 121–136.

Pullen, A. & C. Rhodes (2015). Corporeal ethics and the politics of resistance in organizations. *Organization*, 21(6), 782–796.

Tallberg, L., J. C. García-Rosell, & M. Haanpää (2022). Human–Animal Relations in Business and Society: Advancing the Feminist Interpretation of Stakeholder Theory. *Journal of Business Ethics*, 180(1), 1–16.

Tallberg, L. & P. J. Jordan (2022). Killing them 'softly' (!): Exploring work experiences in care-based animal dirty work. *Work, Employment and Society*, 36(5), 858–874.

Tallberg, L. & L, Hamilton (2022) (Eds.) *The Oxford handbook of organization studies*. Oxford: Oxford University Press.

Tarlow, P. (2005). Dark tourism: The appealing 'dark' side of tourism and more. In M. Novelli (Ed). *Niche tourism: Contemporary issues, trends and cases* (pp. 47–57). Oxford: Elsevier.

Taylor, N. & R. Twine (2014) (Eds.) *The rise of critical animal studies*. London: Routledge.

Thomas, N. (Ed.) (2022). *Animals and Business Ethics*. Cham: Palgrave Macmillan.

Tully, P. A. G. & N. Carr (2021). Farm animals' participation in tourism experiences: A time for proper respect. In J. M. Rickly & C. Kline (Eds.), *Exploring non-human work in tourism: From beasts of burden to animal ambassadors* (pp. 83–100). Berlin: De Gruyter.

Vinding, M. (2014). *Why "Happy Meat" is always wrong*. Scotts Valley: CreateSpace.

Weitzenfeld, A. & M. Joy (2014). An overview of anthropocentrism, humanism, and speciesism in critical animal theory. In A. J. Nocella III, J. Sorenson, K. Socha, & A. Matsuka (Eds), *Defining critical animal studies: An intersectional social justice approach for liberation* (pp. 3–27). New York: Peter Lang

Part III: **Dark tourism and critical memory studies**

Alexis Whitacre

6 Trading paradise for Palestine: Dark tourism to refugee camps in the West Bank

Abstract: In the West Bank, conflict tourism is aided by the proliferation of new media and has become a phenomenon used by Palestinians to invite foreign tourists to actively produce media that constructs or relays particular views about the nature of the occupation of the Palestinian Territories and its effects on life in Palestinian refugee camps. Drawing from disciplines like new media, tourism studies, and conflict studies, this chapter analyzes what compels tourists to visit non-traditional sites like the refugee camp and examines how camp tourists use social media to engage with the traumascape of the camp and represent the Palestine-Israel conflict. Foregrounding camp inhabitants' agency in promoting the camp as a tourist destination, the chapter highlights the complexity of camp tourism and its digital representation and questions whether tourist intervention constitutes exploitation or advocacy. The chapter notes why tourists are encouraged to digitally document camp reality and how tourists' social media representations of the camp help shape perceptions of the complex and enduring Palestinian/Israeli conflict. It also highlights the perceived effects of tourism and new media on local host communities from Palestinian refugees' points of view.

Keywords: dark tourism, spectacle, suffering, authenticity, refugee camp

Introduction

In Palestine, media has become an integral aspect of tourism, as it has around the world. Modern tourists take photographs with smart phones and upload videos to Instagram as proof of having been 'elsewhere' (Nunkoo, Gursoy, & Dwivedi, 2020; Munar & Jacobsen, 2014). Media use by tourists in the West Bank follows such trends as digitally capturing staged performances and posting posed photos of exotic vacations to build social capital (Haldrup & Larsen, 2003; Munar & Jacobsen, 2014). However, media and tourism are complicated by the occupying forces and the increasing trend towards conflict tourism. Whereas tourists in Europe might take a photograph in front of a castle or on a beach, tourists in Bethlehem stand at the entrance to Aida Refugee Camp. Indeed, tours of refugee camps are heavily advertised in Palestine and tourists from around the world can find websites boasting refugee camp tours in Jerusalem, Bethlehem, and Hebron. Local hotels advertise so-called 'alternative' tours of the refugee camp, and tourists often roam the camps documenting for social media their interpretations of the Palestinian-Israeli conflict.

https://doi.org/10.1515/9783110792072-007

The Palestinian movement has become relatively successful by its cooptation of cyberspace. In the transnational dissemination of virtual traumascapes, virtual tourists are invited into the refugee camp, distant spectators of the suffering within. The online campaign has worked so well that new dark tourists – in this case, refugee camp tourists – are seeking out the physical traumascapes of Palestinian refugee camps. These camps have become vacation destinations, and like any vacationing tourist, those in the West Bank document their travels through media. This intervention bolsters the Palestinian national movement, and, as media representations influence perceptions of tourist destinations, tourists' re-presentations of the camps on social media may influence perceptions of the conflict (Kelly 2016; Kelly, 2023; Lund, Cohen, & Scarles, 2018; Stein, 2008; Tham, Mair, & Croy, 2020; Zeitzoff, 2017). How do tourists, and by extension, those in their mediated networks, come to understand and represent conflict and for what purposes? As there is no universal tourist experience, there is a need for more contextualized analyses that incorporate the role of media in tourist imaginaries of the Palestine-Israel conflict and the undeniable role of tourists in media production on tour. The use of new, mobile media, like smartphones and social media, inform tourists' perceptions of Palestine as tourists mobilize and transform conflict space by using mediated systems of representation.

A result of six cumulative months of fieldwork in the West Bank, this chapter explores the social construction of refugee suffering as a form of 'authenticity' for tourists and examines the role social media plays in mediating suffering during political conflict (Isaac, 2010). I examine refugee camp tourism as a form of dark tourism and ask how the human suffering of the camps became a spectacle for the consumption of foreign tourists (Bloch, 2011; Martini & Buda, 2018; Bowman & Pezzullo, 2010). The rise of dark tourism to Palestinian refugee camps has prompted some Palestinians to take advantage and utilize tourism as an activist tool designed to promote solidarity. This kind of alternative tourism explicitly promotes sites of violence that authenticate Palestinian narratives of suffering, which are then transmitted by tourists on social media platforms (Kelly, 2016). Given the success of past social media movements in promoting awareness, social media may also be capable of altering political and social perceptions of the refugee camp (Shirky, 2011).

The success of any media campaign depends on credibility, narrative, and aesthetics. Palestinians have long been stereotyped as uncredible sources and, as a result, their media is sometimes discredited, accused of being biased or doctored (Kuntsman & Stein, 2015; Stein, 2021). Furthermore, censorship, precarity, unpredictability in day-to-day life, power disparities, and lack of political allies are constraining to successful media activism for many Palestinians (Peteet, 2017; Hammami, 2016; Kelly, 2016). Because of this, they have had varying success in advocating for themselves on a global, mediated stage. Conversely, tourists are generally less restricted; they can access spaces barred to Palestinians, document infrastructure of the occupation with relatively little hassle, and more easily access online networks (Bianchi, Stephenson, & Hannam, 2020). By illuminating the complexities of the occupation and demanding international attention, refugee camp tours connect international actors and educate through personal experience on tour.

The politics of pity and the spectacle of suffering

Human suffering-as-spectacle is transmitted to spectators through media and the narrative of suffering elicits an emotional response from viewers (Boltanski, 1999). The suffering of a distant 'Other' is primarily mediated, seen through mediums like television news, documentaries, and photographs (Boltanski, 1999). This mediation creates a spectacle of the suffering, inviting the spectator not just to witness the suffering, but to *gawk* at it.

Eliciting affect from spectators is paramount to the success of the spectacle of suffering (Boltanski, 1999; Chouliaraki, 2006). Pity is a particularly desirable response to witnessing suffering because pity induces action, namely publicly speaking out against the suffering (Boltanski, 1999). However, only suffering that is perceived as undeserved is pitiable, and therefore actionable (Boltanski, 1999). Thus, a 'politics of pity' emerges through the mediated spectacle of suffering (Boltanski, 1999). Spectating audiences are morally obligated to involve themselves socially and politically in the suffering by speaking out about what they witnessed and how they felt watching the spectacle of suffering (Chouliaraki, 2006). With the potential to be a "catalyst for change," the mediated spectacle of suffering is capable of creating a shared sense of responsibility for the distant, suffering 'Other' (Norman, 2009, 252). This cosmopolitanism necessitates meaningful action to relieve suffering, often in the form of publicly speaking out against injustice (Chouliaraki, 2006). Eliciting affect, even when feelings are negative, is crucial to prompt desirable action in response to witnessing a spectacle. As one camp resident informed me, "Feeling sad is a good start. But it doesn't mean anything unless it comes with some kind of action" (interview with author, September 17, 2022, Aida Camp, Bethlehem).

There are two major disadvantages when mediating the spectacle of suffering. Primarily, appropriate actionable responses take place when suffering is made relatable to spectators (Chouliaraki, 2006). The politics of pity is most effective when spectators feel an affinity for the sufferer, and this relatability is best accomplished by establishing at least a perception of proximity (Chouliaraki, 2006). Spectators are inundated with images of suffering, each competing for attention and corresponding action. Because of this saturation of suffering in media, audiences cannot be sure that media portrayals of suffering are *authentic*, yet authenticity is crucial to eliciting pity and encouraging action (Chouliaraki, 2006).

Secondarily, mediation reduces the victims of suffering to 'speechless emissaries' – objects of 'the gaze' (Malkki, 1996; Urry, 1990). Media provides the contact that is necessary for the visibility of suffering and subsequent pity, but the spectacle of suffering manifests a one-way 'gaze' that reproduces the passivity of the victims and the agency of the spectators. Through the media gaze, the spectator objectifies the subject of the medium and, due to this objectification, has no responsibility towards the sufferer (Manlove, 2007; Urry & Larson, 2011). The sufferer-as-object is reduced to nothing more than his suffering through the gaze.

Traumascapes

Bodies in pain resist representation, particularly representation through language (Scarry, 1985). When pain is felt, language cannot accurately articulate the presence of pain. The person in pain is rendered unable to articulate his pain, necessitating the witnessing of the pain by another (Scarry, 1985). Indeed,

> Because the person in pain is ordinarily so bereft of the resources of speech, it is not surprising that the language for pain should sometimes be brought into being by those who are not themselves in pain but who speak on behalf of those who are (Scarry, 1985, p. 6).

However, hearing of pain through an intermediary causes a dilemma: the witness to pain might overstate or understate the severity of the pain because she herself is not experiencing it (Scarry, 1985). Pain's witness is necessary to articulate the existence of pain, but the extent of the pain cannot be known through this proxy. Even through an intermediary, pain cannot be adequately articulated or even authenticated.

However, there are "avenues by which this most radically private of experiences begins to enter the realm of public discourse" (Scarry, 1985, p. 6). Here, the mediation of pain and trauma becomes crucial. Mass media provides the means by which to witness and articulate pain, to store and transmit trauma. Narratives of pain, suffering, and trauma are transformed into testimony through impartial mediums: photography, television, video, etc. (Pinchevski, 2019). Trauma cannot be represented through language, but a picture speaks a thousand words; images articulate and verify the presence of pain and to form a collective consciousness and memory around certain traumatic events. Pain is largely inarticulable, but it is rendered more representable through its mediation, creating a 'traumatography,' a map or authentic representation that both registers and recollects trauma (Pinchevski, 2019). In this way, "[m]edia bear witness to the human failure to bear witness" (Pinchevski, 2019, p. 4).

Culture informs our understanding of trauma. In Western culture, trauma "has become a mark of suffering" that must be diagnosed and treated, and these affirm the authenticity of the suffering (Pupavac, 2008, p. 227). Yet the language used to describe trauma is itself insufficient; trauma itself cannot exist without (mediated) representation. Media technologies are critical for narrating suffering. Virtual traumascapes employ modern media technologies like Internet websites, online photo galleries, and digital tours to broadcast tragedies. These traumascapes attempt to "communicate raw experience[s]" of suffering to widespread audiences (Fassin & Rechtman, 2009, p. 201).

Virtual traumascapes, by virtue of their digital nature, *travel*. The proliferation of virtual traumascapes in the digital age has contributed to increased fascination with atrocity, suffering, and death (Gilbert, 2018; Kaelber, 2007). Virtual traumascapes portray dark sites with traumatic histories and this mediation of suffering is not just newsworthy, but entertaining. The problem, though, is that the trauma presented in virtual traumascapes "can neither be relived nor be vicariously experienced but only encountered in its mediated and imagined forms" (Kaelber, 2007, p. 30).

Humans have always been interested in dark sites, and traveling to places where a disaster occurred is a long tradition (Gilbert, 2018; Kaelber, 2007). But modern technology further piques the curiosity of would-be thanatourists, transforming virtual tourists into physical tourists. For example, the Netflix series *Dark Tourist* documents the most "bizarre, grotesque, and disturbing places in the world," highlighting 'off limits' or dangerous places and portraying them as fun and interesting vacation destinations (Gilbert, 2018, n.p.). Tours of radioactive wastelands and immersive re-enactments of migrants crossing the border into the United States are changing dark tourism practices. The perennial obsession with dark sites has evolved to include not only sites of temporally distant violence but also those of violence acting upon *living* bodies – bodies that suffer. Dark tourists seek to gain proximity to present-day trauma and suffering, but *why*?

Authenticity in tourism

Tourism is perhaps most famously, and controversially, conceptualized as a quest for authenticity (MacCannell, 1976). In an age of hyperreal simulations, modern subjects feel anxious and alienated by the monotony of everyday existence, prompting them to seek true authenticity elsewhere (Eco, 1986; MacCannell, 1976; Rickly-Boyd, 2013; Shepherd, 2015; Xue, Manuel-Navarrete, & Buzinde, 2014). As inauthenticity is a consequence of modernity, authenticity is "thought to be [found] in other historical periods and other cultures, in purer, simpler lifestyles" heretofore untouched by modernization (MacCannell, 1976, p. 3). However, in reality, authenticity is a fantasy and subjects-as-tourists are doomed to search for it endlessly (Knudsen, Rickly, & Vidon, 2016).

Tourist sites are often layered, so it is difficult to categorize any site as entirely authentic or inauthentic. Moreover, authenticity can have many meanings; authenticity can refer to the site itself, the informational content of the site, the artefacts at the site, or tourists' experiences at the site (Rickly-Boyd, 2009; Steiner & Reisinger, 2006; Wang, 1999). Oftentimes, 'absolute authenticity' is less important to tourists than the experiential authenticity established through meaning-making, interpretation, and identity formation at a site (Rickly-Boyd, 2009, p. 8). Essentially, authenticity is socially constructed, and different individuals will define and perceive authenticity differently (Penrose, 2018; Rickly-Boyd, 2009). However, authenticity in some form matters to most travelers, who "value, and are moved by, things and experiences that they believe to be 'real'" (Penrose, 2018, p. 5).

In response to modernity's growing tendency toward simulation, and tourists' heightened awareness of the *in*authenticity of sites, 'post-tourism' has become a new trend wherein authenticity-seekers aim to find non-traditional sites 'off the beaten track' and away from masses of conventional tourists. Post-tourists seek authenticity in their interactions with the 'Other,' rather than in the objective authenticity of a site or an artifact. However, with the acceleration of tourism worldwide, the global tourism industry is prone to marketing and commodifying 'authenticity'; tourists' expectations fuel staged performances designed to make the host destination seem credibly authentic (Edensor, 2000; MacCannell, 1976; Noy, 2004). This, however, prompts tourists to search for the site's 'back stage,' which hosts the *real* performances of truly authentic local life and culture (MacCannell, 1976). Yet as more and more tourists flood the backstage, it is transformed into a 'front stage,' prompting tourists to seek more and more exotic, adventurous, and dangerous sites, like a refugee camp.

To date, most scholarship on dark tourism focuses on sites specifically and uniquely associated with suffering, grief, and death (Martini & Buda, 2018; Seaton, 1990; Sharma & Rickly, 2019; Stone, 2006; Stone, 2012). Palestinian refugee camps, in contrast, are living sites wherein incoming tourists can interact with locals and witness the ongoing violence of the conflict and occupation in person. Tourism to conflict zones like the West Bank contributes to a kind of risk tourism, wherein visitors seek real or simulated physical danger in order to 'feel more alive' (Cater, 2006; Lisle, 2000). Today, many tourists participate in tours that explicitly advertise more violent sites – in Palestine, typically those that emphasize the occupation (Isaac, 2010). Political conflict, then, can be conceptualized as a form of authenticity and refugee camp tourism is emblematic of the recent trend in dark tourism to favor sites of tangible suffering in a contemporary traumascape, like an active conflict-zone.

A site's authenticity, whether objective,[1] constructed,[2] or existential,[3] allows tourists to engage more fully with the site (Rickly-Boyd, 2012). Like any tourist site, the Palestinian refugee camp must be credible, or tourists can question its authenticity and limit their engagement with the site (Rickly, 2009). Social processes and performances authenticate the site as "'original', 'genuine', 'real' or 'trustworthy'" (Penrose, 2018, p. 6). Seen up close and in real-time, the suffering of refugees in the camp is authentic because, in some ways, it 'speaks for itself'. The 'cool authentication' of the camp is "declarative" and "based on [explicit] proof" (Cohen & Cohen, 2012, 1300). Physical evidence – bullet holes, tear gas canisters, UN intervention – abounds in the

1 Genuine, original sites or artifacts (Rickly-Boyd, 2012).

2 Commodified authenticity that fits tourist demand; socially constructed or symbolic authenticity (Heuermann & Chhabra, 2014).

3 Subjective authenticity that arises from emotions felt by the individual on tour; these emotions resulting from on-site experiences are felt to be authentic (Wang, 1999).

camp; these material objects imply the presence of suffering and they exist independent of visitors (Cohen & Cohen, 2012). The effectiveness of the refugee camp's 'cool' authentication "depends on the credibility of the authenticating authority" – the refugees who live there (see Cohen & Cohen, 2012, 1300–1301). 'Hot' authentication is activated and enacted by tourists, themselves, as they engage with and respond to the site and its narratives (see Cohen & Cohen, 2012).

Experiential authenticity

Unlike other refugee camps, Aida is unguarded and open access, and hundreds of tourists flock daily to the camp explicitly for guided tours. Despite being heavily advertised, camp tours do not draw the same kind of suspicion of alteration or inauthenticity as other commodified tourism sites. Indeed, it seems that physical suffering witnessed in the refugee camp is more authentic precisely because it is less advertised, less mediated – a true 'backstage.' Whereas suffering as seen on television can be interpreted as being scripted, the suffering of refugees in the camp cannot be ignored by tourists who occupy the same space. Real refugees act as tour guides, invite tourists into their homes, cook them meals, and even let them stay overnight. Temporal and geographic proximity contributes to feelings of authenticity on-site, as tourists feel like they are living, however briefly, as an actual refugee lives. One tourist from Italy asserted that "the most authentic experience was the visit to Aida camp, because it's the most direct contact that you have with the condition of the Palestinian people living under occupation" (interview with author, September 30, 2022, Aida Camp, Bethlehem).

Camp tourism seeks to incorporate the tourist, as much as possible, into the camp through experiential learning. Mohammed, who lives in Aida Camp, told me, "If you [as a tourist] stay here and live in the camp, you will understand what happens here. You will experience the reality" (interview with author, October 2, 2022, Aida Camp). Many Palestinian refugees believe that it is only by living through the experience that the tourist can truly understand the gravity of the situation on the ground in Palestine. This is perhaps why tourists rent out Airbnb apartments in the camp and tout overnight stays as truly authentic experiences. In visiting the refugee camp, the tourist seeks a kind of 'experiential authenticity,' found in the authentic experiences of others (Cohen, 1979). Experiential tourists, having lost a sense of authenticity in their own daily lives, seek authenticity in the lives of others (Cohen, 1979). For some experiential tourists, the refugee camp is a material manifestation of human suffering and trauma, the epitome of authenticity. In the camp, the search for authenticity is satisfied through embodied engagement and participation in the life of the 'Other' – the Palestinian refugee. Experiential authenticity – the sensations associated or the belief that one is "experiencing something genuine or real" – emphasizes and engages the tourist's senses, or bodily experiences at a site (Penrose, 2018, p. 20). These, in turn, certify a site's reality, its *authenticity*.

Activities like cooking classes, intensive Arabic language lessons, and stays with host families embed tourists in the camp, authenticating camp life. The experimental tourist understands that the suffering and trauma of the refugees are not her own, but the spectacle of suffering is confronted in the camp, sensorily, and experientially (Cohen, 1979). Tourists can touch bullet holes in the walls of houses; they can see surrounding watchtowers, can smell tear gas in the air. As one camp resident noted, "We don't need to lie about the reality of the occupation. You can see it when you come here" (interview by author, September 17, 2022, Aida Camp). Tourists' sensory experiences of the camp – tasting, seeing, touching, smelling – lend credence to the Palestinian claims of suffering and trauma.

Tourists' expectations shape their experiences of a site (Belhassen & Caton, 2006). For some dark tourists, suffering is attractive and satisfying, a morbid form of entertainment (Ashworth & Hartmann, 2005). The representation of suffering in the camp is expected; suffering is considered an authentic marker of 'refugee-ness.' Palestinian tour guides understand that suffering is expected, so it is highlighted for tourists on guided tours. Suffering's emphasis in the camp is a strategic move, as more overt spectacles of suffering engage tourists in a politics of pity. Tourists might be more likely to feel pity and to speak out when suffering appears authentic, and for tourists who are used to seeing mediated spectacles of suffering, more extreme and explicit forms of suffering may be considered more authentic. A group of long-term volunteer tourists staying with host families in Aida camp mentioned that some members of their host families had been arrested and some of their homes targeted in night raids; a few of these tourists had attended funerals for refugees who had been killed in the camp. Several of them had been exposed to tear gas. In these cases, the violence witnessed (or experienced) by tourists matched the narratives of suffering heard on guided tours and contributed to perceptions of the site's authenticity.

In other cases, when expectations of the camp did not match reality – many tourists, for instance, wrongly assume that the refugee camp is constructed of tents (see Kelly, 2023) – the information and knowledge gained from an experience was deemed to be authentic, or at least authentic *enough*. Lina, a young woman from the Netherlands who declared she did not know much of the conflict before visiting, said, "I decided to come to Palestine to try to learn a bit more about it. I came to the camp because I think it's the best place to learn about the conflict from the Palestinian point of view" (interview with author, July 1, 2019, Aida Camp). A pair of college students from Italy who visited several refugee camps in the West Bank noted that their experiences of authenticity, too, were shaped by the knowledge gained on tour. One of these students noted:

> We had a good guide who . . . took us all around the camp explaining a lot of things and we also visited this center [a non-profit organization in the camp] with a lot of information. We've learned a lot (interview with author, September 20, 2022, Al-Arroub Camp).

His friend concurred, adding that the pair had come to the camp to hear the presumably more authentic narratives of Palestinians through personal testimony and first-hand accounts from camp inhabitants.

Narrative framing: A modern battlefield media and tourism in the West Bank

Tourism heavily influences the state's nation-building practices and is used to reify national myths and claims to the land (Abu El-Haj, 2001; Knudsen, Rickly-Boyd, & Greer, 2014; Stein, 2008). For this reason, tourism is a crucial tool in promoting national ideologies and political agendas, particularly in Palestine, which is largely unrecognized as a sovereign state (Cohen-Hattab, 2004; Noy, 2012; Stein, 2002; Yang, 2020). Through tourism, signs and symbols of cultural and historical continuity are established and taught to tourists, who reinforce these narratives (Abu El-Haj, 2001). In this way, tourism is used as a political weapon and as a 'politics of representation' in the ongoing Israeli-Palestinian conflict (Peteet, 2005).

The modern conflict is increasingly being fought as a narrative war between Palestine and Israel and each nation uses its respective tourism industries to advance national narratives. The occupation of Palestine is characterized both by physical violence and by 'digital occupation,' in that technology is increasingly used in conjunction with physical barriers to enclose Palestinians (Tawil-Souri, 2012). In the West Bank, slow internet speeds, lack of communications infrastructure, and censorship are common as new media[4] is used to reinforce the occupation (Tawil-Souri, 2013). However, Palestinians subvert the limits placed on them by certain digital technologies by engaging tourists in a digital representation of the conflict while on tour.

Today, the Palestine-Israel conflict is multimodal, both a physical war and a battle for narrative framing and national legitimacy (Said, 1979). The proliferation of media in tourism industries further contributes to the politicization of the tourist industry and in the West Bank, tourism and media engagement act as forms of modern 'warfare.' Ahmed, a filmmaker, reporter, and resident of Aida Camp told me, "The media is one of our tools [of resistance] and we need to use it" (interview with author, July 8, 2019, Aida Camp). Media has become the primary tool used to create spaces of resistance wherein Palestinians are fighting for the right to define themselves and their struggle through media and are seeking to gain sympathy from global audiences

4 That which can be produced and disseminated digitally.

through the mediatized representation of their suffering. Tourists in the refugee camp document for social media their own interpretations of the Palestinian-Israeli conflict, though many of these narratives have been carefully curated by Palestinian tour guides (Cohen-Hattab, 2004; Brin & Noy, 2010). New, mobile media[5] has become a new-age battlefield and tourists are increasingly used as combatants.

Tourism and media contribute to the national intelligibility of Palestine, and each establishes a network of connections that shape spaces and social processes in the West Bank (Stein, 2008). New media allow tourists and hosts to interact with and make sense of the camp in new ways as social media posts juxtapose physical sites with their own representation. In this way, new media is not separate from the refugee camp but is rather embedded in the interactive encounters, place-making experiences, and narrative storytelling of the camp, and therefore, of the conflict. Palestinians use new media technology to advertise tours and to encourage interactive tourist engagement. Tourism to Aida Camp, surrounded by the Separation Wall, offers tourists an enticing alternative to more mainstream attractions promoted by mass tourism (Isaac, 2009). Such alternative tours critically engage with the politics and violence of the occupation whereas mainstream tours obfuscate the political nature of sites like the camp and the wall (Yang, 2019).

Social media and tourism

Social media broadens the capacity for transnational social participation, as it broadcasts events that might not otherwise receive notable attention (Castells, 2008). Movements like the Arab Spring and the Black Lives Matter movement were mobilized largely through social media and existed in public consciousness because they were mediated. The Palestinian national movement is similarly mediated. Much of the publicity on Palestine comes from social media posts, though not always from Palestinians themselves. Palestinians have learned to utilize transnational networks in unexpected ways in order to gain support (Toenjes, 2014). The Separation Wall, for instance, functions as a global message board that advertises tours and encourages engagement (Larkin, 2014). Tourists' images and discussions of the Separation Wall are promoted on social media, and Palestinian campaigns encourage digital interaction with the messages on the wall. One collaborative initiative used the hashtag #SendMeAMessage and allowed anyone anywhere in the world to virtually post a message on the wall (Larkin, 2014). Social media is crucial to these campaigns because users from around the world utilize these platforms to engage with Palestinians and learn about the conflict, and facilitate dialogue about the occupation (Abu Zayyad, 2015).

5 Media that moves or is able to be transported.

The digital solidarity network expands when travelers in Palestine post accounts of their vacations (Toenjes, 2014). Photographing or filming destinations has long been a ritual practiced by traditional tourists but mobile devices, like cell phones, and social media advertises vacations immediately, on-site. Tourists in the refugee camp can instantly upload a picture of the camp while being guided through the camp. In this way, modern tourists exist and perform in both a corporeal and mediated tourist landscape and for many tourists, maintaining a constant presence in this hybrid – physical and digital – space is a crucial aspect of traveling (Hannam, Butler, & Paris, 2014).

Tourists' use of new media while on tour in the camp is transforming the narrative storytelling of the conflict. The images captured and posted of the sights (and sites) seen on tour are linked through the activities of the tourist, creating a "'proprioception,' an active, embodied engagement" with the camp (Crang, 1997, p. 365). The experiences of the camp's traumascape are broadcasted on social media, reifying a virtual traumascape that allows virtual tourists to experience the camp through its media representation. The conventional boundaries of tourism and the traditional roles of tourists are modified by social media intervention on tour (Hannam, Butler, & Paris, 2014). As tourists engage physically in the camp, they and their peers simultaneously engage digitally with the camp, through comments, re-shares, and 'likes.' Through this engagement, digital citizens become virtual tourists in the camp and physical tourists contribute to the virtual proliferation of the camp-as-traumascape.

Social media as a tool for activism and storytelling

Palestinian media and tourist media re-reproductions redefine the media landscape and how conflict is broadcast on the ground by amateur media content creators – tourists. Tourists are actively invited to produce media that constructs or relays particular arguments about the nature of the occupation, narratives of nation-building, and political legitimacy. For instance, tourists are encouraged to take selfies in front of the Separation Wall, record encounters in the refugee camp, and blog about their exotic vacations.

These new forms of media activity by tourists are both exploitative and advocative, and they can contribute either to activism or normalization of the conflict. On one hand, the act of photographing or recording may implicitly or explicitly "encourag[e] what is going on to keep on happening" by normalizing it or becoming desensitized to it (Sontag, 1977, p. 11–12). On the other hand, social media platforms give voice to marginalized populations barred from other social spaces. However, censorship, lack of communications infrastructure, and barriers to free speech make it difficult for Palestinians to meaningfully engage on social media. Tourists, though, are afforded comparatively greater physical and digital mobility in the West Bank than Palestinians. This necessitates the utilization of tourists' physical and digital mobility by Palestinians by using tourists' media messages to promote Palestinian narratives that travel.

Palestinian alternative tours encourage tourists to document certain sites; indeed, "tourists feel compelled to photograph what has already been introduced, or projected" (Bell, 2013, p. 162). However, as social media use increases, alternative perceptions of place are formulated and disseminated (Bell, 2013). Representation of the camp, through physical tours and through complementary media, informs discourse surrounding the camp, the occupation, and the conflict. Tourists, in effect, authenticate the suffering in the camps by their media dissemination of it. Social media posts are intentionally public-facing and by posting content on social media, tourists frame and interpret events for their followers (Scarles, 2009). In this way, tourists become "players in the game of directed viewing" (Crang, 1997, 370). A college-aged Spanish tourist articulated this, noting, "I just want to document the reality here" (personal communication, September 19, 2022, South Hebron Hills). When asked why he thought it so crucial to film and publish video documentation of the camp, he responded, "I want to challenge the narrative. Palestinians are demonized in Western media. I want to capture the normal life here and talk about Palestinian resilience" (personal communication, September 19, 2022, South Hebron Hills).

Crucially though, tourists' interpretation and documentation of the camp is guided and encouraged by Palestinian refugees themselves. Tourists are guided through the camp by Palestinian guides who point out or stop at noteworthy places. On one private tour, for instance, a sign was posted next to the Separation Wall commanding passing tourists to "Paint the Wall! It's 'not' legal" (guided tour, June 22, 2019, Bethlehem, Palestine) (See Figure 6.1). On a tour with Green Olive Tours, our guide showed us an original Banksy piece and encouraged each member of the group to mimic the stance of the graffitied man in the portrait and pose for a picture. Many tourists comply, taking photographs, uploading them to platforms like Instagram, and reiterating the stories told by their Palestinian tour guides. In this reproduction, tourists follow a prescribed script given to them and, in doing so, ensure that Palestinian stories are publicly repeated in digital tourist circuits (Toxey, 2010). Through media representation, the camp "becomes part of a fluid representational stock of images and experiences that circulate," contributing to collective knowledge about and perceptions of the camp (Jones & Sanyal, 2015, p. 433). Tourists themselves effectively authenticate the Palestinian refugee camp by publicly acknowledging and legitimizing it (Toxey, 2010).

Tourists in Palestine become witnesses to the occupation, and their media content becomes, to an extent, unofficial media coverage of the conflict. Social media is used in the West Bank as an effective tool to critically engage with Palestinian spaces and the politics that established and maintained those spaces. Because Palestinians are outsourcing media production to tourists, tourists have become both consumers and producers of Palestinian national narratives. Palestinians are proving that even despite intense limitations, the suffering of Palestinian refugees is mediated, and this spectacle of suffering can be disseminated in hopes of transforming a space of suffering into a site of resistance. The influx of tourists to spaces like the refugee camp has the potential to radically alter the spectacle of suffering and the politics of pity. Through tourism, tourists can become spectators of suffering where pity can be activated *on the ground* and truth about the camp can be disseminated digitally. And Palestinian refugees are appealing to tourists' sentimentality on tour by incorporating the tourist, as much as possible, into the camp.

The affective storytelling nature of virtual traumascapes is transformed when the witnessed suffering is no longer distant. Now, tourists do not simply passively witness suffering as portrayed through media, but they take part in the documentation of trauma itself. Tourists document their vacations through photography and videography, which provide new, direct opportunities to record and transmit the spectacle of suffering. Therefore, media is capable of redefining tourism in certain spaces as it broadens the confines of traditional tourism in that it allows local tourism sites to be broadcasted globally, transforming the media landscape, and offering new avenues for education, activism, and resistance.

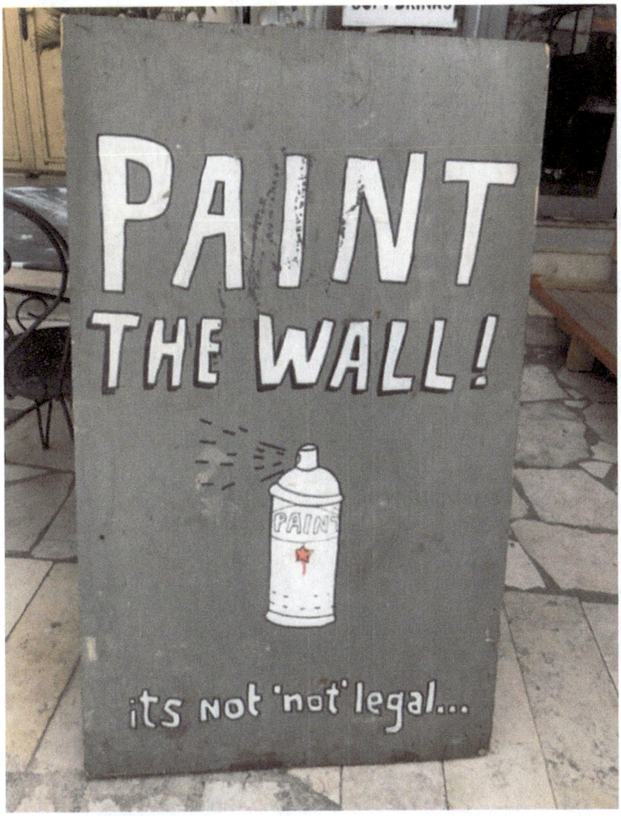

Figure 6.1: A sign outside a shop near the Separation Wall in Bethlehem encouraging tourists to 'paint the wall.' (Source: author).

In the Palestinian refugee camp, media is used both to encourage interaction with the conflict and to disseminate a narrative about the site. Social media posts about the camp enhance the legitimacy of Palestinian testimony, which is always in question (Stein, 2021). Tourists in Palestine become witnesses to the occupation; this witnessing is much more personalized and urgent as tourists meet with Palestinians face-to-face. Palestinians are no longer 'distant others' who can be ignored and tourists' media content becomes, to an extent, unofficial media coverage of the conflict. Tourists' media documentation of the camp accentuates its visibility and produces alternative tourist imaginaries of Palestine.

Conclusion

In their eternal search for some form of authenticity, more and more tourists are seeking out sensational sites for vacation (See Figure 6.2). Tourists are attracted to real-life spectacles of suffering in the camp, which are perceived by tourists and promoted by Palestinians as being truly authentic. "We [Palestinians] want only to show the reality, the truth" of the camp, as one inhabitant disclosed (interview with author,

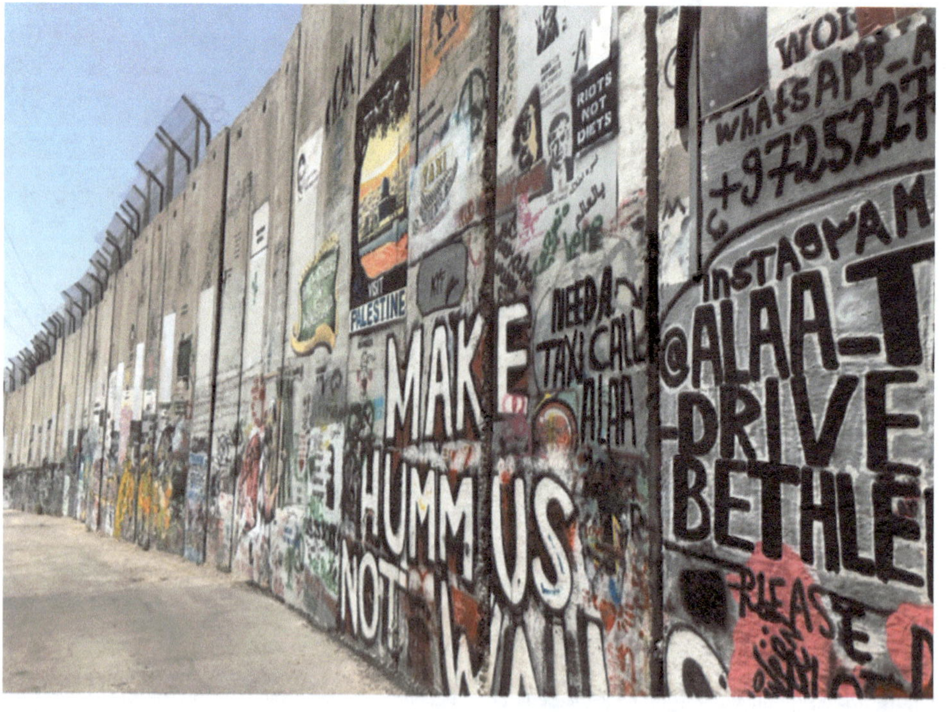
VISIT PALESTINE
RIOTS NOT DIETS
MAKE HUMMUS NOT
NEED A TAXI CALL ALAA
WhatsApp
INSTAGRAM
DRIVE
PLEASE

Figure 6.2: A portion of the Separation Wall in Bethlehem, Palestine. (Source: author).

October 1, 2022, Aida Camp). Refugee camp tours explicitly promote sites of violence that authenticate Palestinian narratives of suffering and tourists' experiences of the camp contribute to the truth of its authenticity (Kelly, 2016).

Dark tourism is critiqued as being a self-absorbed, selfish enterprise wherein tourists appropriate spaces of suffering to witness spectacles for their own morbid pleasure (Korstanje & George, 2017). The 'spectacle of suffering' has always been symptomatic of dark sites, but recently has been appropriated by Palestinians to elicit affect from incoming tourists in the hope that they will carry Palestinian narratives home with them. Tourists are actively invited to produce media that construct or relay particular arguments about the nature of the camp and the authenticity of the suffering therein. Tourists' documentation of the camp creates a virtual traumascape that mirrors the physical and this tourist-made traumatography is seen as impartial, and therefore credible. Perhaps this is why Palestinians have sought to outsource media production to tourists (See Figure 6.3).

The most effective narratives *about* the camp are those informed by experience *in* the camp, the perceived authenticity of which is influenced by experiences had,

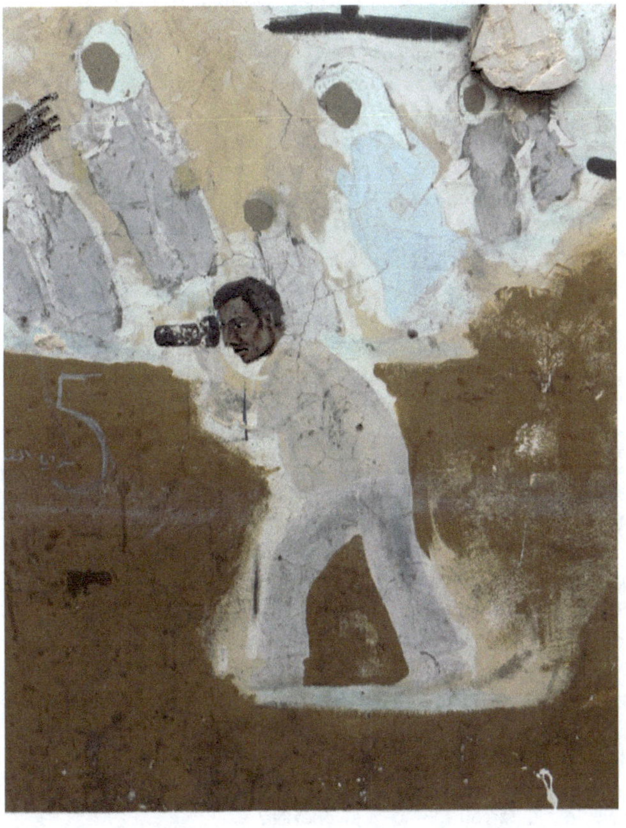

Figure 6.3: A painting of a man holding a camera in Aida camp. (Source: author).

testimony heard, and emotions felt on tour. Unlike in mediated spectacles of suffering – which reduces photographic subjects to objects of the (virtual) tourist gaze and where the objective is (merely) to speak out against suffering – camp tourism allows tourists to engage in concrete action to alleviate suffering through its mediation. Indeed, "[t]he camera is a tool that encourages and even requires active performances", which help to restore some agency to the Palestinians who frame the camp for tourists (Stylianou-Lambert, 2012, p. 1821–1822). Miriam, an Aida Camp resident, informed me, "We [Palestinians] like tourists. They have cameras" (interview with author, October 23, 2022, Aida Camp).

References

Abu El-Haj, N. (2001). *Facts on the Ground: Archaeological Practice and Territorial Self-Fashioning in Israeli Society*. Chicago, Illinois: University of Chicago Press.

Abu Zayyad, Z.K. (2015). Freedom of Expression and Social Media in Palestine. *Palestine-Israel Journal, 21*(5).

Ashworth, G., & Hartmann, R. (2005). Introduction: Managing Atrocity for Tourism. In Ashworth, G. & Hartmann, R. (EdS.) *Horror and Human Tragedy Revisited: The Management of Sites of Atrocities for Tourism* (pp. 1–14). Cognizant Communication Corporation.

Belhassen, Y. & K. Caton. (2006). Authenticity Matters. *Annals of Tourism Research, 33*, 853–856.

Bell, K. (2013). A Comparative Analysis of the Projected and Perceived Images of Gloucester. In J.A. Lester & C. Scarles (Ed.) *Mediating the Tourist Experience: From Brochures to Virtual Encounters*. Ashgate Publishing, Ltd.

Bianchi, R.V., Stephenson, M.L., & Hannam, K. (2020). The contradictory politics of the right to travel: mobilities, borders & tourism. *Mobilities, 15*(2), 290–306.

Bloch, N. (2011). Refugee camp as a tourist attraction: Who and why re(dis)covers Tibetan diaspora? *Ethnografia Polska, 55*, 51–69.

Boltanski, L. (1999). *Distant Suffering: Morality, Media, and Politics* G.D. Burchell (Trans.). Cambridge University Press.

Bowman, M.S., & Pezzullo, P.C. (2010). What's so 'Dark' about 'Dark Tourism'?:Death, Tours, and Performance. *Tourist Studies, 9*, 187–202.

Brin, E., & Noy, C. (2010). The said and the unsaid: Performative guiding in a Jerusalem neighbourhood. *Tourist Studies, 10*, 19–33.

Castells, M. (2008). The New Public Sphere: Global Civil Society, Communication Networks, and Global Governance. *The Annals of the American Academy of Political and Social Science, 616*, 78–93.

Cater, C. (2006). Playing with risk? Participant perceptions of risk and management implications in adventure tourism. *Tourism Management, 27*, 317–325.

Chouliaraki, L. (2006). *The Spectatorship of Suffering*. London, UK: Sage Publications.

Cohen, E. (1979). A Phenomenology of Tourist Experience. *Sociology, 13*(2), 179–201.

Cohen, E., & Cohen, S.A. (2012). Authentication: Hot and cool. *Annals of Tourism Research, 39*, 1295–1314.

Cohen-Hattab, K. (2004). Zionism, Tourism, and the Battle for Palestine: Tourism as a Political-Propaganda Tool. *Israel Studies, 9*(1), 61–85.

Crang, M. (1997). Picturing practices: research through the tourist gaze. *Progress in Human Geography, 21*(3), 359–373.

Eco, U. (1986). *Travels in Hyperreality*. New York: Harcourt, Brace & Javonovich.

Edensor, T. (2000). Staging Tourism: Tourists as Performers. *Annals of Tourism Research, 27*(2), 322–44.

Fassin, D., & Rechtman, R. (2009). Palestine. In D. Fassin & R. Rechtman (Ed.) *The Empire of Trauma: An Inquiry into the Condition of Victimhood* (pp. 189–216). Princeton University Press.

Gilbert, S. (2018). "The Disaster Zone of Netflix's *Dark Tourist.*" *The Atlantic. Retrieved from* https://www.theatlantic.com/entertainment/archive/2018/07/the-disaster-zone-of-netflixs-dark-tourism/565946/.

Haldrup, M., & Larsen, J. (2003). The family gaze. *Tourist Studies*, *3*(1), 23–45.

Hammami, R. (2016). Precarious Politics: The Activism of 'Bodies that Count' (Aligning with those that don't) in Palestine's Colonial Frontier. In Judith Butler (Eds.), *Vulnerabilities in Resistance*. Duke University Press.

Hannam, K., Butler, G., & Paris, C. (2014). Developments and key issues in tourism mobilities. *Annals of Tourism Research*, *44*, 171–185.

Heuermann, K., & Chhabra, D. (2014). The Darker Side of Dark Tourism: An Authenticity Perspective. *Tourism Analysis*, *19*(2), 213–225.

Isaac, R.K. (2009). Alternative Tourism: Can the Segregation Wall in Bethlehem be a Tourist Attraction? *Tourism and Hospitality Planning & Development*, *6*, 24–254.

Isaac, R.K. (2010). Alternative tourism: new forms of tourism in Bethlehem for the Palestinian tourism industry. *Current Issues in Tourism*, *13*(1), 21–36.

Jones, G.A., & Sanyal, R. (2015). Spectacle of Suffering: The Mumbai Slum as a Worlded Space. *Geoforum*, *65*, 431–439.

Kaelber, L. (2007). A Memorial as Virtual Traumascape: Darkest Tourism in 3D and Cyber-Space to the Gas Chambers of Auschwitz. *e-Review of Tourism Research (eRTR)*, *5*(2), 24–33.

Kaelber, L. (2010). Virtual Traumascapes: The Commemoration of Nazi 'Children's Euthanasia' Online and On Site. *Digital Icons: Studies in Russian, Eurasian and Central European New Media*, *4*, 13–44.

Kelly, J.L. (2016). Asymmetrical Itineraries: Militarism, Tourism, and Solidarity in Occupied Palestine. *American Quarterly*, *68*(3), 723–745.

Kelly, J.L. (2023). *Invited to Witness: Solidarity Tourism Across Occupied Palestine*. Durham, NC: Duke University Press.

Knudsen, D.C., Rickly, J.M., & Vidon, E.S. (2016). The Fantasy of Authenticity: Touring with Lacan. *Annals of Tourism Research*, *58*(1), 33–45.

Knudsen, D.C., Rickly-Boyd, J.M, & Greer, C.E. (2014). Myth, National Identity, and the Contemporary Tourism Site: The Case of Amalienborg and Frederiksstaden. *National Identities*, *16*(1), 53–70.

Korstanje M., & George, B. (2017). Concluding Chapter: Dark Tourism and Society. In M. Korstanje & B. George (Ed.) *Virtual Traumascape and exploring the roots of Dark Tourism* (pp. 209–225). Hershey, IGI Global.

Kuntsman, A. & Stein, R.L. (2015). *Digital Militarism: Israel's Occupation in the Social Media Age*. Stanford University Press.

Larkin, C. (2014). Jerusalem's Separation Wall and Global Message Board: Graffiti, Murals, and the Art of Sumud. *The Arab Studies Journal*, *22*(1), 134–69.

Lisle, D. (2000). Consuming Danger: Reimagining the War/Tourism Divide. *Alternatives 25*(1), 91–116.

Lund, N.F., Cohen, S.A., & Scarles, C. (2018). The power of social media storytelling in destination branding. *Journal of Destination Marketing & Management*, *8*, 271–280.

Malkki, L.H. (1996). Speechless Emissaries: Refugees, Humanitarianism, and Dehistoricization. *Cultural Anthropology*, *11*(3), 377–404.

Manlove, C.T. (2007). Visual 'Drive' and Cinematic Narrative: Reading Gaze Theory in Lacan, Hitchcock, and Mulvey. *Cinema Journal*, *46*(3), 83–108.

Martini, A. & Buda, D. (2018). Dark tourism and affect: framing places of death and disaster. *Current Issues in Tourism*, *23*, 1–14.

MacCannell, D. (1976). *The tourist: A new theory of the leisure class*. New York: Schocken Books.

Munar, A.M., & Jacobsen, J.K.S. (2014). Motivations for Sharing Tourism Experiences Through Social Media. *Tourism Management*, *43*, 46–54.

Norman, J.M. (2009). Creative Activism: Youth Media in Palestine. *Middle East Journal of Culture and Communication, 2*, 251–274.

Noy, C. (2012). Narratives and Counter-narratives: Contesting a Tourist Site in Jerusalem. In *Narratives of Travel and tourism*. Routledge Press.

Noy, C. (2004). This Trip Really Changed Me: Backpackers' Narratives of Self-Change. *Annals of Tourism Research, 31*(1), 78–102.

Nunkoo, R., Gursoy, D., & Dwivedi, Y.K. (2020). Effects of social media on residents' attitudes to tourism: conceptual framework and research propositions. *Journal of Sustainable Tourism*, 1–17.

Penrose, J. (2018). Authenticity, authentication and experiential authenticity: telling stories in museums. *Social & Cultural Geography, 21*(9), 1–23.

Peteet, J. (2005). *Landscape of hope and despair: Palestinian refugee camps*. Philadelphia, PA: University of Pennsylvania Press.

Peteet, J. (2017). *Space and Mobility in Palestine*. Bloomington, IN: Indiana University Press.

Pinchevski, A. (2019). *Transmitted Wounds: Media and the Mediation of Trauma*. Oxford University Press.

Pupavac, V. (2008). Refugee Advocacy, Traumatic Representations and Political Disenchantment. *Government and Opposition, 43*(2).

Rickly-Boyd, J.M. (2013). Alienation: Authenticity's Forgotten Cousin. *Annals of Tourism Research, 40*, 412–415.

Rickly-Boyd, J.M. (2012). Authenticity and Aura: A Benjaminian Approach to Tourism. *Annals of Tourism Research, 39*, 269–289.

Rickly, J.M. (2009). The Tourist Narrative. *Tourist Studies, 9*(3), 259–280.

Rickly-Boyd, J.M. (2009). Establishing Authenticity in a Tourist Landscape: Spring Mill Pioneer Village. *Material Culture, 41*(1), 1–16.

Said, E. (1979). *The Question of Palestine*. New York, New York: Times Books.

Scarles, C. (2009). Becoming tourist: renegotiating the visual in the tourist experience. *Environment and Planning D: Society and Space*, (27), 465–488.

Scarry, E. (1985). *The Body in Pain: The Making and Unmaking of the World*. Oxford University Press.

Seaton, A.V. (1990). War and thanatourism: Waterloo 1815–1914. *Annals of Tourism Research 26*(1), 130–158.

Sharma, N., & Rickly, J. (2019). 'The smell of death and the smell of life:' Authenticity, anxiety and perceptions of death at Varanasi's cremation grounds. *Journal of Heritage Tourism, 14*(5–6), 466–477.

Shepherd, R.J. (2015). Why Heidegger did not travel: Existential angst, authenticity, and tourist experiences. *Annals of Tourism Research, 52*, 60–71.

Shirky, C. (2011). The Political Power of Social Media: Technology, the Public Sphere, and Political Change. *Foreign Affairs, 90*(1), 28–41.

Sontag, S. (1977). *On Photography*. New York, NY: Farrar, Straus and Giroux.

Stein, R.L. (2002). 'First Contact' and Other Israeli Fictions: Tourism, Globalization, and the Middle East Peace Process. *Public Culture, 14*(3), 515–543.

Stein, R.L. (2008). *Itineraries in Conflict: Israelis, Palestinians, and the Political Lives of Tourism*. Durham, NC: Duke University Press.

Stein, R.L. (2021). *Screen Shots: State Violence on Camera in Israel and Palestine*. Stanford, CA: Stanford University Press.

Steiner, C.J. & Reisinger, Y. (2006). Understanding Existential Authenticity. *Annals of Tourism Research, 33*(2), 299–318.

Stone, P. (2006). A Dark Tourism Spectrum: Towards a typology of death and macabre related tourist sites, attractions and exhibitions. *Tourism: An Interdisciplinary International Journal, 54*(2), 145–160.

Stone, P.R. (2012). Dark tourism and significant other death: Towards a model of mortality mediation. *Annals of Tourism Research, 39*(3), 1565–1587.

Stylianou-Lambert, T. (2012). Tourists with Cameras: Reproducing or Producing? *Annals of Tourism Research, 39*(4), 1817–1838.

Tawil-Souri, H. (2012). Digital Occupation: Gaza's High-Tech Enclosure. *Journal of Palestine Studies*, *41*(2), 27–43.

Tawil-Souri, H. (2013). Networking Palestine: The Development and Limitations of Television and Telecommunications since 1993. In P. Bauck & M. Omar (Ed.), *The Oslo Accords: A Critical Assessment* (pp. 225–237). The American University in Cairo Press.

Tham, A., Mair, J., & Croy, G. (2020). Social media influence on tourists' destination choice: importance of context. *Tourism Recreation Research*, *45*(2), 161–175.

Thomas, D.A. (2019). *Political Life in the Wake of the Plantation: Sovereignty, Witnessing, Repair*. Durham: Duke University Press.

Toenjes, A. (2014). *This Wall Speaks: Graffiti and the Locations of Transnational Space in Palestine*. Master's Thesis, Illinois State University. Retrieved from https://ir.library.illinoisstate.edu/cgi/viewcontent.cgi?article=1131&context=etd.

Toxey, A. (2010). Via Media: The Circulation of Narratives and their Influence on Tourists' and Residents' Actions and Memories. *Material Culture Review*, *71*, 67–83.

Urry, J. (1990). *The Tourist Gaze*. London, UK: Sage Publications, Inc.

Urry, J., & Larson, J. (2011). *The Tourist Gaze 3.0*. London: Sage Publications, Ltd.

Wang, N. (1999). Rethinking authenticity in tourism experience. *Annals of TourismResearch*, *26*, 349–370.

Xue, L., Manuel-Navarrete, D., & Buzinde, C.N. (2014). Theorizing the concept of alienation in tourism studies. *Annals of Tourism Research*, *44*, 186–199.

Yang, C. (2020). Staging Israel/Palestine: The Geopolitical Imaginaries of International Tourism. *Environment and Planning C: Politics and Space*, *38*(6), 1075–1090.

Yang, C. (2019). Visuality and Violence: Touring the Occupied West Bank. *Geopolitics*, *26*(4), 1175–1195.

Zeitzoff, T. (2017). How Social Media Is Changing Conflict. *Journal of Conflict Resolution*, *61*(9), 1970–1991.

Jonathan Skinner, Magdalena Banaszkiewicz

7 The scope of dark tourism-scapes: Exclusion zones and their creative boundedness from Chornobyl to Montserrat

Abstract: This chapter advances work on the exclusion zone as a dark tourism attraction.[1] It examines the mobile nature of these traumascapes, concentrating on the Chornobyl Exclusion Zone (CEZ) and the Montserrat Volcano Exclusion Zone (MEZ). Both zones have been attraction points that move: they expand and they contract; their influence and significance, impact and riskiness vary according to politics, conflict, science and social scales of tolerance. Drawing upon first-hand, long-term ethnographic research at both very topical sites, these two case studies are used to examine "exclusion" as a dark tourism concept associated with Apocalyptic separation from everyday living. Rather than spaces empty of signification, Chornobyl and Montserrat are represented as places of creativity, and treated as spaces of containment and honoured by artists as Apocascapes linked to revelation – self-destructive, anti-capitalist, exclusive to the wealthy indulging in the post-Anthropocene eco-nightmare. With their ruins and ghost towns, their radioactive and pyroclastic threatenings, and their heavily restricted and policed rules for brief visitings, the sites are more than toxic tourism layovers. These exclusion zones relate to natural and man-made disaster phenomena with the principles of attraction tethered by restraint.

Keywords: dark tourism, traumascapes, exclusion, creativity, Chornobyl

Introduction: Life, death and the exclusion zone

Post-colonial scholar Anthony Carrigan has written of necropower in the testing sites of the Pacific, islands turned into 'toxic exclusion zones' (Carrigan 2010, p. 259) by neocolonial military practices – experiments in the Marshall Islands and Kiribati, the population turned into human guinea pigs. Carrigan was drawing from Mbembe's (2003) work

1 This chapter extends initial research and theorisation in M. Banaszkiewicz and J. Skinner (2022) 'Exclusion Tourism: Sci fi and subjunctive plays in apocalyptic destinations from Chernobyl to Plymouth, Montserrat' in, M. Sigala, I. Yeoman, U. McMahon (eds) *Science Fiction, Disruption and Tourism*, Bristol: Channel View Publications, pp. 213–233. In our writing, we are using the Ukrainian transliteration Chornobyl as opposed to the Russian derived Chernobyl to recognise the contested and neo-colonial dimension of this site. When quoting, we are retaining the original transliteration made by the source.

https://doi.org/10.1515/9783110792072-008

on necropolitics describing tropical locations where populations are subjected to social existence that is barely social or human, where the inhabitants are reduced to 'the living dead' of these 'death-worlds' (Mbembe 2003, p. 39, cited in Carrigan 2010, p. 261). In such neocolonial or even postcolonial environments, the visitors and the visited are suffused in the 'catastrophic histories of violence and exploitation' (Carrigan, 2014, p. 237). This constitutes a form of dark tourism, according to Carrigan. We arrive at it, attracted to the phenomenon by its corona when in fact inside, it is quite literally something bloody awful – blood and awe are constituent parts of dark tourism, after all. Where Mbembe writes of necropolitics as a sovereignty over mortality, one applied by Carrigan to the South Pacific, we can also think more closely to the home of the ghastly 'special military operation' in Ukraine, Putin's synonym for a war made good. Terminology aside, the brutal attempted invasion of Ukraine in February 2022 came largely through the Polesie State Radioecological Reserve and Chornobyl Exclusion Zone, a war machine digging up radioactive dust at what Yankovska and Hannam (2014) refer to as both a 'dark and toxic tourism site' (Carrigan, 2014, p. 932). This is another nuclear necropolitics illustrated as the soldiers are sent to their deaths, losing their lives for an abused notion of imperialism.

In another part of the world, the Soufriere Hills volcano continues to ravage the little Caribbean island of Montserrat, pouring super-heated pyroclastic material down her flanks, still slowly burying the port town Plymouth – now a ghost town or New World Pompeii (cf. Bachelor, 2014; Skinner, 2017). The volcanic eruptions began in 1995 and have established evacuation zones, no-go areas that depend upon a traffic light system of risk (see Skinner & Banaszkiewicz, 2022). The same Carrigan (2011) who wrote about disaster and mortality in the Pacific, examines here a postcolonial ecological life-writing from the island, namely Yvonne Weekes's 2006 memoir *Volcano*, a postcolonial counter to the typical 'erasures' associated with colonialism, deterritorialization and natural disaster. *Volcano* is Weekes's survival voice where, for Carrigan, the volcano kills her but the ash of her death is also an ash of rebirth. In his 'Preface' to the book, writer Kamu Brathwaite uses this metaphor to link to the tectonic birth of the Caribbean chain of islands: Weekes is 'a daughter of the millennium mountain [. . .] the detonations of the heart to heart' (Brathwaite, 2006, p. 7). There is hope in this post-disaster recovery, Carrigan asserts, rather than an apocalyptic ruin for the island and islanders. Disaster stories can be affirming and need not all be 'fatal impact narratives', he states (Carrigan, 2011, p. 121).

Creativity abounds the exclusion zone

Weekes develops an ecological subjectivity as she grew to live alongside the volcano in the south of the island. The mountain inspires her and becomes her muse, but it also overshadows and infects her. Before the volcano (pre-1995), Yvonne worked as

Montserrat's first Director of Culture, and as Director of the Rainbow Theatre Company (JS was with the Company working on a play when the volcano disaster started). During the volcano crisis, she used her theatre arts expertise to bring support to those in shelters in the north of the island whilst she, herself, felt afflicted by "the Montserrat disease".

> [. . .] I am suffering from the Montserrat disease. At night I am haunted by the faces of the people I know who have lost their lives, their homes, their loved ones. I feel helpless and powerless. There is a stillness in me. It is deeper than grief. (Weekes, 2006, p. 72)

It is a bleak time for the islanders suffering an ongoing disaster without relief. The blackness of the imminent threat to mortality and the blackness of the ash-laden sky are akin to the blackness of the Montserratian body, turning Weekes to Jesus (p. 59). It is a time of 'supernatural darkness' for her son (p. 59). There is an ambivalence about Weekes's positionality: the sulphur smell creeping up the ghaut outside like the ghosts of her ancestors (p. 22); the ash falling and creeping into the curtains, stripping the paint from walls, resting on toothbrushes and blowing into the lungs (p. 50). And yet, like other Montserratians, she is absorbed by the volcano, its sublime, raw majesty, following its developments sitting in a line of spectators all in their cars (pp. 21–22). Weekes, other Montserratians and visitors to the island – domestic and international dark tourist voyeurs on an awesome geological, spiritual and supernatural development played out in each of the residential tableaus they explore – are disorientated and unsettled by the volcano and its new landscapes or deathscapes as she dreams of visiting the evacuation zone to find the Evergreen Tree, 'the heart of Plymouth', the roundabout hub of civic life in the capital. All that is left is a carbonized desert with outlier structures presenting the debris of inner living room everyday living circa the late 1990s. Whilst villagers lost their lives to the volcano in the east of the island, there are no records of death in the capital – officially, but there are missing persons presumed to have been evacuated. Her dreams fuse like the twisted glass from the heat of pyroclastic mudflows and ashfalls:

> All I know is that my island is sinking. People I once knew have been burnt beyond recognition. [. . .] A vision of skulls comes to me one night. All the bodies that once lay in their polished mahogany tombs wander the white desert land. Every leaf has been swept away. My spirit wanders through this desert. It tries to find the Evergreen tree, but the earth is melted hot and I cannot find a resting place. I watch helplessly as those skulls are crushed into dust. (Weekes, 2006, p. 86)

Where Carrigan frames Weekes's writing as an ecological subjectivity with this swithering personal sovereignty over mortality, Weekes's work belongs to a growing Montserratian 'survival literature' as islanders turn to narrating their circumstances to gain control over their story (Skinner, 2011). This disaster literature, a dark literary genre, is not new and emerged from a writing tradition on the island from playwrights (George Irish, Yvonne Weekes) to poets (E.A. Markham, Howard Fergus) and performance artists (Edgar Nkosi White, Chad Cumberbatch). Pre-volcano, the Montserrat Writers' Maroon practiced as a collective of resistance writers developing self-determination and promoting postcolonial status for the island (Skinner, 2004). In some way, the disaster frees the mind and facilitates one's imagination, photographer Susan Sontag (1967) proposed, as though great creativity is born from these difficult gestations. Also reviewing Weekes's *Volcano*, Alan Ramon Ward (2014, p. 86) writes of Montserratians' encounter with the volcano as a foundational event, as a new break from the norm, an 'evental disaster' that gives rise to a state of literal, figurative and ontological displacement. Ward is drawing from the philosophy of Alain Badiou (2005) who considers the event an existential rupture in Being that is beyond language and hence beyond articulation. Further to this, for some, a nuclear catastrophe is inexpressible even visually, just as the Holocaust is 'unspeakable' and beyond language (Steiner 1967, p. 163). And yet there are creative attempts to chronicle, visualize and protest that confront this reaction of abjection. Examples are the graffiti found around the site by recent visitors; the photographs of Igor Kostin, the first journalist to reach Chornobyl NPP a few hours after the disaster that have decayed and been destroyed but for fragments by an invisible force; Anaïs Tondeur's rendering of the radioactive wounds in her collaborative 'Chornobyl Herbarium' project – imprints on photosensitive plates of plants that grew in the soils of the Chornobyl Exclusion Zone (Marder with Tondeur 2016). These images are entwined with Michael Marder's poetic fragments to suggest an exploded consciousness. This is a radiated eco-critique on techno-capitalism where, for example, the Chornobyl disaster contributed to a radical revision of established worldviews: "Chernobyl exploded my brain. I started thinking", liquidator Oleg Vorobey reflects in *Voices from Chernobyl*, quoted at the opening of Marder and Tondeur's project (2016, p. 9). They creatively mix genres of text (visual plates, physical plants, oral testimonies) as an artistic rendering of the disaster that defies traditional narratives. It belies an ominous new era that is past the cusp of Modernity identified by Lennon and Foley (2000) in their millennial publication *Dark Tourism*. For *Voices from Chernobyl*, Belarusian journalist and writer Svetlana Alexievich received the Nobel Prize for Literature in 2015. The Nobel Committee justified its decision by awarding the prize for 'her polyphonic writings, a monument to suffering and courage in our time' (The Nobel Prize in Literature, 2015). The polyphonicity of the voices of the victims of the catastrophe can still be heard, as echoes spread through the Zone, which is a desolate place, heritage without heirs.

Chornobyl, Pripyat and Plymouth capital are no longer public places. Both are civic centres that have been emptied of citizens. As urban spaces, they are now people-free. They might be referred to as dead cities, urban landscapes turned into exclusion-scapes. They retain streets that are uncared for, left to decay, empty of the former populations and their everyday living (Dobraszczyk 2010). The signifiers of life's loss intrigue the tourist of the exclusion zone. Some of these visitors feel free to leave their mark, a comment on a place, not being in the hegemony of the monitoring they are used to in livable urban spaces. On Montserrat, abandoned houses have been visited and fingerprints and footprints in the ash can be found throughout the abandoned houses around the former capital Plymouth. On Richmond Hill, guides and "off-piste" tourists have toured private properties, some leaving their names and messages on patio doors, messages of love and self-presence to the future (Skinner, 2016). Equally, Frakic and Kennell (2021) point to the existential dread lying in the interpretations of murals, and street art produced around Chornobyl alluding to the disaster (screaming women, crying babies, unborn children, the bureaucracy of secrecy and cover-up connoting an environment of mad science and the death of civilization). The walls paint a post-disaster world of lost confidence. They are created by the excluded citizens of our urban worlds, as Moreau and Alderman (2011) refer to graffiti artists engaged in illicit aesthetic activity. In Ukraine, they have become doubly excluded in their mural work in an exclusion zone. It is, however, celebrated by visitors and showcased by tour guides. It has become a part of what Hundorova (2019, p. xiii) argues is the postmodern 'atomic plurality of worldview': an event that broke the parameters of Modernity; the catastrophe that ushered in an 'after-modern modernity' (Hundorova, 2019, p. 5). This post-catastrophe that we now face is post-totalitarian and also post-carnivalesque with new forms of humour and post-Bubabist literature (Kyiv-led carnivalesque and ironic, satirical movement from the 1980s) that creatively tackle not just the masks of the Soviet era but also the new invisible diseases and visible 'techno-anthropogenic mutations' (Hundorova, 2019, p. 8) that manifest the environment. When reality is warped, humans respond with a "warped sense of humour".

Of doomscapes and dark tourists

Creative attempts to represent the disaster event represent a coming to terms with the extraordinary: orderly narrating the chaos; fine art interpellating a post-disaster eco-awareness; vernacular 'defanging' the environment as in the case of writing groups in Oakland following the 1991 firestorm (Hoffman, 2002, p. 119). After disaster anthropologist Susanna Hoffman (2002), we learn that audiences develop, even, a jealousy of those who survived the disaster and want to visit and reconstruct aspects of the disaster for real or in their creative imagination whether firestorm, eruption or violent Troubles experience told to offspring as romantic fable. Both types of real or imagined visit are found as 'alternative abreactions of the Chornobyl Trauma' (cf. Lindsay, 2014). They are played out in STALKER texts – whether first-person protagonist computer game or literary narrative. Looking for the place of disaster in the modern humanities reveals the transmission of culture as a process of working with trauma. Literature sublimates trauma (cf. Reiter, 2004, p. 135). These are past accounts of a former time. Reiter was working with the Holocaust memoirs of Binjamin Wilkomirski. Weekes is settling her mind through writing. The comparison between the trauma of the Holocaust and the trauma of Chornobyl is not coincidental. Hundorova (2019), recognizing Chornobyl as a word-symbol, like Auschwitz or Hiroshima, acknowledges that the catastrophe opens a new chapter in postmodern Ukrainian consciousness and literature. but post-catastrophic consciousness proliferates creatively and transforms in successive generations entering the spaces of post-Apocalyptic discourses.

Visitors to Montserrat are voyeurs of the pain looking to their future, dark tourists of an impending Apocalypse, using the exclusion zone as their creative stimulus – a warning space not just for visitors to the area but for wider humanity. Eco-critic Lynn Keller notes the Judeo-Christian thinking behind these dark tourism visits that prefigure the end of times. She re-uses lines from Evelyn Reilly's *Apocalypso* poem in her title that is apt for Montserrat: 'Making Art "Under These Apo-Calypso Rays"' (Keller, 2018, p. 19). This survival writing coming out of the island is a reaction to the Apocalyptic scenes before the writers. They write from the safe spaces in the north of the island, outside of the evacuation zones where life takes on a semblance of normality.

The dichotomy between creativity and destruction, between doomscape of the apocalyptic and carnivalscape with its calypso rhythms, has also been developed in the marketing of the island: a green versus gritty contrastscape between the north and the south (cf. Skinner, 2015). The binary opposition, like the unusual juxtaposition (the Black Irish of Montserrat, or the Rasta with a broad brogue), is the travel writers' eye-catching strapline, just as the (con)fused glass and metal objects stand out in their monstrosityness (cf. Law, 1990). Hundorova's two paradigms of Chornobyl – (non)representation – are not too dissimilar. Chornobyl transforms the catastrophe into a spectacle by performing nuclear sublimation in Stalkerism – illegal exploration of abandoned space in search of new experiences that give meaning to life in the ruins, nature and emptiness of the Zone (Banaszkiewicz, 2022). Chornobyl Stalkerism signifies past-presencing by activities of a new type of witness who is a wanderer of the exclusion zone. An example of this is the travelogue of Markijan Kamysz (2022[2015]), who, coming from a family burdened by the trauma of the catastrophe, searches for places in the Zone that will build his own counter-memory, not traumascape, but pastoral *locus amoenus*. Kamysz (2022) spent hundreds of days in the Chornobyl Exclusion Zone and wrote about his ecstatic reaction to facing oblivion in *Stalking the Atomic City: Life Among the Decadent and the Depraved of Chornobyl*. He is a Stalker and writer attracted to this dystopian reality ('a land of tranquility and frozen time' [2022, p. 4]), currently serving with the Ukrainian military. Reviewers refer to him as the 'nuclear Kerouc' (Rob Doyle) with his gonzo fiction and hallucinatory fact. His work is both spiritual quest and suicide note, drawing from this poisoned well Pripyat (cf. Rees, 2022). Kamysz feels alive only when he has returned from his radioactive urbex quests. His adventuring is more radical than the more brief, temporary and safer visits to Montserrat by the ferry daytrippers, the helicopter flyovers from Antigua, or even the illicit yachters' mooring in the abandoned Plymouth port (Skinner 2018). The luxury of the Kyiv resident is in his ability to visit the exclusion zone, to enter and exit it when he is driven to the experience. The Montserrat residents live a hillside away from the active volcano and can see their abandoned homes in the distance. Plymouth might be just out of their sight, but the volcano – colloquially referred to as "the Beast" – is always living and glowering above them.

Local apocalypses are no less destructive than those macro traumas, such as the 20th-century Holocaust, the Great Terror, the Chinese Cultural Revolution, which affect millions and whose memory is global. They are equally inexpressible, if we use a category taken from Lyotard (1991), because with the destruction of the individual and the world comes the destruction of language. There are no words, no analogies, to name such experience (Aleksievich, 2005), but the world that exists beyond them does not share the radicality of the end – the apocalypse happens far away and its witnesses are mute because their experience is locked in their own microcosm. The arrival of these doom and danger dark tourists has the ability to revitalise that memory, to open up a space to speak out and regain a subjectivity and an agency that had been swept away by the tragedy of the event in the past. Polly Patullo (2005) writes of the 'Last Resorts' tourists in the all-inclusive hotels of the Caribbean as a necessary evil to be endured by the locals. It is the same for many of the Montserratians playing host and attending Montserrat Tourist Board workshops on the history of the island and how to welcome the visitor. It is a similar dialectic in the dark tourism visit from Rojek's (1993, p. 136) 'black spot' tourists, to allude to the hijacking of a disaster.

In his literary analysis of 'Un/Natural Disasters', scholar of travel-writing Graham Huggan (2012, p. 99–102) points to the death zones of Everest or Rwanda and to the extreme pursuits of the visitor creatively wrestling with the sublime. Theirs is an accelerated pioneering, a survival experience and disaster writing reconstruction of fatality. For Huggan, the narrator is the new rugged postcolonial soldier/tourist with their mobile phone. They are not the indigenous, the relocated inhabitants living with local traumas. They are dark tourism spectators on the extreme: the extremities of living and life itself who are being catered for by the fresh victims. Theirs is an interest in the 'simulacral reenactments' of violence in the world (Huggan, 2012, p. 101). It comes, according to Huggan, from what Conrad's Marlow in *Heart of Darkness* defined as 'the fascination of the abomination' (Conrad, [1899]1988, p. 10), cited in Huggan 2012, p. 101), or a century later Lennon and Foley's consumption of 'death, disaster and atrocity' (Lennon and Foley 2000, p. 3 cited in Huggan 2012, p. 101). Huggan (2012, p. 101) contextualises the spectator viewing these sites according to the growing normalization of disaster and the accompanying crisis in masculinity in society. This is particularly the case when the adventurer-explorer visits the heights and depths of the earth's crust on a pilgrimage to the extreme. He also criticizes the overall activity as 'at best morally ambivalent touristic curiosity' (Huggan, 2012, p. 102). This is more so apparent in the "darker locations" carelessly linked to human suffering with little thought for the implications of this labelling: the war zones, disaster spaces, evacuation sites to which we also add the exclusion zone. All are residue spaces of dream worlds to echo Gaston Gordillo's thesis on *Rubble: The Afterlife of Destruction*. Most of these leftover spaces are spaces of negativity where capitalist production has crumbled and the human-made industrial form of these spaces has turned to ruin and unfamiliar shapes and silhouettes (cf. Edensor, 2005). This decay is even hybrid in the twisted melted shapes of superheated material culture. These strange unfamiliar forms challenge what Legg (2018, p. 20), writing about post-conflict, post-industrial landscapes of shipbuilding Belfast refers to as 'the monotony of capital'. There is boredom about these regular and predictable places whereas there is discomfort but intrigue in the distorted. There is, even, an aesthetics of appeal about these dark tourism locations, Rebecca Bathory (2018, 2022) argues in her fine arts photographic tour of the dark tourism locations she visited around the world – from Fukushima to Chornobyl, Pompeii to 9/11 Ground Zero. This sense of difference – visual, haptic, olfactory – provides a unique counterpoint to the quotidian. Within this dark tourism niche, the exclusion zone adds further frisson in the sense of aesthetic chills with prohibition fears. The zones are illicit, (safe)guarded, secure in their perimeter and insecure in their interior. On Montserrat, the zones change with the politics and tectonics of the day (cf. Skinner, 2008), and in Chornobyl, the territory is contested by visitors and invaders. Fukushima is the most stable site in terms of dark tourism afterlife. Fine arts photographer and dark tourist Rebecca Bathory published her exhibition book (*Return to Fukushima*, 2016), creatively drawing visual attention to the well-maintained police lines, and the arcades and views into contemporary bourgeois living (DVD stores, factory workshops, slot machine arcades). Fukushima had bags of radioactive soil in store for decontamination whereas Montserrat is now making use of the pyroclastic mudflow material for sandmining and sinking wells for geothermal renewable energy ("ash to cash" coined by Premier Romeo in 2016 [Schuessler, 2016]).

Zoning laws

In the Chornobyl exclusion zone discourses, anthropologist Sharon Stephens (2002) notes a terminology on radiation and risk in speaking and writing about the status of the area. It also included an assertion of normalcy and control with reference to acceptable standards for consideration and management procedures for visiting. The 'Post-Chernobyl culture' of radiological protection experts (Stephens, 2002, p. 92) is not dissimilar to the risk pronouncements coming from the Montserrat Volcano Observatory on post-eruption Montserrat. There, a traffic light system protects the residents of the island. In both scientific discourses about the disasters, speakers acknowledge areas of uncertainty off-stage or outside of the official communiques but present a contained and bounded scenario to the public (Stephens 2002, p. 95, Skinner, 2008). This ring-fencing or zonation of the landscape separates and contains the area for the visitor and the resident. They cross designated safety thresholds or view the unsafe features of the zone from their position of relative safety. On Montserrat, this entails viewing stations in the south of the island and the balcony of the MVO, both with their fixed telescopes trained on the active volcano. For Chornobyl, the zone is harder to view from afar, and entails time-limited access with dosimeters and initially wearing hazmat suits or, more recently, long-sleeved clothes, trousers and closed-toe shoes.

The rules of the Zone are part of a game of heritage that requires a Byzantine setting. The long list of prohibitions and injunctions that must be signed when entering the Zone sanctions the behaviour of visitors in the Zone. For the organisers, it provides an element of control that self-regulates the movement of human subjects through space. For the subjects of our ethnographies, those spoken with at length or followed during their guided tours, it enriches the experience with a thrill: a fulfilment of the retrospective fantasy of a society of control, offering the possibility of entering a situation of radical subordination in the certainty that it is only an ephemeral gadget, satisfying the desire for submission to unlimited power. No sitting down. No eating. No smoking. No drinking of water. No entering the buildings and no moving at all outside the designated route. The law applies to those who enter and leave whether citizens abiding by legal regimes put in place (http://www.rri.kyoto-u.ac.jp/PUB/report/04_kr/img/ekr009.pdf), or tourists following the rules of the tours (https://realchernobyl.com/en/rules). But is this an abstract formula to those who have returned and stayed? Those who are out-lawed: the self-settlers, a group of people who returned illegally to the zone after its creation.

> We walk over to a house where a relatively young man – sixty, maybe – lives. He works at . While we talk, his chickens run around and his car rubs up against my legs. His dog scratches at fleas. We all munch on the roasted sunflower seeds his wife gives us. [. . .] The man denies there is any radiation. He says the government comes in and checks everything and says everything is normal. [. . .] But as we leave, Victor says the man is lying. What could I expect, that the man would say, "I'm an idiot and I live here even though I know it's going to kill me?" (Cheney, 2006: 164)

Year by year, a dwindling handful of self-settlers lived in the Exclusion Zone with the premise that it is better to die from radiation than starvation . . . or longing . . . Controversially, until the point of invasion, the Ukrainian state has preferred to pretend that they do not exist: several dozen people, neither residents nor displaced live in the zone with an undefined legal status suspended between paragraphs. They die of old age, with the feeling that they have made a free choice as to where they live and, consequently, where they die – no matter the cause. At the age of 80 or 90, in this part of the world, where the doctor comes sporadically, and usually cannot help much anyway, the cause of death remains an abstract need to name fate, the nature of which is universal: we are born, we live and we die, just like the plums from which the best *Polesie samogon* is made. The toxic nature of this exclusion zone need not be from radioactive waste but now also from the competing forces of military complexes. Both combine in a now more effective way of excluding the dark tourist.

Classifying the exclusion zones

We suggest in this chapter that exclusion zones fit into the category of dark tourism, but it is not the most emblematic type of death space. Peter Hohenhaus (2023), the author of a popular dark tourism web portal, places the CEZ (Chornobyl Exclusion Zone) next to 'the very deepest of the dark' such as death camps (Auschwitz-Birkenau), gulags (Magadan), or Ground Zero spaces (Hiroshima and New York's National 9/11 Memorial & Museum). This pooling of dark tourism sites is made according to how emotionally demanding they are for the visitor. Further to this, *I am the Dark Tourist* author H.E. Sawyer (2018) recognises the CEZ as one of his TOP 5 dark tourism sites. Such rankings only demonstrate the difficulty of establishing an objective set of evaluation criteria. In the case of Montserrat and Chornobyl, we are dealing with exclusion zone spaces where historical events involve human casualties. These natural and man-made disasters have ongoing consequences to this day (economic, ecological, medical effects, cultural trauma) and feature universal messages (the risks and rewards of cheap energy and easy living). Being in the Zone, either Zone, is more than being in a state of psychological flow. It involves some risk-taking or even confronting a threat to life due to radiation, the poor material condition of the buildings, or difficult and dangerous to follow routes. It is also an experience of wild nature, whose power is revealed and revelled in the post-catastrophe space. The analysed zones of exclusion at the same time can be referred to as a group of sites described as 'postcolonial, post-conflict and post-disaster' (Séraphin et al. 2019). There, the distinguishing feature is a negative image – the legacy of a history fraught with violence, poverty, and pain.

The uniqueness of an exclusion zone comes from its location off the beaten tourist track. In 2009, in one of its cyclical rankings, *Forbes* ranked Chornobyl as one of 'the world's most unique places to visit', alongside places such as Pyongyang in North Korea or the Takstang Monastery in the Kingdom of Bhutan (In Pictures: World's Most Unique Places to Visit, 2009). The marketing role of discovering interesting destinations has long been taken over by social media, but the classifications used by those wishing to discover secret corners of the world remain the same. They aim to identify "hidden gems", "under-rated destinations", "the most incredible sites". Auschwitz is certainly not a hidden gem. Montserrat made it to *The National Geographic* another year. Neither location would have featured without their traumas. However, the CEZ or Fukushima Exclusion Zone opens up a broad complex of issues related to radioactive waste sites and nuclear heritage, i.e. sites, objects and archives linking the current challenges of nuclear power issues to the history of the last century (Brown 2015, Kaijser et al. 2021). Exclusion zones overlap with dark sites, but they are not just dark sites. The fundamental question then is what makes these excluded areas different? Are there distinct characteristics and is a typology or continuum possible just like there is with dark tourism (cf. Stone 2006; Mitchell, Henthorne and George 2020)? The key to understanding the phenomenon of such places is for us not so much the scale of darkness or the motivation of the consumer vs the producer, but the level of accessibility.

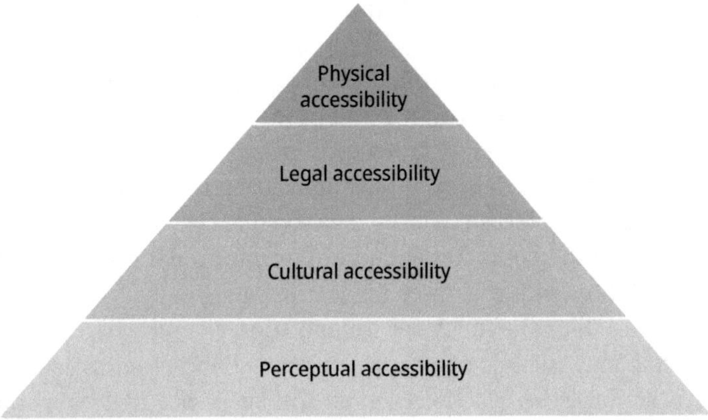

Figure 7.1: Exclusion zone accessibility levels.

In Figure 7.1 we propose that there are four levels of accessibility to consider. These range from the perceptual to the physical in ascending and diminishing order. The physical accessibility quite literally refers to the proprioceptive engagement with the exclusion zone whether legally or illegally. It is about ashy and muddy boots on the ground whether documentary maker Ben Fogle touring Chornobyl and Plymouth for a new documentary (*Inside Chernobyl with Ben Fogle* (2021), *and 'Ben Fogle and the Buried City'* (2023)) or tour guide Sunny Lea driving tourists along the authorised and monitored tourist lines on the outskirts of Plymouth, Montserrat. Exclusion zones, by nature of what they are, have regulations permitting or prohibiting entry. These are maintained legally and enforced. Part of the Stalker experience is to evade capture. On Montserrat, the only road south makes visits containable with a police checkpoint at the entry to the exclusion zone. In terms of accessibility, the exclusion zones operate, then, in the opposite fashion to tourism's heritage destinations. They are closed off rather than opened up. There is no infrastructure within the exclusion zone designed to engage the visitor. The interior of the zone is not traditionally valued in the same way as a heritage structure such as a stately home. Furthermore, the interior nature of structures within the exclusion zone is left unkept. For Deffner et al. (2015), perceptual accessibility refers to the viewers' background. This extends to their practice, their cultural capital – here, a Bourdieusian dark capital from the struggle to be a Stalker.

The exclusion zones are heterogeneous in nature and their accessibility evolves over time. As Banaszkiewicz (2022) describes, the Tourism Area Life Cycle model (Butler, 1980, 2006) can be used to better illustrate the stages of Chornobyl tourism development. With the gradual increase in the accessibility of the Zone (both in terms of the legal status of staying in the Zone and the organisational facilitation resulting from the simplification of procedures and making the range of routes offered more attractive), more and more tourists began to appear in its space. The basic criterion linking the zones in question is the fact that the residents have been displaced and that they are now available to tourists, although this does not limit the number of other spaces of exclusion. Those excluded range from demolition exclusion zones, abortion protest exclusion zones, telecom mast exclusion zones, to licence condition exclusion zones given to prisoners, disease control exclusion zones from bird flu and foot and mouth. Biosecure exclusion zones, personal proscribed exclusion zones and protest zones are spaces visited for non-leisure motivations, even though the thrill or satisfaction associated visiting such places might be perceived as 'leisure' experience by some visitors. They do share the characteristic of authoritarian delimitation and enforcement, and legal regulation with a penalty for infractions. They are not no-go zones such as potentially Free Derry in Northern Ireland (Derry/Londonderry). Nor are they protected no take zones such as conservation protection areas for lobster husbandry in Sainte Luce, Madagascar. The potential no-fly zone lacks the focal point for the visitor's gaze but is a vertical version of the Military Exclusion Zone (a defensive area of public and international interest). The (extended) Demilitarized Zone is a specifically man-made exclusion zone, a thick boundary between two military contestants such as Turkey and Cyprus, North Korea and the Republic of Korea (South Korea). But these typically demilitarized buffers can extend for miles along a border such as the UN Buffer Zone between Turkey and Cyprus, or for miles on either side of a border such as in the case of parts of the Golan Heights, or either side of parts of the northern Syria/Turkey border. The Demilitarised Zone (DMZ) differs from the exclusion zone in that it can contain a living population whereas the exclusion zones we consider are devoid of human inhabitation, or so they should be given that there have been instances of illicit residency in them.

Future proofing the exclusion zone

In recent years, a shift towards a phenomenological approach to dark tourism (Podoshen et al., 2015) has involved investigating the motivations and experiences of visitors rather than the distinctive features of places. Experiences in dark sites can be emotionally engaging (Sigala & Steriopoulos, 2021) and contribute to meaning-making processes they can be spiritual and transformative (Oren et al., 2021) but also edutainment-oriented (Wyatt et al., 2020). Tourism plays an extensive role in the transformation of excluded zones as long as, of course, their exclusion is not total. Even the Stalkers are guilty of self-exploitation as they capitalise on their incursions, tweet, share and comment on their explorations. But are they free in their illicit roaming? The freedom of the CEZ is a freedom from a totalitarian past and – in the context of the current war in Ukraine – a totalitarian future. Though surely the band of photographers on a busman's holiday to compose shots of the abandoned sites is also an example of friends as entrepreneurs filming and testing their projects, their voluntary labour. Philosopher Byung-Chul Han (2017) suggests that this new condition of neoliberal capitalism is the ultimate subjugation because it is desired and self-imposed, a personal panopticon. Performative practices involving tourists in local community or environmental activities known as volunteer tourism (McMorran, 2017) can take the form of strategies of resilience that build around local place-based practices and traditional community knowledge. This shift from dark tourism into blue tourism incorporating non-dark activities enriches the tourist experience by focusing on social and environmental sustainability. It situates post-apocalyptic exclusion zone tourism on the peripheries of the traditionally defined dark site (Lin et al., 2018). Over the past few years, for example, Chornobyl tourism organisers have offered the opportunity to meet with self-settlers (samosely) (people who returned to the Zone after the disaster to live there illegally.) On Montserrat, the work of the Montserrat National Trust has been to open a National Museum with cultural displays including an engagement with the volcano, to develop digital archives and to support STREVA (Strengthening Resilience in Volcanic Areas), a UK-funded international research project drawing attention to citizen science and the arts as an expression of living with a volcanic eruption. STREVA developed pyroclastic poetry materials, a volcano model for the UK and Montserrat and hosted Yvonne Weekes to give a reading from her work. One of the interdisciplinary slogans for the project was as follows: "Montserratians sing the life we live. Montserratians write the life we live." (STREVA, 2019)

This articulates our thesis of resilience and creativity in living with adversity. The consensual hybridisation of the heritage of trauma is also broadening the spectrum of tourist experiences through the thematisation of the offer. Following the spectacular success of the *Chernobyl* series, one Chornobyl tour operator had included a tour in the footsteps of the series in its permanent offer in 2019. The tourist boom of 2019 (over 124,000 visitors), which especially involved non-residents, can be attributed largely to the huge popularity of the series. So, it is not that the cultural message is enough. It shapes the tourist imagination (Salazar & Graburn 2014), further motivating tourists to physically find themselves in the space they have experienced on screen or in reading. This development was also found in the use of parts of the Montserrat Exclusion Zone in the filming of *Wendy*, a post-apocalyptic eco-fantasy spin-off from Peter Pan. Both destinations have become *zeitgeist* film tourism stops.

Critics of this controversial form of dark tourism argue that the narrative of dark sites and related traumas is vulgarised through commodification (Hundorova, 2019), a process that can also be seen for the democratisation of meanings and the opportunity to universalise the message of particular historical events. Mass media techniques expand the community of people who experience the past. Just as the Holocaust is "remembered" through *Schindler's List* (cf. Rapport, 2009), the disaster through HBO's *Chernobyl* series reaches people who, even if they have ever heard of the disaster, did not realise its scale as well as the context in which it occurred. This is intergenerational trauma by association and elicitation. According to Alison Landsberg (2012), mass culture media enables the formation of prosthetic memory. Prosthetic memories do not refer to the memory community of a group based on kinship ties, as in the case of post-memory (Hirsch, 2016), but to the memory of an imagined community that is not limited by gender, class or race. The individual's empathic experience of representations of the past can be made possible by modern technology acting as a medium of the memory itself. This is possible by going beyond previous cultural transmission (such as the written text): the sensory-corporeal experience of the image builds a unique level of engagement with the world. This is especially resonant in the photographic image derived from the camera. In this sense, both exclusion zones are location shoots for this reflexive practice as the Stalker/shooter/photographer "snap and 'shop" their images. Those images are then circulated and published across virtual platforms and physical mediums, often enticing other visitors to the exclusion zones or related dark tourism destinations.

In terms of the future of visits to these exclusion zones, we suggest that the enforced immobility of the pandemic period has recently further stepped up the experience of the world through "simulated" journeys, through the distant lens of an Other. This is despite the virtualisation of tourist experiences and digitisation of tourism services has been one of the most important trends shaping the innovative approaches to tourism development in recent years (Beck et al., 2019; Yung and Khoo-Lattimore, 2017; Loureiro et al., 2020). The gradual shift observed in recent years from online and online tourism to the more technologically complex virtual tourism may play a particular role in relation to exclusion zones as a complement or even substitute for the dark tourism experience. This has already been precipitated by the films, documentaries and computer games related to the CEZ and to a lesser extent the MEZ. Virtual dark tourism, we suggest, can cover a wide range of activities and is growing through the Metaverse. It can include video games, virtual tours, and websites that deal with traumatic events. It can host alternative stories, educate, and serve as a source for cultural resistance (McDaniel, 2018). As Kaelber (2007, p. 27) points out: 'for visiting a physically obliterated traumascape that is difficult or even impossible to access physically, pilgrims and tourists can engage in alternative, technologically mediated appropriation of the darkest tourism sites'. An interesting solution for exclusion zone tourism may be the use of modern technologies such as virtual reality (VR). As Guttentag (2021, p. 150) notes, VR not only can encourage empathy, but it is uniquely useful as an educational technology (see also Rubin, 2020). The Chernobyl VR Project is a documentary virtual experience co-created by The Farm 51 and Carbon Studio implementing the mechanics of interacting with a digitally reconstructed environment through photogrammetry and 3D scanning technology. It has taken on added significance after Russia's attack on Ukraine in February 2022. The added value of projects such as Chernobyl VR is not only the digital preservation of tangible objects or edutainment via Oculus. Heritage Building Information Modelling (H-BIM) is an innovative technology used primarily in the field of the documentation, preservation and management of historic sites – its relevance was witnessed after the great Notre Dame cathedral fire in 2019, and after the Russian attack on Ukraine, the Chernobyl VR project preserves data on objects that have been destroyed by warfare (https://uploadvr.com/chernobyl-vr-project-nuclear-ghost-town/). However, it is difficult to overlook the immense exploration possibilities offered by H-BIM. "Chernobyl VR reproduces physical landscapes in order to offer an experience that is as close as possible to individual exploration of that space, but without the security restrictions that come with their exclusivity." They are modelling the exclusion site for those who remain excluded. Although HBIM is still mainly perceived through the prism of usability from the perspective of architectural structure and materials, the next step – quite literally – is likely to be the ever-expanding metaverse technology that also holds enormous business potential for dozens of industries related to creative industries, tourism and cultural heritage (Zhang et al., 2022). Whether online or offline, the ominous future of the exclusion zone stands to expand exponentially.

References

Aleksievich, S. (2005) *Voices from Chernobyl: chronicle of the future*. Dallas: Dalkey Archive.

Bachelor, B. (2014) 'Montserrat: a modern-day Pompeii in the Caribbean', Fox News 20 February 2014, http://www.foxnews.com/travel/2014/02/20/montserrat-modern-day-pompeii-in-caribbean.html, accessed 1 September 2016.

Badiou, A. (2005) *Being and Event*. New York: Continuum.

Banaszkiewicz, M. (2022) *Tourism and Heritage in the Chornobyl Exclusion Zone*. London: Routledge.

Bathory R. (2022) *Journey into the Dark: The Photographic Practise and Imagery of Dark Tourism*. PhD thesis: University of Roehampton.

Bathory, R. (2018) *Dark Tourism*. London: Carpet Bombing Culture.

Bathory, R. (2016) *Return to Fukushima*. London: Carpet Bombing Culture.

Beck, J., Rainoldi, M. and R. Egger (2019) 'Virtual reality in tourism: a state-of-the-art review', *Tourism Review* 74(3): 586–612.

Brathwaite, K. (2006) 'Preface' in Y. Weekes, *Volcano: A Memoir*, Leeds: Peepal Tree, p.7.

Brown, K. (2015) *Plutopia: nuclear families, atomic cities, and the great Soviet and American plutonium disasters*. Oxford: Oxford University Press.

Butler, R. (2006) *The Tourism Area Life Cycle*. Bristol: Channel View Publications.

Butler, R. (1980) 'The concept of a tourism area cycle of evolution: Implications for management of resources', *The Canadian Geographer/Le Géographe Canadien*, 24(1): 5–12.

Carrigan, A. (2014) 'Dark Tourism and Postcolonial Studies: Critical Intersections', *Postcolonial Studies* 17(3), 236–50.

Carrigan, A. (2011) '(Eco)Catastrophe, Reconstruction, and Representation: Montserrat and the Limits of Sustainability', Postcolonial Islands Special Issue, E. DeLoughrey (Ed.) *New Literatures Review* 47–48: 111–128.

Carrigan, A. (2010) 'Postcolonial Disaster, Pacific Nuclearization, and Disabling Environments', *Journal of Literary and Cultural Disability Studies* 4(3): 255–72.

Cheney, G. (2006) Journey to Chernobyl: Encounters in the Radioactive Zone. Academy Chicago Publishers.

Conrad, J. ([1899]1988) *Heart of Darkness*. New York: Norton Critical Editions.

Deffner, A., E. Psatha, N. Bogiantzidis, N. Mantas, E. Vlachaki, P. Ntaflouka (2015) 'Accessibility to Culture and Heritage: Designing for All', unpublished conference paper, https://www.researchgate.net/publication/280312809, accessed 2 March 2023.

Dobraszczyk, P. (2010). 'Petrified ruin: Chernobyl, Pripyat and the death of the city, *City* 14(4): 370–389.

Edensor, T. (2005) *Industrial Ruins: Space, Aesthetics and Materiality*. London: Bloomsbury Books.

Farkić, J. and J. Kennell (2021) 'Consuming dark sites via street art: Murals at Chernobyl', *Annals of Tourism Research* 90: 103256.

Gordillo, G. (2014) *Rubble: The Afterlife of Destruction*. London: Duke University Press.

Guttentag, D. (2021) 'Digital Destinations and Avatar Tourists: A Futuristic Look at Virtual Reality Tourism and Its Real-World Impacts', in I. Yeoman, U. McMahon-Beattie and M. Sigala (Eds) *Science Fiction, Disruption and Tourism*. Bristol: Channel View Publications, pp. 145–160.

Han, B. (2017) *Psychopolitics: Neoliberalism and New Technologies of Power*. London: Verso Books.

Han, B. (2015) *The Burnout Society*. Redwood City: Stanford Briefs, An Imprint Of Stanford University Press.

Hirsch, M. (2012). The Generation of Postmemory: Writing and Visual Culture After the Holocaust. Columbia University Press.

Hoffman, S. (2002) 'The Monster and the Mother: The Symbolism of Disaster' in S. Hoffman and A. Oliver-Smith (eds) *Catastrophe & Culture: The Anthropology of Disaster*. Oxford: James Currey, pp. 113–142.

Hohenhaus, P. (2023) *Dark Tourism: The guide to dark travel destinations around the world*. Www.dark-Tourism.com. https://www.dark-tourism.com/index.php, accessed 1 March 2023.

Huggan, G. (2012) *Extreme Pursuits: Travel/Writing in an Age of Globalization*, Ann Arbor: The University of Michigan Press.

Hundorova, T. (2019) *The Post-Chornobyl Library: Ukrainian postmodernism of the 1990s*. Brookline: Academic Studies Press.

Kaijser, A., Lehtonen, M., Rubio-Varas, M. and J-H. Meyer (2021) *Engaging the Atom: the history of nuclear energy and society in Europe from the 1950s to the present*. Morgantown: West Virginia University Press.

Kaelber, L. (2007) 'A Memorial as Virtual Traumascape: Darkest Tourism in 3D and Cyber-Space to the Gas Chambers of Auschwitz', *E-Review of Tourism Research* 5(2): 24–33.

Kamysz, M. (2022[2015]) *Stalking the Atomic City: Life Among the Decadent and the Depraved of Chornobyl*. New York: Astra House.

Keller, L. (2018) 'Making Art "Under These Apo-Calypso Rays": Crisis, Apocalypse, and Contemporary Ecopoetics', in A. Hume and G. Osborne (eds) *Ecopoetics: Essays in the Field*. Iowa City: University of Iowa Press, pp. 19–41.

Landsberg, A. (2006) *Prosthetic Memory: the transformation of American remembrance in the age of mass culture*. New York: Columbia University Press.

Law, J. (1990) 'Introduction: Monsters, Machines and Sociotechnical Relations', *Sociological Review* 38(1): 1–23.

Legg, G. (2018) *Northern Ireland and the Politics of Boredom: Conflict, Capital and Culture*. Manchester: Manchester University Press.

Lennon, J. and M. Foley (2000) *Dark Tourism: The Attraction of Death and Disaster*. London: Continuum.

Lin, Y., Kelemen, M., and R. Tresidder (2018) 'Post-disaster tourism: building resilience through community-led approaches in the aftermath of the 2011 disasters in Japan', *Journal of Sustainable Tourism 26*(10): 1766–1783.

Lindsay, S. (2014) *Reading Chernobyl: Psychoanalysis, Deconstruction, Literature*. PhD thesis, University of Stirling.

Loureiro, S. M. C., Guerreiro, J., and F. Ali (2020) '20 years of research on virtual reality and augmented reality in tourism context: A text-mining approach' *Tourism Management* 77: 1–21.

Lyotard. 1991. The Inhuman: Reflections on Time. Stanford: Stanford University Press.

Marder, M. with A. Tondeur (2016) *The Chernobyl Herbarium: Fragments of an Exploded Consciousness*. London: Open Humanities Press.

Mbembe, A. (2003) 'Necropolitics', *Public Culture* 15(1): 11–40.

McDaniel, K. N. (2018) *Virtual Dark Tourism: Ghost Roads*. Basingstoke: Palgrave Macmillan.

McMoran, C. (2017) 'From volunteers to voluntours: shifting priorities in post-disaster Japan', *Japan Forum* 29(1): 1–25.

Mitchell, V., T. Henthorne, and B. George (2020) 'Making Sense of Dark Tourism: Typologies, Motivations and Future Development of Theory', in M. Korstanje and H. Seraphin (eds) *Tourism, Terrorism and Security*. Bingley: Emerald Publishing Limited, pp. 103–114.

Moreau, T. and D. Alderman (2011) 'Graffiti Hurts And The Eradication Of Alternative Landscape Expression', *The Geographical Review* 101(1): 106–124.

Oren, G., Shani, A., and Y. Poria (2021) 'Dialectical emotions in a dark heritage site: A study at the Auschwitz Death Camp', *Tourism Management 82*, 104194.

Pattullo, P. (2005) *Last Resorts: The Cost of Tourism in the Caribbean*. Kingston, Jamaica: Ian Randle publishers.

Podoshen, J. S., Andrzejewski, S. A., Venkatesh, V., and J. Wallin (2015) 'New approaches to dark tourism inquiry: A response to Isaac', *Tourism Management* 51: 331–334.

Ramón Ward, A. (2014) 'Disaster as Event: Yvonne Weekes's *Volcano*', *Moving Worlds: A Journal of Transcultural Writings* 14(2): 84–92.

Rapport, N. (2009) 'Walking Auschwitz, Walking without Arriving', *Journeys* 9(2): 32–54.

Rees, J. (2022) 'Meet the madman who spent 200 days in the Chernobyl Exclusion Zone', *The Daily Telegraph*, 2 July 2022, p.17. https://www.telegraph.co.uk/books/what-to-read/meet-madman-who-spent-200-days-chernobyl-exclusion-zone/, accessed 28 February 2023.

Reiter, A. (2004) 'Memory and Authenticity: the case of Binjamin Wilkomirski', in P. Gray and K. Oliver (ed.) *The Memory of Catastrophe*. Manchester: Manchester University Press, pp. 132–146.

Rojek, C. (1993) *Ways of Escape*. Basingstoke: Macmillan.

Rubin, P. (2020) *FUTURE PRESENCE: how virtual reality is changing human connection, intimacy, and the limits of . . . ordinary life*. New York: HarperOne.

Salazar, N. and N. Graburn (Eds) (2014) *Tourism Imaginaries: Anthropological approaches*. Oxford: Berghahn Books.

Sawyer, H. E. (2018) *I am the Dark Tourist: travels to the darkest sites on earth*. Manchester: Headpress.

Schuessler, R. (2016) 'Ash to cash': Montserrat gambles future on the volcano that nearly destroyed it', *The Guardian*, 3 February 2020 modified from 28 January 2016, https://www.theguardian.com/world/2016/jan/28/montserrat-volcano-british-territory-geothermal-energy-tourism-sand-mining, accessed 21 February 2023.

Séraphin, H., M. Korstanje, and V. Gowreesunka (2020) *Post-Disaster and Post-Conflict Tourism: toward a new management approach*. Apple Academic Press.

Séraphin, H., Zaman, M., & Fotiadis, A. (2019). Challenging the Negative Image of Postcolonial, Post-conflict and Post-disaster Destinations Using Events: The Case of Haiti. Caribbean Quarterly, 65(1), 88–112. https://doi.org/10.1080/00086495.2019.1565223

Sigala, M., and E. Steriopoulos (2021) 'Does emotional engagement matter in dark tourism? Implications drawn from a reflective approach', *Journal of Heritage Tourism* 16(4): 412–432.

Skinner, J. and M. Banaszkiewicz (2022) 'Exclusion Tourism: sci fi and subjunctive plays in apocalyptic destinations from Chernobyl to Plymouth, Montserrat' in, M. Sigla, I. Yeoman, U. McMahon (Eds) *Science Fiction, Disruption and Tourism*. Bristol: Channel View Publications, pp. 213–233.

Skinner, J. (2018) 'Plymouth, Montserrat: apocalyptic dark tourism at the Pompeii of the Caribbean', *International Journal of Tourism Cities*, 4(1): 123–139.

Skinner, J. (2017) '"The smoke of an eruption, and the dust of an earthquake": Dark Tourism, the Sublime and the Re-Animation of the Disaster Location' in, P. Stone, R. Hartmann, T. Seaton, R. Sharpley and L. White (Eds) *Handbook of Dark Tourism Studies*. Basingstoke: Palgrave Macmillan, pp. 125–150.

Skinner, J. (2016) '"Was here": identity traces and digital footprints as survival writing', Terror on Tour – Special Issue, *Liminalities: A Journal of Performance Studies*, 12(5), http://liminalities.net/12-5/washere.pdf. ISSN: 1557–2935 (Online)

Skinner, J. (2015) 'Let's Get Gritty on the Black and Green', *MNIalive.com – Global Caribbean Media*, 21 May 2015, http://www.mnialive.com/articles/let-s-get-gritty-on-the-black-and-green.

Skinner, J. (2011) 'A Distinctive Disaster: Montserrat island under pressure' in, A. Soares and M. McCusker (eds) *Islanded Identities: Constructions of Postcolonial Cultural Insularity*. Amsterdam: Rodopoi, pp. 63–89.

Skinner, J. (2008) 'The text and the tale: the difference between scientific reports and scientists' reportings on the eruption of Mount Chance, Montserrat', *Journal of Risk Research*, 11(1–2): 255–267.

Skinner, J. (2004) *Before the Volcano: Reverberations of Identity on Montserrat*. Kingston, Jamaica: Arawak Publications.

Sontag, S. (1967) *Against Interpretation, and other essays*. New York NY: Farrar Straus-Giroux.

Steiner, G. (1967) *Language and Silence: Essays in Language, Literature and the Inhuman*. New York: Athenaeum.

Stephens, S. (2002) 'Bounding Uncertainty: The Post-Chernobyl Culture of Radiation Protection Experts' in S. Hoffman and A. Oliver-Smith (eds) *Catastrophe & Culture: The Anthropology of Disaster*. Oxford: James Currey, pp. 91–111.

Stone, P. (2006) 'A Dark Tourism Spectrum: towards a typology of death and macabre related tourist sites, attractions and exhibitions', *TOURISM: An Interdisciplinary International Journal* 54(2): 145–160.

STREVA (2019) *Strengthening Resilience in Volcanic Areas*. Information Pamphlet, https://volcanoutreach.uea.ac.uk/wp-content/uploads/sites/2/2019/10/NSF-2019-lanyard-card-Geohazards-Montserrat.pdf, accessed 3 March 2023.

The Nobel Prize in Literature 2015. (n.d.). NobelPrize.org. Retrieved May 12, 2023, from https://www.nobelprize.org/prizes/literature/2015/press-release/.

Weekes, Y. (2006) *Volcano: A Memoir*. Leeds: Peepal Tree.

Wyatt, B., Leask, A., and P. Barron (2020) 'Designing dark tourism experiences: an exploration of edutainment interpretation at lighter dark visitor attractions', *Journal of Heritage Tourism* 16(4): 433–449.

Wyatt, B., Leask, A., & Barron, P. (2020). Designing dark tourism experiences: an exploration of edutainment interpretation at lighter dark visitor attractions. Journal of Heritage Tourism, 16(4), 433–449. https://doi.org/10.1080/1743873X.2020.1858087

Yankovska, G. and K. Hannam (2014) 'Dark and toxic tourism in the Chernobyl exclusion zone', *Current Issues in Tourism* 17(10): 929–939.

Yu, J., and R. Egger (2022) 'Looking behind the scenes at dark tourism: a comparison between academic publications and user-generated-content using natural language processing', *Journal of Heritage Tourism* 17(5): 548–562.

Yung, R., and C. Khoo-Lattimore (2017) 'New realities: a systematic literature review on virtual reality and augmented reality in tourism research', *Current Issues in Tourism* 22(17): 2056–2081.

Zhang, X., Yang, D., Yow, C. H., Huang, L., Wu, X., Huang, X., Guo, J., Zhou, S., & Cai, Y. (2022) 'Metaverse for Cultural Heritages', *Electronics* 11(22): 3730.

Alix Varnajot, Margaréta Pintér, Vesa-Pekka Herva, Albina Pashkevich & Thora Herrmann

8 Exploring the intersections between dark tourism and Arctic traumascapes in the Anthropocene: The case of Finnish Lapland

Abstract: In recent years, an increasing number of people have experienced ecological grief due to significant changes in their environment, mourning the death of more-than-human entities such as glaciers or iconic landscapes. In the southernmost regions of the Arctic, like Finnish Lapland, water and rain is estimated to gradually dominate over ice and snow due to global climate change. However, in the last 40 years, the Arctic tourism industry has grown based on representations of snow and ice, and even today, keeps promoting Finnish Lapland with images of guaranteed white vistas (Herva et al., 2020; Varnajot & Saarinen, 2022). The increasing gap between the dynamic reality and the static promotion of the Arctic in tourism can be understood as the death of the iconic white landscape of Lapland, and, in some cases, leads to the production of Arctic traumascapes. Traumascapes are defined as haunting places "where visible and invisible, past and present, physical and metaphysical come to coexist and share common space" (Tumarkin, 2019, p. 5), and visits to these specific sites of trauma are often referred to as dark tourism (Kaelber, 2007). In the Anthropocene however, dark tourism increasingly encompasses places associated with the death of more-than-human entities, such as the iconic vistas of Lapland (Varnajot & Saarinen, 2021). In line with this, this conceptual chapter investigates the intersections between dark tourism and traumascapes raised by the shrinking cryosphere in the context of Finnish Lapland. Finnish Lapland provides an interesting case where we can already observe some previews of Arctic tourism products being challenged due to changes in seasonality and lack of snow and ice. Therefore, by exploring the production of dark tourism practices in Finnish Lapland, this chapter aims to shed new light on the production of traumascapes in tourism on the one hand and to provide new conceptualizations concerning the idea of 'Arctic traumascapes' on the other.

Keywords: dark tourism, Arctic, traumascape, Anthropocene, cryosphere, Finnish Lapland

https://doi.org/10.1515/9783110792072-009

Introduction

In recent years, an increasing number of people have experienced ecological grief due to significant changes in their environment and have mourned the death of other-than-human entities such as glaciers or iconic landscapes (Westoby et al., 2022). Increasing wildfires and extreme weather events, changing weather patterns, biodiversity loss and accumulating pollution have triggered global concerns about our planet and global ecosystems' productivity (Ceballos et al., 2017; Steffen et al., 2015; Sutton et al., 2016). These experiences of worry about the changing environment can lead to the development of ecological grief, which refers to "grief felt in relation to experiences or anticipated ecological losses, including the loss of species, ecosystems and meaningful landscapes due to acute or chronic environmental change" (Cunsolo & Ellis, 2018, p. 275). Importantly, ecological grief is not solely a response to the loss of iconic landscapes or animal species (e.g., glaciers, coral reefs, rhinos, polar bears), it is also closely tied to environmental changes that impact individuals' local place attachment (e.g., home) (Lewicka, 2010; Mallett, 2004). Indeed, in her seminal work, Canadian researcher and environmental activist Ashlee Cunsolo (2012) gives an account of such a grief experience from her childhood. She writes:

> *When I was five, a pond and thicket area down the street from my house was filled in and leveled while I was away. I remember coming home and finding my beloved ecosystem denuded of all greenery, and completely empty of the beavers and their dam, the minnows, the birds, and the countless rabbits and squirrels that had been a comforting and valued presence. I was devastated. Consumed and overcome by grief and loss. [. . .]. It was the first time in my short life that I became aware of the fragility of life – mine and others – and from that moment, I found myself in a different life-world full of the awareness of the potential for death and injury to befall plants, animals, and ecosystems, aware of the corporeal acuteness of grief and mourning that could emerge from environmental destruction and degradation. This experience was also my first of many moments of environmentally based grief – grief for the loss of non-human bodies, spaces, and places* (p. 137–138).

Ecological grief and worrying for our planet also include concerns for the disappearing cryosphere (Varnajot & Salim, 2024), or the part of the Earth that is seasonally or perennially frozen, encompassing glaciers, sea ice, permafrost, ice sheets and ice caps, river and lake ice, and snow (Dodds, 2018). According to Sörlin (2015), the melting of the (Arctic) cryosphere represents a core event of the Anthropocene, the new epoch in which "[t]he human imprint on the global environment has now become so large and active that it rivals some of the great forces of Nature in its impact on the functioning of the Earth system" (Steffen et al., 2011, p. 842). Although the Anthropocene was first thought of as a geological era, it has now become a bridging concept, encompassing the humanities and social sciences (Gren & Huijbens, 2019). In addition, the Anthropocene is often related to anxiety-driven narratives (Buck, 2015), as well as ruination and post-apocalyptic imaginaries (Bennett, 2020; Huijbens, 2021; Varnajot & Saarinen, 2021).

In the southernmost regions of the Arctic, such as Finnish Lapland, water and rain are estimated to take the place of ice and snow due to global climate change (Varnajot & Saarinen, 2022). However, in the last 40 years, the Arctic tourism industry has grown tremendously based on representations of snow and ice and keeps promoting Finnish Lapland with images of guaranteed white vistas to this day (Herva et al., 2020; Tervo-Kankare et al., 2013). Thus, in this chapter, we argue that this increasing gap between the dynamic reality and the static promotion of the Arctic in tourism can lead to the production of Arctic traumascapes. Traumascapes are defined as "places constituted by experiences of particular [traumatic] events and their aftermath" (Tumarkin, 2019, p. 5). More so, visits to these specific sites of trauma are often referred to as dark tourism (Kaelber, 2007). The melting (Arctic) cryosphere induced by global climate change has been characterized and defined as a slow-onset disaster by the United Nations Office for Disaster Risk Reduction (n.d.). In line with this, authors such as Rucinska (2016), Varnajot and Salim (2024), and Wright and Sharpley (2018) have shown how sites of natural disasters, like scenes of the vanished cryosphere in the Arctic, have arguably become sites of dark tourism. While dark tourism has generally referred to tourism and experiences of places associated with human death and suffering (Stone & Sharpley, 2008), in the Anthropocene, dark tourism increasingly encompasses places associated with the death of other-than-human entities (Craps, 2023; Sideris, 2020; Varnajot & Saarinen, 2021), such as the slowly disappearing wintery landscapes of Finnish Lapland.

This chapter investigates the conceptual intersections between dark tourism and traumascapes raised by the shrinking cryosphere in the context of Finnish Lapland. Finnish Lapland is an interesting case study where we can already preview Arctic tourism products being challenged due to changes in seasonality and lack of snow and ice. Therefore, by exploring the production of dark tourism practices in Finnish Lapland, this chapter aims to shed new light on the creation of traumascapes in tourism on the one hand and to provide new conceptualizations regarding the idea of 'Arctic traumascapes' on the other. The next section provides contextualization on the current practices and meanings of Arctic tourism in Lapland. It is critical to understand the production of Arctic tourism not only conceptually, but also how it manifests in practice since the arguments developed throughout this chapter are highly dependent on how Arctic tourism has been constructed in the past. The following section explores darkness and dark tourism in the Anthropocene while exemplifying these dynamics in the context of Finnish Lapland. The last section discusses the production of Arctic traumascapes through dark tourism practices associated with these other-than-human deaths. This last section also aims to provide a conceptualization of Arctic traumascapes.

Arctic tourism in Finnish Lapland

What is 'Arctic' in 'Arctic tourism'? What is the difference between 'Arctic tourism' and 'tourism in the Arctic', and why is there a need to differentiate these two terms? Tourism in the Arctic is straightforward to define. It is a geographical approach that refers to all forms of tourism taking place within the borders of the Arctic. As such, tourism in the Arctic is not a tourist segment or type of tourism per se. Rather, it encompasses visits to family and relatives, event tourism, adventure tourism, urban tourism, and any number of other tourism types. It is worth noting that this raises the long-discussed issue of where the Arctic begins or ends, but this discussion is beyond the scope of this chapter. Tourism in the Arctic has existed for over two centuries and the first tourists consisted mainly of explorers and wealthy adventurers (Hall & Johnston, 1995). At that time, large areas of the Arctic remained unexplored, and tourism in these circumpolar regions was only a sporadic phenomenon (Varnajot, 2020). Today, however, tourism in the Arctic "starts at the North Pole and quite literally spreads out in all directions from there" (Maher et al., 2014, p. 1), to the southernmost regions of the Arctic, both on land and sea. Tourism in the Arctic now operates year-round and varies from exclusive icebreaker cruises to the North Pole to more accessible and affordable tourism hotspots such as Finnish Lapland (Saarinen & Varnajot, 2019).

In contrast to tourism in the Arctic, Arctic tourism is more complex and necessitates further contextualization. Arctic tourism is grounded in biased and historically constructed representations of the Arctic (Pedersen & Viken, 1996). These representations of the Arctic generally involve images of white, frozen and uninhabited landscapes, thus overlooking other seasons, as well as the climatic, demographic and cultural realities of the region (Saarinen & Varnajot, 2019). As such, Arctic tourism can be defined as "tourism taking place in northern latitudes, where tourists engage in experiences producing and reproducing cryospheric- and winter-based imaginaries" (Varnajot & Lunden, in press). Contrary to tourism in the Arctic, Arctic tourism is more recent and has been growing significantly over the past 40 years in various Arctic destinations due to two phenomena, namely last-chance tourism (LCT) and Arctification (Lundmark et al., 2020). LCT refers to "the desire for tourists to witness vanishing landscapes or seascapes and disappearing species" (Lemelin et al., 2010, p. 477) and has been well conceptualized in the past 15 years, particularly in Polar tourism contexts (Lemelin & Whipp, 2019).

Arctification refers to the production of "particular representations of the North among consumers as well as industry and political stakeholders" (Carson, 2020, p. 6). In tourism, these representations lead to an intensification of stereotypical winter-based imaginaries and standardization of tourism products and experiences engaging with snow and ice (Varnajot & Saarinen, 2022). These stereotypical and standardized activities generally include dog- and reindeer-sledding, snowmobiling, ice-fishing and viewing northern lights (Saarinen & Varnajot, 2019). Viewing northern lights probably provides the most compelling example. Indeed, even if auroras can be observed in late summer and autumn in the southernmost parts of the Arctic, such as Finnish Lapland, they are often associated with snowy and icy landscapes in promotional materials (Herva et al., 2020). Arctification has also reached the accommodation sector. Snow- and ice-castles, and fields of glass igloos, have emerged in several popular Arctic destinations, particularly in the Nordic countries, but also outside the Arctic (e.g., Val Thorens, in the French Alps). While glass igloos draw from Inuit culture; snow- and ice-castles were originally developed through a Swedish initiative. Indeed, the Ice Hôtel of Jukkasjärvi was the first of its kind to have been developed as a tourist attraction where "the unique elements of the Arctic winter were regarded as an asset" (Hall et al., 2008, p. 241).

Besides the various implications for the construction and representations of Arctic tourism, Arctification also dictates adaptation strategies to the increasing lack of snow and ice due to global warming. Indeed, Arctification leads to reactive and technical strategies, mostly involving the production of artificial snow, snow farming, and even domed ski slopes, in order to cope with the lack of cryosphere and the increased climate variability (Varnajot & Lunden, in press). Overall, these strategies aim to make sure tourists' Arctic experiences meet their expectations that have been shaped by the global Arctification phenomenon. From an aesthetic perspective, the preservation strategies set in place to maintain cryospheric conditions can sometimes have an adverse effect than what is desired. Indeed, patches of snow stored under white gauze during summer, or corridors of snow spread on slopes while otherwise being surrounded by green and brown vegetation may, for the critical observer, be jarring. A vivid example of this is the ski resort of Levi, in Finnish Lapland. The resort recently built 'Finland's first glacier' (Snow-Forecast, 2022), using the latest technologies in snowmaking, snow farming, and high-tech insulation during the summer. Although the glacier is permanent, it is only accessible to skiers from early October to early May. These significant changes in the landscape induced by Arctification resonate with the changes in the local pond that led to Cunsolo's (2012) experience of ecological grief during her childhood. Furthermore, these alterations of the Arctic landscape also provide us with an illusion of control over increasing climate and seasonal variability.

The Darkness of the Anthropocene in Finnish Lapland

In recent years, the mourning for disappearing glaciers has become viral in the media and in public discussions, particularly following the mock funeral for Okjokül, an Icelandic glacier that officially vanished – died – in 2014, which was organized by anthropologists Cymene Howe and Dominic Boyer from Rice University (USA) in August 2019 (Árnason & Hafsteinsson, 2020; Varnajot, in press). A commemorative ceremony was organized and a plaque was installed where the glacier used to be, with a letter to the future inscribed on it (see also Bennett, 2020):

> *Ok is the first Icelandic glacier to lose its status as a glacier.*
> *In the next 200 years all our glaciers are expected to follow the same path.*
> *This monument is to acknowledge that we know*
> *what is happening and what needs to be done.*
> *Only you know if we did it.*

Interestingly, following this event for Okjokull, several commemorative ceremonies were organized for vanished – dead – glaciers, like in France, Switzerland, and Oregon (USA) (Varnajot & Salim, 2024). On the one hand, these funerals for other-than-human bodies clearly epitomize broader narratives of the death and ruination associated with climate change, shrinking cryosphere and the Anthropocene in general, and on the other hand, they also demonstrate increasing connections between dark tourism and slow-onset natural disasters such as climate change or the shrinking cryosphere (Varnajot & Saarinen, 2021).

In general, the loss of Earth's cryosphere – not just glaciers – has become an infamous symbol of climate change. In the Arctic, the seas that used to freeze in the winter increasingly remain ice-free all year round, while on land, previously snow-clad landscapes are becoming less so with every passing year. Winters are becoming shorter, lakes and rivers barely freeze, and in mountainous regions, glaciers are retreating, leaving only gray moraines behind (Kleber et al., 2023). The cryosphere is not only of immense ecological value; it is also of great spiritual, economic and aesthetic importance for many local communities (Hovelsrud et al., 2011). For example, glaciers are central to many cosmologies around the world such as in the Himalayas, the Andes or the Saint Elias Mountains in the Yukon (Allison, 2015; Cruikshank, 2012; Gagné et al., 2014). The cryosphere also provides economic opportunities. Indeed, glaciers provide water for electricity production, farming and irrigation (Carey et al., 2022), while also offering unique landscapes for tourism development (Varnajot & Salim, 2024). In Finnish Lapland, iconic white vistas have also become critical elements for both successful and fulfilling Arctic tourism experiences and economically viable winter seasons for tourism operators, communities and municipalities (Herva et al., 2020; Tervo-Kankare et al., 2013, 2018). This situation resonates with the notion of post-Arctic tourism, recently developed by Varnajot and Saarinen (2021, 2022). According to them, post-Arctic tourism is grounded in visions of dystopian and post-apocalyptic Arctic, further connecting with dark tourism.

Mahoney's work on LCT in Antarctica provides one example of the emerging discussion regarding the possibility of darkness in tourism experiences related to other-than-human loss (Mahoney, 2020; see also Dawson et al., 2011). Following this, Varnajot and Saarinen's (2022) claim that the doom and loss semantics associated with LCT embodies anxious narratives specifically related to the Anthropocene. In line with this, Lennon and Foley's (2000, p. 11) argument that dark tourism is an indication of post-modernism is especially relevant to note here, as it acknowledges that darkness in tourism emerges when "objects of tourism themselves appear to introduce anxiety and doubt about the project of modernity." In the context of tourism in Finnish Lapland, the project of modernity may refer to the lengths to which the mass tourism industry goes to maintain the Arctic image as we have come to know it, which in practice speaks to the variety of engineered and technical adaptation strategies put together to cope with the increasing lack of cryosphere. Thus, one could say that the darkness in Arctic tourism in Finnish Lapland refers not only to the more straightforward loss of its cryosphere but can also be understood in terms of the additive measures that have weirded the Arctic landscape in the stubborn efforts to desperately maintain snow and ice.

This leads to an ambivalent situation where the current environmental crisis (i.e., increasing lack of snow and ice) is largely hidden by artificial snow, influenced by Arctification. Indeed, the tourism industry is dedicated to representing Lapland as an otherworldly (cryospheric) amusement park – a glossy surface of a fantasyland. In reality, Lapland winter tourism has for years struggled with the uncertainty of snow availability, especially around the Christmas high tourist season when the presence of pristine snow is most expected (Tervo-Kankare, et al., 2013). With this in mind, the darkness of popular tourist destinations in Finnish Lapland (e.g., Rovaniemi, Levi, Ruka) rests not only in what is present and openly communicated in tourism promotion material but also, and perhaps in greater measure, in what is left unsaid and is actively glossed over. Perhaps in a conventional sense then, tourist destinations in Finnish Lapland would not necessarily qualify as sites of dark tourism per se, where a tragedy directly took place. However, when examined under a critical lens, these efforts to maintain the idea of Arctic tourism feed into a significant amount of dissonance and contested ideals (between the glossed Arctic and the dynamic reality of the region), which trickle into the territory of dark tourism.

For example, in November and early December 2018 – the beginning of the high tourist season in Lapland – the region faced a substantial lack of snow due to mild temperatures. Tourists felt dispirited and disappointed in this experience of a dark Lapland, to such an extent that British tabloids renamed the region 'Crapland' (Varnajot, 2020). In other words, tourists' expectations shaped by Arctification were not met. This incident acutely highlighted the unsustainable tension between manipulated images of the Arctic and climatic realities (see Varnajot & Saarinen, 2022), epitomizing both post-apocalyptic narratives (Varnajot & Saarinen, 2021) and monsters of the Anthropocene (Ulstein, 2017).

Indeed, the sight of snowless tourist destinations in Finnish Lapland may be understood as embodied dystopias, where dying white landscapes are becoming ruins of the Anthropocene, constituting what Bennett (2020, p. 921) terms an "Anthropocene gaze". This dystopic nature of these sites could also be seen as a so-called monster of the Anthropocene, as conceptualized by Latour (2011), and thus connecting Anthropocene issues such as the shrinking cryosphere, to the image of the monster, inspired by

Dr. Victor Frankenstein's monster in Mary Shelley's *Frankenstein*. However, similarly to Shelley's novel wherein one should not fear the monster itself but Frankenstein's negligence and abandonment of his creature, Latour warns us that "just like Dr. Frankenstein, humanity has turned away in dread, shame, and self-righteousness at the birth (and growth) of their own many-headed monsters: global climate change, deforestation, mass pollution, and species extinction (Ulstein, 2017, p. 73)". Ultimately, the Latourian monster is borne out of dominant modernist discourses that equate Science (with a capital S) with progress (Latour, 2011).

With perhaps Levi ski resort currently epitomizing this tendency the most in Finnish Lapland, the struggle to maintain a certain landscape identity is masked by narratives of technoscientific breakthrough and innovation: "Levi ski resort is developing in an unprecedented way" reads a headline from an update on their new artificial glacier, while promising that the new LED technology lighting the slopes will "produce the color of daylight while saving nature." This growing artificialization of Arctic landscapes, may therefore be epitomizing what we term 'Arctic traumascapes'.

Discussion: Dark tourism and Arctic traumascapes

In this context, these tourist destinations of Finnish Lapland may appear as Arctic traumascapes, where the expected white Arctic vistas are replaced by a simulacrum of cryosphere. Traumascapes have been defined as haunting places "where visible and invisible, past and present, physical and metaphysical come to coexist and share common space" (Tumarkin, 2019, p. 5). They are generally characterized as sites where traumatic events and tragedies took place or are ongoing (Tumarkin, 2005), and therefore, are opportunities for dark tourism development (Kaelber, 2007). For example, Varnajot and Salim (forthcoming) claim that sites of slow-onset disasters like vanishing glaciers can be understood as the death of the ice itself (see also Carey, 2007) and have become sites of dark tourism associated with other-than-human deaths. Similarly, in the context of Finnish Lapland, we argue that these sites where landscapes filled with patches of artificial snow that are slowly dominating over white winter landscapes are traumascapes in the making. In this case however, the feelings that feed into these landscapes as potential traumascapes appear when one realizes the shift between one's expectations and the reality of the Arctic, which is a direct consequence of anthropogenic climate change in the region combined with human activity trying to shield itself from said (unwanted) transformations.

The traumascapes found in Finnish Lapland resonate with Derrida's (1994) concept of hauntology. Indeed, these sites of mass tourism are neither dead nor alive, but in a state of in-betweenness, where the natural cryosphere – the white resource attracting tourists – is shrinking and slowly disappearing, but also still very much present thanks to the artificial snow resulting from adaptation strategies. It is important to note that hauntology in the Derridian sense has nothing to do with literal ghosts (Jameson, 1999): rather, these specters refer to a logic transcending all binary opposites such as the self and the other; the presence and absence; the visible and invisible; life and death; the being and nonbeing; or the real and unreal (Derrida & Stiegler, 1996; Harris, 2015).

Furthermore, an awareness of haunting reveals the inescapable troubles that are being reckoned with, it is "that moment [. . .] when things are not in their assigned places, when the cracks and the rigging are exposed, [. . .] when something else, or something different from before, feels like it must be done, and prompts a something-to-be-done" (Gordon, 2011, p. 2–3). In this framing, both trauma and haunting contain an awareness of distress; the difference lies in the clarity with which the specters raised by troubles make themselves visible, and consequently, how much this state of 'something to be done' is activated. Translated into the context of Finnish Lapland, sites that are bent on maintaining their cryospheres in the name of progress are in defensive mode driven by supposed mastery of nature: they are impacted by the effects of climate change, but they are operating based on repression by trying to ignore the issues it brings up until they are unavoidable. On the side of consumption, those who visit these sites in search of a never-ending winter wonderland are allowing themselves to be caught up in a mindset of cognitive dissonance where they separate themselves from the group of potential contributors to an ongoing problem, leaving those critical of such practices embittered by the lack of awareness exhibited by their fellow tourists who willingly subscribe to such fantasies.

Traumascapes linked to dark tourism, much like many forms of ecological grief or feelings of solastalgia, are particularly linked with place and place attachment (see Albrecht 2006; Martini & Buda, 2020). Generally, place attachment refers to "unique emotional experiences and bonds of people with places" (Altman & Low, 1992, p. 2). Sarah Ahmed's (2004, p. 11) insight that "what moves us, what makes us feel, is also that which holds us in place, or gives us a dwelling place," speaks to the highly dynamic ways in which feeling, emotion and affect are embedded into place. The notion that place attachment is such a personal journey may explain why to some, mass tourist sites in Finnish Lapland remain magical and enchanting, while to others, the same landscape can trigger opposite reactions. The lack of coherency in experience speaks to the confusing nature of dark tourism in the Arctic landscape; though it grows increasingly apparent that the landscape is laden with what could be seen as socio-ecological trauma, it is still not as straightforward as other, more universally accepted sites of dark heritage. More so, the study of Arctic traumascapes is critical since in the future, since affects and emotions related to place are different from tourists' and locals' perspectives (Kaltenborn & Williams, 2002). This is particularly relevant in the Arctic, wherein as the ice retreats, there is increased access to new resources, tourist sites and communities, potentially leading to conflicting views regarding the balance between the preservation and utilization of natural and cultural resources in tourism.

Ultimately, Arctic traumascapes appear where the Arctic landscape becomes a Derridean ghost: still there in tourists' expectations and in tourism promotion materials, but in practice, gone and replaced by a simulacrum, an artificial cryosphere. Arctic traumascapes may be sites of vanished glaciers like Okjokűll in Iceland, but also sites where the local tourism industry, municipalities, and actors in general desperately attempt to maintain a "cryospheric gaze", to use Varnajot's (2020, p. 67) words. On the whole, Arctic traumascapes represent our failures in the climate crisis. Traumascapes are "implicated in individual and collective processes of mourning, remembering, and making meaning of specific traumatic events and their legacies (Tumarkin, 2019, p. 4; see also Korstanje & George, 2017). In the context of Arctic traumascapes, Freud's (1957) distinction between mourning and melancholia may help us understand these dynamics further. As recalled by Ahmed (2004), for Freud, mourning is about 'letting go' of the lost object, it is a healthy response to loss, while melancholia is pathological. In a melancholic state, "the ego refuses to let go the object, and preserves the object 'inside itself'" (Ahmed, 2004, p. 159). Following this distinction, in Arctic traumascapes, adaptation strategies focusing on the lack of cryosphere led by processes of Arctification can be associated with a pathological melancholia, where local tourism actors refuse to let go of images of a past glorious Arctic landscape in tourism. In this sense, mourning ceremonies, and mourning in general, appear more ethical (Ahmed, 2004) as they would allow one to refocus on smarter and more responsible adaptation strategies to climate change that do not focus on the lack of cryosphere, but on more diverse Arctic meanings and representations (see Rantala et al., 2019).

That being said, dark tourism at sites of Arctic traumascapes does not have to be only about mourning the death of white vistas and glaciers, as that could lead to an unproductive cycle of perpetual mourning for what is lost. Indeed, dark tourism can also provide educational experiences (Cohen, 2011). As argued by Iliev (2021), a large number of tourists visit sites of dark tourism (including traumascapes) with the objective of learning and understanding what happened at the site. As such, Arctic traumascapes can become opportunities for educational dark tourism, for example, by inviting visitors to learn about climate change implications in the Arctic, but also about what can still be done to safeguard other vulnerable regions across the globe and potentially, to lead people to act more pro-environmentally (Varnajot, in press). The didactic value of Arctic traumascapes therefore may lie in constructing a delicate balance between lamenting the past, acknowledging present challenges, and looking forward to the future. Dark tourism at Arctic traumascapes can therefore transform places of mourning and grieving into places of action.

Conclusion: From dark tourism to dark heritage

The field of dark tourism thus far has mostly concentrated on examining the production and consumption of so-called dark heritage. One could say that all dark tourism contains an element of dark heritage, but not all dark heritage is necessarily explored in terms of (dark) tourism (Roberts & Stone, 2014; Timothy, 2021). Thinking about what makes heritage dark, therefore, adds another layer of understanding to most dark tourism sites. Additionally, the field of heritage, which is "intrinsically reflective of a relationship with the past," provides some insight into how temporality plays into the experience of darkness at certain tourist sites (Harvey, 2001, p. 327). Indeed, to have a constructive discussion about and sound conceptualization of Arctic traumascapes, it is crucial to account for the temporal implications of this notion, even if at first glance it seems more significantly tied to space and place. The passage of time adds context to changes happening in the Arctic, and it is by walking backwards and forwards in time that we can start to notice the changes that are inevitably occurring. The notion that temporality is, and always has been, moldable is a central assumption of the field of critical heritage studies (see Butler, 2006; Harvey, 2001; Smith, 2006).

Therefore, by concerning ourselves with the task of "troubling time", we start to learn how to "stay with the trouble" (Barad, 2017, p. 57; see also Haraway, 2010). When reflecting on the future of dark tourism, Lennon and Foley (2000) remind us that the crux of this sub-category of tourism lies in the understanding that the past is a set of discourses created by a dominant group for the consumption of another. In this chapter we suggest that the temporal element to this quandary can also be inverted while the problematics remain much the same: imagining futures is as much – if not more – a speculative undertaking as the process through which we imagine pasts. Through processes of Arctification, the future that is built up by those in charge of representing Arctic mass tourism sites presently serves to enchant and distract. However, when thinking about the *longue durée* (see Braudel & Wallerstein, 2009) of these sites, their artificially maintained cryospheric conditions are heavily incongruent with their projected fates. "Anthropogenic landscapes are also haunted by imagined futures. We are willing to turn things into rubble, destroy atmospheres, sell out companion species in exchange for dreamworlds of progress," write the editors of *Arts of Living on a Damaged Planet* (Gan et al., 2017, p. G2). Indeed, the darkness of Arctic traumascapes lies precisely in their potential for being haunted by their possible future selves. However, unlike Dickens' Ghost of Christmas Yet to Come, which offers the penny-pinching Scrooge an opportunity for redemption even before what would be lamentable events occur, the changing Arctic landscape seems to have no such luxury of such agency when thinking in terms of its future on a scale of deep-time.

What makes changing landscapes in light of the Anthropocene dark are their self-referentially looping temporalities that enable seemingly infinite possibilities, while at the same time restricting many of those possibilities through ongoing devastations. Pasley's (2022, p. 6) understanding of the Baradian (2010, 2017) concept of temporal im/

possibilities eloquently summarizes this layered conundrum; "pasts that have (not) happened and futures that might (never) be inhabit and coconstitute every moment. Temporality haunts itself." The notion of a haunted temporality becomes especially poignant in the context of the Anthropocene where we are living with the consequences of past transgressions while simultaneously having to reckon with the ghosts of potential futures precisely because of the pervasive presence of these pasts which trickles into present ways of being. Places especially hold tangible proof of these dynamics. In the words of Tumarkin (2005, p. 18), "traumascapes, after all, are precisely places that remind us that the past cannot simply be erased or, for that matter, simply reconstructed." This is echoed by contemporary archaeologist Þóra Pétursdóttir (2016, p. 182) who grounds this idea in the layered sediments of the earth: "the very reason we speak of the Anthropocene is not that we have lost connection with the past but rather that we increasingly are unable to pretend that it's gone. The problem is not that things become buried deep in strata but that they endure, outlive us, and come back at us with a force we didn't realize they had."

It can be said that the Arctic region Is home not only to the effects of Arctic amplification (see Rantanen et al., 2022), but also to the emergent socio-ecological issues in the face of climate change that are magnified at these sites, with the maintenance of certain cryospheric imaginaries epitomizing ongoing incongruencies in sustainability. As mentioned, Arctic traumascapes are currently in the making, and as such, one can only speculate the nature and extent of how these traumatic landscape identities will evolve in this region. Indeed, Arctic traumascapes are not necessarily a reminder of what has been, but rather, what is yet to come, which arguably is all the more terrifying for its lack of closure. For now, we are haunted by the possibilities projected by these landscapes' current state of being, knowing that change is, in fact, inevitable. At its core, the changing nature of Finnish Lapland has spiraled out of humankind's hands. However, Arctic traumascapes present us with the opportunity (or some would say the burden) of choice: to determine how this change is framed, interpreted and *lived within* the coming years.

References

Ahmed, S. (2004). *The Cultural Politics of Emotion*. Edinburgh University Press.

Albrecht, G. (2006). Solastalgia. *Alternatives Journal*, *32*(4–5), 34–36.

Allison, E.A. (2015). The spiritual significance of glaciers in an age of climate change. *Wiley Interdisciplinary Reviews: Climate Change*, *6*(5), 493–508.

Altman, I., & Low, S.M. (1992). *Place attachment*. Plenum Press.

Árnason, A., & Hafsteinsson, S.B. (2020). A funeral for a glacier: Mourning the more-than-human at the edge of modernity. *Thanatos*, *9*(2), 42–71.

Barad, K. (2010). Quantum entanglements and hauntological relations of inheritance. *Derrida Today*, *3*(2), 240–268.

Barad, K. (2017). Troubling time/s and ecologies in nothingness: Re-turning, re-membering, and facing the incalculable. *New Formations*, *92*(92), 56–86.

Bennett, M.M. (2020). Ruins of the Anthropocene: The aesthetics of Arctic climate change. *Annals of the American Association of Geographers*, *111*(3), 921–931.

Braudel, F., & Wallerstein, I. (2009). History and the social sciences: The longue durée. *Review (Fernand Braudel Center)*, *32*(2), 171–203.

Buck, H.J. (2015). On the possibilities of a charming Anthropocene. *Annals of the Association of American Geographers*, *105*(2), 369–377.

Butler, B. (2006). Heritage and the present past. In C. Tilley, W. Keane, S. Kuechler, M. Rowlands, & P. Spyer (Eds.), *Handbook of material culture* (pp. 463–479). Sage Publications.

Carey, M. (2007). The history of ice: How glaciers became an endangered species. *Environmental History*, *12*(3), 497–527.

Carey, M., Barton, J., & Flanzer, S. (2022). Glacier protection campaigns: What do they really save? In K. Dodds & S. Sörlin, (Eds.), *Ice humanities: Living, working, and thinking in a melting world* (pp. 89–109). Manchester University Press.

Carson, D. (2020). Urban tourism in the Arctic: A framework for comparison. In D.K. Müller, D.A. Carson, S. de la Barre, B. Granås, G.Þ. Jóhannesson, G. Øyen, O. Rantala, J. Saarinen, T. Salmela, K. Tervo-Kankare, & J. Welling (Eds.), *Arctic tourism in times of changes: Dimensions of urban tourism* (pp. 6–17). Nordic Council of Ministers.

Ceballos, G., Ehrlich, P.R., & Dirzo, R. (2017). Biological annihilation via the ongoing sixth mass extinction signaled by vertebrate population losses and declines. *Proceedings of the national academy of sciences*, *114*(30), 6089–6096.

Cohen, E.H. (2011) Educational dark tourism at an in populo site: The Holocaust Museum in Jerusalem. *Annals of Tourism Research*, *38*(1), 193–209.

Craps, S. (2023). Ecological mourning: Living with the loss in the Anthropocene. In B.A. Kaplan (Ed.), *Critical memory studies: New approaches* (pp. 69–77). Bloomsbury Academic.

Cruikshank, J. (2012). Are glaciers 'good to think with'? Recognising Indigenous environmental knowledge. *Anthropological Forum*, *22*(3), 239–250.

Cunsolo, A. (2012). Climate change as the work of mourning. *Ethics & the Environment*, *17*(2), 137–164.

Cunsolo, A., & Ellis, N.R. (2018). Ecological grief as a mental health response to climate change-related loss. *Nature Climate Change*, *8*(4), 275–281.

Dawson, J., Johnston, M.E., Stewart, E.J., Lemieux, C.J., Lemelin, R.J., Maher, P.T., & Grimwood, B.S.R. (2011). *Journal of Ecotourism*, *10*(3), 250–265.

Derrida, J. (1994). *Specters of Marx: The state of the debt, the work of mourning and the new international.* Routledge.

Derrida, J., & Stiegler, B. (1996). *Écographies de la television* [Echographies of television]. Galilée.

Dodds, K. (2018). *Ice: Nature and culture*. Reaktion Books.

Freud, S. (1957). Mourning and melancholia. In J. Rickman (Ed.), A general selection from the works of Sigmund Freud (pp. 124–140). Doubleday.

Gagné, K., Rasmussen, M.B., & Orlove, B. (2014). Glaciers and society: Attributions, perceptions, and valuations. *Wiley Interdisciplinary Reviews: Climate Change*, *5*(6), 793–808.

Gan, E., Tsing, A., Swanson, H., & Bubandt, N. (2017). Introduction: Haunted landscapes of the Anthropocene. In A. Tsing, H. Swanson, E. Gan., & N. Bubandt. (Eds.), *Arts of living on a damaged planet: Ghosts of the Anthropocene* (pp. G1–G16). University of Minnesota Press.

Gordon, A.F. (2011). Some thoughts on haunting and futurity. *Borderlands*, *10*(2), 1–21.

Gren, M., & Huijbens, E.H. (2019). Tourism geography in and of the Anthropocene. In D.K. Müller (Ed.), *A research agenda for tourism geographies* (pp. 117–127). Edward Edgar Publishing.

Hall, C.M., & Johnston, M.E. (1995). *Polar tourism: tourism in the Arctic and Antarctic regions*. Wiley.

Hall, C.M., Müller, D.K., & Saarinen, J. (2008). *Nordic tourism: Issues and cases*. Channel View Publications.

Haraway, D. (2010). When species meet: Staying with the trouble. *Environment and Planning D: Society and Space 28*, 53–55.

Harris, V. (2015). Hauntology, archivy and banditry: An engagement with Derrida and Zapiro. *Critical Arts, 29*(1), 13–27.

Harvey, D.C. (2001). Heritage pasts and heritage presents: Temporality, meaning and the scope of heritage studies. *International journal of heritage studies, 7*(4), 319–338.

Herva, V.-P., Varnajot, A., & Pashkevich, A. (2020). Bad Santa: Cultural heritage, mystification of the Arctic, and tourism as an extractive industry. *The Polar Journal, 10*(2), 375–396.

Hovelsrud, G.K., Poppel, B., Van Oort, B., & Reist, J.D. (2011). Arctic societies, cultures, and peoples in a changing cryosphere. *Ambio, 40*, 100–110.

Huijbens, E.H. (2021). The emerging earths of climatic emergencies: On the island geography of life in modernity's ruins. *Geografiska Annaler: Series B, Human Geography, 103*(2), 88–102.

Iliev, D. (2021). Consumption, motivation and experience in dark tourism: A conceptual and critical analysis. *Tourism Geographies, 23*(5–6), 963–984.

Jameson, F. (1999). Marx's purloined letter. In M. Sprinker (Ed.), *Ghoslty demarcations: A symposium on Jacques Derrida's Spectres de Marx* (pp. 26–67). Verso.

Kaelber, L. (2007). A memorial as virtual traumascape: Darkest tourism in 3D and cyber-space to the gas chambers of Auschwitz. *E-Review of Tourism Research, 5*(2), 24–33.

Kaltenborn, B.P., & Williams, D.R. (2002). The meaning of place: Attachments to Femundsmarka National Park, Norway, among tourists and locals. *Norsk Geografisk Tidsskrift, 56*(3), 189–198.

Kleber, G.E., Hodson, A.J., Magerl, L. Schytt Mannerfelt, E., Bradbury, H.J., Zhu, Y., Trimmer, M., & Turchyn, A.V. (2023). Groundwater springs formed during glacial retreat are a large source of methane in the high Arctic. *Nature Geoscience, 16*, 597–604.

Korstanje, M., & George, B. (2017). *Virtual traumascapes and exploring the roots of dark tourism*. IGI global.

Latour, B. (2011). Love your monsters. In M. Shellenberger, & T. Nordhaus (Eds.), *Love your monsters: Postenvironmentalism and the Anthropocene* (pp. 21–44). The Breakthrough Institute.

Lemelin, H., Dawson, J., Stewart, E.J., Maher, P.T., & Lueck, M. (2010). Last-chance tourism: The boom, doom, and gloom of visiting vanishing destinations. *Current Issues in Tourism, 13*(5), 477–493.

Lemelin, R.H., & Whipp, P. (2019). Last chance tourism: A decade in review. In D.J. Timothy (Ed.), Handbook of globalization and tourism (pp. 316–322). Edward Elgar Publishing.

Lennon, J., & Foley, M. (2000) *Dark tourism: The attraction of death and disaster*. Continuum.

Levi. (n.d.). Retrieved from https://www.levi.fi/en/news-and-stories/levi-ski-resort-is-developing-in-an-unprecedented-way

Lewicka, M. (2010). What makes neighborhood different from home and city? Effects of place scale on place attachment. *Journal of Environmental Psychology, 30*(1), 35–51.

Light, D. (2017). Progress on dark tourism and thanatourism research: An uneasy relationship with heritage tourism. *Tourism Management 61*, 275–301.

Lundmark, L., Müller, D.K., & Bohn, D. (2020). Arctification and the paradox of overtourism in sparsely populated areas. In L. Lundmark, D.B. Carson, & M. Eimermann (Eds.), Dipping in to the north: Living, working and traveling in sparsely populated areas (pp. 349–372). Palgrave Macmillan.

Maher, P.T., Gelter, H., Hillmer-Pegram, K., Hovgaard, G., Hull, J., Jóhannesson, G.Þ., Karlsdóttir, A., Rantala, O., & Pashkevich, A. (2014). Arctic tourism: Realities and possibilities. In L. Heininen, H. Exner-Pirot, & J. Plouffe (Eds.), *Arctic yearbook 2014* (pp. 290–306). Northern Research Forum.

Mahoney, S.P. (2020). Behold, the horror of man: Dark tourism in the Anthropocene. *Journal of Tourism and Leisure Studies, 5*(2), 1–18.

Mallett, S. (2004). Understanding home: A critical review of the literature. *The Sociological Review, 52*(1), 62–89.

Martini, A., & Buda, D.M. (2020). Dark tourism and affect: Framing places of death and disaster. *Current Issues in Tourism, 23*(6), 679–692.

Pasley, A. (2022) Trans Im/Possibilities. In L. Allen & M.L. Rasmussen (Eds.) *The Palgrave encyclopedia of sexuality education* (pp. 1–13). Springer Nature.

Pedersen, K., & Viken, A. (1996). From Sami nomadism to global tourism. In M.F. Price & V.L. Smith (Eds.), *People and tourism in fragile environments* (pp. 69–88). Wiley.

Pétursdóttir, Þóra. (2016) Climate change? Archaeology and Anthropocene. *Archaeological Dialogues, 24*(2), 175–205.

Rantala, O., de la Barre, S., Granås, B., Jóhannesson, G.Þ., Müller, D.K., Saarinen, J., Tervo-Kankare, K., Maher, P.T., & Niskala, M. (2019). *Arctic tourism in times of change: Seasonality*. Nordic Council of Ministers.

Rantanen, M., Karpechko, A.Y., Lipponen, A., Nordling, K., Hyvärinen, O., Ruosteenoja, K., Vihma, T., & Laaksonen, A. (2022). The Arctic has warmed nearly four times faster than the globe since 1979. *Communications Earth & Environment, 3*(1), 168.

Roberts, C., & Stone, P.R. (2014) Dark tourism and dark heritage: Emergent themes, issues and consequences (pp. 9–18). In I. Convery, G. Corsane & P. Davis (Eds.) *Displaces heritage: Dealing with disaster and suffering*. Boydell Press.

Rucinska, D. (2016). Natural disaster tourism as a type of dark tourism. *International Journal of Humanities and Social Sciences, 10*(5), 1458–1462.

Saarinen, J., & Varnajot, A. (2019). The Arctic in tourism: Complementing and contesting perspectives on tourism in the Arctic. *Polar Geography, 42*(2), 109–124.

Sideris, L.H. (2020). Grave reminders: Grief and vulnerability in the anthropocene. Religions, 11(6), 293.

Smith, L. (2006). *Uses of heritage*. Routledge.

Sörlin, S. (2015). Cryo-history: Narratives of ice and the emerging Arctic humanities. In B. Evengård, J. Nymand Larsen & Ø. Paasche (Eds.), *The New Arctic* (pp. 327–339). Springer.

Snow-Forecast (2022, February 11). Finnish resort to create glacier for skiers. Retrieved from https://www.snow-forecast.com/whiteroom/finnish-resort-to-create-glacier-for-skiers/

Steffen, W., Broadgate, W., Deutsch, L., Gaffney, O., & Ludwig, C. (2015). The trajectory of the Anthropocene: The great acceleration. *The Anthropocene Review, 2*(1), 81–98.

Steffen, W., Grinevald, J., Crutzen, P., & McNeill, J. (2011). The Anthropocene: Conceptual and historical perspectives. *Philosophical Transactions of the Royal Society A, 369*(1938), 842–867.

Stone, P.R. (2006). A dark tourism spectrum: Towards a typology of death and macabre related tourist sites, attractions and exhibitions. *Tourism: An International Interdisciplinary Journal, 54*(2), 145–160.

Stone, P., & Sharpley, R. (2008). Consuming dark tourism: A thanatological perspective. *Annals of Tourism Research, 35*(2), 574–595.

Sutton, P.C., Anderson, S.J., Costanza, R., & Kubiszewski, I. (2016). The ecological economics of land degradation: Impacts on ecosystem service values. *Ecological Economics, 129*, 182–192.

Tervo-Kankare, K., Hall, C.M., & Saarinen, J. (2013). Christmas tourists' perceptions to climate change in Rovaniemi, Finland. *Tourism Geographies, 15*(2), 292–317.

Tervo-Kankare, K., Hall, C.M., & Saarinen, J. (2018). Costs and benefits of environmental change: Tourism industry's responses in Arctic Finland. *Tourism Geographies, 20*(2), 202–223.

Timothy, D.J. (2021). *Cultural Heritage and Tourism: An Introduction*, 2nd Edn . Channel View Publications.

Tumarkin, M. (2005). *Traumascapes: The power and fate of places transformed by tragedy*. Melbourne University Press.

Tumarkin, M. (2019). Twenty years of thinking about traumascapes. *Fabrications, 29*(1), 4–20.

Ulstein, G. (2017). Brave new weird: Anthropocene monsters in Jeff VanderMeer's "The Southern Reach". *Concentric-Literary and Cultural Studies, 43*(1), 71–96.

United Nations Office for Disaster Risk Reduction. (n.d.). *Disaster*. Retrieved from https://www.undrr.org/terminology/disaster

Varnajot, A. (2020). Rethinking Arctic tourism: Tourists' practices and perceptions of the Arctic in Rovaniemi. *Nordia Geographical Publications, 49*(4), 1–108.

Varnajot, A. (2024). ENlightening dark tourism horizons in a post-apocalyptic Arctic: a geopoetics' approach. In P.R. Stone & D.W.M. Wright (Eds.), The future of dark tourism: Enlightening new horizons (pp. 129–137). Channel View Publications.

Varnajot, A., & Lunden, A. (in press). The short-term future of Arctic tourism: The complexity of seasonal uncertainties for nature-based tourism. In. F. Kock, A. Lindgreen & S. Markovic (Eds.), *Research handbook on tourism, complexity and uncertainty*. Edward Elgar Publishing.

Varnajot, A., & Saarinen, J. (2021). 'After glaciers?' Towards post-Arctic tourism. *Annals of Tourism Research, 91*, 103205.

Varnajot, A., & Saarinen, J. (2022). Emerging post-Arctic tourism in the age of Anthropocene: Case Finnish Lapland. *Scandinavian Journal of Hospitality and Tourism, 22*(4–5), 357–371.

Varnajot, A., & Salim, E. (2024). The hauntology of climate change: glacier retreat and dark tourism. *Tourism Geographies*, 1–18.

Westoby, R., McNamara, K.E., & Clissold, R. (2022). Ways of healing in the Anthropocene. *Climate and Development, 14*(1), 67–74.

Wright, D., & Sharpley, R. (2018). Local community perceptions of disaster tourism: The case of L'Aquila, Italy. *Current Issues in Tourism, 21*(14), 1569–1585.

Alena Pirok

9 "Despicable and disgusting": Emotional labor, and the fear of dark tourism

Abstract: In the early 1990s the historical city of Williamsburg, Virginia entered a period of interpretive change, both in the formal institution that called the city home, Colonial Williamsburg, and in the many small local tour businesses that depended on it. Most notably both entities began to embrace what is now called "dark tourism" offerings, witch and pirate trials, mock hangings, ghost tours, and a slave auction. This chapter will focus on the last two: the ghost tours and the slave auction and illustrate how commodification transformed reality into darkness, and the intentionally dark into an ataractic. Colonial Williamsburg's slave auction was one program within a larger effort by the museum's African American Interpretation Program to address the reality of race and class that the interpreters, and scholars, felt was missing from the institution's predominantly elite white presentation of eighteenth-century Virginia life. These new offerings challenged white visitors who felt that the narrative of slavery sullied the celebration of the United States' intellectual foundations. The Black community expressed a measured acceptance of the new African American cultural programs but found the all-too-realistic presentation of a slave auction inside of the increasingly commercial historical site to be wildly inappropriate. By the end of 1994, it was clear that the reality of slavery was too dark for the American audience.

At the same time, Colonial Williamsburg's interpretive staff were challenging their day-time guests to look directly at eighteenth-century life, private tour companies began offering night-time ghost tours that promised hidden or alternative histories but delivered the familiar, overwhelmingly white, consensus history that the museum's interpreters sought to challenge. In practice, the ghost tours offered guests a way to engage with the eighteenth century under the guise of rebellious dark tourism, without having to face the history that day-time audiences found to be too dark to truly engage with. When placed together the public outcry before, during, and after the mock slave auction, and the popularity of the ghost tours highlight the inherent darkness of critical historical interpretation, and the lightness, or pacifying nature of what is more often deemed dark tourism.

Keywords: dark tourism, emotional labor, slavery, difficult heritage, historical analysis

https://doi.org/10.1515/9783110792072-010

Introduction

In 1993, Colonial Williamsburg's interpretive staff staged a re-creation of an eighteenth-century estate sale. The auction, true to the period, offered up the deceased's real, animal, and human property to pay down debts. The interpreters who planned the event knew that portraying the auction of enslaved people would challenge their audience, but they felt that the re-created event was incomplete, borderline dishonest, if it was scrubbed clean of the emotional horrors of slavery. The institution had previously portrayed difficult life events without issue, and the interpreters did not anticipate negative reactions beyond the bigots who always showed up to mock their work. Most importantly, they had not envisioned a world where the audience would accuse them of mishandling the past. They undertook their work fearlessly but had not considered their audience's perception of the event within the context of an increasingly commercialized institution. Much to the interpreters' surprise, hundreds of protestors converged in Williamsburg to stop the performance. They feared that the slave auction was the institution's attempt to separate gawkers from their money by offering them a glimpse into historical human misery. The people who came to Colonial Williamsburg that day did not have the words to describe what they saw or how they interpreted the 1993 event, but today's scholars would have called it dark tourism.

Colonial Williamsburg's slave auction happened two years before Malcolm Foley and J. John Lennon began to define the category of 'dark tourism', but guests' reactions to the slave auction illustrated a fear, well known to museum professionals today, of commercialism and profit infiltrating educational institutions and a blurring of the distinctions between the two (Foley & Lennon, 1996a). Using a critical historical perspective and testing the concept of dark tourism against this case study, within its historical context, and with a consideration of emotional labor clarifies the concept of dark tourism and reinforces that, in the world of educational institutions, dark tourism is more of a professional fear, than a reality.

More so than in other cases, Colonial Williamsburg's 1993 slave auction illustrates how the public's fear of commercial darkness and historical sites' embrace of difficult histories created what looked like dark tourism developing in an arena where it was powerfully unwelcomed. Situated within its historical context, the case study shows how audience members, as well as Foley and Lennon, mistakenly merged two parallel developments: the increased commercialization at historical sites of the 1990s and public history workers' investment of emotional labor into realistic portrayals of the past, together. Hindsight, and an appreciation for public history's emotional labor, help to unbraid these two movements, illustrating that for professionally curated historical sites, the two did not merge to produce dark tourism, but rather their relative closeness created a fear of dark tourism. This chapter seeks to place dark tourism in its 1990s historical context and offers the story of the slave auction to illustrate how the parallel movements' proximity in Williamsburg created the fear of dark tourism that scholars and professionals have today. In doing so, it offers a vision of dark tourism analysis situated in a historical context that takes public history professionals' motives and emotional labor seriously and provides a tool to differentiate emotionally evocative professional interpretation from dark tourism.

Historical origins of dark tourism

Observing Colonial Williamsburg it is not hard to find the darkness of dark tourism. The prevalence of slavery in the eighteenth-century colony easily qualifies Williamsburg, Virginia, as a potential site of "heritage and atrocity." Foley and Lennon's link between simulations and the development of dark tourism can be applied to Colonial Williamsburg's emotionally evocative first-person interpreters (Foley & Lennon, 1996a; Pirok, 2022, p. 137, 146). It is likewise easy to place Colonial Williamsburg, with its slave auction, court cases, gaol, stocks and pillory, cemetery, and ghost tours into Philip R. Stone's dark tourism spectrum (Stone, 2006; Pirok, 2022, p. 179). However, Lennon and Foley (1996b) made an important distinction in their early work on dark tourism explaining that the central qualifier for dark tourism was not darkness itself but commercial gain.

Exploring the commercialisation or profit motivation in seemingly not-for-profit cultural products was a common scholarly project in the 1990s but failed to provide evidence that professional historical sites had abandoned their academic goals for commercial profits (Carson, 1994). The projects were attempts to exorcise, through exposure, how politics and profit had shaped the way the past was presented to the public (Linenthal & Engelhardt, 1996; Wallace, 1996; Handler & Gable, 1997). It began with a controversy over national history education standards in 1994, that super-charged conservative historical orthodoxy into a powerful political tool (Nash et. al., 2000). As the standards were abandoned, the critical focus turned to museums and historical sites, centering around the Smithsonian's exhibition of The Enola Gay, the plane that dropped the first atomic bomb on Japan (Nash et. al., 2000; Linenthal & Engelhardt, 1996). In each case, critical examinations of the past, and acceptance of historical wrongdoings were labeled as dangerous and threatening by those on the political right.

The matter moved into the popular arena when the Disney corporation stepped directly, and seemingly unknowingly, into the controversy proposing to open a history-themed amusement park on a Civil War battlefield south of Washington, DC. Seeking to avoid claims of sanitizing history from the political left, representatives of the entertainment monopoly promised to "not whitewash history or ignore blemishes" but rather "tell the dark points" of the past by making guests into Civil War soldiers, or having them "feel what slavery was like" in the antebellum south (Synnott, 1995, p. 52). Scholars and members of the public alike found these promises distressing and insensitive.

Faced with the powerful Disney corporation representing itself as a historical authority, scholars redoubled their efforts to protect and affirm their academic credibility and eagerly condemned the influence of profit motive in education. Some, like James Oliver Horton, sought to do both – urging fellow scholars to engage with the history-for-profit world to correct and steer their presentations of the past (Synnott, 1995, p. 57). Others, like Mike Wallace, presented readers with a deeper exploration of the inaccurate and politically powerful heroic myths of US history (Wallace, 1996), while anthropologists Richard Handler and Eric Gable famously battled with Vice President of Research Cary Carson over the extent to which Colonial Williamsburg employees were victims of corporatization or members of an appropriately stratified educational team (Carson, 1995; Handler & Gable, 1997).

Unpacking the complex reality of professionalism, accuracy, and historical truth in an increasingly political and profit-driven world was popular among historians but was largely lost in Lennon and Foley's exploration of historical sites. Rather, their work on sites associated with former US president John F. Kennedy read the "project directors, managers and curators" descriptions of their work as ingenuine (Foley & Lennon, 1996b, p. 210). "What appears more likely," they assumed, in contradiction to the museum workers' assertion, was that the group had "manipulated" the past towards a "tourism/leisure orientation" (Foley & Lennon, 1996b, p. 210).

The pair's method of evaluating historical sites as "more likely" profit motivated, disregarded museum professionals' stated goals, allowing the researchers to read dark tourism's commercial goals into educational institutions and opening the door for other tourism scholars to do the same (Sharply & Stone, 2009; Tinson, et. al., 2015; Fernandes & Jamadagni, 2018; Hartmann, 2013). Omitting curatorial staff members' efforts towards education discounts larger trends of the period, and the emotional labor that public history professionals performed in creating sensitive exhibitions about difficult topics (Oren & Shani, 2012; Martini & Buda, 2020; Tyson, 2013; Tyson, 2008; Waller & Costen, 2012; Welch, 2015). Though the presence of emotional labor does not completely disqualify something from being profit-driven, the consideration of workers' motivations and labors reveals a depth to sites that are easily seen as shallow commercial products and offer a clear delineation between emotionally evocative professional interpretations and dark tourism.

Enter Williamsburg

Colonial Williamsburg is a nationally famous and well-respected educational institution built around the twentieth-century restoration of an eighteenth-century city. The restoration was the brainchild of a local church leader, the reverend W.A.R. Goodwin, who by 1926 had convinced John D. Rockefeller Jr, the son of the wealthiest man in the United States, to purchase the city's old properties and pay for their academically informed restoration (Greenspan, 2009). The project continued throughout the twentieth century and into the twenty-first and now includes 89 original eighteenth-century buildings and hundreds of recreated period structures.

Colonial Williamsburg’s dedication to creating academically informed restorations and recreations included its employees’ research within the larger university-based academic discussions about eighteenth-century North America’s material culture and intellectual writings and made its interpretive experiments models for sites across the United States (Pirok, 2022). In many ways, Colonial Williamsburg of the twentieth century mirrored a university, or the original seventeenth-century museum-as-knowledge-creator model (Bennett, 2004). The institution was careful to protect its educational efforts from its for-profit efforts, and by the mid-twentieth century, the institution had two distinct parts: one a for-profit entity with restaurants and hotels, and the other the original not-for-profit restoration and educational institution.

The twin institution enjoyed a healthy visitor population in the years after World War Two but saw a massive decline in the 1970s (Pirok, 2022). Since then, Colonial Williamsburg’s popularity has risen and fallen alongside the United States’ economic fortunes. The institution saw an increase in guests in the 1990s that coincided with significant interpretive and commercial shifts (Pirok, 2022). These shifts can be seen as efforts to simply regain and remake the restoration’s audience, but that overlooks the internal dynamics at play in this diverse institution. At the same time the for-profit end of the institution attempted to re-make itself into something attractive to vacation-minded guests, employees on the not-for-profit end doubled their efforts to maintain the institution’s educational mission by developing more honest portrayals of the past and deepening their interpretation of emotional power (Pirok, 2022).

In the late 1980s and early 1990s, the institution’s interpretive shifts amounted to an embrace of what was known in historical scholarship as the social history turn. This was a new way of looking at primary source documents that had become popular in academic circles during the 1950s and 1960s. This technique used statistics as historical data and alternative reading methods to highlight the contributions of those who left sparse written records (Appleby, 1998; Bienstock, 1995; Degler, 1980; Gallman, 1977; Moore, 1996). This new method also encouraged scholars to look to contemporary identity groups as sources of information about the past. It was during this time that oral history and folklore research were incorporated into the pantheon of historical sources (Atalay, 2012; Blakey, 1997; Marshell, 2002). These efforts enabled scholars to maintain historical methods while recognizing African Americans, women, immigrants, and ordinary laborers’ contributions to the social, cultural, and economic realities of the past, in ways they had not done before.

The public history world of museums and historical sites embraced this shift a decade later in the 1970s. While arguably late, this shift significantly changed the past that the public interacted with at historical sites. Since the early days of formalized historical tourism in the United States, in the late 1800s, travelers could expect the sites marketed as historical to be shrine-like places of national devotion (Wallace,

1996). Monuments, lovingly restored homes, and memorials recalled simple, often mythic, stories of a heroic American past. Guests were to understand themselves as the proud inheritors of greatness. However, the world and scholarship were changing. The events of the 1960s and the early 1970s, including the Civil Rights Movement, the harsh law and order policies that followed, the war in Vietnam, and the shameful end of the Nixon presidency, exposed inequalities, and deceits within the United States system of governance that challenged the heroic narrative that most historical sites offered (Wallace, 1996).

In response, groups began establishing new sites, like Bootts Mills, which focused on industrial labor, The Angel Island Immigration Station, and the African American Museum of Philadelphia. For many guests, this was the first time they saw people of their race or class celebrated in historical sites. Then, and what concerns this chapter, established historical sites began to think critically about presenting a heroic narrative of the past and expanded their stories to include more complex, and often negative aspects of common people's lives. Topics like injustice, illness, and abuse, were now spoken of in places where only bravery, genius, and hard work had been spoken of before. From this historical vantage point, it is not hard to see where Foley and Lennon were coming from when they observed late twentieth-century sites and described them as "dark tourism," and why historians are deeply uncomfortable with the label.

At Colonial Williamsburg, interpreters aimed not to create dark tourism but to talk accurately about the eighteenth-century residents who lived outside of privilege (Handler & Gable, 1997). The new stories centered on free and enslaved laborers and necessitated engagement with a vision of the past that was grittier than the triumphant revolutionary narrative. Colonial Williamsburg began offering tours like "The Other Half," which focused on enslaved people's lives, their relationship with their enslavers, how their lives differed from free residents and how they sought to push back against abuses (Devlin, 2003, p. 128). Without actively trying to do so, Colonial Williamsburg's embrace of social history brought what guests perceived as, and what later scholars would call, dark tourism to the city.

Of course, Colonial Williamsburg was not the first to pioneer the idea of presenting a vision of the past with all its warts. Plimoth Plantation, now called Plimoth Patuxet Museums, in Massachusetts, USA, was the first to truly embrace the idea of reality no matter how messy. This site was built in 1947 to represent the seventeenth-century English North American settlement of Plimoth. In the 1970s, James Deetz, the assistant director, implemented a new interpretive model that embraced learning and teaching about colonial-era material culture by reproducing them with modern hands, often wearing historical costumes (Rymsza-Pawlowska, 2019). In practice, the interpreters at Plimoth were barefoot, scraggly bearded, and walking through mucky dirt as creatures of all kinds crossed paths and comingled. Guests got to see interpreters do the labor of seventeenth-century English colonists, in an accurate environment. It was not an environment that twentieth-century guests were accustomed to. The interpreters smelled, the site smelled, and one could not avoid getting dirty. Plimoth achieved something accurate and new but learned that guests found *actual* historical realities too distracting. It was certainly not what any scholar would call dark tourism, but it was unpleasant and challenging.

As an educational institution, darkness was never Colonial Williamsburg's intention. The preexisting narrative's effervescent lightness, however, made any realistic recognition of life in the colonial era seem like consumerist macabre by comparison. It was in this context that Colonial Williamsburg began its celebrated first-person interpretive program that sought to "dramatize" the "life and trauma of colonial times" ("News Presented in Brief from All Corners," 1979). This was achieved by having interpreters not only wear period clothing but also adopt well-researched eighteenth-century identities and perform interactive skits. They used primary source materials from the eighteenth century to develop accurate "enactments" that they would perform around the restored buildings ("News Presented in Brief from All Corners,"1979). The performers' goal was not to create dark events but to offer human "insights into 18th-century attitudes, problems, and opinions," joys *and* suffering.

The interpreters could not maintain a celebratory tone when considering the lives of the marginalized residents of the English North American colonies. For most people in eighteenth-century North America, life was unpleasant and filled with suffering. Of the English population in Williamsburg alone over 50% were non-landowners, subject to employer and property owner whims, poverty, the elements, and illness (Lawson, 1995, p. ix). Life stories, though some dotted with triumph and success, were dominated by crushing defeat and created the kinds of tales that contemporary parlance would call "sad" or "dark."

General guest happiness was not a major concern for Colonial Williamsburg before the 1980s, so these early displeasures felt small. The institution was focused on creating an accurate historical environment, interpreted by firm but friendly guides. This changed in the 1980s. Guest engagement and happiness became a critical issue for Colonial Williamsburg and hundreds of other sites throughout the United States after President Ronald Reagan cut the federal funding that many historical sites had depended on to maintain their educational missions (Wallace, 1996). Now that ticket sales were key to sustainability, sites began to assess their offerings in terms of guest satisfaction, some looking to successful commercial offerings for guidance.

In Colonial Williamsburg, the two ends of the institution met the challenge in vastly different ways. The for-profit hospitality-focused departments began advertising the institution as a site for family fun. Offering tours based on American Girl Dolls, and pirate trials (Evans 1991; "Williamsburg Welcoming in Autumn," 1988). The not-for-profit employees sought to attract guests by offering them more realistic and diverse presentations of the past. They doubled down on their educational mission and their dedication to presenting a serious and realistic recreation of the past. This stood in stark contrast to the world of fun that the for-profit end of the institution presented. More so than the years before, Colonial Williamsburg's public history employees were open and honest that the eighteenth century was not *fun* for most people. Making matters more challenging, most guests did not know, or understand, that Colonial Williamsburg was two entities. The combination of commercialism and serious historical reality shared close quarters, creating something guests found suspiciously unappealing – something later scholars would easily label as dark tourism.

The slave auction

No other department within Colonial Williamsburg brought the challenging reality of the past to life at this time like the African American Interpretation Program. Colonial Williamsburg launched the African American Interpretation Program (AAIP) in 1979, the same year they created the broader first-person interpretation program, to produce programing that focused on the lives of eighteenth-century African Americans, and to provide a supportive network for Black interpreters who would invariably be performing as enslaved people (Horton and Horton, 2008; Handler and Gable, 1997). The issues of interpreting slavery as first-person performers were obvious from the beginning. Only a few decades outside of the Jim Crow era, many white guests took the opportunity to verbally assault Black interpreters under a thin guise of using historically accurate language (Pirok, 2022, p. 167). Using historical authenticity as a justification for abusive language was common at historical sites as Horowitz (1999) illustrated at historical reenactments. The creation of the AAIP sought to acknowledge that enslavement was a significantly challenging emotional experience for Black interpreters to present to the museum's audience.

In the early years of the program, interpreters moved forward with caution. The scenes they produced focused on moments of everyday life to highlight the humanity that twentieth-century guests and eighteenth-century enslaved people shared. One of the first performances dramatized a Black overseer coming home to his enslaved wife with conflicted feelings about having beaten a fellow enslaved man for trying to run away ("Combined Talents Create Scenes of Black History," 1980). The performance sought to tackle issues of class within Williamsburg's enslaved population while illustrating that the conflicts of enslaved life included things as simple and universally shared as conversations with partners about ethics and workplace concerns. The AAIP's most popular events, however, were the music programs. Interpreters invited guests to join drum circles, sometimes asking them to take up instruments to experience the music firsthand, and to learn about the community bonds that enslaved people created through "gahu" music ("Colonial Williamsburg's Forgotten Half," 1990; Lawson, 1996, p. 128). These events, both music and otherwise, did not challenge guests. At the most intense, first-person interpreters would express concern about their enslaver selling them or their children or having witnessed a beating, but these scenes were never played out in front of an audience and remained worries or stories, rather than visual realities.

The generally uplifting nature of the music programs should not be understood as a failure to present the past accurately as thoughtfully presenting the pain of slavery is a challenge. Events like the drum circle allowed interpreters to highlight enslaved people's humanity, without having to enact or relive, their enslavers' dehumanization. As senior interpreter Rex Ellis put it; "nobody enjoy[ed] being a slave" ("Combined Talents Create Scenes of Black History," 1980). The AAIP offered African Americans respected, titled positions within an institution that had only hired Black Americans for kitchen and animal husbandry jobs since the 1930s. But the cost was extraordinarily steep. On top of the job's personal and emotional demand to perform as enslaved people, the audiences at the museum were, at times, maliciously cruel. One interpreter recalled that white guests would ask bad faith questions like "slavery isn't so bad, is it," or call female interpreters "Aunt Jemima" or ask them to make demeaning poses in cotton fields for photographs (Jacobs, 2019; Howard, 1995). Some would even use foul language to degrade them asking questions like "how it feels to be an n*****?" ("Combined Talents Create Scenes of Black History," 1980). It was a deeply emotionally challenging job.

The guests' cruel intentions to mock the interpreters' performances and the emotional labor they undertook to present the programing made the truly painful history that they were portraying a real part of their own lives. Even if they wanted to focus on the humanity that enslaved people made for themselves, popular racism in the contemporary United States reminded the workers, and the non-hostile guests, how and why the subject of slavery remained an uncomfortable topic for most Americans.

Despite the abuses that African American interpreters faced from malicious guests, most guests were interested and respectful. Interpreter Shomer Zwelling expressed many of their colleagues' sentiments when they explained in the early 1990s that the "audience was ready" to "understand suffering and living in an uncertain world" ("Combined Talents Create Scenes of Black History," 1980). Far from being an effort to commoditize past people's suffering, as Zwelling explained, interpreters sought to connect personally with the people of the past and bring that shared humanity to their guests.

One of the first controversial programs that the AAIP put together dealt with enslaved marriage, and a white landowner impregnating an enslaved woman ("Slave Auction to Be Re-Enacted," 1994). These programs were carefully crafted by researchers who spent years putting together scenes based on eighteenth-century records and modern historical studies (Pirok, 2022). These programs challenged guests to think about how the legal category of slavery shaped Black Williamsburgers' working and intimate lives. In doing this they brought complication and agency to the image of enslaved Americans. These programs were launched without conflict. Even the program that focused on the rape and pregnancy of an enslaved woman did not cause alarm outside of the performance ("Slave Auction to Be Re-Enacted," 1994). The audience seem to understand rape as a crime and did not find it outrageous to dramatize a discussion of it in the eighteenth century.

After these small successes, the AAIP began to develop a "Publick Times" program. "Publick Times" was a multi-scene performance that had been running in Colonial Williamsburg since the late 1980s and showcased what the capital city was like when the population of the colony would converge in town for judicial, social, and market errands. The AAIP's new scene was described as an estate sale. The premise was that after the death of a white man, Benjamin Powell, his property was put up for auction to pay off his debts. This was a relatively common and relatable premise; Americans in the 1990s were familiar with the idea of selling off a loved one's home or car to cover post-death bills. The difference, of course, was that in the eighteenth century, a white man's property was material, animal, and human. The estate auction featured the sale of various eighteenth-century goods to planted purchasers mixed with the blended twentieth- and eighteenth-century audience. Among those goods were the people that Powell had enslaved.

Like the program about rape, the auction dealt with upsetting events, and the researchers took their task seriously. They built the program out of estate records, and accounts of what auctions were like in the eighteenth century. They believed that accuracy would ultimately make the performance valuable, and they were confident in their ability to present this deeply traumatic scene to the Colonial Williamsburg audience. The group's biggest concern was how they would manage twentieth-century audience members who may try participating in the scene by bidding on the actors ("Slave Auction to Be Re-Enacted," 1994). But overall, they felt positive about the event and had the success of previous programs to confirm their confidence.

When interviewed by National Public Radio (NPR) the head of the AAIP at the time, Cristy Coleman, explained that the group hoped that performing the auction would be an "open call to all educational institutions, museums, schools, colleges, and universities" to "teach history the way it was," so Americans could "understand where" they are currently and where they "need to go next" (Adamas, 1994). Coleman was steadfast in her belief that the unpleasantness of the past should not disqualify it from engagement. She later added that museums in the United States needed to follow the Washington, DC, Holocaust museums' lead and illustrate "the horrors that took place" under North American slavery, to promote a greater understanding of the past and present (Janofsky, 1994). Coleman said that above all else, the group's goal was "to educate" even if it upset "people from time to time" ("Slave Auction to Be Re-Enacted," 1994).

For those on the outside who saw Colonial Williamsburg as more of a tourist attraction than an educational institution, the move was a sharp turn in a new, uncomfortable direction. *Washington Post* writer Tamara Jones wrote that the program represented an "emotional departure" from the institution's regular programing which usually stuck to lighter topics like "How Now, Red Cow: Dairying in the 18th Century," horticulture, and barrel making (Jones, 1994). The slave auction would prove to be a more difficult, and more contemporarily fraught a topic than the institution had tackled before.

Unfortunately, two developments were happening, at Colonial Williamsburg and the United States more broadly in the 1990s that set the slavery program up to be misinterpreted by its audience. First, nationally the American people had grown to distrust institutions. The American conflict in Vietnam, the secret deception revealed by The Pentagon Papers, and the budget cuts and subsequent failure of social programs nationwide made Americans wary of trusting people who presented themselves as officials, or experts. Adding to that, Colonial Williamsburg and historical sites across the nation had historically done a poor job interpreting slavery. For most of post-emancipation US history, historical sites referred to enslaved people as “servants” and placed them in the background of the main narrative of elite white people’s privileged lives. Their oppression was never addressed, let alone alluded to by historical sites (Jay, 2009). Worst still, when white and Black American performers donned the character of an enslaved person, they traditionally did so as a type of clowning called Minstrelsy, or more famously Black Face (Thelwell, 2020). The presence of Black performers in the mocking of enslaved people gave Americans of all races reason to assume that no one could deftly and sensitively perform as an enslaved person. The 1977 television program *Roots* offered one example of a sensitive, humanizing, performance of enslaved life, but the deck was stacked against Colonial Williamsburg’s performers (Berkely, 1977). There was only one *Roots*, only about a decade of the Colonial Williamsburg’s AAIP, and over a hundred years of belittling Black Face performances.

In Williamsburg, at the same time the education department sought to present audiences with a more nuanced and accurate eighteenth-century, the historical institution’s for-profit and market-driven side offered guests “Revolutionary Fun” (Summer Fun 1979, 1979; Straszheim, 1998). After the federal cuts to historical sites in the 1980s, Colonial Williamsburg’s for-profit end took a larger role in the organization to help maintain income where gaps now appeared. The most obvious plan was for Colonial Williamsburg to tie itself to more popular entertainment in the area, notably the thrill park Busch Gardens (Messina, 1997). Ticket deals and advertisements showing the two institutions together led many to understand Colonial Williamsburg in context with the park. While employees at the historical institution saw themselves as working towards a serious and increasingly hard-hitting educational mission, advertisements promised gaiety. Within this context, it is no wonder that the public was horrified by the slave auction. In their eyes, the promise of lightness made the portrayal of historical traumas into dark tourism.

As such, almost immediately after announcing the program, the public began to protest the planned auction (Kolenbrander, 2019; Deviln, 2003). People did not want to see a slave auction and they found the very idea of one being presented to be in poor taste and entirely too inappropriate for the otherwise festive historical site. Newspapers across the nation began interviewing residents for their take on the proposed event, and most did not approve. One resident explained that the “contemporary reality" was "enough" to remind everyone that "the horror of slavery" persisted (Deviln, 2003, p. 56). Another explained that the hopelessness of a slave auction could only stir up unwanted feelings of "shame" and guilt among the African American community (Deviln, 2003). A sympathetic employee of Colonial Williamsburg later explained that the clear injustice and inhumanity of the slave auction made contemporary African Americans feel guilty and weak as if their ancestors "should have done something" like "rose up and rebelled" (Deviln, 2003). Instead of feeling pride from the great actions of the past, the slave auction reminded some viewers of their and their ancestor's powerlessness. Guests did not want to reflect on such a fraught and painful past at Colonial Williamsburg.

The surrounding tourist businesses and advertisements were an inescapably toxic factor for Colonial Williamsburg. People feared that the performance done within Williamsburg would be "trivializing" the enslaved experience (Adamas, 1994). A local pastor said that presenting "the kind of anguish" present at a slave auction for, as he assumed, "entertainment" was "despicable and disgusting" ("Tears and Protest at Mock Slave Sale," 1994). Continuing, he said that the event would produce "the kind of anguish" that Black Americans did not "need to display" ("Tears and Protest at Mock Slave Sale," 1994). Many people called the local branch of the National Association for the Advancement of Colored People (NAACP), a respected legacy institution that has long fought for Black Americans' rights, expressing worry that the museum intended to shock the audience with horror for entertainment and profit purposes – what we would call today dark tourism ("Tears and Protest at Mock Slave Sale," 1994).

One caller shared that they had no desire to see such a "wrenching" event "rehashed again," and could not imagine why any others would ("Tears and Protest at Mock Slave Sale," 1994). A local bricklayer said he found the idea of the event simply "insensitive" ("Tears and Protest at Mock Slave Sale," 1994). Salim Khalfani, the field coordinator of Virginia's NAACP, explained that when "entertainment" was "used to teach history" the "possibility for error or insensitivity and historical inaccuracy" was always present (Smith, 1994). While he planned to attend, to make a judgment call on the performance, the overwhelming consensus before the event was that it was too painful for the museum to present and needed to be stopped.

Despite the ill feelings reported in the newspapers, the event went on as scheduled. The performers had a certain amount of hesitation from all the negative press, but they felt that their careful craft could transform the day into something educational and clarifying (Jones, 1994). As the interpreters prepared to take the stage, they were met by an audience of nearly two thousand people, some supporters, but mostly protestors ("Tears and Protest at Mock Slave Sale," 1994). As the audience swelled, costumed interpreters found themselves impressed into crowd management roles, linking together their eighteenth-century canes and modern umbrellas to create a barrier between the audience and performers. Leaders of the Southern Christian Leadership Committee, a legacy civil rights institution founded by Martin Luther King Jr, joined the crowd, taking seats on the stage steps and challenging the institutions' managers to call the police to have them removed, all while a choir of voices rang out with the classic civil rights era song "We Shall Overcome" ("Tears and Protest at Mock Slave Sale," 1994). It was a powerful scene, but an entirely different kind of power than the interpreters had planned for their performance.

Christy Coleman mounted the stage shortly before the performance began and asked the audience to watch the scene before they rejected it. She pleaded for "indulgence," and the audience settled in and quieted their protests. The auction itself went smoothly, goods were offered and planted costumed audience members bid on them. The dramatic moment came when Coleman's character, who was visibly pregnant at the time, was sold away from her family. Accounts point to Coleman's performance as the audience's turning point. Frustrations and fears seemed to melt away as the weight of the program took its full effect. NAACP's Jack Gravely poetically noted that Coleman's performance illustrated that "pain had a face. Indignity had a body. Suffering had tears" ("Tears and Protest at Mock Slave Sale," 1994). The performers' goals had been met, and the auction made the pain of the past human and brought the reality of enslaved life to Colonial Williamsburg.

However, in the end, the program proved to be too intense for guests and was not repeated. The reaction to the auction suggested that guests did not want historical reality from a visit to Colonial Williamsburg, but they did not want to be lied to either. Most of the callers and interviewees expressed the same idea – that they saw the once respected historical institution as a commercial tourist attraction that could not be trusted with painful pasts. The event and the outcome illustrated the power that the for-profit side of Colonial Williamsburg had over guests' perception of the museum and its educational offerings. The presence, even distant presence, of commercialism dissolved the goodwill and trust that guests had previously given the institution to create a realistic portrayal of the past. Simply put, the fear of dark consumerism jammed public history workers' genuine attempts to connect with their audience.

Conclusion

The idea of dark tourism, though not coined yet, loomed large over the story of Colonial Williamsburg's slave auction. The public's worry, or rather fear, that the parallel developments of commercialism and the field's embrace of historical reality were one, disabled them from appreciating the performance and the interpreters' thoughtful emotional labor. Once coined, dark tourism gave a name to this imagined overlapping of parallel developments at historical sites, giving members of the public something to look for, and historical professionals something to fear.

The fear of dark tourism still lingers in the minds of historical site professionals, and more recently the mouths of their guests. Scores of journalists have penned pieces for *The New York Times, The Washington Post* and other popular news outlets that paradoxically describe dark tourism as an emerging and historical practice undertaken by deviant travelers (Cramer, 2022; Sampson, 2019; Usborne 2019; Kamin, 2014). Their work, in addition to shows like Netflix's *Dark Tourism*, has lent the public an imprecise language to describe sites of history, mourning and memorials that can sow distrust between visitors and public history workers.

Fear of losing their audience's trust motivates many scholars of history to see dark tourism as a problem, and more importantly, something to be cautious about modeling (Moody, 2016; Alderman, 2017; Shrum, 2017; Pedersen, 2016; Dick 2017; Little, 2016; Miles 2015). Just as scholars of the 1990s saw Disney's commercial history as something in crying need of reform, Jessica Moody explained in 2016 that the "distasteful, trivial, or simple unsupported" elements of dark tourism beg historians to engage and counter with "rigorous and serious research" (Moody, 2016, p. 114). Historian Tiya Miles went further explaining that ghost tours, often openly advertised as dark tourism, willfully ignore the social and political complexities of the past in favor of stories that trivialized and demonize real human suffering (Miles, 2015). The commercialization of suffering that dark tourism describes has long irritated historical professionals and museum workers, and its popularity among the broader public has transformed this irritant into the boogieman of the public history profession – that threatens to invalidate their educational aims. However, recognition of professional public history and emotional labor can help to tease commercial dark tourism out from the larger pantheon of historical sites and develop a more precise understanding of commodified pain.

References

Adamas, N. (1994, October). *Slave Auction Re-Enactment Controversy: All Things Considered* [Radio Broadcast]. NPR.

Alderman, D. H. (2017). Tiya Miles. Tales from the South: Dark Tourism and Memories of Slavery. *African American Review*, 50(1), 87–90.

Appleby, J. (1998). The Power of History. *The American Historical Review*, 1–14.

Atalay, S. (2012). *Community-Based Archaeology: Research with, by, and for Indigenous and Local Communities*. University of California Press.

Bennett, T. (2004). *Pasts Beyond Memory: Evolution, Museums, Colonialism*. Routledge.

Berkely, G. (1977, January 30). 'Roots' Recording Breaking Run. *Oakland Post*.

Bienstock, B. W. (1995). Everything Old Is New Again: Social history, the National History Standards and the Crisis in Teaching of High School American History. *Journal of Social History*, 59–63

Blakey, M. L. (1997). Seizing Intellectual Power: The Dialogue at the New York African Burial Ground. *Historical Archaeology*, 31(3), 84–106

Bowman, M. S. and Pezzullo, P. C. (2010). What is so "Dark' about "Dark Tourism'?" Death, Tours, and Performance. *Tourist Studies*. 9(3). 187–202.

Biran, A., Poria, Y., & G. Oren. (2011). Sought Experiences at (Dark) Heritage Sites. *Annals of Tourism Research*, 38(3), 820–841.

Carson, C. (1994). Lost in the Fun House: A Commentary on Anthropologists' First Contact with History Museums. *The Journal of American History*, 81(1), 137–150.
Carson, C. (1995). Mirror, Mirror, on the Wall, Whose History is the Fairest of Them All? *The Public Historian*, 17(4), 61–67.
Carter, B. (1990, September 15). "Civil War" Sets an Audience Record for PBS. *The New York Times*.
Cavalieri, S., Corrizzato, S. & Franceschi, V. (2022). The Dark Past of Slavery in American Plantation Houses: Website Promotion and Perceptions of Visitors I TripAdvisor Reviews. *Zbornik Radova Filozofskog Fakulteta u Prištini*, 52(4). 13–30.
Casbeard, R.& Booth, C. (2012). Post-Modernity and the Exceptionalism of the Present in Dark Tourism. *Journal of Unconventional Parks*, 4(1), 2–8.
Colonial Williamsburg's Forgotten Half. (1990, August). *Southern Living*.
Combined Talents Create Scenes of Black History. (1980, August). *Colonial Williamsburg News*.
Cox, K. (2011). *Dreaming of Dixie: How The South Was Created In American Popular Culture*. University of North Carolina Press.
Cramer, M. (2022, October 28). Beaches? Cruises? 'Dark' Tourists Prefer the Gloomy and Macabre. *The New York Times*.
Dann, G.M.S. & Seaton, A.V. (2002). Slavery, Contested Heritage, and Thanatorism. *International Journal of Hospitality & Tourism Administration*, 2(¾), 1–29.
Degler, C. N. (1980) Remaking American History. *The Journal of American History*. 67(1). 7–25
Deviln, E. K. (2003). *Colonial Williamsburg's Slave Auction Re-Enactment: Controversy, African American History and Public Memory*. [Master Thesis]. The College of William and Mary.
D'Harlingue, B. (2015). On the Plantation with Ghosts: Antagonisms of Slavery Tourism. *Southern Carolina Review*, 47(2), 74–92.
Dick, E. R. (2017). Tales from the Haunted South: Dark Tourism and Memories of Slavery from the Civil War Era. *Journal of American Culture*, 40(3), 294–297.
Evans, F. (1991, August 27). American Girls to Treasure. *Washington Post*.
Fernandes, M. & Jamadagni, R. (2018), The Dark Tours: An Insight into the Appeal of Dark Tourism. *Atithya: A Journal of Hospitality*, 4(2), 41–45.
Foley, M. & Lennon, J. J. (1996a) Editorial: Heart of darkness. *International Journal of Heritage Studies*. 2(4) 195–197.
Foley, M. & Lennon, J. J. (1996b), JFK and dark tourism: A Fascination with Assassination. *International Journal of Heritage Studies*. 2(4). 198–211.
Gallman, R. E. (1977). Some Notes on the New Social History. *The Journal of Economic History*, 37(1), 3–12.
Garrett, B. (2011). Assaying history: Creating temporal junctions through urban exploration. *Environment and Planning D: Society & Space*, 29(6): 1048–1067.
Glassberg, D. (2011). *Sense of History: The Place of the Past in American Life*. University of Massachusetts Press.
Gordon, A. (2008). *Ghostly Matters: Haunting and Sociological Imagination*. University of Minnesota Press.
Greenspan, A. (2002). *Creating Colonial Williamsburg*. Smithsonian Institute Press.
Hartmann, R. (2013). Dark Tourism, Thanatourism, Dissonance in Heritage Tourism Management: New Directions in Contemporary Tourism Research. *Journal of Heritage Tourism* 9. No.2. (2013) 166–182.
Haight O'Connell, L. (1995, October 1). The History Channel and History Education. *Perspectives on History*. https://www.historians.org/research-and-publications/perspectives-on-history/october-1995/the-history-channel-and-history-education
Handler, R. and Gable, E. (1997). *The New History in an Old Museum: Creating the Past at Colonial Williamsburg*. University of North Carolina Press.
Horton, J.O., and Horton, L.E. (Ed.). (2008). *Slavery and Public History: The Tough Stuff of American Memory*. University of North Carolina Press.
Horowitz, T. (1999) *Confederates in the Attic: Dispatches from the Unfinished Civil War*, Vintage.

Howard, S. L. (1995, June 18). Making Colonial Williamsburg Authentic. *Philadelphia Inquirer*.
Inker, P. (2021, December 9). Crime and Punishment . . . and Human Rights. *Colonial Williamsburg*. https://www.colonialwilliamsburg.org/learn/living-history/crime-and-punishment-and-human-rights/.
Jacobs, J. (2019, May 15). Former Historical Interpreters Reflect on Early Days of African American Programming at Colonial Williamsburg. *Chicago Tribune*.
Janofsky, M. (1994, October 8). Mock Auction of Slaves: Education or Outrage. *The New York Times*.
Jay, B. (2009). *The Representation of Slavery at House Museums: 1853–2000* [PhD Dissertation]. Boston College.
Jones, T. (1994, October 11). Living History or Undying Racism? Colonial Williamsburg 'Slave Auction' Draws Protest, Support. *The Washington Post*.
Kamin, D. (2014, July 15). The Rise of Dark Tourism: When War Zones Become Travel Destinations. *The Atlantic*.
Kapsidelis, K. (1996, April 28). Tour Gives Felicity A Starring Role. *Richmond Times-Dispatch*.
Kolenbrander, S. (2019).*"Pain Had A Face, Indignity Had a Body, Suffering Had Tears:" Evaluating The Role of Colonial Williamsburg in Portraying Narratives of Enslavement*. [History Honors Project]. Macalester College.
La Roche, C. J, Blakey, M. L. (1997). Seizing Intellectual Power: The Dialogue at the New York African Burial Ground. *Historical Archaeology*. 31(3) 84–106.
Lawson, A.L. (1995). *"The Other Half": Making African-American History At Colonial Williamsburg*. [PhD Dissertation]. University of Virginia.
Lennon, J. J. and Foley, M. (1999). Interpretation of the Unimaginable: The U.S. Holocaust Memorial Museum, Washington, D.C., and "Dark Tourism." *Journal of Travel Research*. 38(1). 46–50.
Lewis, J. (2003, November 2). Learn the Scary Side of History in Ghost Tours of Williamsburg. *The Plain Dealer*.
Linethal, E. T. and Engelhardt, T. (Ed.). (1996). *History Wars: The Enola Gay and Other Battles for the American Past*. Henry Holt and Company.
Little, R. M. (2016). "Tales from the Haunted South: Dark Tourism and Memories of Slavery from the Civil War Era Tiya Miles. *The North Carolina Historical Review*, 93(2), 230.
Martini, A. and Buda, D.M. (2020). Dark Tourism and Affect: Framing Places and Death and Disaster. *Current Issues in Tourism*, 23(6), 679–692.
Marshall, Y. (2002). What is Community Archaeology. *World Archaeology*, Community Archaeology. 34(2). 211–9.
Messina, D. (1997, June 18). Colonial Williamsburg Hotels Looses Tired to Decline In Visitors. *Virginian Pilot*.
McPherson, T. (2003). *Reconstructing Dixie: Race, Gender, and Nostalgia in the Imagined South*. Duke University Press.
Miles, T. (2015). *Tales from The Haunted South: Dark Tourism and Memories of Slavery from the Civil War Era*. University Of North Carolina Press.
Miles, S. (2014). Battlefield Sites as Dark Tourism Attractions: An Analysis of Experience. *Journal of Heritage Tourism*. 9(2), 134–147.
Moody, J. (2016). Where is "Dark Public History?" A Scholarly Turn to the Dark Side, and What It Means for Public Historians. *The Public Historian*, 38(3), 109–.114.
Moore, L. J. (1996). Good Old-Fashioned New Social History and the Twentieth-Century American Right. *Reviews in American History*. 24(4). 555–573.
Nash, G., C. Crabtree, & Dunn, R. (2000). *History on Trial: Culture Wars and the Teaching of the Past*. Vintage Books.
Nelson, V. (2020). Liminality and Difficult Heritage in Tourism. *Tourism Geography*, 22(2), 298–318.
News Presented in Brief From All Corners. (1979, March 31). *Colonial Williamsburg News*. Visitation Numbers.

Ollove, M. (1996, July 26). As Time Goes By, History Channel Blossoms. *The Baltimore Sun.*

Oren, G., & Shani, A. (2012). "The Yad Vashem Holocaust Museum: Educational dark tourism in a futuristic form". *Journal of Heritage Tourism*, 7(3), 255–270.

Pedersen, A. (2016). Tales from the Haunted South: Dark Tourism and Memories of Slavery from the Civil War Era. *Journal of American History*, 103(3), 773.

Pirok, A. (2022). *The Spirit of Colonial Williamsburg: Ghosts and Interpreting the Recreated Past.* University of Massachusetts Press.

Pitt, H. (2019, July 14). Paradise Lost: Sydney's Forgotten Theme Parks. *The Sydney Morning Herald.*

Rubin, R. L. (2012) *Well Met: Renaissance Faires and the American Counterculture.* New York University Press.

Rymsza-Pawlowska, M. J. (2019). Hippies Living History: Form and Context in Tracing Public History's Past. *The Public Historian*. 41(4). 36–55.

Sampson, H. (2019, November, 13). Dark Tourism, Explained: Why Visitors Flock to Sites of Tragedy. *Washington Post.*

Seaton, A.V. (1996). Guided by the dark: From thanatopsis to thanatourism. *International Journal of Heritage Studies*, 2(4), 234–244.

Shrum, R. (2017). Tales from the Haunted South: Dark Tourism and Memories of Slavery from the Civil War Era. *Journal of Southern History*, 83(1), 240–242.

Slave Auction to Be Re-Enacted. (1994, October 9). *Newport Daily News.*

Sharpley, R., & Stone, P. (2009). Representing the macabre: Interpretation, kitschification, and authenticity. In R. Sharpley & P. Stone (Eds.), *The darker side of travel: The theory and practice of dark tourism* (pp. 109–128). View Publications.

Smith, L. (1994, October 8). Williamsburg Slave Auction Riles VA. NAACP. *The Washington Post.*

Stone, P.R. (2006). A Dark Tourism Spectrum: Towards A Typology of Death and Macabre Related Tourists Sites, Attractions and Exhibitions. *Tourism*. 54(3), 143–160.

Summer Fun 1979. (1979, June). *Colonial Williamsburg News.*

Straszheim, D. (1998, June 20). Pleasant Company Sold to Mattel, CW American Girls Event Unaffected. *Daily Press.*

Synnott, M. G. (1995). Disney's America: Whose Patrimony, Whose Profits, Whose Past?. *The Public Historian*, 17(4), 43–59.

Thelwell, C. (2020). *Exporting Jim Crow: Blackface Minstrelsy in South African and Beyond.* University of Massachusetts Press.

Tinson, J. and Saren, M. A.J., and B.E. Roth. (2015). Exploring the Role of Dark Tourism in the Creation of National Identity of Young Americans. *Journal of Marketing Management*, 31(7–8), 856–880.

Tyson, A. M. (2013). *The Wages of History: Emotional Labor on Public History's Front Lines.* University of Massachusetts Press.

Tyson, Amy. (2008). Crating Emotional Comfort: Interring the Painful Past AT Living History Museums in the New Economy. *Museum and Society*, 6(3), 246–262.

Tears and Protest at Mock Slave Sale. (1994, October 11). *The New York Times.*

Usborne, S. (2019, April 9. Updated 2021, July 15). Dark Tourism: When Tragedy Meets Tourism," *National Geographic.*

Wallace, M. (1996). *Mickey Mouse History and Other Essays on American Memory.* Temple University Press.

Waller, S. N. and Costen, W. M. (2012). Legacy of the Lorraine Motel and the Assassination of Martin Luther King, Jr. *Journal of Unconventional Parks, Tourism and Recreation Research.* 4(1), 9–13

Welch, M. (2015). *Escape to Prison: Penal Tourism and Pull of Punishment.* University of California Press.

Williamsburg Welcoming in Autumn. (1988, October 16). *New York Times*. October 16, 1988.

Yankholmes, A. & McKercher, B. (2015). Rethinking Slavery Heritage Tourism. *Journal of Heritage* Tourism, 10(3), 233–247.

Zaslow, E. (2021). Which Vitamins are in the Chocolate Cake? How American Girl Marketing Has Responded to Shifting Discourses about Gender and Race," *The Public Historian*, 43(1), 18–38.

Florence Smith Nicholls

10 Welcome to Revachol: *Disco Elysium* as virtual dark tourism

Abstract: "When middle-class people talk about foreign places, they like to talk about "contrasts," so begins a devlog for the role-playing video game *Disco Elysium (ZA/UM, 2019)*. Disco is set in Revachol, a fictional city still ravaged by the repression of a communist uprising. You play as Harrier (Harry) Du Bois, a detective who has arguably become a tourist in his own city thanks to drug-induced amnesia. In contrast, his hyper-competent partner Kim Kitsuragi is treated like a tourist in Revachol due to racist assumptions. This chapter considers *Disco Elysium* as a dark tourist experience in line with existing work on the potential of video games to explore digital speculative histories (Milligan, 2018; Smith Nicholls, 2021). Aside from the fictional dark heritage of Disco, the identification (or not) of the player with protagonist Harry will form the second theme of the chapter. Disco is at its heart a role-playing game, and this case study provides an opportunity to examine how the theatricality of dark tourism (Willis, 2014) manifests in this medium. Finally, the dark tourist experience of *Disco Elysium* will be examined using the concept of hauntology and Sara Ahmed's work on queer phenomenology (2006), specifically how the player as Harry is disoriented in a once-familiar world (Sawicki, 2021). The analysis reveals that the game can be understood as haunted on various levels - the video game medium itself, in terms of its post-revolution fantasy-realism setting, and a product of the alleged toxic work environment under which the game was produced.

Keywords: virtual dark tourism, video games, gothic tourism, hauntology, literary analysis

Introduction

Disco Elysium (ZA/UM, 2019) presents a particularly nuanced case study for understanding the potential of virtual dark tourism experiences. There has been limited scholarship into video games as Dark Tourism, and even less on games with fictional settings. This chapter aims to fill that gap, using the literary analysis methodology of close reading to understand Disco Elysium more specifically as a form of gothic tourism, a sub-genre of dark tourism. This study uses Derrida's concept of hauntology (1994) and ideas from queer phenomenology to analyze the game within the context of dark tourism. The analysis reveals that the game can be understood as haunted on various levels: with reference to the video game medium itself, in terms of its post-

https://doi.org/10.1515/9783110792072-011

revolution fantasy-realism setting, and a product of the alleged toxic work environment under which the game was produced.

Background

Dark tourism

Dark tourism, very broadly defined as the deliberate visitation of tourist sites associated with death and disaster, has grown as a niche academic discipline over the last quarter of a century. The coining of the term is often attributed to Foley and Lennon (1996), though there has been scholarship on so-called 'negative sight-seeing' since the 1970s (Nhlabathi & Maharaj, 2020). Isaac (2022) charts a shift in dark tourism scholarship from a focus on sites to experiences in the 2000s as an attempt to understand the demand and motivations for dark tourism. In a survey of dark tourism scholarship, Light (2017) has pointed out that attempts to typologise the field don't contend with the heterogeneous nature of dark tourism, and that there has been limited critical engagement with its political implications.

A more recent paper by Nhlabathi and Maharaj (2020) goes against the grain by arguing that the field of dark tourism emerged out of a neoliberal restructuring of higher education from the 1980s onwards, with academics using the term 'dark tourism' as a brand to market themselves and their work. This argument is at least partly reinforced by Light's (2017) assertion that dark tourism has gained wider media attention beyond academia. Nhlabathi and Maharaj (2020) draw from the results of interviews conducted at dark tourist sites in South Africa, concluding that there was more evidence that visitors were motivated to pay respect and learn rather than be voyeuristic. This is in contrast to Korstanje and George (2018, p. 16), who also envisage dark tourism as a product of neoliberalism, but rather as one which encourages "the supremacy of liberal cultural values enrooted in late-capitalism". Overall, dark tourism continues to be a niche but a lively field, and one which must consider the political and ethical considerations of not only its subjects but also of itself.

Virtual dark tourism

There has been a wide range of scholarship on the intersection of video games and tourism. The majority of recent work in this area has focused on the simulation of real-world tourist sites in games (Banaszkiewicz & Duda, 2019) and video game-induced tourism (Bowman et al., 2023; Champion, 2022; Dubois & Gibbs, 2018). Earlier work within the broader field of games studies considered the affordances of the medium to provide escapist tourism fantasies and the reenactment of colonial narratives

(Fuller & Jenkins, 1995; Schwartz, 2006; Miller, 2008). There has been less work considering video games as a tourist experience from a *design* rather than a consumption perspective (Lamerichs, 2018). However, the idea that tourism itself is a form of play has considerable precedent (Cohen, 1985) and environmental storytelling techniques that are commonly used in video games draw from the constructed landscapes of one of the world's most famous tourist sites: Disneyland (Jenkins, 2004).

The majority of dark tourism scholarship pertains to analogue sites, but there has been a steady increase in work related to virtual dark tourism over the last decade. However, as early as 2002, Miles (2002, p.1177) writes that "as sensory cognition evolves in relation to progressive computerization, however, longstanding psychological distinctions between real and virtual, here and there, subject and object may themselves loosen. If so, then the dark cyber tourist may not in fact sense a substantial difference between walking and browsing through Auschwitz".

Miles anticipates the slippage between the so-called 'real' and 'virtual' which characterises not just contemporary digital dark tourism studies, but wider conversations around the digital and authenticity. This is a strand that I picked up in my work (Smith Nicholls, 2018) on digital dark tourism and the re-creation of a real-world heritage site, the Ospedale Psichiatrico di Volterra, in the video game *The Town of Light* (LKA, 2016).

Furthermore, I argue that video games marketed as being set at such sites associated with difficult heritage can be understood through the lens of the commodified experience of sites associated with death and disaster – the very definition of dark tourism. Harrer and Pichmair's article is notable for not only critiquing the player as a coloniser-tourist in Resident Evil 5 but also placing it within the colonial history of the Herrensafari as a white male leisure activity in 1950s America (2015, p. 3).

Korstanje (2014, p. 8) differentiates between "tourism online, online-tourism and virtual tourism", the last of which he describes as the visitation of digitally reconstructed sites. The edited volume *Virtual Dark Tourism: Ghost Roads* (McDaniel, 2018) also discusses literary and film tourism under the rubric of virtual dark tourism. More specifically, it includes chapters on alternate history games (Milligan, 2018) and fictional history in EVE Online (Fandino 2018). Both chapters explore the agency of virtual tourists to navigate and interpret digital worlds. These two pieces are unusual in that they focus on video games depicting fictional settings that arguably still provide a dark tourism experience. This is an area that remains understudied, perhaps because the labelling of these fictional examples as dark tourism could be seen as less legitimate than the representation of non-fictional tourist sites in digital media.A recently edited volume related to virtual dark tourism, *Difficult Heritage and Immersive Experiences* (Bernadou and Droumpouki, 2022), generally takes an experiential approach to the topic, including virtual and augmented reality studies. Though there have been discussions of virtual dark tourism since the nascence of the field, there is still limited scholarship in this area, especially regarding fictional game worlds. This chapter provides a new case study for virtual dark tourism studies, drawing on the sub-field of gothic tourism and hauntology.

Gothic tourism and Gothic gaming

One of the most prolific researchers of gothic tourism is Emma McAvoy (2016, p. 5), who defines it as: tourism that is intimately connected with the Gothic narrative, its associated tropes, discourses, and conventions.

The Gothic, rather like dark tourism, is notoriously difficult to define. It can be "more accurately reflected as a tendency than a coherent movement" (Stevens 2000, p. 31) that is rooted in the 18th-century trend across art, literature and architecture that reacted against neo-classical ideas of order and taste based on rationalism (Stevens 2000, p. 10). McEvoy (2016, p. 5) contends that tourism has always been integral to the gothic aesthetic.

McAvoy's definition of gothic tourism has been critiqued for being too vague and better defined as a form of literary tourism, or a 'lighter' form of dark tourism (Light, Richards, and Ivonova, 2021), perhaps akin to the 'Dark Fun Factories' that Stone (2006) identifies in a potential spectrum of dark tourist sites. However, in an earlier piece on 'Dracula tourism' in Romania, Light (2017, p. 127) observes that "it is a ludic form of tourism with a strong affective dimension based on horror, dread, thrills, frights and a delight in the uncanny and unknown. In particular, Gothic tourism involves a theatrical delight in creating or entering imaginary (or imaginative) worlds." I would argue that Gothic tourism can be considered a subset of dark tourism that is particularly well-suited to contextualising video games within this field, precisely because it is associated with the ludic and the imaginary. Furthermore, there is a strong body of literature on the gothic qualities of the video game medium itself.

Much like McAvoy's (2016) definition of gothic tourism, Krzywinska (2015) identifies gothic video games as those that display the classic tropes of the literary genre, such as the false hero or a haunted setting. However, Krzywinska (2015, p. 32) goes beyond gothic representation and aesthetics to consider the video game itself as a gothic medium: "In a Gothic context, a game's algorithmic system potentially accrues a mysterious, godlike power that steers choice, behaviour and morality through arrays of determinants". Kirkland (2022, p. 638) also contends that "video games have always been gothic" in that the literary gothic genre itself is ludic, playing with reader expectations. Furthermore, the video game medium embodies the doubling trope of gothic fiction through the player-avatar relationship, and a sense of perpetual uncertainty in that every playthrough will be different (Kirkland, 2022, p. 636). Hancock (2016, p. 166) also draws parallels between gothic fiction and video games, pointing out that both the early gothic novel and video games have been the focus of moral panics. Circling back to the theme of neoliberalism touched on before, and linking this up with the gothic: "Video games are the uncanny symptom of the neo-liberal subject's recognition of its own lack of self" (Hancock, 2016, p. 167).

Hancock (2016, p. 167) argues that the medium of video games can highlight the lie of rational choice under neoliberalism, by presenting free choices to the player while ultimately constraining them within the logic of the game. This intertwines with McLachlan's (2022) thesis that the Gothic communicates a feeling that something is wrong with the world. This also echoes McEvoy's (2016) emphasis that gothic tourism can be identified by its affective qualities, and work by Martini and Buda (2020) on dark tourism and affect. On a meta level, video games as a medium can communicate that something is very wrong with our neoliberal world, haunted as they are by the broken promise of simulated fantasy.

Disco Elysium

The role-playing video game *Disco Elysium* (ZA/UM, 2019) is arguably very much concerned with the failure of neoliberalism, taking place in a fantasy realist world that draws on the history of our own. The player character is Harrier (Harry) De Bois, an amnesiac detective tasked with solving a murder alongside fellow investigator and narrative foil Kim Kitsuragi. The game takes place in Martinaise, a poor coastal district of the city Revachol. Martinaise is scarred by a failed communist revolution half a century prior, with Revachol now under the control of an alliance of capitalist nations known as the Coalition. Gameplay mainly involves interacting with non-player characters and objects in the world, along with skill checks based on random dice rolls. Furthermore, the protagonist has 24 skills organised around four different abilities (Intellect, Psyche, Physique, and Motorics) which can modify dice rolls and be upgraded throughout the game. Not only do the skills have a mechanical significance, but a rhetorical one as they speak directly to Harry as part of the dialogue.

Perhaps unsurprisingly given the themes of the game, much of the existing academic literature is related to political themes and the fractured nature of the protagonist's identity. In terms of the former, several researchers (e.g., Gekker & Joseph, 2021; Ozimek, 2021) have written about the political economy of the game's development, first in Estonia and then in the United Kingdom. Case (2018, p. 79) comments on how the skill checks and dice rolls constantly allude to alternate experiences of the game, and by extension alternate versions of the protagonist. Belmonte (2021) emphasises the tension between choice, failure, and the memory of the player, who has the ability to re-load saved files after a failed skill check but will still remember past playthroughs even if the game itself does not. Vella and Cielecka (2021) also focus on memory, though in their case they comment on Harry's amnesia as one way in which *Disco Elysium* presents a protagonist with an inherently fractured sense of self. Conversely, Khamis (2021) argues that it is this memory loss that allows Harry to potentially find a new perspective on a disturbing phenomenon in the fictional game world known as "the Pale," a sort of incomprehensible anti-matter that some people think is man-made "rarified past," to quote one non-player character in the game (ZA/UM, 2019).

Another set of scholarship is themed around how the game conveys meaning spatially as well as temporally. Kłosiński (2021, p. 58) points out that although time passes during conversations, it is not affected by the player exploring the game space. Other scholars have also written about how the spatial organisation of the game relates to the internal cognition of the protagonist (Medvedeva, 2022; Tamahori, 2022).

Tying together these themes of the fractured self and an unstable present is Novitz's piece (2021). This argues that *Disco Elysium* can be considered a piece of gothic fiction on the basis that the game has an unreliable narrator, a sense of disorientation due to a surfeit of information, and "the city as an environment where the past constantly intrudes upon and threatens the present" (Novitz. 2021, p. 38). Novitz draws on Derrida's theory of hauntology (2021, p. 40), which forms a key theoretical framing for his chapter. Though the majority of academic work on *Disco Elysium* does not explicitly reference the gothic, Novitz's piece demonstrates that many of the qualities of the game emphasised in the literature are essentially gothic tropes, inviting an analysis through the lens of gothic tourism.

Hauntology

The theoretical lens through which *Disco Elysium* as a gothic and dark tourism experience will be explored is hauntology. The term was coined by the philosopher Jacques Derrida in Spectres of Marx (1993). To summarise, hauntology presupposes that ideas from the past persist or 'haunt' the present. One of the most renowned applications of this theory has been Mark Fisher's (2014) work on the hauntology of music stuck in nostalgia for imagined futures that never arrived. In What is Hauntology? (2012) Fisher argues that by the mid-2000s electronic music had stagnated in terms of technical innovation, no longer futuristic but instead defined by a future that never came to be.

Hauntology has been widely cited in dark tourism studies. Buser (2017) applies hauntology to the development of an augmented reality game as Bodlam Castle, which draws upon the indeterminacy of the ruined site and its contemporary interpretation and presentation to the public. Hasian and Paliewicz (2021) draw on hauntology to discuss the radical political potential of dark tourism in relation to the National Memorial for Peace and Justice (NMPJ) and Legacy Museum in Montgomery, Alabama, which centres on the history of racism in America. Goulding and Pressey (2023) consider the hauntology of Dachau as a site layered with multiple histories. A theme shared by all this research is the political potential of inciting hauntology: "the word itself is less important for such work than the constant mode of self-critique it invokes" (Sterling, 2021, p. 83).

Applying hauntology to *Disco Elysium* as a *virtual* dark tourism site takes on additional significance when considering that Fisher's (2012, p.16) influential article was very much concerned with critiquing "the digital cul-de-sacs of the twenty-first century" and the video game as haunted medium will be expanded upon below. Apart from Novitz's (2021) work on Disco Elysium as gothic fiction, there has yet to be significant academic engagement with the game from a hauntological perspective. In contrast, there have been several pieces of non-academic writing on this subject (DuBois, 2020; Howe, 2020; Matta, 2021). These pieces will be drawn upon in the following hauntological close reading of the game.

Methodology

Close reading

This chapter uses the method of close reading to explore *Disco Elysium* as a dark tourism experience through the lens of the gothic and hauntology. Close reading is a method that originally came from literary theory and has been adapted to other forms of media, involving a detailed deconstruction of a specific text (Bizzocchi & Tanenbaum, 2011, p. 289). In discussing the close reading of video games, Bizzocchi and Tanenbaum (2011, p. 299) refer to the indeterminacy of the medium in that individual 'readings' will vary. In this sense, close reading has to contend with one aspect of video games which is also a common aspect of the gothic genre. For Stang (2022, p. 233), the intimacy and subjectivity of close reading are powerful in challenging traditional stereotypes about gaming culture. As Stang (2022, p. 234) puts it: "our work on games must be grounded in a consideration of the social, cultural, and historical contexts of their production and reception and we, as researchers subject to the same power relations we are critiquing."

This chapter embraces the inherent subjectivity of the close reading methodology as a strength rather than a weakness, especially as it provides another layer of gothic indeterminacy. Though close reading is derived from literature studies, it will be important to engage with the mechanics of the case study in order to further reflect on how "vastly different playthroughs and experiences are possible" (Yang, 2009, n.p.). Fittingly, this approach also echoes the hauntological one that Goulding and Pressey (2023) take at Dachau, in which they emphasise the importance of individual subjective experiences.

Analysis

The video game as a haunted medium

Beyond looking at specific video games from a hauntological perspective, the video game medium itself can be understood as haunted. In 'Ghosts of the Present Past', Janik (2019, p. 11) discusses how games are haunted by past playthroughs:

> If we have made the wrong choice and we have loaded a previous save to fix it, our new actions are clearly inspired by the past, which has "not yet" materialized and "no longer" exists.

Atkins (2007) also focuses on how players' memory of previous playthroughs becomes an 'Other' to which they compare themselves. In *Horror Games and the Idea of Haunted Media*, Schwartz (2019, p. 22) poses that the classic 'gameplay loop' involves repeated actions in specific locations which could be seen as a kind of haunting. Though not explicitly from a hauntological perspective, Mukherjee (2017, p. 60) considers that players are conscious of not only their own previous playthroughs in a game but a collective memory of the player community as well.

With the hauntology of games, there is a tension between the representation of an imagined future that will never come and the cultural past that the medium inevitably draws upon. In this way, "like any archaeologist, the gamer theorist treats these ruins of the future with obsessive care and attention to their preservation, not their destruction" (Robertson, 2013, p. 16). On an even broader level, games are haunted by the past work they reference (Grace, 2019). The hauntology of games links back with the neoliberalism of dark tourism discussed earlier. In a piece on *The Games Industry: Accelerationism and the Hauntological in Microcosm* (XENOGOTHIC, 2020), the author contrasts the constant desire for technological progress within the games industry with the continual nostalgia for older game titles, leading to remakes. In this way, games are a "microcosm of neoliberalism" (XENOGOTHIC, 2020).

To illustrate the hauntology of the video game experience, I can use some examples from my playthroughs of *Disco Elysium*. In their article on close reading, Bizzocchi and Tanenbaum (2011, p. 9) consider that a researcher should construct the phenomenological experience of an imagined naive player. However, given the importance of memory in the hauntology of games, I will instead be leaning into my personal phenomenological experience of *Disco Elysium*.

I played the game on the Nintendo Switch and ended up restarting it several times. In my first attempt, I made the mistake of min-maxing (a strategy of maximising a specific attribute at the expense of others) the protagonist's abilities so that he had incredibly high Intellect and Physique but very low Psyche and Motorics. This made passing some skill checks incredibly difficult, so I had to restart and 'remake' my character, though my first experience influenced all subsequent ones, as I continually reflected on what skills would be optimal for the 'ultimate' playthrough of the game. Protagonist Harry can die if his Health reaches zero, or essentially lose the will to live or continue the investigation if his Morale is depleted. There were several times in early playthroughs of the game when Harry's Morale was unexpectedly affected by a conversation and the game ended with me losing a considerable amount of progress. Though *Disco Elysium* has an autosave function, it is only triggered sporadically, so without manually saving frequently players are likely to lose a lot of progress if they fail. This means that in a literal sense, I retained memories of playing the game which my console did not, linking back to the idea that games are a medium haunted by memory on numerous levels. From a dark or gothic tourism point of view, this also indicates how the video game medium itself can provide a disconcerting metanarrative experience for the player.

The Pale

One aspect of the fictional world of *Disco Elysium* is particularly relevant to the meta-discussion of the video game as a haunted medium: the Pale. The world in which *Disco Elysium* is set consists of land masses that are isolated from each other by a separative tissue known as the Pale. It does not have a discernible appearance and its "fundamental property is the suspension of properties: physical, epistemological, linguistic" (ZA/UM, 2019, n.p.). Overexposure to the Pale can lead to brain damage as "the human mind becomes over-radiated by past" (ZA/UM, 2019). The Pale covers 72% of the known world, and it is expanding. Reflecting on the hauntology of Disco Elysium and the Pale, "It is filled with information from the past, but none that is clear instead degraded like that of the damaged tapes found in the game" (DuBois, 2020, n.p.).

The Pale, characterised as it is by memory loss and the corrosion of reality, can be considered a metaphor for multiple crises in our world: climate change, collective trauma and capitalism. On another meta-level, the Pale is a manifestation of the limits of and eventual degradation of all video game media. Consider that, according to one Non-Player Character:

> The further into pale you travel, the steeper the degree of suspension. Right down to the mathematical – *numbers* stop working. No one has yet passed the number barrier. It may be impossible (ZA/UM, 2019).

This mention of the breaking down of numbers is akin to the gradual process of data degradation that happens due to an accumulation of non-critical failures in different forms of data storage, commonly known as bitrot. This provides yet another layer to the interpretation of the video game as a gothic medium haunting itself.

The Indeterminacy of *Disco Elysium*

A character who perhaps best encapsulates the indeterminacy of *Disco Elysium* is the Novelty Dicemaker, Neha. The Dicemaker's way of life offers an alternative future on several levels, not just in terms of how she lives but what her craft represents. Dice are an analogue procedural generation system, an answer to the problem of trying to generate a seemingly infinite amount of content (a concern for the in-game failed development of Wirrâl Untethered, discussed below). They also represent the tension of indeterminacy, as the Dicemaker says:

> It's like every time you cast a die, something disappears. Some alternative ending, or an entirely different world [. . .] (ZA/UM, 2019).

Focusing on the Dicemaker is not to say that the analogue is superior to the digital, but that perhaps the digital has not yet reached the promised future for dark tourism that Miles (2002) identified twenty years ago, of the dark cyber tourist not being able to distinguish between either. That being said, not all hauntings are a loss – the failure of digital dark tourism to fully materialise along with seamless technological advancement is perhaps not a failure at all. After all, time is out of joint "where ghosts have not been exorcised by the need to tell a singular narrative" (Buser, 2017, p. 9). This echoes González-Tennant's (2015, p. 171) assertion that the indeterminacy of the digital allowed him to present the town of Rosewood while avoiding stereotypes that it was "simply a site of death and tragedy by collapsing the town's history into a single event". Alternative experiences may haunt us, but they also represent possibilities beyond futures already imagined. Thus, the indeterminacy of the virtual dark tourism experience has political significance.

Disco Elysium as a gothic tourism destination

"Welcome to Revachol!"

The Map of Martinaise in *Disco Elysium* bears the following text description:

> A worn and torn map of the Martinaise area, dating from '48. A title on the top reads: Bienvenue à Revachol. It's a bit out of date, as it was originally created by a design studio in a failed attempt to spruce up Martinaise and turn it into a fancy tourist location (ZA/UM, 2019).

Martinaise is the poverty-stricken coastal district of Revachol in which the game is set. It bears the scars of a failed communist revolution but is also haunted by the promise of the tourist resort it never became. It would be difficult to argue that the developers of the game are explicitly referencing the meta-touristic experience of *Disco Elysium* through this text description. However, the title "Bienvenue à Revachol" holds particular significance in that it echoes an infamous line spoken by a Non-Player Character named the "Racist Lorry Driver." He greets your partner and Revachol local Kim Kitsuragi as if he were a tourist: "Welcome to Revachol!" (ZA/UM, 2019) on the basis that he is of mixed ethnicity. What could be a sincere welcoming remark is warped into racist microaggression. Writer Helen Hindpere also said in an interview that the name 'Revachol' is a deliberate misspelling of the French anarchist François Claudius Koenigstein's nom de guerre "Ravachol," which features in the lyrics of Estonian punk band Vennaskind's song 'Welcome to America' (Dimopoulos, 2021). Thus, the title "Bienvenue à Revachol" is haunted by its associations both inside and outside of the game world. Mechanically, the Map of Martinaise allows Harry to fast travel within different locations; the theme of convenient travel is thus also woven into the mechanical affordances of the object in the game world. There remains the implicit knowledge that convenient travel around Revachol is available only for certain kinds of 'tourists'.

Perhaps the most hauntological objects in *Disco Elysium* are a series of discarded postcards that can be found at different locations. The postcards depict locations across Revachol, and mostly they date prior to the revolution, such as the "Postcard Couron '33":

> This one has 'HELL' written on its back. It could not be further from the truth. It's the boom years, and Couron, the nicest district in Revachol West, is enjoying a sun-drenched day (ZA/UM, 2019).

The idealised views that these postcards depict are indicative of what Urry and Larsen (2011) call the "tourist gaze", which orders an environment according to the romanticised view of the tourist, compartmentalising anything that does not fit. One postcard, "Postcard Boogie Street '46", can be considered a more explicit materialisation of the 'dark tourist gaze':

> This crumpled up postcard depicts an open air market in Boogie Street ~5 years ago. A vendor smiles as dead roosters line his stalls – hung by their feet from the canopy. Red blood flows onto the muddy street, blurry shadows of people pass (ZA/UM, 2019).

There is a voyeurism in the description of this postcard, which in its depiction of dead roosters veers into the macabre spectacle that so often characterises cynical ideas of dark tourism. In a post on Steam titled "Welcome to Revachol!" by the game writer Robert Kurvitz (2019):

> When middle-class people talk about foreign places, they like to talk about "contrasts" . . . And what they mean by "contrasts" is that most people are pornographically poor while a few are obscenely wealthy.

The postcards, with their idealised sun-drenched views or depiction of poverty porn, reveal this contrast through the eyes of the wealthy middle class who can afford to commemorate their visits. Mechanically, the postcards have no function other than to be sold at the Pawn Shop, "just assets to be liquified to build your portfolio and energize the economy, or something like that," as one tongue-in-cheek writer puts it (Kelly, 2021). That being said, they do function as a kind of epistolary worldbuilding device in the gothic tradition. In this way, numerous items in *Disco Elysium* explicitly reference tourism and implicitly implicate the player as a tourist themself, both within and without the fictional game world.

Feld

Disco Elysium contains hauntings that are far more direct than just the idea of the past haunting the present. To the northwest of Martinaise, there is a derelict building that before the revolution was owned by FELD, a computer engineering business. They were developing a state-of-the-art tape-based computer before their assets were liquidated by the revolutionary government. This history alone makes the FELD building a perfect candidate for a hauntological analysis. There is a further meta-layer to the FELD haunting as well- the dialogue interface for *Disco Elysium* is designed to look like the tape that the device ran on. As Krzywinska (2015, 72) points out, the Gothic regularly deploys technology as a way to try and understand or control the Other, especially in video games. In *Disco Elysium*, the Other is the player who is accessing the game using a technology that, according to its narrative, should not exist.

Turning back to more obvious ghosts, there is one particular scene of interest which is triggered when Harry interacts with a building covered in bullet holes near the FELD building. If he passes a Visual Calculus check, he can see:

> A row of ghostly shades stand facing the wall . . . Ten metres away – other shades are lined up in an orderly manner, automatic rifles primed (ZA/UM, 2019).

The game visualises these 'shades' as opaque orange figures. They represent an execution that happened after the fall of Martinaise, but it is unclear who is involved. This 'impossible' view of the past in the present brings to mind Ahmed's (2006, p. 258) argument that "social conflict can be experienced as being "out of time" as well as "out of place". With the identities of the people involved never resolved, *Disco Elysium* is prepared to give the player an uncomfortable experience in which not every mystery can be solved. This use of a ghostly tableau is also reminiscent of the audio installation at Bodiam Castle and its "attempt to destabilise visitors' sense that the past is fixed or inert" (Buser, 2017, p. 11).

The ghost of ZA/UM

The Doomed Commercial Area

There are other ghostly presences in Martinaise, with perhaps the best-known being associated with the so-called "Doomed Commercial Area" (DCA). The DCA has been home to numerous businesses which have all failed due to a rumoured curse. Investigating further into the DCA as I played, I found the experience to be in keeping with many of the classic gothic and horror tropes one might expect in a video game. Harry has to use a flashlight to illuminate the labyrinthine rooms behind the bookshop, containing strange artefacts of failed businesses past. The soundtrack for this area contains mechanical noises, suggesting interference, which works thematically well with one of the most pertinent failed companies in the DCA-Fortress Accident.

Fortress Accident was a studio working on a radio roleplaying game called "Wirrâl Untethered." The DCA contains the remains of their former office, including a radio computer. The game was overly ambitious and was eventually dropped due to a compiling error and no off-site back-up. If Harry finds the "Production Schedule Filament Memory," for Wirrâl Untethered and accesses it via the computer, more background is revealed:

> S. Luukanen-Kilde, the lead programmer of Fortress Accident: "The off-site copy was on-site because there was no *off-site* anymore, not for me, not after eight months of crunch (ZA/UM, 2019).

Gualeni and Fassone (2023, p. 177) consider Wirrâl Untethered to be a "satirical mise en abyme", an alternate version of ZA/UM, the studio which developed *Disco Elysium*. There are many ways in which Fortress Accident can be considered a key part of the gothic tourism experience of *Disco Elysium*. For one, we learn about it through the epistolary form of the aforementioned Filament Memory, and its fate is tied to the theme of lost memory which pervades so much of the game. Beyond this, Fortress Accident functions as a doppelganger for *Disco Elysium's* own development studio, revealing beyond the humour a potential dark reality of video game production involving compulsory overtime (the aforementioned "crunch"). Thus, the game is a dark tourism site because it was produced in a toxic work environment.

ZA/UM

In October 2022 Martin Luiga, an editor on *Disco Elysium* and a co-founder of the ZA/UM cultural association (separate from the main company) posted a now infamous Medium post claiming that three of the original founding members of ZA/UM were no longer working at the company and "their leaving the company was involuntary" (Luiga, 2022, n.p.). After a lot of speculation, ZA/UM itself confirmed that:

> the dismissed employees had limited to no engagement in their responsibilities and work, created a toxic work environment, demonstrated misconduct towards other employees including verbal abuse and gender discrimination, and attempted to illegally sell ZA/UM's intellectual property. (Partis 2022, n.p.).

However, in November 2022, former game director Robert Kurvitz and art director Aleksander Rostov (two of those founding members dismissed) posted on *Medium* stating they were pursuing legal action against Ilmar Kompus and Tõnis Haavel, the majority shareholders who they claim have acted fraudulently and pushed them out of the company (Kurvitz & Rostov, 2022). They point out:

> Until now, we've refrained from speaking out. This has been entirely voluntary, out of consideration for the people still working at ZA/UM – and for our mental health (Kurvitz & Rostov 2022, n.p.).

It appears that one lawsuit against Kompos has been dropped, while "one of those ousted founding developers told PC Gamer that their fight is far from over" (Litchfield, 2022, n.p.). Perhaps one of the most telling comments reported in the press is a ZA/UM source reported as saying there was "CEO corporate scheming on one side, a toxic auteur on the other" (Partis, 2022, n.p.). This seems to be confirmed by a documentary on ZA/UM published by People Make Games (2023), in which current and former employees of the studio were interviewed.

It is not the place of this chapter to speculate on these events, but instead to reflect on them as the wider context of the labour that went into *Disco Elysium*. After all, "like any type of tourism, game tourism is not only a type of leisure but involves economic structures and labour" (Lamerichs, 2018, p. 622). Haunted as it is now by these accusations of a toxic work environment, *Disco Elysium* is now a dark tourist experience of the game industry in a microcosm (Smith Nicholls, 2021). It is hard to imagine being able to play the game, especially the sections about ZA/UM's digital double Fortress Accident, without wondering what exactly was lost in terms of human dignity in the process of making it.

Conclusion

Throughout this piece, whether in regard to discussing gothic tourism, hauntology, or *Disco Elysium*, there have been three consistent themes: the indeterminacy of the video game medium, unstable memory, and the cultural corrosion of neoliberalism. Using close reading as a methodology has proved to be particularly relevant to a study of gothic tourism in games, especially as both stem from literary studies and also stress the inherent subjectivity of interpretation. Reflecting on the writing of this piece, I am drawn to Kirkland's (2021) comment that the research process itself can take on a gothic form. The epistolary nature of games research, using Let's Play archives (Arist, 2021) and fan wikis (Disco Elysium Wiki, n.d.) as aides memoires alongside my screenshots was another way in which the fallibility and plurality of memory were woven even into the labour of this piece itself.

Disco Elysium is a dark tourism experience as a hauntological game on at least three different levels. Firstly, the video game medium itself is haunted by its capacity to create an experience of doubling between the player and protagonist and to provide multiple versions of the same title through different playthroughs that coexist in the memory of the player, if not the game. Secondly, the fictional gameworld of *Disco Elysium* is haunted not just by a failed communist revolution, but by the promise of futures never realised, the technological brilliance of the Feld radio computer and the misguided creativity of Wirrâl Untethered snuffed out like a candle in the wind. Thirdly, the shadow of ZA/UM's alleged toxic working environment is now cast over the game, forever throwing its contents into a new light. Thus, the game is a fantastic example of digital dark tourism, or more specifically, the potential of Gothic tourism as seen through the lens of digital games.

References

Ahmed, S. (2006). *Queer Phenomenology: Orientations, Objects, Others*. Durham: Duke University Press.

Arist (2021) *Disco Elysium*. lparchive. https://lparchive.org/Disco-Elysium/ (accessed 31 December, 2022)

Atkins, B. (2007). Killing time: Time past, time present and time future in Prince of Persia: The sands of time. In T. Krzywinska, & B. Atkins (Eds.) *Videogame, Player, Text*, pp. 237–253. Manchester: Manchester University Press.

Banaszkiewicz, M., & Duda, A. (2019). To be a S.T.A.L.K.E.R. on architecture, computer games and tourist experience in the CEZ. In M. Gravari-Barbas, N. Graburn, & J-F. Staszak (Eds.) *Tourism Fictions, Simulacra and Virtualities*, pp. 197–210. London: Routledge.

Belmonte, J.F. (2021). The hanged rhizome on the tree: Arborescence and multiplicity in. *Baltic Screen Media Review*, *9*(1), 44–54.

Benardou, A., & Droumpouki, A.M. (Eds.) (2022). *Difficult Heritage and Immersive Experiences* (1st ed.). London: Routledge.

Bizzocchi, J., & Tanenbaum, J. (2011). Well read: Applying close reading techniques to gameplay experiences. In D. Davidson (Ed.) *Well played 3.0: Video Games, Value and Meaning*, pp. 262–290. Pittsburgh: ETC Press.

Bowman, N.D., Vandewalle, A., Daneels, R., Lee, Y., & Chen, S. (2023). Animating a plausible past: Perceived realism and sense of place influence entertainment of and tourism intentions from historical video games. *Games and Culture*. https://doi.org/10.1177/15554120231162428

Buser, M. (2017). The time is out of joint: Atmosphere and hauntology at Bodiam Castle. *Emotion, Space and Society*, *25*, 5–13.

Case, J. (2018). Our bodies, our incoherent selves: Games and shifting concepts of identity and narrative in contemporary storytelling. *Storyworlds*, *10* (1/2), 71–93.

Champion, E. (2022). Swords, sandals, and selfies: Videogame-induced tourism. In E. Champion, C. Lee, J. Stadler, & R.M. Peaslee (Eds.) *Screen Tourism and Affective Landscapes*, pp. 238–252. London: Routledge.

Cohen, E. (1985). Tourism as play. *Religion*, 15(3), 291–304.

Derrida, J. (1994). *Specters of Marx: The State of the Debt, the Work of Mourning, and the New International.* London: Routledge.

Dimopoulos, K. (2021). Disco Elysium: Designing the city of Revachol. *Wireframe Magazine.* https://wireframe.raspberrypi.com/articles/disco-elysium-designing-the-city-of-revachol (accessed 31 December, 2022)

Disco Elysium Wiki (n.d.). https://discoelysium.fandom.com/wiki/Disco_Elysium_Wiki (accessed 31 December, 2022)

Dubois, L.E., & Gibbs, C. (2018). Video game–induced tourism: A new frontier for destination marketers. *Tourism Review*, 73(2), 186–198.

DuBois, R. (2020, March 23). One Day I Will Return to Your Side: Disco Elysium and Hauntology. *Medium.* https://medium.com/@rose.elizabeth.dubois/one-day-i-will-return-to-your-side-disco-elysium-and-hauntology-619a6654f16a (accessed 31 December, 2022)

Fandino, D. (2018). Remembering fictional history and virtual war in *EVE Online*. In K.N. McDaniel (Ed.) *Virtual Dark Tourism: Ghost Roads*, pp. 287–308. Cham: Springer.

Fisher, M. (2012). What is hauntology? *Film Quarterly*, 66(1), 16–24.

Fisher, M. (2014). *Ghosts of My Life: Writings on Depression Hauntology and Lost Futures*. London: Zero Books.

Foley, M., & Lennon, J.J. (1996). JFK and dark tourism: A fascination with assassination. *International Journal of Heritage Studies*, 2(4), 198–211.

Gekker, A., & Joseph, D. (2021). Selling Elysium: The political economy of radical game distribution. *Baltic Screen Media Review*, *9*(1), 20–31.

González-Tennant, E. (2015). Resurrecting Rosewood: New heritage as applied visual anthropology. In A. Gubrium, K. Harper, & M. Otañez (Eds.) Participatory Visual and Digital Research in Action, pp. 163–177. London: Routledge.

Goulding, C., & Pressey, A. (2023). A palimpsestic analysis of atmospheres at dark tourism. Annals of Tourism Research, 101, 103577.

Grace, L.D. (2019). *Hauntology, the Penumbra, and the Narratives of Play Experience.* Paper presented at the 25th International Symposium of Electronic Art, Gwangju, South Korea, July 2019.

Gualeni, S., & Fassone, R. (2023). *Fictional Games: A Philosophy of Worldbuilding and Imaginary Play.* London: Bloomsbury Academic.

Hadden, A. (2019). A Storm Is Blowing from Paradise: Disco Elysium on the Past and Present. *Medium.* https://alastairhadden.medium.com/a-storm-is-blowing-from-paradise-disco-elysium-on-the-past-and-present-e2fff5d629be (accessed 31 December, 2022)

Hancock, M. (2016). Doppelgamers: Video Games and Gothic Choice. In J. Faflak & J. Haslam (Eds.), American Gothic Culture: An Edinburgh Companion, pp. 166–184. Edinburgh: Edinburgh University Press.

Harrer, S, & Pichlmair, M. (2015). Black skin white guns: Becoming colonizer in Resident Evil 5. Paper presented at the Philosophy of Computer Games Conference, Berlin, Germany.

Hasian, M., & Paliewicz, N.S. (2021). The national memorial for peace and justice, dark tourist argumentation, and civil rights memoryscapes. *Atlantic Journal of Communication*, 29(3), 168–184.

Howe, B. (2020, December 5). The Future Echoes of Disco Elysium. *Blood Knife*. https://bloodknife.com/future-echoes-disco-elysium/ (accessed 31 December, 2022)

Isaac, R.K. (2022) Introduction to dark tourism. In R.K. Isaac (Ed.) *Dark Tourism Studies, pp. 1–12.* London: Routledge.

Janik, J. (2019). Ghosts of the present past: Spectrality in the video game object. *Journal of the Philosophy of Games*, *2*(1), 1–22.

Jenkins, H. (2004). Game design as narrative architecture. *Computer*, 44(3), 118–130.

Jenkins, H., & Fuller, M. (1995). Nintendo and new world travel writing: A dialogue. Cybersociety: Computer-mediated Communication and Community, 61, 18.

Kelly, R. (2021, April 2). Disco Elysium: How to Make Money. *TheGamer*. https://www.thegamer.com/disco-elysium-money-making-guide/ (accessed 31 December, 2022)

Khamis, D. (2021). Disco Elysium as Philosophy: Solipsism, Existentialism, and Simulacra. In D.K. Johnson, D.A. Kowalski, C.Lay and K.S. Engels (Eds.), The Palgrave Handbook of Popular Culture as Philosophy, pp. 1865–1882. Palgrave Macmillan, Cham.

Kirkland, E. (2022). Gothic Gaming, Queer Mash-Ups, and Gone Home. In N. Neill (Ed.) *Gothic Mash-Ups: Hybridity, Appropriation, and Intertextuality in Gothic Storytelling*, pp. 205–223. London: Lexington Books.

Kirkland, E. (2021). *Videogames and the Gothic*. London: Routledge.

Kłosiński, M. (2021). The object gives rise to thought: Hermeneutics of objects in Disco Elysium. *Baltic Screen Media Review*, *9*, 56–66.

Korstanje, M. (2014). Conceptual discussion of dark tourism: Suffering, egoism and the depersonalization of death. Paper presented at the conference, Globalization of Tourism: Opportunities and Challenges, Goa, India. 2–3 May 2014.

Korstanje, M., & George, B. (2018). Emotionality, reason, and dark tourism: Discussions around the sense of death. In M. Korstanje, & B. George (Eds.) *Virtual Traumascapes and Exploring the Roots of Dark Tourism*, pp. 1–25. Hershey, PA: IGI Global.

Krzywinska, T. (2015). Gamification of Gothic. In M. Fuchs (Ed.) *Diversity of Play*, pp. 21–38. Lüneburg: Meson Press.

Kurvitz, R. *Welcome to Revachol!* (2019). Available at: https://discoelysium.com/devblog/2019/10/08/welcome-to-revachol (Accessed: 13 December 2021).

Lamerichs, N. (2018). Hunters, Climbers, Flâneurs:How video games create and design tourism. In C. Lundberg, & V. Ziakas (Eds.) *The Routledge Handbook of Popular Culture and Tourism*, pp. 161–169. London: Routledge.

LKA (2016). *The Town of Light*. Florence: LKA.

Light, D. (2007). Dracula tourism in Romania cultural identity and the state. *Annals of Tourism Research*, 34(3), 746 –765.

Light, D. (2017). Progress in dark tourism and thanatourism research: An uneasy relationship with heritage tourism. *Tourism Management*, *61*, 275–301.

Light, D., Richards, S., & Ivanova, P. (2021). Exploring “gothic tourism”: A new form of urban tourism? *International Journal of Tourism Cities*, 7(1), 224–236.

Litchfield, T. (2022). $4.8 million paid to ZA/UM and one lawsuit dropped as the battle over Disco Elysium continues. *PC Gamer*. https://www.pcgamer.com/dollar48-million-paid-to-zaum-and-one-lawsuit-dropped-as-the-battle-over-disco-elysium-continues/ (accessed 31 December, 2022)

Luiga, M. (2022). *THE DISSOLUTION OF THE ZA/UM CULTURAL ASSOCIATION*. Medium. https://medium.com/@martinluiga/the-dissolution-of-the-za-um-cultural-association-779788390a03 (accessed 31 December, 2022)

Nhlabathi, S.S., & Maharaj, B. (2020). The dark tourism discipline: A creative brand in a competitive academic environment? *Current Issues in Tourism*, *23*(19), 2428–2439.

Novitz, J. (2021). Disco Elysium as Gothic fiction. *Baltic Screen Media Review*, *9*, 32–42.

Martini, A., & Buda, D (2020). Dark tourism and affect: Framing places of death and disaster. *Current Issues in Tourism*, 23(6), 679–692.

Matta, D. (2021, November 1). *Disco Elysium: Ghosts of a lost future*. Honi Soit. https://honisoit.com/2021/11/disco-elysium-ghosts-of-a-lost-future/ (accessed 31 December, 2022)

McDaniel, K.N. (Ed.) (2018). *Virtual Dark Tourism: Ghost Roads*. Cham: Springer.

McEvoy, E. (2016). *Gothic Tourism*. Cham: Springer.

McLachlan, E. (2022). *AdvX 2022 – Eve McLachlan – Dark Passages: Interactive Fiction and the Gothic*. https://www.youtube.com/watch?v=lPcKf-GZETY (accessed 31 December, 2022)

Medvedeva, A.R. (2022). Urban shivers: Recoding actual space in Disco Elysium. *Galactica Media: Journal of Media Studies*, *4*(3), Article 3. https://doi.org/10.46539/gmd.v4i3.318
Miles, W. (2002). Auschwitz: Museum interpretation and darker tourism. *Annals of Tourism Research*, 29, 1175–1178.
Miller, K. (2008). The accidental carjack: Ethnography, gameworld tourism, and Grand Theft Auto. Game Studies, 8(1), 147.
Milligan, C.A. (2018). Virtually historical: Performing dark tourism through alternate history games. In K.N. McDaniel (Ed.) *Virtual Dark Tourism: Ghost Roads*, pp. 265–286. Cham: Springer.
Mukherjee, S. (2017). Re-membering and dismembering: Memory and the (re)creation of identities in videogames. *Sessões do Imaginário*, *22*(38), 53–63.
Ozimek, A. (2021). Production of game making spaces: Disco Elysium and the game making community in Estonia. *Baltic Screen Media Review*, *9*, 6–18.
Partis, D. (2022). *Disco Elysium studio ZA/UM confirms former employees were fired for misconduct.* GamesIndustry.Biz. https://www.gamesindustry.biz/disco-elysium-studio-zaum-confirms-former-employees-were-fired-for-misconduct (accessed 31 December, 2022)
People Make Games (2023, May 29). Investigation: Who's Telling the Truth about Disco Elysium? [Video] YouTube https://www.youtube.com/watch?v=JGIGA8taN-M&t=6s (accessed 12 July 2023)
Price, R. (2021). *A Year Later, I Still Can't Stop Thinking About Disco Elysium*. Kotaku. https://kotaku.com/a-year-later-i-still-cant-stop-thinking-about-disco-el-1847585413 (accessed 31 December, 2022)
Robertson, A. (2013). Gaming with Ghosts: Hauntology, Metanarrative and Gamespace in Video Games. Unpublished master's thesis, Carleton University, Canada
Rostov, A. (2022). TO FANS OF DISCO ELYSIUM, CONCERNING THE SITUATION AT ZA/UM. *Medium*. https://medium.com/@artofrostov/to-fans-of-disco-elysium-concerning-the-situation-at-za-um-3e6bc46ea9c (accessed 31 December, 2022)
Sawicki, E. (2021) '"FAILURES OF THE WORLD, UNITE!"', *Medium*, 19 October. https://medium.com/@eryk.sawicki/failures-of-the-world-unite-fc1def0c6056 (accessed 31 December, 2022)
Schwartz, L. (2006). Fantasy, realism, and the other in recent video games. Space and Culture, 9(3), 313–325.
Schwartz, Ł. (2019). Horror Video Games and the Idea of Haunted Media. Unpublished master's thesis, University of Silesia in Katowice, Poland.
Smith Nicholls, F. (2021). Picture imperfect: Photography, dark tourism and video games. *Historical Games Network*, 11 August. https://www.historicalgames.net/picture-imperfect-photography-dark-tourism-and-video-games/ (accessed 31 December, 2022)
Smith Nicholls, F. (2018). Virtual dark tourism in The Town of Light. In E. Champion (Ed.) *The Phenomenology of Real and Virtual Places*, pp. 223–237. New York: Routledge.
Stang, S. (2022). Too close, too intimate, and too vulnerable: Close reading methodology and the future of feminist game studies. Critical Studies in Media Communication, 39(3), 230–238.
Sterling, C. (2021). Becoming hauntologists: A new model for critical-creative heritage practice. *Heritage & Society*, 14(1), 67–86.
Stevens, D. (2000). *The Gothic Tradition*. Cambridge: Cambridge University Press.
Stone, P.R. (2006). A dark tourism spectrum: Towards a typology of death and macabre related tourist sites, attractions and exhibitions. *Tourism*: An International Interdisciplinary Journal, 54(2), 145–160.
Tamahori, M. (2022). *Beyond the Pale: Exploring the Spatial, Temporal, and Characterization Mechanics of the Detective Videogame Disco Elysium*. Unpublished thesis, University of Auckland, New Zealand.
Ting, T. (2019). *Game Level Design, Gay Cruising and the Queer Gothic in The Rawlings*. Unpublished master's thesis, OCAD University.
Urry, J., & Larsen, J. (2011). *The Tourist Gaze 3.0*. London: SAGE
Vella, M., & M. Cielecka. (2021). "You Won't Even Know Who You Are Anymore": Bakthinian Polyphony and the Challenge to the Ludic Subject in Disco Elysium. Baltic Screen Media Review, 9, 90–104.

Willis, E. (2014). *Theatricality, Dark Tourism and Ethical Spectatorship: Absent Others*. London: Palgrave Macmillan.

XENOGOTHIC (2020). *The Games Industry: Accelerationism and the Hauntological in Microcosm*. Xenogothic. https://xenogothic.com/2020/06/07/the-games-industry-accelerationism-and-the-hauntological-in-microcosm/ (accessed 31 December, 2022)

Yang, R. (2009) *How to Close Read Video Games*. https://www.blog.radiator.debacle.us/2009/12/how-to-close-read-video-games.html (accessed 31 December, 2022)

ZA/UM Studio (2019). *Disco Elysium*. London: ZA/UM Studio.

Part IV: **Dark tourism, power and identity**

Maximiliano E. Korstanje

11 Sites of (dark) consciences: Investigating dark tourism cosmologies in a post-colonial landscape

Abstract: Although dark tourism has captivated the attention of scholars over recent years, part of the specialized literature overlooks the interplay between dark tourism and politics. Dark tourism and politics are inextricably intertwined. As Joy Sather-Wagstaff noted, dark heritage can be politically and ideologically manipulated to protect some interests; on occasions, affirming long dormant neocolonial discourses negating the ethical liabilities of European nations in their abuses during the colonial period (Korstanje & Baker 2018). This book chapter holds that dark tourism is aimed at commoditizing history that tells visitors only a partial truth of the real story. It engages with critical theory as the touchstone of its analysis while laying the foundations towards a new understanding of dark tourism. Centered on the assumptions that dark tourism looks to consume the "Other`s pain" for narcissistic reasons, the material asymmetries between the Global North and South persist. Nonetheless, dark tourism offers a fertile ground to provide a lesson to society enhancing resiliency and adaptation to traumatic events. Having said this, dark tourism helps to understand bloody events which should not be repeated in the future. This book chapter discusses critically the contributions and limitations of dark tourism theory in a postcolonial context.

Keywords: dark tourism, capitalism, colonial exploitation, Postcolonialism, trauma

Introduction

Dark tourism is undoubtedly a fascinating topic of study and a buzzword that has captivated the attention of scholars worldwide. Aside from this, the term has ignited a hot debate these days in academic circles (Podoshen, 2018). Some scholars agree that dark tourism is a form of reflexivity provided by "the Other´s" death. As Stone (2012) eloquently discusses, dark tourism acts as an instrument that helps visitors contemplate their own finitude through the "Other`s death" (Stone, 2012). This academic school is known as the "thanaptopic tradition". Scholars who embrace this conceptual paradigm hold that thanatosis, which means a much deeper anthropological attempt to understand one's own life through the lens of the "Other`s death", is a key factor in the formation of dark sites (Stone, 2012; Seaton, 1996; Miles, 2014). Contrary to that, other studies signal towards the phenomenon as a form of new macabre heritage that helps understand traumatic events (Cohen, 2011; Korstanje & Ivanov, 2012; Jordan &

https://doi.org/10.1515/9783110792072-012

Prayag, 2022). The heritage-based paradigm emphasizes the importance of dark tourism to understand not only a bloody history or dissonant heritage but also in constructing a lesson that re-memorizes the traumatic event (Heidelberg, 2015; Ivanova & Light, 2018). Many other academic paradigms debate on the nature and evolution of dark tourism, typically in a state of conceptual fragmentation (Hooper & Lennon, 2016). Each academic school tells only a part of the story (Sharpley, 2009; Biran & Hyde, 2013). Further, dark tourism exhibits a place of consumption that is marked by a great tragedy, or mourning which includes sites of genocide, mass death, or destruction without mentioning natural or man-made disasters and political violence. In dark tourism sites, visitors look to feel what the victims felt, being close to their last days (Hartmann, 2014; Wight, 2006). As Peter Tarlow puts it, dark tourism speaks to us of a type of nostalgia for death evoked to understand our present (Tarlow, 2007).

In recent years, some critical voices have focused on the limitations and methodological problems in dark tourism research. To the classic epistemological dispersion, which means the proliferation of similar terms and theories (Hooper & Lennon, 2016) one must add emerging narratives orientated to protect the status quo or the current political interests of the ruling elite (Potts, 2012; Korstanje 2016; Tzanelli 2016). Dark tourism gives a lesson about dark events which sometimes are politically manipulated or distorted to protect specific interests (Sather Wagstaff, 2016; Bowman & Pezzullo, 2009). Although this is a case easily found in many tourist destinations not directly related to dark tourism consumption in the strict sense of the word, the truth is that beyond dark tourism, lies a history of trauma and loss. This sentiment often derives from a state of conflict or the local discontent which is directed against the authorities. When this happens, authorities devote efforts to reshape the re-memorizing process while imposing their own interpretation of the reasons behind the disaster (Sather Wagstaff, 2016; Korstanje, 2016).

Under some conditions, which range from political intervention [as clarified earlier] to the creation of light spectacles to amass further profits, the real reasons for the disaster are commoditized or biased increasing the odds of the same disaster repeating in the short run (Stone, 2006; Korstanje, 2016). The opposite is equally true; some dark allegories are carefully designed to silence some peripheral voices (Miles, 2015; Busby & Devereaux, 2015) or at least to cover the material asymmetries between the center and its periphery (Sharpley, 2009). At a closer look, the dismantling of European Empires [just after WWII ended] and the passage from the decolonial period to a global post-colonialism opened the doors to an amnesia for the crimes committed by European powers. Part of the political instability or ethnic genocides has been determined by European occupation. Nowadays, dark tourism alludes to a dissonant heritage in peripheral nations where not all voices are taken into consideration in the re-memorizing process. The official discourse not only affirms the status quo but also ignores a significant part of historical pastime. Nicolle Guidotti-Hernandez coins the term “unspeakable violence” to denote these types of discursive amnesias oriented to protect the interests of the privileged elite. As the author eloquently notes, political violence is often repressed or silenced for the next generations but in some cases, it is spectacularized to be consumed by tourists. According to her viewpoint, tourists never look at the truth, but a fabricated sense of truth that legitimate their emotional world previously constructed in their urban metropolises (Guidotti-Hernandez, 2011). Of course, this moot point will be placed under the critical lens of scrutiny in the next sections.

In a seminal book entitled *Thanatourism and cinematic representations of risk*, Tzanelli (2016) describes the philosophical dilemmas revolving around dark tourism consumption as well as its connection with neoliberalism and neo-colonialism. From her standpoint, dark tourism sites offer a commoditized message to visitors who are looking for consuming stories of mass death and human suffering. Thousands of European tourists visit former colonies to hear the stories of genocides and ethnic cleansing. Although these tourists are sympathetic to the "Other′s pain", they are unfamiliar with the moral responsibilities of their states in the colonial expansion as well as the cruelty and violence exerted in the colonies. For some authors, this occurs simply because dark tourism – far from healing historical wounds affirms the old center-periphery dependency (Tzanelli, 2016; Light, 2017). Those voices that embrace enthusiastically that dark tourism replicates the basis of the old colonialism are dubbed as "the critical turn" (Korstanje, 2020). In consonance with this, Dang (2021) argues convincingly that some dark tourism sites are mainly linked to spaces of suffering or mass death but also replicate the perspectives of the Anglo-American cosmology or the Anglophone world. As Tzanelli (2016) concludes, dark tourists are not familiarized with the crimes committed by their states in the colonial period. Dark consumption, in this way, only tells a partial truth which is coincidental with Western cultural values. To some extent, there is a selective memory that remembers only a version of the historical facts. In a doctoral dissertation, Keira Smalley (2021) sheds some light on the problem of coloniality and dark tourism consumption. As per her stance, dark tourism consumption alludes to the commercialization of the "Other" though this point is never questioned (at least in the specialized literature). Basing her point using psychoanalytical theory, she explores how dark tourism evokes a spectral interruption in the present silencing or distorting the bloody past. In other terms, as she observes, the white tourist is valorized as a rational and democratic agent interested in a bloody story. At another corner of the square ring, we find the bestial black or "non-Western Other" whose bestiality or criminality is narrated and circulated through different discourses and stereotypes. What is more important is that dark tourism should be conceptualized as a racially charged encounter where human suffering is marketed to be consumed by a white audience. This mourning, which evokes an early loss, not only becomes a commodity but a criterion of attraction. These racialized spaces are systematically constructed by the gravitation of authorities and dark site managers. Dark tourism offers some fabricated fantasies that help reproduce the technology of whiteness which is related to a much deeper colonial genealogy.

As previously argued, this book chapter interrogates further the problems of current dark tourism research, more oriented towards dark tourism management, while laying the foundations to expand the impacts of dark tourism in neo-colonial landscapes. Hence, this chapter explores the political nature of dark tourism as well as its intricacies in the configuration of (neo) colonial cosmologies.The goals of this editorial project are twofold. On one hand, we provide the next steps in the research agenda for the decades to come. On another, we focus on the complex current limitations of dark tourism studies nowadays. Having said this, the first section offers a discussion on the current limitations of dark tourism research today. These limitations include the proliferation (if not fragmentation) of definitions as well as an excessive valorization of tourists´ expectancies. A historical sweep fills the gap left by the literature. In the second section, we scrutinize the role played by political violence and trauma during the colonial period. European powers launched to colonize the world re-educating the "non-western people in the Western mainstream cultural values. This process – far from being peaceful- recreated serious financial asymmetries and social maladies which today are consumed by rich European tourists. Complementarily, the third section ignites a hot debate revolving around the intersection of dark tourism and the colonial genealogy which means the set of stereotypes, discourses and narratives oriented to describe the "Non-Western Other". The fourth section contains the steps towards a future epistemological agenda in dark tourism studies. Here, critical theory occupies a central position in discussing to what extent dark tourism heals or affirms the dominant discourses forged during colonial rule.

Methodological problems in dark tourism studies

As stated in the introductory section, dark tourism has gained traction as an area of study over the years. This led invariably to a knowledge fragmentation where each author defines the issue following different guidelines (Hooper & Lennon). Some studies, headed by Sharpley and Stone emphasize dark tourism as a reflexive attempt to understand one's own life through the Other´s death (Stone & Sharpley, 2008; Shapley & Stone 2009). This definition includes a lot of activities at sites of mass death, destruction or disaster as well as prisons, exhibitions or concentration camps. To give a more accurate classification, Philip Stone offers a model which ranges from the lightest to darkest spectrum of dark tourism practices (Light 2017; Stone 2013; Timothy 2021). Whereas the former signals to spaces of cultural entertainment and consumption, the latter points towards places mainly marked by extreme suffering and pain (Stone 2006; Strange & Kempa 2003). Other works focus on the historical lesson dark tourism sites provide. For these scholars, dark tourism should be defined as a form of heritage offered to visitors interested in historical facts (Biran, Poria & Oren, 2011; Collins-Kreiner, 2016). For these studies, authenticity occupies a central position in the configuration of dark tourism sites (Cohen 2011; Hartmann, 2014; Magee & Gilmore 2015). For the sake of clarity, scholars acknowledge that dark tourism rests on the thanaptopsis (or thanaptopic process) which means the possibility for the visitors to experiment his-her own finitude through the "Other´s death" (Seaton, 1996; Stone 2012).

A new horizon of interesting research explores dark tourism as a continuation of collective unconsciousness or death drives. Based on Freud´s contributions, Buda (2015) argues that dark tourism should equate to the collective drive for death which enhances social resilience. According to her argument, dark tourism should be studied according to new methodological paradigms which accept the advances of the psychoanalytical model as well as the power of emotions in consumers´ behavior (Buda 2015; Cave & Buda, 2018; Martini & Buda, 2020). After all, death is a creative force that brings all of us together. Dark tourism recycles spaces of mass destruction that otherwise would remain uninhabitable (Korstanje & Ivanov 2012; Buda 2015). Applications of dark tourism theory have been successfully adopted in post-disaster recovery studies worldwide (See Martini & Sharma, 2022). The global risks such as terrorism, natural disasters or the current ecological crisis without mentioning the recent COVID-19 pandemic have pushed the tourism industry to the brink of collapse. Dark tourism studies adopt innovative models that mitigate the effects of risk while accelerating the recovery timeframe (Stone 2011; Tucker, Shelton & Bae, 2017; Lin, Kelemen & Tresidder, 2018). Needless to say, dark tourism studies have some methodological limitations that deserve some critical discussion.

At first glimpse, dark tourism research is strictly based on what A. Franklin (2007) dubbed as "tourist-centricity" which means the obsession to take what tourists say as the only source of valid information. Although the applied research is certainly based on extensive samples, the questionnaires conducted are limited to describing the visitors` psychological motivations as well as their experience and expectancies. Methodologically speaking, sometimes interviewees lie to protect their interests or simply are unfamiliar with their inner world and emotions. Men are educated to repress their emotions. What is more important, interviewees engage positively with the fieldworkers negating their inappropriate answers and feelings. How would a gangster respond if we ask: what is your profession? Surely, he would reply: I am a businessman; so the moot point is, is this true?

The second associated problem lies in the negotiations and struggles of stakeholders to impose their narratives, worries and explanations about the original event. When the real causes of the disasters are distorted, the possibilities for the event to be repeated are significant (Korstanje 2015; Korstanje & George 2015; Olsen & Korstanje 2019). By the same token, Bowman & Pezzullo (2009) interrogate further the ethical dilemmas and socio-anthropological dimensions of darkness. Since the concept of darkness is opposed to light, authors acknowledge that Western researchers have adopted a negative image of dark tourism as strictly associated with mass death, massacre, or everything that should be devoid. Dark also denotes a dark (bad) side that attracts us. Hence over the years, researchers tried to respond to the motivations of dark tourists to visit these spaces of mourning and pain. More prone to creating a subdivision of the phenomenon instead of understanding its nature dark tourism researchers embraced the thanaptopic model. This invariably means that tourists are looking to experience their own finitude through the "Other`s death". Authors question to what extent is anxiety the main factor that guides tourism consumption in dark sites, and anxiety to what? is the question that immediately surfaces. Dark tourism should be seen as a ritual that negotiates and helps deal with human pain and the emptiness left by the atrocity. Through these rituals, survivors and visitors meet with the new four stages of creation and accommodation: sanctification, designation, rectification and obliteration. Rites of passage put people in a liminoid space where their identities are unfixed as well as their rules for life. It is difficult to resist the impression that rituals are always transformative of the biographical self and performative reminding precisely death is not an event of the past, but rather, what shapes the present and future. Bowman & Pezzullo go on to write: *"Rather than seeing tourist sites and practices as products, destinations, or consumption that always-already interpellates us as 'tourists,' we might instead, as Löfgren (1999, p. 7) puts it, imagine tours 'as a cultural laboratory where people have been able to experiment with new aspects of identities, their social relations or their interactions with nature and also to use the important cultural skills of daydreaming and mind-travelling.'* (Bowman & Pezzullo, 2010, p. 197)"

Last but not least, an emerging body of critical theorists has lamented the lack of interest of dark tourism researchers to discuss social injustices and asymmetries in the past (Tzanelli, 2016; Sather Wagstaff, 2016; Sharma & Martini, 2024). The former colonial exploitation practices are ideologically silenced by the formation of global discourses where the "Other" is reduced to being a victim. But beyond this sentiment, there is no remorse for the crimes committed by European states during the colonial period over locals in the former colonies. In films, novels and TV programs, locals are portrayed as mere individual victims whose suffering is derived from some cultural social maladies enrooted in their societies. These maladies include corruption, civil wars, genocide or cleansing and even poverty. In these ideological compositions, there is no mention of the extractive practices and institutions that violated natives` human rights in the overseas colonies (Tzanelli, 2016; Korstanje, 2016; Sather Wagstaff, 2016; Carrigan, 2014). Carrigan (2014) holds that dark tourism leaves spaces of symbolic conflicts, bloody legacies, and trauma because of the actions of colonial powers. The sense of trauma appears to be a concept very hard to operationalize empirically (Carrigan, 2014; Tumarkin, 2001).

The critical turn offers a fertile ground to decipher the repressed forms of domination that characterized the center-periphery dependency in the past (Lemelin et al, 2013). In an interesting book titled *Writing the dark side of Travel*, Jonathan Skinner (2012) questions to what extent experts can decide what a site of suffering is or define an event as darker than others. Furthermore, dark tourism engages –as a type of pilgrimage- with the "Other's death" but in multiple ways and shapes. Dark tourism mediates between citizens, their states (laws) and death. Skinner overtly recognizes that these sites are organized to offer a cultural spectacle that says nothing about the real causes behind the disaster. Ethnographers who are interested in dark tourism issues often allude to documenting (in writing) what they observe, the outcomes are written according to their idiosyncrasy. Often dark tourism practices are controlled by dominant groups who push some other voices to the periphery, as Skinner adheres. To fill the gap, researchers should examine the politics of dark tourism in the years to come. Skinner's text begs us to reflect on some intriguing questions such as who can define whether Alcatraz is a space of pain or simply a space of discipline? Is the tourist's morbid taste the key factor that defines dark tourism? Or are there scientific methods that help understand the pain or at least how it is re-memorized?

The present book chapter adopts a historical sweep to answer part of the above-referenced questions as well as laying the foundations towards a new understanding of dark tourism as a phenomenon culturally enrooted in the political process of European colonialism. The chapter also interrogates further on the political nature of dark tourism as an instrument of legitimacy cemented by a fabricated past. The term fabricated here does not denote any positive or negative assertion, it rather means a social construction or dissonance that does not always meet with the historical facts.

Colonialism and trauma

Doubtless, there is no other moment of trauma in human history than European colonialism. In this respect, Tumarkin (2001) coins the term "traumascape" to denote the human capacity to deal with and re-memorize traumatic experiences in the present. Traumatic experiences are often forgotten or repressed to achieve a mental balance. The same applies in the social sphere, where traumas are silenced. The concept of traumascape is associated mainly with a bloody past or a disaster where society gradually recovers. In the recovery, the event cannot be memorized as it happened, also it is evoked according to what society offers as a narrative to visitors and tourists. Hence, traumascape exhibits the encounter of the traumatic past with the present time offered as a form of spectacle; as she recognizes, any attempt to re-memorize tragedies calls for a partial reliving of an unspoken, negated, or unassimilated past. Tragedies –like colonialism- have the potential to create spaces of trauma and mourning which transform the territory where the event occurs (Tumarkin, 2001; 2005). In addition, Gagne (1998) speaks of trauma as a psychological shock that brings not only emotional damage but also durable effects on the mind or culture. She analyses the roles of colonialism leading to a much deeper sentiment of dependency in the colonies marked by racism, genocides and alcoholism. According to her viewpoint, the economic dependency associated with social maladies (maelstrom) is the key factor of social deviation in former colonies. Today, peripheral nations or former colonies offer social degradation, certainly accelerated by European occupation, as a form of embellished spectacle which is consumed by first-world tourists. This spectacle is centered on local criminality, ethnic cleansing, or genocides perpetrated during wars or coups. The climate of political instability is seen as a sign of inferiority or cultural incapacity of locals to embrace democracy and stability. This Eurocentric discourse however has little to say about the crime of European countries during the colonial period. This suggests that the tourist product [or dark spectacle] serves as an ideological instrument of subordination and indoctrination. In consonance with this, the political external structures have imposed the center to prevent the economic progress of the peripheral nations while protecting the proper (colonial) interests. The connection between the center and periphery never breaks while mutating to new forms in the threshold of time. We could say that colonialism constitutes a cultural bereavement that exhibits long-lasting cycles of viciousness and maladies including suicide, poverty, alcoholism or drug addiction and crime (Czyzewski, 2011; Miller, 2020). In this vein, Braithwaite & Lee (2006) argue convincingly that dark tourism offers a fertile ground for reconciliation in destinations characterized by durable political violence, slavery, and economic deprivation. The psychological violence left by decades of exploitation or political violence can be healed while introducing dark tourism. Other studies say that the reconciliation process, stimulated by tourism, is successfully achieved when hosts and guests pass from intense hate to empathy and practical forgiveness leaving behind the dark clouds of conflict and violence (Braithwaite & Lee, 2006). Under some conditions of stability, which means the suspension of political violence as the main requisite, dark tourism enhances social cohesion while placating rivalries or sentiments of discontent among groups. These rivalries have been fostered in the past according to unresolved conflicts or wars. Once the community is pacified, dark tourism plays a leading role in sanitizing not only the economy but also the nagging wounds so that survivors can be placed in equal conditions before the law. Clarke, Dutton & Johnston (2014) use the term 'dark travels' to the itineraries, cultural practices and derived experiences in zones of extreme mourning and pain, or spaces devastated by traumatic experiences. Dark travels are not an object of study in the strict sense of the word but dispositions finely enrooted into post-colonial studies. In these dark landscapes, visitors engage with a commoditized space mainly traversed by colonial exploitation, mistrust, and discontent.

Dark tourism in a postcolonial landscape

As debated, dark tourism provides a fresh insight into reconciling resentment in post-conflict destinations (Causevic & Lynch, 2011; Mitchell, Henthorne & George, 2020). Under some conditions, dark tourism may very well potentiate the material inequalities generated by European colonialism at the destinations. One of the methodological problems of dark tourism applied to the postcolonial context seems to be related to the distortion of the narratives revolving around the dark sites (Tzanelli, 2016; Korstanje,

2016). In the context of recovery or post-disaster, some political groups or pressure groups offer a biased description of the reasons behind the tragedy. They often not only silence some actors relegating them to a peripheral position, but also some discourses forged in the colonial period are valorized. These discourses are based on the incompatibilities of local cultural values with democracy and prosperity. The effects of disaster are potentiated in poor nations historically marked by political instability or political conflict. Echoing this Eurocentric discourse, aboriginal (local) cultures are unable to adopt democratic institutions. As a result of this, the disaster is the consequence of local incapacity to foster strong institutions. The interplay between prosperity and Europeanness is engulfed in the core of colonialism (Potts, 2012; Tzanelli, 2016; Sather Wagstaff, 2016). In 2014, Joachim Ntunda published *Investigating the Challenges of promoting Dark Tourism in Rwanda.* He started from the premise that dark tourism takes many forms and shapes depending on the hosting culture. What is equally important, is that actors struggle with their own interpretations and meanings around the reasons why the disaster happened. Mainly involved in an ongoing state of conflict, bloody cleansing, and warfare, Rwanda is the perfect example of how dark tourism may heal past wounds. Regardless of this fact, the author finds structural problems such as the lack of skilled staff and infrastructure to develop dark tourism in the country. In the case of former colonies, tourism often fails to provide efficient poverty alleviation. As Ntunda eloquently stresses, subject to years of violence, Rwanda faced countless coups that devastated the local economies.

Dark tourism offers a fertile ground for economic maturation in a long-distant future. Tzanelli (2016) explains that dark tourism reflects the radical mutations of the tourism industry to new forms. In various of her books, Tzanelli does not agree that dark consumption should be defined as an ideological mechanism of control. Rather, as she adheres, dark tourism corresponds with a creative destruction process culturally enrooted in global capitalism, where death (destruction) is the epicenter of something new. Disaster is not the end, but the start of a new cosmology. Through dark tourism, devastated areas are finally recycled in months and adapted to be consumed by external visitors. However, this does not imply that dark tourism acts as a pedagogic instrument of heritage reproduction. Though these areas can be recycled following various models, as Tzanelli adheres, in the post-recovery facet original dwellers are pushed to live in peripheral neighborhoods. The foreign investors not only take the lead in the reconstruction stage but also press the authorities to raise the local taxes. The city downtown is reserved for luxury projects or leisure activities, while the dwellers who cannot pay the new taxes are pushed to the margins. Against the previous backdrop, dark tourism sites result from zones of extreme poverty whipped by political violence and colonial exploitation. It is important not to lose sight of the fact that these zones are packaged to be consumed through different media, which includes TV programs, novels, and of course cinema.

Tzanelli uses the term *cinematic representation* to denote the fabrication of ideologies and narratives oriented to interpret colonialism or at the least the crimes perpetrated by the European powers over locals. These interpretations are in favor of a Eurocentric discourse where the local is seen as an irrational agent that needs re-education. This opens the doors to a paradoxical situation simply because many of the dark sites today located in the former colonies (like Africa, or Asia) have been generated by the European occupation or internal ethnic wars during the colonial period. Paradoxically, first-world tourists are interested in these types of sites while they are not familiarized with the responsibilities of their states. (Tzanelli, 2013; 2016; 2018; 2021), At this point, postcolonialism should be understood as a state of capitalism where human suffering is commoditized as a criterion of attractiveness and curiosity as never before (Tzanelli & Korstanje, 2019).

Although dark tourism has captivated the attention of scholars over the recent years, no less true is that publications are not approaching the connection of the phenomenon with politics. As Joy Wagstaff (2016) puts it, under some conditions dark heritage is politically manipulated, or echoing Rodanthi Tzanelli (2016), it affirms the long-dormant discourses originally forged in the colonial period. On occasions, not only dark tourists are unfamiliar with the role played by their nations in the colonial expansion, but in others, they also replicate involuntarily much deeper material asymmetries between the Global North and South. Dark tourism tends to commoditize history to tell visitors only a part of the real story. The present book chapter ignites debate revolving around critical theory as the touchstone of its analysis while laying the foundations towards a new understanding of dark tourism. Based on the preliminary assumptions exhibited in the rise of Thana Capitalism and Tourism (Korstanje, 2016), we hold that dark tourists look to consume the "Other´s pain" to feedback a strange narcissism that reminds the so-called Western superiority over other cultures.Dark tourists look to embrace their political institutions as well as look for a reason to feel special. The "Other", like a child irrational and uneducated, represents not only how important the triumph of capitalism and democratic lifestyle is over other forms of government but also the European mainstream cultural values. As Tzanelli noted, in doing so, they misjudge the responsibilities of their governments in the sorrow over former colonies during the colonial period even to date. This argument raises some vexed questions: what do Belgian or French tourists know about the crimes perpetrated by Belgium and France in Congo or Algeria? What motivates Britons to visit India or South Africa?

The injustices and bloody past that mainly mark European colonialism are systematically neglected by dark tourists. However, it is safe to say that dark tourism offers a fertile ground to give a lesson to society enhancing resiliency and adaptation to traumatic events. From this perspective, dark tourism helps to understand bloody events which should not be repeated in the future. This chapter discusses critically the contributions and limitations of dark tourism theory for a future research agenda in a post-colonial context.

Critical theory and future research agenda

In the preface of their recent book, Stone et al. (2018) call attention to setting a new agenda for dark tourism research. Over more than 20 years, theorists have combined different disciplines and theoretical models [which include thanatology, anthropology and sociology] to define the nature of dark tourism. To date, dark tourism has been recognized internationally as an activity limited to those who travel to difficult heritage sites or at least linked to mass death. This conception divides voices to agree on a consensus in practical and empirical fields. But at a closer look, dark tourism says more about the life and the living than the dead. Dark tourism intersects with culture, as well as dissonant heritage without mentioning the intricacies of political injustices. Critical theory takes the lead introducing readers to a critical reflection on dark tourism and the colonial legacy (Jamal & Lelo, 2010). Iliev (2020) sheds light on the new direction the discipline should follow. His finding reveals that dark sites are formed according to what tourists want to gaze at, but it is rarely articulated according to the presence of history, death, thanatopsis or heritage. Rather, dark sites offer experiences though they cannot be labeled as dark. Tourist behavior seems to be more complex and dynamic than what researchers acknowledge. For that reason, future research needs a post-disciplinary approach integrating various sub-disciplines and methods.

As per the previous argument, critical theory assists in deciphering the ideological discourses widely framed during colonialism leading society towards a climate of harmony and re-conciliation. How this happens is a good point to be carried out in future layouts. Last but not least, critical theory stimulates critical thinking to imagine dark tourism beyond the already-existent cosmologies. The word critical does not mean that the theory lacks of a specific theoretical framework. Over the years, critical studies have exerted a caustic critique in various fields of tourism research without providing a fresh model to illustrate future generations of researchers.

Conclusion

The present book chapter explores the methodological problems and limitations of current dark tourism studies. Over the years, dark tourism studies have emphasized the dark-site formation as well as tourist motivation factors. This position led scholars to minimize the critical theory as a fertile ground for new epistemological models to understand dark tourism. Having said this, the colonial legacy has left a climate of extreme competition, mistrust, and hate in former colonies. This means that dark tourism is running short to conciliate disrupting attitudes among locals and foreign tourists. Some critical voices have alerted on the importance of analyzing and deconstructing the allegories created in the colonial period. The European travelers were often portrayed as educated men dotted with fine skills and versed in the excellence of European culture. Rather, locals –treated as naïve children- were seen as irrational and uneducated. The cultural factor served as a key factor that explained the local backwardness in the colonies. In so doing, the responsibilities of European Nations in the ethnic cleansing and genocides were overlooked. The different ethnic cleansing, as well as inter-kinship wars and conflicts, have been ultimately defined as the cultural impossibilities of natives to negotiate their interests. The same dichotomies persist in dark tourism studies where researchers devote their efforts to exploring the tourists` behavior and psychological motivations while the past crimes of European nations are systematically negated. In this vein, dark tourists –who are in quest of something different that makes them feel more special – ideologically accept the social institutions of the cultures where they come from. In so doing, the ethical liabilities for colonial abuse remain beyond any serious discussion.

References

Biran, A., & Hyde, K. F. (2013). New perspectives on dark tourism. *International Journal of Culture, Tourism and Hospitality Research*. 7(3): 191–198.

Biran, A., Poria, Y., & Oren, G. (2011). Sought experiences at (dark) heritage sites. Annals of tourism research, 38(3), 820–841.

Bowman, M. S., & Pezzullo, P. C. (2009). What's so 'dark' about 'dark tourism'?: Death, tours, and performance. *Tourist Studies*, *9*(3), 187–202.

Buda, D. M. (2015). The death drive in tourism studies. *Annals of Tourism Research*, *50*, 39–51.

Braithwaite, D., & Lee, Y. L. (2006). Dark tourism, hate and reconciliation: The Sandakan experience. *International Institute for Peace Through Tourism Occasional Paper*, 8: 1–15.

Busby, G., & Devereux, H. (2015). Dark tourism in context: The diary of Anne Frank. *European Journal of Tourism, Hospitality and Recreation*, *6*(1), 27–38.

Cave, J., & Buda, D. (2018). Souvenirs in dark tourism: Emotions and symbols. In *The Palgrave handbook of dark tourism studies* (pp. 707–726). Palgrave Macmillan, London.

Carrigan, A. (2014). Dark tourism and postcolonial studies: Critical intersections. *Postcolonial Studies*, *17*(3), 236–250.

Causevic, S., & Lynch, P. (2011). Phoenix tourism: Post-conflict tourism role. *Annals of Tourism Research*, *38*(3), 780–800.

Czyzewski, K. (2011). Colonialism as a broader social determinant of health. *International Indigenous Policy Journal*, *2*(1): 1–9.

Clarke, R., Dutton, J., & Johnston, A. (2014). Shadow Zones: Dark travel and postcolonial cultures. *Postcolonial Studies*, *17*(3), 221–235.

Cohen, E. H. (2011). Educational dark tourism at an in populo site: The Holocaust Museum in Jerusalem. *Annals of tourism research*, *38*(1), 193–209.

Collins-Kreiner, N. (2016). Dark tourism as/is pilgrimage. *Current Issues in Tourism*, *19*(12), 1185–1189.

Dang, T. K. P. (2021). Tourism imaginaries and the selective perception of visitors: Postcolonial heritage in Con Dao Islands, Vietnam. *Island Studies Journal*, *16*(1), 249–270.

Franklin, A. (2007). The problem with tourism theory. *The critical turn in tourism studies: Innovative research methodologies*, Altejvic I, Pritchard, A & Morgan N, Oxford, Elsevier, 131–148.

Gagné, M. A. (1998). The role of dependency and colonialism in generating trauma in First Nations citizens. In *International handbook of multigenerational legacies of trauma* (pp. 355–372). Danieli Y (eds) Boston, Springer.

Guidotti-Hernández, N. M. (2011). Unspeakable violence. *Remapping US and Mexican national imaginaries*. Durham, Duke University Press.

Hartmann, R. (2014). Dark tourism, thanatourism, and dissonance in heritage tourism management: New directions in contemporary tourism research. *Journal of Heritage Tourism*, *9*(2), 166–182.

Heidelberg, B. A. W. (2015). Managing ghosts: Exploring local government involvement in dark tourism. *Journal of Heritage Tourism*, *10*(1), 74–90.

Hooper, G., & Lennon, J. J. (Eds.). (2016). *Dark tourism: Practice and interpretation*. Abingdon, Routledge.

Iliev, D. (2020). Consumption, motivation and experience in dark tourism: a conceptual and critical analysis. *Tourism Geographies*, 23(5–6): 963–984.

Jamal, T., & Lelo, L. (2010). Exploring the conceptual and analytical framing of dark tourism: From darkness to intentionality. In *Tourist experience* (pp. 49–62). R. Sharpley & P. Stone (eds). Abingdon, Routledge.

Jordan, E. J., & Prayag, G. (2022). Residents' cognitive appraisals, emotions, and coping strategies at local dark tourism sites. *Journal of Travel Research*, *61*(4), 887–902.

Korstanje, M. (2015). The anthropology of dark tourism. Exploring the contradictions of capitalism. CERS, Repository of University of Leeds.

Korstanje, M. E. (2016). *The rise of thana-capitalism and tourism*. Abingdon, Routledge.

Korstanje, M. E. (2020). The dark tourist: Consuming dark spaces in the periphery. *Tourism, terrorism and security*. Korstanje M & Seraphin H. (135–150). Bingley, Emerald

Korstanje, M. E., & Baker, D. (2018). Politics of dark tourism: the case of Cromañón and ESMA, Buenos Aires, Argentina. *The Palgrave handbook of dark tourism studies*, Stone et al (ed). 533–552. Basingstoke, Palgrave Macmillan.

Korstanje, M. E., & George, B. (2015). Dark Tourism: Revisiting Some Philosophical Issues. *E-review of Tourism Research*, *12*.(1–2): 127–136

Korstanje, M. E., & Ivanov, S. H. (2012). Tourism as a form of new psychological resilience: The inception of dark tourism. *CULTUr-revista de Cultura e Turismo*, *6*(4), 56–71.

Miller, M. C. (2020). 1 Trauma, Colonialism and Post-Imperial Ideology. In *Wronged by Empire* (pp. 7–34). Stanford, Stanford University Press.

Mitchell, V., Henthorne, T. L., & George, B. (2020). Making Sense of Dark Tourism: Typologies, Motivations and Future Development of Theory. In *Tourism, Terrorism and Security*. Korstanje M & Seraphin H (eds), Bingley, Emerald Publishing Limited

Ntunda, J. (2014). *Investigating the challenges of promoting dark tourism in Rwanda*. Anchor Academic Publishing (aap_verlag).

Lemelin, R. H., Thompson-Carr, A., Johnston, M., Stewart, E., & Dawson, J. (2013). Indigenous people: discussing the forgotten dimension of dark tourism and battlefield tourism. In *New Issues in Polar Tourism* (pp. 205–215). Springer, Dordrecht.

Light, D. (2017). Progress in dark tourism and thanatourism research: An uneasy relationship with heritage tourism. *Tourism Management*, *61*, 275–301.

Lin, Y., Kelemen, M., & Tresidder, R. (2018). Post-disaster tourism: building resilience through community-led approaches in the aftermath of the 2011 disasters in Japan. *Journal of Sustainable Tourism*, *26*(10), 1766–1783.

Ivanova, P., & Light, D. (2018). 'It's not that we like death or anything': Exploring the motivations and experiences of visitors to a lighter dark tourism attraction. Journal of Heritage Tourism, 13(4), 356–369.

Magee, R., & Gilmore, A. (2015). Heritage site management: from dark tourism to transformative service experience?. *The Service Industries Journal*, *35*(15–16), 898–917.

Martini, A., & Buda, D. M. (2020). Dark tourism and affect: Framing places of death and disaster. *Current Issues in Tourism*, *23*(6), 679–692.

Martini, A., & Sharma, N. (2022). Framing the sublime as affect in post-disaster tourism. *Annals of Tourism Research*, *97*, 103473.

Miles, S. (2014). Battlefield sites as dark tourism attractions: An analysis of experience. *Journal of Heritage Tourism*, *9*(2), 134–147.

Miles, T. (2015). *Tales from the haunted south: Dark tourism and memories of slavery from the Civil War era*. Durham, UNC Press Books.

Mitchell, V., Henthorne, T. L., & George, B. (2020). Making sense of dark tourism: Typologies, motivations and future development of theory. In Tourism, terrorism and security (pp. 103–114). Emerald Publishing Limited.

Olsen, D. H., & Korstanje, M. E. (Eds.). (2019). *Dark tourism and pilgrimage*. Walingford, CABI.

Podoshen, J. S. (2018). Dark tourism in an increasingly violent world. *The Palgrave handbook of dark tourism studies*, 173–187, Stone et al (ed). Basingstoke, Palgrave Macmillan.

Potts, T. J. (2012). 'Dark tourism'and the 'kitschification'of 9/11. *Tourist Studies*, *12*(3), 232–249.

Sather-Wagstaff, J. (2016). *Heritage that hurts: Tourists in the memoryscapes of September 11*. Abingdon, Routledge.

Sharma, N., & Martini, A. (2024). Dark tourism geographies: ontological, epistemological and axiological perspectives. *Tourism Geographies*, 1–10.

Sharpley, R. (2009). Dark tourism and political ideology: Towards a governance model. The darker side of travel: The theory and practice of dark tourism, 145-163. Sharpley R & Stone P (eds) Bristol, Channel View

Sharpley, R., & Stone, P. R. (Eds.). (2009). *The darker side of travel: The theory and practice of dark tourism*. Bristol, Channel view publications.

Seaton, A. V. (1996). Guided by the dark: From thanatopsis to thanatourism. *International Journal of Heritage Studies*, *2*(4), 234–244.

Skinner, J. (2012) *Writing the dark side of travel*. New York, Berghahn Books.

Smalley, K. (2021). *Raising the spectre of race: phantoming and phenomenologies of whiteness in dark tourism* (Doctoral dissertation, University of British Columbia).

Stone, P. R. (2006). A dark tourism spectrum: Towards a typology of death and macabre related tourist sites, attractions and exhibitions. *Tourism: An International Interdisciplinary Journal*, *54*(2), 145–160.

Stone, P. R. (2011). Dark tourism: Towards a new post-disciplinary research agenda. *International Journal of Tourism Anthropology*, *1*(3–4), 318–332.

Stone, P. R. (2012). Dark tourism and significant other death: Towards a model of mortality mediation. *Annals of tourism research*, *39*(3), 1565–1587.

Stone, P. (2013). Dark tourism scholarship: A critical review. *International Journal of Culture, Tourism and Hospitality Research*. 7(3): 307–318

Stone, P., & Sharpley, R. (2008). Consuming dark tourism: A thanatological perspective. *Annals of tourism Research*, *35*(2), 574–595.

Stone, P. Seaton T, White L, Hartmann R. & Sharpley R. (2018). "Dark tourism themes and consequences: a preface". In The Palgrave Handbook of Dark tourism Studies. (Stone et al) eds. Basingstoke, Palgrave Macmillan. Vii-X

Strange, C., & Kempa, M. (2003). Shades of dark tourism: Alcatraz and Robben Island. *Annals of tourism research*, *30*(2), 386–405.

Tarlow, P. (2007). Dark tourism–the appealing 'dark'side of tourism and more. In *Niche tourism* (pp. 61–72). Novelli M (ed) Abingdon, Routledge.

Timothy, D. J. (2021). 21 Dark Tourism: Atrocity and Human Suffering. In *Cultural Heritage and Tourism* (pp. 483–516). Timothy D (ed). Bristol, Channel View Publications.

Tucker, H., Shelton, E. J., & Bae, H. (2017). Post-disaster tourism: Towards a tourism of transition. *Tourist studies*, *17*(3), 306–327.

Tumarkin, M. (2001). 'Wishing you weren't here . . .': Thinking about trauma, place and the port Arthur massacre. *Journal of Australian Studies*, *25*(67), 196–205.

Tumarkin, M. M. (2005). *Traumascapes: The power and fate of places transformed by tragedy*. Melbourne, Melbourne Univ. Publishing.

Tzanelli, R. (2013). *Heritage in the digital era: Cinematic tourism and the activist cause*. Routledge.

Tzanelli, R. (2016). *Thanatourism and cinematic representations of risk: Screening the end of tourism*. Abingdon, Routledge.

Tzanelli, R. (2018). *Cinematic tourist mobilities and the plight of development: On atmospheres, affects, and environments*. Abingdon, Routledge.

Tzanelli, R. (2021). Colonial heterotropics and global heritage aesthetics in Roundhay's Tropical World, Leeds. *Experimental Museology*, 83.

Tzanelli, R., & Korstanje, M. E. (2019). On killing the 'toured object': Anti-terrorist fantasy, touristic edgework and morbid consumption in the illegal settlements in West Bank, Palestine. In *Tourism and hospitality in conflict-ridden destinations* (pp. 71–83). Abingdon, Routledge.

Wight, A. C. (2006). Philosophical and methodological praxes in dark tourism: Controversy, contention and the evolving paradigm. *Journal of Vacation Marketing*, *12*(2), 119–129.

Sarike van Slooten

12 Towards a postcolonial museum? Experiencing legacies of colonialism in dark tourism museum exhibits

Abstract: The awareness of the legacies of colonial histories and difficult heritage has grown significantly in public and academic debates over the past two decades with the majority of debates revolving around issues concerning the acknowledgement of, and accountability for, the enduring impacts of colonisation. Narratives about colonisation include prevailing notions of civilisation and citizenship, while narratives of slavery and less victorious aspects of colonisation are often silenced. A prevailing sentiment about the acknowledgement and accountability of the enduring impact of colonisation within public representations increasingly challenges museums to rethink representations of colonial pasts in the present. This chapter seeks to identify how museums can connect better to contemporary debates of colonialism, particularly relevant in the context of dark tourism that often deals with legacies of the trauma of colonialism such as slavery, genocide and human oppression.

Keywords: dark tourism, museum, postcolonial, new museology, trauma, visitor experience

Introduction

Over the past two decades, awareness of the legacies of colonial histories has grown significantly in public and academic debates. Most of these debates revolve around issues concerning the acknowledgement of, and accountability for, the enduring impacts of colonisation. Hamilton et al. (2012) use the term 'transnational phenomenon' to describe this outburst of academic and public debate about how narratives of colonisation are represented through slavery heritage and museum exhibitions.[1] The controversial representation of the celebrative tradition 'Saint Nicholas' [Sinterklaas] and 'Black Pete' [Zwarte Piet] is a Dutch example of such debate. That Black Pete is represented as stereotypical of an enslaved man, and that the social hierarchy between him and Saint Nicholas resembles former racial structures and propagates racial disparity is seen as problematic.[2] As the relevance of slavery heritage sites and museum

1 Scholars such as Violi (2012, pp. 37–44) and Onega et al., (2017, pp. 1–9 and 311–313) have confirmed this.

2 For a comprehensive explanation of this perceived problematic representation, see Rodenberg & Wagenaar (2016) and Sahadat, (2019).

https://doi.org/10.1515/9783110792072-013

exhibits for dark tourism lies in how we understand and negotiate colonial legacies and difficult heritage, this chapter seeks to explore how the legacies of colonialism are experienced by visitors through museum exhibitions in various colonial geographies. This exploration seeks to identify how museums can connect better to contemporary debates of colonialism, which is particularly relevant in the context of dark tourism that often deals with legacies of the trauma of colonialism such as slavery, genocide and human oppression.

Internationally, debates about the legacies of colonial histories have led to global activism and protest against the public glorification of historic figures that symbolise a memory characterised by human oppression, slavery, and racism.[3] This outburst as described by Hamilton et al. (2012) further aligns with a worldwide fixation on the awareness and commemoration of our national pasts in narratives of colonisation.[4] Particularly in Western societies, narratives about colonisation unswervingly include prevailing notions of civilisation and citizenship, while narratives of slavery and less victorious aspects of colonisation are silenced. A prevailing sentiment about the acknowledgement and accountability of the enduring impact of colonisation within public representations increasingly challenges museums to rethink representations of colonial pasts in the present. Dark tourism as a tool for creating awareness and personal learning plays a significant role in this sentiment, as more awareness of the impact of colonisation through colonial representations, particularly those engaged in the trauma of slavery, can be realised. This directs my imagination of the (im)possibility of the construction of a postcolonial museum, which connects museums better to contemporary society's debates on colonialism. More specifically, this chapter seeks to yield an understanding of the (im)possibilities of the construction of a postcolonial museum through the visitors' perception and experience of museum exhibitions in relation to colonial histories along the trans-Atlantic geography. In the following, I will reflect on current academic debates about the concepts relevant for the context of this chapter: colonialism and colonial histories, dark tourism, the museum, new museology and the visitor experience.

About forty years ago, Ronald Horvath (1972) described the academic literature about colonialism as both increasingly rich and lacking common ground as to how it can be defined.[5] Regardless of this inconsistency, a universally agreed notion of colonialism does exist: the domination and control by individuals or groups over territory

3 For example, statues, memorials, monuments, street names and public buildings. The most prominent protest in Western societies in recent years has been #Black Lives Matter – https://blacklivesmatter.com/.

4 For other studies that confirm this claim, see Bhatia (2009, pp. 1–7) and Nettleback (2012, pp. 40–46).

5 In his article 'A Definition of Colonialism' (1972).

and/or behaviour of other individuals and groups (Horvath, 1972).[6] Many attempts to define colonialism depart from the search for power and expansion that can be characterised by the migration and settling of people from the colonising geography to the colony. Williams and Chrisman (1994, p. 24) argue that theorising colonialism raises various questions in relation to the definition and function of the nation and national culture, concepts of time and place, types of colonialisms and their effects on the colonised and cultural identity. These questions produce concerns and critiques in the conceptualisation of colonialism, colonial subjectification, and the legacies of colonialism for individuals and societies today. For example, Sunderason (2020) argues that departures of various colonising powers from the colonies during the twentieth century left imprints of war, genocide, famines, partitions and displacements within these geographies, and shaped new transnational frames and spatial imaginaries. These concerns and critiques are at the heart of the literary body of postcolonial literature today, which started to emerge and intensify halfway through the twentieth century.[7] Postcolonial literature variously deals with legacies of colonialism. It acknowledges the uniqueness of each colonial experience and "shares only the original subjugation by the imperial power, meaning that any generalisation across colonial experiences would miss the "uneven development" inherent in the colonial experience as well as its aftereffects" (Scanlon and Kumar, 2019, p. 203).

My discussion of colonial histories as histories shaped by colonialism is informed by Ania Loomba's *Colonialism/Postcolonialism: The New Critical Idiom* (2015) and John McLeod's *Beginning Postcolonialism* (2010, p. 7–40). These colonial histories are characterised by seizure and control over lands, goods, and people across times and places by European colonisers roughly between the 1500s and 1900s.[8] They shaped the beginning of a global multicultural society that is Eurocentric and upholds a European un-

6 Although colonialism and imperialism are discussed in literature as closely related yet distinct concepts (i.e., see Horvath, 1972; Williams and Chrisman, 1994; Loomba, 2015; McLeod, 2010), I am not distinguishing between these conceptualisations in my discussion about colonialism.

7 See Williams and Chrisman (1994), Child and Williams (1997), Moro-Abadía (2006), Harrison and Hughes (2010) and Nebbou (2018) for a clear overview of the development and differences between the colonial discourse and the postcolonial discourse. Important writings that address the concerns and critiques in postcolonial literature, and have inspired many postcolonial writings and writers, are Edward Said's *Orientalism* (1978) and *Culture and Imperialism* (1994), Gayatri Chakravorty Spivak's *Can the Subaltern Speak?* (1985) and Homi Bhabba's *Location of Culture (*1994). Another valuable contribution to postcolonial writing from various theoretical and geographical perspective is the *Postcolonial Studies Reader* (1995), edited by Bill Ashcroft, Gareth Griffiths, and Helen Tiffin.

8 I am aware that colonialism is neither a linear nor an identical process between times and geographies, and that colonisation reaches beyond the 15th century (i.e. see Harrison and Hughes, 2010). However, this study frames colonialism as the seize and control over lands and goods that occurred parallel to the development of modernism and the creation of a capitalist Western Europe from the 15th century during which the trans-Atlantic slave trade played a crucial role (Loomba, 2015; McLeod, 2010). A justification for this demarcation is connected to the construction of contemporary society. European colonialism from the 15th century ushered in significant societal, cultural, and political

derstanding of history inside the museum.[9] Thus, they are also shaped by the events of European colonisation in which various geographies were engaged that, particularly from the sixteenth century, ushered in significant societal, cultural, and political changes to global society, and left various legacies that are noticeable today. With regard to the sociocultural legacies of colonialism, Loomba (2015) argues that complex and traumatic relationships in human history, as the result of European colonisation, are still prominently visible within societies and communities. In fact, public debate has become more aware of the relationship between current day societal turmoil around racial discrimination and unequal power dynamics and the colonial experience. Human knowledge mostly evolved through the documentation of information based on the colonial experience from a European, colonising perspective. As such, writings and documentation (i.e., travel writings, scientific writings, logbooks, archives, etc.) have been regarded as authoritative and as producing distinctive conceptions and modes of language that we still use and debate today.[10] This Eurocentric understanding of history is problematic for any form of postcolonial travel (Light, 2017), such as dark tourism. It directs visitors' meaning-making of history from a colonial perspective that is based on a system of classification, ordering, hierarchy, and superiority instead of a postcolonial, contemporary perspective that upholds the values of multiperspectivity, social justice, diversity, equality, and mutual respect.[11] Hence, a more inclusive tourist experience can be realised by enriching the Eurocentric perspective with postcolonial perspectives. This study contributes to this realisation, as it explores and compares the visitors' experience of colonial legacies through museums at various colonial geographies,

Karwan Fatah-Black (2021) discusses the intellectual legacy of colonialism. He remarks that much contemporary understanding of the relationship between colonialism, specifically slavery, and civilisation is formed through the frames of the 'grand narrative'. He describes this narrative as an overarching interpretation of the past that enables societies to express the core values underlying [national] culture, and that legitimises a historic, cultural identity. In this light, Loomba (2015) and Stoler (2007) also assert that

---

changes to global societies. An insight into the legacies of the trans-Atlantic slave trade and contemporary society is provided in the following paragraphs.

9 Dussel, Krauel and Tuma (2000), Ashcroft, Griffiths and Tiffin (2007, pp. 84–85 and 103–104) and Mignolo (2011) discuss the conceptual development of Eurocentrism in the modern world in more detail, connected to the events of modernity. Jörgen Tjon a Fong discussed eurocentrism in more detail in relation to the museum at the symposium 'Wiens Gouden Eeuw?' organised by the Amsterdam Museum on 29 September 2019 as a response to the museum's decision to replace the term 'Golden Age' with '17th Century', (Amsterdam Museum, 2019 and NOS, 2019). I refer to Ashcroft, Griffiths and Tiffin (2007, pp. 84–85 and 103–104), Mignolo (2011, pp. 2–152) and Hupperetz (2022, p. 28) for a conceptual analysis of modernity and in relation to the museum.

10 Examples of these concepts are 'nation' and 'national culture', 'identity', 'race and stereotypes'.

11 For comprehensive insights into the connection between dark tourism and postcolonialism, see the studies of Carrigan (2014) and Clarke, Dutton and Johnston (2014).

history as experienced, documented, and dispersed by the colonising powers, is history embedded in Fatah-Black's 'grand narrative'. It traditionally excludes other historic experiences but focuses on the European/Western experience established in archival history.[12] Thus, the intellectual property of the grand narrative re-creates a nation-state based on the experience of Western, colonial domination.

Colonial legacies in the museum: A challenging field?

Hopefully it has become clear from the above that colonisation has left numerous legacies in our present.[13] McLeod (2010, p. 7–40) argues that these legacies continue to influence how history and culture are represented and experienced today, for example through dark tourism.

> Visits to historical sites, including those that portray events associated with human suffering and mass death have become a significant aspect of tourist visitation (Austin, 2002, p. 447).

Lennon and Foley coined the concept of dark tourism in 1996 in academic discourse, exemplifying tourist performances at historical and ancient sites or attractions that were allied to pain, death, atrocity and tragedy "which continue to impact our lives" (Tarlow, 2005, p. 48).[14] But what we perceive as painful and tragic, or what we perceive as significant to our lives, depends on who has the power to represent and the politics of remembering within society (Alderman, 2010). In the words of Alderman (2010, p. 90), "what is defined as memorable or historically significant is open to social control, contest, and negotiation. Places of memory narrate history in selective ways that not only contribute to the process of remembering, but also the process of forgetting".

Since dark tourism attained prominence at the end of the 20th century, gradually more and more places and sites were declared as dark heritage sites. It is an increasingly significant niche that steers economic growth, and educational awareness and enables

12 See Said (1978), Anderson (1991, Introduction), Cain (2011, pp. 105–109), and Onega et al. (2017, pp. 1–9 and 311–313) for further insights into grand narrative.

13 Tangible legacies, for example buildings, art, education, cultural and natural landscapes, and artefacts. Intangible legacies, for example, knowledge, values, customs, language, identity, nation-making, diaspora, and trauma.

14 Before Lennon & Foley coined the concept 'dark tourism' in academic discourse in 1996, this form of travelling had in all scholastic literature, relentlessly, been referred to as 'black-spot tourism' (Rojek, 1993), 'milking the macabre' (Dann, 1994), 'thanatourism' (Seaton, 1996), 'morbid tourism' (Blom, 2000) and, more recently defined as 'political tourism' (Simone-Charteris & Boyd, 2011).

personal reflection on death and dying through the visitor experience (Boateng et al., 2018; Xingyang, 2022). This increase could arguably be attributed to "the contemporary, western fascination with death, real or fictional, media inspired or otherwise" (Stone & Sharpley, 2008, p. 147) and to the increasing mass tourism that dominates the late 20th century. Though it is widely accepted that dark tourism has grown substantially over the past two decades, research on how visitors experience dark heritage sites remains limited (Stone, 2011; Yan et al., 2016; Podoshen et al., 2018; Boateng et al., 2018; Xingyang, 2022). Slavery heritage in particular has become a main reason for travel, which makes destinations connected to slavery and the slave trade an important aspect of the dark tourism activity (Mowatt & Chancellor, 2011). This importance can be attributed to the traumatic and dark character of history related to slavery, for which slavery exhibitions and trauma objects serve as direct reminders of this history, "as well as reservoirs for heritage and information" (Mowatt & Cancellor, 2011, p. 1410). This chapter contributes to the call for research into the visitor experience at dark heritage sites and seeks to gain academic insights related to the 'darkness' of colonialism and slavery through the eyes of visitors within a postcolonial, contemporary context.

Besides (dark) tourism, Loomba (2015) argues that every branch of knowledge, educational programme, or academic discipline has been affected by European knowledge-making. This might not come as a surprise, given the production, collection, documentation and dissemination of information and materials from the lands and peoples beyond Europe by the European colonisers during colonisation, and the conservation of this information in the archives.[15] This knowledge informs current-day interpretations of history, which is reflected by the grand narrative presented in museums.[16] Alderman's (2010) earlier claim about what parts of history are remembered is decided by those in power to represent, is particularly challenged in light of colonial history and slavery heritage. However, minorities, marginalised and diasporic groups increasingly challenge historical representations that are informed by the grand narrative. For example, the narrative of slavery and slave trade at Kura Hulanda Museum in Willemstad (Curaçao) is informed by the Dutch colonial experience and excludes the Afro-Carribean experience. As a result, the exhibition contains a chronological storyline about slavery and slave trade on the island from the perspective of the Dutch colonising power.

I discuss the museum as a cultural, educational, and scientific institution that produces and represents the knowledge that is generated through documenting, collecting, archiving, conserving, and representing national history. Museums that represent national history – national museums – principally represent the origins and evolvement of a nation and culture in contrast to other cultures through the grand narra-

---

15 Stoler (2002, 2007) and Turner (2020) provide a more critical insight into this claim.

16 Stoler (2002) provides a deeper insight into the authoritative role and uses of the colonial archive as a databank upon which an understanding of history is perpetuated from a Western, colonial perspective.

tive.[17] Smith (2010) refers to these museums as the 'Authorized Heritage Discourse' [from here AHD] and explains that heritage [museum and exhibitions] is described as materialistic, monumental, grand, representing 'nation' at its best through a framed system of representation that aims to direct visitor responses. Luepken (2011) describes the value of the museum collection, in line with Smith's ADH, as typically based on scientific knowledge. Objects have gone through processes of appropriation to integrate the object within the parameters of the grand narrative. I further consider the museum as an institution of perceived authority, geared to representing a national identity that is anchored in the grand narrative, which may or may not be state-funded and/or governed.[18] I also perceive the museum as an institution created under the eye of modernity that reflects a national culture and identity according to the grand narrative.[19] I relate this argument to the claims of Said (1978) and of Anderson (1992/2016). Both of them have stressed that cultural representations include an evident imagined sense of nation and identity of the superior West, which, as I would like to argue, is also reflected in, or is characteristic of, the grand narrative and describes the nature of the national museum.

As national museums represent an imagined sense of nation and identity through the grand narrative, they also materialise the narrative through, mostly, objects and artefacts connected to colonisation. Hicks (2020) argues that the museum justifies the grand narrative through a 'Euro-pessimistic' material representation, which suggests an understanding of history and culture through objects that coincides with the knowledge produced during colonisation. This makes the grand narrative exclusive and, consequently, exhibitions become exclusive spaces of representation. Bennett (1995, p. 9) already addressed nearly thirty years ago that "[. . .] there should be parity of representation for all groups and cultures within collecting, exhibition and conservation activities of museums, and the demand that the members of all social groups should have equal practical as well as theoretical rights of access to museums". In other words, the call upon museums to create exhibitions that are more inclusive about collecting and representing is not a new twenty-first-century phenomenon; it is

17 For relevant studies about the museum in connection to nation, see Bennett (1995), Trotter (1998, pp. 48–58). Lleras (2017's use of 'master narrative' is similar to the conception of the 'grand narrative'. Hence, I do not distinguish between these two terms.

18 For relevant discussions in relation to this claim, see Luepken (2011, pp. 157–173) and Andermann & Arnold-de Simine (2012, p. 1–3).

19 As proposed by Walter Mignolo in *The Darker Side of Western Modernity* (2011, pp. 2–152), I view modernity as the start of the Western expansion that formed a Eurocentric logic through the course of colonisation. Colonisation and modernity are inherently connected forms of logic that place the Western experience at the centre of the representation of history and culture in museums. Since I use modernity as a context closely related to colonialism, I will not enter a historic, semantic, and political discussion of this concept in relation to colonialism and museums. For relevant studies that discuss the national museum, see Trotter (1998, p. 48–58), Van der Laarse (2005, pp. 1–17), Luepken (2011, pp. 157–173), Cain (2011, pp.105–109), Mignolo (2011), Levitt (2015, pp. 6–7), Tolia-Kelly (2016, pp. 896–904), and Hicks (2020).

an ongoing business as it were. Although Hupperetz (2022) considers inclusiveness as a 'game changer' within the heritage industry, Abungu (2018) argues that museums, particularly in the West, are known to be inclusive, but mostly in theory rather than in practice.[20] This is particularly valid for what he calls 'flagship museums', which I argue can be classified under Smith's AHD. They are museums that narrate national history.[21] I explore museums typified by Smith's ADH that represent colonial collections and objects connected to the trauma of slavery. These collections fall under Dann's (1998) 'Themed Thanatos' as a collection constructed around life and death, and Stone and Sharpley's (2008) 'Dark Exhibitions' that typifies a predominant educational focus in a collection that revolves around death and trauma.

New museology and visitor experiences

Over the nineteenth and twentieth centuries, the relationship between the museum and society, as well as the value of the museum within contemporary frames of society, began to be questioned. This movement revised the meaning and role of the museum and generated the 'new museology'. New museology is the response to the call for a changing role of the museum alongside changing societies (Vergo, 1989).[22] Stam (1993) asserts that the new museology rhetoric calls for a change in value, meaning, control, interpretation, authority and authenticity within museums, as well as a curatorial redistribution. This required museums to transition from the paradigm in which museum practices were embedded in the Western colonial experience, to a paradigm of diversity and multi-perspectivity that represents history and culture from a more contemporary, societal perspective.[23] In light of dark tourism, new museology is essential to encourage a more inclusive visitor understanding of colonial history and the trauma of slavery that moves away from a sole meaning-making based on the Western, colonial experience, to a meaning-making that reflects a diversity of perspectives, including those found in the diasporic memory. This new paradigm implies that narratives should become more subjective based on personal and individual experiences of being, becoming, and belonging. New museology asks museums to reflect on contemporary debates of colonialism in their representation that encourages the capability of communities to live in a cross-cultural and multi-ethnic environ-

20 Although Abungu's claim is specifically directed to museums in the West, this is not unique to museums in the West as museums in non-Western geographies generally represent the national narrative, for example, through disregarding the former dominant perspective.

21 Abungu's 'flagship museums' are known to exhibit artefacts and narratives from 'great' explorations and within the period of colonisation and focus on the representation of culture and place.

22 Peter Vergo discusses the second museum age and new museology in more detail in his book *The New Museology* (1989).

23 For an insight into the paradigm of diversity, see Tolia-Kelly (2016, pp. 896–904).

ment. It invites museums to enrich their representation and implement a variety of interpretation methods that allow for active participation, multiple meaning-making, and learning (Luepken, 2011, p. 157–173). Consequently, representations have become more diverse, transferrable and self-reflective and contest the exclusive character of the museum as a nineteenth-century institution. Instead, the museum has become a 'contact zone' (Naguib, 2013b, p. 82) or a 'space of difference' (Lord, 2006, p. 5) for interaction, dialogue, and reflection.[24] Additionally, meaning-making occurs in the connection between the object and the context in which it is represented, rather than through an understanding of the object itself.[25] Although contemporary societies are culturally pluralistic, they cannot realise social change if the representation of the out-group's culture remains excluded or un(der)-experienced. Even though various authors called for change nearly twenty-five years ago, Cain (2011) argues that cultural exclusion in the museum space remains evident and should be criticised.[26] This critique leads me to explore the relationship between museums and contemporary debates on colonialism through the visitor experience.

According to Falk and Dierking (2013), the visitor experience in the museum is a complex process of interaction across personal, social, and physical contexts that starts prior to the visit and continues after. While Roederer and Filser (2018) argue that the museum experience is merely an interaction between visitor, object, and museum, Falk and Dierking (2013, p. 23–33) define it more comprehensively: a holistic phenomenon comprising "[. . .] the totality of the experience, from the moment the thought occurs to someone that visiting a museum might be a good idea, through the visit itself, to the recollection of the experience days, weeks and even years later" (2013, p. 23).[27] It is an interaction between three intersectional fields: personal, sociocultural, and physical context. They argue that the personal context is the unique set of prior knowledge, prior experiences, personal interests, and needs that shape the individual visitor experience. The sociocultural context is defined by the sociocultural background of the visitor as well as the social environment of the visit.[28] The physical context comprises an experience through the physical environment of the exhibition and the emotional understanding of the building of the museum or location of the exhibition. Finally, Falk and Dierking (2013) mention time, which they reason is a silent context that undeniably impacts the visitor experience across personal, sociocultural, and physical contexts. Scholars in various academic debates have detected that people have a growing need for an authentic experience in a

24 more studies that argue this development, see Thomas (2009, pp. 125–133) and Nettleback (2012, pp. 40–46).

25 For example, Lord (2006, p. 1–11) and Black (2011).

26 See Simpson (1996, pp. 7–76) and Trotter (199, pp: 48–58). Cain's argument is confirmed by Coleman (2018, pp 39–51).

27 The notion of the visitor experience as a holistic process is confirmed in more studies, such as Palese (2018, pp. 2–19) and Vermeeren et al. (2018, pp. 1–16).

28 For relevant studies about this context, see Hamilton et al. (2012, pp. 1–4).

world in which culture has become increasingly plural, artificial, and imaginary.[29] Visitors have become more critical and knowledgeable over the years, which contributes to this need and confronts museums with a quandary. Larsen and Svabe (2014) argue that the visitor experience is shaped by the expectation of visual enjoyment and intellectual understanding. Here, the visitor experience is conceptualised as a visually active and physically passive act and limits the experience by excluding multiple senses. Their conception contradicts the advancement of visitor expectations as discussed by various scholars earlier, as visitors expect experiences through educational, emotional, immersive, and multi-sensory representations.[30] According to Light et. al (2018), museums have increasingly become visitor-centred, which constitutes a transition from experiences that are created top-down to co-created experiences in which the visitor plays a key role in the design of exhibitions.[31] The latter mainly aims for an immersive, engaging, interactive, and edutaining experience. The co-creational and participative aspect of such an experience calls for alternative methods of interpretation that promote what McCarthy and Ciolfi (2008) have termed a 'dialogical experience'; interpretation formed through the dialogue between the visitor and the exhibition.[32] In other words, the museum experience is shaped through the dialogue between and interaction with the visitors, the objects, and the museum. Similarly, Polese (2018) perceive the visitor experience as a holistic process shaped by the sum of all aspects described above, including the type of visitor, expectations, personal identity-related motivation, the interplay of interaction between the visitor and the museum across personal, sociocultural, and physical contexts, time, and the pre-visit, on-site visit, and post-visit. With these various notions of the visitor experience in mind, this concept is challenging for academics and practitioners to explore and map, yet validates the need for more explorative research. This chapter responds to this need.

Experiencing colonial histories in slavery exhibitions

Based on how the triangular trading route in the trans-Atlantic region steered a mass relocation of enslaved people from Africa to the Americas and Europe over the course of centuries, and profoundly impacted and reformed global society, I have chosen museum exhibitions of colonial histories in various geographies along this route: Curaçao, Eng-

29 For relevant studies about the need for an authentic visitor experience, see Urry (1990), MacCannell (1999), Urry and Larsen (2011), Pine and Gilmore (2007, pp.1–4), and Hede et al. (2013, pp. 1395–1398).

30 Studies that confirm this claim and discuss the advancement of visitor expectations and demand, see Falk and Dierking (2013, pp. 23–299), Dal Falco & Vassos (2017, pp. 3975–3980), Vermeeren et al. (2018, pp. 1–16) and Antón et al. (2018, pp. 1406–1412).

31 For relevant studies that confirm this claim, see Vermeeren et al. (2018, pp. 1–16) and Polese (2018, pp. 2–19).

32 For insights into dialogical engagement of the visitor experience, see McCarthy and Ciolfi (2008, pp. 247–253) and Vermeeren et al. (2018, pp. 1–16).

land, Ghana, and the United States of America.[33] The experiences of the museums and exhibitions explored in these geographies are (1) the Rijksmuseum's permanent exhibition of seventeenth-century Dutch art and (2) the 'Slavery' exhibition (Amsterdam, The Netherlands), (3) the Tropenmuseum's former permanent exhibition 'Netherlands East Indies' and (4) 'Afterlives of Slavery' exhibition (Amsterdam, The Netherlands), (5) the International Slavery Museum's permanent exhibition (Liverpool, England), (6) Cape Coast Castle Museum's full exhibition and guided tour through the castle (Cape Coast, Ghana), (7) the National Museum of African-American Culture and History's full exhibition (Washington DC, United States of America), (8) the Museum of London's (London, England) permanent galleries from 'Expanding City Gallery' until 'World City', and (9) the Kura Hulanda Museum's exhibition about the trans-Atlantic slave trade (Willemstad, Curaçao).[34] The visitors' experiences are explored through a qualitative survey with visitors between 2017 and 2020.[35]

The visitors' perspective in relation to the permanent collection of the Rijksmuseum was evaluated through a qualitative survey with 15 visitors in May 2017, and for the 'Slavery' exhibition, I analysed several interviews in the media with the head of history in the period 2019–2020, the 'Slavernij' museum publication of 2021 and the presentations of the curators at the symposium 'Sources of Slavery and Slave Trade' that was hosted by the Rijksmuseum on 23 April 2021.[36] The visitors' experiences and perspectives in the 'Netherlands East Indies' exhibition was explored with 30 visitors in May and June 2017, and with 7 visitors in March 2020 at the 'Afterlives of Slavery' exhibition.[37] A qualitative

33 Without downplaying the slave trade around Asia and the impacts of slavery and slave trade on Asian societies or diasporic communities connected to this experience, it seems to have left fewer sociocultural legacies within the geographies selected for this study.

34 The Museum of London has several locations. This research took place at the Museum of London in central London, which focuses on the development of London city and the people (Museum of London, n.d.). The research at Kura Hulanda Museum and the 'Slavery' exhibition at the Rijksmuseum were not possible to conduct onsite due to enduring measures against Covid-19.

35 As Kura Hulanda museum and the Rijksmuseum were closed in the midst of the Covid-19 pandemic, I was not able to explore the visitors' experience through a qualitative survey. Therefore, I based my analysis of the visitors' perspectives and experiences on existing TripAdvisor reviews from visitors who had visited the exhibition prior to the pandemic at Kura Hulanda Museum, and on an envisaged visitor experience according to the curatorial team at the Rijksmuseum.

36 The 15 visitors were individual visitors, 18+ years with the Dutch nationality. The media interviews include NPO Radio1 on 4 December 2019, De Volkskrant on 2 July 2020, the University of Leiden on 17 September 2020, Historisch Nieuwsblad on 27 January 2021 and Het Parool on 6 February 2021, Wiegman (2021, February 6).

37 The visitors at the 'Netherlands East Indies' exhibition were individual visitors, 18+ years with Dutch nationality. 7 visitors were willing to participate in the survey at the 'Afterlives of Slavery' exhibition. This number limits the reliability of the visitors' perspective due to limited visitor participation and researcher's availability, instead of reaching saturation (Richards, 2015, pp. 154–159). These visitors were individual visitors, 18+ years with the Dutch nationality. In total, 4 participants that represent the perspective of the institution of the museum and 52 visitors were included in this research.

survey with 27 visitors was conducted in May 2018 at Cape Coast Castle to evaluate the visitors' perspectives and experiences in relation to the permanent collection in the museum as well as the guided tour experience. The visitors' perspectives and experiences at the International Slavery Museum were explored with 7 visitors in August 2018.[38] The visitors' perspectives and experiences at the NMAAHC were evaluated through a qualitative survey with 10 visitors in October 2018, and the analysis of the visitors' experience at Kura Hulanda Museum is based on TripAdvisor reviews of visitors who visited the Kura Hulanda Museum between 2019 and 2021.[39] All visitors were asked the same eighteen questions in relation to their perception of the narrative, the exhibition, their pre-visit experience, onsite-visitor experience and post-visitor experience (i.e., *Could you shortly summarise the narrative of the exhibition? How did you experience the exhibition? Could you describe the exhibition in three words?*).

An inclusive visitor experience through multiple perspectives

The following insights are based on the visitor experience at the Rijksmuseum and Tropenmuseum in 2017, 2020 and 2021. As both museums were revising their permanent collection and exhibition in 2017, a comparative analysis of the visitor experience took place in 2017 and 2020–2021 in which their newest exhibitions were hosted called 'Slavery' at the Rijksmuseum and 'Afterlives of Slavery' at the Tropenmuseum. This comparison seeks to provide new and different insights into how these museums can create a more inclusive visitor experience.

38 7 visitors participated in this survey. This number limits the reliability of the visitors' perspective. Saturation could not be reached due to the limited willingness of participants and researcher's availability, instead of reaching a point of saturation (Richards, 2015, pp. 154–159). These were individual visitors, 18+ years, with British and international nationality.

39 At the NMAAHC, 10 visitors participated in this survey. This serves as a limitation to the research reliability with respect to the visitors' perspective. Due to limited visitor participation and researcher's availability, a saturation point was not realised (Richards, 2015, pp. 154–155). The visitors were Afro-American women of different ages. As I do not involve gender as a criterion for the visitors' experiences and perspectives, I consider the female visitor reflections as the visitors' experiences and perspectives in this case study. At Kura Hulanda Museum, saturation was reached after 24 reviews, as similar experiences started to appear at a time when no new descriptions were posted. This selection of reviews serves as the representative of the overall museum experience, as suggested by Miguéns, Baggio & Costa (2008, pp. 2–3).

Reflections of visitors of the permanent collection at the Rijksmuseum and Tropenmuseum's 'Netherlands East Indies' permanent exhibition in 2017

In 2017, both museums show similar perceptions among visitors. Visitors of the Rijksmuseum perceived the art collection as 'spectacular, interesting, unique and powerful' and believed that the collection clearly represents a Dutch history of wealth through art.[40] They indicated that the collection creates a sense of (be)longing to the Dutch culture, but within the frames of how the Rijksmuseum represents this culture. Many visitors enjoyed the 'grand' art collection, but some of them indicated they missed an inclusive representation of Dutch colonial history through art, for example by depicting less glorious sides of the Dutch Golden Age. Visitors missed narratives of trauma, counter-perspectives and themes as race and migration.[41] They further reflected the collection as a one-sided, historic representation of Dutch colonial history, without any connection to the difficult situations at plantations and colonies voiced by the then colonised. Many visitors believed that the collection spotlights a history of wealth and prosperity and neglects the history of hardship and trauma, which amounts to an outdated account of Dutch history and culture (Hall, 1994, pp. 222–237). Regardless of an expressed need, by some visitors, to showcase a more inclusive representation of Dutch colonial history through art that is connected to Dutch colonisation, the majority of the visitors seemed to have been satisfied with the uniqueness of the collection, which created a sense of nationhood. Nevertheless, remarks about the collection strongly address a perceived exclusion in the collection, for the majority believes there is a clear focus on the rich side of The Netherlands.

Visitors at the Tropenmuseum described their visit as 'informative', 'interesting', and 'complete', but indicated that they had mixed perceptions of the permanent exhibition 'Netherlands East Indies'.[42] While some visitors experience the exhibition as interesting, impressive, and interactive, others mentioned they find it a distinct, yet confronting, exhibition that represents Dutch colonial history in the East Indies and Asia from a European perspective.[43] Some of the visitors indicated they left the exhibition with mixed feelings. On the one hand, they appreciated the attempt to create awareness of Dutch interference in life overseas. On the other hand, they felt disgusted and embarrassed by this interference. Just like the visitors at the Rijksmuseum, most visitors at the Tropenmuseum had noticed an overexposure of a Dutch coloniser's perspective within the exhibition. "The big success of The Netherlands with a *black* side can be more exposed" (anonymous, 31 May 2017) or "more attention to Dutch interference in Indonesia" (anonymous, 31 May 2017) are just a few examples of

40 Anonymous visitors, personal communication, 30 May 2017.

41 Counter-perspectives are perspectives that are not represented in the grand narrative

42 Interviewee 4, personal communication, 20 June 2017.

43 Anonymous visitors, personal communication, 31 May 2017.

visitor remarks that indicate the need to foreground 'first voices' and the Indonesian perspective.[44] Generally, visitors perceived this exhibition as a significant contributor to the memory of colonisation, the heritage of multiculturalism and their personal identity formation.

Reflections of visitors of the 'Slavery' Exhibition at the Rijksmuseum 2021 and the 'Afterlives of Slavery' Exhibition at the Tropenmuseum in 2020

The Rijksmuseum aimed for visitors to the 'Slavery' exhibition to have a dialogical, co-creational, inclusive, immersive, and multi-sensory experience.[45] A dialogical experience, as visitors are invited to share their experience and thoughts with the museum at the end of the visit to produce ten new narratives. Consequently, these new narratives aim to create a wider image of shared ancestors who individually took part in the system of slavery.[46] An inclusive experience is therefore promoted and founded on the conviction that a combination of a tangible representation with oral history and personal storytelling provides a broader and balanced understanding of Dutch slavery and the slave trade that is a shared experience.[47] The immersive and multi-sensory experiences are believed to be based on the various personal stories and memoires and rooted in the variety of interpretation methods.

Visitors at the Tropenmuseum perceived the 'Afterlives of Slavery' exhibition as an intellectual and emotional experience.[48] Apart from a more prominent emotional experience at the 2020 exhibition, visitors in 2017 and 2020 indicated a comparable experience (i.e., 'impressive' and 'interesting'). However, in 2020 visitors used descriptive words that indicated an emotional experience stressing *tacit* understanding, such as 'intense', 'painful', 'reflection', 'dull', 'shame', 'incomprehension', 'dark', 'sad', 'amazed', 'fascinating', 'arousing', 'uncomfortable', 'heavy loaded', 'horrible' and 'lurid' (anonymous, personal communication, 7 March 2020).[49] A clear contrast with the 2017 visitors' perceptions is connected to multi-perspectivity, as visitors in 2020 perceived the exhibition as visibly narrated from the personal accounts of the 'first voices' and a non-dominant cultural perspective (i.e., Caribbean and Suriname). This enabled visitors to

---

44 Interviewee 4, personal communication, 20 June 2017.

45 Due to Covid-19 measures, the exhibitions were not open to the public, hence no direct data was available on the visitors' perspectives and experiences. Consequently, I approached the visitors' perspectives and experiences as 'envisaged' based on the perceptions of the institution of the museum.

46 This is confirmed in Sint Nicolaas and Smeulders (2021, pp. 8–21).

47 This was discussed in NPO Radio 1 (2019), Het Parool (2021), Wiegman (2021, February 6) and Interviewee 3, personal communication, 23 April 2021.

48 Anonymous visitors, personal communication, 7 March 2020.

49 Hooper-Greenhill (2000, pp. 1–162) describes tacit understanding as emotional and intangible.

relate the exhibition to contemporary problems such as racism and the impacts of the Dutch slave system on society today, which suggests that the museum connected new museological values with contemporary societal issues that increased the museum's societal relevance.[50] They particularly valued the (audio)visuals and personal objects (i.e., photos and clothing), as well as authentic objects related to the trauma of colonisation (i.e., shackles). However, what is remarkable is that, despite a seemingly increased contemporary relevance and the perceived multi-perspectivity, most of the visitors also indicated that the exhibition was lacking in multi-perspectivity. They missed other perspectives from other contexts, such as slave traders, different 'types' of the enslaved, the descendants of the enslaved, the Dutch, the global slave system, the East Indies, and other locations in The Netherlands apart from Amsterdam. Whereas the museum was perceived as primarily representing the white colonising perspective in 2017, the museum was still perceived as exclusive in 2020.

Material displays and storytelling as contributors to an authentic experience

The following insights are based on the visitor experience at Cape Coast Castle and the International Slavery Museum. The visitors at Cape Coast Castle and the International Slavery Museum showed similar experiences in 2018. Visitors of the International Slavery Museum (Liverpool) understood a Western perspective of the slave trauma and narrative in Europe a, while visitors of Cape Coast Castle (Ghana) understood the trauma from an African American and Africanperspective.[51] This latter perspective was partly shaped by the physical location of the museum and the events that occurred there in relation to the slave trade, but also by their understanding of the material display, as it was described as mostly African-centred and focussed on the African–American experience. Regardless of the differences in their perspectives, visitors to both museums generally perceived the exhibitions as emotional, educational, and confrontational representations of the trauma. They learned about other experiences of the trauma through personal storytelling, individual experiences and perspectives, which were considered valuable for their contemporary relevance. This relevance was simultaneously supported by a feeling of empathy with the people who endured the trauma and a feeling of urgency to understand its impact on the present.

At Cape Coast Castle, visitors indicated they had gained a more profound understanding of "[. . .] life before the whites came" (anonymous, personal communication,

50 For new museological values, for example emotion and affect (Tolia-Kelly, 2016, pp. 896–904). Examples of societal issues are racism and migration.

51 Anonymous visitors, personal communication, 3 and 4 August 2018 and anonymous visitors, personal communication, 3 and 4 May 2018.

3 and 4 May 2018) from a perspective they had not encountered before. They mentioned that "slavery is the reason for brothers of diaspora to visit" (anonymous, personal communication, 3 and 4 May 2018), which shows that slavery has become a key motivator for global travel.[52] At the International Slavery Museum, visitors indicated that they had gained a complete notion of the impacts of slavery as it "[. . .] filled in gaps" (anonymous, personal communication, 3 and 4 August 2018) and it created empathy with the experience of trauma, as the representation "[. . .] put you into other people's shoes" (anonymous, personal communication, 3 and 4 August 2018).

Visitors at both museums mentioned different significant contributors to their experience. At the International Slavery Museum, most of the visitors indicated that the overall feeling of cruelty, the personal stories and experiences, and the diverse interpretation methods typically contributed to their understanding of the trauma and of the implications this trauma has had on their current social environment.[53] At Cape Coast Castle, most of the visitors indicated that the combination of the material and textual display of the slave trade typically contributed to their understanding and constructed their overall experience, which was strongly shaped by the guided tour.[54] It was striking that all visitors of Cape Coast emphasised combined material and textual/verbal interpretation methods as a strong feature of their meaning-making process. At both museums, they indicated that they had appreciated the connection between the narrative and the implications of trauma on today's society.[55] Hence, meaning-making seems relational, based on the relation between the material display, textual display, and the context of the narrative, as already suggested by Hooper-Greenhill (2000).

With respect to the experience of the material display by visitors, I would like to draw attention to two remarkable outcomes. First, at Cape Coast Castle, visitors indicated that the interpretation outside the museum space was perceived as essential for an emotional understanding of the trauma of slavery. For example, slave cells and sculptured faces of enslaved men and women on the floor of the cells, the 'door of no return', the guided tour and the authenticity of the site. This indicates that the visitors' experience at Cape Coast Castle is based on a predominantly cognitive understanding inside the museum and an emotional understanding outside the museum. A second remarkable outcome relates to the reflection of visitors at the International Slavery

52 See also Araujo (2010, pp. 145–173), Light (2017, pp. 276–285), and Gravari-Barbas (2018, pp. 173–176).

53 Anonymous visitors, personal communication, 3 and 4 August 2018.

54 Anonymous visitors, personal communication, 3 and 4 May 2018.

55 Examples of this understanding, at Cape Coast Castle, are such expressions as "freedom-fighting", "American civil rights leaders", and "impacts of slavery on the country" (anonymous visitors, personal communication, 3 and 4 May 2018). Examples of this understanding, at the International Slavery Museum, are such expressions as "stories of people nowadays", "quotes", "personal experiences of people of the last century" and "people's most recent understanding" (anonymous visitors, personal communication, 3 and 4 August 2018).

Museum that informative objects and personal storytelling through audio and video, and authentic objects, were chief contributors to their meaning-making process. In contrast, visitors at Cape Coast Castle valued the powerful objects, such as images and pictures of the trauma, and authentic objects as chief contributors to their meaning-making process. In both cases, shackles were variously mentioned as powerful, authentic objects, for they bear direct evidence of the trauma. Additionally, visitors in both museums indicated ethnic objects as being significant to their understanding of the overall narrative of life before, during, and after slavery (i.e., African artwork, African jewellery and Chiefs' staffs). Although these objects are not directly related to the trauma of slavery, their significance plays a role in a holistic experience. This suggests that the whole representation can only be understood through the consideration of its smaller parts – the ethnic objects that are not related to the trauma of slavery – and their relationship with the whole.

Representations of diasporic memory, imperial grandeur and value perceptions

The following insights are based on the visitor experience at National Museum of African-American History and Culture [NMAAHC] and the Museum of London. The experience of visitors at the NMAAHC and the Museum of London suggest somewhat remarkable, but perhaps expected discrepancies. Visitors at the NMAAHC mostly indicated that a diasporic memory was represented, as American history was presented through personal narratives from an African-American perspective, and the African diaspora. They further indicated that new perspectives on slavery and the significance of slavery for today's society, as well as the brutalities of slavery and how it shaped African-American culture, were portrayed.[56] Visitors at the Museum of London indicated that they experienced a chronological (hi)story of London and the British Empire, including aspects of daily life, city expansion, colonisation, and slavery.[57] It became obvious that visitors mostly experienced the British grand narrative, with limited references to contemporary British society, whereas visitors at the NMAAHC indicated that they experienced a diasporic memory and a relevance of this memory to today's American society.

Visitors at the NMAAHC expressed their experience mostly using positive adjectives, which describe an educational experience through an emotional state of mind, such as 'uplifting', 'inspirational', 'informative', 'mind-changing', 'impressive' and 'moving' (anonymous, personal communication, 10 October 2018). They further per-

56 Anonymous visitors, personal communication, 10 October 2018.

57 Personal communication, 29 and 30 June 2017.

ceived the museum as a place for connecting people and a place of wider significance. Despite the size of the museum, visitors also experienced their visit as cramped and crowded, which endorsed their feeling of incompleteness. It had prompted some to curtail their visit as it affected the quality of their experience.[58] Visitors at the Museum of London indicated a variety of different experiences, for which they used adjectives that describe a rational, emotional, and educational experience, such as 'fun', 'lovely', 'nice', 'mysterious', 'dark', 'awkward', 'helpful', 'informative', 'entertaining', 'incomplete', 'disjointed' and 'exhausting' (anonymous visitors, personal communication, 29 and 30 June 2017). Strikingly, various visitors introduced their experience with 'interesting, but . . .' and 'nice, but . . .', followed by signs of incompleteness, confusion, and one-sidedness.[59] This can be attributed to a potential mismatch between the representation of the British grand narrative and the knowledge, experiences, and memories carried by the visitor(s).

The objects that contribute significantly to the understanding of visitors at the NMAAHC are the pictures, personal and authentic objects, political and symbolic objects and regional objects.[60] Visitors at the Museum of London mostly listed the representational panels, such as a chronological timeline and a map of the British Empire, combined with the interactive interpretation methods as significant contributors to their understanding (i.e., game panels and screen-installations that take visitors back in time). Several visitors indicated various specific trauma and authentic objects (i.e., objects in relation to slavery and the narrative of Olaudah Equiano) and personal objects (i.e., shoes, clothes and a dolls house) as significant contributors to their meaning-making.[61] Although visitors at both museums implied similarities in the perceived significance of authentic, personal and regional objects, there are notable differences in what they perceive as most valuable in the representation. Whereas visitors at the NMAAHC focus more on the objects, visitors at the Museum of London focus more on the interpretation method of the exhibition which they regard *as* an object. This is remarkable as the NMAAHC includes a wide range of digital and interactive representation methods, and the Museum of London has authentic and symbolic artefacts on display as well. However, visitors at the NMAAHC seem to find the objects more significant in their descriptions of the exhibition, while the visitors at the Museum of London indicate a stronger significance as to how the narratives were represented.

58 Anonymous visitors, personal communication, 10 October 2018.

59 Anonymous visitors, personal communication, 29 and 30 June 2017.

60 Personal and authentic objects are, for example, African-American artefacts in time of slavery. Political and symbolic objects are, for example, objects related to the American Revolution, Civil Rights Movement, and segregation. Regional objects are, for example, Oprah Winfrey's studio and objects from African-American inventors. Personal communication (10 October 2018).

61 Personal communication (29 & 30 June 2017).

Authenticity as influenced by Eurocentric representations

The following insights are based on the visitor experience as reviewed on TripAdvisor at Kura Hulanda Museum. To connect the TripAdvisor reviews to Falk and Dierking (2013), Falk (2016, p. 17–91) and Vermeeren et al. (2018, p. 1–16) in relation to the visitor experience, a total of five types of experiences become evident. The experience of the Kura Hulanda Museum varies from educational, authentic, physical, and emotional to engaging experiences. The educational experience is supported by descriptions such as 'informative,' 'learning' and a 'new glimpse on Curaçao'. Other visitors indicate a perceived authentic experience as they interpreted the exhibition as 'true', 'real' and 'historical', which is a contradicting experience for several reasons.[62] Although the visitors did not specify which parts of the exhibition were experienced as true, real and historical, it cannot be determined that this is an outcome of the narrative, material display, exhibition or location, or a combination of these. In terms of the narrative, an authentic experience is most likely based on a Eurocentric notion of this history and connected to the visitors' prior knowledge. This leaves an opportunity for the museum to encourage a wider interpretation that retains a perceived authenticity but pursues a more inclusive and holistic experience by introducing more perspectives into this narrative through multiple interpretation methods. Although Cape Coast Castle and the Kura Hulanda Museum can both be perceived as sites of trauma that directly bear witness to the trauma of slavery, visitors at Cape Coast Castle signified this as valuable for the experience, while no reflection of this is traceable in the physical experience of visitors.[63] Visitors seemed to have experienced a profound, mental involvement during the exhibition that left them impressed and prompted them to recommend it to others.[64] The reviews also imply that the visitor experience included tacit and verbal understanding as visitors perceived their visit as "moving", "disturbing", "heavy", and "a reality check". However, reflections of a multi-sensory, participatory and inclusive experience are absent, which suggests room for improvement in the journey towards creating a contemporary visitor experience that considers the new museological values and visitor needs.[65]

---

62 The study of Hede et al. (2013, pp. 1395–1399) discusses the perceived authentic experience in more detail.

63 It must be remarked again that there is no archaeological proof of this assumed authenticity for the Kura Hulanda Museum (Interviewee 10, personal communication, 8 April 2021). Examples of these broad descriptions are "an exceptional collection", "it was nice", "well-presented" and "well-designed".

64 Example descriptors in these reflections are "impressive" and "must-see".

65 For an overview of objectives related to new museology, see McLean (2005, p. 1), Luepken (2011, pp. 157–173) and Naguib (2013a, pp. 2178–2182), Naguib (2013b, pp. 77–84).

Conclusion: Towards a postcolonial museum?

How can museums connect better to contemporary debates of colonialism through the consideration of the dark tourism visitor experience? In light of dark tourism, I argue that slavery has become one of the main reasons for travelling by diasporic communities who are seeking to explore the routes and roots of their identity. This visitor experience is manifested in the need to experience the trauma of slavery in an authentic, co-creative and interactive manner, in which the visitor is invited to engage in the representation through multiple interpretation techniques, personal storytelling and personal reflection. Representing colonial collections from a postcolonial, contemporary context is essential for creating an inclusive, co-creative and authentic dark tourism experience that fosters multivocality and social justice. In light of museum exhibitions, I argue that museums can start by choosing an appropriate paradigm and pedagogy, or a combination of these, to construct a contemporary visitor experience. The contemporary visitor experience upholds new museological values and visitor's needs and asks for a visitor experience that is inclusive, co-creational, authentic and interactive. In line with the contemporary visitor experience, museums that uphold a paradigm of diversity, approach the exhibition from a popular education pedagogy, which allows them to represent colonial history as a subjective, individual experience.[66] For museums in formerly colonised geographies, a combination of the popular education pedagogy and trauma pedagogy invites local visitors to bring in personal memories, memoirs, and experiences to the exhibition and summons visitors from various cultural backgrounds, minorities, and the diaspora to bring in their perspective.[67] Furthermore, a contemporary visitor experience requires a multitude of interpretation methods and sources of data as this strengthens the multivocality in exhibitions, and facilitates a perceived inclusive experience for a wider target market. As part of the contemporary visitor experience, multiple perspectives reflected through a combination of oral and written history must be experienced. For museums in formerly colonised geographies, it is particularly vital to bring forward the local perspective in the representation and narrative through a new type of knowledge. This new type of knowledge should be created from a local or regional, non-Eurocentric perspective (i.e., from an Afro-Curaçaoen perspective), and brought forward through multiple types of data and sources that reflect concepts such as creativity, emancipation, diversity, dignity, and cultural respect. For local visitors, this perspective could strengthen self-awareness and contextual learning. For museums in

66 The popular education pedagogy embraces the visitor as the receiver and sender of information, which creates a framework for inclusive learning, according to Dorfsman and Hrenczyk (2018: 171–175).

67 The trauma pedagogy engenders understanding through the connection of tangible objects and their significance to people who endured the trauma, which 'encircles' the trauma in the representation. For a relevant study that argues the pedagogy of trauma, see Onega et al. (2017: 1–9 and 311–313).

formerly colonising geographies, it is particularly vital to represent a shared notion of history through a reflection of diversity and multivocality through multiple interpretation methods, types of data and sources. Here, concepts of trauma and migration from a counter-perspective within the grand narrative must be reflected, as this can construct a counter-balance in the reflection of nationalism that is experienced in the grand narrative. A balance between these can enhance a shared notion of history, culture, and identity. Considering the contemporary visitor experience from the notion of the experience economy, visitors profoundly engage with exhibitions that include various types of sources and data through multiple and multisensory interpretation methods. This arrangement does not only allow for multiple meaning-making, but it also enables critical questioning with visitors and steers a relational understanding of history. Such experience variously steers a rational, emotional, interactive, and contextual meaning-making of history.

References

Abungu, G.O. (2018). Connected by History, Divided by Reality. Eliminating Suspicion and Promoting Cooperation between African and European Museums. In Laely, T., Meyer, M. and Schwere, R. (eds.) *Museum Cooperation Between Africa and Europe. A New Field for Museum Studies*, pp. 25–41. Germany: Transcript Verlag.

Alderman, D.H. (2010). Surrogation and the politics of remembering slavery in Savannah, Georgia (USA). *Journal of Historical Geography*, 36, 90–101.

Amsterdam Museum. (September 2019). *Amsterdam Museum Gebruikt Term 'Gouden Eeuw' Niet Meer.* Retrieved from https://www.amsterdammuseum.nl/nieuws/gouden_eeuw.

Andermann, J., & Arnold-de Simine, S. (2012). Introduction: Memory, Community and the New Museum. *Theory, Culture and Society*, 29(1), 3–13.

Anderson, B. (1991/2016). *Imagined Communities: Reflections on the Origin and Spread of Nationalism.* London: Verso / New Left Books.

Antón, C., Camarero, C. & Garrido, M.J. (2018). Exploring the Experience Value of Museum Visitors as a Co-Creation Process. *Current Issues in Tourism*, 21(12), 1406–1425.

Araujo, A.L. (2010). Welcome to the Diaspora: Slave Trade Heritage Tourism and the Public Memory of Slavery. *Ethnologies*, 32(2), 145–178.

Austin, N. K (2002). Managing heritage attractions: Marketing challenges at sensitive historic sites. *International Journal of Tourism Research, 4(6)*, 447–457.

Ashcroft, B., Griffiths, G., & Tiffin, H. (2007). *Post-Colonial Studies: The Key Concepts, 2nd Edn.* London: Taylor & Francis.

Bennett, T. (1995). *The Birth of the Museum: History, Theory, Politics.* London: Routledge.

Bhabba, H. (1994) *The Location of Culture.* London: Routledge.

Bhatia, S. (2009). *Postcolonial Diasporas and Globalization: Reconstructing Culture, Identity and the Practice of Psychology.* Paper presented at Implications For Psychology conference, Clark University, Massachusetts, USA. Abstract retrieved from https://www.clarku.edu/micro/freudcentennial/pdfs/Bhatia.pdf.

Black, G. (2011). Museums, Memory and History. *Cultural and Social History*, 8(3), 412–427.

Blom, T. (2000). Morbid Tourism: A Postmodern Market Niche with an Example from Anthorpe. *Norwegian Journal of Geography*, 54(1), 29–36.

Boateng, H., Okoe, A.F., & Hinson, R.E. (2018). Dark tourism: Exploring tourist's experience at the Cape Coast Castle, Ghana. *Tourism Management Perspectives*, 27, 104–110.

Cain, A. (2011). Representations of Africa and the Diaspora in European Museums. *Human Architecture: Journal of the Sociology of Self-Knowledge*, 9(4), 105–115.

Carrigan, A. (2014). Dark Tourism and Postcolonial Studies: Critical Intersections. *Postcolonial Studies*, 17(3), 236–250.

Childs, P., &Williams, P. (1997). *An Introduction to Postcolonial Theory*. London: Routledge.

Clarke, R., Dutton, J., & Johnston, A. (2014). Shadow Zones, Dark Travel and Postcolonial Cultures. *Postcolonial Studies*, 17(3), 221–235.

Coleman, L.E. (2018). *Understanding and Implementing Inclusion in Museums*. New York: Rowman & Littlefield.

Dal Falco, F. & Vassos, S. (2017). Museum Experience Design: A Modern Storytelling Methodology. *The Design Journal*, 20(1), 3975–3983.

Dann, G. (1994). Tourism: The Nostalgia Industry of the Future. In Theobald, W. (Ed.). *Global Tourism: The Next Decade*, pp. 55–67. Oxford, Butterworth Heinemann.

Dann, G. (1998). *The Dark Side of Tourism*. Aix-en-Provence: Centre International de Recherches et d'Etudes Touristiques.

Dorfsman, M.I., & Horenczyk, G. (2018). Educational Approaches and Contexts in the Development of a Heritage Museum. *Journal of Experiential Education*, 41(2), 170–186.

Dussel, E.D., Krauel, J., & Tůma, V. (2000). Europe, Modernity, and Eurocentrism. *Nepantla: Views from South*, 1, 465–478.

Falk, J. H. (2016). *Identity and the Museum Visitor Experience*. London: Routledge.

Falk, J.H. & Dierking, L.D. (2013). *The Museum Experience Revisited*. London: Routledge.

Fatah-Black, K. (2021). *Slavernij en Beschaving. Geschiedenis van een Paradox*. Amsterdam: Ambo|Anthos Uitgeverij.

Gravari-Barbas, M. (2018). Tourism as a Heritage Producing Machine. *Tourism Management Perspectives*, 25, 173–176.

Hall, S. (1994). Cultural Identity and Diaspora. In Williams, P. & Chrisman, L. (Eds.) *Colonial Discourse and Post-Colonial Theory: a reader*, pp. 391–401. New York: Columbia University Press.

Hall, S. (1997). The Work of Representation. In *Representation: Cultural Representations and Signifying Practices* (pp.15–69). London: Sage.

Hamilton, D., Hodgson, K., & Quirk, J. (2012). Introduction: Slavery, Memory and Identity National representations and Global Legacies. In Hamilton, D., Hodgson, K. and Quirk, J. (Eds.) *Slavery, Memory and Identity*, pp. 1–14. London: Routledge.

Harrison, R., & Hughes, L. (2010). Heritage, Colonialism and Postcolonialism. In Harrison, R. (ed.), *Understanding the Politics of Heritage*, pp. 234–269. Manchester: Manchester University Press.

Hede, A.M., Garma, R., Josiassen, A. & Thyne, M. (2013). Perceived Authenticity of the Visitor Experience in Museums. Conceptualization and Initial Empirical Findings. *European Journal of Marketing*, 48(7), 1395–1412.

Hicks, D. (2020). *The Brutish Museums. The Benin Bronzes, Colonial Violence and Cultural Restitution*. London: Pluto Press.

Hooper-Greenhill, E. (2000). *Museums and the Interpretation of Visual Culture*. London: Routledge.

Horvath, R. (1972). A Definition of Colonialism. *Current Anthropology*, 13(1), 45–57.

Hupperetz, W. (2022). *Museums, Heritage and Digital Curation. Theory and Practice at the Allard Pierson*. Leiden: Sidestone Press.

Larsen, J. and Svabo, C. (2014). The Tourist Gaze and "Family Treasure Trails" in Museums. *Tourist Studies*, 14(2), 105–125.

Levitt, P. (2015). *Artifacts and Allegiances: How Museums Put the Nation and the World on Display*. Los Angeles: University of California Press.

Light, D. (2017). Progress in Dark Tourism and Thanatourism Research: an Uneasy Relationship with Heritage Tourism. *Tourism Management*, 61, 275–301.

Light, B., Bagnall, G., Crawford, G., & Gosling, V. (2018). The Material Role of Digital Media in Connecting With, Within and Beyond the Museum. *Convergence: The International Journal of Research Into New Media Technologies*, 24(4), 407–423.

Lleras, C. (2017). National Museums, National Narratives, and Identity Politics. In Hamilton, P. & Gardner, J.B. *The Oxford Handbook of Public History*, pp. 349–368. Oxford: Oxford University Press.

Loomba, A. (2015). *Colonialism/Postcolonialism: The New Critical Idiom*. London: Routledge.

Lord, B. (2006). Foucault's museum: Difference, representation, and genealogy. *Museum and Society*, 4(1), 11–14.

Luepken, A. (2011). Politics of Representation – Normativity in Museum Practice. *Journal of Religion in Europe*, 4, 157–183.

MacCannell, D. (1999). *The Tourist: A New Theory of the Leisure Class*. Los Angeles: University of California Press.

McCarthy, J., & Ciolfi, L. (2008). Place as Diaologue: Understanding and Supporting the Museum. *International Journal of Heritage Studies*, 14(3), 247–267.

McLean, F. (2005). Museums and National Identity. *Museum and Society*, 3(1), 1–4.

McLeod, J. (2010). *Beginning Postcolonialism*. Manchester. Manchester University Press.

Mezzadra, S., & Rahola, F. (2006) The Postcolonial Condition: A Few Notes on the Quality of Historical Time in the Global Present. *Postcolonial Text* 2(1), 1–13.

Miguéns, J., Baggio, R., & Costa, C. (2008). Social media and Tourism Destination: TripAdvisor Case Study. *Proceedings of the* IASK *Advances in Tourism Research 2008* (ATR2008), *Aveiro, Portugal*, 26–28 May, 194–199.

Mignolo, W.D. (2011). *The Darker Side of Western Modernity*. Durham, NC: Duke University Press.

Moro-Abadía, O. (2006). The History of Archaeology as a 'Colonial Discourse.' *Bulletin of the History of Archaeology*, 16(2), 4–17

Mowatt, R.A., & Chancellor, C.H. (2011). Visiting Death and Life: Dark Tourism and Slave Castles. *Annals of Tourism Research*, 38(4), 1410–1434.

Museum of London. (n.d.). About Us. Retrieved from http://www.museumoflondon.org.uk/corporate/about-us/who-are-we/.

Naguib, S.A. (2013a). Museums, Diaspora and the Sustainability of Intangible Cultural Heritage. *Sustainability*, 5, 2178–2190.

Naguib, S.A. (2013b). Collecting Moments of Life: Museums and the Intangible Heritage of Migration. *Museum International*, 65(1–4), 77–86.

Nebbou, A. (2018). The Colonial Discourse Versus the Anti-Colonial. *Scholars World Net*, 1(3).

Nettleback, A. (2012). Remembering Indigenous Dispossession in the National Museum: The National Museum of Australia and the Canadian Museum of Civilization. *Time and Society*, 21(1), 39–54.

NOS. (May 2021b). *NOS Opening Slavernij Tentoonstelling Rijksmuseum*. Retrieved from https://www.npostart.nl/nos-opening-slavernijtentoonstelling-rijksmuseum/18-05 2021/POW_04900767.

NOS. (September 2019). Amsterdam Museum Neem Afscheid van 'Gouden Eeuw.' *NOS*. Retrieved from https://nos.nl/artikel/2301454-amsterdam-museum-neemt-afscheid-van-gouden-eeuw.html.

Onega, S., Del Río, C., & Escudero-Alías, M. (2017). Introduction. In Onega, S., Del Río, C. and Escudero-Alías, M. (Ed.), *Traumatic Memory and the Ethical, Political and Transhistorical Functions of Literature*, Palgrave Studies in Cultural Heritage and Conflict

Polese, M. (2018). *The Museum Experience in the 21st Century. The Expectations of the Potential Audience and the Experiences Designed by Museum Professionals: The Case of Boijmans van Beuningen Depot.* Unpublished Master's Study. Erasmus University, Rotterdam.

Phillips, R. (2005). Re-Placing Objects: Historical Practices for the Second Museum Age. *The Canadian Historical Review*, 86(1), 83–110.

Pine, J. and Gilmore, J.H. (2007). Museums and Authenticity. *Museum News*. Retrieved from https://northernlight.nl/wp-content/uploads/Pine-and-Gilmore-Museums-and-Authenticity.pdf.

Podoshen, J.S.,Yan, G., Andrzejewski, S.A., Wallin, J. and Venkatesh, V. (2018). Dark Tourism, Abjection and Blood: A Festival Context. *Tourism Management*, 64, pp. 346–356.

Richards, L. (2015). *Handling Qualitative Data. A Practical Guide (3rd ed.)* London: Sage Publications.

Rodenberg, J. & Wagenaar, P. (2016). Essentializing 'Black Pete': competing narratives surrounding the Sinterklaas tradition in the Netherlands. *International Journal of Heritage Studies*, 22(9), 716–728.

Roederer, C., & Filser, M. (2018). Revisiting the Museum Experience. *Qualitative Market Research:An International Journal*, 21(4), 567–587.

Rojek, C. (1993). *Ways of Escape*. Basingstoke: Macmillan.

Sahadat, I. (September 2019). Heleen Schols bestudeerde vier jaar het Zwarte Pieten-debat: 'De vraag zou moeten zijn: als dit een kinderfeest is, voor welke kinderen is het dan een feest?.' *De Volkskrant*. Retrieved from https://www.volkskrant.nl

Said, E.W. (1978). *Orientalism*. London: Routledge & Kegan Paul.

Said, E.W. (1993). *Culture and Imperialism*. London: Random House.

Sandell, R. (2007). *Museums, Prejudice and the Reframing of Difference*. London: Routledge.

Scanlon, L.A. & Kumar, M.S. (2019). Ireland and Irishness: The Contextuality of Postcolonial Identity. *Annals of American Association of Geographers*, 109(1), 202–222.

Schoenberger, E. (June 2020). *What does it Mean to Decolonize a Museum?* Retrieved from http://www.museumnext.com/article/what-does-it-mean-to-decolonize-a-museum/

Seaton, A. (1996). Guided by the Dark: From Thanatopsis to Thanatourism.*International Journal of Heritage Studies*, 2(4), 234–244.

Simone-Charteris, M.T. & Boyd, S.W. (2011). The Potential for Northern Ireland to Promote Politico-Religious Tourism: An Industry Perspective. *Journal of Hospitality Marketing & Management*, 20(3–4), 457–483.

Simpson, M. (1996). *Making Representations. Museum in the Post-Colonial Era*. New York: Routledge.

Sint Nicolaas, E. and Smeulders, V. (2021). Slavernij een Meerstemmig Tentoonstelling. In: Archangel, S., Fata-Black, K., Gosselink, M., Holtrop, M., Lambrechts, L., Sint Nicolaas, E. and Smeulders, V. (Eds.) *Slavernij*. Amsterdam: Atlas Contact.

Smith, A. D. (1991). *National identity*. London: Penguin.

Smith, L.J. (2010). 'Man's inhumanity to man' and other platitudes of avoidance and misrecognition: an analysis of visitor responses to exhibitions marking the 1807 bicentenary. *Museum & Society*, 8(3), 193–214.

Spivak, G.C. (1985). Can the Subaltern Speak? In Spivak, G.C. & Loaiza, E.P. (eds). *Can the Subalterns Speak?* Berlin: Verlag der Buchhandlung Walther Konig,Germany.

Stam, D. (1993). The Informed Muse: The Implications of 'The New Museology' for Museum Practice. *Museum, Management and Curatorship*, 12, 267–283.

Stoler, A.L. (2002). Colonial Archives and the Arts of Governance. *Archival Science*, 2, 87–109.

Stoler, A.L. (2007). The Pulse of the Archive. *Ab Imperio*, 2007(3), 225264.

Stone, P. & Sharpley, R. (2008). Consuming Dark Tourism: A Thanatological Perspective. *Annals of Tourism Research*, 35(2), 574–595.

Stone, P. (2011). Dark tourism: Towards a new post-disciplinary research agenda. *International Journal of Tourism Anthropology*, 1 (3–4), 318–332.

Sunderason, S. (2020). Trans-Imaginaries of Decolonization: Three Frames of the Art of Locus: Afro-Asian Writings. In Amanshauser, H. and Bradley, K. (Eds.), *Navigating the Planetary*, (pp.131–147). Vienna: Verlag für moderne Kunst.

Sussman, N.M. (2000). The Dynamic Nature of Cultural Identity Throughout Cultural Transitions: Why Home is not so Sweet. *Personality and Social Psychology*, 4(4), 355–373.

Tarlow, P. (2005). Dark Tourism: The Appealing 'Dark' Side of Tourism and More. In: Novelli, M. (Ed.). *Niche Tourism: Contemporary Issues, Trends and Cases*. Oxford, Elsevier.

Thomas, D. (2009). Museums in Postcolonial Europe: an introduction. *African and Black Diaspora: An International Journal*, 2(2), 125–135.

Tlostanova, M. (2019). The postcolonial condition, the decolonial option and the postsocialist intervention, In Albrecht, M. (ed.), *Postcolonialism Cross-Examined: Multidirectional Perspectives on Imperial and Colonial Pasts and the Newcolonial Present*. London: Routledge.

Tolia-Kelly, D. (2016). *Feeling* and *Being* at the (Postcolonial) Museum: Presenting the Affective Politics of 'Race' and Culture. *Sociology*, 50(5), 896–912.

Trotter, R. (1998). The Changing Face and Function of Museums. *Media International Australia Incorporating Culture and Policy*, 89, 47–61.

Turner, H. (2020). *Cataloguing Culture. Legacies of Colonialism in the Museum Documentation.*Vancouver: University of British Columbia Press.

Urry, J. (1990). *The Tourist Gaze: Leisure and Travel in Contemporary Societies*. London: Sage.

Urry, J., & Larson, J. (2011). *The Tourist Gaze 3.0*. Los Angeles: Sage.

Van Der Laarse, R. (2005). *Bezeten van Vroeger: Erfgoed, Identiteit en Musealisering*. Amsterdam: Het Spinhuis.

Vergo, P. (1989) *The New Museology*. London: Reaktion Books.

Vermeeren, A.P.O.S., Calvi, L., Sabiescu, A., Trocchianesi, R., Stuedahl, S, Giaccardi, E., & Radice, S. (2018). Future Museum Experience Design: Crowds, Ecosystems and Novel Technologies. In Vermeeren, A., Calvi, L. and Sabiescu, A. (eds.) *Museum Experience Design. Crowds, Ecosystems and Novel Technologies*. Cham, Switzerland: Springer.

Violi, P. (2012). Trauma Site Museums and Politics of Memory. *Theory, Culture & Society*. 29(1), 3675.

Wiegman, C. (2021, February 6). Hoofd geschiedenis Rijksmuseum: 'Ik wil mensen hun naam teruggeven'. *Het Parool*. https://www.parool.nl/ps/hoofd-geschiedenis-rijksmuseum-ik-wil-mensen-hun-naam-teruggeven~b274072f/

Williams, P., & Chrisman, L. (1994). *Colonial Discourse and Postcolonial Theory. A Reader*. London: Routledge.

Xingjang, L., Ruihua, L., Shuangyu, X., Jiaojiao, S., & Yang, Y. (2022). Exploring Visual Embodiment Effect in Dark Tourism: The Influence of Visual Darkness on Dark Experience. *Tourism Management*, 89, 1–14.

Yan, B.J., Zhang, J., Zhang, H.L., Lu, S.J. & Guo, Y.R. (2016). Investigating the Motivation Experience Relationship in a Dark Tourism Space: A Case Study of the Beichuan Earthquake Relics, China. *Tourism Management*, 53, pp. 108–121

Cecilia de Bernardi, Bailey Ashton Adie, Esther Snell

13 Exhibiting power: Dark tourism and crime in the police museum

Abstract: This chapter discusses the representations of crime in state-run police museums, which are found around the world with varying foci. As state institutions, these museums function as an expression of official narratives of justice, control, and state-sanctioned morality, all of which come in the guise of edutainment. The approach taken here is a critical stance on ideologies, hegemony, and power. Methodologically, this chapter employs critical discourse analysis to appraise how information is presented within three diverse contexts: the Polismuseet in Stockholm, Sweden; the Police & Justice Museum in Sydney, Australia; and the Police Museum in Hong Kong, China. Through a comparative analysis, this chapter critically engages with the dichotomy inherent in crime as an attraction within the context of state power.

Keywords: dark tourism, hegemony, Police Museum, discourse analysis, power

Introduction

Dark tourism spans the spectrum of leisure activities, from those designed for pure entertainment, i.e. the London Dungeon (Ivanova & Light, 2018; Stone, 2009) to sites of profound human tragedy, such as the Auschwitz-Birkenau concentration camp (Dalton, 2015). Sites and spaces dealing with criminal acts would then similarly fall across this dark tourism spectrum dependent on the emphasis within the site narrative. However, when this narrative is filtered through a museum space, the museological drive towards edutainment (Huey & Broll, 2017; Thurston, 2017) places these spaces firmly in the middle of this spectrum. Surprisingly, however, there has been relatively little engagement with crime as a dark tourism topic (Adie & Snell, 2021). To that end, this chapter discusses the representations of crime in state-run police museums, which are found around the world with varying foci. As state institutions, these museums function as an expression of official narratives of justice, control, and state-sanctioned morality, all of which come in the guise of edutainment. The approach taken here is a critical stance on ideologies, hegemony, and power. Methodologically, this chapter employs critical discourse analysis to appraise how information is presented within three diverse contexts: the Polismuseet in Stockholm, Sweden; the Police & Justice Museum in Sydney, Australia; and the Police Museum in Hong Kong, China. Through a comparative analysis, this chapter critically engages with the dichotomy inherent in crime as an attraction within the context of state power.

https://doi.org/10.1515/9783110792072-014

Dark tourism and crime

Dark tourism has been investigated across multiple types of sites, but predominantly those witness to the following: mass murder (Dalton, 2015; Kang et al., 2012), disasters (Yoshida, Bui, & Lee, 2016), terrorism (Frew, 2017), slavery (Hanna, Alderman, & Bright, 2018; Rice, 2009), war (Baldwin & Sharpley, 2009; Vanneste & Winter, 2018), genocide (Ashworth & Tunbridge, 2017; Friedrich, Stone, & Rukesha, 2018), and assassinations (Foley & Lennon, 1996). However, to date, there has been relatively little discussion of crime within the dark tourism literature. Those studies that do engage with crime as an element of dark tourism have predominantly discussed it in the broader sense, focusing on atrocities and sites of mass murder (see Dalton, 2015; Lennon, 2010), with individual crime and the penal system receiving significantly less attention. This is particularly interesting as Timothy (2018, p. 386) highlighted that "people are morbidly fascinated by mass murders and serial killings." Therefore, the overall lack of understanding of this element of dark tourism warrants further investigation, particularly given the broad array of sites that attract dark tourists with an interest in crime.

Public interest in crime, particularly violent crime, is visible both in terms of historical mobilities (Gibson, 2006) as well as in the modern incidental development of tourism at sites of gruesome murders, as was observed in Snowtown, Australia (Kim & Butler, 2015) or Amityville, USA (Heidelberg, 2015). In both of these cases, as well as in others, the rise of crime-related tourism has brought unwanted attention to the local area and caused distress to victims' families and local communities, many of whom view the dark crime tourism activities as callous (Kim & Butler, 2015). In other contexts, particularly those where there is a modicum of temporal distance from the crimes, organized dark tourism is more common, as can be observed in the development of murder walking tours. For example, Jack the Ripper tours in London are quite popular with visitors (Powell & Iankova, 2016; Wilbert & Hansen, 2009). In comparison to other forms of organized dark tourism where the victims are the key focal point, these tours frequently memorialize the criminals while simultaneously minimizing the victims, even to the point of dehumanization (Adie & Snell, 2021; Wilbert & Hansen, 2009). Interestingly, crime sites whose narratives are driven by the concept of "punishment" are equally as likely to glorify and dehumanize, but these sites are often deemed acceptable as the criminals are the degraded party while law enforcement are the heroes.

The museum context

Hegemony, power, and the museum

According to Gramsci, hegemony is not taken by force but instead is established with the consent of subordinate classes, due to a variety of factors, including indoctrination, false consciousness, and "ideological predominance" (Im, 1991, p. 124). The basis for establishing hegemony is economic wherein all elements of the state apparatus must be moulded so as to promote this underpinning, and silent, economic consensus. Therefore, everything, including museums, must promote this class compromise, which in turn aids in cementing the existing hegemonic apparatus and the dominance of the ruling class (Im, 1991). The state, as the key element which reinforces the dominance of one class over the rest, also organises consent (Im, 1991). In Gramsci's conceptualisation, the state apparatus extends to civil institutions such as the press, as one of its core functions is to adapt cultural and value systems in line with capitalist economics (Im, 1991). Museums, then, particularly those owned and operated by the state, are not only key to the reinforcement of current hegemonic systems but also function as loci of state narratives of self, effectively symbols of power and authority (Tsai, 2016). They do this through the careful curation of their collections, which Bennet (1995) notes is a discursive display of power, building on Foucault's theories on punishment. According to Bennett (1995, p. 66), "museums, galleries, and, more intermittently, exhibitions played a pivotal role in the formation of the modern state and are fundamental to its conception as, among other things, a set of educative and civilizing agencies." This builds on Gramsci's view of the state as "an educator" (Gramsci, 1971, p. 247, as cited in Bennett, 1995, p. 91).

This educative modus operandi is inherent in the museum's position as an ostensibly public good wherein collections, some of which were previously inaccessible in the hands of private owners, are displayed for the benefit of the public as a means to "regulate" the working class (Bennet, 1995, p. 73). Furthermore, Bennet (1995) highlights that the narrative presented is not stagnant as certain attractions shift from the fringe to the mainstream narrative through the exercise of official control. State museums are often the conduit through which official "history" is presented to the general populace, and thus it is important to look into who participates in the construction of narratives, who is and is not represented, and which relations are constructed (Bennet, 1995). For example, Bennet (1995) highlights that representations of the working class in museums are often idealized interpretations of working-class culture and history as viewed by the middle classes, for example through myths of resilience and eccentricity. However, the expressions of hegemony within the museum context extend beyond the development of collection narratives, particularly as museums are designed as spaces of interaction where visitors engage with content, museum staff, and other visitors. Building again on the Gramscian idea of hegemony by consent, the manner in which these interactions are controlled, for example through exhibit design, is a subtle exertion of state power through which the working class both consumes and becomes part of the dominant narrative. In this way, the state, through the museum, assimilates the working class into its narrative through a more technical and ideological display of power as opposed to that shown by force (Bennett, 1995).

Curating crime: Power, morality, and justice in the museum

Given the importance that public museums have in the maintenance and promotion of state-driven hegemonic discourse, it is perhaps unsurprising that there has been a rise in state-managed police and crime museums over the last century. While criminal activity has been of public interest for centuries, as evidenced by the popularity of public executions and even records of prison tours from the 19th century, the rise of the modern crime or police museum can be traced back to the turn of the 20th century, due in part to the development of the field of criminology (Chazkal, 2012). This intersection between the scientific treatment of crime and museological interest in the subject has led to a strong connection between curation practices and the scientific understanding of criminality (Ystehede, 2016). For example, the use of skulls in exhibitions has sparked a significant amount of controversy, echoing the conversations visible in the field of anthropology, around the ethics of displaying remains instead of returning and/or burying them (e.g., Meloche, Spake, & Nichols, 2020; Squires, Errickson, & Márquez-Grant, 2019). However, behind this sheen of scientific inquiry, museological displays of crime are, in many ways, the modern, and more socioculturally acceptable, incarnation of public displays of punishment that were popular in the past, such as public executions (Bennett, 1995; Ystehede, 2016). Thus, the crime museum provides space for visitors "to explore fears in ways that are not only physically and ontologically safe but also allow for the conversion of fear into pleasure" (Huey, 2011, p. 397).

Within the context of penal- and crime-related museums, hegemonic discourse is particularly visible due to the clear narrative depictions regarding what is and is not appropriate under the existing legal system. However, these narratives are not consistent as the representations of crime can vary significantly depending on how victims and perpetrators are described and presented, where certain crimes may even be "excused", dependent on the circumstances behind the illegal act. Therefore, it becomes relevant to look into how all elements of crime, including the investigative process, punishment, as well as the criminals themselves, are portrayed. This is part of what Bennet (1995, p. 95) describes as "a museological trope" in which punishment is displayed with great detail and where the state sits in a position of absolute dominance. This is, in many ways, a necessity, particularly in police museums, which can be viewed as symbolic representations of the moral authority of the state (Tsai, 2016).

The very existence of these institutions requires the positioning of police in opposition to criminal activity in order to "justify the history and the contemporary presence of the police by developing and characterising both sides of this binary" (Pauls, Walby, & Piché, 2022, p. 4). In some cases, as was observed in Texas, inmates are presented as a dangerous, almost animalistic, potential threat that is effectively neutralised by the prison system (Thurston, 2017). In comparison, law enforcement, i.e. police, prison guards, and wardens, are shown as morally strong individuals who truly care about the criminals in their care and only use morally justifiable violence (Thurston, 2017; Walby, Piché, & Friesen, 2018). In this particular narrative, incarceration is shown as a necessity, with punishment highlighted as a just response to the prisoners' crimes, effectively justifying punitive measures (Barton & Brown, 2012; Regener, 2003; Thurston, 2017).

More frequently, police museums have been developed in order to address public opinion of policing activities, sanitizing and mythologizing the history of policing efforts. These narratives often draw a line between past, perhaps questionable practices by the police force and modern policing activities, emphasizing the importance of progress (Murphy & Chang, 2022; Walby & Piché, 2011; Ystehede, 2016). In Mexico, for example, Buffington (2012, p. 160) notes that local police museums have sought to counteract public distrust in law enforcement by

> forg[ing] a new collective memory for embattled police officers that studiously avoids any mention of police malfeasance past or present – not to invent traditions or construct histories but to cleanse collective memories and, by extension, the police culture that those memories reflect and shape.

Buffington (2012) also highlights that certain police museums in Mexico may effectively only have the current police force in mind as a potential audience when designing exhibitions as their intrinsic purpose is less educative and more intrinsically memorializing, showcasing an idealized interpretation of policing designed to be aspirational. Of course, it would be incorrect to assume that all museums discussing crime are inherently supportive of the hegemonic status quo. For example, Eastern State Penitentiary Museum in Philadelphia, USA, has made it their mission to turn a critical lens onto the modern justice system through historical narrative, effectively questioning the hegemonic discourse (Bruggeman, 2012).

It should be noted, however, that even though the mission of Eastern State Penitentiary is not in line with the hegemonic discourse around policing, the overall narrative is still disconnected from the realities of incarceration and the local context, in part as the museum was developed and is run by non-community heritage activists (Bruggeman, 2012). This has a direct impact on its audience's ability to absorb and critically engage with its message as these museum spaces are intrinsically interactive, often fluctuating between education and entertainment (Regener, 2003; Thurston, 2017; Ystehede, 2016). While museums that over-emphasise the entertainment element can be problematic, visitors who connect to the educational elements can become heavily engaged and have their views of the justice system altered through their visit, as was observed by Knackmuhs, Farmer, and Knapp (2020). This is particularly relevant as police museums frequently have an additional raison d'être, namely the reinforcement of state-defined justice and morality in contrast to deviance as represented by the criminals. Nonetheless, this may lead to complications when there are drastic socio-cultural shifts in terms of how criminality is viewed. Nowhere is this clearer than in the case of the South African Police Museum, which was a popular attraction when it was first opened but became a contested space due to its ties to the colonial past, as well as its outdated institutionalised representations of race (Comaroff & Comaroff, 2006). Thus, it could be argued that modern police museums not only memorialise but also reinforce the existing justice system while simultaneously hiding the realities of modern crime and punishment from visitors.

Discourse analysis: Not a theoretical framework or method

Given the emphasis on power and the resulting imbalanced relationships associated with the concept, discourse analysis has been selected as the most appropriate framework through which to analyse the selected case studies. Norman Fairclough (2001, p. 121) proposed an approach to discourse analysis based on a series of steps, and he criticised the concept of 'method', stating that Critical Discourse Analysis (CDA) is

> as much theory as method – or rather, a theoretical perspective on language and more generally semiosis (including 'visual language', 'body language', and so on) [. . .] which gives ways of analysing language or semiosis within broader analyses of the social process.

Thus, theory and method are seen as being in dialogue with each other, with studies using CDA focusing on anything that can be meaning-making, from visual images to body language (Fairclough, 2001).

Fairclough (2001) describes social life as a network of different social practices, all with their own semiotic element. For example, language is integral to the quotidian human existence, and this language is used and processed in specific ways. Furthermore, representations of practice, which are recontextualized, are also elements of semiosis as are performances, which are reliant on an individual's role within the performance process. Semiosis can then be grouped into genres, which are "different ways of acting, producing social life, in a semiotic mode" (Fairclough, 2001, p. 123). For example, conversations, websites, and videos on TikTok are all different genres. Finally, there are discourses, which are positioned representations of social life (Fairclough, 2001). As with our analysis of crime, people who are in disadvantaged positions are represented in different ways through discourses in the social practices related to crime. These discourses will be dependent on the institution, i.e. the state or the medical field. Social actors enact different roles depending on their positions, and performed positions are referred to as styles.

Fairclough (2001) then explains how social practices are networked together, constituting the social order. The aspect that relates to signs, which Fairclough (2001) calls semiotic, is called the order of discourse. Connecting back to Gramsci, when a group achieves dominance and power, the discourse is ordered in a way that makes it possible to maintain their dominant position. In Fairclough's (2001, p. 124) words, "some ways of making meaning are dominant or mainstream in a particular order of discourse; others are marginal or oppositional." Thus, hegemony is a good word to describe when an order of discourse achieves a dominant position (Fairclough, 2001).

The framework proposed by Fairclough (2001) begins with a focus on a social problem that includes a semiotic element. In this chapter, the websites of crime-related museums managed by the state have been selected. The identified social problem is how crime is presented to uphold and reinforce the hegemonic dominance of certain groups. The museum websites under study in this work were selected through convenience and maximum variation sampling processes. The convenience sampling was the result of limitations in relation to language comprehension, and thus only websites in which the authors could read the source language or for which there was a comprehensive English page were selected. Furthermore, websites had to contain details on exhibitions and/or museum contents, which precluded many police museum websites. Maximum variation sampling through a global search was also undertaken in order to ensure greater generalizability, as well as to avoid biases towards specific contexts. Once there was a saturation of data through which to conduct a satisfactory discourse analysis, this search ceased as discourse analysis requires an in-depth study wherein fewer cases may be studied in more detail (Tsui, 2012).

The second phase sought to identify the obstacles to the solution to the selected social problem. To do this, Fairclough (2001) proposes a series of steps in which the discourse and its relationships to other practices and other discourses are analysed. To this end, the selected websites have been analysed in relation to wider discourses around state power, morality, and justice within a museum context. As these websites have varying structures, there was a focus on the home page and other sections that related to exhibitions, both temporary and permanent, which are relevant to the analysis. Following the multimodal discourse analysis method of Hallett and Kaplan-Weinger (2010), the websites were each navigated and subsequently analysed as if the researchers were tourists. Detailed information about the analysis is provided in each case's subsection wherein the presented social problem is discussed in relation to why this problem is 'needed'. Fairclough (2001) explains that social problems are often not solved because it is in some dominant group's interest for things to remain as they are. Therefore, this aspect is appraised through a discussion, both in the analysis and conclusion, as to why the websites are structured as they are in order to illustrate how dominant groups exercise power by perpetuating certain discourses about state power, morality, and justice. Finally, recommendations are made on how to circumvent the identified obstacle, and an iterative process of self-reflection on the conducted analysis is undertaken.

Analysed cases

Polismuseet, Stockholm, Sweden

The Polismuseet (Police Museum) in Stockholm is part of the Swedish Police Authority and, according to the website, has been in its current form since 2007. In 2019, the museum had about 76,000 visitors. Their mission is described as being the same as the police authority: to fight crime and increase safety in society (Polismuseet, n.d.-a). The website of this museum is available in both English and Swedish, but a large amount of information is available only in Swedish. Therefore, the Swedish version will be the one analysed, as one of the authors is fluent in Swedish.

Analysis

First, it is important to discuss the goal of the museum as stated on the website. The purpose is to fight crime and increase safety, which is the same as Swedish Police Authority, albeit in a completely different style. This is particularly interesting as it illustrates the variety of ways that discourse can be conveyed across styles and genres (Fairclough, 2001). This is a statement of relative neutrality in comparison with the glorification visible in previous studies (Buffington, 2012; Thurston, 2017; Walby, Piché, & Friesen, 2018). Interestingly, though, when looking at the museum's homepage (Polismuseet, n.d.-b), the narrative shifts to one that more actively presents a positive view of the police force and is especially aimed at children. The main picture, which occupies the entirety of the screen horizontally, illustrates a lighter, even funny, interpretation of police officers, with a laughing policewoman, a police dog, and what appears to be a police diver. The accompanying text talks about "a bigger task" (original: en större uppgift) and about the variation in everyday police work. Further down the page, different temporary exhibitions and materials specifically meant for schools are listed. Thus, the museum's purpose appears to be to function as a conduit between the police and younger generations, as well as to give legitimacy to police work, in line with previous research (Pauls, Walby, & Piché, 2022; Thurston, 2017; Walby, Piché, & Friesen, 2018).

For this chapter, one temporary exhibition, "150 years of Police Photography", is of particular interest (Polismuseet, n.d.-b). Unlike the museum's homepage, which is designed to be educational, the temporary exhibition information page is more focused on entertainment value, highlighting how police artefacts can be interesting due to their connection to crime. This emphasis on entertaining content supports the idea of police museums as spaces of edutainment (Thurston, 2017), which places this museum in Fairclough's (2001) network of practices, which in this context are tied to the crime museum as an institution. The edutainment dimension within the discourse here is part of a wider network of genres and styles, not merely those related to museums. In particular, media discourse around crime uses similar edutainment elements (Adie & Snell, 2021), as was observed by McCabe (2022) in relation to Netflix true crime documentaries. The discourse inherent in Nordic Noir, a popular genre of crime fiction in Sweden, follows similar patterns (Bergman, 2014).

The temporary exhibition page emphasises the importance of the camera as a police tool but stresses the importance of the photograph subjects as well (Polismuseet, n.d.-b). For example, the exhibition page notes that visitors to the exhibition will have the opportunity to look at historic Swedish "mugshots" (in English in the original), as well as see evidence from crime scenes, both physical and photographic. The text shows a concerted effort by the author(s) to underscore the importance of the identity and lived experiences of the subjects of the photos, but, when compared with the sensationalist text, the impact of this effort is minimized. Given the importance of language within CDA (Fairclough, 2001), the language used here is important, particularly given the tendency towards sensationalism in this type of museum (Huey & Broll, 2017). In the photography exhibition information, mugshots and *uppmärksammade* (famous) Swedish crimes are mentioned several times, at one point noting that the exhibition includes photographs and objects from "Sweden's most famous criminal cases in modern history." These include homemade bombs and other items from the world-famous bank robbery that led to the identification and discussion of Stockholm syndrome (De Fabrique et al., 2007). This reinforces the entertainment element of this edutainment exhibition while simultaneously disregarding the importance of the photograph's subjects after the initial sentence.

Justice & Police Museum, Sydney, Australia

The Justice & Police Museum in Sydney, Australia, is part of a group of 12 different museums, including historic houses and gardens. Established in 1980, their purpose is "to enrich and revitalise people's lives with Sydney's living history, and to hand the precious places in our care and their collections on to future generations to enjoy" (Sydney Living Museums, n.d.-a). The page also provides additional background on the museum's history and values as a way to build trust with potential visitors. While this page illustrates a genuine attempt to emphasise the learning element of edutainment through expertise, in line with Regener (2003), it is not easily accessible. In order to find it, visitors need to scroll to the bottom of the homepage to reach a small text link in the right-hand corner. Its minimisation is important as it has been noted that website architecture is highly important in CDA, particularly when discussing what is prominent and what is hidden (Saichaie, 2011).

Analysis

The homepage opens with a large multimedia slideshow, including photographs of exhibits and galleries, as well as videos of visitors, which is then followed by general visitor information, such as opening times, prices, and museum location (Sydney Living Museums, n.d-b). Further down the homepage, visitors find large font text that invites them to "step into the dark side of Sydney's past" while also mentioning "crooks," "drifters," "the guilty," and "the innocent." The museum promises its visitors a look into the world of "crime, punishment and policing, from bushrangers, sly grog and razor gangs to forensics." In comparison with the relatively mild sensationalism found in the Swedish Police Museum, the Justice & Police Museum in Sydney relies heavily on sensationalist tropes, drawing attention to the moral aspects of criminal activity wherein there is an overt focus on the crime itself over the investigative and punitive elements seen in other museums (Thurston, 2017).

In line with the analysis of the Polismuseet, the Forensic archive, which contained a strong photographic element, was next to be analysed (Sydney Living Museums, n.d-c). The archive page is fairly similar in style to the Polismuseet photo page in that there is again a focus on sensationalism, but, in contrast, in the Sydney museum, the subjects of the displayed photos are not mentioned at all. This page begins with a presentation of the number of photographs within the collection before shifting to a presentation of the exhibition collection. Within this description, Sydney is called "Sin City", and the exhibit highlights the city's "people, their misfortunes and their crimes". Similarly to the homepage, there is an element of moralizing through a discussion of people suffering from "misfortune" and thus committing "crimes". This reinforces the concept of criminal deviance arising from specific circumstances within the exhibition narrative, which can be understood as providing a template as to how to avoid suffering the same fate and separating the visitor from the criminal (Pauls, Walby, & Piché, 2022).

Further down the page, there are links to additional information on the website, including the New South Wales Police Photography Archive and a collection of negatives (Sydney Living Museums, n.d.-c). Here too there is an emphasis on sensationalist vocabulary. For example, the photograph collection is described as "eclectic" and "remarkable". In comparison, and similarly to the Polismuseet, the description of the negatives collection is dedicated to explaining the technological development of forensic photography, shifting back, albeit briefly, towards an educative focus. However, there is a quick shift back to entertainment-driven content, including an "underworld blog" and various subpages focused on a variety of cases, criminals, and events. The use of blogs in this context is illustrative of a different style through which to disseminate the museum's discourse. As blogs are more informal forms of text, they can be viewed as another edutainment tool. This webpage also contains links to related exhibitions that again rely heavily on sensationalist phrasing, with titles such as "City of Shadows" and "Notorious Criminals." Finally, and similarly to the Polismuseet website, visitors who arrive at the bottom of the webpage are greeted with a large collection of mugshot thumbnails which can be clicked to read more about the subject. The data provided varies by photo, but most contain the date of the photo, the individual's name, and the crime for which they were arrested, with some containing considerably more detail than others in regard to the details of the crime.

Overall, and in contrast to the Polismuseet, the Justice & Police Museum has a significant number of collections and archival material available online. As discourse can take a variety of forms through styles and genres (Fairclough, 2001), the multitude of online content not only has an edutainment focus but also a marketing function. It is also important to note that although both the Polismuseet and the Justice & Police Museum are publicly managed, the Justice & Police Museum is managed through a heritage-focused state organization as opposed to being managed by the police directly. This may account for the breadth of archival coverage as well as the digitization of content. However, as has been observed, many aspects, particularly around the dichotomy between crime and justice, are similar.

Police Museum, Hong Kong, China

The Police Museum in Hong Kong is part of the Hong Kong Police force and was initially developed in 1964. Over its history, it has been expanded, moved, and refreshed several times with the most recent of these beginning in 2020 and only reopening to visitors in September 2022. The current museum houses four galleries: the Orientation Gallery, Thematic Gallery, Serious Crime Gallery, and the Triad Society Gallery (Police Museum, 2022a). This website differs slightly from the previous two cases, and thus the analysis focuses on the homepage (Police Museum, 2022b) and on the virtual visit (Police Museum, 2022c). Additionally, due to language limitations, this website was analysed in English, but, given a comparison of the website in all languages available, it is clear that the information provided is similar in length. Thus, it is possible that some nuance may be lost, but the basic information should remain the same.

Analysis

Unlike the other two examples, there is no clear mission statement on the museum's homepage, but the museum's tagline, "eyewitnessing the force's century-old glory", overlaying an artistic image of the museum, is prominent at the top of the site and clearly indicates a historical and memorialising focus (Police Museum, 2022b). Moving past this image and a partial view of the "about us" information, visitors are shown images of the galleries and key points of interest within the exhibitions. This is followed by a discussion on the use of technology in the newly renovated museum, which has been introduced to "increase its attractiveness and enhance visitors' understanding of the history and work of the Hong Kong Police Force" (Police Museum, 2022b). Technological elements highlighted include a digital map that traces the history of the Hong Kong police force, life-size holograms of various branches of the force, and a digital photo booth that allows visitors to "try on" uniforms from throughout police history. While quite different in terms of implementation, this is very similar in essence to the design of the Polismuseet's child-friendly design developed to showcase the quotidian police experience (Polismuseet, n.d.-b). Similar to the Swedish case, the Hong Kong museum is managed by the Hong Kong police force and thus seeks to legitimise police work while also showing the advancements made through the use of, and emphasis on, technology (Murphy & Chang, 2022; Thurston, 2017; Walby & Piché, 2011; Ystehede, 2016).

Similarly to the other case studies, there is also a focus on edutainment. This is visible in the final section of the homepage where visitors can find links to dramatizations of famous past cases (Police Museum, 2022b). As previously noted, the popularity of crime documentaries has been on the rise (McCabe, 2022), and thus this style of discourse transmission can be viewed as an attractor to entice visitors to the museum. Interestingly, this differs from the Swedish case in that there is a significantly stronger historical narrative element than was observed in Sweden (Polismuseet, n.d.-c). However, there is also a clear element of police memorialization. For example, in the virtual visit, viewers, upon entering the first gallery, can see text noting that the police "has an important duty of safeguarding and protecting the life and property of the citizens of Hong Kong, upholding the rule of law, and maintaining law and order" (Police Museum, 2022c). In addition, there is also a newly added memorial wall to remember those who have given their lives in the line of duty. This is notably different from the other two cases but is in line with what has been observed at other penal and police museums (Pauls, Walby, & Piché, 2022; Thurston, 2017).

The most striking aspect of the Hong Kong case is the focus on new technologies as both a pedagogical and a marketing tool (Police Museum, 2022b). These technologies are particularly evident in the virtual visit, which follows two visitors as they explore the new museum and engage with the various technological tools on offer. Viewers observe these two actors engaging with interactive videos describing investigative methods for capturing murderers and engaging with pedagogical activities such as studying fingerprints (Police Museum, 2022c). These galleries are full of positive descriptions of the police force, calling them "outstanding criminal investigators" and "sensational" (Police Museum, 2022c). This represents a clear overlap between all the cases in relation to sensationalist language. Additionally, and possibly due to a translation issue, one element of the crime gallery text refers to a prostitute as a "compensated-dating girl" (Police Museum, 2022c). In line with previous discussions regarding morality in crime and penal museums (i.e. Thurston, 2017; Walby, Piché, &

Friesen, 2018), a potential explanation for this "incorrect" terminology is that the curators have attempted to avoid specific terminology to maintain decorum.

Conclusions

Police museums, especially those run by the state as seen in this chapter, are inherently spaces of hegemonic discourses that are supported through displays of idealized righteousness in the face of criminal deviance. As dark leisure spaces, they function as an educative and often moralizing actor, curated to reinforce existing power dynamics. The cases presented here all exhibit similar genres of discourse, albeit in very different styles, for example the emphasis on the history of the police force in the Hong Kong case. However, cumulatively, the overall discourse on crime as well as the police force themselves exhibit commonalities. In particular, there is a strong emphasis on sensationalisation of content, often dehumanizing the criminals under discussion (Thurston, 2017; Walby, Piché, & Friesen, 2018). This sensationalism is often used to add the entertainment value to the museum's edutainment offer. In fact, in all three museums, there was a clear emphasis on entertainment, either through the already mentioned sensational language as was seen in the Sydney case, or fun, interactive technology in the case of Hong Kong. In all cases, the entertainment emphasis was ostensibly developed in order to increase foot traffic.

However, building on Gramsci's discussion of civil institutions (Im, 1991) and Bennet's (1995) more specifically on museums, entertainment-heavy edutainment could also be viewed as an easily consumable medium through which a state-driven apparatus inculcates mediated understandings of law, order, and "right" in the general public. This is then buttressed through the glorification via memorialization of police activities, cementing the dichotomous view of good (police) and evil (criminals) noted by Pauls, Walby, & Piché (2022). This is what constitutes the obstacle in Fairclough's (2001) analysis. To move past these hegemonic representations, police museums need to not only acknowledge past policing mistakes as an accountability mechanism but also to illustrate how policing has and is evolving and improving. This, in combination with a refocus on the educative element would enhance the overall impact of these museums and allow for greater nuance. However, as symbols of state moral authority (Tsai, 2016), it is unlikely for a state-run institution to ever manifest in such a self-critical way without risking its own raison d'être.

This chapter has endeavoured to discuss the intersection of hegemony and discourse within the context of state-run police museums as dark leisure spaces. While there has been a concerted effort to provide an in-depth discussion of the cases in question, the study was limited due to the emphasis on website content. Future research should include analyses of museum layouts and actual visits as website and on-site curation practices may differ. There is also a need to undertake a more inclusive analysis, not only in terms of geography but also in relation to public/private ownership as well as the typology of museums to ensure full coverage of the global museological discourse on crime. In addition, and given the focus here on hegemony and power, it would be of interest to undertake more focused research on the museological discourse on crime and how this intersects with the politics of justice, potentially charting the shifting attitudes towards curation practices from a dark tourism perspective. Finally, and given the emphasis on the creation and dissemination of discourse in this work, future research should also include discussions with the visitors to these dark tourism spaces to understand how they are interpreting the edutainment that they are consuming, particularly as it relates to morality and justice and their own positionality.

References

Adie, B.A. & Snell, E.J. (2021). Touring female crime: power and perceptions. *Journal of Heritage Tourism*, 16(4), 382–394.

Ashworth, G.J. & Tunbridge, J.E. (2017). Death camp tourism: Interpretation and management. In G. Hooper & J.J. Lennon (Eds.). *Dark Tourism: Practice and Interpretation* [pp. 69–82]. Abingdon, UK: Routledge.

Baldwin, F. & Sharpley, R. (2009). Battlefield tourism: Bringing organised violence back to life. In R. Sharpley & P.R. Stone (Eds.). *The Darker Side of Travel: The Theory and Practice of Dark Tourism* [pp. 186–206]. Bristol, UK: Channel View Publications.

Barton, A., & Brown, A. (2012). Dark tourism and the modern prison. *Prison Service Journal*, 199, 44–49.

Bennet, T. (1995). The birth of the museum. *History, theory, politics*. London: Routledge.

Bergman, K. (2014). Swedish crime fiction: The making of Nordic Noir. Swedish Crime Fiction, 1–191.

Bruggeman, S.C. (2012). Reforming the carceral past: Eastern State Penitentiary and the challenge of the twenty-first century prison museum. *Radical History Review*, 113, 171–186.

Buffington, R.M. (2012). Institutional memories: The curious genesis of the Mexican police museum. *Radical History Review*, 113, 155–169.

Chazkal, A. (2012). Police museums in Latin America: Preface. *Radical History Review*, 113, 127–133.

Comaroff, J., & Comaroff, J. L. (2006). Criminal Obsessions, after Foucault: Postcoloniality, Policing, and the Metaphysics of Disorder. In J. Comaroff, & J. L. Comaroff (Eds.). *Law and Disorder in the Postcolony* (pp. 273–298). University of Chicago Press.

Dalton, D. (2015). *Dark Tourism and Crime*. Abingdon, UK: Routledge.

De Fabrique, N., Romano, S. J., Vecchi, G. M., & Van Hasselt, V. B. (2007). Understanding stockholm syndrome. *FBI L. Enforcement Bull., 76*, 10.

Fairclough, N. (2001). Critical discourse analysis as a method in social scientific research. In R. Wodak & M. Meyer (Eds.), *Methods of critical discourse analysis* (pp. 122–138). SAGE.

Foley, M. & Lennon, J.J. (1996). JFK and dark tourism: A fascination with assassination. *International Journal of Heritage Studies*, 2(4), 198–211.

Frew, E. (2017). From living memory to social history: Commemoration and interpretation of a contemporary dark event. In G. Hooper & J.J. Lennon (Eds.). *Dark Tourism: Practice and Interpretation* [pp. 160–173]. Abingdon, UK: Routledge.

Friedrich, M., Stone, P.R. & Rukesha, P. (2018). Dark tourism, difficult heritage, and memorialisation: A case of the Rwandan genocide. In P.R. Stone, R. Hartmann, T. Seaton, R. Sharpley, & L. White (Eds.). *The Palgrave Handbook of Dark Tourism Studies* [pp. 261–289]. London: Palgrave Macmillan.

Gibson, D.C. (2006). The relationship between serial murder and the American tourism industry. *Journal of Travel & Tourism Marketing*, 20(1), 45–60.

Hallett, R. W., & Kaplan-Weinger, J. (2010). *Official tourism websites: a discourse analysis perspective* (Vol. 23). Channel View Publications.

Hanna, S.P., Alderman, D.H. & Bright, C.F. (2018). Celebratory landscapes to dark tourism sites? Exploring the design of southern plantation museums. In P.R. Stone, R. Hartmann, T. Seaton, R. Sharpley, & L. White (Eds.). *The Palgrave Handbook of Dark Tourism Studies* [pp. 399–421]. London: Palgrave Macmillan.

Heidelberg, B.A.W. (2015). Managing ghosts: exploring local government involvement in dark tourism. *Journal of Heritage Tourism*, 10(1), 74–90.

Huey, L. (2011). Crime behind the glass: Exploring the sublime in crime at the Vienna Kriminalmuseum. *Theoretical Criminology*, 15(4), 381–399.

Huey, L., & Broll, R. (2017). Punishment as sublime edutainment: "Horrid Spectacles" at the Prison Museum. In *The Palgrave handbook of prison tourism* (pp. 517–539). Palgrave Macmillan, London.

Im, H. B. (1991). Hegemony and counter-hegemony in Gramsci. *Asian Perspective*, *15*(1), 123–156.

Ivanova, P., & Light, D. (2018). 'It's not that we like death or anything': Exploring the motivations and experiences of visitors to a lighter dark tourism attraction. *Journal of Heritage Tourism*, 13(4), 356–369.

Kang, E.-J., Scott, N., Lee, T.J. & Ballantyne, R. (2012). Benefits of visiting a 'dark tourism' site: The case of Jeju April 3rd Peace Park, Korea. *Tourism Management*, 33(2), 257–265.

Kim, S. & Butler, G. (2015). Local community perspectives towards dark tourism development: The case of Snowtown, South Australia. *Journal of Tourism and Cultural Change*, 13(1), 78–89.

Knackmuhs, E., Farmer, J., & Knapp, D. (2020). Addressing contemporary criminal justice issues as interpretive outcomes at a prison museum. *Visitor Studies*, *24*(1), 1–16.

Lennon, J. (2010). Dark tourism and sites of crime. In D. Botterill & T. Jones (Eds.). *Tourism and Crime: Key Themes* [pp. 215–228]. Oxford: Goodfellow Publishers Ltd.

McCabe, R. (2022). Conversations with a killer: the Ted Bundy tapes and affective responses to the true crime documentary. *Studies in Documentary Film*, *16*(1), 38–54.

Meloche, C. H., Spake, L., & Nichols, K. L. (Eds.). (2020). *Working with and for Ancestors: Collaboration in the Care and Study of Ancestral Remains*. Routledge.

Murphy, H., & Chang, Y-L. (2022). Saints and ghosts: Nation-building and narratives of punishment in Taiwan's prison museums. *International Journal of Tourism Cities*. https://doi.org/10.1108/IJTC-02-2022-0025.

Pauls, H., Walby, K., & Piché, J. (2022). Regimes of representation in Canadian police museums: Othering, police subjectivities, and gunscapes. *Crime Media Culture*, 1–21. https://doi.org/10.1177/17416590221086543.

Police Museum (2022a). About us. Available at: https://www.police.gov.hk/museum/en/intro.html.

Police Museum (2022b). Home. Available at: https://www.police.gov.hk/museum/en/index.html.

Police Museum (2022c). Virtual visit. Available at: https://my.matterport.com/show/?m=nnXjeFwZkgz

Polismuseet (n.d.-a). Om Polismuseet. Available at: https://polismuseet.se/om-polismuseet/

Polismuseet (n.d.-b). Start. Available at: https://polismuseet.se/

Polismuseet (n.d.-c). Polishistoria. Available at: https://polismuseet.se/veta-mer/polishistoria/

Powell, R. & Iankova, K. (2016). Dark London: Dimensions and characteristics of dark tourism supply in the UK capital. *Anatolia*, 27(3), 339–351.

Rice, A. (2009). Museums, memorials and plantation houses in the black Atlantic: Slavery and the development of dark tourism. In R. Sharpley & P.R. Stone (Eds.). *The Darker Side of Travel: The Theory and Practice of Dark Tourism* [pp. 224–246]. Bristol, UK: Channel View Publications.

Regener, S. (2003). *Criminological museums and the visualization of evil* (Vol. 7, No. 1, pp. 43–56). Droz.

Saichaie, K. (2011). *Representation on college and university websites: An approach using critical discourse analysis* (Doctoral dissertation, The University of Iowa).

Squires, K., Errickson, D., & Márquez-Grant, N. (2019). Ethical approaches to human remains. *A global challenge in bioarchaeology and forensic anthropology*. Cham: Springer Nature.

Stone, P. R. (2009). 'It's a bloody guide': Fun, fear and a lighter side of dark tourism at The Dungeon visitor attractions, UK. In R. Sharpley & P. R. Stone (Eds.), *The darker side of travel: The theory and practice of dark tourism* [pp. 167–185]. Channel View Publications.

Sydney Living Museums (n.d.-a). About us. Available at: https://sydneylivingmuseums.com.au/about-us

Sydney Living Museums (n.d-b). Justice & Police Museum. Available at: https://sydneylivingmuseums.com.au/justice-police-museum

Sydney Living Museums (n.d-c). NSW Police Forensic Archive. Available at: https://sydneylivingmuseums.com.au/justice-police-museum/forensic-archive

Thurston, H. (2017). Museum ethnography: Researching punishment museums as environments of narrativity. *Methodological Innovations*, *10*(1), 2059799117720615.

Timothy, D.J. (2018). Sites of suffering, tourism, and the heritage of darkness: Illustrations from the United States. In P.R. Stone, R. Hartmann, T. Seaton, R. Sharpley, & L. White (Eds.). *The Palgrave Handbook of Dark Tourism Studies* [pp. 381–398]. London: Palgrave Macmillan.

Tsai, G. (2016). Morality of state symbolic power. *Social Theory and Practice*, 42(2), 318–342.

Tsui, A. B. (2012). Ethnography and classroom discourse. *The Routledge handbook of discourse analysis*, 383–395.

Vanneste, D. & Winter, C. (2018). First World War battlefield tourism: Journeys out of the dark and into the light. In P.R. Stone, R. Hartmann, T. Seaton, R. Sharpley, & L. White (Eds.). *The Palgrave Handbook of Dark Tourism Studies* [pp. 443–467]. London: Palgrave Macmillan.

Walby, K., & Piché, J. (2011). The polysemy of punishment memorialization: Dark tourism and Ontario's penal history museums. *Punishment & Society*, 13(4), 451–472.

Walby, K., Piché, J., & Friesen, B. (2018). ". . . they didn't just do it because it was a job": Representing wardens in Canadian penal history museums. *International Journal of Law, Crime and Justice*, 53, 1–8.

Wilbert, C. & Hansen, R. (2009). Walks in spectral space: East London crime scene tourism. In A. Jansson & A. Lagerkvist (eds.). *Strange Spaces: Explorations into Mediated Obscurity* [pp. 187–204]. Farnham, UK: Ashgate.

Yoshida, K., Bui, H. T., & Lee, T. J. (2016). Does tourism illuminate the darkness of Hiroshima and Nagasaki? *Journal of Destination Marketing & Management*, 5(4), 333–340.

Ystehede, P. J. (2016). Contested Spaces: On Crime Museums, Monuments, and Memorials. In P. Knepper & A. Johansen (Eds.). *The Oxford Handbook of the History of Crime and Criminal Justice* (pp. 338–352). Oxford University Press

Rebecca Finkel and Katherine Dashper

14 Representations in UK witches tours: Walking over the roots of misogyny

Abstract: This chapter focuses on issues of gender in dark tourism, a topic the field has barely addressed. Based on feminist approaches, this chapter explores the ways in which witches, and related dark histories of misogyny and violence, are represented in witches tours in Britain. Witches tours are a popular tourist attraction in places that once held witch trials and executions. We seek to examine how those historically accused of being witches, who were mainly older or independent women, are portrayed in contemporary times and what gendered narratives this promotes and emphasizes. Methods include ethnographic techniques of participant and direct observation of witches tours to be immersed in the visitor experience including how these tours are advertised and how so-called witches are represented and to examine how the historic persecution of (some) women has been commercialised and sanitised for touristic consumption. How we view the past often influences how we see things in the present, and even tourist attractions based loosely on historic events can have an impact on re/constructing and reinforcing gendered narratives. The ways these witches tours are presented online suggests that they can be interpreted as one of the 'lightest' forms of dark tourism in that they are oriented for edutainment in a Disney-fied vein.

Keywords: dark tourism, witchcraft, feminism, gender, misogyny, edutainment

Introduction

Dark tourism is still an emerging scholarly subject specialism that draws upon cross-disciplinary literatures and methodologies to provide deeper critical understandings of the less salubrious aspects of visitor attractions, place-based destinations, and travel and tourism industries. As with any emerging subject, this often means there is scope to develop investigations into more marginalized subjects and topics, as the initial focus is often on mainstream and dominant groups to set the context for further conceptualizations. Although research has been published on dark tourism as it relates to identity and geographies of belonging (e.g., White & Frew, 2013), much of the literature still focuses on disparate case study examples (e.g., Lennon & Foley, 2000; Stone et. al., 2018), which help to define and indicate types of dark tourism in a more generalized way. This chapter draws upon this body of work to focus more distinctly on issues of gender in dark tourism. Although there is attention surrounding commercial sex tourism (e.g. Carr & Berdychevsky, 2021; Hall & Ryan, 2001), gendered inquiry

https://doi.org/10.1515/9783110792072-015

is an area that the field of dark tourism has barely addressed. Based on feminist approaches, this chapter explores the gendered experiences of witches tours throughout Britain. Witches tours are a popular tourist attraction in places that once held witch trials and executions. We seek to examine how those historically accused of being witches, who were mainly older or independent women, are portrayed in contemporary times and what gendered narratives this promotes and emphasizes.

According to the National Museum of Scotland, "In the late 16th-and 17th-century Scotland, between three and four thousand people were tortured and executed as 'witches', a group identified as threatening social stability" (NMS, H.MR 43), around 85% of whom were women (Goodare et al., 2003). About 500–1000 people, 90% of whom were women, were put to death in England between the 15th and 18th centuries. Additionally, approximately 40,000 people, of whom 80% were women, were killed in Western Europe at that time under suspicion of witchcraft (Hutton, 2010). Folklore has sprung from these misogynistically-motivated systemic mass murders, and accusations of witchcraft have long been used to discipline and control women's behaviour. Although there are a variety of cultural representations, serious literature, and other historically informed texts about witch trials and executions, tourism attractions have mainly veered towards an emphasis on the occult, magic, and almost cartoonish popular cultural portrayals of witches for entertaining experiential purposes. Whilst edutainment is an important aspect of many tourism attractions, including many dark tourism experiences (Wyatt et al., 2021), there is a danger that the underlying historical details and uncomfortable truths become sanitized and forgotten.

How we view the past often influences how we see things in the present, and even tourist attractions based loosely on historic events can have an impact on re/constructing and reinforcing gendered narratives. In this chapter, we examine the ways in which witches, and related dark histories of misogyny and violence, are represented in witches tours in Britain.

Understanding dark tourism in the experience economy

Dark tourism is "a highly complex and multidimensional phenomenon involving visits to real and recreated places associated with death, suffering, misfortune, and the seemingly macabre" (Wyatt et al., 2021, p. 434). Sites, attractions, and events associated with war are enduringly popular (Cakar, 2020), as are those associated with slavery (Hanna et al., 2018) and genocide (Lischer, 2019). Whilst these sites are undoubtedly connected to death and suffering, some other dark tourism sites may be associated less directly with death and more with punishment, such as infamous prisons (Strange and Kempa, 2003), or even fantastical representations in literature and popular culture, such as Dracula. Thus, Stone (2006, p. 146) argues, there are "various shades of darkness" along a "fluid spectrum of intensity", which is "dependent upon various defining characteristics, perceptions and product features." Miles (2002) makes a distinction "between sites associated *with* death and suffering, and sites that are *of* death and suffering" (cited in Stone, 2006, p. 151). On this spectrum, the 'lightest' dark tourism sites focus on heritage topics that are loosely based on macabre historical events but are presented more as entertainment, where visitors seek "to experience fear and thrill in a safe context" (Norfelt et al., 2023, p. 454). In many respects, witches tours are similar to this, as they weave stories loosely based on actual grisly place-based historical events in an informative yet theatrical manner that is similar to the 'true crime' genre of media entertainment in a tourism environment.

When interpreted in this way, dark tourism attractions can be understood within current cultural-economic frameworks. Sharpley (2009, p. 7) argues that there is a "relationship between dark tourism and the cultural conditions and social institutions of contemporary societies." Therefore, it can be seen that witches tours are operating within a societal context that emphasizes entertainment-focused experiences of a destination. Stone (2006, p.150) draws from Seaton's (1999) work, which argues that "production of the dark and disturbing past is not only driven by consumer tastes, which are often media-influenced, and by commercial marketing ploys on behalf of the supplier but is also subject to changes in the wider political and cultural climate." As Finkel and Platt (2020) reflect, the city is often treated as a 'theme park' (Sorkin, 1992), as part of discourses surrounding the Disneyization of society (Zukin, 1993), driven by cultural commercialization and the experience economy (Pine and Gilmore, 2011). Events and tourist sites tend to be commodified (Waitt, 2008) to create an urban space in which the middle classes can consume in comfort and safety (Zukin, 1993). This connects with Debord's (1994) argument that "the spectacle can be considered a commodity in contemporary society because of its ubiquitous production and rigorous marketing [. . .]. The spectacle is the chief product of present-day society" (cited in Finkel & Platt, 2020, p. 5). Therefore, an uneasy balance emerges between historical accuracy and experiential entertainment in the storytelling of the past in order to engage with contemporary audiences.

Dark tourism, representation, and edutainment

All tourism sites, attractions and experiences involve representation; historical and contemporary sites, events, groups and individuals are represented for tourist consumption and understanding. Wyatt et al. (2021) discuss the challenges in balancing the management of ethical issues with the representation of past tragedies for packaged tourism purposes. Tourism is a commercial enterprise, and attractions seek to entice tourists to visit and spend money. Consequently, many sites have embraced edutainment as a means to appeal to visitors, including children (Seraphin & Yallop, 2020).

Edutainment is an important aspect of many contemporary tourism attractions, combining education and learning with fun, through exploration and interactivity (Pratt & Suntikul, 2016). Although edutainment has been widely adopted in the heritage tourism industry (Hertzman et al., 2008; Luo, 2021), its use in dark tourism is more controversial. For example, Potter et al. (2020) argue that the use of edutainment options at plantation sites in the southern United States may well attract a greater number and more diverse range of visitors, but at the same time risks erasing the trauma and pain associated with slavery at these sites. However, Oren and Shani (2012) argue that careful theming, an aspect of edutainment, can be an important means to engage visitors emotionally in difficult histories, such as those presented at the Yad Vashem Holocaust Museum in Jerusalem.

Despite the potentially problematic implications of deploying edutainment in dark tourism, its use is widespread. Bristow and Jenkins (2020) discuss the popularity of fright tourism in urban centers, where visitors seek to engage with dark, supposedly haunted or otherwise frightening locations for fun, seeking a balance between fear and excitement. Similarly, Powell and Iankova (2016) identified 'light dark tourism' attractions, such as the London Dungeons, as popular within London's touristic offering. This kind of attraction "imagines and recreates historical events for the undiluted purposes of providing entertainment" (Powell and Iankova, 2016, p. 347). Those historical events usually relate to the pain and suffering of real people, often involving torture and death, but their representation repurposes these historic and gruesome experiences and practices as fun and safe entertainment for contemporary tourists.

As these sites and historical events are reconstructed for commercial benefit, selective storytelling is enacted. As Lennon (2017, p. 26) suggests, dark tourism sites are a

> meeting place for history and visitation where questions of authenticity and fact are sometimes juxtaposed with the operation of tourism facilities. What is celebrated, interpreted, and developed is often selective, and dilemmas of commemoration of the unacceptable and acceptable are reflected clearly in the condition, nature, and content of these sites.

Therefore, mainstream stories from hegemonic groups and dominant perspectives are those that are more prevalent throughout dark tourism narratives. Indeed, Adie and Snell (2021) found that there exists a 'significant gap' in relation to the discussion of dark tourism activities with engagement with gender at these sites, meaning that "the tourist activities that revolve around dark heritage sites, especially those that deal with violent criminal activity, reinforce gendered stereotypes around 'acceptable' transgression" (p. 382).

Dark tourism, gender, and witchcraft

There has been minimal scholarly attention paid to the ways in which dark tourism is gendered. Some studies have explored gender differences in tourists' knowledge of and interest in dark tourism. Magano et al. (2022) found that women were more likely than men to know about dark tourism, whereas Bhati et al. (2021) found no differences between male and female interest in and willingness to travel for dark tourism. In contrast, Urbonavicius (2021) found motivational differences between men and women in visiting Chernobyl, with females driven by more novelty-seeking and escape motivations and males by ego-enhancement and prestige.

However, the gendered aspects of dark tourism go beyond the demographics and motivations of tourists and also encompass the representation of dark tourism sites and the historical events and people with whom they are associated. To our knowledge, there has not yet been any examination of the ways in which many dark tourism sites, such as those associated with war, represent gendered discourses related to men and masculinities. As most dark tourism sites are related to the acts of mainly men (such as war and genocide, the commercial elements of the slave trade, and mass murderers, among others), this is a significant omission. There have been a few considerations of dark tourism sites associated with women, although these rarely employ gender or feminist theory in analysis. For example, Busby and Devereux's (2015) study of associations between tourists' motivations to visit the site of Anne Frank's house in Amsterdam and whether or not they had read her diaries identified differences between men and women in this way, and the importance of literature to dark tourism, but did not employ a gender lens to consider how this site and Anne Frank herself are represented, or why female tourists may be more likely to have read the diaries prior to visitation. Similarly, Palleiro and Peltzer's (2023) interesting evaluation of narratives around the 'lady ghost' in Argentina does not consider the gendered discourses mobilized within these representations of dead women.

An exception to this is Stone and Morton's (2022) examination of the female dead. They note that men and women are not treated the same in death, or in dark tourism. They argue that the female dead are exploited through dark tourism, subject to a variety of forces of Othering, erasure, voyeurism, misogyny, and sexualization, perpetuated by a dominant male gaze. These insights are highly relevant to how women (real and imagined, historical and contemporary) are represented through witches tours.

This limited engagement with gender analysis in examining dark tourism sites and experiences is reflective of a wider trend in tourism studies that considers gender a niche subject, rather than being central to understanding the field. There are some notable exceptions where critical gender theory has been utilized to explore issues ranging from tourism work (e.g., Costa et al., 2017) to violence (e.g., Eger, 2021) and debates around sustainability (e.g., Alarcón & Cole, 2019). However, Pritchard (2018) argues that there is inadequate interaction between tourism studies and feminist inquiry, and feminist methods and approaches struggle for legitimacy in a field dominated by post-scientific paradigms. Dark tourism studies is increasingly engaging with critical theories, such as those of postcolonialism (Carrigan, 2014), morality, (Chen & Xu, 2021), and affect (Martini & Buda, 2020). There is, therefore, scope for much greater engagement with critical gender and feminist theories and approaches.

Witches, witchcraft, and witch trials provide a source of dark tourism in many locations and rely on gendered histories of misogyny. Associated sites draw on historical tales of (mainly) women who were persecuted as witches in the 18th century. For example, Kužnik and Veble (2018) found that witches and witchcraft were used in dark tourism in the city of Krsko, Slovenia. Also, Trasmoz, Spain, has capitalized on its 'cursed' village brand by using its dark history to attract tourists. Over 6,000 tourists attend its lighthearted witchcraft festival, *Feria de Brujería*, each year (Kassam, 2021). Heidelberg (2015) discusses Salem, Massachusetts, the site of the notorious Witch Trials in 1692. The story of these Witch Trials has been retold many times, across different media platforms, from books to movies and television dramas. Heidelberg (2015) argues that modern Salem embraces its historic notoriety with both local government and businesses using imagery, stories and locations associated with the Trials to entice tourists, 330 years later. Whilst contemporary attractions are based on historical events, the horrific persecution of those found guilty and hanged (14 women and five men) are repackaged, sanitized and commodified for tourists. For example, each year the Salem Haunted Happenings festival, which takes place over the month of October, is presented as "a festive celebration of Halloween and fall in New England" aimed at families interested in visiting the "Witch City" (Haunted Happenings, 2022). The event's website uses stereotypical tropes associated with witches, such as silhouettes of women on broomsticks, with pointy hats, sitting on the moon. The only mention of the dark history that has made Salem (in)famous comes in a section called "Facts & Fun – History" and includes just two sentences about the Trials and the deaths of 19 innocent people. Further, although five men were also executed as part of the Trials, all witch-related imagery used relates to women, illustrating the gendered nature of representations of witches and witchcraft wherein only women are associated with this persecuted identity.

Robison-Greene (2021) also draws on Salem in her discussion of the ethics of dark tourism. She discusses the Salem Witch Dungeon as a site ostensibly created to educate tourists about the Trials, and the imprisonment and execution of those who were accused of witchcraft. However, she goes on to note some of the problematic issues that arise when dark tourism meets edutainment, describing the Dungeon as being "more like a haunted house than it is a respectful educational opportunity" (p. 2), meaning that the tragic and dangerous history of the site, and those who were persecuted and executed, is easily overlooked by tourists when "people wearing spooky makeup are hired to generate screams" (p. 2).

Witches and witchcraft thus make an important element of dark tourism and provide an opportunity to explore the ways in which gendered narratives are deployed in contemporary representations of a gruesome past in which (mainly) women lived under fear of accusation of being witches and subsequently persecution and often execution. We draw on insights from feminist perspectives of the representation of strong or unconventional women as witches, which continue to be mobilized to undermine women's power and positions in society. As Rosen (2017, p. 22) argues, the image of the witch is still used contemporarily to "reinforce gender inequality and marginalize women who push back against patriarchal societies", and witches tours play an important, if usually unacknowledged, role in this public misogyny.

Research methods

In this project, we were interested in investigating how witches and witchcraft are represented through edutainment to attract and entertain, possibly educate, tourists across Britain. We analyzed online materials associated with the tours (websites and social media) to evaluate the representation of witches, women, the tours, tour participants, and associated gendered narratives, including how these tours are advertised and how so-called witches are represented to examine the ways in which the historic persecution of (some) women has been commercialized and sanitized for touristic consumption. Case study examples of the tours were selected by geography to have a representation from different areas of the country as well as the necessity of a social media presence. Independent tours, the ones not associated with bundled entertainment sites, were selected to focus on witches tours as stand-alone experiences more specifically.

Our analysis in this chapter is based on four commercial witches tours run by three different companies, focusing on the formal representation of these tours on the associated websites. We present each as a short case study before discussing shared themes and their implications in relation to the gendered discourses (re)presented and (re)packaged through this form of dark tourism.

Case One: Witches & history walking tour, Edinburgh

Including 'history' in the name of the tour positions this tour as providing a reliable and educational form of touristic leisure setting up expectations that this will be an informed tour based on historical records and perhaps artifacts. This does not appear to be the case upon further investigation into the website. For example, the homepage features a stereotypic depiction of a witch silhouetted by a full moon with outlines of recognizable landmarks of Edinburgh dotted around on the sides. The 'witch' has a pointy hat and broom and is in a power pose with an arm bent at the hip. The tag line – "Discover a wicked history" – perhaps plays on the popular musical theater show, *Wicked*, whose protagonists are the two witches from the *Wizard of Oz*. The 'Book Now' buttons utilize a dripping effect to resemble blood, giving it a 'spooky' vibe. Despite claims to be historic, no names of actual people arrested or tried as witches or even the names of witch hunters or judges are mentioned at all. Humanity is not what is on display here. Representations are squarely in the Halloween camp. The connotation here is that the subject matter is transgressive, but in a fun way without risk or actual danger and very much situated in the contemporary popular culture of witches rather than unsettling past events.

A search for more information brings a page where words like 'spellbinding', 'enchanting', and 'bewitching' are used often. Among these 'magic' phrases are also reassurances that this is a 'historical' and 'factual' tour of the city. Although it may appear incongruent to have hints at the occult with a credible record, the website dares us, "Are you ready to learn historical facts? Are you ready to be thoroughly entertained?" In this way, the tours are positioning themselves as both performance and instructive narrators of the past. Witch hunts are called 'infamous', an 'injustice', and the tours promise to help attendees "learn from the past". This is not expounded upon, but it can be surmised that it is a reference to 'witch hunts', which implies accusations without validity, and that these acts of violence are not condoned. However, the site also states that the tours will "bring to life the stories of Edinburgh's real-life witches", which is problematic in that it portrays people condemned as witches to be 'Other' and not actual women (and, in fewer cases, men). 'Real life witches' is used perhaps as a device to distance the tour from the horrific treatment that occurred at the time and the underlying misogyny that propelled such acts, as it implies such things were happening to supernatural creatures or dangerous beings rather than ordinary, often marginalized and vulnerable, human beings. At the bottom of the page, there is the ubiquitous nod to Edinburgh-specific popular culture with *Harry Potter* and *Outlander* references. This, again, sets the tone to be light, entertaining, and family-friendly in a way that spectacle-izes and commercializes a past of gruesome torture, misogynistic oppression, and state-sanctioned femicide.

Case Two: Witches & history tour, York

The same company also runs tours in York and London. The York version is particularly notable, in terms of how it deploys entertainment and cultural tropes of magic and witches in its package and marketing of the tour. The York tour includes an extra element – "a magical potion-making experience". Tourists are invited to "Unleash your own magic as you enter the secret potion room and lose yourself in an immersive Potion Making Experience." This feeds directly into fantastical representations of witches. There is no attempt to link this immersive experience with historical facts or the women accused of witchcraft in York. It is purely about entertainment, aimed primarily at children and families.

The imagery on the website supports these magical and ahistorical representations of witches. A silhouette of a witch is presented, through the tropes of a pointy black hat and long black cloak, looking into a lit-up shop called 'The Potions Caldron'. Tourists are invited to participate and to "Dare to join the coven". Unlike both the Edinburgh and London versions of this tour, there is no attempt to link the York tour with historical facts about the city and its treatment of those accused of witchcraft, completely detaching the tour from the historic reality and relying solely on fictional and fantastical representations of witches and magic. Rather, tourists are invited to "Join a characterful witch who will captivate you with this engaging, often enlightening and ultimately uplifting experience". That this tour is described as "ultimately uplifting" belies the dark histories on which it is loosely based, erasing the pain and suffering of the many women (and some men) who were persecuted and executed as witches in and around York.

Case Three: The Newcastle Witchery tour

This tour, organized by Newcastle Ghost Walks & Tours with the strapline "Gruesome Geordie Histories & Ghost Walking Tours", makes more explicit references to the historical events that inspired the tour, promising to take tourists back to "the old folkloric days of the Newcastle Witchcraft Trials of 1649 and 1650". The website presents the tour as an opportunity to engage with sites around the city that are related to the Trials, comparing it to the more well-known Pendle Witch Trials of 1612 and even to the Salem Witch Trials and "the innocent people that were executed all over the world". The image on the website shows a woman dressed in historical garments with fingers pointing at her, evoking a sense of public shaming, persecution, and desperation on her face. Although the website only ever uses the term 'witches', with no use of pronouns, the choice of a woman in the top image directs tourists' sympathies towards women accused as witches and involved in these trials, with frequent reference to the historic events that inspired the tour.

There are many associations made between witches and evil on the website for this tour. A historical image shows witches riding broomsticks alongside the devil, or "the witch father", with the accompanying text prompting tourists to question whether it is true that witches give themselves to the devil and if they eat babies. Further associations with the occult and evil are made through the use of terms like "very sinister looking" and frequent associations between witches and spirits, which are presented as witches' "familiars" who "do their bidding". Witches are also referred to as "cunning folk" who would meet "the man in black" (i.e., the devil), making pacts with him to gain their powers. In such ways, the tour builds upon historic associations to amplify the dark side of witchcraft, building suspense and probably some nervous anticipation in tourists through evoking discourses of evil and the supernatural.

Unusually in our sample, this tour is led by a man who is presented as "a real folk witch", disrupting the commonsense association between witches and women. The tour guide is said to be not Wiccan or pagan but a practitioner of folkloric witchcraft, which is the kind that Newcastle witches were accused of practicing and that led to the deaths of 28 people, tying the tour to the historical events on which it is loosely based. At the same time, however, the commercialized elements of edutainment are never far from the surface as the witch guide – presented as being able to prove his witchy ancestry through ownership of certain historical artifacts that he will display for visitors on the tour – is also presented as a palm reader and tea leaf reader, and tourists can purchase these services at an extra price (£25 per reading). The witch guide is also presented as carrying with him vials of herbs for sale for just £5 that can be used for "protection to love, cursing and more", maximizing opportunities to elicit more money from tourists through engagement in magical experiences.

The representations of this tour certainly invoke historical narratives, but present a somewhat ambivalent view of witches as both unfairly persecuted victims and as agentic beings actively seeking out associations with the devil, evil, and the occult. The gendered representations are complex, as both women (in the imagery) and men (through the guide) are associated with witchcraft, although it is the contemporary male witch who is credited with powers that can help and inform tourists (at an extra price, of course), and it is the historical female witches who are associated with evil and the devil.

Case Four: Hex and the City, London

Herstorical Tours runs a Hex and the City walking tour focusing on telling "the story of London's witches." The name of the tour is a play on the popular TV show, *Sex and the City*, and it is therefore implied that the focus is on independent women. Indeed, the emphasis on the website is to highlight "forgotten women" by telling their stories. The banner of the website includes Wiccan symbols, such as the Pentecostal star, and other images on the website are of the tour guide dressed in a big coat and floral headwear. There are no stereotypic witch material culture or traditional Halloween images.

The site states, "Explore London's witch-ridden, pagan past on our immersive theater walking tour." The images of the tour guide making grand gestures make more sense given the inclusion of the word "theater" to explain the tour. The guide, the website states, "welcomes you to her coven and unveils to you the dark, devilish and downright unjust history of witchcraft in London." It promises a "spooky and moving" experience. This illustrates two main themes – the devilish and spooky badges of a so-called witch, as well as the injustice and moving experiences that the women accused of witchcraft had to suffer. It can be seen to be attempting to bridge the entertainment aspect with the upsetting reality of what occurred by mentioning both aspects equally throughout the site. The site also features quotes from feminist figures, such as "Well-behaved women seldom make history" by Laurel Thatcher Ulrich, and "When a man gives his opinion, he's a man. When a woman gives her opinion, she's a bitch" by Bette Davis, among others. This sets a more contemporary feminist tone, hinting at the unjust treatment of women and the ways in which accusations of witchcraft have long been used to control and contain outspoken women.

Discussion and conclusion

The ways these witches tours are presented online suggests that they can be interpreted as one of the 'lightest' forms of dark tourism in that they are oriented for edutainment in a Disneyfied vein, in ways similar to other visitor attractions based very loosely on dark historical events, such as the London Dungeons (Powell & Iankova, 2016). In many respects, location is not a particularly important factor for marketing most of these tours, as there is a tangential connection to witch trials in all of these cities, and the tours are packaged as part of the wider generic urban tourism offering. Based on the imagery, these tours are family-friendly, fun and playful, and mainly aligned with the 'spooky' interpretation of witchcraft centering on the occult, supernatural, and popular cultural representations of the materiality of witches, such as broomsticks, pointy hats, long cloaks, and black cats. It is also notable that these witches tours are private commercial enterprises, not run by historical societies or councils, and thus rely on selling tickets. Also, they will be reliant on social media reviews and recommendations to sustain a steady flow of business, which means customer service and satisfaction is of importance. Therefore, historical accuracy is not the top priority. And, to be fair, the tours are not claiming that it is. They will be providing what participants seek out from such a tour – to be informative, perhaps, but mainly to curate a good time. The tours are packaged as a night out, not a history lecture.

Gendered narratives are (re)presented in different ways in these tours. For the Halloweenesque tours in Edinburgh and York, gender is used as a stereotypic trope to sell the experience. Witches are associated through imagery and language with women only, through 'spooky' comparisons and feminine tropes such as pointy hats. In Newcastle, gendered images based on fantastical representations of women witches are employed as well, but the male tour guide shifts the perspective and acts as a reminder that women were not the only ones embroiled in this injustice. However, his self-proclaimed expertise in witchcraft does come at an extra price to tourists. The London tour claims to support a feminist position, which focuses on the gendered violence of these acts victimizing women. Yet, it also approaches this with trappings of the occult and paganism, which lean toward the theatrical. Such performances seemingly seek to empower but also can be seen to profit from the historical pain and suffering inflicted on all those accused of witchcraft.

The case study examples support Stone and Morton's (2022) work with regard to problematizing how the female dead are represented. Women as so-called witches featured in the tours' online materials are not given a voice and sometimes not even given a face. The ways that these women are portrayed are as Other, if not otherworldly. The motifs conveyed can be viewed through the lens of objectifying women who were cruelly maltreated by the dominant (white, male, elite) class at a dangerous time in history. In some respects, it could be interpreted that these tours legitimize the exploitation of these women in the past by weaving tales of diabolical encounters with magical exoticism, as well as in the present by profiting from their misfortunes (often their executions) by turning them into a tourism product without adequately acknowledging their suffering. When the histories of witches and witch trials are reappropriated in contemporary tourism, the real and harrowing stories of the women (and men) who suffered at the hands of puritanical powers are erased. Witchcraft becomes something that is fun, exciting, and possibly a little mysterious, rather than a violent example of how women's behaviors and presence in society were controlled and disciplined.

The ways in which women are represented as witches in the tours reflects an underlying mistrust, even misogyny, that continues to pervade contemporary society. Women who are seen as strong, independent, old, 'difficult', powerful or in any way different risk being derided as witches, as Rosen (2017) explains in relation to Hilary Clinton and Margaret Thatcher. The image of the witch is still used to undermine and disempower women who step out of line and challenge acceptable roles available to them in patriarchal societies. Although women in the twenty-first century are unlikely to be executed for witchcraft, they may be hounded online and silenced through unflattering associations with stereotypical imagery of witches, as evident in the witches tours in this study. As Siapera (2019) notes, the contemporary witch hunt has moved largely online but still operates to coerce women to conform and to exclude them from active participation in the online community. The witches tours in this study may appear benign and unrelated to these obvious expressions of misogyny, yet they contribute to a wider pervasive public discourse that continues to control women's behaviours, appearance and action in the public realm.

However, it is worth noting that more respectful approaches to honoring the memory of the victims of witch hunts have been enacted through historical societies and women's groups in the past few years. Witches of Scotland, for example, is leading a campaign for a legal pardon and apology for those – mostly women – convicted of witchcraft and executed in Scotland from 1563–1736 (Brooks, 2022). Nevertheless, these movements are not part of the experiential economy and the appropriation of the history of witches and witch trials through tourism is largely ahistorical and entertainment focused. Clearly, the tours examined in this chapter are supposed to be fun, and they do not claim to offer any depth of insight into the historical tragedies on which they are loosely based. Yet, this does not mean that they need to ignore historical insight completely and can instead combine fun with informative insight that does some justice to the real people who were persecuted as witches. Perhaps edutainment enterprises can learn about embracing more sensitive approaches to gender representation and responsibility from these serious pursuits. Further consideration could be given to the narratives that witches tours reiterate and reinforce about gendered themes that still thread throughout our culture and society. Witch trials made a spectacle of executions, and although the death penalty is fortunately absent from contemporary British public life, witches tours are still making a spectacle of these deaths, even when they occurred hundreds of years ago. Stone and Morton (2022, p. 12) call for incorporation of "narratives of empathy into interpretations of the female dead for more sympathetic and realistic dark tourism experiences", which, based on the case study examples presented here, we agree is long overdue.

Tourists want to be entertained, but this does not also have to be at the expense of erasing information. Witches tours provide an opportunity for remembering the many women (and some men) who were persecuted several centuries ago, challenging gendered narratives that associate witches with (a certain type of) women and reclaiming the myth of the witch in more positive and empowering ways (Zanette et al., 2023). Contemporary women who identify as witches are reclaiming their identity as positive and powerful, resisting historic associations that labeled strong and independent women as witches and therefore as evil outsiders to be mistrusted and punished (Quilty, 2020). The figure of 'the witch' can be seen as a source of common identification with the historical oppression of women and can be repositioned as a powerful form of feminist mythology. Witches tours have the potential to contribute to this shifting discourse, combining education and fun, in the spirit of edutainment. In so doing, dark tourism attractions, even those at the 'lighter' end of the spectrum, can help inform and educate tourists, challenging gendered stereotypes, and ensuring that the stories of those who suffered are not forgotten.

References

Adie, B.A., & Snell, E.J. (2021). Touring female crime: Power and perceptions. *Journal of Heritage Tourism*, 16(4), 382–394.

Alarcón, D.M., & Cole, S. (2019). No sustainability for tourism without gender equality. *Journal of Sustainable Tourism*, 27(7), 903–919.

Bhati, A., Agarwal, M., Tjayaindera, D.N., Aung, R., Thu, M., & Nguyen, T.M.T. (2021). Dark tourism in Southeast Asia: Are young Asian travelers up for it? *International Journal of Hospitality & Tourism Administration*, 22(5), 550–566.

Brooks, L. (2022). Calls for Scotland to pardon witch-hunt victims gather pace. *The Guardian*. 13 March. Available from: https://www.theguardian.com/uk-news/2022/mar/13/calls-scotland-pardon-witch-hunt-victims-gather-pace [Accessed 8/12/22].

Bristow, R. S., & Jenkins, I.S. (2020). Geography of fear: Fright tourism in urban revitalization. *Journal of Policy Research in Tourism, Leisure and Events*, 12(2), 262–275.

Busby, G., & Devereux, H. (2015). Dark tourism in context: The diary of Anne Frank. *European Journal of Tourism, Hospitality and Recreation*, 6(1), 27–38.

Çakar, K. (2020). Investigation of the motivations and experiences of tourists visiting the Gallipoli Peninsula as a dark tourism destination. *European Journal of Tourism Research*, *24*, 2405–2405.

Carr, N., & Berdychevsky, L. (2021). *Sex in Tourism: Exploring the Light and the Dark*. Bristol: Channel View Publications.

Carrigan, A. (2014). Dark tourism and postcolonial studies: Critical intersections. *Postcolonial Studies*, *17*(3), 236–250.

Chen, S., & Xu, H. (2021). The moral gaze in commercialized dark tourism. *Current Issues in Tourism*, *24*(15), 2167–2186.

Costa, C., Bakas, F. E., Breda, Z., Durão, M., Carvalho, I., & Caçador, S. (2017). Gender, flexibility and the 'ideal tourism worker'. *Annals of Tourism Research*, *64*, 64–75.

Debord, G. (1994). *Society of the Spectacle*. New York: Zone Books.

Eger, C. (2021). Gender matters: Rethinking violence in tourism. *Annals of Tourism Research*, *88*, 103143.

Finkel, R. & Platt, L. (2020). Cultural festivals and the city. *Geography Compass*, 14(9), e12498.

Goodare, J., Martin, L., Miller, J., & Yeoman, L. (2003). *The Survey of Scottish Witchcraft*. Edinburgh: University of Edinburgh. Available from: https://www.shca.ed.ac.uk/Research/witches/ [Accessed 2/10/2022].

Hall, M., & Ryan, C. (2001). *Sex Tourism: Marginal People and Liminalities*. Abingdon: Routledge.

Hanna, S.P., Alderman, D.H., & Bright, C.F. (2018). From celebratory landscapes to dark tourism sites? Exploring the design of southern plantation museums. In P.R. Stone, R. Hartmann, T. Seaton, R. Sharpley, & L. White (Eds.) *The Palgrave Handbook of Dark Tourism Studies*, pp. 399–421. London: Palgrave Macmillan.

Haunted Happenings (2022). Haunted happenings. Available from: https://www.hauntedhappenings.org/ [Accessed 08/12/22].

Heidelberg, B.A.W. (2015). Managing ghosts: Exploring local government involvement in dark tourism. *Journal of Heritage Tourism*, 10(1), 74–90.

Hertzman, E., Anderson, D., & Rowley, S. (2008). Edutainment heritage tourist attractions: A portrait of visitors' experiences at Storyeum. *Museum Management and Curatorship*, 23(2), 155–175.

Hutton, R. (2010). Writing the history of witchcraft: A personal view. *The Pomegranate: The International Journal of Pagan Studies*, 12(2), 239–262.

Kassam, A. (2021). Excommunicated Spanish 'witch' village turns curse into tourist cash. *The Guardian*. 22 August. Available from: https://www.theguardian.com/world/2021/aug/22/excommunicated-spanish-witch-village-turns-curse-into-tourist-cash [Accessed 8/12/22].

Kužnik, L., & Veble, N. (2018). Into the dark–dark stories in the cities of Brežice and Krško in Slovenia as a basis for the future dark tourism products. *International Journal of Tourism Cities*, *4(1)*, 40–53.

Lennon, J. (2017). Dark tourism. *Oxford Research Encyclopedia of Criminology*. Available from: https://oxfordre.com/criminology/view/10.1093/acrefore/9780190264079.001.0001/acrefore-9780190264079-e-212 [Accessed 5/12/2022].

Lennon, J., & Foley, M. (2000). *Dark Tourism*. Boston: Cengage.

Lischer, S.K. (2019). Narrating atrocity: Genocide memorials, dark tourism, and the politics of memory. *Review of International Studies*, 45(5), 805–827.

Luo, Y. (2021). Safeguarding intangible heritage through edutainment in China's creative urban environments. *International Journal of Heritage Studies*, 27(2), 170–185.

Magano, J., Fraiz-Brea, J. A., & Leite, Â. (2022). Dark tourists: Profile, practices, motivations and wellbeing. *International Journal of Environmental Research and Public Health*, 19(19), 12100.

Martini, A., & Buda, D. M. (2020). Dark tourism and affect: Framing places of death and disaster. *Current Issues in Tourism*, *23*(6), 679–692.

Miles W.F.S. (2002). Auschwitz: Museum interpretation and darker tourism. *Annals of Tourism Research*, 29(4), 1175–1178.

National Museum of Scotland (nd). *Witches and Witchcraft*. Exhibit H.MR 43. Available from: https://www.nms.ac.uk/explore-our-collections/stories/scottish-history-and-archaeology/witchs-iron-collar/ [Accessed 2/10/2022].

Norfelt, A., Kock, F., Karpen, I., & Josiassen, A. (2023). Pleasure through pain: An empirical examination of benign masochism in tourism. *Journal of Travel Research*. 62(2), 448–468.

Oren, G., & Shani, A. (2012). The Yad Vashem Holocaust Museum: Educational dark tourism in a futuristic form. *Journal of Heritage Tourism*, 7(3), 255–270.

Palleiro, M. I., & Peltzer, M. E. (2023). 'The lady ghost' in the Recoleta Argentinian graveyard: Dark tourism and ghostly narrative itineraries. *Journal of Tourism and Cultural Change*, 21(2), 223–236.

Pine, J., & Gilmore, J. (2011). *The Experience Economy*. Cambridge, MA: Harvard Business Review Press.

Potter, A. E., Hanna, S. P., Carter, P. L., & Modlin, E. A. (2020). "Give them more and more for their dollar": Searching for slavery amongst the plantation edutainment complex. In J. Micieli-Voutsinas, & A.M. Person (Eds.) *Affective Architectures*, pp. 9–39. Abingdon: Routledge.

Powell, R., & Iankova, K. (2016). Dark London: Dimensions and characteristics of dark tourism supply in the UK capital. *Anatolia*, 27(3), 339–351.

Pratt, S., & Suntikul, W. (2016). Can marine wildlife tourism provide an "edutaining" experience? *Journal of Travel & Tourism Marketing*, 33(6), 867–884.

Pritchard, A. (2018). Predicting the next decade of tourism gender research. *Tourism Management Perspectives*, *25*, 144–146.

Rosen, M. (2017). A feminist perspective on the history of women as witches. *Dissenting Voices*, *6*, 21–31.

Quilty, E. (2020). Letting the juices flow: Reclaiming the body through witchcraft. In S. Page, & K. Pilcher (Eds.) *Embodying Religion, Gender and Sexuality*, pp. 95–109. Abingdon: Routledge.

Robinson-Greene, R. (2021). The Ethics of Dark Tourism. *The Prindle Post*. April 7.

Siapera, E. (2019). Online misogyny as witch hunt: Primitive accumulation in the age of techno-capitalism. In D. Ging, & E. Siapera (Eds.) *Gender hate Online: Understanding the New Anti-Feminism*, pp. 21–43. London: Palgrave Macmillan.

Seaton, A.V. (1999). War and thanatourism: Waterloo 1815–1914. *Annals of Tourism Research*, 26, 130–158.

Sempruch, J. (2004). Feminist constructions of the 'witch' as a fantasmatic other. *Body & Society*, 10(4), 113–133.

Seraphin, H., & Yallop, A. (2020). An analysis of children's play in resort mini-clubs: Potential strategic implications for the hospitality and tourism industry. *World Leisure Journal*, 62(2), 114–131.

Sharpley, R. (2009). Shedding light on dark tourism: An Introduction. In R. Sharpley, & P. Stone (Eds.) *The Darker Side of Travel: The Theory and Practice of Dark Tourism*, pp. 3–23. Bristol: Channel View Publications.

Sorkin, M. (1992). *Variations on a Theme Park*. New York: Hill and Wang.

Stone, P. (2006). A dark tourism spectrum: Towards a typology of death and macabre related tourist sites, attractions and exhibitions. *Tourism*, 54(2), 145–160.

Stone, P., Hartmann, R., Seaton, T., Sharpley, R., & White, L. (2018). *The Palgrave Handbook of Dark Tourism Studies*. London: Palgrave Macmillan.

Stone, P.R., & Morton, C. (2022). Portrayal of the female dead in dark tourism. *Annals of Tourism Research*, 97, 103506.

Strange, C. & Kempa, M. (2003). Shades of dark tourism: Alcatraz and Robben Island. *Annals of Tourism Research*, 30(2), 386–405.

Urbonavicius, S. (2021). Chernobyl: Analysis of young travellers' motivations to visit a unique dark tourism destination. *Tourism*, 69(1), 127–139.

Waitt, G. (2008). Urban festivals: Geographies of hype, helplessness and hope. *Geography Compass*, 2(2), 513–537.

White, L., & Frew, E. (2013). *Dark Tourism and Place Identity: Managing and Interpreting Dark Places*. Abingdon: Routledge.

Wyatt, B., Leask, A., & Barron, P. (2021). Designing dark tourism experiences: An exploration of edutainment interpretation at lighter dark visitor attractions. *Journal of Heritage Tourism*, 16(4), 433–449.

Zanette, M.C., Rinallo, D., & Mimoun, L. (2023). Reclaiming the witch: Processes and heroic outcomes of consumer mythopoesis. *Marketing Theory*, 23(1), 163–182.

Zukin, S. (1993). *Landscapes of Power: From Detroit to Disney World*. Oxford: Blackwell.

Nitasha Sharma, Annaclaudia Martini & Dallen J. Timothy

15 Critical theories in dark tourism: Over the years and beyond

The chapters in this volume have highlighted different issues of contemporary relevance in dark tourism studies and theoretical perspectives related to affect and emotions, critical animal studies, critical memory studies, identity, power, and ideology. In doing so, they draw attention to pertinent issues in dark tourism that are often overlooked such as climate change, misogyny, emotional labor, refugees and migration, animal ethics, colonial legacies, and power hierarchies. In the future, we anticipate more studies on dark tourism from across the globe that contribute to theoretical progress, methodological advancements, and pragmatic solutions, and we hope this edited volume can be a starting point for future reflections. The Introduction chapter provides a broad compilation of critical theories that have been used to examine dark tourism and lays the foundation for future theoretical advancements. This final chapter reflects on some of the key underlying themes that have emerged from the current chapters that shed light on how the theoretical foundations of dark tourism have shifted and are likely to change in the coming years.

Critical approaches, as addressed in this book, not only seek to identify hierarchies of power and systems of power differentials in dark tourism but are also nested within a tradition of critical thought that advocates subjectivity and reflexivity. These approaches are open to inquiry, self-reflection, inclusivity, accountability, and ethical imperatives, thereby allowing a language that combines critique, as well as future possibilities. Simultaneously, we also recognize the different paradigmatic and theoretical entanglements that come along when using critical theories such as the debates around theory and praxis, issues around the term 'critical', disparities between critical theory and constructivist/interpretative approaches in relation to ontology and differences between critical theory and critical realism. While disentangling these theoretical entanglements deserves writing a separate book altogether, based on some recently published literature and in line with the critical perspectives used in the chapters, we argue that we must be open and willing to move beyond these critical entanglements and disparities, and instead recognize the existence of multiple ontologies that can coexist in their specificity with their cultural, social and political peculiarities. This further reinforces Sharma and Martini's (2024, p. 7) point about "accepting dark tourism with its fuzzy, mobile, and fluid boundaries".

Although we did not address it in the introductory chapter, the use of phenomenological approaches merits a good discussion despite phenomenology and critical theory being two different traditions with their entanglements and divergences and therefore, little engagement with each other. However, the two traditions display several affinities, especially in terms of the "constitution of meaning, the relational struc-

https://doi.org/10.1515/9783110792072-016

ture of experience, and the intersubjective conditions for engaging with the world, oneself, and others" (Procyshyn, 2020, p. 670) and these affinities are enough to open a dialogue and bridge the gap between the two traditions. Several dark tourism studies have applied phenomenological approaches in the past (See Swer, 2023; Podoshen, et. al, 2018; Boateng, et. al., 2018). While a group of phenomenologists are strict about the methodological applications, other scholars, particularly feminists such as Sara Ahmed, Lisa Guenther, Amy Allen and others have used an approach known as 'critical phenomenology' to address issues like racism, sexism, colonial heritage, discrimination and social injustice.

It is interesting to note that from an epistemological and ontological perspective, several latent themes emerge from the current chapters and recently published studies in tourism and other areas of study. A notable theoretical stance or an increasingly influential philosophical school of thought in the social sciences that warrants a mention is critical realism, the application of which has been recently observed in several studies of dark tourism (See Israfilova & Khoo-Lattimore, 2019; Kerr, Stone, & Price, 2022; Dresler, 2024). As pointed out by Sharma and Martini (2024), critical theory has a complex relationship with ontology and critical realism attenuates the perennial debate between critical theory and pragmatism. It should be noted, however, that not all chapters in this book are committed to the adoption of a critical realist philosophical framework. However, all of them demonstrate the potential of a theoretical engagement with it paving the way for future conversations between critical realists and critical theorists despite the complexities associated with the two streams of thought.

Critical theory and realist approaches

Critical realism has emerged as an influential school of thought spanning multiple disciplines and empirical phenomena (Bhaskar, 1975, 1979). Shannon-Baker (2016) and Maxwell and Mittapalli (2010) note that critical realism is contextualized within the traditional realist ontology where reality can exist beyond individual perceptions. According to Stutchbury (2022, p. 113), "critical realism combines a realist ontology (there is something to find out about) with a relativistic epistemology (different people will come to know different things in different ways)". Although there may be multiple perspectives on a single event or object (Healy & Perry, 2000), critical realism also recognizes that there are unknown realities (Guba, 1990), and therefore, since theories are only "impartial representations of reality" (Shannon-Baker, 2016, p. 329), a critical realist uncovers the invisible or underlying structures and discourses in both the natural and social worlds that consist of the domain of the real (Bisman, 2010). The invisible social structures underlying human interactions create a reality that transcends individual belief (Tinsley, 2022). A complete understanding of the empirical is not possible by dismissing these invisible social structures or mechanisms or without acknowledging the domain of the real. For example, colonialism may produce visible and invisible phenomena such as acts of violence, microaggressions, transgressive tourist behavior and an increased Othering of death. In dark tourism, it may manifest in events, tourist experiences, behaviors and site representations through multiple ways in which death and the Other are perceived temporally and spatially. Just because the underlying mechanisms through which they manifest are invisible does not mean that they do not exist. A good case exemplifying this is the Western tourist response to the death-related rituals of the Aghori sect in India (Sharma, 2021).

In her chapter 'Interrogating the 'Critical' in Critical Approaches to Tourism Research, Donna Chambers mentions that most of what is categorized as critical theory "borrows from constructivist/interpretative approaches such as poststructuralism, postmodernism, postcolonialism, and feminism" (p. 115) and highlighted few of the ontological disagreements between critical theory and those of constructivist/interpretative approaches. She points out that approaches such as feminism, postcolonial theory, etc. consider a relativist ontology or plural perspectives and deny the existence of one single reality which contradicts the emancipatory objective of critical theory because according to her, if "all truths are equally valid then within what context can emancipation take place?" (p. 115). These theoretical questions and dilemmas are worth pondering in the way death and death-related rituals or issues such as crime, punishment, war, and memorialization are perceived across different cultures.

However, recent studies reveal that there are ways to overcome these entanglements, and points of convergence between critical theory and critical realism are worth exploring. For example, Tinsley (2022) suggests the use of postcolonial critical realism (PCR) as an ontological framework that explains the structuring relationship between racialized, colonial discourses and the social world. Such a framework is not only useful in exploring global issues of importance such as climate change but also "anticolonial thought in the social sciences, as well as social movements", demonstrating how PCR can be a point of convergence between critical realism and critical theories such as postcolonialism and yet maintaining the objective of emancipation. As Varnajot and Salim (2024) critically argue when exploring the complex connections between dark tourism, glacier retreat, and spectral geographies, framing glacier tourism as dark tourism can improve tourists' pro-environmental behavioral changes, as well as expand climate change discourses, ethics, and politics. In this case, a critical theoretical perspective such as hauntology brings with it an ontology that is reminiscent of critical realism with its de-prioritization of actualism and presence (Wood, 2023) with the concept of "haunting" being used for understanding how the effects of social violence and abusive systems of power in the past are "real, felt and sensed yet not always empirically evident; they are hidden in plain sight" (Parr, 2024, p. 5; Lea, 2020).

Let us consider, for example, the silent and erased histories and experiences of enslaved people in the plantations of the American South, the absence of dark tourism studies, and the impacts on victims or those belonging to the subordinate category or an absence of African voices in dissonant heritage assessments and dark travel. Indeed, we have failed to realize how dark tourism can provide us with an effective platform to confront the racialization and colonial and postcolonial configurations of power because the legacies of colonialism play out in unintended and invisible ways. To that end, critical realist perspectives, when combined with environmental humanities can prove to be effective tools for analyzing dark tourism, providing greater insight into the context of post-disaster tourism (oil spills, Fukushima, etc.), especially in light of neo-colonial racial capitalism.

Further, Kanth (2004) points out critical realism's ontological similarities to Asian philosophies such as the Vedas and other pre-modernist traditions, thereby offering an opportunity to include non-Eurocentric ontologies of death and death-related rituals that challenge generalizations in dark tourism frameworks and classifications.

Another example is the convergence of critical realist interventions with gender studies and feminism with feminist theorists becoming slowly interested in issues of ontology, materiality, and nature and critical realists also realizing how their field has remained masculine in nature (Gunnarsson, Dy & Van Ingen, 2018). Several scholars have combined critical realist perspectives with feminism and intersectional approaches (Gillman, 2016; Griffiths, 2018; Smirthwaite & Swahnberg, 2016). There are two takeaways from these studies, which can be effectively considered as conversations or productive dialogues between critical realism, gender and feminism. First, it alleviates Chambers' (2007) earlier concerns and second, the foregrounding of ontology and new forms of realism emerging within the current 'new materialist' turn (Alaimo & Hekman, 2008; Coole & Frost, 2010), a trend which is increasingly gaining traction in dark tourism studies. A critical realist intersectional perspective may provide a lot of answers in examining how the perception of dark tourism products differs spatially and across cultures, societies, and races.

A significant point that deserves mention is the idea of inclusion in dark tourism research such as that on disability and accessibility, particularly that of children at dark tourism sites (Kerr, Stone & Price, 2022; Dresler, 2024). Accessibility is a critical feature of inclusion, particularly in tourism research and in light of recent technological developments and a possible future where dark tourism goes virtual, the concept of inclusion is of vital importance. Burnett (2007) pointed out that critical realism may provide a framework and a philosophical 'compass' (Egbo, 2005) to address complex issues around inclusion and disability.

In addition, Skrede (2020) also argues that Critical Realism (CR) as a philosophy of science may serve as a platform "where non-representational and representational approaches can meet to more fully grasp how we represent and respond to heritage" (p. 88). While there have been several studies on difficult and dark heritage (Smith & Campbell 2015, p. 449), he suggests that the emotional side of heritage encounters, without rejecting the relevance of representations, could provide an important supplement to other ways of "reading" heritage.

Critical realism can also prove to be an effective approach in critically evaluating the recent 'digital turn' in dark tourism focusing on future technologies about AI, robotics, and dystopian attractions and increasingly leading to a blurring of the real and the virtual world. The recent discussions and developments on immersive virtual, augmented, and mixed reality experiences in dark tourism raise issues about the ethical implications of using such technologies with little being known about the impact of immersive experiences on children, young and psychologically vulnerable people such as those who have experienced some trauma in the past. Although there are studies that have discussed how digital platforms such as vlogs, blogs, and related online forums can foster and develop information-sharing and research collaboration in the realm of dark tourism (Bolan & Simone, 2018), their unethical use, cultural consequences, and role of "influencers" are yet to be critically explored. For example, a YouTube star, Logan Paul, in 2018 was highly criticized for posting a video that reportedly showed a suicide victim's body hanging from a tree in Japan's Aokigahara Forest. Wheaton and Kreps (2023) explore the detrimental consequences that can arise from digital transformation (DT) using a critical realist approach. Without any doubt, the application of critical theories is imperative and holds more relevance in the context of this 'future world' of dark tourism, especially in terms of facilitating a deeper understanding of the underlying, generative mechanisms and promoting a wiser and ethical approach.

Therefore, such thematic alignments not only demonstrate the emancipatory and inclusive potential of critical theories but also how critical theories can play a key role in understanding and enriching the quality of dark tourism studies. In the next section, we discuss the recent shift in dark tourism towards a posthuman ontology.

From an ontology of the self towards a posthuman ontology

Stone (2012) highlighted the role of dark tourism as a "(new) mediating institution within secular death-sequestered societies, which not only provides a physical place to link the living with the dead, but also allows a cognitive space for the Self to construct contemporary ontological meanings of mortality" (p. 1565). A key point to be noted here is how dark tourism so far, has always remained anthropocentric in character with a strong focus on emancipation and ontological meanings of death for the human "Self". The ideas of early critical theorists such as Descartes (1998) and Locke (1847) on subjectivity could be considered partly responsible for this denial of non-human subjectivity and agency along with an exclusion and marginalization of all other beings as a consequence. In a similar vein on the concept of humanism, Gunkel (2014, p. 7) says that "it has always been a way of excluding others, whether they were African peoples, whether they were Aboriginal peoples, whether they're women, whether they are animals, there is a way in which the concept of the human has been a way for one group in power to disempower others". However, recent critical studies in dark tourism using posthumanist approaches demonstrate a shift in axiological perceptions and a broadening of agency for the more-than/non-human world and environmental formations such as glaciers (See Varnajot & Salim, 2024; López-López & Venegas, 2021). Ivic (2022) notes how a posthuman ontology opens up the possibility for new identity politics and ethics based on an idea of "responsibility to otherness" (Gibbons, 1991).

These posthumanist ideas apply to virtual dark tourism too, if we consider how posthumanism can include overcoming the limitations of the human body through virtual immortality, as well as going beyond humanism and anthropocentrism. However, as immersive experiences and technological interventions such as AI and robots in dark tourism may lead to a blurring of boundaries between the technological and the human, the human and non-human, the natural and artificial, they also raise several ethical concerns and ontological issues around moral agency, privacy, digital trauma, personal identity (e.g. creation of hybrid identities), and the social community. Fisher and Bolter (2018) in pointing out the increased use of augmented reality (AR) tourist experiences at dark tourism sites, note that the ethical impact, design, and development of such dark AR experiences have not received critical attention as they ideally should have. VR nudges such as the use of empathy-enhancing simulations or "empathy enhancers" have been criticized and therefore, their use in the context of dark tourism, calls for further critical inquiry.

Lastly, critical theory has always acknowledged the importance of situated knowledge so that reality may be better understood. We hope that this book prompts its readers to think how multiple critical perspectives when placed in conversation with each other, can help us to achieve a synergetic end and not only engage with dark tourism at a deeper level but also explore its transformative and emancipatory potential in society. Although there are some empirical aspects to the pieces that have been included, the contributions in this volume primarily have a critical thrust. We also made a minuscule attempt at ground-clearing by discussing some existing theoretical entanglements and pointing out convergences, emerging trends, and signposting promising future paths. The critical theories discussed in this book are not exhaustive; it does, however, tell us about the epistemological and ontological transformation of dark tourism over the years. We highly encourage an exploration of the potential use and application of critical psychological and sociological perspectives in dark tourism. Needless to say, the potentialities of dark tourism are yet to be actualized and therefore, we hope that the chapters in this book will encourage new and stimulating forms of theoretical and empirical research in this field balancing ethics with future creative scenarios.

References

Alaimo, S., & Hekman, S. J. (Eds.). (2008). *Material feminisms.* Indiana University Press

Bhaskar, R. (1975). *A realist theory of science.* Routledge.

Bhaskar, R. (1979). *The possibility of naturalism: A philosophical critique of the contemporary human sciences.* Routledge.

Bisman, J. (2010). Postpositivism and accounting research: A (personal) primer on critical realism. *Australasian Accounting, Business and Finance Journal, 4*(4), 3–25.

Boateng, H., Okoe, A. F., & Hinson, R. E. (2018). Dark tourism: Exploring tourist's experience at the Cape Coast Castle, Ghana. *Tourism management perspectives, 27,* 104–110.

Bolan, P., & Simone-Charteris, M. (2018). "Shining a digital light on the dark": Harnessing online media to improve the dark tourism experience. In P. R. Stone, R. Hartmann, T. Seaton, R. Sharpley, & L. White (Eds.), *The Palgrave handbook of dark tourism studies* (pp. 727–746). Palgrave Macmillan.

Burnett, Nick B. (2007) *Critical Realism: The required philosophical compass for inclusion?* In Proceedings Australian Association of Research in Education: Research Impacts: Proving or improving? Fremantle, Western Australia.

Chambers, D. (2007). Interrogating the 'Critical' in Critical Approaches to Tourism Research. In I. Ateljevic, A. Pritchard, & N. Morgan (Eds.) *The critical turn in tourism studies: Innovative research methodologies* (pp. 105–119). Routledge.

Coole, D., & Frost, S. (Eds.). (2010). *New Materialisms: Ontology, Agency, and Politics.* Duke University Press.

Descartes, R. (1998). Discourse on method and meditations on first philosophy (DA Cress, Trans.). *Indianapolis, IN: Hackett,* 59–103.

Dresler, E. (2024). Children picturing suffering in dark tourism: the use of photo-elicitation method. Current Issues in Tourism, 27(2), 184–199.

Egbo, B. (2005). Emergent Paradigm: Critical Realism and Transformative Research in Educational Administration. *McGill Journal of Education,* 40(2), 267–284.

Fisher, J. A., & Bolter, J. D. (2018, October). Ethical considerations for AR experiences at dark tourism sites. In *2018 IEEE International Symposium on Mixed and Augmented Reality Adjunct (ISMAR-Adjunct)* (pp. 365–369). IEEE.

Gibbons, M. T. (1991). The ethic of postmodernism. *Political theory, 19*(1), 96–102.

Gillman, L. (2016). Critical realist and postpositivist realist feminisms: Towards a feminist dialectical realism. *Journal of critical realism, 15*(5), 458–475.

Griffiths, D. A. (2018). Queer genes: realism, sexuality and science. In L. Gunnarsson, A. Martinez Dy, & M. van Ingen (Eds.) *Gender, Feminism and Critical Realism: Exchanges, challenges, synergies* (pp. 79–97). Routledge.

Guba, E. (1990). The Paradigm Dialog, Sage.

Gunkel, D. (2014). *Do machines have rights? Ethics in the age of artificial intelligence.* Aurora Online with David Gunkel, interview by Paul Kellogg. http://aurora.icaap.org/index.php/aurora/article/view/92/114. Accessed 15 April 2024.

Gunnarsson, L., Martinez Dy, A., & van Ingen, M. (2018). Critical realism, gender and feminism: Exchanges, challenges, synergies. In L. Gunnarsson, A. Martinez Dy, & M. van Ingen (Eds.) *Gender, Feminism and Critical Realism: Exchanges, challenges, synergies* (pp. 1–7). Routledge.

Healy, M., & Perry, C. (2000). Comprehensive criteria to judge validity and reliability of qualitative research within the realism paradigm. *Qualitative market research: An international journal, 3*(3), 118–126.

Ivic, S. (2022). Posthuman Ethics: The Priority of Ethical Over Ontological Status. In Tumilty, E., Battle Fisher, M. (eds) *Transhumanism: Entering an Era of Bodyhacking and Radical Human Modification.* The International Library of Bioethics, vol 100. Springer, Cham.

Israfilova, F., & Khoo-Lattimore, C. (2019). Sad and violent but I enjoy it: Children's engagement with dark tourism as an educational tool. Tourism and Hospitality Research, 19(4), 478–487.

Kanth, R. (2004). Eurocentrism, realism and the anthropic cartography of emancipation. In J. Joseph & J. M. Roberts, eds. *Realism, Discourse and Deconstruction*, pp. 171–179. London: Routledge.
Kerr, M. M., Stone, P. R., & Price, R. H. (2022). Young tourists' experiences at dark tourism sites: Toward a conceptual framework. In M.M. Kerr, P.R. Stone, & R.H. Price (Eds.) *Children, young people and dark tourism* (pp. 19–39). Routledge.
Lea, T. (2020). *Wild policy: Indigeneity and the unruly logics of intervention*. Stanford University Press.
Locke, J. (1847). *An essay concerning human understanding*. Kay & Troutman.
López-López, Á., & Venegas, G. J. (2021). Animal dark tourism in Mexico: Bulls performing their own slaughter. In C. Kline & J.M. Rickly (Eds.) *From beasts of burden to K-9 security: The working animals of the tourism industry*, pp. 69–82. De Gruyter.
Maxwell, J. A., & Mittapalli, K. (2010). Realism as a stance for mixed methods research. In Tashakkori, A. & Teddlie, C., (Eds.) *SAGE handbook of mixed methods in social & behavioral research*, *2*, (pp. 145–168). Thousand Oaks: Sage.
Parr, S. (2024). Hauntology: The Emotional Costs of Social Policy for Mothers Experiencing Homelessness. *Housing, Theory and Society*, 1–18.
Podoshen, J. S., Yan, G., Andrzejewski, S. A., Wallin, J., & Venkatesh, V. (2018). Dark tourism, abjection and blood: A festival context. *Tourism Management*, *64*, 346–356.
Procyshyn, A. (2020). Phenomenology and critical theory. In Santis, D. De, Hopkins, B. C. & Majolino, C. (Eds.), *The Routledge Handbook of Phenomenology and Phenomenological Philosophy* (pp. 670–683). Routledge.
Shannon-Baker, P. (2016). Making Paradigms Meaningful in Mixed Methods Research. *Journal of Mixed Methods Research*, *10*(4), 319–334. https://doi.org/10.1177/1558689815575861
Sharma, N. (2021). Dark tourism and moral disengagement in liminal spaces. In R. Bristow, & I.S. Jenkins (Eds.) *Liminality in Tourism: Spatial and temporal considerations*, (pp. 55–79). Routledge.
Sharma, N., & Martini, A. (2024). Dark tourism geographies: ontological, epistemological and axiological perspectives. *Tourism Geographies*, 1–10.
Skrede, J. (2020). Discourse analysis and non-representational theories in heritage studies: a non-reductionist take on their compatibility. *Journal of Cultural Geography*, *37*(1), 88–108.
Smith, L., & Campbell, G. (2015). The elephant in the room: Heritage, affect, and emotion. In Logan, W., Craith, M.N., & Kockel, U. (Eds.) *A companion to heritage studies*, (pp. 443–460). Wiley-Blackwell.
Smirthwaite, G., & Swahnberg, K. (2018). Comparing critical realism and the situated knowledges approach in research on (in) equity in health care: An exploration of their implications. In L. Gunnarsson, A. Martinez Dy, & M. van Ingen (Eds.) *Gender, Feminism and Critical Realism: Exchanges, challenges, synergies* (pp. 44–61). Routledge.
Stone, P. R. (2012). Dark tourism and significant other death: Towards a model of mortality mediation. *Annals of tourism research*, *39*(3), 1565–1587.
Stutchbury, K. (2022). Critical realism: an explanatory framework for small-scale qualitative studies or an 'unhelpful edifice'? *International Journal of Research & Method in Education*, *45*(2), 113–128.
Swer, G. M. (2023). Towards a Phenomenology of Dark Tourist Experiences. In *Tourism and Culture in Philosophical Perspective* (pp. 153–166). Cham: Springer International Publishing.
Tinsley, M. (2022). Towards a postcolonial critical realism. *Critical Sociology*, *48*(2), 235–250.
Varnajot, A., & Salim, E. (2024). The hauntology of climate change: glacier retreat and dark tourism. *Tourism Geographies*, 1–18.
Wheaton, J., & Kreps, D. (2023). Towards a critical realist approach to the dark side of digital transformation. *Frontiers in Human Dynamics*, *5*, 1252458.
Wood, M. A. (2023). Communing with the many shades of Ghost Criminology. *Crime, Media, Culture*, *19*(3), 404–409.

List of contributors

Duncan Light is a Senior Lecturer at Bournemouth University, Department of Tourism Management, UK. He is a cultural geographer with his research focusing on two broad areas. First, he is interested in the relationships between tourism, heritage and identities. His recent research has explored these issues with reference to Dracula tourism in Romania and holidaymaking in socialist Romania. Second, his research examines relationships between urban space, power, identity and memory in socialist and post-socialist contexts. He is particularly interested in urban place names.

Derek H. Alderman (he/him) is Professor of Geography and former Department Head at University of Tennessee. Alderman is a past President of the American Association of Geographers (2017-2018). He is a cultural geographer focused on the role of memorial landscapes, heritage tourism, and the politics of place-naming and mapping in struggles over race, rights, and public space–often in context of the African American Freedom Struggle. He is the founder of Tourism RESET (tourismreset.com). With affiliated researchers and industry specialists from over twenty-five universities and organizations, RESET is on the leading edge of studying and challenging racial inequalities in travel and tourism. Dr. Alderman is (co)author of over 170 articles and book chapters along with the award-winning book Civil Rights Memorials and the Geography of Memory (2008), the co-edited *The Political Life of Urban Streetscapes: Naming, Politics, and Place* (2018) and the co-authored book R*emembering Enslavement: Reassembling the Southern Plantation Museum* (2022) The latter advocates for a more inclusive interpretation of plantation museums and provides ethical-practical guidance to site staff that centers the difficult history of slavery and the experiences of enslaved people rather perpetuating a romanticization of the Old South. Alderman frequently moves beyond academia to contribute to the national dialogue about commemorative, cultural, and tourism issues. He has provided unpaid assistance to dozens of agencies, community organizations, and diversity initiatives and journalists have quoted or interviewed him over three hundred times. The National Science Foundation and the National Endowment for the Humanities have funded his work. Dr. Alderman is the recipient of over twenty-five university, regional and national awards for excellence in teaching and mentorship, distinguished research, and public outreach. Since 2019, Stanford University has included him in its annual list of the top 2 percent of scientists in world based on research citations.

Ethan Bottone is an Assistant Professor of Geography at Northwest Missouri State University, where he teaches courses in cultural geography and sustainability. He received his Ph.D. from the University of Tennessee, which explored landscapes and mobility networks of the Green Book, a Jim Crow-era travel guide developed and used by Black travelers. His current research interests focus on critical aspects of tourism, particularly in relation to race, ethnicity, and disability. He also has interests in the intersections of tourism with sustainability and environmental justice. Bottone is a research fellow with Tourism RESET, an interdisciplinary research and outreach initiative that seeks to identify and challenge patterns of social inequity in the tourism industry. He also serves as the editor of Material Culture, a peer-reviewed journal published by the International Society for Landscape, Place, and Material Culture (ISLPMC). In his spare time, Ethan enjoys traveling to "off-the-beaten-path" tourism destinations and minor league baseball games with his spouse.

Stefanie Benjamin (she/her) is the Co-Founder of CODE (Collaborating on Dialogue & Equity) and Associate Professor of tourism studies at the University of Tennessee Knoxville. Her research seeks to challenge existing paradigms and traditional perspectives, offering fresh insights and transformative perspectives to the tourism field. With an extensive publication record, Dr. B has published numerous academic journal articles amplifying counter-narratives and disseminating this research within popular press pieces inclusive of *AFAR Travel Magazine*, *The Conversation*, and *Conde Nast Traveler*. Beyond her

https://doi.org/10.1515/9783110792072-017

academic pursuits, Dr. B actively engages in community outreach and collaboration with industry leaders and organizations striving to bridge the gap between academia and the tourism industry. Driven by a deep-rooted commitment to disrupting dominant ideologies, Dr. B continues to make 'good trouble' through her research, teaching, and service. Her critical scholarship serves as a pedagogical framework, shedding light on how oppressive systems must be dismantled to reimagine a more inclusive and sustainable academic and touristic world.

Sarah Frankel (she/they) is an adjunct of retail, hospitality and tourism management at the University of Tennessee Knoxville. Currently they are collecting information to archive a detailed account of gnome cultures and have little interest in the affairs of mankind.

Rami K. Isaac was born in Palestine and did his undergraduate studies in The Netherlands and graduate studies in the U.K. He earned his PhD from the University of Groningen, in Spatial Sciences, in The Netherlands. He is an associate professor in tourism teaching at the undergraduate and postgraduate levels at the Academy for Tourism at Breda University of Applied Sciences in The Netherlands. In addition, he is an associate professor at the Faculty of Tourism and Hotel Management at Bethlehem University, Palestine. Currently, he is the Vice-President of the Research Committee 50 on International Tourism, International Sociologist Association ISA (2018-2025). His research interests are in tourism development and management, critical theory, and political aspects of tourism. He published numerous articles and co-edited books on tourism and political (in)stability, occupation, tourism and war, dark /heritage tourism, violence and transformational tourism.

José-Carlos García-Rosell is a Professor of Business Ethics at Oulu Business School, University of Oulu, Finland. Additionally, he holds the position of visiting scholar at the University of Lapland within the Faculty of Social Sciences, at the Multidimensional Tourism Institute (MTI). He also serves as an Associate Professor in Corporate Social Responsibility in Tourism at Tampere University, Finland, and the University of Maribor, Slovenia. He works in the fields of corporate social responsibility, business ethics, and responsible management education. His current research agenda focuses on human-animal relations, responsible tourism experiences and experiential learning. He has published in a variety of journals such as *Journal of Business Ethics, Management Learning, Journal of Marketing Management, Journal of Sustainable Tourism, Tourism Geographies, Tourism Recreation Research*, and *Journal of Teaching in Travel & Tourism*. He has also co-authored several chapters for books published by Routledge, Palgrave McMillan, Springer, and DeGruyter.

Philip Hancock is a Professor of Work and Organisation Studies and a member of the Centre for Work, Organisation and Society at Essex Business School, University of Essex, UK. Along with Melissa Tyler, he is a coordinator of the Centre's 'Future of Creative Work' cluster. His primary research interests include the affective and atmospheric dimensions of work and its organisation, the critical theory of Axel Honneth, and work in the performing and creative arts. His research has been published in a number of leading scholarly journals, including Organization Studies, Human Relations, Work, Employment and Society, and Organization. His book *Organizing Christmas* was published by Routledge in 2023, while 2024 will see the publication of his co-authored monograph with Melissa Tyler provisionally entitled *Performing Artists and Precarity – Work in the Contemporary Entertainment Industries*, which is based on a two-year study of the experiences of freelance and self-employed performers during and in the wake of the COVID-19 pandemic.

Sarike van Slooten is a lecturer at the undergraduate programme 'International Tourism Management' and the postgraduate programme 'International Leisure, Tourism and Event Studies' at NHL Stenden University of Applied Sciences. Besides lecturing, Sarike is a researcher at the *European Tourism Future*

Institute (ETFI) for which she explores ways to connect the heritage sector, and specifically the museum sector, better to contemporary society in relation to colonial history, multivocality and inclusiveness. As an ETFI researcher, she also seeks to find ways on how to make the heritage, museum and cultural sector more meaningful and resilient through the use of scenario-planning and strategic foresight. Her academic background started in Leisure & Tourism Studies, for which she developed a personal and academic appetite for Heritage in relation to identity formation and memory, and Dark Tourism. She followed her doctorate research at the University of Amsterdam's research school 'Amsterdam School of Heritage, Memory and Material Culture, for which she explored opportunities for the (im)possibility of the construction of a postcolonial museum. She started a post-doctorate study in February 2024 for which she explores opportunities to make Unesco World Heritage Sites in the Kingdom of the Netherlands more multivocal and inclusive in their representation, meaning-making and visitor experience.

Alexis Whitacre is a PhD Candidate in the Department of Geography at Indiana University (IU) in Bloomington, IN. After receiving a B.A. in International Studies from the University of Evansville in 2018, she graduated with a master's degree in Geography from IU in 2020. She is currently working as an Assistant Professor at IU, and her research focuses on the interconnections between refugee studies, tourism studies, and media studies. Her forthcoming doctoral dissertation centers around the phenomenon of tourism to refugee camps in the West Bank and examines how the perceived authenticity of real-life spectacles of suffering contributes to camp tourism, which, in turn, redefines conceptualizations of 'camp-ness' itself.

Magdalena Banaszkiewicz is an Associate Professor of Cultural Anthropology at the Institute of Intercultural Studies at the Jagiellonian University in Krakow. Her research focuses upon the interpretation of heritage in the context of tourism development in Central and Eastern Europe. She has published three monographs, including *Tourism and Heritage in the Chornobyl Exclusion Zone* (Routledge 2023, OA), and tens of articles. She has co-edited several anthologies, such as *Anthropology of Tourism in Central and Eastern Europe. Bridging Worlds* (Lexington Books, 2018). In addition, she is a co-founder of the flagship project of the Critical Heritage Studies Hub (https://crihestu.id.uj.edu.pl/) and represents the Jagiellonian University in the steering committee of Una Europa in the field of cultural heritage.

Jonathan Skinner is Reader in the Anthropology of Events in the Department of Hospitality and Events at the University of Surrey. He has an active interest in tourism and tour guiding, exclusion zones and their representation and governance since he lived through the initial volcanic eruptions on the British island of Montserrat in the Eastern Caribbean in 1995. He has written articles and book chapters about the disaster and its developments and authored the book *Before the Volcano: Reverberations of Identity on Montserrat* (Arawak Publications). He has general teaching and research interests in tourism, social dance and leisure practices from Carnival to St Patrick's Day, and the creative use of research methods such as interviewing using digital glasses.

Maximiliano Korstanje is Reader at Economics Dep University of Palermo, Argentina. He serves as book Series editor of Advances in Hospitality, Tourism and the Services Industry (IGI Global) and Tourism Security-Safety and Post Conflict Destinations. He was Visiting Professor at University of Leeds, The University of Las Palmas de Gran Canaria and University of Habana.

Alena Pirok is Associate Professor of History at Georgia Southern University. Her research focuses on the history of museums, and the place of lore, rumor, and memory in historical interpretation. Her work with ghost stories, rumors of haunting, and sites of violence, places her work aside dark tourism. She has pieces in *The Public Historian*, *The Florida Historical Quarterly*, and *Southern Cultures*. Her first book *The Spirit of Colonial Williamsburg: Ghosts and Interpreting the Recreated Past* (2022) illustrates how people's talk of ghosts and hauntings has structured the idea of historical place and historical experience at Colonial Williamsburg since the early twentieth century. In her forthcoming chapter "Oaks of Ill Repute" in Branching Out: The Public History of Trees Pirok explores how local-tour guides have used fabricated tales of ageless hanging trees to bring the factual history of Jim Crow violence to Savannah, Georgia's pleasant yet false vision of the past. Her next book, Cell Block Revival, traces how late-twentieth century ideas of safety and justice have shaped the creation and interpretation of U.S. prison museums. In addition to her research Pirok is an active member of the National Council of Public History, serving on the Environmental Sustainabiltiy Committee as well as chairing the Labor taskforce.

Katherine Dashper, PhD, is Professor and Director of Research Degrees in the School of Events, Tourism, and Hospitality Management at Leeds Beckett University. Her research applies a critical sociological lens to examine practices of work and leisure, particularly focusing on gender issues and interspecies encounters in events, tourism, and hospitality. She has co-edited five books: *Leisure in the Pandemic* (2022, Routledge); *Sport, gender and mega-events* (2021, Emerald); *Humans, horses and event management* (2021, CABI); *Rural tourism: An international perspective* (2014, Cambridge Scholars); and *Sports events, society and culture* (2014, Routledge). She has published numerous articles in peer reviewed journals across Leisure Studies, Sociology, Tourism, and Event Studies, and a research monograph (Human-animal relationships in equestrian sport and leisure, 2017, Routledge).

Rebecca Finkel, PhD, is Professor of Critical Event Studies and Director of Research Centre for Culture in Society at Queen Margaret University, Edinburgh. Research situates events and festivals within social justice, gender in/equality, and cultural identity frameworks. Published in sociology, gender studies, cultural management, urban geography, leisure, tourism, events journals and books, including co-editing special issues on EDI-related topics. Co-Editor of *Routledge Critical Event Studies Research Book Series* as well as *Creative Research Methods for Critical Event Studies* (2024, Routledge); *Leisure in the Pandemic* (2022, Routledge); *Multispecies leisure: Human-animal interactions in leisure landscapes* (2021, Routledge); *Gendered Violence at International Festivals* (2020, Routledge); *Accessibility, Inclusion, and Diversity in Critical Event Studies* (2018, Routledge); *Research Themes in Events* (2014, CABI).

Cecilia de Bernardi holds a PhD in Tourism research from the University of Lapland (Finland). Her publications concentrate mostly on the conceptualization of authenticity in indigenous tourism, especially regarding marketing communication. This is the topic that has inspired her studies on discourse analysis and different critical theories on representation. She has also published on policy, sustainability, events, Airbnb, and animal tourism, among others. Cecilia has several research interests, both related to tourism, but also just pertaining to the philosophical approach of critical realism. Her latest work has focused on the policy terrain concerning the sustainability of different sport and outdoor activities.

Bailey Ashton Adie is a Postdoctoral Researcher in the Geography Research Unit at the University of Oulu, Finland. Her research interests include World Heritage, heritage tourism, community resilience, community-based tourism, natural hazards and tourism, tourism and development, second homes, film tourism, and dark tourism. Her work has been published in book chapters as well as in leading journals, including *Annals of Tourism Research*, *Current Issues in Tourism*, and the *Journal of Sustainable Tourism*. She is also the author of the book *World Heritage and Tourism: Marketing and Management* (2019) and co-editor of *Second Homes and Climate Change* (2023). She sits on the editorial boards of the *Journal of Heritage Tourism*, *Tourism Geographies*, and *Tourism Management Perspectives*. She is the Chair of the Leisure Studies Association and Director of Communications for the Recreation, Tourism and Sport Specialty Group (RTS), part of the American Association of Geographers.

Nitasha Sharma is a lecturer at the Department of Geography, University of Alabama (USA). She is a tourism geographer whose research broadly examines the multiple and contested representations of place and spatial behavior through projects situated in critical tourism studies. She specializes in the perception of authenticity, dark tourism, folklore and heritage, magical tourism, rituals, pilgrimage and sacred spaces. Her other research interests include moral and ethical issues in tourism and decolonial studies.

Annaclaudia Martini is an assistant professor at the University of Bologna, Italy. Her research interests include critical geography, geographies of affect, tourism and heritage studies, and qualitative and creative methods using affects and emotions. Having worked with disaster-hit communities in Japan, she also has a keen interest and commitment in methods and frameworks for social participation, and engagement outside academia.

Dallen J. Timothy is Professor of Community Resources and Development, and Senior Sustainability Scientist at Arizona State University. He also holds visiting professorships in Mexico, China, Spain, and South Africa. His current tourism research in Africa, Asia, North America, Europe and the Pacific islands includes perspectives on geopolitics and globalization, international borders, pilgrimage, heritage management, retail consumption, human mobility, and sense of place.

Esther Snell is Senior lecturer in criminology. After completing a BA (Hons) History and Music at Canterbury Christ Church University, Esther gained her History PhD from the University of Kent. Before coming to Southampton, she worked as a lecturer at Canterbury Christ Church and also Oxford Brookes universities. Esther then had a brief stint as a research assistant at the Open University, specializing in the history of crime and punishment and mentalities in the early modern period. Esther's research is particularly interested in the representations of criminality and justice in the media.

Florence Smith Nicholls is a PhD student at Queen Mary University of London, specialising in digital archaeology and game AI research. They focus on generative archaeology games, featuring procedural content, that invite players to archaeologically record and interpret them. Prior to their doctoral research, they worked as a field archaeologist and heritage consultant, including a position at Museum of London Archaeology. They are also a narrative designer and have worked in the writers' room at the independent games studio Die Gute Fabrik on the adventure game Saltsea Chronicles. Furthermore, they have collaborated with the British Library on a project to collect contextual information for narrative mobile apps. They are particularly interested in creative approaches to games preservation, queer games and dark tourism.

Alix Varnajot is a postdoctoral researcher at the University of Oulu, Finland, affiliated with the History, Culture and Communications Research Unit and the Biodiverse Anthropocenes (ANTS) program. He holds a PhD in Human Geography. His research interests include tourism geographies of the Arctic and Antarctica, dark tourism, last chance tourism, and tourism adaptation to climate change in the Anthropocene. His most recent work also involves the study of interrelations between science and expedition cruise tourism in the Polar regions.

Margaréta Pintér is an emerging researcher currently undertaking a PhD fellowship based at the Saxo Institute at the University of Copenhagen, where she is affiliated with both the UCPH School of Archaeology and the Centre for Sustainable Futures. Since completing her MA in Aarhus University's Sustainable Heritage Management programme in 2022 most of her work sits in the environmental humanities, contemporary archaeology and critical heritage studies nexus. Her doctoral work focuses on a specific drystone wall, the so-called Sheep Dyke on the island of North Ronaldsay (Orkney, Scotland), and examines interactions and assemblages with this shifting structure through the lens of more-than-human agency, temporal entanglement and care ethics. Using ethnographic methods to study this archaeological object, her work aims to understand the at-time conflicting values, identities and politics embedded into the wider heritage landscape of the island, which has been greatly shaped by the presence of the wall. Margaréta often works interdisciplinarily, and has worked both independently and collaboratively on a number of research projects that spanned across various academic fields. An advocate of combining robust theory with creative methods, much of her work tries to expand on heritage theory, specifically thinking with the notion of time, change and care obligations.

Vesa-Pekka Herva is Professor of Archaeology at the University of Oulu, Finland. His research interests encompass material culture, human-environment relations and cosmology in the European high North from the Neolithic to the present day. He has studied the European (sub-)Arctic as a material and symbolic resource space with a focus on the multiple entanglements of tourism, extractivism and cultural heritage, particularly as related to long-term perceptions and cultural ideas of Finnish Lapland and northernmost Fennoscandia. Vesa-Pekka is currently working on the cultural and cosmological aspects of contemporary extractive industries in relation to long-term human engagements with the subterranean world and is Principal Investigator of the Academy of Finland funded research project "Extractive Industries as Engagement with the Extraordinary Subterranean: Culture, Heritage and Impact of Resource Extraction in Northernmost Europe" (Academy of Finland, 2021-2025). He has published on a wide range of topics from the dynamics of Neolithization to the dark heritage of the Second World War and the uses of cultural heritage in Lapland Christmas tourism and is the author, with Antti Lahelma, of *Northern Archaeologies and Cosmologies: A Relational View* (Routledge, 2020).

Albina Pashkevich is Associate Professor in Tourism Studies in the Centre for Tourism and Leisure Studies (CeTLeR), School of Culture and Society, Dalarna University. Her research interests in tourism include destination development of Arctic territories, institutional settings and barriers for the tourism development of peripheral regions, maritime and coastal cruise tourism development in the Arctic, and uses of cultural and natural heritage in tourism and leisure activities.

Thora Herrmann is a Professor of socio-environmental sustainability within the Biodiverse Anthropocenes Research Programme at the University of Oulu, Finland. She collaborates with First Nations, Inuit and Sámi communities and organizations in action-research projects on human-environment interactions, socio-ecological changes in polar regions, community-based environmental monitoring, and biocultural approaches to conservation. She has a strong interest in art-based methodologies, working with community filmmaking and photovoice, and also interactive mapping. She strongly advocates for decolonial and co-creative research methodologies and for inclusive collaborations in research.

David A. Fennell is a Professor at Brock University who researches mainly in the areas of ecotourism, tourism ethics, and moral issues tied to the use of animals in the tourism industry, and sustainability. A major thrust of his research involves the use of theory from other disciplines (e.g., biology, philosophy) to gain traction on many of tourism's most persistent issues and problems. He is the founding Editor-in-Chief of the *Journal of Ecotourism*.

Bastian Thomsen is a Research Affiliate in the School of Anthropology & Museum Ethnography at the University of Oxford, and a Lecturer (Assistant Professor) of Sustainability at the University of Sydney Business School. He is a member of The Ethno-ornithology World Atlas Research Group at the University of Oxford and a member of the Sydney Environment Institute at the University of Sydney.

Samuel R. Fennell is a PhD student at Oregon State University. He has interests in cultural anthropology and social psychology as they relate to the causes and consequences of human behavior in natural settings.

List of figures

https://doi.org/10.1515/9783110792072-018

Index

https://doi.org/10.1515/9783110792072-019